RA395.A3 S76 1988
The bitter pill : tough choices in

THE BITTER PILL

Tough Choices in
America's Health Policy

RICHARD SORIAN

McGRAW-HILL BOOK COMPANY
Healthcare Information Center

New York   St. Louis   San Francisco
Colorado Springs   Oklahoma City   Washington, D.C.

THE BITTER PILL
Tough Choices in America's Health Policy

Copyright © 1988 by McGraw-Hill, Inc. All rights reserved. Printed in the United States of America. Except as permitted under the United States Copyright Act of 1976, no part of this publication may be reproduced or distributed in any form or by any means, or stored in a data base or retrieval system, without the prior written permission of the publisher.

123456789 DOC DOC 8921098

ISBN 0-07-059736-7

This book was set in Times Roman by the McGraw-Hill Book Company Publishing Center in cooperation with Monotype Composition Company; the sponsoring editor was Deborah Glazer; the production supervisor was Robert R. Laffler. The jacket and cover were designed by Eileen Burke. Project supervision was done by Harriet Damon Shields & Associates. R. R. Donnelley & Sons Company was printer and binder.

Library of Congress Cataloging-in-Publication Data

Sorian, Richard, date–
The bitter pill : tough choices in America's health policy / Richard Sorian.
    p.   cm.
Includes index.
ISBN 0-07-059736-7
1. Medical policy—United States. 2. United States—
    Politics and government—1981–   I. Title.
RA395.A3S76   1988
362.1'0973—dc19   88-12830

To my parents.

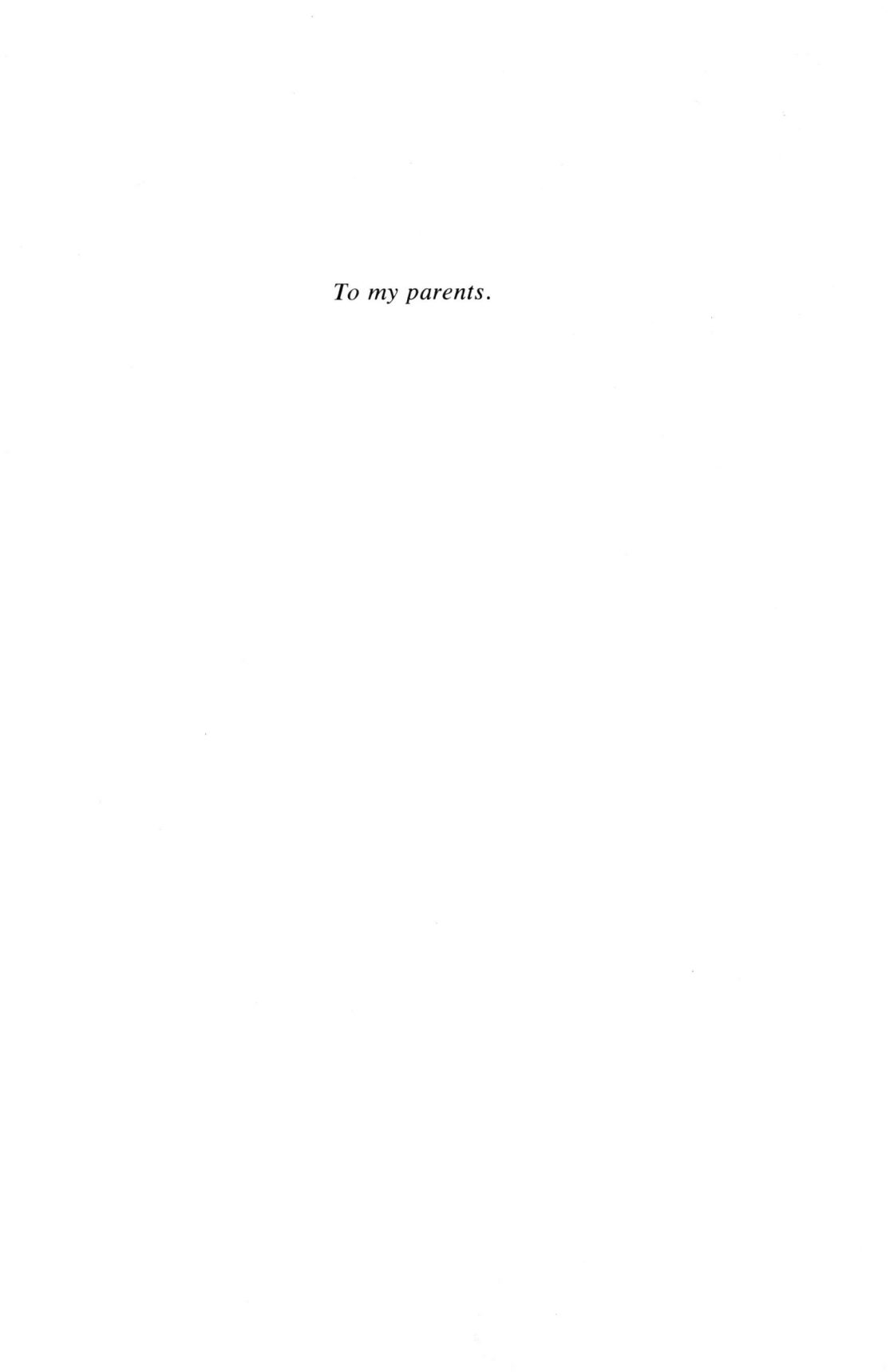

Contents

Foreword   vii

Acknowledgments   xi

1 / **Reagan's Revolution**   1

2 / **Medicaid**   17

3 / **Block Grants**   37

4 / **Reagan's Health Secretaries**   57

5 / **Unemployed, Uninsured**   75

6 / **The Medicare Mess**   89

7 / **The Party's Over**   105

8 / **The Social Agenda**   123

9 / **Deregulation?**   141

10 / **Vouchers**   155

CONTENTS

11 / **Catastrophic Insurance**   177

12 / **AIDS**   203

Index   239

Foreword

When Ronald Reagan was elected President, Richard Sorian had been a health reporter for exactly seven months. As the newest cub reporter for McGraw-Hill's Washington health newsletters, he asked for the unpopular assignment of covering the Reagan "transition team" at its daily 8 a.m. meetings. Most health reporters ignored the transition team, figuring it was routine, at best a story for the political beat. But Sorian saw those breakfast meetings as a way to get to know the people who were going to select the men and women who would shape policy in the new administration.

His reporter's instincts served him well. During the Reagan administration, health care has undergone incredible changes, going from an inflationary system where doctors prescribed and the government and private insurance companies paid, to a business where doctors and hospitals often find themselves on opposite sides of the bottom line.

In the ensuing years, no one has covered health care policy developments in Washington more thoroughly and consistently than Richard Sorian. Readers of *Medicine & Health* know that what happens in Washington Friday afternoon that affects health policy will be in the newsletter on Monday morning, weeks, sometimes months, before other reporters have caught on to the significance of the event. Officials within the Department of

Health and Human Services, the Office of Management and Budget, and the White House have said that they have to read *Medicine & Health* to find out what's happening in their own administration. On Capitol Hill where information provides access, health committee staffers have been known to read and then hide the newsletter so they can provide personal "insights" to their congressmen.

In 1986, the *National Journal* recognized the value of *Medicine & Health* and the skills that Richard Sorian brings to that publication by including him in a list of 20 media members who "Make A Difference" in Washington policymaking. Sorian is "first to report a lot of breaking news in the health policy arena; keeps an eye on the whole gamut of health legislation and regulation; occasionally gives a reading on the impact of various policies; considered must reading among health policy makers."

Despite the recognition that his reporting has brought, there has been an increasing sense of frustration. Quick and concise are the hallmarks of newsletter journalism, yet much of the story of the changes being wrought in Washington was neither. Richard would come back from the Hill, write his news story, and then, at the end of the day, share with his colleagues some of the stories behind the story. "Can't we get some of that in the newsletter," someone would inevitably ask. "No, it would take too much space to explain," he would reply with regret. Over the years, through special reports and in numerous speeches before health care groups Sorian has found ways to tell parts of that story. Readers and audiences always wanted more.

In newsletter journalism we use a device we call the "fishback," a parenthetical reference to alert the reader to an earlier news story. In many ways, this book is a whopper of a fishback, as the author pulled together the many, many stories that collectively represented a 180-degree turn in national health policy.

The Bitter Pill chronicles the dramatic changes in federal health care policy in the 1980s. It portrays the policies, the politics, and the personalities that produced those changes. It examines the shifts in the way the government pays for hospital care of the elderly and health care for the poor, the creation of new state-run block grants, the dismantling of federal regulatory programs, the impact of the "religious right" on federal health policy, the evolution of catastrophic insurance for the elderly, and the nation's battle with the AIDS epidemic.

Where we are as a nation always reflects where we have been. *The Bitter Pill* not only tells how we got where we are in health care, it also provides important insights into where we are going. As Washington and the nation prepare for a new President and a new turn in health policy, this book provides a road map of where we are, where we've been, and where we are going. This is Richard Sorian's first book. I am sure it will not be his last. The revolution in American health care is not yet over.

Lucigrace S. Koizumi
Publisher and Editor in Chief
Healthcare Information Center
Washington, D.C.

Acknowledgments

To write a book tracing nearly eight years of dramatic change in federal health policy, a reporter depends on scores of individuals and organizations. For many of them, anonymity is preferred and provided. In my daily work as editor of *Medicine & Health* and in this past year's work on this book, I have relied on a broad range of elected and appointed officials and their staffs to gain information and insight into the workings of the federal government. To them, I offer my thanks and my respect for the difficult and important work that they do.

This book could not have been written—and surely not completed—without the intellectual, emotional, and spiritual support of my editor and mentor, Lucigrace Koizumi. She has given her time, her eyes, her mind, and, most importantly, her heart to this work.

My thanks also go to Karen Glenn, my colleague and my guidepost, for reading draft chapters while commuting between New York and Washington and keeping me on the right path while steering me clear of the wrong ones. At McGraw-Hill, I offer my thanks, too, to Susan Namovicz and Karen Migdail for many tedious but vital services. My special thanks to my sponsoring editor, Deborah Glazer, who guided this product from beginning to end and put up with my endless queries.

Insights were provided by some of the people who helped to

shape the nation's health policy. Special thanks go to Jack Ebeler and Glenn Markus, of Health Policy Alternatives, for their patience and assistance in educating me about the ins and outs of Medicare and Medicaid. Thanks also to Richard Froh, of Kaiser Foundation Health Plans, Inc., for his assistance and his friendship.

1
Reagan's Revolution

It was the "Reagan Revolution": a sudden and dramatic turn to the political right, a wave of conservative values—both fiscal and social. Ronald Reagan would use his two terms in the White House to alter the American landscape; nowhere was that more evident than in America's health policy. A new era of fiscal constraint tightened the belts of U.S. hospitals, doctors, and nursing homes. A government policy of deregulation and market-oriented policies put an end to nearly two decades of federal expansion in health care delivery and insurance. Federal policymakers shifted their interest from expansion of access to health care services to containment of health costs.

It was budget government, a time when the bottom line was the only line. Unprecedented government retrenchment caused a program's worth to be measured more often by its cost than by the people it served. A president with strong antipathy toward government programs and the largest federal budget deficits in history left lawmakers little room to expand the government's role in health care delivery. Instead, the nation saw year after year of constriction. Health programs, used to an ever-increasing federal budget, suddenly were forced to fight for their very existence. Some fell by the wayside; others continued with a more limited agenda.

Reagan's fight to reduce federal spending seemed, to many

Americans, a distant battle that had little or no effect on their lives. But because of the government's dominant role in American health care, changes made in Washington did have an effect on the lives of all Americans, rich and poor, young and old, black and white. In some cases, the people suffered along with the programs. America's success in combating infant mortality and teenage pregnancy slowed. The eradication of such childhood diseases as measles, mumps, and diphtheria—a goal that seemed within reach when Reagan took office—seemed to slip away. America's infant mortality statistics, the best measure of a nation's health care system, began to show disturbing trends: Lines that had been running steadily downward began to flatten out, some even turned upward. The percentage of Americans living in poverty increased, after nearly a decade of progress. The percentage of those poor people receiving medical assistance from the government also dropped. The number of Americans without health insurance began to rise for the first time in more than a decade. And while the government geared to reduce its role in health care, the country faced a new nemesis—acquired immune deficiency syndrome (AIDS)—an epidemic that threatened to wipe out thousands, if not millions, of American lives at a time when government action was needed more than ever.

Budget government had its positive sides as well. Years of ignoring the escalation of health care costs forced Washington policymakers to rein in the cost of such programs as Medicare and Medicaid. Congressmen who previously could not muster the political will to face down health care provider lobbyists found the budget crunch a convenient excuse to crack down on what had become a fat and wasteful health care system. The government's open-wallet health care policy came to a crashing close. Regulatory programs that had, in some cases, become ways to support the regulators, were forced to prove their worth. Some failed that test; others saw their mission significantly altered.

The government's reordering of priorities had widespread effects on America's health care institutions. Hospital mergers increased and providers began to diversify into other businesses. Some hospitals closed their doors, others began to lay off thousands of nurses, orderlies, and support staff. Patients who used to be treated in a hospital were cared for in an outpatient department and sent home to recover. Patients who were admitted to the hospital were released much sooner than previously. Physicians began to consider the cost of lab tests before ordering them. Private health care insurance companies took a close look at their own policies and began to mimic the government's moves. Employers, tired of paying a bigger and bigger insurance bill, began to pressure insurers to cut their rates.

The decline of traditional medical care also led to a rise in the use of health maintenance organizations, a prepaid form of health care delivery that stressed less use of health care services. Across the country, the practice of medicine began to change in response to cost-containment moves by the government. But despite these reforms, health care spending continued to grow in the United States from about $360 billion per year when Reagan took office to more than $500 billion when he left. The rate of growth was lower than it had been in the 1970s, but it still exceeded the annual growth in consumer prices by nearly two to one.

The changes made in Washington affected the people as well. America's pluralistic health system had always left many of its citizens without the protection of health insurance or government programs. Decades of debate over a national health insurance system had run aground during the Carter administration and drew scarcely a mention in the Reagan years. The "private sector" would take care of the problem, the new government in Washington assured its citizens. But the private sector did not, perhaps could not, handle a swelling number of uninsured Americans. The economic recession of 1981 to 1983 put millions out of work, costing them their health insurance along with their jobs. The recovery that followed replenished the job supply but not the insurance rolls. Companies replaced full-time workers who were required to be insured with part-time employees who were not. Service sector jobs replaced those lost to closed factories, but health insurance didn't follow. By the end of 1986, the number of uninsured Americans had risen from thirty-one million when Reagan took office to thirty-seven million, the first increase in number since corporate America and the government began working to provide health coverage.

The budget government of the 1980s followed the era of high inflation and economic turmoil in the 1970s. Health care costs, which had always risen faster than the general economy, were jumping by double digits at the end of the 1970s. The economic disaster led to Ronald Reagan's decisive victory over President Jimmy Carter in 1980 and helped to shape the new president's domestic agenda. Reagan took office with five major domestic policy goals: to quickly bring down the double-digit inflation rate, to reduce soaring interest rates, to increase defense spending, to cut personal and corporate income taxes, and to decrease social program spending. Those issues dominated the national policy agenda throughout the 1980s as Reagan and his supporters prodded a reluctant Congress to reorder domestic priorities and reduce the government's role in American's lives.

When it came to health care, the Reagan administration had two basic goals; sometimes they were complementary, other times contradictory. They wanted to reduce the government's spending on health care programs and increase the power of market competition in the health care industry. The theory behind both these policies was simple: Americans were using too much health care and were insulated from its cost by government programs and private insurance. As a result, health care providers felt free to raise their prices and expand the volume of services they gave to their patients. Employer-paid health insurance had immunized Americans to the cost of care; doctor and hospital bills were simply sent to the insurance company, the patients often didn't even see them. No questions were asked of doctors who prescribed numerous expensive diagnostic tests; hospitals weren't asked to explain why patients were kept in their facilities after they were ready to go home. Government incentives were skewed toward encouraging more care, whatever the expense.

In the 1970s, as lawmakers and economists watched the rapid rise in health costs, federal lawmakers turned to regulatory solutions. Washington tried to regulate the growth of hospitals, the incomes of physicians, and the amounts each charged. These early attempts at cost containment were coupled with government attempts to regulate the quality of health care. Scandalous stories of substandard care in the nation's nursing homes had led Washington to apply a heavy dose of regulation.

Reagan's arrival in Washington was hailed by the politically conservative leaders of the nation's health care lobbying machine. The President-elect's talk of getting the government off the backs of U.S. business and depending on "competitive" forces to control the health care industry produced glee in corporate health care board rooms. More than a decade of Washington debate about regulatory control of health care providers had left many feeling chafed. Reagan's promise of a hands-off approach to regulation sounded too good to be true. Reagan said he would allow the marketplace to decide the order of things. Physicians and hospital administrators salivated.

The central player in the Reagan Revolution was Budget Director David Stockman, a young and brash politician whose credo could best be summed up as, "the best government is no government." That philosophy matched that of his new boss and the traditional core of the Republican party. Stockman would cleverly match his ideology to the calls from the new Republican recruits from the fundamentalist right to reduce government's interference in the lives of the American people.

Following Reagan's election, Stockman and Republican New York Congressman Jack Kemp put together a list of policy moves that they pressed on Reagan. At the top of that list was a call for cuts in federal spending. The U.S. economy, Stockman and Kemp warned, was facing an "economic Dunkirk" that could be avoided only by quick action to curb spending and cut taxes.

Reagan named Stockman director of the Office of Management and Budget (OMB) in December of 1980. The nominee wasted no time in assembling a "hit-list" of domestic programs that he wanted eliminated or pared. While other Reagan nominees to the Cabinet prepared for their congressional confirmation hearings, Stockman locked himself away with the budget books. By getting the jump on his fellow administration officials, Stockman cemented a central role for himself in the first year of

Reagan's administration. By the time the rest of the Cabinet got around to the business of running the country, Stockman was running rings around them. His hard work paid off. When Reagan took office in January, Stockman clearly was the lead figure in the new government. His budget became the centerpiece of Reagan's 1981 legislative agenda and that pattern would be locked in place for most of Reagan's eight years in Washington.

The selection of Stockman for the key Cabinet post was pushed by Reagan's most conservative supporters. During his three terms in Congress, Stockman had been one of the brightest and quickest minds in the phalanx of young conservative Republicans. During the campaign, Reagan spoke little about the drastic cuts in domestic spending he would request once in office. The most the Republican candidate would say was that he would cut out "waste, fraud, and abuse" in federal programs. Reagan's promise to cut taxes, raise defense spending, and balance the federal budget had been derided by his opponents as "smoke and mirrors" and "voodoo economics." That last appellation—coined by Reagan's future Vice President, George Bush—would prove quite prescient.

Reagan's numbers just didn't add up. The new President could not cut taxes and raise defense spending without increasing the size of the deficit. To cut enough out of domestic spending programs to achieve Reagan's promise of a balanced budget would require too much pain. Stockman knew the problem Reagan faced, but he also knew the solution was beyond both men's grasp. Reagan would not alter his priorities or his rhetoric. In 1981, Congress approved a three-year 25 percent tax cut, a five-year $1 trillion defense spending plan, and $35 billion in domestic spending cuts. While Reagan and Stockman were hailed as miracle workers in 1981, their success would prove to be a Pyrrhic victory. Rather than balancing the budget, Reagan's economic policies would create the largest budget deficits in the history of the country.

But those very deficits helped to cement Stockman's hold on domestic policy decisions. By running the deficit so high, Stockman was able to preempt any attempts by congressional Democrats—and perhaps any President who would follow Reagan into the White House—to forge new health care programs or to invigorate those left lifeless by the Reagan budget cuts.

The deficit created problems for Stockman and his budget team, but it also provided them with new ammunition in the battle to cut domestic spending. Large deficits gave Congress little room to expand existing programs and created pressure to reduce spending year in and year out. The size of the federal budget deficit became the overriding issue in domestic policymaking in the Reagan era.

Stockman was given a free hand in designing the Reagan budgets. He and his young team at OMB were granted unprecedented authority to set budgets and to oversee the workings of the federal departments and agencies. The Office of Management and Budget had seen its power increase sharply in the decade before Reagan took office, but Reagan and Stockman would go much further. David Stockman would be the most powerful budget chief in the nation's history. While OMB had always had control over government budgets, Reagan extended that purview to the murky area of federal regulations. In past years, Cabinet secretaries who had lost their budget battles found ways to advance their agenda through regulations, masking a major shift in policy in the pages of the *Federal Register*.

When Reagan took office he decried the amount of federal red tape. In his first week in office, Reagan signed an executive order granting OMB the power to review all regulations promulgated by all departments and agencies. By extending Stockman's power to the regulatory arena, Reagan effectively gave him carte blanche to run federal domestic policy.

The rise of OMB was one of the least noticed aspects of the Reagan Revolution. Stockman's budget brilliance was noted by the daily press coverage of the budget battles, but few reporters and few in government noticed the sway that OMB had over the rest of the Reagan Cabinet.

Ronald Reagan professed a passion for what he called "Cabinet government." The members of his Cabinet were to make policy and go about implementing it. In some ways there was

Cabinet government during the Reagan era; the problem that was some Cabinet officers were more equal than others. In the health arena, Stockman was king. The Department of Health and Human Services (HHS), which had traditionally had final say on federal health programs, was purposely downgraded under Reagan. Richard Schweiker, Reagan's first health secretary, spent much of his two years in the Cabinet fighting Stockman's budget attacks; most of the time he lost. Schweiker brought with him a policymaking team that tried to fight off OMB, but once a frustrated Schweiker left office in 1983, his successors, Margaret Heckler and Otis Bowen, had little firepower to fight Stockman and his successor, James Miller. During Heckler's reign, OMB was literally setting and implementing federal health policy. That power grab had a greater effect on health programs than many understood at the time. By holding up needed regulations, OMB was able to thwart domestic initiatives by Schweiker, Heckler, and Bowen. Legislation enacted by the Congress over the President's objections was often subverted by OMB's regulatory delays. Many times the HHS secretaries were forced to pull back their plans or make changes to satisfy the OMB regulatory overseers. A key question about the post-Reagan era will be whether OMB retains its authority or returns to its former role as the government's accountants.

Stockman's most successful year by far was 1981, during Reagan's honeymoon with the Congress. While later years would see Congress rediscover its backbone, 1981 was all Reagan. He pushed through a tax cut and a budget that challenged many of the entrenched domestic programs of the 1970s, programs begun under Richard Nixon and continued under Gerald Ford and Jimmy Carter. On the chopping block were the Civilian Employment and Training Act (CETA), school lunch programs, loans to college student, mass transit supports, general revenue sharing, farm supports, Amtrak, and dozens of others. Stockman launched a frontal attack, arguing for the total elimination of nearly two dozen programs and the virtual elimination of scores of others.

On the health care front, Stockman's number one target was Medicaid, the joint federal-state health program for the nation's poor. In the fifteen years since Congress created the program, Medicaid spending had grown rapidly. Congressional committees held scores of hearings to look into the inflationary aspects of the program but had done relatively little to constrain those costs. At the same time, despite its expense, Medicaid still failed to cover millions of people living at, or below, the federal poverty line. Stockman, picking up an old rallying cry of the Nixon and Ford administrations, fought to cap the federal share of the program and put permanent limits on its future growth. On another front, Stockman asked Congress to do away with federal administration of two dozen small-, medium-, and large-sized grant programs, leaving those functions to the states. The "block-grant approach" was, again, nothing new; it had been tried unsuccessfully under Nixon and Ford. But Stockman coupled his proposal with a plan to slash spending on such programs as childhood immunization, family planning, and community and migrant health centers by 25 percent.

Reagan would wait until 1982 to begin the longest assault of his presidency: the fight to reverse the runaway costs of Medicare, the health insurance program for America's elderly and its disabled. This would be Reagan's greatest triumph, and the budget deficit would work in his favor. Medicare was the government's second largest domestic program. With an annual budget that would top $80 billion by the time Reagan left office, it was a prime target for overhaul. Created in 1965, Medicare remained virtually untouched until 1972 when preliminary cost-containment efforts were made. But beginning in 1982, Reagan and the Congress began enacting major changes.

The assault on Medicare was a well-planned and executed effort to revamp a payment system that had, almost from the beginning, encouraged American hospitals to provide too much care to the elderly while expanding their operations to the point of excess.

It is quite possible that many, if not all, of Reagan's efforts on the health care front would have failed but for the cooperation of Congress. Stockman's budget scenario leaned heavily on Congress' agreement to package all of Reagan's domestic policy initiatives into an omnibus bill. Going into the 1981 budget battle, Reagan and Stockman figured they could count on the support of the newly elected Republican leaders in the Senate. Majority Leader Howard Baker, Budget Committee Chairman Pete Domenici, and Finance Committee Chairman Robert Dole were united behind the administration's push for budget cuts. They insisted, in fact, that the budget cuts be enacted before they would take up Reagan's tax bill. The White House expected stiff resistance from the Democrats in the House, but the Democrats were a no-show. Speaker of the House Thomas "Tip" O'Neill, Jr. didn't want his party labeled as obstructionist, so he agreed to accept the omnibus approach. In doing so, he sealed the fate of many of the programs he and Democrats would vainly fight to preserve. But O'Neill's strategy also absolved Democrats of much of the blame for the effect of Reagan's policies. In the congressional elections of 1982, 1984, and 1986, Democrats reaped the spoils of those policies by increasing their majority in the House of Representatives and gradually regaining control of the Senate.

The omnibus bill approach to domestic policy would continue throughout the Reagan years. It had attractive elements for all concerned. The White House knew that it could not win a series of showdown votes on domestic policy changes. It had watched Carter's domestic agenda picked apart by Congress. On Capitol Hill the omnibus-bill approach served to protect legislators from voters' wrath. A congressman facing an angry constituent could say he too opposed the item that upset the voter but had to vote for the overall bill to cut the budget. To paraphrase Senator Russell Long, legislators were able to tell their constituents: Don't blame you, don't blame me, blame that fella behind the tree.

Congress would take the one bill, one vote approach to its extreme. Year after year major domestic policy decisions were made with little attention to the detail of the legislation, few public hearings, and little debate. It is difficult to assess blame—or credit—to any one legislator for the actions of the congresses of the 1980s. Voting records are almost impossible to analyze when most of the major decisions of the day were buried in bills that ran from 500 to 600 pages each.

The move to consolidate most major domestic policy changes in giant bills also cut down on the public's ability to influence the course of those policies. Where in previous years important pieces of legislation would be introduced months before they were to be considered, now they were unveiled only hours before a committee vote. The opportunity to lobby for changes in the legislation was lost. While this helped to weaken the power of the "special interest" lobbying groups, it had the same effect on groups representing the people served by such programs as Medicare and Medicaid. Omnibus bills also led to sloppy legislating. Errors in legislation, which previously would have been caught by watchful lobbyists, now found their way into law. Seemingly minor changes in law slipped into an omnibus bill would come back to haunt congressmen who had voted for them; a second bill often was necessary to correct problems in the first one.

Stockman wasn't the only player in the health care reform game. Schweiker's policy team at HHS worked hard in 1981 to come up with a blueprint that would form the basis for the actions taken in 1982 and beyond. A team led by Dr. Robert Rubin, Schweiker's assistant secretary for planning and evaluation, began work shortly after Reagan took office to come up with what became known as the administration's "competition-based health policy." Reagan's advisers borrowed liberally from competitive theories developed in the fifteen years between enactment of Medicare and Reagan's 1980 election. The HHS competition team studied federal programs (Medicare, Medicaid, veterans health programs), the private sector, and the U.S. tax code. The administration remained remarkably consistent to those themes throughout the next eight years.

While Rubin and his HHS team were at work, the administration was getting important outside help from one of the unknown warriors of the health care reform battle. David Winston, a former Reagan aide in California and Schweiker's chief health adviser in Congress, could have had any post he wanted in the administration. The soft-spoken Winston instead chose to turn to the private sector. But he retained close ties to Schweiker at HHS and the new management team at the White House. Winston helped to recruit Schweiker's team at HHS and would bridge many communication gaps between HHS and the White House while steering administration health policy.

Winston's work began before Reagan took office. The Heritage Foundation, a heretofore unknown conservative think tank, gathered a group of top GOP thinkers to come up with a battle plan for the new president and his administration. After eight years of watching moderate Republicans dominate the Nixon and Ford years and liberal Democrats control the capital for the past four years, the Heritage boys wanted to provide the Reagan administration with advice whether asked for or not.

Winston headed up the health division of the Heritage Foundation effort. In 1981 Heritage released a monumental 1093-page report, *Mandate for Leadership*. Winston's chapter on health laid the groundwork for Rubin's work at HHS and Stockman's work at OMB. In it he called for the elimination of several federal grant programs that had outlived their usefulness, repeal of regulatory controls on health care providers, and a new emphasis on market-oriented policies.

As the Reagan team began its work, Schweiker asked Winston to form an external advisory group to recommend strategies to carry out the competition model. The Winston task force operated separately from the Rubin group but came to many of the same conclusions. But Winston's group was not handcuffed by the political concerns of a new administration. While Rubin had to watch his every step so that he did not trigger a public relations land mine for the new secretary and the President, Winston was free to develop a report that could be embraced or ignored by the new government.

Winston's work did not end with the report his task force issued late in 1981. While he continued to refuse to take a formal role in the government, Winston was a key—if not *the* key—adviser in the first Reagan term. Tragically, Winston's life ended in 1986 in a bizarre incident following an argument between Winston and a passing motorist in San Francisco. A punch to the jaw resulted in Winston hitting the pavement with such force that he suffered irreparable brain damage and died within days.

In 1981, Winston's views of the health care system in America were being embraced by Reagan, Schweiker, and Stockman. Winston's vision of the future became the foundation of the changes to come in American health policy. In the view of Winston and his conservative colleagues, America's health system was big, fat, and out of control. Government programs had been allowed to grow indiscriminately without ensuring that the United States got its money's worth when it bought health care services for the people it served. United States tax laws were skewed to provide incentives for overutilization of health services while leaving important gaps for those with catastrophic illnesses. The government bureaucracy had grown too. They believed many programs had been created in the 1970s with little thought to their need. Those that had been useful had lost their purpose as the country changed. Meanwhile, the giant federal government in Washington had robbed the states of most control over the delivery of health care services in their own towns and cities.

Reagan would call for a total reordering of government policies. The federal government would become a "prudent purchaser" of health care services; tax laws would be changed to encourage Americans to buy their health services in a similar manner. States would regain control over the health care delivery system and the federal government would drop its regulatory strangle hold on the U.S. health care system.

In 1981 Reagan would ask Congress to eliminate two dozen federal grant programs and replace them with a pair of state-run block grants. Regulatory programs that sought to control health care utilization and capital expenditures would also be repealed under the Reagan plan. Medicaid—the health benefits program for the poor—would absorb the biggest spending cut via a federal cap on Medicaid dollars.

It would take another year of internal debate before the administration settled on the outline of its competition package. On February 28, 1983, Reagan transmitted a message to Congress laying out that plan. Reagan criticized what he called the "perverse incentives" in the existing U.S. health care system, including cost-based reimbursement of providers, poorly structured cost-sharing for patients, and an open-ended tax subsidy for employer-provided health insurance.

"Health care costs are climbing so fast that they may soon threaten the quality of care and access to care which Americans enjoy," Reagan told Congress. Federal outlays for Medicare and Medicaid had risen 600 percent between 1970 and 1983, Reagan noted. Health care costs were consuming a growing portion of the nation's gross national product (GNP). In 1982, health care spending comprised 10.5 percent of GNP; the average hospital stay cost Americans $2168 in 1981. Rising costs hurt everyone, the President said. The elderly who depended on Medicare faced the threat of catastrophic illness with no Medicare coverage; the poor on Medicaid had seen coverage reduced by states; workers with employer-paid health insurance were receiving lower wages. Health care costs also were built into the prices of other goods and services bought by American consumers.

Reagan's Health Incentives Reform package proposed replacing Medicare's cost-based provider reimbursement system with a prospective pricing system; the open-ended tax subsidy for employer-paid health insurance would be capped; the elderly would be encouraged to leave Medicare and enroll in private health insurance plans; cost-sharing for health care services would gradually be increased; and Medicare would provide protection against "catastrophic" medical bills.

Reagan's 1983 message to Congress laid out the administration's market-oriented policies. To a remarkable degree, the administration stuck to those policies throughout Reagan's two terms in office. But budget deficit problems of the 1980s forced some important departures from the text. Most significantly, the administration that condemned overregulation by its Democratic predecessors turned to the regulatory solution to get a grip on rising Medicare costs.

Reagan would not have an easy time doing away with the status quo. Many in Congress from both political parties had participated in the building of that system. Sure it had its faults, they would say, but let's not throw the baby out with the bath water. Democrats on Capitol Hill were, however, deflated by the 1980

1 / Reagan's Revolution

election results. Not only had Reagan driven Carter from office but he had brought with him the first Republican Senate in twenty-six years. Key committee chairmanships had changed hands overnight. Some Democrats decided to sit by and watch Reagan have his way, believing—or hoping—that the failure of those policies would then help their party regain its prominence. Others tried to beat Reagan at his own game. If the voters wanted lower taxes, Democrats would go further than Reagan. If voters wanted a bigger defense budget, they would get it. If Americans were tired of the welfare state, they would pare back the programs. Still another group of Democrats in Congress wailed and flailed at Reagan's budget proposals but were ineffective in their attempts to defeat him.

But Reagan may have met his match in the person of a four-term Democratic congressman from his home state of California. Congressman Henry Waxman of Los Angeles, a dyed-in-the-wool liberal Democrat, would play the key role in fighting the Reagan mandate. Like Reagan, Waxman believed health care cost too much for the average American to afford. In 1979, he had led the unsuccessful effort in Congress to pass President Carter's hospital cost-containment bill. But, while health care costs concerned Waxman, he was more bothered by his belief that the U.S. health care system contained too many holes through which many of its poorest citizens were falling. The job of improving access to health care was not done, in Waxman's eyes. But over the next eight years, the clever California congressman would find himself fighting what was often a very lonely fight against the conservative tides that had swept Reagan into office.

The role would not be unfamiliar to Waxman; he had chaired the health committee in the California state legislature when Reagan was governor. Now in Washington, as his Democratic colleagues were being steamrollered by the Reagan budget machine, Waxman would be one of the few members of Congress who would successfully stand in the President's way. Waxman would fight to convince Congress that Reagan was going too far in dismantling the health care programs that he and his colleagues had worked so long to create.

Waxman's successes—and there were several—came about because of his strategy of compromise. While condemning Reagan's policies and vowing to fight them tooth and nail, Waxman also sought a middle ground where some programs would be sacrificed but others would be protected. Waxman liked to call his approach "damage control," but many others credited him with saving a large portion of the American health care state.

But even Waxman's victories over Reagan came at a price. In order to stave off the most draconian cuts in federal health spending, Waxman had to accept budget cuts that would make his attempt to patch the holes in the system that much more difficult. For Waxman, and for Reagan and his followers, the 1980s would be a time of tough choices, a balancing of the economic needs of the country as a whole and the health care needs of its citizens. It was a time when the government and the people it served had to swallow a bitter pill to cure what ailed it.

2

Medicaid

As with the rest of Reagan's domestic policy victories, 1981 would be the turning point in reform of health care coverage for the poor. Riding the wave of his sweeping victory over Carter, Reagan planned to make the most of the six- to nine-month "honeymoon" period granted him by Congress and the public. Never again would Reagan hold such sway on Capitol Hill.

The focus of Reagan's 1981 domestic agenda was the tax cut and cuts in domestic spending. At the Office of Management and Budget, Stockman was busily at work rewriting Carter's budget plan sent to Congress just before Reagan's January 20 inauguration. As was the custom, Carter had sent his final budget to Capitol Hill in January before leaving office. In past years, new presidents had done little to change the budget sent to Congress before the inauguration but focused instead on developing budget proposals for the following year. The deteriorating U.S. economy would not allow Reagan to wait. Stockman began work on a revised FY82 budget three months before taking office. By February Reagan was ready to announce the broad details of his budget revisions, and in March the first Reagan budget was sent to Congress.

* * *

Reagan and Stockman would not go it alone in the battle over the budget. Reagan's electoral sweep in 1980 carried along several GOP senatorial candidates who defeated entrenched Democratic incumbents. The result: the first Republican Senate majority in twenty-six years. Out were such veteran Democrats as George McGovern of South Dakota, Frank Church of Idaho, Warren Magnuson of Washington, Birch Bayh of Indiana, Herman Talmadge of Georgia, and Gaylord Nelson of Wisconsin. In total, twelve Democratic Senate seats changed hands. Along with control of the Senate, the Republicans also gained control of the Senate committees. Most of the new committee chairmen were men with lengthy experience but none were used to the job of proposing legislation and pushing it through to enactment. Some would prove quite adept at the job; others would be dismal failures. Some of the new class of senators had served in the House of Representatives, others were neophytes to the congressional scene. Ever conscious of how much their electoral success had been linked to Reagan's, these new senators would march in lockstep behind the President's lead. They would be the loyal foot soldiers in Reagan's fights with Congress.

Over in the House, the Republicans remained a minority party. But the elections had increased the number of Republican House members, bringing the GOP closer in number to the Democrats than they had been in nearly two decades. At the same time, the number of conservative Democrats, mainly in the south, also increased, giving the conservative forces a working majority in the House. The swelling of ranks gave the House Republican leadership new energy and a faint hope that they could follow the Senate's lead and take over in 1982. That hope also helped to cement the Republicans into a solid phalanx ready to carry Reagan's flag on Capitol Hill.

Leading the Reagan side in the Senate were Majority Leader Howard Baker of Tennessee, Budget Committee Chairman Pete Domenici of New Mexico, and Finance Committee Chairman Robert Dole of Kansas. Baker and Dole were well known on the national scene. Baker made his reputation in the congressional Watergate hearings with his now famous question: "What did the President know, and when did he know it?" Since that time he had risen in the ranks of Senate Republicans until he won election as minority leader. With the Republicans in charge, Baker was now the man who controlled the Senate's calendar and was responsible for bringing the divergent views of the GOP into line.

Dole caught the nation's attention as President Gerald Ford's 1976 running mate. While Ford whiled away the election in the White House Rose Garden, Dole crisscrossed the country slashing away at Democrats Jimmy Carter and Walter Mondale. In the losing effort, Dole severely damaged his reputation. By 1981, he had begun a remarkable repair process, fashioning a reputation as a capable, powerful, sometimes self-deprecating committee chairman.

In contrast, Domenici was hardly known outside his home state of New Mexico. Since his election to the Senate in 1972, Domenici had been a quiet behind-the-scenes Senator. But in 1981, he became chairman of the Senate Budget Committee. In the 1980s the Budget Committee would be the focal point of all major legislation in Congress.

Baker, Dole, and Domenici would prove to be the keys in Reagan's successful march through Congress in 1981. Baker, the soft-spoken Tennessean, would create the Republican unity needed to overcome Democratic opposition; Domenici would take the President's budget outline and press it into law early in the year; Dole would provide the legislative skill needed to enact the specific changes in law needed to make Reagan's proposals law.

The Republicans in the Senate got an important helping hand from their counterparts in the House. After a quarter-century in the minority, many House Republicans were used to sitting on the sidelines and watching the Democrats run the show. The new House Minority Leader, Bob Michel of Illinois, used the carrot of future majority status to prod reluctant Republicans into line behind Reagan's policies. If Reagan succeeds, Michel argued, we may be able to take control of the House in 1982 the way we did the Senate in 1980. As a result, Michel was able to fashion an almost unheard of unity in his party. House Republicans voted with the Reagan positions in lockstep in 1981.

On health issues, Michel turned to fellow Illinois Republican, Edward Madigan. Madigan had been in the House for eight years before Reagan took office; his involvement in health issues had been minimal. In 1981, he became the senior Republican member of the House Energy and Commerce Subcommittee on Health and the Environment. From that post, Madigan would try to push the President's health care agenda. His knowledge of health programs could not compare with that of Subcommittee Chairman Henry Waxman, but Madigan's knowledge of the political process gave him an ability to get things done. Over the course of the next two years, Madigan quietly would play one of the key roles in development of the health care revolution.

* * *

Medicaid was at the top of Stockman's list of domestic programs in need of budget surgery. Picking up an idea first presented by Nixon, Stockman would ask Congress to place a cap on the federal share of Medicaid and force the states to change their eligibility and coverage rules to live within the new budget.

As Reagan took office, Medicaid was celebrating its fifteenth birthday. Created in 1965, as almost an afterthought to Medicare, the program had grown quickly and had a remarkable effect on the health of poor Americans. Until Medicaid was created the poor in America had little access to the U.S. health care system other than through the door of the local hospital's emergency room. Poor people saw doctors less often than healthier middle- and upper-income Americans. Conditions related to poverty—poor nutrition, substandard housing, and lack of quality education—worked against the poor getting a fair shake. Children born to poor families had less of a chance of getting through their childhood without suffering a disabling disease.

In the years since Medicaid was created, the health status of poor Americans had improved. By 1981, the poor saw doctors more frequently than the nonpoor; the infant mortality rate among the poor had dropped dramatically. But with the blessings came some curses.

Medicaid established two categories of mandatory eligibility—recipients of Aid to Families with Dependent Children (AFDC) and of Supplemental Security Income (SSI). States were encouraged to extend coverage to many of the near poor in their midst through optional eligibility. A basic benefit package covering hospital and physician care as well as nursing home care was mandated from Washington; again states were encouraged to expand on that package.

By linking Medicaid eligibility to AFDC and SSI, Congress assured a continuation of the varied systems of health coverage that existed before Medicaid. A person or family considered poor in one state was unable to qualify for Medicaid in another. States with large tax bases were quick to expand coverage to many of the optional groups; states that were reluctant to tax their citizens were forced to construct very limited welfare and Medicaid programs. Without federal standards the poor are subject to a patchwork health care system that has left many Americans uncovered. In Texas, the state offers Medicaid coverage to a large number of its citizens but provides coverage of so few benefits and pays so little for those benefits that the poor of that state have some of the worst coverage in the country. In New York, by contrast, eligibility standards are among the most liberal in the country, benefits are extensive, and payment levels sometimes approach those offered by insurers and Medicare.

Even with its holes, Medicaid proved to be a financial problem for lawmakers in Washington and in the state capitals. Within a year of its enactment, Congress began to worry that it had created a fiscal monster. The original estimate that Medicaid would cost about $3 billion in 1966 was not breached; the problem was that only six states were participating. Those first states took full advantage of the optional eligibility rules by covering people earning far above the poverty line. When the other states joined—and all but two did within two years—the cost estimates of 1965 would be thrown out the window. To partially stem the flow, Congress enacted its first Medicaid cost-containment measure in 1966, voting to limit optional eligibility to those earning less than 133 percent of the federal poverty level.

Costs would continue to bother policymakers in Washington

but so would the many holes in the Medicaid fabric. Jimmy Carter tried to patch the program. He sent Congress Medicaid reform legislation that would have set uniform national income standards for eligibility and improved the basic benefit package all states are required to offer. Carter's Child Health Assurance Program (CHAP) was debated and dissected for two years by Congress but was never enacted because of strong opposition from southern states with skimpy Medicaid programs. The chairman of the Senate Finance Committee, Democrat Russell Long, continually stalled the CHAP bill in his committee until Carter's popularity had sunk and Congress was unwilling to consider expansion of the federal welfare network. Long's state, Louisiana, has one of the worst Medicaid programs in the country despite having some of the poorest people.

In 1981 Stockman's concern was not with the holes in Medicaid, but with costs. In Stockman's eyes, the federal government was spending too much on Medicaid and the open-ended payment system was encouraging states to be spendthrifts. The solution: a permanent cap on the size of the federal contribution. No longer would the federal government match each dollar the states spent on health care for the poor. Instead, each state would get a lump sum to spend any way it saw fit. Federal spending on Medicaid had reached $17.2 billion in 1981; states were spending almost as much. Under Carter's budget, the federal share would hit $18.8 billion in 1982. Stockman wanted to hold the increase in the federal share to 5 percent in 1982, a cut of $1.3 billion from Carter's budget. In future years, Medicaid spending from Washington would rise only as fast as the gross national product deflator. In total, over five years, the Medicaid cap would pare nearly $20 billion from the federal budget.

* * *

Before he could get a Medicaid cap in place, Stockman had to convince Congress to accept Reagan's entire budget plan. As a junior member of Congress during the Carter administration, Stockman had learned well the price of sending domestic policy to Capitol Hill in pieces; it came back in even more pieces. Carter's domestic policy initiatives were so chopped and pureed by legislators that the final product bore little resemblance to what was originally sent. Members of Congress complained that Carter would not set priorities and concentrate his efforts on one thing at a time.

Reagan and Stockman would not make the same mistake. Instead of identifying all that was wrong with domestic programs and pursuing solutions in separate bills, the new administration declared that economic recovery was the country's greatest illness and budget cuts were the cure. Stockman's plan was to bundle all the domestic initiatives into one big bill and push it through Congress before Reagan's popularity began its inevitable decline.

Stockman chose to manipulate the Congress' own budget process to give him the vehicle he needed to gain passage of the domestic policy changes. In 1974, Congress had passed the Congressional Budget and Impoundment Control Act setting up its own annual budgeting system. The act was passed in reaction to Richard Nixon's perceived abuses of the President's impoundment authority. Nixon simply refused to spend money that Congress had appropriated for program's that he did not like. In fighting Nixon, Congress sought for itself a greater role in determining the budget priorities of the country in the coming year. The budget act called for Congress to pass its own budget resolution at the beginning of each year after it received a "budget message" from the President. The budget resolution set spending limits on each category of federal spending—defense, education, health care, agriculture. Those limits would guide the congressional committees in passing legislation that would commit the government to spend money. If, later in the year, those committees breached the limits set earlier, Congress would begin a "budget-reconciliation process" to cut spending to bring the budget within limits.

Stockman would turn the congressional budget lion on itself, and senators and congressmen would be licking their wounds for years to come. Stockman's notion, shared by Senate Budget Committee Chairman Domenici, was to start the year with a budget bill that would force legislators to reel in government spending. The resolution would include specific instructions to each committee to reconcile its spending with the new budget. This budget-reconciliation process would become the driving force behind nearly every major health policy decision in the 1980s.

Congress agreed to Stockman's budget scheme with surprising alacrity. House Democrats, still shocked over Carter's overwhelming defeat, were in no mood to challenge Reagan so soon after he took office. "Let Reagan have his way," Democrats said; that way he would get the blame. But, by accepting the revised budget system, members of Congress also were committing themselves to tremendous budget cuts in the domestic programs that served so many poor Americans.

Over in the Senate, Domenici pushed through the Reagan budget line for line, and Democrats just rolled over. In the House, new Budget Committee Chairman Jim Jones of Oklahoma wanted to refashion the Reagan budget to stress traditional Democratic programs, including health care. The Jones budget adopted Reagan's overall budget total but moved the money around to give less to defense and more to domestic programs. Instead of the $1.3 billion cut in Medicaid called for in the Reagan budget, Jones asked for only $1 billion in Medicaid cuts.

The Jones budget plan reached the House floor in June. The White House had enlisted the help of two House members—one Democrat and one Republican—to offer a bipartisan alternative to Jones. Republican Delbert Latta of Ohio and Democrat Phil Gramm of Texas offered a substitute to the Jones budget that closely resembled the Reagan budget with its $1.3 billion Medicaid spending cut. In an historic test of Reagan's strength, the House approved the Gramm-Latta substitute by a narrow margin.

Once Reagan's budget outline had been endorsed by Congress, Stockman still had many battles to win on the legislation to carry out that budget. Democrats who lost the first battle were determined to win the war, and they nearly did. The new Democratic strategy was to structure the budget cuts in such a way that while programs would endure some immediate pain, the basic structure would remain in place in hope that economic and political tides would turn and money could be restored. Stockman, no babe in the woods when it came to legislative trickery, knew that he could only truly win his fight if he got the basic structure of the programs changed.

Stockman's Medicaid cap proposal would be central in the budget battle of 1981. While the budget chief asked for a 5 percent Medicaid cap in 1982, Stockman really didn't care how high the cap was set. The key to the plan would be the future limits on growth. Once the federal Medicaid contribution became a fixed amount, budget fights would be over the size of the annual increase, not over eligibility and benefits. States would be left to live within a fixed Medicaid budget and would therefore make the difficult choices of who would continue to receive coverage and who would become uninsured. Stockman's plans for Medicaid would meet with stiff opposition from the nation's governors, both Democrats and Republicans.

The leader of the opposition would be Henry Waxman. Stockman and Waxman knew each other well from their days together in the House. More than any other member of Congress, Waxman knew the ins and outs of Medicaid and most of the other health programs within his panel's jurisdiction. He also had at his side a pair of Congress' most able aides: Karen Nelson, subcommittee staff director and Andreas Schneider, counsel. Nelson had spent many years in the Department of Health, Education, and Welfare (HEW) bureaucracy learning the details of Medicaid and other welfare programs. Schneider cut his teeth advocating health issues for the poor at the National Health Law Program. Among the three of them, no Medicaid stone remained unturned. They knew the program and they could match Stockman and his crew tit for tat when it came to twisting the legislative system to their advantage.

Waxman had to come up with a counterproposal to the Stockman Medicaid cap. Because Reagan's budget had been ratified, Waxman was locked into finding about $1 billion in Medicaid savings for 1982. Waxman, Nelson, and Schneider sat down to map out a strategy to beat Reagan and Stockman. They constructed a labyrinth of proposals that would, on paper, achieve the $1 billion in budget savings but keep the program structurally unchanged. Waxman's "3-2-1 plan" was to reduce federal payments to each state by 3 percent in 1982, 2 percent in 1983, and 1 percent in 1984. States could still spend as much as they wanted on the poor but would get 97 cents on the dollar in 1982, 98 cents in 1983, and 99 cents in 1984. But in 1985, everything would return to normal, and the federal government would go back to paying its full share of the bill. Stockman's plan meant permanent change; Waxman's was only temporary pain.

* * *

As chairman of the House Subcommittee on Health and the Environment, Waxman is one of the most visible spokesmen on health issues in Congress. An unabashed liberal, Waxman is a strong supporter of national health insurance and believes the federal government must play a central role in health care delivery. He came to Washington in 1975 as part of the "Watergate baby" class of freshmen Democrats elected to Congress in the wake of the scandal that swept President Richard Nixon from office. But Waxman's election was not a product of the Nixon woes; he had spent six years in the California Assembly, chairing its reapportionment committee and later its health committee. In that capacity he helped frame the response to the program of Governor Ronald Reagan.

Once he reached Capitol Hill in 1975, Waxman wasted no time moving up the political ladder. He quickly landed a prime seat on the Energy and Commerce Committee (then known as the Interstate and Foreign Commerce Committee) and a slot on its health subcommittee. By 1978, Waxman decided that he had paid his dues and readied a challenge for the subcommittee chairmanship. With the unexpected retirement of subcommittee Chairman Paul Rogers, Waxman had his shot. To get to the top, however, Waxman had to jump over several more senior Democrats on the panel. His chief opponent was a quiet-spoken, respected former judge, Richardson Preyer of North Carolina. Preyer was second in seniority to Rogers on the subcommittee and the obvious successor. Waxman, then 39 years old, was not content to wait his turn while Preyer ran the subcommittee for another half-dozen years. As many of his young House colleagues did, Waxman decided to buck the congressional seniority system and take Preyer on head to head.

The Waxman-Preyer fight was one of the key battles of the young Watergate class for power in Congress. Until the late 1970s, Congress was a bastion of seniority; senators and representatives often served in their seventies, eighties, and even nineties. But things began to change in the mid-1970s, as the younger generation of members began to assert itself. A series of successful challenges to senior House members for leadership jobs led many other veteran legislators to voluntarily lay down their weapons before some Lancelot pierced their armor. By the end of the 1970s the face of Congress had changed dramatically. Gone from the halls of the Capitol were the aged veterans. In their place was a new crop of young, ambitious legislators with their eyes on the television cameras and the newspaper headlines. In some ways the new breed of congressmen brought some fresh ideas and new energy to national policymaking; in other ways the change of generations robbed Congress of the knowledge and experience needed to judge the merit of those ideas and the institutional memory to recall similar proposals that were rejected in years past.

The Waxman-Preyer fight shaped up as a generational battle. In winning his fight with Preyer, Waxman employed tools that have become commonplace in today's political arena but were, in 1980, unfamiliar to many in Congress. He used his political base in California to lock up the California Democratic delegation. He used his fundraising base in his Hollywood district to create his own political action committee, or PAC. In the post-Watergate period, Congress had limited personal contributions to political campaigns for Congress and the presidency, thereby effectively setting the stage for enormous growth in PAC giving. Until 1974, PACs were mainly creatures of the labor movement. After 1974, corporate America embraced the PAC concept and began to exert its political influence through their own PACs.

Waxman was one of the first national politicians to create his own PAC. The informally christened Wax-PAC used leftover campaign money to help other liberal-leaning politicians who had tougher races than Waxman did. During his campaign for the subcommittee chairmanship, Waxman handed out political campaign contributions to many of the Commerce Committee members who would later vote for him. In 1978, this was an unusual practice; two years later most major politicians had set up PACs of their own and were handing out money right and left.

Waxman was not averse to some old-fashioned political maneuvering. Besides feathering the nests of his committee colleagues, Waxman made sure to remind those weighing the Waxman-Preyer choice that Preyer represented the interests of North Carolina tobacco growers, a dubious association for a man seeking to head up a panel dealing with health care issues. Preyer also had ties to the pharmaceutical industry, which the subcommittee regulates. When push came to shove, Waxman carried the day and was elected chairman of the health subcommittee by a fifteen to twelve margin.

After defeating Preyer, Waxman kept a low profile, working to patch relations with his defeated rival and his supporters. Before he lost his House seat in the 1980 Reagan sweep, Preyer had become one of Waxman's closest allies. Along the way, Waxman turned into one of the House's most effective legislators.

* * *

Waxman was not the only opponent to the Medicaid cap in Congress. Republicans in the House and Senate were getting strong messages from officials in their state capitals that the plan would sap their ability to care for the poor and force them to make many unpopular decisions on eligibility and benefits. Still the Republican-dominated Senate was ready to bite the bullet and go along with Stockman and the Medicaid cap. The administration tried to garner support from the governors by adding proposals to expand state "flexibility" in running Medicaid. But the governors saw the proposals as a smoke screen hiding a substantial and permanent reduction in federal spending on health care for the poor. To cement his hold on the governors, Waxman also added flexibility provisions to his Medicaid plan, including new authority for states to place the elderly in home- or community-based care programs instead of institutionalizing them in hospitals or nursing homes. While Stockman wanted to eliminate a federal rule requiring states to provide the poor with the freedom to choose their providers, Waxman offered a waiver of that authority if a state could prove to the government that it was necessary.

The Republican Senate stayed strongly behind Reagan, but even its leaders had some doubts about the Medicaid cap. Finance Committee Chairman Dole went along with the plan but upped the cap from 5 percent to 9 percent. Dole also proposed to drop the minimum federal matching rate from 50 percent to 40 percent, a move that would have a tremendous negative impact on large states like New York and California. Stockman was perfectly happy to accept the 9 percent limit, figuring he could come back later and fight to lower future increases. The principle of the cap was the thing, the size of the first-year limit was relatively meaningless to the budget chief.

Over in the House, Stockman's dream of a Medicaid cap was beginning to fray. While Reagan had pulled out an incredible victory by gaining House passage of a Republican substitute budget blueprint, the defeated Democrats were determined to shape the required cuts so that the damage would be temporary and reparable. Time after time, the Democratic led House committees were structuring their budget-reconciliation packages to frustrate Stockman's goals. In the House Commerce Committee, Henry Waxman's Medicaid plan was kept close to the vest until just before his health subcommittee was ready to vote.

While Waxman had the Democratic votes to push through his package in committee, he felt he had to gain Republican support in order to prevent another Reagan ambush. He and Edward Madigan began a series of meetings to hammer out a package that would be acceptable to both while meeting the strictures of the budget resolution. Madigan, ever the pragmatist, pushed as hard as he could to advance the Reagan agenda but when faced with outright Waxman opposition, Madigan chose to negotiate, to compromise. Together the two men shaped a package of block grants and Medicaid spending cuts that would meet the budget resolution's orders and advance some of the Reagan agenda.

But Madigan had moved far out in front of Stockman and his budget staff. While Madigan felt he had the green light to negotiate with Waxman as long as the budget cuts ordered in the budget resolution were achieved, Stockman wanted the cuts made the way he proposed them. Stockman's insistence angered Madigan, who, while often appearing placid, even laconic, in public, had a sharp temper and could explode in private. Explode he did.

On the day the Commerce health subcommittee was to meet to vote on the compromise package ironed out by Waxman and Madigan, Dave Stockman was on the telephone. Waxman watched as Madigan left the hearing room to take one, two, then three phone calls from the budget director. When he returned from the last call it was obvious to reporters at the press table that Madigan was no longer keeping his cool. He and Waxman left the room together and didn't reappear for nearly thirty minutes. When they did return, the air was heavy with disappointment. Stockman had ordered Madigan to call off the deal; he was to stick to the Reagan line. Madigan's jaw was set, his teeth grinding.

Waxman opened the session with a statement explaining that weeks of negotiations with Madigan had culminated in an agreement. He made no mention of Madigan's enforced change of heart. Madigan, however, was ready with a statement of his own. Making no mention of Stockman, Madigan said he had to oppose the Waxman package. Waxman would go it alone; he introduced his package and called for votes. Republican members, no longer constrained by Madigan's deal, began hacking away at the Waxman plan. But Waxman was determined to get the bill approved that afternoon. He used his parliamentary powers to push through the bill over Madigan's objections. When the day was done, the bill was approved. Madigan stormed out of the room, complaining to reporters that he "had been rolled." Of course, it turned out that the roller was Stockman, not Waxman.

Waxman's package survived the full Commerce Committee despite cries of outrage from conservative Republicans like Thomas Bliley of Virginia and William Dannemeyer of California. Throughout the House, similar bills were being cleared and readied for a single up or down vote on a budget-reconciliation package. Democrats felt they had triumphed over Reagan and Stockman by playing the budget game by their rules. But the President and his budget director had a trump card to play.

Stockman planned to repeat his victory on the budget resolution when the House took up the reconciliation package. Instead of allowing the Democrats to push through their budget proposals, Stockman began assembling a substitute bill to be offered by congressmen Phil Gramm, a Democrat from Texas, and Delbert Latta, an Ohio Republican. It was the same Gramm-Latta pairing that had brought Reagan's budget blueprint to victory earlier in the year.

Stockman hoped to put together a package of law changes that would mirror the Reagan budget submitted to Congress in March. Even though the Republican Senate had already changed much of the Reagan plan, Stockman wanted to be a purist in the House. But GOP support for the specifics of the Reagan health budget was spotty. Pressures from home-state governors and legislators made House members very resistant to the Medicaid cap. Stockman knew he would have to compromise with the GOP if he was going to beat the Democrats again.

In mid-summer, Stockman told House Republicans he could live with a 6 percent Medicaid cap instead of the 5 percent plan sent to Capitol Hill in March. That wasn't good enough for the balking Republicans; Stockman soon moved up to 7 and finally to 7.5 percent. At the same time, he was negotiating changes in other parts of the package to gain support from moderate Republicans. Many of the moderates were from the northeast. To differentiate themselves from the southern conservative "Boll Weevils," these moderate Republicans called themselves "Gypsy Moths." They wanted changes in the Reagan proposals to slash mass transit support, energy support, and Medicaid; on other issues, they were willing to accept Stockman's dictum.

Quietly, health programs were moving to the center of the dispute between Stockman and the Gypsy Moths. Health, energy, and transportation programs all lay in the jurisdiction of the Commerce Committee. Stockman began negotiating two packages: One, Gramm-Latta II, would include the bulk of the Reagan budget; the other would encompass programs in the Commerce Committee. It would be sponsored by the committee's ranking Republican member James Broyhill of North Carolina. Broyhill was a traditional Republican conservative with doubts about the policies of the brash young budget chief. After all, less than a year before, Stockman had been one of the committee's junior members, following Broyhill's orders. The stately Broyhill did not like to see the tables turned.

Broyhill, the Gypsy Moths, and Stockman negotiated for nearly a week. As the Friday-night House vote on the budget package neared, Stockman still believed he had the votes for the Medicaid cap. But support was weak and Republican governors kept up a drumbeat of opposition. On the eve of the vote, Stockman knew he had lost the support he needed. When the House took up the budget bill it narrowly supported the Gramm-Latta substitute. But to the surprise of Waxman and the Democrats, Broyhill withdrew his amendment and the Democrats' health package was approved without a fight. So confusing was the House floor action that newspapers reported the next day that the House had approved a Medicaid cap. By Monday, after the dust had settled, it was clear that while Reagan had won a major victory on the budget, he had been beaten on the key issue of health programs.

Waxman's Medicaid plan still had to survive the House-Senate conference meeting on the budget, but once he had won on the House floor, he was on a roll. Dole, never a big fan of the Medicaid cap, was more than happy to drop his 9 percent cap in favor of a modified version of the Waxman 3-2-1 plan. The final compromise called for a 3 percent cut in federal Medicaid payments in 1982, a 4 percent cut in 1983, and a 4.5 percent chop in 1984. States hard hit by unemployment would get back 1 percent of the cut. States also could earn back some of the lost money if they had a health care cost-containment system in place or saved money by combating fraud and abuse. The bill also eased Medicaid rules to allow states to make changes in their programs. New innovations in home health care delivery, health maintenance organization enrollment, and other programs would result. But states also would have to live with less money, at least for the next three years. The cut in federal support would result in a loss of more than one million Medicaid recipients, many of them children. But the changes enacted in 1981 would have some positive effects. The new home- and community-based waiver program allowed thousands of elderly people to avoid life in nursing homes and to continue to live on their own without losing Medicaid coverage.

The defeat of Reagan's Medicaid cap was a victory for the Democrats, but the poor did pay a price. As a result of the three-year reduction plan and a corresponding set of changes in the welfare programs, the number of Medicaid recipients dropped in 1982 even as the nation was plunging into an economic recession. Despite that drop, Reagan came back in later years to press again for his Medicaid cap. But never again during the Reagan years would Congress agree to cut so deeply into Medicaid spending. As Reagan's 1981 mandate faded into the history books, Congress began to slowly repair the damage by expanding coverage of pregnant women and young children.

Beginning in 1985, and continuing through the rest of the Reagan years, Waxman would turn the budget-reconciliation process to his advantage. While Waxman would never like reconciliation and its penchant for packaging major policy decisions in one large bill, he knew how it could work for him. Legislation improving Medicaid coverage would almost certainly be vetoed by Reagan if it made it to his desk. In addition, Waxman constantly worried about giving conservative congressmen any opportunity to add restrictive language to the Medicaid statute barring federal payment for abortions. While Congress had been annually barring such funding for more than a decade, Waxman was determined not to allow that ban to become permanent. A freestanding Medicaid bill would certainly attract such an amendment, but budget bills were considered on the House floor under a "closed rule" that prohibited such amendments from even being offered. By packaging Medicaid improvements in the budget bill, Waxman would protect the program from antiabortion amendments and make it difficult for Reagan to veto the changes.

Waxman's strategy for building up Medicaid was almost as clever as his successful plan to fight off the Medicaid cap. Over the period of four years, Waxman sought to put into law as many pieces of Carter's Child Health Assurance plan. Its major component—federal income eligibility rules to replace the fifty individual state standards—was clearly out of reach. But CHAP's other elements, which sought to guarantee Medicaid coverage of pregnant women and of young children, were possible. In 1984, Waxman pushed through mandatory coverage of all pregnant women living in families below the poverty line. In addition, he required states to cover first-time pregnant women below the poverty line. While forty-three states already offered such coverage, seven states provided no coverage until the child was born, thus depriving the mother of insurance coverage for critical prenatal care. The 1984 law required states to begin covering young children in families below the federal poverty line.

In 1985, 1986, and 1987, Waxman came back with further expansions of coverage for women and children. States were given the option of covering any pregnant woman even if she were in a two-parent family, as long as the income earned by the parents fell below the state's poverty line. Families with an unemployed primary breadwinner were granted coverage too. Coverage of young children was extended to age 8. States were given the chance to extend Medicaid coverage to families with income as high as 185 percent of the federal poverty line. If states took Waxman up on his offer, nearly two million families living in poverty would gain health insurance.

The Reagan administration fought Waxman tooth and nail each time he pressed for these Medicaid expansions. But the President's own reliance on omnibus legislation to get his way forced him to accept Waxman's legislation and sign it into law. By 1987, state-federal Medicaid spending was rising at nearly 11 percent per year; not quite back to the days of 15 percent growth before

Reagan came to Washington, but considerably higher than the 5 to 7 percent growth of the first half of the 1980s.

But the budget constraints of the 1980s hampered Waxman's efforts to patch the Medicaid holes. Between 1975 and 1985, the percentage of American's who were living under the federal poverty line and qualified for Medicaid dropped from 78 percent to 48 percent. Millions of Americans who could not afford to pay their monthly food bills, much less skyrocketing hospital and doctor bills, were left without health insurance. The effect of that growing number of uninsured Americans was manifold. United States hospitals were burdened with a greater and greater share of uncompensated care. By the time Reagan would leave office, hospitals would be providing nearly $7 billion in free care to people who couldn't afford to pay their bills.

But even more troubling was the effect on people who couldn't get care—free or not. In modern society, health care experts have tended to measure the success of the medical care system by the progress the country made in combating infant mortality. Beginning in 1966, the year after Medicaid was enacted, the infant death rate in the United States had dropped sharply. But shortly after Reagan's administration began, that rapid rate of descent began to slow. In 1983, Dr. Edward Brandt, Reagan's assistant secretary for health, warned that American progress on infant mortality was in danger of grinding to a halt. The culprit: cuts in Medicaid and in programs aimed at serving poor women and their children. Reagan and the Congress ignored that counsel as they pursued budget cuts to reduce the budget deficit. By 1985, Brandt's prediction came true; progress on infant mortality stopped and the rate of deaths among black infants actually began to rise. Fewer and fewer women in America received early and adequate prenatal care; as a result, their babies were more often born underweight and in danger of health problems that would either kill them or leave them partially disabled for the rest of their lives. The changes in Medicaid law that Waxman pushed through Congress over Reagan's objections in the latter half of the 1980s may help to stem that tide of bad news.

3

Block Grants

The second key health battle of 1981 would be fought on two fronts: the familiar budgetary line, and a more complex argument over the role of the federal government versus that of the various states. The debate would involve the future of nearly two dozen small-, medium-, and large-sized health programs that served the needs of millions of Americans, many of them poor.

The list of federal health programs had been growing steadily since the early 1930s when Congress created the Maternal and Child Health program. The number grew rapidly in the 1960s as President Lyndon Johnson's "Great Society" programs became law. The 1970s showed no slowdown. Democrats in Congress worked with Republican presidents Nixon and Ford to expand the federal health role (the pace grew so rapid that Washington wits began talking about the "disease-of-the-month club").

The programs addressed such needs as the lack of health care clinics in poor neighborhoods, the absence of health facilities to treat migrant workers in America's farmland, the necessity for contraceptive services for poor young women, and the need for prenatal and postnatal care for pregnant women and their new children. Many of the programs served useful purposes and helped to improve the health of America's poor. But some of the programs outlasted their usefulness while others were overly limited from the outset.

In the 1970s, a perceived problem was met with a real program. But, when the problem went away the program didn't. The government was handing out grants to local governments, local charitable organizations, and individuals to fluoridate water, control rats, and encourage Americans to take exercise. Along the way, legislators in Washington lost sight of their compatriots at the state level.

Some of these programs were quite successful. Take for example, the Childhood Immunization program. In the 1960s, America's children still were being ravaged by diseases that could be prevented by early vaccination of school-age and preschool children. The vaccines were available, yet millions of families were going unprotected and children were suffering. Measles, mumps, diphtheria, pertussis, tetanus, and other ailments were more common than American medical experts believed was necessary. Congress responded with a new federal program that would channel millions of dollars into the purchase of vaccines and the early vaccination of the nation's children. States began requiring children to be vaccinated before they could begin school. Assembly-line type vaccination days were held, and millions of children were protected. Over the course of the following two decades the incidence of once-common childhood diseases dropped dramatically. By the time Reagan took office, measles was nearly eradicated and other diseases were increasingly rare.

Equally successful, but much less popular was the Community Health Centers (CHC) program. America's medical establishment was one of the most advanced in the world. The United States had the best trained doctors, the finest facilities, the most up-to-date equipment, and the world's leading scientists achieving breakthrough after breakthrough. And yet millions of poor Americans were unable to avail themselves of these services. Many doctors did not want to practice medicine and settle down in poor inner-city and rural areas. Others who did practice in those areas simply saw no purpose in treating patients who could not pay their bills. So Congress voted to open government clinics, known as community health centers, and staff them with newly graduated doctors who had received scholarship assistance from the government through another federal program, the National Health Service Corps. Within a few years, the poor, who had been among the lowest users of the U.S. medical system, became the highest users. Infant mortality, disabling diseases, and other health problems that had unnecessarily plagued the poor began to abate, at least somewhat.

Community health centers also had their detractors. The American Medical Association, for example, viewed the CHCs and their corps of government-paid doctors as an incursion into the private sector; it lobbied hard against the program and later unsuccessfully sought veto power over the placement of the new clinics. Local communities were not always happy with CHCs either. The federal government had opened these clinics to serve the poor and the migrant workers—hardly a popular group of people. During the 1960s, as the plight of migrant workers became known to the general public—chiefly through some highly publicized hearings by then-Senator Robert Kennedy of New York—Congress acted to protect the workers. State and local governments had little interest in spending their own money to aid these workers, since they were not residents and would only be in their states for short periods of time. A federal role was needed to provide at least a minimal level of health care.

But the community and migrant health center programs had as many foes as they did fans. While the centers brought needed health care services to poor and isolated rural communities, they also brought political activism that bothered local government officials. The centers, staffed by young activist physicians, often became centers of action at the local level to carry Johnson's Great Society message. Governors and local politicians were, needless to say, loathe to allow the federal government to spread its message on their turf. Ironically, the clinics also became centers of the movement against Johnson's Vietnam war effort.

Equally controversial was the federal Family Planning program. Enacted in 1970, the Title X program provided federal grants to local clinics to counsel poor men and women on the ways to prevent unwanted pregnancy. For many young adults and maturing teenagers, these federal clinics were the sole source of contraceptives. While the clinics helped to contain the burgeoning epidemic of teenage pregnancy, their advocacy of contraception angered conservative politicians and their followers. Concerns expressed by the then-young antiabortion community led Congress to explicitly ban use of federal family planning money for abortions. But the abortion issue would stick to the program for years to come. Again, the federal government was stepping into the local scene and using its financial clout to alter the landscape.

Conservative Reagan supporters wanted the Family Planning program repealed. Lacking the political muscle to achieve that aim, they chose instead to fight for the program's inclusion in a new health block grant that would be under state control. Antiabortion groups have historically been stronger at the state level than in Washington. By adding family planning to a block grant, antiabortion groups hoped to chip away at the program state by state.

Reagan wanted to turn control of most federal health programs over to the states in the form of two large block grants. As a former governor, Reagan was determined that his administration would reassert the role of the states in delivery of health and other social services. As part of a policy that he called "New Federalism," Reagan proposed in 1981 to establish a series of block grants to the states that would pay for a range of services. But the money would no longer be handed out from the government in Washington; instead, the pay window would shift to the state capitals.

Congress had dabbled with the block-grant notion as far back as 1967, when it bundled a group of disease prevention programs into a single grant program known as 314(d). Consumer groups had argued against creation of 314(d) under the Johnson administration but had lost. Their thirteen years of experience with that block grant taught them to be leery of Reagan's new proposals. Funding for 314(d) had remained stagnant for nearly a decade. Federal lawmakers lost touch with the constituencies served, and therefore, were slow to respond to calls for more money. These same groups worried that Reagan's block grants would follow the same track. Money given to the states would be considered a federal handout; federal legislators would no longer connect the dollars with the people they served.

Reagan may have won his block grants if Stockman had not muddied the waters with a push for a 25 percent reduction in funding. In his last budget message to Congress, Carter had requested $1.7 billion for these programs; Reagan wanted only $1.4 billion. The $300 million cut, Reagan argued, would not affect services; it would come out of "administrative savings."

Reagan's budget called for creation of two health block grants that would combine twenty-five categorical grants programs. According to administration arguments, it did not make sense for the federal government to be awarding millions of dollars in grants to local organizations. Instead, the money would go from the federal government in Washington to each state. Governors and state legislatures would decide who got the money and how it was distributed. The health services block grant would include community and migrant health centers, black-lung treatment clinics, maternal and child health services, and mental illness, alcoholism, and drug abuse programs. A separate block grant would include politically hot programs like family planning, childhood immunization, adolescent pregnancy prevention, and venereal disease (VD) prevention and control; also included were efforts to fluoridate water, prevent lead-based paint poisoning, control rats, and reduce high blood pressure. In proposing his block grants, Reagan noted that 1600 federal employees managed the programs, 235 pages of federal rules regulated them, and 365,000 man-hours were needed to write required reports. More than 12,000 individual groups got money from Washington to carry out the programs. "Day-to-day management has developed into a costly bureaucratic morass of planning, regulating, and reporting at the federal, state, and local levels," Reagan told Congress.

Reagan's argument was not one that many in Congress could argue against. In 1981, Congress included numerous former governors and state legislators; they were sympathetic to local legislators' cries for more control over the goings-on in their states and communities. At the same time, some members of Congress were not crazy about block grants to the states. While a combination of programs would surely simplify the national legislative process, giving up control of the federal purse strings to the governors and state legislators did not sit well with many on Capitol Hill.

Health lobbyists didn't like the idea of block grants at all. They were used to lobbying in Washington; they knew the key members of Congress and could easily press their case. If the money went to the states, organizations would have to lobby in fifty different capitals and the chances of success would be that much smaller. The history of 314(d) haunted them too.

But Reagan's popularity meant the Congress couldn't ignore the block-grant plan. Some form of program would have to be fashioned. Again, California's Henry Waxman was at the center of the opposition. In the House, Waxman's Commerce Committee would have jurisdiction over the health block-grant proposals.

Waxman was an opponent of the block-grant ideology, fearing that pressures on state and local governments would result in money being shifted away from small health programs toward larger ones, or, even more worrisome, to other areas like education and road construction. An all-out effort to defeat Reagan's block grants would be fruitless, so Waxman came up with a strategy that would appear to go along with the President while actually undermining the block-grant effort.

Waxman was aided in his effort by Stockman's insistence that the funding for the programs be cut 25 percent. While many in Congress agreed with Stockman that they had been overly generous with funding of the various programs to be included in the blocks, a 25 percent cut seemed too large. Waxman sought to draw his colleagues' attention to individual programs. Rather than talking about an overall 25 percent cut, Waxman wanted the congressional dialogue to center on the effect of a 25 percent cut in funding for childhood immunizations, family planning services, community health centers, and so forth. Witness upon witness was called before Waxman's subcommittee to testify about the coming devastation if the Reagan plan were adopted. There was little talk about the block-grant concept but lots of debate about the size of the budget.

Waxman's approach appeared to be paying off. Nervous Republicans in Congress went to Stockman about possible compromise cuts, but he held out for the full 25 percent reduction. When GOP legislators asked Stockman to consider exempting some of the more sensitive programs from the cuts or the blocks, Stockman again refused.

Waxman countered the Reagan-Stockman plan with a series of bills of his own. He proposed establishing three, not two, block grants. A prevention block would be similar to that proposed by Reagan, but instead of the health services block, Waxman proposed creating two other blocks—one for maternal and child health services and one for alcohol and drug abuse prevention. In all, Waxman would lump seventeen programs into the three blocks. But, more important than what Waxman did include in his three blocks were the programs that he left out. Community and migrant health centers, family planning clinics, mental health clinics, childhood immunization, and VD control would remain federal programs. Again, to make a showing of his spirit of cooperation, Waxman proposed to cut the spending for each of these programs but staggered his cuts to protect favored programs. Waxman had made himself look like the conciliator granting some of the administration's wishes but not all of them.

While Waxman appeared to be giving ground in agreeing to establish block grants and turn over their control to the states, his legislation had some well-hidden strings that would bind the hands of governors and state legislators so that the federal money would be spent the way Washington intended.

Over in the Senate, the block-grant issue was shaping up into one of the most interesting battles in the new Republican era. The battle over the blocks would pit a veteran liberal Democrat—Edward "Ted" Kennedy of Massachusetts—against a young up-and-coming conservative Republican—Orrin Hatch of Utah.

Hatch was still in his first Senate term when he was elevated to the chairmanship of the Senate Human Resources Committee. He had come to the Senate in 1976, after winning a close race for the Republican nomination and upsetting incumbent Democratic Senator Frank Moss. Hatch ran in 1976 as a Reagan backer and was gleeful when his political mentor rose to the White House in 1981. At 46 years old, Hatch saw a bright political future ahead. Hatch and his supporters had dreams of the White House. As chairman of one of the Senate's most prestigious committees, Hatch would make his mark. The human resources panel, after all, held sway over many of the nation's key health, education, and welfare programs. Hatch would help bring Reagan's dream to fruition. He would be Reagan's loyal warrior.

But Hatch's performance in 1981 would prove an embarrassment to him and his party. Hatch clearly was unprepared to assume the leadership of the Human Resources Committee. While he and Kennedy were close in age, Kennedy had been in the Senate since 1963 and was schooled in its rules. Hatch had barely had time to get his feet wet. The Human Resources Committee was not the most attractive assignment for a conservative Republican like Hatch.

In the 1970s, under the leadership of Kennedy and New Jersey Democrat Harrison Williams, the panel had shaped many of the categorical grant programs now being attacked by Reagan. In those days, conservative Republicans shunned the panel because to serve would have meant to cast numerous votes against these attractive programs. In 1980, the committee had two kinds of Republican members. Moderate-to-liberal Republicans like Jacob Javits of New York saw the committee as a plum assignment, but conservatives stayed away from the panel. Even veteran moderates like Robert Stafford of Vermont and Lowell Weicker of Connecticut had, in earlier years, passed on the committee, choosing other panels first, and only later, reluctantly agreeing to join Human Resources. Ironically, through the 1970s, it was Richard Schweiker of Pennsylvania who had led the Republican forces on the committee. For years Schweiker worked with Williams and Kennedy to shape compromise legislation; as Reagan's first HHS Secretary, he would work to dismantle it. But beyond the moderates like Stafford and Weicker, the committee was now populated by a young cadre of ultraconservative Republicans led by Orrin Hatch. Hatch's group came to be called the "down-in-flamers" for its penchant to oppose any legislation sponsored by the Democrats or that expanded the government's scope.

In 1981, Javits had been defeated and Schweiker had retired his Senate seat and joined Reagan's Cabinet; the unexpected rise of the Republican party to majority status landed Hatch in the chairman's seat. Stafford and Weicker held seats on the committee but were ineligible to become chairman because they already led other committees. (Senate rules limited each senator to the chairmanship of one full committee and one subcommittee.)

After becoming chairman, Hatch was faced with an immediate choice: Retain Kennedy's health subcommittee, or eliminate it. If the health subcommittee remained, Kennedy would probably be replaced as chairman by ultraconservative Gordon Humphrey of New Hampshire. Humphrey, a former airline pilot, was even too conservative for Hatch. Besides, Hatch wanted to go head-to-head with his old nemesis, Ted Kennedy. In what turned out to be a display of hubris, Hatch felt he could beat Kennedy and get the Reagan election "mandate" turned into law. The health subcommittee was disbanded and health matters were to be considered at the full committee level.

Hatch assembled a small, inexperienced staff from leftover members of Schweiker's old staff and health advisers to the down-in-flamers. Like Hatch, his staff was used to opposing legislation, not proposing it. They would prove to be the new chairman's Achilles' heel.

Hatch introduced the Reagan block grants and sought to push them through the committee as quickly as possible. But he neglected to do some simple head counting on his own committee. To maintain control of the sixteen-member committee, Hatch needed nine votes. On the surface, that seemed an easy task. After all, Hatch had nine Republican votes on the committee while Kennedy had only seven Democratic votes.

But Hatch couldn't rely on blind support from his GOP members. Six of Hatch's eight fellow Republicans were new to the committee and of a conservative bent. Newly elected freshmen Dan Quayle of Indiana, Paula Hawkins of Florida, Jeremiah Denton of Alabama, and John East of North Carolina and Don Nickles of Oklahoma joined with Gordon Humphrey to form a conservative phalanx with Hatch. Stafford and Weicker became the focus of the battle for control. They would be the swing votes on any issue of controversy. It would take some clever negotiating to keep the Republicans in line.

The first job of a good chairman and his staff is to find out the priorities of each of his committee members, particularly those on his side of the aisle. Hatch knew he could count on the support of his conservative colleagues. But aides to senators Stafford and Weicker, both veteran legislators with a vested interest in many of the programs that Reagan sought to abolish, say Hatch and his staff *never asked* about their bosses' priorities, they simply assumed that all Republicans would go along with the Reagan mandate. Hatch and his inexperienced staff got little assistance from the Reagan White House in making the case for the block grants; Kennedy had the help of a legion of health care lobbyists to argue against the block-grant scheme.

Stafford, a respected and soft-spoken man, was most concerned with Reagan's plan to cut funding to community health centers, an important source of health care for many of the rural areas of Vermont. Otherwise, Stafford's main concerns were in the area of education. Weicker was similarly concerned about proposed cuts in programs to aid the handicapped and the developmentally disabled. Weicker, as the father of a child with Down's syndrome, had a particular sensitivity to those programs.

Hatch ignored those concerns and continued to press ahead. But Hatch's insistence on pure Reagan philosophy chased Stafford and Weicker into Kennedy's camp. With their support, Kennedy could defeat Hatch's proposals and gain victory for his own. Hatch delayed the committee's consideration of the bills and went to Stafford and Weicker to try to change their minds, but found them in no mood to bargain with their chairman. Instead, they stuck with Kennedy, even going to the point of granting Kennedy the power to vote in their absence. Traditionally, senators grant that right, the proxy vote, to their own party leader. When the committee finally met, Hatch was forced to accept a watered-down pair of block grants that would retain existing funding patterns and retain categorical grants for several programs. Hatch declared a "moral victory," but the White House complained that the block grants were merely "categorical grants in disguise." When all was said and done, Hatch had lost, and lost badly.

Meanwhile, over in the House, Waxman's proposals to create three block grants got a lukewarm reception from the Republican members of his committee, led by Illinois' Edward Madigan. Madigan was pleased with Waxman's acceptance of the block-grant concept but felt he didn't go far enough in cutting funding for the programs. Waxman's 15 percent cut contrasted with Reagan's request for a 25 percent slash.

But Waxman and Madigan developed a good working relationship in 1981 and sought to work out a compromise. Madigan, using his political instincts, felt he had the latitude to negotiate a deal with Waxman if the dollar savings matched up to the Reagan request. Waxman was more interested in preserving the character of the programs involved and was willing—although reluctantly—to accept a deep funding cut, figuring the money could be restored in later years when the impact of the reductions was felt.

Waxman and Madigan worked out a compromise, shaped by Waxman's original blueprint, setting out three distinct block grants and preserving the federal nature of the remaining programs. But Madigan was again receiving mixed signals from the administration. Over at HHS, Schweiker told Congress it was all right to exclude the childhood immunization program from the blocks. According to Schweiker's word, it was the dollar cuts that were most important. But at OMB, Stockman was holding the line for the block grants. Like Waxman, Stockman knew creation of the blocks would be the best tool to cut the support out from under the programs. Lobbyists could never replicate their successful efforts on Capitol Hill in the state capitols. State legislatures and governors had too many local concerns to worry about. To Stockman, the important thing was what went into the blocks. The dollar savings were minimal compared to the big ticket items he was pressing, like the Medicaid cap.

When Waxman and Madigan emerged with their political deal, the results were pleasing to Schweiker but displeasing to Stockman. In an early signal of who was calling the shots, Stockman shot down the Madigan deal and ordered him to vote against the proposal he had just finished negotiating with Waxman. An angry Madigan complied with Stockman's orders, but the deal he had made with Waxman would prove to have more staying power than the budget director believed.

Waxman's interest in preserving the categorical nature of programs like community health centers and family planning clinics was a repeat of past congressional battles over the nature of those programs.

Waxman's determination to preserve those programs was met by similar conviction by Stockman to reduce them. After the Waxman-Madigan deal fell through, Waxman pushed his own bills through the Commerce Committee, over the objections of conservative Republicans led by William Dannemeyer. Dannemeyer, whose Orange County district is solidly Republican, is one of the odder members of Congress. His conservative credentials are sterling, but his ability to get his views heard and reflected in legislation are almost nil. Dannemeyer frequently takes ultraconservative stances in situations where a somewhat more moderate position might have won the day; instead, his right-wing proposals are easily defeated while more liberal proposals are adopted. In 1981, Dannemeyer was no match for Waxman in the Commerce Committee. If Stockman was to win his block grant fight, he would have to go to the House floor to do it.

Stockman put together an alternative block-grant proposal that would have used Waxman's three-block structure but included twenty-four of the twenty-five programs originally slated for the blocks by the Reagan budget. (Stockman bowed to Schweiker's demand that the childhood immunization program be kept out of the blocks.) But Stockman again insisted on the 25 percent budget cut Reagan had requested. Again, moderate and liberal Republicans balked at the size of the cut.

The health block grants were to be packaged with the Medicaid cap and other Commerce Committee programs in a floor amendment offered by Congressman James Broyhill, a Republican from North Carolina. But objections from moderate Republicans convinced Broyhill to drop his effort at the last minute and allow Waxman's proposals to be adopted by the House.

Waxman's surprising victory was not the end of the fight. He still had to face Hatch over a House-Senate conference committee table. Hatch, not yet over the embarrassment of losing his committee's biggest fight of the year, was determined to yield no further ground in his discussions with Waxman and the House.

Because the massive budget-reconciliation bill affected so many programs, congressional leaders appointed nearly a score of conference subcommittees to work out compromises on the differing House and Senate bills. The health block grants would be worked out by members from the House Commerce and Senate Human Resources committees. Waxman and Hatch would head their respective teams.

Having lost his first round of fights in the Senate, Hatch wanted to avoid further defeat by making sure he had a loyal team of negotiators behind him when he began bargaining with Waxman. More specifically, he wanted to make sure Stafford and Weicker would be nowhere near the negotiating table. Weicker helped matters when he chose to concentrate his work on disability programs and did not join the health subconference. But Stafford wanted a seat at the negotiating table.

Hatch went to Senate Majority Leader Howard Baker to try to get out of this problem. Hatch and Baker cooked up a plan that would effectively exclude Stafford from the health subconference. The new Hatch-Baker "rule" would limit a full committee chairman to serving on only one subconference panel outside of his own committee. Since Stafford was chairman of the Senate's Environment and Public Works Committee, he would be able to choose only one subconference panel. Stafford also chaired the Human Resources Education Subcommittee and wanted to participate in the House-Senate negotiations over education programs. Hatch's strategy seemed to have succeeded until Stafford announced that he would temporarily give up his chairmanship of the Environment Committee for the course of the conference negotiations. This would free him up for service on both the education and health subconferences.

Hatch went back to Baker's office and they came up with a second new rule. Under this plan, senators would be limited to one subconference panel unless they were the chairman of the full committee. Again, Stafford would be forced to choose between education and health. This time, Stafford blew his top. He stormed into Baker's office and demanded an explanation of all of these new rules. Baker was forced to back down and Stafford was allowed to serve on both the education and health panels. But the damage was done. Not only did Hatch have a disloyal member on his health negotiating team, but he also had managed to alienate Stafford just in time for the conference to begin.

Hatch entered the negotiations as the nominal head of the Senate's team. He came to the first negotiating session with a list of "nonnegotiable" demands. The block grants approved by the Senate would be as far as Hatch was willing to go. This unusual negotiating style had no effect on Waxman, who was not about to cave in to the demands of a chairman who had no one behind him. Waxman decided to wait Hatch out.

While Waxman and Hatch waited, the other House-Senate negotiators were finishing up their business and readying the massive bill for final House and Senate votes so that it could be sent to Reagan for his signature. But the bill couldn't go to Reagan until a decision was made on the health block grants. Hatch's intransigence was holding up the ballgame, so he was sent to the bench. Baker and Senate Budget Committee Chairman Pete Domenici stepped in and negotiated a deal with Waxman without Hatch's help.

The deal set by Baker, Domenici, and Waxman closely resembled the plan set out months before by Waxman and Madigan. During the weeks of back-and-forth negotiations with Hatch, Madigan had quietly suggested that his old plan might be the perfect middle ground. The plan called for creation of four health blocks.

A prevention block would contain many of the programs suggested by Reagan—rat control, water fluoridation, emergency medical services, home health training, and hypertension control. While states would get control of the money, Congress added some strings requiring them to keep spending the money in the same way the federal government had spent it. Protections were built in for politically sensitive programs combating hypertension and providing local emergency medical services.

A maternal and child health services block grant would lump together seven categorical grant programs—an existing state-run block grant, financial aid for handicapped children, and programs for genetic research, adolescent pregnancy prevention, sudden infant death syndrome, hemophilia research, and lead-based paint poisoning prevention.

An alcohol, drug abuse, and mental health services block would combine three programs—community mental health centers, alcohol abuse clinics, and drug abuse clinics. Waxman wound some federal strings around this block, requiring states to maintain current efforts for three years and barring clinic closures for two years.

Finally, the fourth block grant contained only the community health center program. But this block was the product of another Waxman maneuver. To qualify for block-grant money, a state would be required to provide matching funds from their own treasuries. If a state didn't want to contribute its own money, its community clinics could continue to receive their money directly from Washington. In the three years of this program's existence only West Virginia tried to gain control of the money, but a court struck down its plan to contribute other federal dollars to the effort. Congress repealed the program in 1986 and community health centers continued just as they had before.

An unhappy Reagan administration tried to cut down the size of the CHC program by closing down dozens of the clinics across the country and by shutting down the pipeline of young doctors who worked at the clinics. In 1982, the year after the block-grant effort failed, the administration sought to eliminate clinics by redefining areas that qualified as "medically underserved." Congress once again stepped in to block the White House, but clinics still were faced with a dwindling supply of doctors.

Congress had created a federal aid program for medical students aimed at enlarging the medical school classes and providing a supply of doctors to areas that could not attract or hold their own physicians. The National Health Service Corps offered medical students scholarship money in return for a promise to serve in government-designated areas. With the cost of medical school climbing and more and more middle- and lower-class youngsters looking to go into medicine, the Corps flourished and provided a steady supply of doctors to the new community clinics. When Reagan took office, he sought to plug that pipeline and cut off all future scholarship money. Congress refused Reagan's request to repeal the program, but money for it dried up even as the size of medical student debt grew to historic levels.

Six other programs targeted for block-grant status in the Reagan budget survived and continued as categorical programs. Family planning, childhood immunization, migrant health centers, venereal disease prevention, tuberculosis control, and primary care research were retained.

Again, Reagan didn't stop trying to get his way. In each of its remaining years in office, the administration asked Congress to add the remaining categorical grant programs to the blocks created in 1981; again and again Congress refused. Family planning clinics, particularly those that ran separate abortion clinics, came under repeated attack by administration conservatives.

In 1983, just before he left the administration, Schweiker signed a set of regulations that would have required federally funded clinics to notify the parents of any teenage girl who received contraceptives that their daughter was taking "the pill" or using a diaphragm. The so-called squeal rule was challenged in court and thrown out. Legislative attempts by Hatch and others also failed. But the controversy over the issue kept the program in a state of flux and kept its funding frozen even as thousands of American teenagers were becoming mothers before they left high school.

Congress created a new categorical-grant program in 1981 that is quite a story in itself. Formally called the Adolescent Family Life Act, the program is more commonly referred to as the "chastity bill." It was the brainchild of freshman Republican Senator Jeremiah Denton of Alabama. When Denton introduced his plan early in 1981 it drew giggles from liberals and huzzahs from conservatives. The program would "promote chastity" among America's teenagers for an investment of $30 million per year. But the Denton dream would become a reality because of some unusual circumstances, the most prominent of which were the views of the older sister of a key Democratic senator.

Democrats looked to Ted Kennedy to defeat the Denton proposal, but Kennedy's hands were tied by his allegiance to his sister, Eunice Shriver. Shriver was a firm believer in Denton's philosophy of government championing of chastity. She privately pressed her brother to support Denton and help his bill become law. Kennedy and Denton spent months negotiating some compromises. Most important to Kennedy was the removal of a proposal that would require parental consent before a teenager could get assistance from the program. Denton agreed to water down that provision. But the bill's final push into law was Waxman's assent from the House side. Waxman was no fan of the chastity bill, but he knew a good political chip when he saw one. Waxman was more concerned about preserving the Family Planning program than he was in defeating Denton. He agreed to support Denton if Denton would agree to support him on family planning; a deal was made and it stuck.

The aftermath of the block-grant fight was played out over several years. The fears of lobbyists that the blocks would lead to the dismantlement of many programs proved to be unfounded. States and local governments were reluctant to cut off money to groups that had been on the federal dole, so, many of the funding patterns remained the same.

But the funding cuts that accompanied the new block grants would take their toll. Creation of the Alcohol, Drug Abuse, and

Mental Health block grant came less than a year after Congress had painstakingly completed action on the Mental Health System Act of 1980. Behind the strong leadership of Rosalyn Carter, the First Lady, Congress had come up with a comprehensive plan to offer community-based mental health services to the thousands of people who had been released from state-run mental institutions in the 1960s and 1970s. Many of those people needed to stay on a regimen of medication that allowed them to function in everyday life. The block grant repealed the Mental Health Systems Act, and the budget cuts forced closure of scores of local centers; many others were never opened. Later, as America faced a sharp increase in the number of homeless people, administration officials turned their criticism on the "do gooders" who had released these people from mental institutions in the first place.

Budget cuts also strained the resources of local drug abuse clinics. Again many clinics shut down and others never got off the ground. In 1984 the President and Nancy Reagan, the First Lady, launched a "war on drugs" but found there were not enough clinics to handle the thousands of Americans who sought treatment.

In other areas, the budget cuts meant more cases of lead-based paint poisoning, tuberculosis, and teenage pregnancy. More tragically, the U.S. infant mortality rate, which had been dropping rapidly since the mid-1960s when most of these programs were enacted, stagnated in the mid-1980s.

Politically, Hatch never recovered from the losses he suffered in 1981. His six-year stint as committee chairman was marked by few successes and many stalemates. Early in 1982, I went to his office to conduct a scheduled interview on the coming year's health agenda. With him in his office were seven staff members, and on Hatch's lap was a binder three inches thick, crammed with briefing papers. Now it was not unusual for a member of Congress, particularly a senator, to need a little help answering reporters' questions. Most had their top aide and, perhaps, a press secretary sit in on interviews. Most also had a briefing paper noting key points the legislator ought to raise during the interview. But the scene in Hatch's office was not the usual.

Clearly, the chairman of one of the Senate's major committees was not "up" on the issues at hand, and, more clearly, he couldn't rely on any one staffer to help him through the interview. During the hour-long meeting, Hatch never looked up from that book as he read his staff-prepared answers to my questions. When a follow-up question got too specific for the chairman, he turned to his staff members, who proceeded to argue over the answer.

A more telling incident happened before the interview began. Hatch was late; he was running about thirty minutes behind schedule. Waiting in his reception room, I grew restless and glanced around the room. The walls were lined with framed copies of bills Hatch had introduced along with White House pens. (Traditionally, the White House gives a pen to the author of a bill that the President has just signed.) Most of the bills on Hatch's walls were unfamiliar to me, but a few were health related. Looking closer, I realized these health bills were the original block-grant bills Hatch had introduced early in 1981. Not only were these bills dramatically changed over Hatch's objections, but the measure Reagan eventually signed was an omnibus bill that had been sponsored by one of Hatch's colleagues. I realized those framed bills said a lot more about Hatch than any speech, floor statement, or vote he had made or would make.

4

Reagan's Health Secretaries

The selection of members of a president's Cabinet is always a tricky process. The choices that are made seldom have much to do with the competence of the individuals or their suitability for the post. More often than not, appointments are made to settle old political debts. Other times, the selections are dictated by the president's own political weaknesses; Cabinet members often serve as gestures to political constituencies. Others serve as peacemakers, replacing controversial predecessors to restore harmony to a department rocked by controversy.

Ronald Reagan had the opportunity to pick three secretaries for the Department of Health and Human Services, the largest of the federal departments and agencies. Former Senator Richard Schweiker of Pennsylvania, former Congresswoman Margaret Heckler of Massachusetts, and former Governor Otis Bowen of Indiana could not be more different. Each represented one of the Cabinet types just described.

Reagan's first health chief, Secretary Schweiker, certainly fell into the category of settling a political debt. When he was picked, Schweiker had recently ended a twenty-year career in Congress, capped by two terms in the Senate. His career on Capitol Hill was not marked by any major legislative achievements. For much of his career, Schweiker was considered a moderate-to-liberal northeastern senator. His voting record in Congress had earned him fair marks from the liberal Americans for Democratic Action and poor grades on conservative scorecards, but all that changed in 1976.

In 1976, former California Governor Reagan challenged incumbent President Gerald Ford for the Republican nomination for President. Ford had succeeded Richard Nixon in 1974, when the thirty-seventh President resigned in the wake of the Watergate scandal. After promising not to run for a term of his own, Ford grew to like the presidency and its trappings. His decision to run again spoiled the plans of many Republicans—Reagan included—who had been waiting in line for the end of Nixon's second term. Most GOP contenders stepped aside when Ford announced his change of heart, but Ford's decision did not deter Reagan. Concerned with what he perceived as a moderate tilt in Ford's administration, Reagan challenged the incumbent for the nomination.

Reagan's challenge started slowly. A narrow Ford victory in February's New Hampshire primary was followed by commanding victories in several northern states. As the two men got ready for the North Carolina primary, Reagan was on the ropes and many political pundits expected a polite withdrawal after yet another Ford victory. But Reagan tapped a lode of conservative Republican opposition to Ford's administration and won handily in North Carolina. The fortunes of the two men began to seesaw as they evenly divided the remaining delegates to the Republican convention in Kansas City.

When Reagan reached Kansas City he trailed Ford by a narrow margin. Both camps carefully were counting heads and concluded that absent a Ford faux pas or a Reagan roundhouse, the incumbent would be nominated for another term. Reagan huddled with campaign manager John Sears. A veteran Republican political operative, Sears had shaped the Reagan campaign from day one and now was faced with his greatest challenge. What could be done to put the former governor over the top?

The Sears strategy was simple. Reagan would name his vice presidential choice before the nomination for President was settled. To counter his conservative credentials and shore up support in northeastern states, Reagan would reach out to the moderate wing of the Republican party. Sears chose Pennsylvania Senator Richard Schweiker. The allure of the Schweiker selection was clear, at least to Sears. He would help bring some moderate GOP delegates over to the Reagan camp.

But more importantly, the ploy of announcing a vice presidential nominee before the presidential nomination was decided would force Ford to make a similar move. Ford had already ruled out running with his Vice President; Nelson Rockefeller, former governor of New York, was anathema to the Reagan wing of the party, and Ford dumped him from the ticket before he got to Kansas City. With Reagan moving to Schweiker, Sears figured Ford would move to the right to balance his ticket with a conservative. Sears and Reagan's other advisers hoped the President would stumble and make a bad selection, thus pushing some of his delegates to desert to the Reagan side.

But Sears did not count on the uproar that erupted on the Reagan side when Schweiker was picked. Conservative Reagan supporters were outraged that their leader would bring a moderate into the picture. Schweiker, to them, was nothing more than another northeastern Republican from the Rockefeller-Javits wing of the party. Moreover, Sears hope of attracting moderate Republican delegates to Reagan's side failed. Ford's delegates stayed put and Reagan gained no ground. With the political wind now against Reagan, Ford could sit back and reject Reagan's demand that he name his choice for Vice President. In a last ditch attempt to win the nomination, Reagan asked the convention to change its rules and force Ford to name his vice-presidential choice. Once that effort failed, Reagan's chances were shot. Ironically, Ford later picked acerbic conservative Senator Robert Dole of Kansas to run with him, a move that could have cost him some of his moderate delegates if announced before his nomination.

Schweiker came away from Kansas City damaged goods. He had lost his standing with moderate Republicans, who branded him a traitor. His new conservative friends didn't trust him either. When he returned to the Senate in 1977, Schweiker embarked on a curious journey of political repositioning. His voting record turned noticeably conservative and his staff took on a California tint with other former Reagan aides joining the Schweiker office. Former Reagan adviser David Winston joined Schweiker in Washington to run his minority staff on the Senate Labor and Human Resources Committee. Winston, it was said, was the Reagan spy in Schweiker's camp. He would keep an eye on the converted conservative.

Schweiker's job as the "good soldier" paid off when Reagan won the presidency in 1980. After the damage done in 1976, Schweiker didn't dare run for another term in the Senate from his moderate-to-liberal state of Pennsylvania. Instead, he announced his retirement from the Senate in 1980 but had no plans for the future. Schweiker was the clear choice for HHS once Reagan had won. No other candidate was even considered. The job was Schweiker's if he wanted it; and he did.

The announcement of Schweiker's selection surprised few observers in Washington. For the last four years of his term in the Senate, Schweiker had been the ranking Republican on the Senate's Labor and Human Resources Committee and the Subcommittee on Appropriations of the Labor-HHS-Education Committee. In holding both posts, Schweiker had much to say about the formulation of American health and welfare policy and its financing. Traditionally, authorizing and appropriations committees in Congress are at odds over federal policies. Turf battles between competing chairmen often delay legislation for months or years. By holding the top Republican posts on both the authorizing and appropriations committees, Schweiker was able to increase his influence over the shape of the policies and the amount of money they received. As is almost always the case with former members of Congress who are nominated for Cabinet posts, Schweiker sailed through his confirmation hearings, and his nomination was approved by the Senate.

At HHS, Schweiker modeled his staff after his Senate office. His management team was headed by Chief of Staff David Newhall, while his policy team was run by Dr. Robert Rubin, a nephrologist, who had advised Schweiker on health policy in the Senate. But the real power behind the throne was David Winston.

Winston chose not to stay in government; instead he became an unpaid adviser on all issues. Winston played the central role in development and implementation of Reagan health policies: Besides his service to Schweiker, Winston advised the White House on HHS issues and personnel. His close ties to Reagan's California administration served Schweiker well. At times Winston served both as the White House eyes at HHS and Schweiker's ears at the White House. Winston used his position to push his agenda of competition-based health care financing, reduced federal regulation and staff, increased state control, and creation of state-run block grants. Those were the key elements of the first term Reagan health policies.

Shortly after taking office, Schweiker found that he would not have the dominant role in developing administration health policy. That job would go instead to Reagan's budget director, David Stockman, a two-term congressman from Michigan who came to be the most powerful member of the Reagan Cabinet during the President's first term. With his mastery of domestic spending programs and his ability to get the President's ear on key issues, Stockman was able to blow away all challengers in the early administration budget fights. Soon after his selection as director of the Office of Management and Budget, Stockman set to work on a sweeping review of federal spending policies. He assembled "Stockman's black books"—a set of proposals to dramatically reduce domestic spending. It included cuts and reform of many of the programs in Schweiker's domain.

A natural resentment arose among the newly selected Cabinet members but Stockman was able to trump their complaints with his bleak forecasts for the U.S. economy and the federal budget deficit. Some of the cuts Stockman demanded were easy to accept in Schweiker's HHS, others were not. As the two men engaged in a back-and-forth debate over health priorities, Stockman won most of the battles. Schweiker and his advisers viewed OMB as a "numbers crunching outfit" with little sense of the nation's health needs. Stockman's crew thought Schweiker was captured by the special interest lobbying groups dependent on government largess for much of their income.

Although Stockman won most of the budget fights in 1981, Schweiker was able to save face by protecting a select few programs from the budget ax: biomedical research at the sprawling National Institutes of Health, and childhood vaccinations. But Stockman came back to fight many of those battles again in 1982 and Schweiker found himself losing more often than he won.

Late in 1982, Schweiker decided he had had enough and told the White House he was ready to leave. The Schweiker resignation was announced in January 1983 as he joined the American Council on Life Insurance as its president. The cushy $200,000 job would seem even easier since he would no longer have to face the scowling Stockman over the budget table.

Schweiker's departure followed on the heels of the first midterm congressional elections of the Reagan presidency. Republicans took a beating in 1982 due to the economic recession and high unemployment. A total of twenty-six Republican House seats were taken by Democrats.

While the White House had expected to lose seats in Congress in 1982 because of the recession, its postelection polls showed a disturbing trend. Women were increasingly turning against GOP candidates. While men continued to back Reagan and support his policies, a majority of women thought the President was wrongheaded in his approach to domestic and foreign policy issues. The White House labeled this trend the "gender gap." With Reagan already looking ahead to his own 1984 reelection bid, the White House wanted action to improve the President's standing with women. One solution, they decided, was to appoint women to the Reagan Cabinet. During his first two years in office, Reagan had only one Cabinet-level woman in his administration—Jeanne Kirkpatrick, the ambassador to the United Nations. In 1983 he would name two more.

The perception that Reagan needed to place women in high-profile positions of responsibility, combined with the President's own feeling of responsibility to help the defeated GOP House members find employment, resulted in one of the worst personnel decisions of Reagan's first term.

In Massachusetts, Congresswoman Margaret Heckler lost her

House seat to Congressman Barney Frank. A redistricting plan by the Massachusetts legislature pitted the two congressional incumbents. Heckler had been in the House for sixteen years; Frank for two. But the new district leaned toward Frank. The Heckler-Frank campaign was one of the nastiest of 1982. Believing Frank's bachelorhood could be used against him, Heckler campaigned around the sprawling district with her husband, John, and their children. The message to the voters was clear: Heckler was a family person, Frank was not. (In 1987, Frank made clear what Heckler was hinting at in 1982, revealing in a *Boston Globe* interview that he is homosexual.) But the voters did not buy Heckler's Frank-bashing. Frank beat Heckler over the head with her own voting record. The Republican paid the price for her loyalty to Reagan in 1981 on budget cuts and tax cuts. Frank reminded the voters that Heckler had supported Reagan's economic policies and claimed that deep recession and unemployment were the result. Frank won 60 percent of the vote, defeating Heckler by nearly 39,000 votes.

Heckler wanted a job in the administration. She reasoned that it was only right that the President she had defended and lost her seat for should give her a job. She wanted the vacant number two job at HHS. When she arrived at the White House for her job interview, however, interesting news awaited her: Schweiker was resigning as HHS secretary. Would Heckler consider the job? Stunned, she quickly accepted.

Heckler's choice made lots of sense at the White House. By picking a woman, Reagan could begin to bridge the gender gap. (At almost the same time, Reagan named Elizabeth Dole to head the Department of Transportation, a good choice for a job she was well suited to hold.) Reagan also was a loyal Republican who rewarded good soldiers. When his chief of staff, James Baker III, handed the President the short list of candidates to replace Schweiker, Reagan made clear how well he knew his new secretary: "Let's go with that woman from Massachusetts," the President said.

Unfortunately, the White House neglected to check with some of Heckler's recent House colleagues before naming her to the Cabinet. If they had asked, the President's men would have found that Heckler was an erratic member of the House, switching major committees on whim and discarding staff assistants at a remarkable pace. Even members of the Massachusetts delegation, some of whom she had served with in Congress for sixteen years, held Heckler in low esteem. Republican Congressman Silvio Conte, for years the only other GOP member from Massachusetts, openly disliked Heckler's taste for "photo opportunities." "Margaret would walk a mile for a camera," Conte quipped.

The White House had no illusions about Heckler's ability to handle the difficult job of running HHS. It never intended to have the new secretary take on the nuts and bolts of managing the department and its policies. The plan called instead for newly selected Under Secretary Jack Svahn to handle those duties. Secretary Heckler would be the public face for the department and Reagan's message to American women that he cared.

But the White House failed to tell Heckler about this arrangement. Some quiet behind-the-scenes negotiations with the secretary-designate may well have ended in an agreement to allow Svahn to take the lead on policy matters while Heckler served as the spokesperson for the nation's downtrodden. But Heckler was faced instead with an embarrassingly public division of duties. The implication that she would simply be a figurehead while Svahn ran the department was too much for the proud Irishwoman.

Heckler's back went up and stayed that way for much of her tenure at HHS. The situation was not helped much by Svahn's personality—described by friends as grating, by others as obnoxious. Svahn was a member of Reagan's California administration. He served two years under Schweiker as commissioner of the Social Security Administration. After presiding over the administration's campaign to purge the disability rolls of those considered healthy enough to work, Svahn felt ready for a promotion. He yearned to be HHS secretary but that job was out of his reach. Svahn's controversial tenure at the Social Security Administration was bound to turn any Senate confirmation hearing on his nomination for secretary into a forum on Reagan's disability policies.

The Heckler-Svahn feud was one of the worst-kept secrets in Washington. Both parties took every opportunity to trash the other. Heckler, in the Svahn camp, was known only as "that woman." The HHS under secretary and his minions regularly leaked unflattering stories about Heckler's performance and personality. Heckler was no innocent; she hadn't spent twenty years in politics for nothing. But Svahn had her at a disadvantage. Heckler came to HHS with few allies. Many of her staff members were holdovers from the Schweiker regime; none were too interested in helping her fight off Svahn. Svahn, on the other hand, had numerous allies in the department and at the White House. Many of the assistants Heckler inherited from Schweiker had more allegiance to Svahn than they did to their new boss.

Heckler's first move after taking office was to jettison Schweiker's management team. Chief of Staff David Newhall, rather than being kept on to help with an orderly transition, was given twenty-four hours to clean out his desk. In his place, Heckler hired George Siguler, a Boston lawyer and an associate of John Heckler, the secretary's husband. Siguler had no experience in federal government or in managing an organization as vast as HHS. Other Schweiker-appointed managers were let go in a relatively short time.

The Schweiker policymaking team did stay in place, but it was not trusted by the new secretary. Heckler had to keep them on to finish the work begun before Schweiker left. Sensitive negotiations on Capitol Hill on the shape of Medicare's new hospital payment system were the administration's number one health priority. Heckler, already paranoid about her situation with Svahn, trusted no one in her department. Schweiker's policymakers were kept busy in 1983 gaining congressional enactment of the administration's Medicare reforms and writing the regulations needed to implement those changes. By 1984, the remains of the Schweiker team left.

Beginning in 1984, Heckler began to dig her own grave. With Schweiker's team gone, and Svahn in a period of quiescence, Heckler had the opportunity to install her own policymakers. But Heckler was plagued by constant worry about being undercut by those who knew more than she did; that kept her from choosing a team that could put her stamp on the department. Posts central to the development and implementation of the administration's revolutionary changes in national health policy remained vacant for embarrassingly long periods because of Heckler's indecision. (So many posts were held by officials on an "acting basis" that HHS became known as the "thespian society.") The personnel issue—humorous at times, aggravating at others— would prove to be Heckler's downfall.

One of Heckler's problems seemed solved in 1984 when Svahn left HHS. Svahn had grown tired of fighting Heckler, and she had effectively closed him out of all top-level policy discussions. But Heckler's nemesis landed solidly on his feet at the White House as President Reagan's chief domestic policy adviser. From his new post, Svahn intensified his war of words and deeds with Heckler. From within the White House, Svahn also could point out the personnel problems at HHS.

To compound Heckler's problems, Svahn's promotion to the White House coincided with the arrival at HHS of a new chief of staff. Siguler, once Heckler's closest adviser, was out—a victim of the newly revealed marital difficulties between Heckler and her husband. John Heckler filed for divorce in Virginia; he revealed that the pair had not lived together in nearly twenty years. The messy divorce trial would drag on for months and was played out in the press. Because the chief of staff was an old friend and associate of Heckler's estranged husband, Siguler lost access to and influence with his boss. Excluded from the inner circle of advisers, Siguler submitted his resignation. In one associate's words, "John Heckler got custody of George Siguler."

Siguler was replaced by C. McClain "Mac" Haddow, a political ally of Senator Orrin Hatch, Republican of Utah. Haddow had served a short while in the Utah state legislature and hosted a television talk show. Most recently, he had served as a special adviser to Heckler. Heckler's choice of Haddow to replace Siguler earned her one important political friend—Hatch —and many, many enemies. It was probably the worst decision she was to make at HHS.

Haddow was a classic Washington operator. As chief of staff, he felt he had found the stepping stone he needed to a position of power and authority, and he didn't care who he stepped on to get there. He planned to whip the department into shape and make Margaret Heckler a star. In the meantime, he would polish his own reputation.

Haddow's methods often were crude and ineffective. Having observed from afar the success of Washington insiders in manipulating the press to make their case, Haddow became "Mr. Accessible." Any reporter's call was promptly returned, and the chief of staff was quite willing to talk about any subject raised. He often was willing to raise subjects himself, providing reporters with juicy "exclusive" stories on policy and personnel moves being made at HHS. What Haddow didn't understand was that others had succeeded at the Washington game by providing accurate information that truly was exclusive for the reporter involved. Haddow's exclusive stories were often incorrect. A favorite Haddow trick was to "leak" Heckler's choice of a new top policymaker. But many times the selection had not been approved by the White House. On at least one occasion, Haddow and Heckler had not even bothered to inform one of these choices of his selection. He, in fact, had turned down an earlier offer and told the White House he would never go to HHS as long as Heckler was secretary and Haddow ran her staff. Haddow operated on an assumption shared by a few misguided bureaucrats that if the press reported something as fact, the opponents of that decision would cave in and accept it. He was, of course, wrong. Reagan's White House staff was much smarter than Haddow—all of Heckler's choices were put on hold. An eighteen-month standoff began.

Haddow was also unskilled in managing the giant HHS bureaucracy. With a manner that often resembled a bulldog, Haddow sought to bully his troops into allegiance with the embattled Heckler. He was not successful. In 1985, Haddow boasted to a group of reporters that he had recently fired two secretaries in Heckler's office for participating in a betting pool. The secretaries were betting on the date on which Heckler would be fired or would resign. Haddow's purpose seemed to be a show of force—

his; instead, it gave reporters a perfect example of how low the secretary had sunk.

After Heckler's departure from office in 1985, Haddow experienced a quick fall from grace. Within months of his own departure from HHS, he was the target of an FBI investigation into allegations that he had helped set up a private charitable foundation to encourage handwashing by children in hospitals and had funneled more than $30,000 to his wife, Alice, by ordering the foundation to pay a Washington secretary to perform public relations duties. The secretary dutifully sent the money, minus a 10 percent commission, on to Mrs. Haddow. A similar deal had been struck by Haddow and two Washington speech writers. In 1986, Haddow pled guilty to charges of conflict of interest, and was sentenced to one year in a federal prison.

Despite all of her weaknesses, Heckler could have been a good HHS secretary. Her years in Congress had trained Heckler to have a nose for issues. Shortly after she took the HHS job, Heckler began pressing the White House to back off from its controversial hard-line stand on review of government benefits for disabled individuals. The administration's campaign to strip the disability lists of those who could work had become an embarrassment both to the White House and GOP members of Congress. Heckler had been involved in the fight in Congress to put a halt to the disability reviews, and she carried that fight with her to HHS. Several months after she took office, Heckler helped negotiate a deal with Congress that placed a temporary moratorium on disability reviews.

Heckler also was quick to identify the significance of the AIDS epidemic as a public health and political issue. Schweiker paid little attention to AIDS, choosing to leave it in the able hands of the assistant secretary for health, Dr. Edward Brandt, Jr. Heckler moved AIDS to the front burner and declared it her department's "number one public health priority." But Heckler did little to back up her words on AIDS with action.

Heckler was more successful in her efforts to identify the issue of child support enforcement. While at the helm of HHS, Heckler helped move legislation through Congress that increased government efforts to force absent fathers to pay the child support they owed. New penalties and greater government policing helped to sharply reduce the unpaid bills.

Despite these accomplishments, Heckler must be considered one of the least successful HHS secretaries. Her inability to get along with the Reagan White House and her selection of such managers as Haddow led to her downfall in 1985. The beginning of the end came for Heckler in December 1984, two months after Reagan's election to a second term. Heckler had hoped to stay at the helm through the rest of the Reagan administration. But in December 1984, Heckler lost one of her few allies in the White House when Chief of Staff James Baker III and Secretary of the Treasury Donald Regan switched jobs. With Baker out and Regan in, Heckler not only lost a friend but gained an enemy in Reagan's inner circle. In their few dealings with each other at Cabinet meetings, Secretary Regan and Secretary Heckler did not usually see eye to eye. Regan regarded Heckler as a lightweight on politics and policy. He also did not view her as a team player. Regan, on the other hand, was the ultimate team player.

In the wake of President Reagan's sweeping reelection victory over Democrat Walter Mondale, the White House began reassessing the Cabinet. Top members of the Reagan White House staff and Cabinet began to return to the private sector. Regan was in charge now and it was clear he wanted Heckler out. In March, Regan and his staff made quiet inquiries of Heckler and her aides about the possibility of Heckler becoming U.S. ambassador to Ireland. But Heckler got her Irish up and declined the offer. Her refusal to go quietly kicked off nearly a year of open warfare between the powerful White House chief of staff and the HHS secretary.

Regan put a hold on any and all political appointments at HHS. While Heckler went about interviewing prospective candidates for the many vacant posts in her department, Regan was passing the word that none would get the jobs they wanted until Heckler was safely on her way to Ireland.

Regan made his campaign public in October 1985 by leaking

to the press his desire to get Heckler out of the Cabinet. Having given Heckler the chance to depart with her dignity intact, Regan now was determined to get rid of her in the most humiliating fashion. Regan's leak was followed by denials from Heckler and the White House. But the White House chief of staff noted the absence of any public hue and cry in Heckler's defense. In fact, the only defender Heckler could muster was Senator Hatch, who was called to arms by his former aide, Haddow. In the absence of any strong Heckler supporters, Regan let the press know about his offer of the ambassadorship. When asked about the offer, Heckler called it "a nice job—for someone else." But by then her fate was sealed. Regan got the President to call Heckler to the White House and make the ambassadorial job offer directly. Heckler, still hoping she could survive the onslaught, asked the President for a few days to think it over. But twenty-four hours later Reagan and Heckler stepped before the cameras in the White House pressroom to announce the HHS secretary's "promotion" to the ambassadorial post. A grim-faced Heckler appeared on the brink of tears; Reagan didn't look much happier.

With the deed done, Regan was now faced with the task of finding a successor to Heckler. In most cases, when the White House forces a Cabinet secretary to resign, a replacement is ready to be announced on the same day, thereby deflecting the public's attention to the newcomer. But, in his haste to rid himself of Heckler, Regan had not yet begun the process of selecting a successor.

A two-month search for a new HHS chief ended with the selection of former Indiana Governor Otis Bowen, M.D. White House aides crowed that Bowen was a "triple crown" cabinet selection. As a former governor, state legislator, and physician, Bowen would bring administrative skills, legislative knowledge, and a medical background to one of the toughest jobs in Washington. The 67-year-old Bowen was beyond reproach. His kindly bedside manner turned angry congressmen into pussycats. No one criticized the selection and confirmation was assured.

Bowen's mild-mannered countenance fooled many observers into believing he was a caretaker secretary. But during his sixteen years in the Indiana state House of Representatives—including six years as speaker of the house—Bowen was an able legislator and leader of the Indiana Republican party. Later, during two four-year terms as governor of Indiana, Bowen presided over an economic boom that saw lower taxes and economic growth. Many in the state say Bowen could have been governor for life, but he chose to retire in 1982, following the lengthy and painful death of his first wife, Elizabeth, from cancer. As a physician and loving husband, Bowen was rarely away from his wife's side during her extended illness. It was during this time that Bowen began to think about the need for insurance coverage for catastrophic illness.

After he left the governor's mansion, Bowen planned a restful retirement. He had remarried in September 1981 and was happy with his part-time teaching position at the University of Indiana. In 1982, however, Secretary Schweiker asked Bowen to chair an advisory commission charged with studying Medicare and coming up with ways to preserve the program's fiscal solvency. Government actuaries had estimated that the rising cost of medical care, combined with the projected increase in the number of elderly Americans in the latter part of the twentieth century, would leave Medicare bankrupt by the 1990s.

As chairman of the Medicare commission, Bowen was given a thankless task. Any proposals to save Medicare from bankruptcy would involve reduced benefits for the elderly, higher taxes for working Americans, or both. Nevertheless, Bowen set to work on a year-long project, determined to come up with an acceptable report. At his side was a veteran government bureaucrat, Thomas Burke. Burke, who had previously worked at the Department of Defense and at HHS, became Bowen's chief adviser and unofficial guide through the federal maze. When the commission completed its work, it came up with a lengthy report that recommended a combination of reduced federal support for certain medical procedures, a delay in eligibility for Medicare benefits, and increased taxes.

Because the Bowen commission report was completed almost at the same time that Congress was enacting a new hospital payment system for Medicare, its recommendations—including the suggestion that Medicare provide catastrophic illness insurance for the elderly—got little attention.

Two years later, as the White House looked to sweep Margaret Heckler out the door, Bowen's name rose to the top of a list of candidates for the HHS job. Oddly enough, he advanced without any effort of his own. In fact, Bowen told his supporters that he would prefer to remain semi-retired in Indiana and did not relish the idea of coming to Washington to finish out the Reagan term. But Bowen's friends in Washington—Indiana's two Republican senators, Dan Quayle and Richard Lugar, in particular—convinced the former governor to take the job.

Once he was in place, Bowen was given an opportunity to fill the many vacant posts in his new department, although the White House kept close tabs on most selections. Bowen named Burke, who had helped him get through the Medicare commission days, as his chief of staff. For his under secretary, Bowen turned to Donald Newman, an old Indiana colleague. Newman had come to Washington twelve years earlier when then-Governor Bowen named him the state's lobbyist in Washington. In theory, Newman was to be in charge of policy development at HHS, while Burke was in charge of management. But because of his more forceful character and his close allegiance with Bowen on the catastrophic issue, Burke proved to be a powerhouse at HHS.

Bowen immediately began calm the roiling waters at HHS. In an effort to restore morale, he made a walking tour of the giant headquarters, wishing all employees a happy holiday. For many, Bowen's appearance was the first sight they had had for many years of an HHS secretary.

Bowen was determined not to serve as a caretaker secretary during the final two years of the Reagan administration. He wanted to leave his mark before returning to Indiana for what he believed would be his retirement. As any smart politician would do, Bowen set himself an agenda. On that list were items that he knew the White House would want him to pursue—a campaign against drug abuse, for example. But the core item on the list was Bowen's dream of a Medicare catastrophic health insurance plan. Bowen was convinced that the government should provide some peace of mind and financial protection to the elderly who face lengthy illness and enormous medical bills. It would take a long, hard fight against the conservative advisers to Reagan in the White House, but Bowen would win presidential support for his initiative and eventually see it become law (see Chapter 11).

5

Unemployed, Uninsured

The economic recession of 1981 and 1983 gave Democrats in Congress another chance to pursue their expansionary health care philosophy. From the outset of President Reagan's administration, the national agenda was dominated by a concern to reduce the historically high levels of inflation and to bring down high interest rates. To bring down inflation, Reagan worked with the Federal Reserve Board to tighten the supply of money. With less money to spend, consumers bought less. With customers buying less, companies had to cut their prices. The result was a rapid decline in the rate of inflation from nearly 12 percent in the last year of Jimmy Carter's administration, to just over 4 percent in the first year of Reagan's first term.

But Reagan's tight money policy had its natural and expected negative effects on the economy as well. Companies had to balance their loss of revenue due to lower prices with a cut in their own costs, which led to enormous worker layoffs. As a result, the U.S. unemployment rate skyrocketed in 1982 and 1983 to 10.4 percent. A larger percentage of workers were unemployed in 1983 than in any year since the Great Depression. At the same time, Reagan's tight money policy helped to keep interest rates near their historic levels.

The high unemployment rate made for some very nervous Republicans in the White House and, particularly, on Capitol Hill.

Unlike Reagan, Republican congressmen had to face the voters in 1982. The prospect of campaigning on an economic "success" that resulted in millions of unemployed and continuing high interest rates did not please the GOP senators and representatives who had to run for reelection that November.

At the midpoint of his first term, Reagan asked his GOP supporters in Congress to stick with him; to a remarkable degree, they did. Reagan's Republican support in Congress did not wane in 1982 despite rising unemployment and the worsening recession. But Republican legislators paid the price at the polls in November. The GOP lost twenty-six seats in the House, effectively erasing the working majority the Republican party had forged with conservative southern Democrats. In the Senate, the losses were not nearly so bad, mainly because Republicans had to defend only twelve of the thirty-three Senate seats up for grabs. Yet the GOP nearly lost its majority. Republicans lost only one incumbent—first-termer Harrison Schmitt of New Mexico—but came close to losing half a dozen others. Veteran Republican senators Robert Stafford of Vermont, John Danforth of Missouri, and Lowell Weicker of Connecticut came within a hair's breadth of losing their seats. Other senior GOP senators were running scared up until election day but won reelection with fairly comfortable margins. Their Democratic opponents hammered on the issues of high unemployment and interest rates. Ironically, moderates like Stafford, Danforth, and Weicker had voted against many of Reagan's economic policies.

It was a wary 98th Congress that convened in January 1983. Reelected Republican senators were no longer willing to march in lockstep with the President. The nineteen GOP senators facing reelection in 1984 had concluded that loyalty to the White House could add them to the unemployment rolls. In the House, Speaker Thomas "Tip" O'Neill, Jr. was reveling in his reborn Democratic majority. From 1981 to 1983, O'Neill was forced to take a back seat to the new President, as Reagan shaped a bipartisan majority in the House and Senate combining nearly unanimous Republican support with the backing of one- to two-dozen conservative southern House democrats (the Boll Weevils). Now, with the Democrats regaining twenty-six seats in the House, the two-year reign of the Boll Weevils was over. Democrats moved quickly to cement their new power with committee appointments. O'Neill was determined not to make the same mistakes twice; Reagan was not going to end-run the Speaker in 1983.

House Democrats wasted little time in putting their new power to use. Early in 1983, the Democratic caucus met to chart the party's legislative initiatives. High on the list of domestic issues was help for the unemployed. Acting on O'Neill's orders, the House Budget Committee made room in the fiscal 1984 budget for a $1.8 billion program of health insurance benefits for unemployed workers. The announcement by Budget Committee Chairman James Jones of Oklahoma touched off a year-long debate that at times appeared headed toward the creation of a new health care entitlement program. Sponsors of the legislation had the public's support and were riding the crest of a political wave. But proponents of health insurance for the unemployed failed to ride the wave to shore; instead, they crashed on the rocks. The failure of the Congress to enact such a program demonstrates how much Reagan had changed the political landscape in just two years in office. It also is a prime example of how congressional egos can get in the way of policy.

Democratic leaders realized that they had only a small window of opportunity to enact legislation to help the unemployed. But their agenda was packed with items, many of them shopworn proposals from years past. Weeding out the items that were possible from those that were merely pipedreams wasted months of precious time. A limited program of health insurance for the unemployed did remain on the agenda.

Because the United States relies on a patchwork of government programs—primarily Medicare and Medicaid—and private health insurance to provide health benefits to its people, many Americans are still without adequate coverage, millions more have no insurance at all. From the mid-1940s on, Congress after Congress rejected the national health insurance models that had been adopted in Europe and other parts of the world. When employers began buying private health insurance as a fringe benefit for their workers in the 1950s, federal lawmakers saw a way around the issue of national health insurance. By granting employer-paid insurance a full exemption from federal taxation, the government took a giant step toward protecting Americans against the cost of health care. Employers could provide billions of dollars in health insurance coverage and not a dime of that expense would be taxed. At the same time, workers—particularly those in labor unions—could receive a valuable benefit that, unlike salary, was untaxed. The government's move paved the way for a massive expansion of employer-paid health insurance benefits for working Americans. In 1965, Congress stepped in to fill some of the gaps in that system by creating Medicare to insure elderly retirees and Medicaid to protect the poor. Gaps, however, were not completely eliminated. Congress left Medicaid coverage decisions to the states; the result is a widely varying system in which a poor family in one state gets comprehensive health care coverage, while another family in the same straits but a different state gets a bare-bones insurance policy. One of the most gaping holes was, and still is, the lack of protection for laid-off workers. When health insurance became a privilege of the working class, it became yet another deprivation for those who are out of work. Many policymakers thought Medicaid would catch those who fell through the social safety net, but Medicaid was not designed to help.

The plight of the unemployed aroused concern in Congress during the economic recession of 1975 and 1976. Congress briefly toyed with the idea of creating a federal health care entitlement program to provide temporary insurance coverage for those out of work. But Congress became caught in a bind that would prove to delay many needed repairs to the U.S. health care system. Proponents of national health insurance—primarily organized labor—would not brook enactment of a program just to aid the unemployed. If Congress was to address the health care needs of the nation, then it would have to go all the way with national health insurance. While policymakers argued this point, the national unemployment rate began to drop. As unemployment flagged, so did congressional interest in a new program.

5 / Unemployed, Uninsured

In 1983, Washington experienced a bout of déjà vu. Democrats launched the new year with ambitious plans for a new program of health insurance for the unemployed. At the height of the recession, an estimated 10.7 million Americans were out of work and out of luck because their health insurance had expired. Congressional hearings were held, featuring victimized unemployed workers, overburdened corporate leaders, concerned health care providers, profound health care policy analysts, and photogenic legislators. Once the hearings were out of the way, Congress got down to the work at hand—drafting legislation.

California Congressman Henry Waxman was the first to come forth with a proposal to provide health insurance benefits to unemployed workers. As a liberal chairman in a conservative era, Waxman more often than not confounded his political opponents by getting legislation enacted that moderated Reagan policies or expanded programs in the face of administration opposition. Waxman carefully built alliances with key members of the House, including Speaker Tip O'Neill and Rules Committee Chairman Claude Pepper, of Florida. But Waxman's success also earned him some foes within his own party. Chief among these is Dan Rostenkowski, chairman of the Ways and Means Committee.

Rostenkowski is an old-time Chicago politician, raised by the political machine of the late mayor, Richard Daley. He spent six years in the Illinois legislature before being elected to Congress in 1958. Rostenkowski is one of the most powerful members of the House. In 1981, he was faced with the difficult choice of taking the chairmanship of the House Ways and Means Committee, with its control over national tax policy and much of the federal social welfare budget, or remaining in the House Democratic leadership as the majority whip, the third ranking position behind the Speaker of the House and the majority leader. By staying in the leadership, Rostenkowski would have put himself on track to become Speaker near the end of the twentieth century. Instead, he heeded the call of his fellow Democrats and took the Ways and Means post, thus effectively sacrificing his chances at the Speaker's chair. His early tenure at Ways and Means was not promising. In 1981, Rostenkowski got into a bidding war with

President Reagan over tax cuts. The result: a tax bill that gave away billions in federal revenue. Rostenkowski was determined to repair his wheeler-dealer image and prove his mettle as a substantive legislator.

Rostenkowski did not look kindly on the new generation of upstart congressmen. He and Waxman could not be more different. Rostenkowski is big and brusque; Waxman is short and shy. The natural tensions between the two men were heightened by their rivalry as chairmen of competing House committees. The Waxman-Rostenkowski rivalry also is based on the division of authority over health programs in the House. In the Senate, jurisdiction over health programs is clearly split. Authority of the giant Medicare and Medicaid programs rests solely with the Finance Committee; work on public health programs is done by the Labor and Human Resources Committee. Over in the House health issues are divided in a rather haphazard manner between the Commerce and Ways and Means committees. While Commerce has total control over Medicaid and public health programs, the two panels split work on Medicare. Ostensibly, Ways and Means has control over Medicare's hospital insurance program and a piece of Medicare's physician insurance program. The rest of the physician insurance program lies with Commerce. The division of labor creates friction between the two panels that often delays progress on legislation.

Waxman proposed a broad new program that would set national standards for eligibility and benefits. Patterned after the Medicaid program, Waxman's proposal would have created a third new federal health care entitlement program. Under the terms of the proposal, any worker who was laid off by his employer would be automatically eligible for up to one year of government-provided health insurance. Employers would be required to provide three months of coverage, and the government would pick up the tab for the remaining nine months. The federal price tag on Waxman's bill was $1.8 billion in the first year and $5.5 billion over three years. The most prominent feature of Waxman's bill was its entitlement nature. Laid-off workers would not have to prove that they could not afford to buy insurance;

the only criteria for qualifying was loss of a job. With eligibility and benefits set in advance, there would be little ability on the part of the federal government to control its costs.

Rostenkowski, whose committee was regularly struggling to control runaway Medicare costs, was not about to accede to Waxman's wishes and create another locomotive to drive health care inflation. He openly opposed the Waxman approach and offered instead to create a state-run block-grant program in which the federal government would hand the states $1.8 billion a year to cover the costs of health insurance for unemployed workers. Under Rostenkowski's plan, states would decide who is eligible for the benefits and what type of benefits would be provided. If costs exceeded the $1.8 billion the federal government provided, states would have to come up with the additional money on their own. Continuing disagreement between Rostenkowski and Waxman served to delay House approval of legislation until late in the summer, a stall that would prove fatal to the bill.

Not all the blame lies with the Democrats. Congress still could have passed a health benefits bill for the unemployed if not for some clever political maneuvering by the Reagan White House and the Republicans running the Senate. The 1982 election had hammered home the political price of laid-off workers. In the Senate, Republican leaders felt compelled to follow the lead of the House and come up with a plan to provide health insurance benefits to the unemployed. At first, the White House said it wanted no bill, but that approach proved unpalatable on Capitol Hill. Following the 1982 election, Senate and House Republicans would prove much less willing to listen to White House marching orders.

The White House went into Washington's version of the "big stall." Budget Director David Stockman was opposed to creation of a new health care entitlement program. Stockman knew that if he could stall Congress long enough, the unemployment rate would begin to come down and political pressure for action would ease. Stockman pressured Senate Republicans to slow down their rush to pass legislation. Early efforts by Senate Finance Committee Chairman Robert Dole were thus thwarted by Stockman.

Dole hoped to attach his own health insurance proposal to a major bill to reform the nation's Social Security system. The Social Security package was the product of two years of intense negotiations. It was must-pass legislation and Dole's idea to pin on the health insurance measure could have guaranteed quick passage. Stockman hit the roof and insisted that Dole back off. Instead, Stockman promised to come up with an administration proposal that he would bring to Congress in the summer. A reluctant Dole agreed to hold off on his legislation.

Stockman never intended to come up with a viable proposal to insure the unemployed against huge medical expenses. In mid-April, Stockman brought a plan before the President's Cabinet that he knew could not fly. The budget director said that the private sector—employers, health insurers, and others—should bear the cost of insuring the unemployed. Stockman asked HHS Secretary Margaret Heckler to carry his plan to Capitol Hill; Heckler refused. In a series of Cabinet-level meetings, Stockman was forced to back off from his "private sector only" proposal. For Stockman, it was back to the drawing board. While publicly dismayed that his proposal was shot down, Stockman was privately gleeful because the Cabinet's refusal played into his plan to continue stalling the congressional effort to pass legislation in 1983.

A frustrated Dole decided to go ahead without Stockman and the administration and introduced his own $1.8 billion health insurance package, building on the existing Medicaid program. At first, Dole proposed to limit the program to states with high unemployment. When senators from the seven states that would fail to qualify said they would vote against any bill that excluded their constituents, Dole capitulated because he couldn't afford to lose fourteen votes on such a critical issue.

Stockman had to act fast to cut Dole off at the pass. He quickly dropped his private sector option and came up with a new approach: The federal government would provide health insurance to unemployed workers, but, in return, employed workers would pay a tax on their own insurance. Stockman had long favored a limit on the federal tax exemption for employer-paid health insurance. He argued that the exemption led companies to buy "Cadillac insurance" for everyone rather than limiting insurance to high medical costs. As a member of Congress, Stockman had proposed limiting the exemption to the first $100 or so per month in insurance premiums. All premiums that exceeded that cap would be taxed. Organized labor, health insurers, and employers all opposed Stockman's so-called tax cap. The United Auto Workers (UAW), representing the millions of employees of Ford, General Motors, and Chrysler, were vehemently opposed to the tax cap idea. Their opposition was easily understood—the average auto worker had health insurance valued at more than $300 per month. Auto workers, unlike most Americans, paid no deductibles, paid no coinsurance, and had coverage for everything from eyeglasses and dental care to psychiatric therapy. For the UAW, the tax cap meant big bucks out of their members' pockets. Stockman put the auto workers on the spot with his challenge to labor that those who were working should help those who were out of a job. Although the tax cap had few supporters in Congress, Dole was among them. By linking the health insurance for the unemployed issue to the tax cap, Stockman succeeded in again slowing action in the Senate.

The key to Stockman's delaying tactic in the Senate was continued foot-dragging in the Democratic House. Stockman sought to maintain the rift between Waxman and Rostenkowski by backing Rostenkowski. That move angered Waxman and hurt Rostenkowski's efforts to gain liberal Democratic support. After all, if David Stockman liked the idea, it couldn't be any good, many House Democrats believed. Stockman's carefully crafted strategy may have come apart when Waxman reached out to moderate Republican Congressman Edward Madigan of Illinois. As the ranking Republican member of Waxman's subcommittee and a part of the Republican leadership team in the House, Madigan held sway on many health issues. Despite Stockman's pleas, Madigan conducted a month-long negotiation with Waxman on the terms of a compromise health insurance bill. When they announced their agreement, the logjam in the House seemed broken. To gain Madigan's support, Waxman agreed to slightly modify his original proposal so that benefits would end in 1986 and assistance would be limited to states with high rates of unemployment. These were safe sacrifices for Waxman to make because he could be relatively sure that the Senate would insist on covering all states and that Congress would be unlikely to allow a program to die even if the number of unemployed dropped.

The Waxman-Madigan deal angered the White House. Until that point, Madigan had been the White House's fair-haired boy on health issues. Madigan's efforts on the President's behalf had earned him no help from the White House and no affection from his constituents. When Madigan joined forces with Waxman in 1983, the White House washed its hands of him. But House Republicans continued to respect and support their soft-spoken, sardonic colleague. With Madigan's support, Waxman's bill was approved by the House Commerce Committee at the end of May by a thirty-four to eight margin.

Waxman's success made Stockman's job all the more difficult. With the House legislation seemingly on a fast track, the budget chief had to slow the Senate and hope for an improvement in the unemployment rate. By the summer of 1983, the national unemployment rate had steadied at about 10 percent and showed signs of dropping. Manufacturers, taking advantage of the tax breaks provided by Congress in 1981, began expanding their plants and hiring back many of the laid-off workers. But Stockman needed another month or two to ensure his plan would work. Stockman got his break when Rostenkowski blocked Waxman's bill from reaching the House floor.

Rostenkowski took advantage of an obscure House procedure allowing committee chairmen to claim jurisdiction over the work of other committees. Waxman's bill contained a mandatory deduction from federal unemployment compensation checks to pay for part of the health insurance coverage. Rostenkowski's committee was responsible for the unemployment insurance program so he claimed jurisdiction. Waxman's bill was referred to the Ways and Means Committee in June, with strict orders that it was to move to the House floor by the end of the month. But Rostenkowski had no intention to restrict his action to the unemployment compensation portion of the Waxman bill. He used his time to drastically alter the entire bill, replacing Waxman's open-ended entitlement with his own state-run block grant.

Waxman was incensed by Rostenkowski's power grab. He dug in his heels. In the words of one Waxman aide, Rostenkowski wanted to "put $1.8 billion on a tree stump and let the states do with it what they will." Waxman wanted federal standards for eligibility and benefits; Rostenkowski wanted none. Stockman looked on with glee as the Waxman-Rostenkowski feud continued.

Meanwhile, back in the Senate, Dole's plan was on hold. At Stockman's prompting, Dole had agreed to hold off on any action until the fight in the House was completed. But Dole's decision did not bind the hands of yet another congressional committee. Over in the Senate's Labor and Human Resources Committee, Dan Quayle, a Republican from Indiana, and Ted Kennedy, a Democrat from Massachusetts, worked out their own deal and introduced legislation calling for a partnership between the private and public sectors. Employers would be asked to continue insuring their workers for ninety days; after that time, laid-off workers could buy their own insurance at the company's cheaper group rate. For workers unemployed for more than six months, a new federal program would provide insurance. The Quayle-Kennedy plan was approved by the committee at the end of June and was seemingly on the way to the Senate floor. The bill never reached the floor. To protect his turf, Dole placed a parliamentary hold on the legislation.

Finally, in early July, Rostenkowski and Waxman took off their boxing gloves. Waxman gave in to Rostenkowski's demands, and a $1.8 billion block-grant program was approved by Ways and Means by a twenty-one to eleven margin. It was another month, however, before the bill reached the House floor. In early August, the House voted 252 to 174 to approve the Rostenkowski plan. The standoff between Waxman and Rostenkowski had lasted almost three months and wasted the momentum built up behind the issue in the early part of 1983. By the time Waxman backed off, the national unemployment rate had begun to edge downward and political support began to evaporate.

Dole was now out of excuses and was forced to lift his hold on the legislation. Nevertheless, by the time the Senate was free to consider health insurance for the unemployed, the urgency behind the issue was gone and the legislation withered. One last effort was made late in the year as Senate proponents introduced a scaled down $900 million program, but even that plan lacked enough support to risk a vote. When Congress adjourned in December, no action had been taken. Stockman's strategy worked; by slowing the congressional freight train, the budget director had staved off what would have been a budget-busting new program.

The story of health insurance for the unemployed shows how political egos often can get in the way of good policy. Unemployed workers need health insurance just as much—in fact, more than—those who have a job. With the United States continuing to rely on a patchwork system of insurance, it is the unemployed who suffer. In the succeeding years, the price of the Congressional failure of 1983 became clear. While employment rose and the number of out-of-work people fell, the number of Americans without health insurance stayed high. Many of the workers who lost their jobs in the recession of 1982 and 1983 went back to work but never regained their health insurance. They were hired back by companies that didn't offer insurance or took part-time jobs that did not carry insurance. By 1986, the number of uninsured Americans hit thirty-seven million, up nearly 20 percent from 1980.

While the number of uninsured grew, the Reagan administration insisted that indigent health care was a "state and local government problem." No federal assistance was forthcoming. But congressional health policymakers didn't agree. A bipartisan effort continued after the death of health insurance for the unemployed to put into law pieces of a national policy that relied on the private sector but used government's economic clout to make sure it worked.

In 1985, Congress passed legislation that required employers to offer continued health insurance coverage to laid-off workers for a period of eighteen months. Unlike the earlier bill, the new law required the workers to pay for the coverage themselves—in fact, they were required to pay a premium equal to 102 percent of the group rate paid by their former employer. But even that rate was considerably lower than the individual insurance policy charges unemployed workers and their families faced before the law's enactment. The bill, sponsored by Democratic Congressman Fortney "Pete" Stark of California, Republican Representative Bill Gradison of Ohio, and Republican Senator Dave Durenberger of Minnesota, also provided coverage to the divorced spouses of workers and the widows of workers who died while still employed; they were able to buy group-rate insurance for thirty-six months.

But even those steps only covered a small proportion of the uninsured. Two-thirds of the uninsured during the Reagan years were working Americans and their families; one-third were children under age 18. Many companies had taken advantage of the opportunity provided by the recession to eliminate health insurance coverage for the dependents of the workers they hired back during the recovery. This new and vexing problem demanded new solutions. In 1987, an answer was put forward by Massachusetts Senator Ted Kennedy. Kennedy's plan: to require all employers to provide health insurance coverage to all full-time workers. Like the minimum wage law, Kennedy's plan would cover all companies large and small. Kennedy's plan was put forward near the tail end of the Reagan years with little hope for enactment before the President left office. But Kennedy, whose liberal credentials give him great influence in the course of Democratic policies, was laying the groundwork for the possibility of a new Democratic president in 1989. By staking out the health insurance issue early, Kennedy was steering the Democrats in his direction for the future. Early in the 1988 presidential campaign, several of the Democratic hopefuls embraced the Kennedy plan and promised to press for its enactment once they were in office.

6
The Medicare Mess

By the time Reagan took office, Medicare was in a state of economic chaos. Created in 1965 to help the nation's elderly pay for needed hospital and physician services, Medicare had grown rapidly in the fifteen years preceding Reagan's presidency. By the time Reagan took office, Medicare's Hospital Insurance trust fund was fast approaching bankruptcy. Medicare's economic crisis presented both a dilemma and a challenge to the new President and his advisers. It was a challenge that the administration would meet head on, with significant assistance from the leaders in Congress.

Reagan's Medicare solution would exact a heavy price from the U.S. health care industry. Medicare had fed a voracious appetite in America's hospitals, nursing homes, and doctors' offices. During the late 1960s and throughout the inflationary 1970s, the U.S. health care industry experienced unprecedented growth, fueled by an open-checkbook policy of government reimbursement. By the end of Reagan's term in office, hospitals were no longer a financially secure business and many of the less stable facilities were threatened with closure.

Medicare's growth was not merely an economic phenomenon; it also changed America's downtrodden and often impoverished elderly into a constituency to be reckoned with. The rise in status for the elderly is one of the real success stories of Lyndon Johnson's Great Society. In the twelve years between the Johnson and Reagan administrations, the elderly, once one of the nation's poorest and least cared for groups, reached a level where they could go through their daily lives with a roof over their heads, food on their tables, and a doctor who would care for them when they were sick. While many in America now take this for granted, it was not too long ago that things looked quite bleak for an American who reached his or her retirement years.

Enactment of Medicare in 1965 climaxed two decades of national debate. When he signed it into law in Independence, Missouri, President Johnson said, "No longer will older Americans be denied the healing miracle of modern medicine. No longer will illness crush and destroy the savings that they have so carefully put away over a lifetime so that they might enjoy dignity in their later years. No longer will young families see their own incomes, and their own hopes, eaten away simply because they are carrying out their deep moral obligations to their parents, and to their uncles and to their aunts."

Johnson had achieved what his Democratic predecessors, Harry Truman and John Kennedy, had failed to do. He convinced Congress to overcome the opposition of America's health care providers—most particularly the American Medical Association (AMA)—to a national program of health insurance for the elderly. Medicare's enactment also marked the end to a string of victories by the powerful AMA, which had lambasted all proposals for government-paid health insurance as "socialized medicine."

Congress had debated a government health insurance program as early as 1912. During the Great Depression, President Franklin Roosevelt nearly included such a plan in the 1935 Social Security Act but decided to wait until the end of World War II to press his case. Roosevelt didn't live to see that day, and it was up to Truman to pick up the fallen torch.

While many in Washington expected Truman to steer clear of the health insurance issue, the feisty President waded in with his hip boots on. Truman spent much of his first term pressing for a national health insurance system; but by 1952, as his second term drew to a close, he narrowed his focus to the elderly, asking Congress to enact a program he called Medicare. But Truman was out of time and his successor Dwight Eisenhower wanted no part of Medicare or national health insurance. Eisenhower did take one action that eventually helped the Medicare cause; he created the Department of Health, Education, and Welfare (HEW). The AMA, which had opposed creation of a federal health department, agreed to back Eisenhower's HEW in return for the President's continued opposition to a national insurance program. Ironically, the groundwork for Medicare was done at HEW during Eisenhower's years in office. Arthur Flemming, Eisenhower's third HEW secretary, publicly opposed Medicare but privately supported it. Once he was freed from the bonds of Republican service, Flemming became an outspoken advocate.

When John Kennedy took office in 1961, the country was ready for Medicare, and the young President felt a debt to the elderly. Kennedy's razor-thin election margin in 1960 was helped by the strong support he received from the emerging "gray vote" from America's elderly. Organized labor also had backed Kennedy and hoped to convince him to make Medicare an early priority. Labor and the Democratic National Committee combined forces to form the National Council of Senior Citizens, one of the first consumer lobbying groups for the elderly. But the Congress was not ready for Medicare. Kennedy faced a determined opposition, prodded by the AMA, that included the leaders of the two congressional committees that would have to vote on Medicare first. Both men were from Kennedy's own Democratic party. House Ways and Means Committee Chairman Wilbur Mills of Arkansas and Senate Finance Committee Chairman Harry Byrd, Sr., of Virginia.

The narrow nature of Kennedy's election victory worked against him taking on Mills and Byrd during his first term. Kennedy figured he could wait out the opposition and push Medicare through in his second term. But, like Roosevelt before him, Kennedy wouldn't live to see a second term. His 1963 assassination put Lyndon Johnson in the White House.

Johnson too was committed to Medicare, but even with the sympathy derived from Kennedy's death, Johnson was not able to convince Mills and Byrd to support Medicare. Administration supporters in the Senate went around Byrd in 1963 to attach a streamlined Medicare program to a bill to raise Social Security retirement benefits, but Mills killed the plan in the House-Senate conference.

Years of frustration ended on election night in 1964. Lyndon Johnson's sweeping reelection brought an infusion of new Democrats to the House and Senate. Now the Congress, like the people, was aligned in favor of Medicare. Mills and Byrd knew their fight was over; neither man liked to lose, so both decided it was better to join Johnson than try to beat him.

The AMA was not prepared to give up the fight; after all, its leaders had committed millions of dollars and built their own reputations on a determined battle against "socialized medicine." But the AMA also knew that they couldn't beat Johnson outright. In 1965, AMA leaders switched gears; rather than criticize Medicare for going too far, they charged Johnson with not going far enough. Johnson offered sixty days of hospital care insurance along with extended-care coverage in skilled nursing facilities and home health agencies. Johnson did nothing about the elderly's doctor bills. The AMA put forward its own alternative, "Eldercare," which would provide government subsidies to the elderly to purchase private health insurance.

But Mills, once AMA's ally and now its enemy, knew a trump card when he saw it. When Ways and Means met to consider the Johnson plan in early 1965, Mills announced that he agreed with the AMA: Johnson's plan didn't go far enough. He offered a single bill with three parts. The first would embrace the Truman-Kennedy-Johnson hospitalization plan. The second would expand Medicare to include an optional program of doctor bill insurance. The third would expand an existing program of health benefits for the poor—known as Kerr-Mills for Senator Robert Kerr, a Democrat from Oklahoma, and Mills himself. The new program, dubbed Medicaid, would provide more benefits for more people. Mills' "three-layer cake" sailed through the Ways and Means Committee with barely a word of objection from AMA supporters. (Eldercare had at least one well-known supporter: Retired actor Ronald Reagan recorded an appeal to the wives of AMA members, calling on them to oppose Medicare and support Eldercare in letters to Congress. "If you don't do this, one of these days you and I are going to spend our sunset years telling our children and our children's children what it once was like in America when men were free.")

Johnson didn't even wait for Mill's bill to clear the House before he went to work on Byrd. At a nationally televised press conference, the President was joined by Mills, House Speaker John McCormack of Massachusetts, House Democratic Whip Hale Boggs of Louisiana, Byrd, Senate Majority Leader Mike Mansfield of Montana, and Vice President Hubert Humphrey. Most were there as window dressing; Byrd was there for "the Johnson treatment." Johnson was worried that Byrd would tie up the bill in his committee, and the President didn't want to trust matters to a private conversation. With the nation watching, Johnson turned to Byrd and said: "I know that you will take an interest in the orderly scheduling of this matter and giving it thorough hearing. Would you care to make an observation?" Byrd answered: "There is no observation I can make now because the bill hasn't come before the Senate. Naturally I'm not familiar with it. All I can say is...I will see that adequate and thorough hearings are held on the bill." Johnson continued, "And you have nothing that you know of that would prevent that coming about in reasonable time—there is not anything ahead of it in the committee?" Byrd responded: "Nothing in the committee now." Johnson pressed Byrd: "So, when the House acts and it is referred to the Senate Finance Committee you will arrange for prompt hearings and thorough hearings?" Byrd: "Yes."

Johnson had his promise and he got it in front of millions of Americans. Byrd could no more hold up the Medicare bill than he could hold up the local bank. The Medicare bill moved quickly through the Finance Committee and the Senate. By summer, a compromise measure had been hammered out in conference between the House and Senate and the bill was sent to Johnson for his signature. The President took the bill to Missouri to sign it with Harry Truman at his side.

Part A of the new program, scheduled to begin July 1, 1966, provided sixty days of hospitalization coverage, with the beneficiary paying $40, or the cost of the first day. Another 100 days of extended care would be provided, as would as many as 100 home health visits a year. To pay for the program, working Americans would absorb a 0.35 percent increase in their Social Security payroll tax (about $1.50 per month); employers would pay an equal amount. The services of a physician would be covered under Medicare's optional supplemental medical insurance program, Part B. Those elderly who chose to buy such coverage would pay a monthly premium financing half the cost ($3 in 1966). For that premium, Medicare would pay 80 percent of each doctor bill submitted.

But Congress made a lot of compromises to ensure passage of the Medicare law. Some of those compromises would come back to haunt the authors and confound their successors. Hospital payments, for example, were to be based on costs. Whatever bill a hospital presented, Medicare would pay. In fact, just to make sure hospitals would participate, the government added a 2 percent bonus. Physicians were given even more latitude. Rather than having the government set fees for doctors, Medicare would base each physician's fees on past billing history. And, if doctors did not like the amount Medicare offered, they could refuse to accept that assigned amount and bill the patient directly for the difference. Many other deals cut in 1965 created a payment system that was generous to a fault.

The cost of that generosity was evident not long after the Medicare program began operating. When Congress enacted Medicare in 1965, it estimated the Part A program would cost $3.1 billion by 1970; instead, costs jumped to $5.8 billion. The estimate for 1975 was $4.3 billion but turned out to be $7.6 billion. Part B costs also had jumped: The 1967 estimate of $623 million had escalated to $1.245 billion by 1970.

Congress had already raised the Medicare tax once in 1967 and increased the amount of income that was taxed from $6600 to $7800 per year. But even that increase did not appear to be sufficient. In 1969, President Richard Nixon asked Congress to raise the Medicare tax again, this time to the tune of $135 billion over the next twenty years. Nixon's Social Security actuaries told him such an increase would restore fiscal solvency to the program. But new Finance Committee Chairman Russell Long thought higher taxes weren't the answer. He worried that the program would just continue to skyrocket and bigger and bigger tax hikes would be needed. A shrewd politician, Long knew that the American people would take only so much before turning against the fledgling program. In 1969, Long asked his staff to begin a one-year study of the Medicare and Medicaid programs to report on their effectiveness and check on their fiscal health.

On February 9, 1970, the staff report was delivered to Long. Its findings were shocking: Costs for hospital and physician care had escalated so rapidly in the first three years of the program that it was estimated the Part A Hospital Insurance Trust Fund would be bankrupt by 1973. To keep the program solvent, the government would need to raise payroll taxes by $136 billion over the next twenty-five years. Raising those taxes, the staff report noted, would sap the government of any source of money for expansion of Medicare.

Cost increases also were having their effect on the pocketbooks of the elderly. The Part A deductible, which started at $40 in 1966, went to $44 in 1969 and $52 in 1970. The Finance Committee staff predicted the deductible would zoom to $60 in 1971, $68 in 1972, $76 in 1973, and $84 in 1974. The Part B premium, which had started at $3 per month in 1966, was already up to $4 in 1969 and scheduled to go to $5.30 in 1970.

Rather than relying solely on tax increases, the Finance Committee staff recommended "making reasonable costs more reasonable." Nixon and Congress already had taken one step to contain hospital costs. In 1969, Medicare's 2 percent bonus to hospitals was eliminated and providers were paid only their costs. But still the system was overcompensating. The Finance staff said the payment method was "encouraging duplication, overlapping, and unnecessary expansion of facilities and services and created an unhealthy economic incentive to maximize operating costs."

One solution put forward in the 1970 report was revolutionary for its time. The staff suggested that the government begin comparing one hospital to another and judging whether one provider was overcharging. Until that time, hospitals did not have to worry what their competitors down the street or across town were charging; Medicare would simply pay whatever bill it was sent. Medicare payments should be "limited to no more than a reasonable difference above costs for comparable care and services in a similar, less expensive, institution in the area," the report recommended.

On the physician side, the report found that HEW had broadly interpreted the 1965 Medicare statute and was paying physicians too much. The broad interpretation was deliberate; Johnson's HEW didn't want to alienate an already angry physician community by appearing to clamp down on physician payments. By paying high fees, Medicare assured that threats of physician boycotts of the program were just that, threats. "As a consequence, Medicare generally allows payments for the aged which are substantially higher than those paid under Blue Shield's most widely held contracts for the working population," the report found. Again the Finance staff suggested that Medicare begin comparing doctors' fees and limiting the annual increase in fees to some standard related to what the doctors in a certain area were charging. To cut down on abuses in the system, the report also suggested that Medicare pay reduced fees when a doctor saw more than one patient on a trip to a hospital or nursing home; payments for routine lab tests also should be cut. In a more far-reaching recommendation, the report said Medicare should limit the difference in fees across the country. No doctor should be paid more than 15 percent more than a physician in another part of the country. The report also suggested incentives to get doctors to join what it called a "participating physician program" of doctors who would accept Medicare's fees as payment in full and not try to charge the elderly a higher amount.

Finally, the report found that internal utilization review had been "of a token nature and ineffective as a curb to unnecessary use of institutional care and services." It recommended establishment of external review panels made up of physicians from the community to check on the work and the billings of the providers in the Medicare program.

The Finance Committee report went relatively unnoticed in the daily press but it caught the attention of hospital and physician lobbyists in Chicago and Washington. The very idea of comparing one provider to another and setting limits on Medicare fees provoked an outcry from the American Medical Association and the American Hospital Association. Once again, shrieks of "socialized medicine" rang in the halls of Congress and on the editorial pages of many of the nation's newspapers.

But the Finance Committee report was only the opening volley in a two-year battle to place some limits on the open-ended Medicare reimbursement system. It would take until 1972 for Congress to pass legislation implementing a few of the Finance staff's suggestions. But even then, the bill was sweetened with numerous give-aways to quiet the opposition and to attract support from others. After all, in 1972, consumer groups like the National Council of Senior Citizens and the American Association of Retired Persons (AARP) were not much concerned with Medicare's skyrocketing costs. Even with the rise in premiums and deductibles, Medicare was a bargain compared to the private insurance that the elderly had been buying; it was certainly a better deal for those who couldn't afford private insurance in the first place.

So Congress traded support for new Medicare cost controls for an expansion of the coverage base to the thousands of Americans suffering from kidney disease and requiring dialysis to survive. Recent medical advances had enabled doctors to vastly prolong the lives of these people and allow them to function in the world. But the treatment was expensive and could not be stopped without leading to death. In one of the more dramatic episodes in the 1972 fight over Medicare, the House Ways and Means Committee sat and watched as a doctor dialyzed a patient in the panel's hearing room. Medicare's financial advisers warned that the costs of a Medicare kidney dialysis program would zoom out of control, but were ignored.

But the real sweetener in the pot had nothing to do with Medicare. Republican legislators, tired of the Democrats in Congress gaining electoral support by voting an increase in Social Security benefits each election year, proposed to make such hikes automatic: An annual cost of living adjustment (COLA) would be added to the Social Security program so that benefits kept up with inflation. In those years of low inflation, such a proposal was not very costly but politically was very attractive.

While Congress was being so generous to the elderly, it decided to go one step further. Medicare's Part B premium also was rising quickly. The 1965 law required the premium to bring in enough money to pay for half of the Part B program. That linkage was forcing the premium higher and higher. So Congress voted to limit the annual increase in the premium to the Social Security COLA. The change had its desired effect; the rapid increases in premiums were slowed but the rise in Part B costs was not. As a result, by the time Reagan took office, the premium was bringing in about 22 percent of Part B costs and the federal treasury, that is, the taxpayers, was paying the rest.

All the costly window dressing worked to attract the support needed to carry the Medicare payment reforms through Congress. and legislators did adopt many of the suggestions made in the Finance Committee report. Those changes had to be scaled back to soften the impact on providers. Still, Congress did establish a system of cost controls on hospital room and board charges that limited increases to a percentage of the national average. These so-called Section 223 limits were set too high to effect payments, but they did establish the principle of comparison shopping.

Policymakers were less successful on the physician side of the program. Congress rejected the idea of fee schedules or broad fee comparisons. Instead, it voted to limit the rise in many doctors' fees to a new measure known as the Medicare Economic Index (MEI). The MEI purported to measure the cost of doing business for the typical physician. It included such things as overhead, nurses' salaries, equipment costs, and insurance premiums paid for malpractice coverage and the like. Beginning in 1973, the MEI would work to hold down increases by the higher paid doctors in the country. Again, the lenient limits had little effect on the majority of doctors, but they did establish the principle of comparing one doctor to another.

Congress did follow the advice of the Finance staff in establishing an independent review body to check on provider behavior. The new Professional Standards Review Organizations (PSROs) program would police the industry to check for overcharging and overutilization. The PSROs would number more than 200 by the end of the 1970s and would prove to be an enormous thorn in the AMA's side. Despite the fact that PSROs were supposed to be staffed by physicians, most of the work was done by nurse reviewers who didn't have quite the same level of adoration for M.D.s. The fight between AMA and PSROs would carry over into Reagan's administration, and he would call for repeal of the program.

The bottom-line result of the 1972 amendments was an expansion of the inflationary program begun in 1966. The kidney dialysis program would grow quickly, reaching $2 billion per year by the time Reagan reached Washington. The cost controls placed on hospital room and board charges and on physician fees had little effect in controlling those budgets. The PSROs were a nuisance to many providers but lacked the teeth needed to take a real bite out of costs.

The 1972 reforms did little to slow the escalating cost of health care in the United States. President Nixon's 1973–1974 wage and price controls did, however, slow the rate of growth in hospital charges. But once the controls were lifted, costs resumed their meteoric rise. By the time Jimmy Carter entered the White House in 1977, health care costs were becoming a major public policy issue.

Carter took office as a political outsider. His election was largely a result of public antipathy toward Washington that had built up during the Nixon years and the Watergate scandal. But once in office, Carter needed to reach out to the political establishment. One way he did that was to embrace the long-time Democratic call for a national health insurance program. Carter promised to press for enactment of such a system and directed his HEW secretary, Joseph Califano, to put together a proposal.

But Carter and Califano were determined that before national health insurance could become a reality, the United States must get a handle on health care costs, particularly those in hospitals. In 1979 Carter set up an ambitious hospital cost-containment scheme that would have applied government limits to the annual rise in each hospital's revenue. The proposal drew immediate condemnation from the increasingly influential hospital lobby. The American Hospital Association, representing most U.S. hospitals, and the Federation of American Hospitals, lobbying for more than 1000 investor-owned for-profit facilities, launched a joint all-out attack on Carter's regulatory solution to health care inflation. The pair also called on the AMA to return the favor they had granted during the original fight against Medicare, asking the doctors to lend AMA's might to the effort.

Carter drew support for his effort from organized labor, but got little backing from such lobbying giants as the American Association of Retired Persons and the National Council for Senior Citizens. Despite the fact that rising health care prices were draining the bank accounts of many elderly Americans, groups representing senior citizens were more concerned by Carter's lack of progress on national health insurance. Yet Carter almost pulled off his cost-containment challenge.

Carter relied on the legislative leadership of a pair of liberal Democrats in the House—representatives Paul Rogers of Florida and Henry Waxman of California. Rogers chaired the House Subcommittee on Health and the Environment of the Interstate and Foreign Commerce Committee; Waxman, with only two terms under his belt, was the panel's rising star, destined to succeed Rogers when the chairman retired. Both liked the regulatory approach to cost-containment. But the Commerce Committee wasn't the only panel with jurisdiction over Carter's proposal. Because of its impact on Medicare spending, the bill also had to clear the Ways and Means Committee. There, the health subcommittee chairman, Dan Rostenkowski, a Democrat from Illinois, did not like Carter's approach. Over in the Senate, Carter had support from the health subcommittee chairman, Edward Kennedy of Massachusetts, but got no help from the finance panel leader,

Russell Long. If he were to win, Carter would have to go over the heads of these powerful congressional leaders and gain strong public support for the fight against escalating health care costs.

But Carter's agenda was divided into many pieces. The President still was pressing his war on energy prices, dealing with sharp increases in the cost of oil bought from members of the Organization of Petroleum Exporting Countries (OPEC). Carter's political support, so strong when he took office in 1977, was growing weaker. By the time he launched his cost-containment fight, the public had grown weary of the President's calls for help to fight the special interest lobbyists in Washington. Carter got support for his effort on the editorial pages of many of the leading newspapers, but his fight generated little interest among the general populace.

Still, Carter came darn close to winning. Rogers and Waxman defeated attempts in the Commerce Committee by a young congressman from Michigan named David Stockman to water down Carter's plan. Over at Ways and Means, Rostenkowski stalled and kept the bill bottled up for months, but eventually he released his grip and allowed the measure to move to a momentous showdown vote on the House floor. Busy hospital lobbyists raced all over Washington lining up opposition to Carter's plan. In addition to Rostenkowski and Stockman, the industry won over another young congressman, a Democrat from St. Louis, Richard Gephardt. Gephardt disliked the regulatory approach taken by Carter but knew that to defeat the President he had to present an alternative. He and Stockman sat down with hospital lobbyists and drew up their battle plan. "Competition" would be their buzzword as they argued against an interventionist government and in favor of market forces. Hospitals, they argued, simply needed some incentives to control their own costs. They put forward what became known as the voluntary effort (VE), in which hospitals would gradually slow their inflationary pace without government controls.

The voluntary effort—devised by a group of hospital industry leaders led by lobbyist Michael Bromberg—was a stroke of brilliance. Hedging legislators now could confidently vote against

Carter because they had an alternative to support. In that way, if Carter and his supporters blasted them for their opposition, cost-containment foes could hold up their vote for the voluntary effort as evidence of their concern. When Gephardt offered the voluntary effort on the House floor as an alternative to the Carter plan, he was victorious. Carter had lost one of his biggest domestic policy battles; a year later his attempt to phase in a national health insurance scheme went down in flames as he and Kennedy readied for a bitter primary fight for the Democratic presidential nomination.

The defeat of Carter's cost-containment plan was a high point for hospital lobbyists. An industry used to divisiveness and infighting had united against a common enemy and won. At a victory celebration, the lobbying forces gathered around an ice sculpture in the shape of the letters "VE." But the unity among hospitals began to melt almost as soon as the sculpture. The VE was a hollow promise by the industry to control costs. A one-year dip in the inflation rate for hospital costs proved illusory. When the fight over cost containment had receded into the history books, hospitals took up where they left off and began hiking their prices once again.

Hospitals were cheered by Reagan's election in 1980; they had feared that a reelected Carter would press his cost-containment bill again and win. Reagan's campaign rhetoric against government regulation and the selection of his advisers once he was in office were good signs for industry officials. In many ways, hospitals were lulled into a sense of security. They looked forward to the lifting of the fairly minor regulatory controls that had been placed on them by the government.

But economic forces were working against those who liked the status quo. Reagan came to Washington determined to conquer the inflation "monster" that he had used to slay his predecessor. His efforts to control federal spending would bring his administration into direct conflict with health care industry leaders.

Still, the sense of complacency among industry leaders continued in 1981 as Reagan concentrated his health care reform efforts on Medicaid and a raft of categorical grant programs. Medicare was placed in what Reagan called his "social safety net"—a group of programs that he said would be untouched by budget cuts. Reagan was true to his word for only one year. In 1982 the health care industry's honeymoon was over. Hospitals and physicians soon found themselves longing for the days when they were relatively free of government regulation.

7

The Party's Over

Beginning in 1982, health care providers—hospitals, in particular—came under constant attack by the government in Washington to change their behavior and lower their costs. For almost as long as the government had kept track of such things, health care prices consistently rose more than the general rate of inflation. Because the government was so heavily invested in health care services—paying nearly half of the nation's health bill—the rise in health care costs had a direct effect on the federal budget. In fact, because most Americans were shielded from the direct cost of health care through employer-paid or government-provided health insurance, Washington felt the pinch of health care costs more than the American public.

The health care industry's defenders, including many of the top policymakers in the Reagan administration, were embarrassed by the failure of the hospitals' voluntary effort and were not prepared to fight attempts to enforce government cost controls. Stockman and his budget team at OMB knew that health care was one area of the budget they must attack if they were to bring the looming budget deficits under control.

Reagan had left Medicare alone in 1981. Most of the budget cuts of the President's first year in office had been aimed at the welfare state—Medicaid, AFDC, food stamps, and so forth. When Reagan was feeling the heat of the public reaction to those budget cuts, he announced that he would spare a group of programs that he labeled America's "social safety net." Included were Social Security, Medicare, veterans' benefits, Head Start, SSI, and summer job programs. Oddly, despite the fact that most of these programs served the middle-class and the programs targeted for budget cuts served the poor, the public and the press bought the White House's safety-net defense.

But by 1982, the safety net—if it ever existed—had dissolved under a wave of mounting budget deficits. Now, no programs were off limits, and Medicare topped the list of entitlement programs that would be cut under Reagan's fiscal 1983 budget that went to Capitol Hill early in 1982. Congressional Democrats had stolen a little of Reagan's thunder in 1981 by enacting a handful of Medicare changes, including a $15 increase in the annual Part B deductible paid by the elderly before Medicare coverage kicked in. A retiree would pay the first $75 per year instead of $60. Those moves frustrated Stockman because they were made instead of cuts in welfare programs; besides, Stockman had counted on such Medicare savings for the second round of the budget battle.

Stockman and his budget-writing team began work on the fiscal 1983 budget late in 1981. With many of the "easy" domestic cuts made in 1981 the Reagan team had a fairly limited "menu" of programs to select from for the new cuts. Medicare, with its $70 billion annual budget, was a prime target. From his days leading the opposition to Carter's hospital cost-containment program, Stockman was well acquainted with the ins and outs of Medicare. He knew the program's faults and how to get the savings he needed to cut the deficit.

When it came time to decide which cuts Reagan would send to Congress, the administration was being pulled in two directions. Stockman knew that the quickest way to budget savings was regulatory controls over what Medicare paid for various services, because such controls yielded immediate savings. But Reagan had been elected, at least partly, on his call for less government regulation. How would it look, then, if his administration came forward with more regulation, not less?

In the first go-round of budget talks Stockman's OMB favored imposition of new controls over what Medicare paid hospitals for the thousands of tests and procedures performed by doctors and labs. These so-called ancillary services formed the core of the Medicare cost problem. Section 223 of the 1972 Medicare amendments limited what Medicare paid for room and board. While those limits had been left loose, they had established an important precedent that would form the basis for the 1982 amendments. The process of comparing hospitals' costs around the country began with the Section 223 limits. Section 223, in effect, said the government would take a national average of costs and hold all providers to a percentage of that. For the first time, the government began comparing what one hospital charged to that of its competitor down the block, across town, across state, and, even, across country.

In 1982, Stockman wanted to extend the Section 223 limits to ancillary services; by controlling both parts of the hospital billing ledger, Medicare could force some real economies. But the Stockman plan ran into opposition from the purist wing of the administration. Heavy-handed government regulation would not be proposed by this administration, Stockman was told. Competition was the name of the game; the "invisible hand" of the free market was going to do the trick.

Hospital lobbyists were similarly upset. They worried that Section 223 limits on ancillary services would harden into a regulatory iron fist and sought to persuade the administration to take another tack. Leading the charge was Michael Bromberg, head of the Federation of American Hospitals—one of the country's top lobbyists. Bromberg had spent years railing against government regulation of the health care system; he had led the fight and built his reputation in the defeat of Carter's hospital cost-containment plan. He would be damned if he would see the first antiregulation administration in memory turn around and slap such a system on his industry. His solution: Rather than having the government decide what it would pay for each test and each procedure, why not get the savings the administration needed by a simple across-the-board cut in payments.

Under Bromberg's alternative, the government would pay 98

cents on the dollar. His fellow hospital lobbyists were at first slow to follow Bromberg's strategy. Shortly after he circulated his notion, a fellow lobbyist printed up facsimiles of a dollar bill with Bromberg's face in place of Washington's. In the corners, the bogus bill read "98 cents." An embarrassed Bromberg promptly denied authorship of the plan.

But Stockman knew an out when he saw it. Faced with almost united opposition to his Section 223 plan, Stockman adopted Bromberg's "2 percent solution" as his own. When Reagan sent his budget to Congress in February of 1982, he called for a 2 percent reduction in all hospital payments.

The reaction to Stockman's plan on Capitol Hill was mixed. Congressional leaders of both parties privately were glad to see the President taking on Medicare. Legislators who had been through the 1972 Medicare reforms and the 1979 battle over cost containment knew that Congress had done only half the job. With Reagan's support, they believed Congress would overcome the special interests of the health care lobbyists and enact cost controls that worked.

Congress approved Reagan's call for deep cuts in Medicare as part of the fiscal 1983 budget resolution. At the same time, however, Congressional policymakers voiced their discontent with the 2 percent plan and indicated a desire to find an alternative.

Senate Finance Committee Chairman Robert Dole of Kansas would be the key figure in the congressional consideration of the 1982 Medicare amendments. Dole was ably assisted by his health adviser, Sheila Burke, who had earned her wings working with the people who had earlier helped write the Medicare law and the 1972 amendments. Burke was one of the masters of Medicare policy on Capitol Hill. She had planned to leave Dole's staff after the 1980 election to pursue a graduate degree at Harvard University. When the surprise election results elevated Dole into the key post of Finance Committee chairman, Burke agreed to stay on Capitol Hill while commuting on weekends to Boston to finish her course work. Remarkably, the determined Burke was able to handle both tasks.

Burke was aided in her efforts by a former Democratic staffer

John Kern, who earlier had worked for Senator Herman Talmadge in the 1970s when the latter was chairman of the Finance health subcommittee. Kern had helped shape a bill introduced in the mid-1970s by Talmadge, calling for expansion of Section 223 limits to ancillary services. In 1982, Talmadge was back in Georgia but his bill would become the basis for the second major overhaul of Medicare's payment system.

Almost from the moment Reagan's 2 percent reduction proposal reached Capitol Hill, insiders knew it didn't stand a chance. Congressional leaders felt a simple across-the-board reduction in payments would provide no incentives to hospital administrators to change their ways. Many feared hospitals would absorb the cut without structurally changing their operation and hope that full payments would be restored once the political winds had changed. Instead of the 2 percent cut, Congress wanted to change Medicare's payment system in a permanent way that would force hospitals to cut their costs and watch future inflation. Section 223 limits were the favored course.

Some thought that Stockman had sent the plan to Congress knowing full well that it would be rejected in favor of the Section 223 limits he favored; the wily Stockman would never admit to such a strategy, at least not publicly. But once Congress began rewriting the Reagan budget, little objection was heard from the other end of Pennsylvania Avenue. In fact, officials from Reagan's Health Care Financing Administration helped Burke and Kern fashion the legislation to impose such limits.

The plan devised by the Finance Committee was masterful. The bill called for imposition of Section 223 limits on ancillary charges that would gradually get tighter and tighter. Unlike the 1972 limits placed on room and board charges, the new controls would take a real bite out of hospital revenues. The limits started off relatively high—in 1983, limits would be set at 120 percent of the national median. But that limit would drop the next year to 115 percent, then to 110 percent, and finally to 105 percent. By the end of the four-year transition, no hospital would be paid more than 5 percent above a national median. In addition, Medicare would set limits on how much it would pay per case with an adjustment for each hospital's mix of cases. Hospitals that were able to keep their costs under the limits would be eligible for a bonus, but the extra cash would be limited to 5 percent. Hospitals that exceeded the limit would lose money, and there would be no limit on that loss.

The Finance Committee plan sent hospital lobbyists into a tizzy. But the problem was one of their own making. By opposing Carter's cost-containment plan in 1979 and letting the voluntary effort slide, hospitals spent their political capital and had little left to aim at the Section 223 limits. The budget politics of the 1980s meant opposition to one plan had to be accompanied by support for another. With Congress voting to make Medicare cuts, the hospital industry had to come up with a plan that would achieve the savings demanded in the budget resolution without exacting the kind of pain that the Section 223 limits threatened.

A worried group of hospital lobbyists gathered to discuss what to do about the Finance Committee plan. Clearly they could not fight off the Section 223 limits. The House Ways and Means Committee was ready to act on a similar package within weeks. But the idea of permanent regulatory controls on all aspects of their business appalled the industry leaders. They needed to come up with a workable alternative that Congress could accept and that would appease their angry association members.

Hospital industry leaders met with Dole and Burke to talk about their concerns. Dole said he was willing to entertain alternatives as long as they met two basic criteria: First and foremost, they had to achieve the budget savings required under the budget resolution; second, and more important to Dole, they had to create incentives for a change in behavior.

Hospitals came back with a plan that they all could support. They would accept the Section 223 limits in 1983—after all the ceiling was up at 120 percent of the median—but they wanted a commitment from congressional leaders that they would consider replacing the regulatory system with an approach that would allow hospitals to share in the savings they achieved by containing costs.

Dole agreed. He would add language to his bill that called on

HHS to come up with a prospective pricing system for hospitals under Medicare and deliver it to the Congress by January 1, 1983. Congress would then consider the alternative early in 1983, in time to replace the Section 223 limits before they got too tight. Dole's compromise was acceptable to the House and was included in the law Reagan signed later that year.

Hospital lobbyists were happy with the compromise. They could go back to their members and say the Section 223 limits were only temporary and would be replaced with a competitive scheme before they did any real harm.

Some believe hospitals overreacted to the Section 223 limits and painted themselves into a corner with their call for a prospective pricing system. But in 1982, the industry had little choice. Budget government had achieved what Carter could not; hospitals had accepted government controls on Medicare revenues that would force revolutionary changes in their business.

The 1982 Tax Equity and Fiscal Responsibility Act—known as TEFRA—ended nearly fifteen years of profligate spending by Medicare on hospital services. It also paved the way for permanent reforms that, to many people's surprise, were enacted just one year later.

The call for a new prospective payment system for Medicare became a clarion at HHS. Secretary Richard Schweiker organized his troops for an all-out effort to devise a system that would be acceptable to hospitals and to Congress. Schweiker's team had less than six months to complete the report that Congress requested.

Schweiker and his advisers were determined to complete the report on time. For the first time since they took office, the HHS policymakers were in control of developing a major health care policy. Development of the prospective payment system was placed squarely in the hands of the department, Stockman and OMB were not involved. This would be the chance for Schweiker to leave his mark on federal health programs and to implement his much-talked-about competitive health policy.

In December 1982, Schweiker delivered his report to Congress. He called for creation of a prospective pricing system based on diagnosis-related groups (DRGs). Medicare would limit what it paid for the care of a patient to an average price for the treatment of the illness that caused the patient to be admitted to the hospital. Every hospital would be paid the same basic amount no matter its costs. An adjustment would be allowed, however, for the differing costs of labor.

In his report, Schweiker sharply criticized the cost-based reimbursement system used by Medicare since 1966. "The present system...has been one of the major contributors to high rates of inflation. By reimbursing, essentially, incurred costs at any level, this system does not provide incentives for hospitals to manage their operation in a cost-effective manner. The greater a hospital's costs, the larger its Medicare reimbursement. Thus, well-intentioned hospital managers face pressure to spend more. This system contributes to the depletion of the Hospital Insurance Trust Fund, a situation which threatens the security of present and future beneficiaries. It defies control and makes predictability of payments uncertain, at best. Clearly, reform is required."

Schweiker noted that Medicare hospital payments had been increasing at an average rate of 19 percent since 1972. Even in 1982, when overall inflation had dropped to 5 percent, hospital costs rose 15.5 percent. Schweiker praised the 1982 TEFRA amendments but noted that even those per case limits did nothing to encourage hospital administrators to cut costs. By setting a ceiling and allowing only a limited bonus to those who kept costs below the limit, the government still was encouraging low-cost hospitals to raise their rates up to the limit and providing little incentive to high-cost hospitals to cut their costs below the limits.

Under the proposed DRG system, all hospitals would have incentives to control their costs. For high-cost hospitals the government waved a big stick—administrators would have to swallow any cost above the limit. For low-cost hospitals the government offered a carrot—they could keep the difference between their costs and the limits. In the meantime, Schweiker said, Medicare would become a "prudent buyer" of medical services.

While Schweiker's plan would apply only to Medicare patients, it would provide a clear invitation to other payers—Medicaid, Blue Cross-Blue Shield, and private insurers—to follow suit. For years Medicare had set the pace for an inflationary health insurance market; now Schweiker wanted to lead the country in the opposite direction.

Schweiker's choice of DRGs was a wise one. The government had been experimenting with DRGs since 1972 when HEW signed an agreement with researchers at Yale University to develop and test the system. New Jersey had adopted DRGs as the payment mechanism in their cost-containment system applied to all payers. Experience in New Jersey provided Congress with a record of achievement. As in most cases, Washington followed the lead of the states in reforming federal health programs.

Being a smart politician, Schweiker knew that pure DRGs wouldn't fly in Congress. His plan offered exceptions for certain sensitive types of hospitals—long-term facilities, children's hospitals, and psychiatric hospitals—that would have little ability to change behavior to cut costs. He also excluded medical education costs—the training of interns and residents in major teaching hospitals—and capital costs—for construction of new buildings, renovation of existing facilities, and purchase of new medical equipment. Again, these were areas that did not open themselves to rapid cost containment. All other hospital costs would be placed under the DRG system by October 1, 1983.

Schweiker's report arrived on Capitol Hill in December 1982 while Congress was still in recess. Following the 1982 election, Democrats had strengthened their control over the House by reclaiming twenty-six seats taken by Republicans in Reagan's 1980 landslide. Republicans had maintained control over the Senate, but several senior members squeezed by in unexpectedly close races. Schweiker's team was nervous about the DRG plan's chances on Capitol Hill.

But as Congress got ready to consider the Schweiker plan, the administration gained new ammunition in its battle to control Medicare costs. In February, the trustees of the Medicare Hospital Insurance Trust Fund issued a shocking report: High rates of inflation threatened to plunge Medicare into bankruptcy.

The public was used to such proclamations from Washington. Many such reports had been issued in the years since the 1965 enactment of the program. But those reports always put bankruptcy ten, or even twenty, years in the future, not enough to worry members of Congress who only tend to think as far ahead as their next election. But this report was different. The trustees said that if Congress didn't act, and act fast, the program would go belly up by 1987—a short five years away. The reason: rising hospital costs. In 1982, while inflation dropped to 3.9 percent—its lowest point in over a decade—hospital charges rose 12.6 percent. A growing elderly population and a rise in use of health care services by the elderly added to the program's woes.

The financial ills facing Medicare were not temporary. The Congressional Budget Office (CBO) estimated that the deficits would grow "rapidly." By 1995, outlays from the Medicare trust fund would exceed tax revenues coming in by two-thirds. In fact, the actuaries could not find a point at which the gap would begin to narrow. With more and more Americans reaching retirement age as the "baby boom" generation of the 1950s matured, there would be fewer and fewer working Americans left to finance costly programs like Medicare and Social Security.

The Medicare mess had uncanny parallels with the economic problems being experienced with the Social Security retirement program. As 1983 began, Congress was preparing to deal with the most difficult domestic issue of the 1980s—the bankruptcy of the Social Security trust fund. In 1977 Congress had voted to raise payroll taxes to fill the trust fund that paid retirement benefits to the elderly. But those tax increases proved to be insufficient to restore Social Security to fiscal health. Shortly after Reagan took office, the Social Security actuaries reported that the trust fund once again faced bankruptcy within five years. The cause: record increases in benefits due to the 1972 law that indexed benefits to the Consumer Price Index.

Reagan ordered Schweiker to come up with a Social Security rescue plan that avoided new tax increases. Candidate Reagan had campaigned against Carter by criticizing what he called "the largest tax increase in history," namely the Social

Security hike of 1977. The new President could not turn around and propose yet another increase in those payroll taxes without looking like a hypocrite.

Schweiker and his advisers followed orders and put together a package of reforms that would erase the trust fund deficit without increasing taxes. But the path to solvency was studded with controversial plans to reduce benefits to early retirees, delay the age-65 eligibility date, and eliminate benefits for those over age 18. Somehow Schweiker's years of experience on Capitol Hill seemed to fail him; he unveiled the Social Security plan without a hint of any awareness of the political fallout that would ensue.

Democrats swooped down on the Schweiker plan like buzzards. House Speaker Tip O'Neill and Florida Congressman Claude Pepper lambasted the Secretary and the President for their "callous" call for reduced Social Security benefits. The plan was immediately withdrawn, and Reagan later named a bipartisan commission to study the program. In the meantime, Democrats pounded their GOP opponents in the 1982 midterm elections helping to win twenty-six House seats and almost retaking control of the Senate.

After the election, the commission issued its report, recommending a combination of tax increases and benefit reductions and a one-time delay in the annual cost of living adjustment. The Social Security rescue plan became the first priority for the 97th Congress when it opened in 1983. Having cut the political deals necessary to fix Social Security, neither party wanted to delay any longer for fear the deal would unravel.

The fate of the Social Security rescue plan would, surprisingly, become joined with that of Schweiker's DRG proposal. But Schweiker would not be around to see it. In February, the HHS chief surprised most of Washington with his announcement that he was resigning to take over the American Council of Life Insurance. Reagan nominated former Republican Congresswoman Margaret Heckler of Massachusetts to replace Schweiker (see Chapter 4). But Schweiker's policymaking team would remain on the job to see the plan through to passage.

Congressional committees began hearings on the DRG plan

shortly after the New Year. Most witnesses were supportive in their testimony—hospital groups embraced Schweiker's plan but reserved judgment on the timing of its implementation. Only the American Medical Association opposed the plan, but its opinion did not carry nearly the weight it had in the 1960s during the original Medicare debate. Since the plan was considered a "hospital issue," AMA's opinion didn't matter much on Capitol Hill.

But the seeming support for the DRG plan would not lull legislators into a sense of complacency. Many of the leaders in Congress in 1982 had seen the effectiveness of the health care lobby in the 1970s. They did not want to run the risk that the support hospitals gave the DRG plan in January would give way to internal bickering and outright opposition later in the year when votes would be taken. Instead, House Ways and Means Committee Chairman Dan Rostenkowski decided he would tie the DRG plan to the Social Security rescue plan. The Social Security bill was destined to move through Congress quickly with no crippling amendments. Rostenkowski figured if he attached DRGs to the bill he would preempt any lobbying effort by opponents.

Over in the Senate, Dole was wary of Rostenkowski's plan. Debate over the DRG proposal could break down much in the same way the 1979 debate over Carter's cost-containment plan. Dole didn't want anything to slow the progress of the Social Security bill; his party had taken enough knocks on Social Security in the 1982 election. He wanted to leave no chance that his party could be blamed for blocking the rescue package. Rostenkowski, on the other hand, believed the momentum behind the Social Security rescue package was just the thing he needed to ensure that hospitals could not change their mind and seek to block the DRG bill. Dole eventually gave way when Rostenkowski promised he would drop the DRG portion from the Social Security bill if delays occurred. With Dole and Rostenkowski in agreement, the way was clear for quick passage of the DRG plan.

But before Congress could vote on the Schweiker DRG plan it needed some changes. Schweiker had proposed a nearly pure system that would begin immediately and included no adjustments for the variations in health care costs across the country. In the report, Schweiker noted that Medicare now paid anywhere from $1500 to $9000 to a hospital to treat a patient after a heart attack. Similarly, payments for hip replacement surgery varied from $2100 to $8200, and payments for cataract removal ran from $450 in one hospital to $2800 in another. DRGs were meant to do away with such price swings, but many felt that hospitals could not survive long if prices were unified all at once.

The most important testimony heard during the congressional hearings on Schweiker's plan came from the Congressional Budget Office. Paul Ginsburg, CBO's chief health care policy analyst, was one of the most respected health care experts on Capitol Hill. His opinions represented no group, no party, and no particular ideology. No one could call Ginsburg a liberal or a conservative—he was neither. In the world of Washington policymaking, people like Ginsburg were indispensable because they offered advice that could be accepted by both parties and would not be challenged as biased by the interest groups lobbying for or against a bill.

Ginsburg analyzed the Schweiker DRG plan and presented Congress with his findings. If Schweiker's plan went into effect unchanged, Ginsburg predicted that 34 percent of hospitals would lose money on Medicare patients; only 4 percent would profit; the rest would break even. Large urban hospitals, because of their higher than average costs, would fare worst; small rural facilities, which had much lower costs on average, would fare best. Small hospitals—particularly those with fewer than 100 beds, would earn a windfall profit of 23 percent above costs. Hospitals with 300 or more beds would lose 6 percent. Teaching hospitals, which tend to treat the sickest patients, would lose under the DRG system, Ginsburg warned.

Ginsburg's analysis opened the door for a series of changes to the Schweiker plan to make it more equitable to hospitals and to ease the impact on any particular region. The problems he outlined presented policy and political problems. No congressman wanted to shortchange the hospitals in his district or state. Political considerations moved to the forefront. Ways and Means

Chairman Rostenkowski wouldn't vote for a plan that would harm his Chicago hospitals. Dole wanted protection for large rural hospitals in his home state of Kansas. Other congressmen holding seats on Ways and Means and Finance committees also had their price for support of the DRG plan. Texas Congressman J. J. "Jake" Pickle, for example, wanted to help Anderson Hospital, Houston's premier cancer treatment center; he got an exemption for cancer hospitals. Minnesota Senator Dave Durenberger wanted to protect the Mayo Clinic; Congress added a provision exempting that facility (a rule later known as "hold the Mayo"). The end product resembled the Schweiker plan but bore the imprint of political maneuvering.

To smooth out some of the other rough edges in Schweiker's plan, Ways and Means and Finance each voted to phase in the system over four years. Separate rates would be set for urban and rural hospitals and for nine regions of the country. Over the course of the transition period, payments would be a blend of a hospital's costs and the average for the region. A separate fund was created to pay additional amounts for particularly costly cases, known as "outliers," and payments for medical education costs and capital projects would continue to be made on a cost basis. The final bill exempted long-term care hospitals, children's hospitals, rehabilitation hospitals, and psychiatric hospitals.

Once the changes were made and the deals were cut, the way was cleared for quick congressional action. Late in March, the House and Senate approved the compromise bill and on April 20, 1983, President Reagan signed it into law.

The quick passage of the DRG bill—a scant four months after Schweiker delivered his report—caught most hospitals by surprise. They spent weeks pouring over the massive bill, trying to make head or tail of it. They didn't have much time, however; the system was to be up and running by October 1, the beginning of fiscal 1984. The industry's initial reaction was one of joy. After all, the new system offered efficient hospitals the opportunity to reap a profit on Medicare business. Under the new system, if a hospital cut its costs Medicare wouldn't automatically cut its payments. Incentives for change were strong. But others worried that the four-year transition wouldn't be enough time to make the changes needed to take advantage of the new system.

The rush to judgment on Capitol Hill achieved its purpose—quick passage—but also led to some sloppy law writing. Congress couldn't decide on a base year from which to compute the new payment system. Lawmakers left that up to the Reagan administration. Over at HHS, the Health Care Financing Administration (HCFA) went into overdrive to produce the reams of regulations needed to implement the law. The regulations had to be issued by September 1, only four months after Reagan signed the bill into law. The Health Care Financing Administration had to make some quick decisions, the most important of which was the base year for DRG payments. To avoid underpaying hospitals—a move that could threaten the success of the system—HCFA chose to base the payments on unaudited hospital cost reports. That was a risky move for both parties, government and hospitals. If the unaudited cost data proved to be an overstatement of actual costs, the government would lose millions; if the data was an understatement of costs, hospitals would lose.

Hospitals took another gamble in 1983 as Congress was considering the DRG system. An important issue was how the DRG rates would be increased each year to handle inflation. Hospitals argued that the rates should automatically increase to cover the rise in costs incurred by hospitals for goods and services. Medicare had been measuring those cost changes as part of what is called the hospital marketbasket. Industry lobbyists wanted DRG rates to rise each year by the increase in the marketbasket plus an additional one percent to cover the cost of new medical technology.

In his report, Schweiker had proposed that the authority to increase rates should be left with the secretary of HHS. An automatic increase such as the one supported by the industry would get Medicare in the same kind of mess that the Social Security COLA index had caused in the retirement system.

Congress split the difference: For the first two years of the system the rates would be increased automatically by the rise in the marketbasket plus one percent for technology. But beginning in fiscal 1986, the secretary of HHS would have the power to set the increase. Hospitals bought that deal; a decision that its leaders would regret.

Once the DRG system was in place, the administration and the Congress had run out of the "easy" changes in Medicare law that would yield large budget savings. With hospital costs under control, there were few places to turn for further economies. The administration would continue to propose significant increases in patient premiums, deductibles, and coinsurance, but Congress was unwilling to reach into the pocketbooks of the elderly to exact those savings. Instead, hospitals remained the prime target for budget cutters. In 1985, Reagan announced he would freeze hospital payments at the 1984 levels. Hospitals rose in anger at what they called an abuse of the discretionary authority granted to the HHS secretary to set the annual rates. Congressional leaders, too, were upset at the freeze plan. In retaliation, Congress took back the authority to set the annual rates. But instead of protecting hospitals from the Reagan budget ax, Congress simply took on the role itself. From 1984 to 1988, per-case hospital payments under Medicare rose an average of 2 percent per year, significantly less than the rate of inflation in hospital costs.

Hospitals were able to absorb the first and second round of those cutbacks because the original DRG rates were set too high. Hospitals reaped profits averaging from 14 to 15 percent in 1984 and 1985. Those profits led Congress to clamp down even harder in 1986 and 1987. The result: Many hospitals, particularly those in rural areas of the country, found themselves losing money on Medicare and threatened with bankruptcy. In 1986, a record seventy-one hospitals closed their doors; more than half of them were rural providers.

The battle to control health care costs in America certainly hasn't been won, but creation of Medicare's DRG system was a major step toward that goal. The program paid immediate dividends; within a year of its creation, the system had forced hospitals to cut the average hospital stay from nine days to seven. Hospitals began laying off workers for the first time in recent history. In 1984 alone, hospital staff shrank 2.6 percent. Hospital admissions also began to drop. Where the average hospital had a 72.6 percent occupancy rate in 1983, by 1987 that rate had dropped to about 60 percent. Hospitals began to eliminate unneeded beds; in 1986, 2.2 percent of hospital beds were closed.

Diagnosis-related groups also paid off for Medicare's fragile trust fund. The savings accrued from those cost-saving moves staved off the predicted 1987 Medicare bankruptcy. In 1987, Medicare's trustees were predicting the program would remain in the black into the twenty-first century. Unlike the Social Security program, Congress had not waited until the very last minute to pass a massive "rescue" plan that imposed harsh cuts on beneficiaries and high taxes on workers. Instead, working together, Reagan and the Congress had taken a gradual approach that pushed back the sea of red ink.

Imposition of DRG cost controls on Medicare represented a dramatic move away from the administration's competition-based health care policies. While the original DRG system included incentives for hospitals to cut costs and make a profit, the cranking down of the payment rates in subsequent years has turned the system into a heavy-handed regulatory tool. By the late 1980s, administration officials were already disillusioned with DRGs but knew they had nowhere to turn for the kind of budget savings they needed to control the federal budget deficit. By the end of Reagan's term, his policymakers were looking for ways to move away from the regulatory DRG system toward the free-market approach to health care that Reagan had promised back in 1981.

8

The Social Agenda

From the beginning of his administration, President Reagan found himself pulled in opposite directions by his conservative supporters. On one side were the economic conservatives pressing their case for budget and tax reductions; on the other, the social conservatives pressing their agenda of changes in laws that they believed were rending America's moral fiber. The economic conservatives had always formed the backbone of the Republican party; the social conservatives were the newcomers who, in many ways, had given Reagan his margin of victory in the 1980 election.

During his 1980 campaign against Carter, Reagan had received unprecedented support from fundamentalist religious groups. With the backing of such religious leaders as Moral Majority founder Jerry Falwell, Reagan offset Georgian Carter's regional support to win several key southern states. While Reagan had always toed the conservative line in his past state and national election bids, in 1980 his campaign rhetoric was carefully designed to appeal to the newly active religious right. Reagan appealed to those groups with his new stand against abortion, calling for a reversal of the 1973 Supreme Court decision legalizing abortion in the United States. Reagan also called for an emphasis on "family values," including a return to school prayer and the elimination of government programs and regulations that came between parents and their children.

But once he was in office, Reagan often had to choose between his two corps of supporters. Any new President has a honeymoon period during his first year in office during which Congress tries to accommodate the agenda that the voters had so recently ratified. But as the experience of his predecessor had shown only too well, the presidential honeymoon was growing shorter with each successive presidency. Reagan and his advisers knew they would have less than a year before Congress would begin to reassert its political muscle. To gain the economic policy victories he wanted, Reagan had to concentrate the attention of the Congress on budget and tax cuts. Senate Majority Leader Howard Baker of Tennessee cautioned Reagan against a detour into a debate over the divisive social issues of abortion and school prayer. Like Baker, most of the new Senate Republican leaders and committee chairmen were from the traditional wing of the GOP; their chief concern was to shape up the economy.

In 1981, when his influence was at its greatest, President Reagan convinced the social conservatives to put their agenda on hold while the administration pursued its economic policies. When that fight was over, Reagan promised, the social agenda would move to the forefront. That was a promise Reagan never would keep.

For most of his two terms in the White House, Reagan sided with the budget cutters, relegating the social agenda to a back burner. Despite two terms under one of the most conservative presidents in recent history, fundamentalists were unable to achieve a single major victory on the national scene. When Reagan entered office, the social conservatives were perhaps at the acme of their political strength, by the time he would leave, the conservatives were steadily losing power. Still the political clout of the social conservatives forced Reagan to pay at least lip service to their causes. Most of Reagan's attempts to change laws and government regulations to reflect the wishes of the social conservatives were rebuffed, either on Capitol Hill or in the courts.

The abortion issue was at the center of most of the social policy debates of the Reagan years. Anger over the Supreme Court's 1973 decision in *Roe v. Wade* had been steadily growing. By the time Reagan was elected, that anger was palpable. Since 1973, the ranks of the grassroots antiabortion, or "right-to-life," movement had swelled and grown more politically active. From its onset, the antiabortion movement had been aligned with no party; there were just as many Democrats as Republicans who found the Court's decision repugnant. In 1976, Jimmy Carter received a great deal of support from the fundamentalists. Born-again Carter was viewed as a foe of abortion, but he did not press that issue during his four years in Washington. With Reagan's embrace of their cause in 1980, the antiabortion community became more and more an arm of the GOP.

In the 1978 congressional elections, the antiabortion groups got their first taste of the fruits of their labor. Democratic senators Dick Clark of Iowa and Thomas McIntyre of New Hampshire were defeated in close races that featured active campaigning by the right-to-life groups in those states. In 1980, Reagan became the first presidential candidate since the court's decision to campaign against legalized abortion. His victory was accompanied by a string of Republican wins over incumbents who favored legally available abortion—the "pro-choice" forces. While many factors led to the defeat of those liberal incumbents, opposition from the antiabortion groups was considered a major reason for their defeats.

Despite their gains, the antiabortion forces were still short of a majority in Congress. But the electoral trends left lawmakers leery of crossing the right-to-life groups. As often as possible, Congress would avoid taking votes on the abortion issue. But antiabortion forces wouldn't let Congress ignore their feelings. In 1976, Illinois Republican Congressman Henry Hyde pushed through the first of what would be an annual series of amendments to government funding bills banning federal support of abortions. The Hyde amendment, as it became known, had its chief effect on Medicaid. Under its terms, no abortions could be paid for under Medicaid unless the pregnancy was the result of rape or incest or would endanger the life of the woman if carried to term.

In the 1970s debate over the Hyde amendment was fierce. Each year, appropriations bills for the Department of Health, Education, and Welfare were held up as Congress fought over the abortion issue. Pro-choice groups took the issue to the courts, but in 1980 the Supreme Court upheld the constitutionality of the Hyde amendment. That decision seemed to take the starch out of the amendment's foes. By the time Reagan took office, the fight was over the edges—whether or not to retain the three exemptions for rape and incest victims and women who faced a life-or-death decision when they became pregnant. Once Reagan took office, the rape and incest exceptions fell by the wayside.

Right-to-life groups wanted to take a quantum leap beyond the Hyde amendment by enacting a constitutional amendment reversing the Supreme Court on *Roe v. Wade*. Hyde and Republican Senator Jesse Helms of North Carolina introduced such an amendment and pressed Reagan for his support. On January 22, 1981, two days after his first inauguration, Reagan met with antiabortion protesters gathered in Washington to observe the seventh anniversary of the high court's decision in *Roe v. Wade*. The new President pledged his support for a constitutional amendment. But that promise was put on hold while the administration pursued its budget and tax cuts.

Hyde and Helms weren't happy with the delays in carrying out the social agenda. They reluctantly went along with Reagan's decision to wait until 1982 but began pressing for strong presidential leadership. While they waited, Hyde and Helms also fiddled with the constitutional amendment idea. Both men knew that they did not have the two-thirds majority in both houses of Congress needed to amend the Constitution. If pressed, they thought they could round up a simple majority in each house. Hyde and Helms began searching for another solution to the abortion problem that would need only that majority margin. Early in 1982 they settled on a plan that called for enactment of a statute that simply declared that human life began "at the moment of conception." By so defining life, Hyde and Helms figured on outlawing abortion without going through the cumbersome and iffy process of a constitutional amendment.

The Hyde-Helms human life statute divided the right-to-life movement in the United States. Half of these groups wanted to continue pressing for a constitutional amendment; they feared the statutory approach would not stand up in court. The rest backed the new approach, hoping to gain quick congressional approval. Helms sought the assistance of freshman Senator John East of North Carolina. East had been elected in 1980 with the backing of Helms' political machine in North Carolina. After taking his seat in the Senate, East was made chairman of the Senate Judiciary Committee's Subcommittee on Separation of Powers. He quickly scheduled hearings on the Helms-Hyde bill. Early in 1981, East's subcommittee approved the Helms bill by a four to two margin, but it would be months before the full Judiciary Committee would take up the matter.

One of the votes for the Helms bill in subcommittee was that of Orrin Hatch of Utah, chairman of the Judiciary Constitution Subcommittee. Hatch was a strong proponent of the right-to-life position and the sponsor of a constitutional amendment to reverse *Roe v. Wade*. He also considered himself an expert on the Constitution. In voting for the Helms bill, Hatch expressed concerns about its constitutionality. By the time the measure was ready for full committee consideration, Hatch was convinced the Hyde-Helms approach was not constitutional. Hatch's opposition effectively killed the Helms bill. He blocked full committee consideration of the Helms bill and instead the Judiciary Committee approved Hatch's antiabortion constitutional amendment and sent it to the Senate floor for a vote. As Helms predicted, the Hatch plan failed to gain the two-thirds majority it needed. In fact the Senate approved the amendment with barely a majority of its members.

While attempts to directly ban abortion were thwarted in 1982, the right-to-life community did not let up in its pressure on the Reagan White House. Reagan continued to call for a constitutional amendment banning abortion throughout his two terms. Each year the President would include the obligatory call in his

State of the Union address; each year Congress paid him little mind. Disappointed antiabortion groups looked for other ways to stem the number of abortions in the United States. They turned their attention to other federal programs, looking to stamp out any signs of government support of abortion. These ideological battles would tie the Congress in knots and ensnare several established health programs in their net. Chief among those was the Family Planning program.

Family planning clinics had survived Reagan's block-grant attack of 1981, emerging with reduced federal funding but protected from state attacks on their independence. In 1983, the clinics would face another battle. Only days before he left office, HHS Secretary Richard Schweiker signed proposed regulations that would embroil the Family Planning program in controversy for the rest of Reagan's administration. Schweiker had been a right-to-life supporter in Congress, voting for the Hyde amendment and supporting a constitutional amendment to reverse *Roe v. Wade*. Once he joined the Reagan administration, Schweiker too pledged his support to stamping out abortion. His swan-song regulations had that goal in mind.

What Schweiker proposed was to require all federally funded family planning clinics to notify the parents of any teenager who received prescription contraceptives. Clinics that refused to follow that rule would lose all of their federal funds. Schweiker's squeal rule drew an angry reaction from clinic operators and leading members of Congress, but they drew an equally strong huzzah from the right-to-life community. Antiabortion forces had argued for most of the eight years since the federal program was created that government support of contraception was encouraging teenagers to engage in premarital sex. Parents, they felt, were squeezed out of the equation when their children could go to federally funded clinics and get birth control pills, condoms, diaphragms, and intrauterine devices (IUDs).

When Congress enacted the Family Planning program (Title X of the Public Health Service Act) in 1974, antiabortion forces then in Congress raised strong objections. To calm their concerns the original legislation specifically barred use of federal funds to pay for abortions. In 1981, as Congress was rejecting Reagan's block-grant request, it agreed to add language to the Title X statute calling on clinics to "encourage" parental involvement in the care of their teenagers. In his regulation, Schweiker chose to interpret "encourage" as broadly as he could. Clinics would be required to involve the parents whenever contraceptives were prescribed to teenage girls—the squeal rule was aimed only at them.

In crafting the regulation, Schweiker satisfied the concerns of some in the antiabortion movement but not all. A large segment of the community believed that parents should be involved before contraceptives were provided. They wanted to require clinics to notify parents when their teenage children requested contraceptives. Only with parental approval would pills, diaphragms, IUDs, or condoms be distributed to those under age 18. Schweiker rejected that counsel and was condemned in some quarters of the movement he was trying to serve.

Schweiker's last action as secretary left his successor, Margaret Heckler, with a problem. Before she lost her seat in the 1982 election, Heckler, as a member of the Congressional Women's Caucus, had signed a letter to Schweiker urging him not to place a parental notification requirement on family planning clinics. Heckler had passed the abortion litmus test that was applied to all top HHS officials during Reagan's term. She was opposed to abortion but believed that if the operation was legal, then all women should have access to it. Now, as the newest member of the Reagan Cabinet, Heckler had to swallow that opposition and back the squeal rule.

Publication of the squeal rule touched off a battle in Congress and one in the courts. Family planning groups promptly took the government to court seeking to overturn the regulation. A federal judge granted an immediate injunction suspending enforcement of the rule while the case made its way through the courts, eventually reaching the Supreme Court. The high court ruled that Schweiker had overstepped his bounds in interpreting the 1981 congressional language. The rules were thrown out but the fight was not over.

Once again disappointed, antiabortion groups carried their fight to Capitol Hill. Hatch and Helms this time were on the same side. They were determined to add statutory language to Title X that would require federally funded clinics to notify parents of teens who got contraceptives. But again these two leaders of the conservative cause in the Senate would fail. Liberals Henry Waxman and Ted Kennedy would face down Helms and Hatch and refuse to add such restrictions. The result was a stalemate in Congress that would last until the end of the Reagan administration. But in the meantime lawmakers would keep the program running. Hatch, who had failed in 1981 to put the program in the hands of the governors, was particularly embarrassed this time around because his home state of Utah had passed a law requiring government-funded clinics to notify parents. Because of Hatch's failure in Washington, Utah's health department found itself stripped of federal funds because its parental notification policy clashed with the federal statute. Instead, the federal dollars would go to private groups in Utah.

By the time the family planning flap had run its course, the social conservatives were beginning to feel quite downtrodden. The elections of 1982 did not prove to be nearly as successful for antiabortion candidates as had those of 1978 and 1980. To some in Washington, the political rise of the right-to-life movement was beginning to look like a temporary phenomenon; its leaders were determined not to permit that.

In 1982, antiabortion groups found a new cause that would again embroil health care providers in controversy. This fight was touched off by the birth of a severely handicapped child in Bloomington, Indiana. The infant, identified as "Baby Doe," was born with Down's syndrome and other defects requiring surgery. His parents faced the most difficult decision any mother and father could face: Should they fight to keep their son alive with artificial means, knowing that the child would likely lead a short painful life, or should they withhold treatment and allow the child to die?

The dilemma faced by Baby Doe's parents in 1982 is one that faces many more parents today than ten or twenty years ago.

Medical skills and technology continue to advance in the United States at amazing rates. For millions of Americans those advances bring health and joy. For others, like the parents of Baby Doe, it forces horrible decisions. If Baby Doe had been born in 1972 instead of 1982 his parents would have had no decision to make. The medical personnel in Bloomington would have been able to do nothing to save Baby Doe, and he would have died within days, if not hours, of his birth. But the very advances that breathed life into other infants only promised to prolong a life that some thought was not meant to be.

Little could those sad parents in Bloomington know that their difficult decision would create a national controversy that would end up on the docket of the Supreme Court. For when those parents decided to forego treating the multiple medical problems their baby was born with and to withhold nutrition that would have extended his painful life, the antiabortion community rose in anger. In Washington, the Reagan White House, already sensitive to charges that it had abandoned the social conservatives, responded quickly.

Within weeks after Baby Doe's death, President Reagan ordered HHS to issue a directive to all U.S. hospitals saying the withholding of medical treatment on the basis of an infant's handicap was illegal. Shortly thereafter, Reagan ordered Schweiker to develop regulations that would prevent hospitals from following the wishes of the parents of future Baby Does. Development of those rules would take nearly a year. In March of 1983, with HHS now under Heckler, the first set of Baby Doe regulations were published.

In 1983, HHS declared that hospitals could not withhold medical treatment from any patient because of a handicap. While the rules were broadly written, they clearly were aimed at cases involving newborn handicapped infants. The government ordered hospitals to post conspicuous notices in their waiting rooms informing the public that "Discriminatory failure to feed and care for handicapped infants in this facility is prohibited by federal law." The notice announced the opening of a new federal telephone hotline. People who suspected a hospital was withholding treatment from a handicapped infant could anonymously notify the government; it would send a team of investigators. The rule, HHS said, was immediately in effect.

Health care provider groups immediately took the government to court. A suit filed by the American Academy of Pediatrics, the National Association of Children's Hospitals and Related Institutions, and the Children's Hospital Medical Center in Washington, D.C. accused the administration of once again stretching the meaning of federal statutes. This time, HHS hooked its regulatory claim to the 1973 Rehabilitation Act, which barred discrimination against the disabled. The rules, the groups charged, would "insert federal investigators into pediatric wards in a way that is dangerous to the health and lives of seriously ill infants."

A federal judge threw the 1983 Baby Doe regulations out. But Judge Gerhard Gesell did not rule on the claim that the administration had overstepped the bounds of the 1973 law; instead, he ruled that it had violated the older Administrative Practices and Procedures Act, which requires the government to give the public sufficient time to comment on proposed rules before they go into effect. By rushing the rules into effect, HHS had suffered another defeat. In June of 1983, the government published another set of Baby Doe rules and gave the public sixty days to offer its comments.

Not surprisingly, the critics of the first set of Baby Doe rules were no happier with the second set. The same groups that sued HHS in March went back to court in June. This time they were joined by the American Medical Association and the American Hospital Association. Combined, the litigants represented the wide sweep of medical providers. Together, they also had a legal war chest that would assure the government would be in court for some time.

While the second Baby Doe court fight was waged, HHS began work on a third set of regulations. This time, the effort was led by U.S. Surgeon General Dr. C. Everett Koop. Koop came to the administration in 1981 under strained circumstances. As a pediatric surgeon in Philadelphia, Koop had built an international reputation in the field of infant care, but he also had been an early enlistee in the fight against legalized abortion. In speeches, books, and films, Koop had compared abortion to euthanasia and to the Nazi attempt to exterminate the Jews of Europe. When Reagan named him surgeon general in 1981, pro-choice forces balked. Confirmation of his nomination was held up for nearly a year. Because Koop was 64 years old when Reagan nominated him, he exceeded the mandatory retirement age for the Public Health Services corps. Congress would have to change that law before he could become surgeon general. Democrats also argued that Koop did not have the public health experience needed to run the corps. They wanted to add such requirements to the law before they eliminated the outdated retirement rule. It was not until late in 1981 that Koop's way was cleared as part of a political deal on a budget bill.

Koop was determined to shed his "right-wing crazy" image. He worked diligently at the Baby Doe regulations trying to come up with a compromise that would satisfy his colleagues in both the antiabortion movement and the health care industry.

While Koop was at work, the government began to use its new Baby Doe authority. In New York an infant was born with spina bifida (an open spinal column); her parents decided that "Baby Jane Doe" would not benefit from life-prolonging surgery. Local right-to-life groups learned of the decision. They went to court to get an order for the hospital to perform the surgery her parents did not want. In Washington, the Reagan administration went to court trying to obtain Baby Jane's medical records. Once again, the courts said no.

Koop's work with the medical organizations seemed to be paying off. The pediatricians, children's hospitals, and the Association of Retarded Persons issued what they called the "Principles of Treatment of Disabled Infants." It said, "When medical care is clearly beneficial, it should always be provided. Considerations such as anticipated or actual limited potential of an individual and present or future lack of available community resources are irrelevant. The individual's medical condition should be the sole focus of the decision." The groups went on to say, "It is ethically and legally justified to withhold medical or surgical procedures which are clearly futile and will only prolong the act of dying. However, supportive care should be provided, including sustenance as medically indicated and relief of pain and suffering."

Koop lifted much of that language and included it in his Baby Doe regulations issued in January 1984, the government's third try. Koop's Baby Doe rules also would require hospitals to post notices announcing the illegal nature of withholding treatment. But instead of requiring a poster sized notice to be tacked up in the waiting room—possibly needlessly worrying expectant parents—Koop required a five-by-seven-inch notice to be posted in areas visible only to nurses and doctors. Gone was the confrontational language of the early notice. Koop's notice would read, "It is the policy of this hospital, consistent with federal law, that nourishment and medically beneficial treatment (as determined with respect for reasonable medical judgments) should not be withheld from handicapped infants solely on the basis of their present or anticipated mental or physical handicap." The notice would direct people with complaints or questions to call the hospital, a state agency, or the federal hotline.

Koop added another ingredient to his regulatory cake: He directed all hospitals to establish ethics panels that would advise physicians who are confronted with the kind of dilemma that faced the doctors treating Baby Doe in Indiana and Baby Jane in New York. The idea of institutional ethics panels wasn't new; many hospitals already had them. A 1980 presidential commission had urged creation of such panels across the country to help with the cases like Baby Doe as well as those involving "Grandpa Doe," an aged parent nearing death whose life could be extended by medical technology but whose family did not want to prolong the act of dying. Some hospitals had responded to that suggestion, but many others still did not have an established method to deal with these modern dilemmas.

Koop's regulations continued to draw legal fire. Provider groups still were unhappy with the notion of the federal government creating an authority to monitor medical decisions. Beneath all of Koop's compromise language there remained a government police unit in Washington that could swoop down on a hospital and order it to change a medical treatment plan. Hospital and doctor groups went back to court and the Koop rules were thrown out. The administration would carry its effort to the Supreme Court but would again be rejected.

The Baby Doe battle was not over, it simply shifted to a new arena. Antiabortion groups turned to Congress to enforce the kind of rules Koop had drafted. They found a welcome reception from conservative lawmakers. Senator Jeremiah Denton of Alabama introduced legislation that would amend the Child Abuse Prevention and Treatment Act to require states to set up Baby Doe units. Denton was a freshman senator elected in 1980 on Reagan's coattails. Before taking office, Denton's reputation was shaped around his incarceration in a North Vietnamese prisoner of war camp. Upon his triumphant return to the United States, Denton had become involved in the fundamentalist movement in Alabama. In his first try at electoral politics, Denton was swept into office. The first three years of his term had been marked mainly by continuous turnover on his Senate staff and his successful effort to pass the chastity bill in 1981 (see Chapter 3). Denton also had acquired a reputation as an "oddball." Departing staff told of three-hour harangues from their boss on the dangers of communism and the powers of Jesus Christ. But in 1984, it was Denton who would head the Baby Doe fight on Capitol Hill.

The House approved a Baby Doe bill in February that would require states to police hospitals. During its debate, the House considered a proposal crafted by representatives Rod Chandler of Washington, a Republican, and Henry Waxman of California, a Democrat. The Chandler-Waxman plan, crafted with the help of the AMA and others, would have left decisions up to hospitals. In return, hospitals would be required to set up review committees to help guide decisions in future Baby Doe cases. The House narrowly rejected that plan, but, as with many legislative fights, the defeated plan would later come back to help shape the final compromise.

Once the court had thrown out the last set of HHS regulations, Denton pressed ahead with his legislation. Denton's bill, however, was too closely related to the regulations. Provider groups worked with Orrin Hatch of Utah and Alan Cranston of California to shape a compromise that would give states less power to police hospitals but would ensure that oversight would occur. In August, with the 1984 election quickly approaching, the Senate unanimously approved a compromise measure crafted by Denton, Hatch, Cranston, and others. By the end of the year a final version was put into law.

Although it is rare for today's federal government to track how a law it creates actually works, it did so in the case of the Baby Doe law of 1984. In 1987, HHS Inspector General Richard Kusserow and his staff visited a handful of states to see how the Baby Doe law was working. To their surprise they found very few cases had been referred to the new state regulatory offices. In the first fifteen months after the law was enacted, a total of five cases had been taken to the states; in only two instances had the states intervened to force a hospital to change its treatment plan. The five-case total was nearly identical to the total in the fifteen months before the law was passed. So a question must be asked: Was the three-year fight in the courts and the halls of Congress much ado about nothing? Probably so.

Right-to-life forces were still unhappy with their lack of progress in Washington. Family planning clinics continued to operate unhindered by new federal requirements and Congress had slowly increased funding so that the Title X budget was approaching the pre-Reagan level. By 1987 time was running out.

Reagan and his antiabortion supporters would take one last run at family planning and the abortion issue in 1987. Antiabortion groups had long complained that while Title X grantees abided by the letter of the law that prohibited use of federal funds to pay for abortions, they were making a mockery of the spirit of the law. Federally funded family planning clinics were operating side by side with privately funded abortion clinics. Counselors in one clinic were advising pregnant women to go down the hall to obtain an abortion.

Conservative ire was most heated when it came to clinics

run by the Planned Parenthood Federation of America and its subsidiaries. While many of the pro-choice organizations had chosen to ride out the Reagan storm, Planned Parenthood took the antiabortion movement head on. A woman's right to choose what to do with her body had been recognized by America's highest court and Planned Parenthood was determined to preserve that right. Its success only raised the blood pressure on the right; conservatives were determined to get their revenge. Their goal was to throw Planned Parenthood out of the Title X program.

Schweiker's squeal rule had been only the first attempt the administration would make to get rid of Planned Parenthood. With its failure, antiabortion groups would turn to other methods. In 1986, they began pressing new HHS Secretary Otis Bowen to rewrite federal family planning regulations. First they wanted him to bar any clinic that operated an abortion clinic in the same facility. Not only would that get rid of Planned Parenthood, which operated some one-third of the federally funded Title X clinics, it also would have booted out nearly 100 clinics operated in hospitals. Second, they called on Bowen to block federally funded clinics from advising pregnant women of the availability of legal abortions or from directing them to an abortion clinic if they sought one. In other words, having lost the fight for a squeal rule, they now wanted a "gag rule."

Bowen resisted the call of the antiabortion groups. Like Schweiker and Heckler, Bowen opposed legalized abortion, but his background as a physician led Bowen to also oppose government interference in medical decisions. He would spend nearly a year quietly resisting the conservative's pressure.

Antiabortion groups turned once again to Capitol Hill for assistance. Late in 1986 they found help from conservative Republican Congressman Jack Kemp of New York. Kemp, who was readying a 1988 run for the Republican presidential nomination, wanted to shore up his support among the social conservatives. Kemp rushed forward to sponsor the gag rule in Congress, seeking to attach it to the HHS appropriations bill, much like Hyde had done a decade earlier. Kemp would lose his bid; in fact, his effort never got out of committee. Antiabortion groups turned back to the White House.

By 1987, the social conservatives were running out of patience. Their powerful leader in the White House hadn't redeemed any of his 1980 promises to them. Moreover, Ronald Reagan's clout in Washington was growing weaker as the end of his two terms approached. Time was running out.

Antiabortion groups went back to Bowen and asked him again to change Title X rules to ban abortion counseling. Again Bowen turned a deaf ear, but within his department, the right-to-lifers found a sympathetic ear. JoAnn Gasper, a graduate of the antiabortion movement, was in charge of administering Title X. She was appointed by Heckler following the resignation of Marjory Mecklenburg, an advocate of the squeal rule. (Mecklenburg quit amid allegations that she had spent more time traveling the country meeting with her conservative supporters and watching her son play football than she had in Washington doing her job.) Gasper began complaining to her bosses that the antiabortion movement deserved their support. Her pleas were ignored.

In January 1987, after meeting with antiabortion groups in her office, Gasper shocked her superiors by issuing an unauthorized memorandum to her regional offices ordering them to cut off funding to Planned Parenthood. Gasper claimed Planned Parenthood clinics were "promoting" abortion as a means of contraception, an act in violation of federal rules. One day later, HHS Assistant Secretary for Health Robert Windom, Gasper's immediate boss, issued his own memo overruling Gasper. Gasper was reprimanded, but the fight was far from over. Windom's reprimand touched a nerve in the conservative movement. They asked the White House to reinstate Gasper's memo and reprimand Windom and his boss, Bowen. The White House remained mum, hoping the latest flap would blow over.

But Gasper was determined not to let the issue die. In March, she refused to approve contract extensions for grants to two Planned Parenthood groups in Minnesota. First Windom, and then Bowen, ordered her to sign the contracts; she refused, and Bowen fired her for insubordination. The antiabortion movement had its martyr. Gasper quickly appeared on Capitol Hill at the side of Republican Senator Gordon Humphrey of New Hampshire; Humphrey demanded her reinstatement and the publication of the gag rule.

Within weeks, the White House responded. At a meeting with his right-to-life supporters, Reagan announced that he was ordering Bowen to publish regulations that would bar abortion counseling at Title X clinics and require physical and financial separation of family planning and abortion clinics. Having little choice in the matter, Bowen complied, but he would not hire Gasper back; instead, she was added to the payroll of the Department of Education.

Republican Senator Lowell Weicker of Connecticut tried to block the Reagan gag rule but was thwarted by Congressman Hyde. Early in 1988, the administration published final rules and was promptly taken to court by family planning advocates.

9

Deregulation?

Ronald Reagan's 1980 campaign pledge to "get the government off the people's backs" was warmly received in the health care industry, where government rules and regulations often dictated who was hired, how much they were paid, and the hours they worked. The government told hospitals what they could build, when they could build it, and how much it could cost. It told nursing homes how many nurses they needed on staff, how clean their rooms should be, and how much they could charge for care they provided. Physicians too were bound by rules that sought to define quality health care and by committees that looked over their shoulders to make sure they were providing the right kind of care.

Decades of federal involvement in paying for health care for the nation's elderly and its poor had resulted in reams of federal regulations. Using the leverage provided to them by the dollars they spent through Medicare and Medicaid, government policymakers created a new golden rule: "He who has the gold, makes the rules." When it came to health care, the government had the gold and it made lots of rules. By 1980, Medicare was providing, on average, 40 percent of each hospital's revenue, Medicaid another 15 percent. For nursing homes, Medicaid paid 50 percent of the bill. When Washington said, "jump," providers asked, "how high?" When Reagan took office, the health care industry was one of the most regulated industries in the nation.

Providers had a "hit list" of federal regulations that they wanted Reagan to wipe off the books. Hospitals sought repeal of a 1974 law regulating construction and modernization of their facilities and the purchase of expensive new medical equipment. Physicians trained their sites on a 1972 program setting up squads of their peers to oversee their work on Medicare and Medicaid patients. Nursing homes wanted a rollback in federal and state regulations regarding health and safety requirements utilizing state-run inspection teams that swooped down every year to check for compliance.

The health care industry found a welcoming ear in Reagan's Washington. On the day of his inauguration, Reagan announced that he would put the kibosh on a list of regulations promulgated by the Carter administration between the time Reagan had won the election and the time he took office. These "midnight regulations" included a set of rules that would have beefed up nursing home safety standards. Within the month, President Reagan appointed Vice President George Bush to head a task force that would study all government regulations and identify those that were superfluous or overreaching and find ways to eliminate or pare them back. The "Bush brigade" identified three health areas: health planning regulation of capital projects, Professional Standards Review Organizations (PSRO), and nursing home quality standards.

Bush's call for the elimination of health planning and PSROs fit in nicely with Stockman's budget cutting effort over at OMB. President Reagan's first budget message to Congress called for a three-year phaseout of both programs.

In proposing elimination of federal health planning support, Reagan said, "This program represents an effort to impose a complex national health regulatory program on states and localities. Moreover, it has not proved effective in controlling costs on a national basis, and it inhibits market forces needed to strengthen competition and provide less costly services." Under the Reagan budget, support for planning agencies would drop from $153 million in fiscal 1981 to $115 million in FY82, $43 million in FY83, $25 million in FY84, and zero thereafter.

The health planning program was created on Richard Nixon's watch, as the federal government began to get truly concerned by the continuous rise in U.S. health care costs. Under its terms, hospitals, nursing homes, and other providers would be required to submit their capital expansion plans to local and statewide agencies that would decide whether the project could begin. Through the local Health Systems Agency (HSA) and Statewide Health Planning and Development Agency (SHPDA) programs, certificates of need (CON) would be issued to projects judged worthy; but if the planning folk said no, the project would come to a screeching halt.

From the beginning, providers were unhappy with this intervention into their business. Their discontent grew worse when HSA and SHPDA began to be employment havens for social advocates who used the CON power to leverage hospitals into changing their business practices. Hospital construction projects, in effect, were often held hostage to the demands of the growing staffs of the planning agencies. From the industry's point of view, health planning was unjustified invasion of the government into their business. From consumer groups' viewpoint, planning was a way to press their case for expanded access to health care services for the nation's most vulnerable citizens, the poor and the uninsured.

Hospital and physician groups had periodically called for repeal of health planning during the Ford and Carter administrations, but to no avail. With Reagan in the White House, they smelled blood; in 1981 they moved in for the kill. While health care industry lobbyists worked against many of the Reagan-Stockman budget cuts, they offered their full support for the health planning repeal effort.

But again, Stockman would come up against the willful Henry Waxman. Waxman entered Congress shortly after the planning law was enacted but he had become a strong supporter of it. What's more, one of his key staff advisers, Dr. Brian Biles, had written much of the original law when he was an aide to Kansas

Democrat Bill Roy. Waxman and Biles would work to thwart the administration's wishes once again. As in his other fights with Reagan over Medicaid and health block grants, Waxman again used his strategy of appeasement to beat the President. While refusing to agree to the administration's repeal request, Waxman sharply scaled back the planning program by eliminating many of its smaller duties and focusing its efforts on capital growth control. The number of HSAs began to shrink, but the program continued.

Provider groups would not give up the fight and neither would the administration. While Waxman won the first battle in 1981, Stockman came back year after year with the same request of Congress: Repeal health planning. Remarkably, Waxman continued to stave off the hounds for five years.

Several times, Waxman came close to preserving the planning program into the 1990s but each time he fell short. For such a small program health planning would take up more congressional debate time than many of its bigger brothers. Using all of his legislative skills, Waxman tried to fashion a compromise that would cede more control over planning decisions to the states but retain a federal role. Waxman figured if he could save the framework of a federal planning program through the Reagan years, he could rebuild what was lost if and when the political tides turned in his direction. But Waxman was unable to fashion that final compromise; in 1986, after five years of stalemate, a decimated planning program was repealed.

But the five-year delay in carrying out Reagan's repeal request had enabled many planning agencies to line up support from private businesses concerned about rising health care costs and from state governments who wanted to keep a lid on their health budgets. At the same time, the boom in health care construction that threatened to escalate costs in the 1970s had waned in the 1980s as hospital beds stood empty and the demand for expansion evaporated.

Physician groups were less successful in their quest to get rid of PSRO program. Started in 1972 when Congress began to consider ways to hold down Medicare costs, PSROs had never been

9 / Deregulation?

popular with physicians. While the concept of peer review appeared to guarantee a voice for organized medicine in its own oversight, the PSRO system tended to be a thorn in doctors' sides. Physicians had always been independent, strong-willed sorts, unused to government regulation interfering with the practice of medicine. But now nearly every doctor had government-paid physicians looking over his shoulder, judging whether care that had been provided was justifiable. The PSRO program had a negligible effect on medical costs but its mere existence stuck in medicine's craw.

Reagan said repeal of PSRO would "substantially reduce federal regulation of health care services." He argued that the review boards weren't saving the government money; in fact, they were raising health care costs. "The cost of the nationwide system of hospital utilization review organizations exceeds the resulting savings achieved by reductions in length of hospital stay and lower admission rates," Reagan said. Stockman argued that even the savings achieved by PSROs were passed on to patients by doctors intent on collecting their fees.

But Reagan's repeal request would run into bipartisan opposition on Capitol Hill. This time, opposition to the Reagan plan came from the Republican Senate. PSROs found a champion in the new chairman of the Senate Finance Committee's Subcommittee on Health, David Durenberger of Minnesota. Durenberger was a rarity in the Senate, a man who knew the intricate details of the programs he was in charge of overseeing. Durenberger came to Congress with experience in the health care field, thanks to his work in Minnesota government as a top aide to then-Governor Harold LeVander and later as an executive with H. B. Fuller Company, a plywood manufacturer. His surprise election to the Senate in 1978 gave the Senate a leading voice on health policy that would be heard often and listened to throughout the Reagan years.

While Durenberger was most often found in the Reagan camp on budget matters, he took a separate path in 1981 on PSRO. Peer review had worked well in his home state of Minnesota, a state that in many ways had been a microcosm of the competitive market that was soon to describe the American health care system. But Durenberger believed what was wrong with the review organizations was that they didn't have any incentive to achieve results. Federal grant funds continued to flow to nearly 200 PSROs, no matter their effectiveness. Durenberger decided they needed a healthy dose of competition. But he didn't quite have his ideas fleshed out in 1981, so he came up with a plan to scale back the number of PSROs by about one-third while he went to work on his reform plan.

In 1982, Durenberger had his plan in hand. Along with Democratic Senator Max Baucus of Montana, Durenberger proposed replacing the PSRO network with a system of 50 statewide Peer Review Organizations (PRO). Each PRO contract would be awarded through competitive bidding and every two years they would be put up for bids again. If a PRO was successful in holding down health costs it would win another two-year contract; if not, anyone would be free to bid for the government's money. Taking advantage of the omnibus-bill approach adopted by Congress, Durenberger and Baucus were able to push through their reforms over Stockman's objections.

But the PRO system wouldn't gain its real power until 1983, when Congress created Medicare's prospective payment system (see Chapter 6). The new payment system would create incentives for hospitals to bend the rules in their favor. While the old system encouraged hospitals to keep a patient in a bed as long as possible and provide as many services as they could, the new system favored short hospital stays and a minimum of services. The best way for a hospital to make money under Medicare now would be to admit more patients and keep them in the hospital for less time.

During the debate over Medicare's payment system Durenberger pushed a major role for his PRO program. Hospitals, he argued, would take advantage of the government unless someone was keeping an eye on them. The Sherlock Holmes of his choice: PRO. As part of the 1983 Medicare reforms, Durenberger required hospitals to sign contracts with the PRO in their state and submit their records for review. Peer review organizations were empowered to deny payment for entire cases—a potential loss of thousands of dollars at a time.

The enhanced power of the PROs went unnoticed by health care lobbyists as their attention was turned to the larger context of Medicare payment reform. By the time the AMA and other lobbying giants had noticed, Durenberger had pulled a fast one. He had repealed PSROs, just as the AMA and Stockman asked, but in place of those paper tigers were fifty tigers with real teeth to take a bite out of hospital revenues.

Reagan's 1982 attempt to reform federal nursing home regulations would get him into hot water. The administration, still caught up in its feeling of invincibility, did not expect the outpouring of opposition that its proposals would bring. More than one million Americans were living in nursing homes when Reagan took office; millions of other senior citizens lived in almost daily fear that their weakening health would lead them to a nursing home door. Almost every American worried that someday a parent or relative would be confined to a nursing home.

Most of these Americans had not forgotten the nursing home scandals of the 1970s. Investigations had revealed that many homes, particularly those serving the poor, were nothing more than holding pens for the elderly, offering not care and comfort but squalor and disease. State and federal policymakers worked to clean up the nursing home mess by instituting new rules and regulations and empowering squads of investigators to visit homes and check the conditions.

At the federal level, there were two sets of nursing home regulations. Medicare's "conditions of participation" set the standards for all nursing homes to meet. It provided rules on cleanliness, staffing, medical care, and safety. Failure to meet these conditions would result in a home being expelled from Medicare and Medicaid. Nursing homes depended on Medicaid for a large portion of their revenue.

To check on nursing home compliance with Medicare's conditions, the federal government established an annual system of nursing home inspections, known as "survey and certification." States were given federal dollars to pay the salaries of their inspectors. If an inspection revealed health or safety problems, a home would be threatened with expulsion. Homes were given ninety days to clean up their act before the inspectors returned for a second visit.

Consumer groups believed the federal rules needed improvement. The conditions of participation put too much emphasis on what these groups called "bricks and mortar" issues; not enough attention was paid to the quality of the care given to residents and the quality of their lives. They pressed Carter to improve the conditions by adding new rules regarding patient health. Carter's second HEW secretary, Patricia Harris, drafted such regulations, but they were held up in bureaucratic and political haggling until only a month before Reagan took Carter's place. Once in office, Reagan quickly dropped Carter's rules.

Consumer groups also argued that the federal rules were too inflexible. By requiring miscreant homes to be kicked out of Medicare and Medicaid, the rules presented states with an impossible choice. If a home was deficient and was kicked out, none of its residents would get care. If the problems were ignored, the quality of their care would continue to deteriorate. Consumers sought a system of "intermediate sanctions" that would temporarily suspend a home from participation in Medicare and Medicaid; if problems persisted, a permanent expulsion would be in order. Nursing homes, happy with the emasculated rules on the books, opposed creation of such sanctions, fearing they would put real teeth in the rules.

Following Bush's recommendation that Medicare's conditions of participation and survey and certification rules be revamped, Schweiker's HHS undertook a massive study. By the end of 1981, Schweiker concluded that the conditions should not be changed; in fact, he believed they needed improvements much like those Harris had proposed, but in this antiregulation administration he dared not propose such a move. Instead, Schweiker had to fight a bitter battle to keep the current conditions in place.

But Schweiker's fight wasn't over yet. Under pressure from Bush's group and the new regulation masters at OMB, he was asked to consider changes in the survey and certification rules.

9 / Deregulation?

In May 1982, the White House forces prevailed and HHS published proposed changes in the inspection rules.

Under the Schweiker plan, nursing homes would no longer be inspected every twelve months; inspectors would have the option of checking on homes as infrequently as once every twenty-four months. Follow-up visits would no longer be required; if an inspection team wanted to check, it could telephone the home to see if the problems had been cleared up.

The angry reaction from consumers and members of Congress surprised the administration. Within weeks of their publication, four members of Congress introduced bills calling for their withdrawal. Opponents included Republican Senator John Heinz of Pennsylvania, the chairman of the Senate's Special Committee on Aging, and Democrats Senator David Pryor of Arkansas, Ohio Congresswoman Mary Rose Oakar, Connecticut's William Ratchford, and House Committee on Aging Chairman, Claude Pepper of Florida. More than fifty members of Congress signed letters to Schweiker, asking him to kill the regulations.

The reaction in Congress was atypical. After all, Congress had been in a "deregulation" mood for several years, dating back to Carter's administration. But nursing home issues touched a special spot in the hearts of these congressmen. Pryor, for example, had been a two-term governor of Arkansas when that state cleaned up its nursing homes. Ratchford had led a similar effort in Connecticut's state government before he came to Washington. Heinz, Pepper, and Oakar had spent years on congressional committees dealing with the issues of aging; they had listened to the testimony in the 1970s nursing home hearings. None of them could believe the problems they had confronted less than a decade before could have been eliminated so thoroughly that the federal rules could be relaxed in this manner.

Opposition to the Schweiker rules built during the summer of 1982. By fall, Congress passed a bill setting aside the rules for one year while an independent study of federal and state nursing home rules would be conducted by the prestigious National Academy of Sciences' Institute of Medicine (IOM). The Department of Health and Human Services signed a contract with IOM in 1983.

The IOM study would take more than two years; in the meantime the federal rules remained unchanged. The IOM appointed a twenty-member committee chaired by Sidney Katz, associate dean of medicine at Brown University in Providence, Rhode Island. In March 1986, the panel unveiled its findings.

The IOM report was a sweeping rejection of the Reagan philosophy on nursing home regulation. Rather than agreeing with the administration that nursing homes were overly regulated, the IOM said federal and state regulations weren't tough enough. The majority of care provided in America's nursing homes was "substandard," IOM said. Federal regulations paid too much attention to procedures and not enough attention to the care being provided to elderly and disabled nursing home residents, it added. The IOM called for an overhaul of federal and state nursing home rules, with a new emphasis on the quality of care provided and the quality of life that resulted.

IOM rejected Reagan's proposed twelve- to twenty-four-month inspection cycle. Instead, it recommended that homes be inspected as often as every nine months—for homes with poor compliance records—and no later than once every fifteen months. Every state should have an average inspection cycle of twelve months, IOM said, but the annual inspection cycle had become "too predictable." By varying the cycle, homes could not prepare for inspectors by patching holes and cleaning up; surprise inspections would be a truer test of a home's performance. The report called for inspectors to talk to the residents of each nursing home to get a first-hand report on the quality of care and life in an institution. More emphasis was to be given to the human side of nursing care; less would be paid to bricks and mortar.

But the IOM didn't stop at the inspection rules. The report called for a rewriting of Medicare's conditions of participation. A new set of standards would emphasize patients' rights and seek to guarantee the residents of nursing homes a quality of life that they should have been able to expect. A federal nursing home residents' "bill of rights" would be added to the regulations. Every nursing home resident should be guaranteed care "in such an environment as will promote maintenance or enhancement of their quality of life without abridging the safety and rights of other residents."

Rather than eliminating federal nursing home staffing requirements, IOM said the government should expand those rules to require a licensed nurse on duty twenty-four hours a day. Nurses' aides, the front line defense for nursing home residents, should have at least eighty hours of preservice training, IOM said. It shouldn't matter what kind of home the government was regulating, all rules should be equal. For years, many states in the south had evaded federal rules by classifying their nursing homes as "intermediate care facilities," or ICFs. Federal rules were much tougher on "skilled nursing facilities," or SNFs, which were supposedly providing a higher level of care. But some states were calling nearly all of their homes ICFs to avoid the staffing requirements leveled on SNFs. The IOM report said the regulatory distinctions between SNFs and ICFs should be eliminated.

Many nursing homes failed to assess the needs of a new resident and come up with a plan of care. The IOM report said an assessment should be made of every resident within the first two weeks of a stay. Based on that assessment, a home should come up with a care plan for each resident.

The Institute of Medicine was concerned about a growing tendency by nursing homes to discriminate against their poor patients. Because Medicaid payments for nursing home patients were notoriously low, homes preferred to admit patients who paid their own bills. Discrimination against Medicaid recipients was wrong, IOM said, and it should be eliminated. The report also weighed in against the practice used by some homes of trying to discharge residents who became eligible for Medicaid after they had been admitted. At times homes would send such a resident to a hospital for special care; when the patient was ready to return, his bed would be filled. That practice should be outlawed, IOM said.

The Institute of Medicine report created a groundswell of support for stronger, not weaker, regulation of nursing homes. Congressional leaders who had put a stop to the 1982 HHS regulations, now introduced legislation to carry out the IOM's recommendations.

Over at HHS, Schweiker was long gone; in fact HHS was on its third secretary, Dr. Otis Bowen. At the Health Care Financing Administration there was new leadership as well. Carolyne Davis, who had run HCFA when Schweiker's rules were published, left in 1985; her replacement was Dr. William Roper. Roper had spent three years in the White House as the President's health policy adviser. While Roper and Bowen also toed the administration's antiregulation line, they weighed in strongly in favor of implementing the IOM's recommendations. Both men were doctors—Bowen a family physician, Roper a pediatrician. Both had spent time in state government when nursing home scandals had rocked the state capitals. And both men knew very well what life in a nursing home could be like—each man's mother was confined to a home.

Roper spent nearly a year drafting regulations to carry out many of the major recommendations in the IOM report. His work was spurred by congressional interest in legislation introduced by representatives Dingell and Waxman and Senator George Mitchell of Maine, the new chairman of the Senate Finance health subcommittee. Roper wanted to beat Congress to the punch and repair the administration's tattered reputation on nursing home regulation.

But Roper and Bowen would run into opposition to their plan from OMB. While Stockman was gone (he left the Cabinet in 1985 to join a Wall Street firm), his successor, James Miller, was just as opposed to government regulation. HHS proposed round-the-clock nursing for all homes; OMB wanted to require "sufficient nursing." HHS wanted a nine- to fifteen-month nursing home inspection schedule; OMB wanted to stick with a six- to twenty-four-month cycle. But with Congress on their side, Bowen and Roper would prevail.

Reagan's attempt to reduce regulation of the health care industry most certainly failed. While the administration succeeded in repealing the federal health planning statute, states kept up the program with their own funds. By the time planning bit the

9 / Deregulation?

dust, the economic health of so many health care providers had deteriorated to the point that they were rarely planning major expansions. When PSROs metamorphosized into PROs, regulatory clout far eclipsed that of their predecessors. Nursing homes were more regulated by the time Reagan was ready to leave office than they were when he was elected. The administration learned a key lesson: When it comes to health care, Americans want more regulation, not less.

10

Vouchers

While much of the Reagan administration's competitive strategy for health care got lost in the search for budget savings, one tenet of the original plan laid out in 1981 by the Winston and Rubin task forces remained a central part of the Reagan policies from the beginning to the end of his two terms. That idea was to enroll Medicare-eligible senior citizens in private health insurance programs through a voucher program. By doing so, the administration hoped to reduce the amount of direct government involvement in health care. Vouchers were the purest form of market-oriented competition. In fact, in its early years, the Reagan administration proposed use of vouchers for several social programs, including education and housing.

As with many of the other policy initiatives taken by the Reagan administration, the Medicare voucher concept was not new. Congress and the Department of Health, Education, and Welfare had been experimenting with prepaid health care for seniors since the early 1970s. Proponents of the idea in Congress ranged from liberal Democrats like Henry Waxman of California to conservative Republicans like Phil Gramm of Texas and Dave Durenberger of Minnesota. But voucher proponents came to their position for very different reasons. Conservatives saw vouchers as a way to save the government money and to limit government regulation; liberals saw them as a way to expand benefits to the elderly without costing the government more money.

Representatives of the then-fledgling prepaid health care industry pressed Congress in 1965 to allow its members into the Medicare ballgame. But Congress rejected the idea because of concern that prepaid plans like health maintenance organizations (HMOs) would attract only the healthiest seniors, leaving the traditional Medicare program to serve only the sickest retirees. Health maintenance organizations were allowed to continue caring for their members after they reached age 65, but were paid under normal Medicare rules. Lobbyists continued to press for expansion of Medicare to cover HMOs but ran into a brick wall in the Senate Finance Committee, where staff chief Jay Constantine adamantly opposed such a move. In 1972, Congress did agree to a slight modification to Medicare law that allowed HMOs to participate in the program, but limits on profits kept most plans from joining; only Oregon's Group Health Cooperative of Puget Sound signed a contract under the 1972 rules.

In 1979, under the Carter administration, Medicare used its authority to conduct demonstration projects by signing up five plans in Oregon, Minnesota, Washington, and Massachusetts. Under those contracts, HMOs were paid a predetermined premium to care for Medicare patients.

The voucher concept evolved slowly during the 1970s and continued to change during the Reagan years. When Reagan came to office, his policymakers envisioned a broad voucher program in which the elderly would be handed a government chit that could be exchanged for a private health insurance policy. The elderly would shop for a plan and buy private insurance, much like employers shop for the best deal in buying health insurance for their workers. The existing Medicare program offered the elderly no choice; every senior was given the same benefit package at the same price without regard to their needs. An elderly American who needed more home health coverage and less acute care insurance could not make that kind of tradeoff. As a result, some people got more coverage than they needed while a lot of others got much less than they needed. With a voucher program, the elderly could shop for the health insurance plan that best met their needs. Voucher proponents within the Reagan administration believed that health insurers would lower their premiums and offer the elderly additional benefits to attract their business. In turn, insurers would pressure health care providers to cut their charges so that the lower premiums would cover their costs. In this roundabout way, the competition theory advanced by the administration would bring down health care prices.

Critics of the voucher concept worried that the elderly would fall prey to insurance scams. Administration officials claimed their opponents were underestimating the intelligence of the elderly, and argued the elderly were quite capable of choosing the kind of insurance they wanted.

Voucher supporters compared their vision to the existing health insurance program for federal employees. Under that program, federal workers chose among more than 400 private health insurance plans. Some of the offerings were quite liberal in the kind of services they covered, but charged higher premiums. Others included a fairly limited benefit package but charged a low premium. Federal employees and their families would choose the plan that best fit their medical and financial situation. For example, a couple that intended to have a child in the coming year would choose the "high option" plan that included broad coverage of maternity benefits. A couple with several children would choose the plan that offered the best coverage of pediatric care. A single worker would be likely to opt for the "low-option" plan with limited benefits and low cost-sharing.

Reagan administration officials who supported the Medicare voucher concept believed that the elderly could make the same judgments that working Americans did each year. They saw no logic in the current Medicare system in which all beneficiaries were given the same benefits at the same price.

Congressional skeptics feared the administration would use the voucher system to eventually dismantle the existing Medicare program. Under Reagan's original proposal, the voucher system would be voluntary up to a certain point. When—or more likely, if—50 percent of the Medicare population enrolled in a private health insurance program, the rest of the elderly would be required to join such a plan. Critics of the Reagan plan also were wary of the seemingly generous payment level offered by the administration. They worried that while Reagan now said the government would pay 95 percent of average costs, a universal voucher system would be an easy target for across-the-board reductions in premiums.

The broad Reagan Medicare voucher plan could not fly in Congress. Too many questions remained unanswered. Could the elderly make intelligent choices when it came to health insurance or would they be susceptible to scurrilous salesmen who would sell them the most expensive plan? Experience with the private health insurance industry indicated that free choice for the elderly could be anything but free.

In the 1970s, private insurers offered supplemental coverage to beneficiaries to cover what Medicare did not. These policies filled the gaps in Medicare's benefit package—hence the term "Medigap insurance." For many elderly people Medigap insurance served a useful purpose. But for some the business of buying Medigap insurance was quite confusing. It is often said that elderly Americans have two chief concerns: their health and their wealth. The worry is which one will fail first. A combination of those two fears left many senior citizens vulnerable to unscrupulous insurance salesmen. In a series of major congressional hearings in the 1970s, lawmakers found that some insurers had declared open season on the elderly, selling them as many overlapping health insurance policies as they could. One woman told a congressional committee that she had purchased fourteen separate Medigap policies, thus exhausting her life savings and providing her with little extra coverage and certainly no additional peace of mind. The Medigap insurance scandals led Congress to enact legislation authored by Montana Senator Max Baucus that offered government certification to Medigap insurers in return for their meeting a series of standards. By providing this kind of "Good Housekeeping Seal of Approval," the government hoped to knock out some of the disreputable insurance firms. The widespread fraud in Medigap insurance abated, but investigators today still find examples of fraud and abuse directed at the vulnerable elderly.

For those reasons, and many others, Congress was not ready to adopt the broad voucher program the administration wanted in 1982. Waxman, for one, was leery of the idea of turning over care for the nation's elderly to businessmen intent on earning a profit. Waxman's caution was not unfounded. In his stint in the California legislature, Waxman presided over an investigation into a scandal-ridden experiment with vouchers under the state's Medicaid program for the poor. California's then-Governor Ronald Reagan had set up a program known as "Prepaid Health Plans," or PHP, to provide managed-care services for the poor. Without getting the legislature's approval, and without issuing any regulations, Reagan's health department began signing contracts with private HMOs to care for the poor in southern California. A series of exposés in the *Los Angeles Times* and other papers revealed that several HMO owners were getting rich on the program. One plan in particular had aggressively signed up Medicaid recipients via door-to-door marketing and free chicken dinners. But many of California's poor weren't getting health care under the plan. Working with the California Rural Legal Assistance Corporation and the National Health Law Program, Waxman fashioned legislation to regulate the program. While the California program later folded, its problems left an indelible imprint on Waxman when he went to Congress in 1974.

Waxman was intent that President Reagan wouldn't be given the same leeway with the Medicare voucher that Governor Reagan got in California with Medicaid. He pressed for a much more limited program that offered the elderly the opportunity to voluntarily enroll in private HMOs. The legislation offered a fixed premium to HMOs that agreed to participate. The government would pay a premium equal to 95 percent of the average cost of serving a Medicare beneficiary in a geographic area. If the cost of care for an individual proved to be higher than that premium, the HMO would take the loss. But if the costs proved to be lower than the premium, the HMO earned a limited profit. In effect, Waxman's plan was to limit the profit an HMO could make on

Medicare patients to the same percentage it made on its other patients. Meanwhile, the government would reap a small savings because it paid HMOs a discounted price.

Administration officials opposed the Waxman plan, preferring to push instead for their broader voucher scheme. They got support for their plan from a pair of House Ways and Means Committee members—Democrat Richard Gephardt of Missouri and Republican Bill Gradison of Ohio. In a closed-door committee session, the two men made their case for the administration's voucher plan. Ways and Means members weren't biting. They instead adopted a slightly modified version of the Waxman plan. Waxman's Energy and Commerce Committee added its approval and sent the bill on to the Senate.

Over in the Senate, the modified voucher plan ran into trouble in the Finance Committee. Constantine had left the panel by then but his successor, Sheila Burke, and her boss, Chairman Robert Dole of Kansas, shared Constantine's antipathy for the voucher plan. Committee members John Heinz, a Pennsylvania Republican, and Minnesota's Durenberger favored the concept. They introduced a plan that was similar to the Waxman proposal. But it looked like the bill would go nowhere until Heinz pulled a rabbit out of his hat. In a closed meeting of Finance Committee Republicans, called to discuss the panel's budget bill, Heinz announced that he would trade his vote in favor of all the proposals to raise cost-sharing for the elderly if Dole would back the voucher bill. A surprised Dole agreed to the swap and the measure was included in an omnibus budget bill.

With Finance on board, it was clear to the HHS lobbyists that their broader voucher proposal would not fly. Rather than work against the limited voucher, they pressed Heinz and Durenberger to expand the scope of the program slightly beyond HMOs so that it would include what they called "competitive medical plans." The two senators agreed and so, later, did Waxman. The administration figured it would get its foot in the door with the limited voucher program and work to broaden its scope in future years.

Waxman built specific safeguards into the new voucher law

to guard against some of the abuses he had seen in California with the Medicaid voucher fiasco. His chief worry was that the lure of Medicare payments would attract "Johnny-come-lately" entrepreneurs into the HMO industry. Waxman's rules were designed to limit the size of profits and to guard against entry into the program of new companies that weren't tested in community service. No HMO would be allowed to participate if more than 50 percent of its members were Medicare or Medicaid recipients. The idea behind the 50-50 rule was that private-sector enrollment would guarantee the performance of an HMO because employers could pull out all their members if the HMO had a poor showing. Waxman insisted on his proposal to limit the size of profits earned on Medicare patients; all excess profits had to be plowed back into the program in the form of additional benefits or lower cost-sharing for patients. This "adjusted community rate" system would prevent HMOs from offering too many benefits to the elderly to draw them into their plan only to find the company couldn't keep its promises to provide those services. Health maintenance organizations also were barred from discriminating against sickly Medicare beneficiaries, misleading consumers through advertising, or dropping a Medicare member whose health care costs proved to be too high.

Congress passed the legislation setting up the voucher system in 1982, but HHS took nearly two years to complete the regulations needed to implement the system. The reason: a family feud between HHS and OMB. The Health Care Financing Administration at HHS completed the first set of draft regulations in mid-1983 but they sat and waited in Secretary Margaret Heckler's office for nearly six months. Decisiveness was not one of Heckler's strong points. During her first year in office, regulations piled up on Heckler's desk while "Madame Secretary" weighed the pros and cons. With her tenuous hold on power, Heckler was wary of signing any regulation that could cause a public relations problem for the administration. Heckler's political instincts told her that she, not the White House, would be the one to take the heat for such screwups. As a result, the regulations backlog became overwhelming.

Heckler finally signed the draft HMO regulations early in 1984 and sent them to OMB for final approval, where Director Stockman held up publication of the regulations until midyear because of his belief that the new program would add to the Medicare budget. Stockman was upset to learn that HHS had been signing up HMOs under demonstration contracts and paying them a higher rate than the new law would allow. Converting those contracts to the new program would cost the government even more.

But power, not money, was the real reason for Stockman's delay of the voucher regulations; HHS and OMB were locked in a battle for control of health policymaking in the Reagan administration. Like a pack of wolves attacking a lame lamb, Stockman and his minions at OMB went in for the kill when Heckler's weaknesses were exposed. By holding up the voucher regulations, OMB could force Heckler to capitulate to its views. But the HHS secretary decided to draw the line on the HMO issue. She directed the HCFA administrator, Carolyne Davis, to resist OMB demands for information about HMOs.

Stockman told his health care assistant, John Cogan, to look into the "mess at HHS." Cogan was a bright, ambitious, and energetic disciple of Stockman's brand of budget government, who had little regard for Heckler and her team at HHS. He pressed Davis for the documents on the Medicare demonstration contracts with HMOs. With Heckler's blessing, Davis demurred. When Cogan turned up the heat through a series of demanding and angry memos, Davis wrote, and leaked, a memo of her own, labeling OMB's efforts a "power grab." In the Washington world, leaked memos are nothing new, but Davis made a classic mistake; she leaked her memo before it had arrived on Cogan's desk. The memo heightened the tension between the two agencies. An angry Stockman demanded that the White House force Heckler to comply with the request; it did, and she did.

Once Cogan got his hands on the incriminating evidence, it was clear heads would roll. Surely Heckler would not go down because of Davis' mistake, and Davis wasn't about to be forced out if she could blame someone on her staff. That someone was the director of HCFA's Office of Research and Development,

Bryan Luce. Davis' staff was furious; they had warned her that she would have to go to the mat once she decided to leak the memo, and she had promised she was ready to do just that. But when push came to shove, it was Luce, not Davis, who took the fall.

In the meantime, Stockman and Cogan slapped a freeze on new HMO demonstration projects and forced Heckler and Davis to agree to a schedule to move the existing demonstration plans to risk contracts within one year.

Once the administration battles were over, the government published final rules in early 1985 and Medicare began signing up HMOs soon thereafter. Most of the early recruits were the plans already serving Medicare patients under demonstration project contracts. Growth in the program was quick; by the end of 1985, nearly 775,000 Medicare beneficiaries were enrolled in HMOs. Voucher supporters at HHS were excited by the early success of the voucher program, but officials close to the program were beginning to worry about problems at the biggest HMO in the system—Florida's Miami-based International Medical Centers Inc. (IMC).

The trouble that inflicted the Medicare voucher program in 1986 was a homemade product; built brick by brick by overly zealous proponents of the administration's competitive policy. The frustrating thing for voucher proponents was that all the trouble could have been avoided if the administration had stuck to the rules laid down by Congress. Instead, Reagan regulators waived the rules set by Congress to protect the elderly.

The trouble actually began in early 1982, a few months before Congress enacted the Medicare voucher bill. The owner of a small health maintenance organization based in Miami was watching the Congressional debate very closely. Miguel Recarey, Jr. had bought International Medical Centers in 1980. It was his first venture into health care. Recarey was a Cuban refugee who had built a successful business in Florida and become active in state and national politics. Until 1982, he hadn't done much to expand IMC but he had big plans for the future.

Back in Washington, Reagan administration officials were anxiously watching the debate on Capitol Hill. Although their quest for a broad Medicare voucher was destined for failure, they hoped to take full advantage of the limited program that Congress seemed sure to approve. By making a success of the limited voucher program, they figured their case for a broader plan would gain acceptance in Congress. The key to success was quick growth and a rising number of Medicare beneficiaries enrolled in prepaid health plans.

In 1982, as Congress debated the voucher plan, HCFA signed twenty-three demonstration contracts with HMOs; among those was Recarey's IMC. Recarey's contract hadn't come easily. When his application arrived at HCFA headquarters in Baltimore, Maryland, career agency officials were appalled. Recarey had only two years of experience in the HMO field and was operating a very small firm with no proven track record of service in the community; there was no evidence that the company could take on the task of serving the elderly population of southern Florida. The career staff at HCFA recommended that Davis reject the proposal. Their advice was to give IMC a few years to prove itself, and then reconsider the application.

Like any good bidder on a government contract, Recarey and his people had their eyes and ears open in Washington and knew that IMC's application was in jeopardy. The IMC brass met with HCFA officials to press their case but seemed to get nowhere. Recarey was unwilling to wait two years to resubmit his application; he wanted a Medicare demonstration project contract now. He was determined to get the administration in Washington to change the HCFA decision.

Until Reagan's 1980 election, Recarey's political activism was strictly a Democratic affair. He contributed generously to the Democratic National Committee and to local Democratic elected officials. But after 1980, Recarey switched his allegiances to the Republican party; his money started going to the Republican National Committee and to GOP candidates. The only Democrat he continued to support was Miami Congressman Claude Pepper.

When Recarey found himself stymied at HCFA in 1982, he began spending some of his money on outside lobbying help. He signed up the first of a string of high-powered, politically connected lobbyists—former Reagan campaign director John Sears. Besides his service as Reagan campaign chief in 1980 and 1984 (he was fired after the New Hampshire GOP primary after a falling out with Reagan's other advisers), Sears had scores of connections with establishment figures in Washington, including many of the top figures in the new administration. In 1982, Sears was running his own lobbying firm and signing up many of the country's biggest accounts. Ordinarily, the affairs of a small Florida HMO would not interest Sears, but Recarey was no ordinary businessman. He offered Sears $250,000 to lobby the administration for IMC's contract.

At the same time, Recarey asked Pepper and freshman Florida Republican Senator Paula Hawkins to use their influence in the administration to help the waiver along. Sears, Pepper, and Hawkins were a formidable lobbying team; HCFA officials were inundated with calls from the trio and their White House contacts.

Davis was unprepared, and perhaps unwilling, to withstand the pressure brought to bear on her and her agency in 1982. Prior to joining the administration, Davis had been dean of nursing at the University of Michigan. She got the HCFA job through Michigan Republican Congressman Carl Pursell. She had little experience with Medicare and Medicaid—the two programs HCFA was responsible for administrating—and no experience running a huge bureaucracy like HCFA's 1200 employees. Some believed she got the job because the new administration was determined to downgrade HCFA and leave most of its authority with the budget offices of HHS and OMB. Davis caved in to the lobbying pressure, and IMC got its contract and joined Medicare late in 1982, as the ink was drying on the new voucher law. However, that was not the end of the political maneuvering on IMC's behalf.

Recarey was a smart businessman. He could easily decipher the new voucher law and determine where the money was going to be. Because the voucher program would pay HMOs based on average local Medicare costs, Florida's Dade County—home to Miami and IMC—would be the highest paid area in the country.

If IMC could keep its costs below the average, it would make a profit; but if costs exceeded the average, IMC would lose money. The way to keep costs low was to reduce utilization of services. HMOs traditionally have succeeded by lowering the use of hospitals and doctors' offices. To attract members, HMOs use the savings from lower utilization of hospitals to eliminate coinsurance and deductible charges and to pay for additional optional services like outpatient prescription drugs, eyeglasses, home care, and the like.

Recarey didn't build his business in the traditional HMO fashion. In fact, very little about IMC was traditional when it came to health care delivery. Whereas most HMOs either place physicians on salary or contract with a network, or group, of physicians, IMC signed up nearly 200 "subcontractors," who owned and operated clinics throughout southern Florida. Recarey patterned his company after the medical care delivery system in his native Cuba. But Floridians—even Recarey's fellow Cuban refugees—were not used to Havana health care. The storefront clinic approach used by many of IMC's subcontractors did not please the plan's new elderly enrollees.

The elderly were pleased, however, with the wide array of services IMC offered. In his aptly named "Gold Plus Plan," Recarey offered the elderly free prescription drugs, free dental care, free eyeglasses, and home care at reduced cost. Elderly members of Gold Plus also paid no deductibles, no coinsurance, and no copayments. Unlike most other HMOs in the voucher system, IMC charged no additional premium to cover the cost of these additional services. Astonished onlookers wondered how IMC could afford to pay for the expected demand for such services. Instead of reducing utilization, IMC's benefit package promised to increase the amount of services each member would use. The plan's design seemed to be a prescription for disaster.

Problems began soon after Recarey signed his Medicare contract: IMC could not offer Gold Plus to the working residents of Miami and the rest of Florida. To offer such a plan, IMC would have to charge a premium so high that no firm would think of enrolling its workers. Employers were trying to cut their health care costs in 1982, and the way to do that was to limit fringe services and impose higher cost sharing. International Medical Centers was caught in a conundrum: If it offered Gold Plus to local workers at the same price Medicare was paying, it would lose money; if it offered a cheaper package to the nonelderly, Medicare rules called for a reduction in voucher payments.

But Recarey had to increase his non-Medicare enrollment. Medicare rules limited the number of Medicare members to 50 percent of total membership. At the pace IMC was going, the rule would be breached by the end of its first year of operation. These two rules—commonly referred to as the 50-50 rule and the adjusted community rate (ACR)—would be IMC's biggest obstacles to success. To meet the 50-50 rule, IMC had to enroll local workers; to live by the second, it had to charge a premium that was so high that no workers would enroll.

Recarey's answer was that HCFA should waive the 50-50 rule and the ACR. That way IMC could enroll thousands of Medicare members without risking a cut in Medicare payments. Recarey promised to meet the rules at a later date. Career officials at HCFA again strongly advised Davis to reject the waiver requests. Recarey sent Sears, Hawkins, and Pepper back to their telephones. Davis approved the waivers. Now IMC was really in business, and Medicare was really in trouble.

Beginning in 1983, IMC took full advantage of the waivers Davis had granted. It launched a concerted recruiting campaign among Florida's elderly population. Its sales personnel went door to door telling elderly residents they could have free eyeglasses, dentures, and prescription drugs at absolutely no cost if they joined IMC. Who could resist? Few did. To entice other residents, Recarey took to the airwaves with commercials featuring such senior-citizen heroes as George Burns. Happy Reagan administration officials watched as the voucher program took off in Florida. By 1986, 170,000 of Florida's senior citizens had joined IMC.

Down in Florida, IMC's success wasn't spreading joy and happiness among the state's health care providers. Because IMC's clinics were poorly staffed and equipped, patients often had to wait days, or even weeks, for an appointment. Many patients were being referred to doctors and hospitals that were not part of IMC, and providers were waiting as long as three months to get paid. As a result, some doctors and a few hospitals began to turn away IMC patients unless there was a medical emergency.

For Recarey, business was booming. IMC was cashing a monthly check from HCFA for a cool $30 million. Business was so good that in 1985 Recarey called HCFA with one more waiver request. He wanted to expand his business to Philadelphia and southern California. Could HCFA extend the waiver of the 50-50 and ACR rules to those new sites?

By the time Recarey's latest waiver request arrived, HCFA was in a state of transition. After four and one-half years of constant pounding, Davis had quit. At HHS, Secretary Heckler was in the midst of another power struggle with the White House; her choices for the growing number of vacant posts in her department were rejected by the White House and she in turn refused White House-based choices. As a result, when Davis left late in 1984, Heckler named her staff chief, C. McClain Haddow, as acting HCFA administrator. It would be up to Haddow to rule on the IMC waiver request.

Recarey left nothing to chance. He added to his lobbying stable of Sears, Pepper, and Hawkins former White House adviser Lyn Nofziger and former HHS general counsel Juan del Real. Del Real, who was named IMC chief of staff, was the latest in a line of former HHS officials to go to work for IMC after leaving government service. Recarey also hired Hawkin's daughter—perhaps for good luck. The IMC lobbying machine didn't need to exert much effort to convince Haddow to approve the waiver. The new HCFA chief was looking to curry favor with a White House that seemed determined to get rid of his boss, Heckler. Anything that would keep the White House happy was fine with Haddow. Once again, a Reagan political operative overrode the objections of HCFA's career staff and approved the IMC waiver request.

But the problems of late payments and a lack of doctors to treat IMC members began to attract the attention of lawmakers in Washington. The chairman of the House Ways and Means health subcommittee, California Democrat Pete Stark moved to block the waiver expansion with legislation. He added a provision to a pending budget bill that would reverse Haddow's decision. But before the bill could reach the House floor, it had to go through the House Rules Committee and its chairman, Claude Pepper. Pepper told Stark his bill would never reach the House floor unless the offending provision were removed. Stark knew he was outmatched, and dropped the provision. (The waiver was later rescinded by Haddow's successor at Stark's request; IMC never expanded beyond Florida.)

By the end of 1985, HCFA investigators began to conclude that something had to be done about IMC. But the administration's commitment to the voucher program tied its hands. The sheer number of IMC Medicare members worked against any drastic actions. Revoking IMC's waivers would close its doors. Forcing 135,000 Medicare beneficiaries to look for a new health care provider and depriving them of the attractive additional benefits IMC promised would make the administration look like Scrooge and could undermine confidence in the entire voucher program. "We'd have been called a bunch of pointyheaded bureaucrats," one HCFA official said when asked why the government didn't put a halt to IMC in 1985.

Instead, HCFA began pressuring IMC to gradually increase its private membership. Recarey promised to comply; he never did. In fact, a 1986 General Accounting Office report to Congress showed that IMC's private membership was gradually shrinking as unions withdrew their members; meanwhile, IMC continued to enroll elderly Florida residents.

At the end of 1985, Heckler's fight with the White House was over and she had lost. Reagan "promoted" her to U.S. ambassador to Ireland. In her place was Dr. Otis Bowen, former governor of Indiana. Haddow too was gone, shown the door not long after Heckler's plane landed in Dublin. Haddow now was a private "consultant." His first (and only) client was IMC. The new HCFA administrator was Dr. William Roper who had been a White House health policy adviser to President Reagan since 1982 and a strong proponent of the voucher system. He also was a man of strong moral principles; what he saw at IMC made him sick. But Roper knew there were no quick solutions to the Florida fiasco.

By mid-1986, complaints from Florida health care providers about IMC's nonpayment of bills and evidence that IMC had begun to "encourage" the disenrollment of some of its sickest—and most costly—members brought investigators from HCFA, the Justice Department, the FBI, and the Florida State Insurance Commissioner's office. By now the IMC imbroglio was daily news in Florida's newspapers and had begun to seep into the national papers.

Some of the "business practices" that investigators found at IMC were particularly disturbing. Since an HMO only makes money on patients who do not use too many services, IMC had reasons to want to enroll only the healthiest seniors in town. One way IMC managed that was to put enrollment offices on the third floor of buildings with no elevators. Another method was holding enrollment dances for senior citizens. After all, a sick elderly person isn't likely to attend a dance, but a healthy senior is.

Even with such "fail-safe" mechanisms in place, IMC worried that it might wind up with costly members. Federal investigators found an unusual number of IMC members had been treated by IMC doctors before enrolling in the HMO. Those doctors had performed a wide array of screening tests to see if there might be a person with high blood pressure, heart disease, or some other disabling illness that might require more than the usual amount of care once they were enrolled. Recarey's IMC couldn't lose under this arrangement. Healthy patients who were encouraged to enroll in IMC already had a series of costly tests performed, and those costs were not chalked up against the voucher payment IMC would receive; sickly patients were not encouraged to join. The problem was that all of these practices were patently unethical; many were illegal.

The Reagan administration could no longer deal quietly with the IMC mess. Public headlines demanded public solutions. Roper had barely gotten his feet wet at the HCFA, when he had to deal with the crisis building in Florida. He dispatched an investigation team to Miami to look at IMC's files and to interview IMC employees and members. Physicians and hospital administrators in Florida had been contacting HCFA officials on their own throughout 1985, and complaints from IMC patients gave HCFA's team an idea of where to look. But when the team arrived, they found IMC corporate officials sitting in on many of the interviews they had arranged. Some were asked to leave and did; others kept an eye and an ear on the interviewees. At least one interview subject canceled at the last minute.

What the investigators found was shocking. Not only was IMC late in paying its bills—now as much as ninety days behind schedule—but the company itself was in the red. It had been losing money for some time, but some of those losses were expected as the plan expanded to handle the growing number of Medicare members it enrolled. In 1981, its books showed a "working capital deficit" of $2.5 million; another $4.4 million shortfall was reported in 1982; and $6.8 million was lost in 1983. By 1984, IMC should have been earning a tidy profit, but losses jumped to $18.2 million; in 1985, losses totaled $22 million. Yet Medicare was still sending a $30 million monthly check to Recarey.

Florida Insurance Commissioner Bill Gunter ordered Recarey to obtain $9.1 million in outside capital to shore up IMC's bank account and pay off those late bills. Recarey got the money; but it was transferred from other family holdings.

Congress too was looking into the IMC situation. Florida Congressman Dan Mica and Ways and Means Health Subcommittee Chairman Stark intensified their efforts to get to the bottom of the problem. Mica and Stark urged Roper to cut off any new Medicare enrollment in IMC until the situation could be resolved; Roper said he lacked such authority. Despite the newspaper headlines, Florida's elderly continued to sign up with IMC.

By June, Roper's investigation was complete. The HCFA found IMC "out of compliance" with federal Medicare law and regulations. Among its findings: IMC lacked the "personnel and systems sufficient to organize, plan, control, and evaluate the health services aspects of the HMO." Roper criticized IMC's system of 200 separate "affiliated provider centers" that had little communication with IMC headquarters in Miami; HCFA was most critical of IMC's failure to pay its bills on time. As of March 1986, 53 percent of IMC claims were ninety days past due; 34 percent were sixty days old. Despite promises to the contrary, Roper found "IMC has no organized approach to address this problem."

But Roper had no power to force Recarey to fix the problems, short of throwing the HMO out of Medicare, and that still was out of the question. To evict Medicare's largest HMO would likely have ended any chances of expanding the voucher program during Reagan's years. Stark already was at work on legislation that would give HCFA the power to suspend an HMO like IMC from further Medicare enrollment and to fine the owners of any plan that fell behind in its bill payments. But the IMC situation couldn't wait for Stark's legislation; something had to be done.

Recarey recognized the mess he was in. If he persisted in expanding his business in Florida, Roper might be left with no choice but to boot him out of the program no matter what the effect on the administration's voucher policy. On June 12, Recarey announced that he was "voluntarily" capping the number of Medicare members in IMC at 137,500.

In effect, it seemed that Recarey was voluntarily doing what Mica and Stark had asked Roper to do: halting Medicare enrollment. But in reality by promising to "cap" Medicare enrollment, Recarey retained the right to enroll new members to replace those that dropped out or died. Medicare enrollment continued for months after Recarey's promise. In July, Roper gave Recarey ninety days to clean up his company or face termination of his Medicare contract.

While Roper was issuing his ultimatum, Recarey was busy offering a deal of his own: He put IMC up for sale to the highest bidder. Despite the mounting financial and legal problems the company faced, IMC was an attractive purchase. With its 137,500 Medicare enrollees and $360 million in annual Medicare income, a new owner could earn a nice profit if management controls could be achieved. Recarey announced in July he would sell IMC to Humana Inc., a proprietary health care company based in Louisville, Kentucky. Roper and his HCFA team breathed an audible sigh of relief. The IMC mess was over; at least, so it seemed.

The agreement between IMC and Humana called for completion of the deal by November 1986. Humana would buy not only IMC but also Miami General Hospital, a 400-bed acute care facility also owned by Recarey and used to treat many IMC members. The purchase price: $60 million.

The announcement of IMC's imminent change of ownership quieted the din surrounding the voucher program. As the headlines began to fade and the congressional inquiries were wrapped up, things seemed to return to normal. In October, Congress enacted legislation giving HCFA the authority to suspend Medicare enrollment in an HMO that was consistently late in paying its bills. Stiff federal penalties were set up for plans that tried to discourage the sickly elderly from joining or tried to force costly patients out. Most importantly, Congress voted to require Medicare peer review organizations—the government's health care watchdogs—to begin looking into the business and medical practices of the HMOs participating in the voucher system. In effect, IMC's behavior brought about a slew of new regulatory requirements that quickly made the program less attractive to the honest HMOs.

By November, Humana's bookkeepers had gotten a good look at IMC's financial records; the legal department also had looked into the possible lawsuits the new owner of IMC would face if it acquired the company. Humana chiefs began to have second thoughts; the scheduled purchase date was pushed back to "sometime by the end of the year." The delays didn't seem to raise any eyebrows in Washington; most assumed the deal would go through, but would take a little longer than expected. The same held true when the purchase date was delayed again to "the end of February" in 1987, and again when it became "this spring."

Meanwhile, Recarey and other IMC officials were doing very little to change their behavior. Bills still were behind schedule, and patients continued to have a hard time getting care. The HCFA officials, happy that Humana was about to solve their problems, returned to the lackadaisical oversight style of the early years of the voucher program. "Why pressure Recarey to fix things when Humana is going to change everything once they take over?" one HCFA official explained.

What HCFA didn't realize was the Humana-IMC deal was falling apart. The more Humana's legal and accounting departments looked at the IMC books—what books they could get their hands on—the worse the deal seemed. Humana stood to lose millions if it acquired IMC's debts along with its assets, and no one could put a finger on how high those debts could go. At the same time, negative newspaper headlines had cost IMC thousands of Medicare members. No new seniors were signing up to take their place.

By March 1987, the situation had worsened considerably. Two of Recarey's subcontractors were indicted on charges of defrauding Medicare of more than $100,000 and ordering extensive and expensive diagnostic tests for people who expressed interest in enrolling in the HMO. While the Justice Department stressed that IMC headquarters had "cooperated fully" with its investigators and had nothing to do with these cases, the smell of smoke began to rise.

In April, the Humana deal began to crumble. Recarey began courting other buyers; he wanted someone who would buy both his assets and his debts. There were some takers but, like Humana, the new suitors lost interest when they got a look at IMC's books.

On April 22, the bottom fell out. Recarey and his brother were indicted on federal racketeering charges related to attempts to bribe local union officials to offer IMC coverage to their members. Ironically, one of Recarey's attempts to increase non-Medicare enrollment—albeit a highly illegal one—caused his downfall.

While the Justice Department was moving in on one front, Roper and his HCFA team were moving in on another. The ninety-day deadline Roper had set for change at IMC back in

July had long passed; HCFA had deferred action while the Humana negotiations were going on, but now Roper had no choice but to take action. On April 15, HCFA notified IMC that it would terminate its Medicare contract within ninety days unless changes were made—$8 million in outside capital, and new leadership; Recarey was to separate himself from the management team running the company. When Recarey could not come up with the money in time to meet HCFA's May 14 deadline, Roper notified IMC that he was moving to terminate its contract as of July 1.

Roper's move served as a gust of wind through the house of cards that Recarey had constructed in Miami. Without a Medicare contract and the $30 million per month in income it brought, Recarey's business had nowhere to go. State Insurance Commissioner Gunter announced that Florida would temporarily take over management of the company until a buyer could be found. One week later, a U.S. court declared IMC insolvent, a move that cleared the way for any buyer to obtain only its assets, not its debts. Two weeks of heavy bidding ended with Gunter's announcement that Humana had won with a $40 million bid. Miami General Hospital would be sold by the state to help pay IMC's creditors.

The Reagan administration paid a heavy price for the Florida fiasco known as IMC. Its credibility suffered the most; congressional advocates of a broader voucher backed off, and opponents honed their arguments. Attempts by the administration to broaden the voucher program were summarily rejected on Capitol Hill. In 1987, when Roper sought to expand the program to include employers with large numbers of Medicare-eligible retired workers, Congress clamped down with new requirements. Concern that Roper's idea would result in "another IMC" pervaded the debate.

Other HMOs paid a price, too, even though they were essentially innocent bystanders. Many plans had joined the voucher program because they saw it as an attractive alternative to the regulation-heavy traditional Medicare program and as more consistent with the way they operated. With the advent of the IMC controversy, that was no longer true. Congress enacted severe new restrictions on HMOs and required greater oversight than ever before. That regulation, combined with tighter and tighter budget constraints on Medicare, led more than two dozen HMOs to drop out of the program at the end of 1987, leaving 80,000 of the one million HMO enrollees out in the cold. Although HCFA officials sought to downplay the desertions, it was clear that Medicare's voucher experiment would take several years to recover from the problems caused by IMC; another battalion of Reagan revolutionaries found themselves disheartened.

11

Catastrophic Insurance

Six years of incessant budget cutting left federal health policymakers with a yen to do "something positive." While many in Washington correctly defended the cuts they made in Medicare as necessary to restore the program's fiscal solvency, they could not escape the feeling that they needed to send some positive message to the elderly and to working Americans who were worried that all the talk of impending bankruptcy might mean there would be no protection available by the time they retired.

Medicare had some gaping holes. One of the biggest gaps was the limits on coverage of hospital stays. A senior citizen was required to pay for the first day of hospitalization, but Medicare picked up the tab for the next fifty-nine days. Medicare offered only limited coverage of days sixty-one to ninety and required a beneficiary to dip into an additional sixty-day lifetime reserve if a hospitalization lasted more than ninety days. But if a beneficiary were unfortunate enough to need more than 150 days of care, Medicare paid none of the additional bill. Even for that 150-day stay, out-of-pocket costs to the patient could run as high as $18,000.

As they cut the growth in Medicare's budget, the administration and the Congress did little to address the program's shortcomings. Small improvements were enacted along the way to cover such things as hospice care for the critically ill and payment for pneumonia vaccinations to prevent one of the leading causes of illness in the elderly. But basic problems were never addressed. As the Reagan years wore on, however, lawmakers were nervously looking for something to pass that could show their constituents they had improved their lot.

*   *   *

Earlier in his administration, President Reagan had proposed a Medicare catastrophic insurance bill that would have eliminated the sixty-day limit on hospitalization insurance. But in return, Reagan asked Congress to impose a new coinsurance on the first thirty days of hospital care. The catch was that the revenues from that coinsurance would have far exceeded the cost of the new coverage offered to those with catastrophic insurance bills. Democrats in Congress rightly identified the plan as a poorly disguised way to increase government revenue without giving the elderly much in return. The idea fizzled and was later dropped.

Reagan's record on catastrophic insurance wasn't always so poor. During his tenure in the California governor's mansion, he proposed what many called an innovative policy to address catastrophic illness costs for all citizens of his state. Reagan wanted to require all employers in that state to extend catastrophic coverage and to create a state insurance pool that would offer cut-rate insurance policies to those who couldn't get insurance elsewhere. Unfortunately, the Reagan plan foundered.

In the late-1980s federal policymakers would "find" the catastrophic insurance issue once again. The catalyst would be Reagan's third health secretary, Dr. Otis Bowen. Bowen's selection in December 1985 capped a year-long battle to displace HHS Secretary Margaret Heckler (see Chapter 4). The former Indiana governor was a popular choice. His experience as a state executive would help him run the large HHS bureaucracy; his tenure as speaker of the Indiana House of Representatives would aid in relations with Congress; and his career as a family doctor would help ease tension between the administration and organized medicine.

Unlike his two predecessors, Bowen came to HHS with an agenda—albeit a short one. A catastrophic health insurance program for the nation's elderly topped his list of priorities. Bowen's awareness of the lack of catastrophic insurance stemmed from his first wife's two-year battle with cancer, his career as a family physician, and his one-year stint as chairman of a presidential commission that studied the Medicare program in 1983. Bowen also was a smart politician who knew a popular issue when he saw it.

Like so many other health policies that came to fruition during the Reagan years, catastrophic insurance was not a new concept. Lawmakers knew from the moment they enacted Medicare in 1966 that they were leaving a gaping hole. Senators Russell Long of Louisiana and Abraham Ribicoff of Connecticut tried to convince the Senate to drop the sixty-day limit on hospital coverage but were defeated. Labor leaders, the driving force behind Medicare at the time, opposed Long and Ribicoff because they feared the costliness of the expansion would cause the program's defeat. Long was, until the last moment, an opponent of Medicare, so his motivation was questioned. Medicare supporters believed they could come back later and patch the holes.

Long, who later replaced Virginia Senator Harry Byrd, Sr. as chairman of the powerful Finance Committee, proved his 1965 doubters wrong by retaining his interest and commitment to catastrophic insurance to the end of his career in the Senate in 1986. Several times throughout the 1970s, Long led efforts to provide catastrophic coverage to the elderly through Medicare and to the rest of the nation through their employers. But Long's efforts were thwarted by the opposition of organized labor and other national health insurance proponents who believed enactment of a separate catastrophic insurance bill would weaken their case for a national program.

By the time Bowen took office in December 1985, the debate over national health insurance was past, and its proponents were in a state of political retreat. Not since 1980, the year before Reagan took office, had the leading proponent of national health insurance, Senator Edward Kennedy of Massachusetts, even introduced such a bill. Kennedy and his supporters in the labor movement were ready to accept the piecemeal approach that catastrophic insurance represented.

*   *   *

Bowen's arrival in Washington couldn't have been timed better for proponents of catastrophic insurance. When he left the Indiana statehouse in 1980, Bowen had planned a quiet retirement to his home in Bremen, Indiana; he had not campaigned for the Cabinet post. So he hadn't watched his words and deeds in the months before Reagan asked him to come to Washington. Less than two weeks after Reagan tapped Bowen to head HHS, some of those words came to the public's attention.

Together with Tom Burke, his staff chief on the presidential Medicare commission and later his chief aide at HHS, Bowen had written a four-page article for *FAH Review,* the in-house magazine of the Federation of American Hospitals, a trade organization representing proprietary hospitals. The article, entitled "Cost Neutral Catastrophic Care Proposed for Medicare Recipients," was a call for creation of a new Medicare benefit for those few elderly who faced the cost of catastrophic illness.

Bowen and Burke wanted to drop the limits on hospitalization coverage and place a $350 cap on out-of-pocket spending for physician services. Total out-of-pocket costs would not be allowed to exceed $750 per year. To pay for such coverage, they said, the elderly should pay a monthly premium estimated at $12, or $144 a year. In that way, the cost of the new coverage would be spread over Medicare's estimated thirty-one million elderly and disabled members.

Bowen and Burke also proposed a way to help working Americans lessen the threat of economic catastrophe due to the need for nursing home care. The government should allow tax-free deposits into "Individual Medical Accounts," or IMAs. Like Individual Retirement Accounts (IRAs), IMAs would be used to save money for a person's old age; money would be withdrawn at that time to pay costly nursing home bills.

"The proposal is intended to be provocative," Bowen and Burke quite correctly predicted. "The acid test of any idea is whether it will stand up to the close scrutiny of other professionals in the field. It is being presented with that objective in mind. If it does weather the close examination of others, perhaps it then would be given careful consideration by our nation's policymakers."

Bowen almost certainly had not written that article with the knowledge that he would soon be in position to do something about it, but when given the opportunity, would prove to be a man of his word.

Shortly after he arrived in Washington, Bowen began pressing to have his catastrophic insurance plan included in Reagan's fiscal 1987 budget due for submission in early February 1986. Bowen made quick progress; he secured a promise from Reagan that the catastrophic insurance matter would make it into the State of the Union address. Bowen wanted to nail down a presidential commitment to send legislation to Congress in 1986. The late date made Bowen's task difficult. White House aides asked him if he would settle for a promise to submit legislation later in the year. Bowen said that would be all right with him as long as the President made such a promise in the State of the Union.

Bowen came remarkably close to gaining Reagan's blessing in early 1986. Up until a week before the President's speech, Bowen and his aides were confident the State of the Union would include a promise to send legislation to Capitol Hill by year's end.

Insurance companies went on "red alert" when the Bowen-Burke catastrophic insurance proposal hit the streets in December. They realized that creation of such a Medicare benefit would quickly eat into the estimated $8 billion in Medigap insurance premiums they collected each year. Medigap salesmen had capitalized on the elderly's fear of catastrophic illness, often selling a retiree more coverage than was needed.

But insurers had to find a way to present their case against the Bowen plan without being viewed as "granny bashers." They seized on the administration's own rhetoric about the role of government. The health insurers said the Bowen plan was anti-private enterprise, ran counter to Reagan dogma, and would "federalize" the Medigap business.

Insurers did not have much time to make their case. Bowen's late 1985 arrival meant a decision on the issue had to be made within six weeks. There wasn't enough time for the usual "education campaigns" run by large trade groups like the Health Insurance Association of America. Instead, individual insurers called out their hired guns. Mutual of Omaha, one of the nation's largest Medigap insurers, called on Washington lobbyist Robert Gray. Gray was one of the growing legion of lobbyists who capitalized on their personal relations with the new power brokers in the White House. Where most lobbyists would take weeks, if not months, to gain access to a high-level White House aide, Gray could pick up his phone and have an appointment within minutes. Gray picked up that phone and began calling his friends at 1600 Pennsylvania Avenue, asking them to stop Bowen's plan before it was too late.

Gray couldn't kill the Bowen plan; Reagan had already promised to call for some kind of plan in the State of the Union. White House officials were fairly sure that if the catastrophic insurance idea was shot down, Bowen would quit and the administration would be faced with an embarrassing situation. So instead of killing the plan, the White House agreed to Gray's request to slow the process. Rather than promising to send catastrophic insurance legislation to Capitol Hill in 1986, Reagan would announce in his State of the Union message that he was asking Bowen to study the issue and report back to him by year's end.

To many, Reagan's announcement represented a defeat for Bowen. In Washington, often the easiest way to kill an idea is to "study" it. Hopefully, by the time the study is finished, the political will and popular support will have diminished, and public policymakers will have gone on to something else. But Bowen would confound the odds makers.

Rather than let the year's delay sap the support for his plan, Bowen kept up a quiet campaign for public support. As the newest Reagan Cabinet member, Bowen was the subject of numerous profiles in newspapers and magazines in which the health chief would press his case for catastrophic insurance for the elderly. As he had done throughout his political career in Indiana, Bowen cleverly used his "good guy" image to garner sympathy and support. The press was not used to an administration member pressing for creation of a new program; Schweiker and Heckler had spent much of their time trying to convince the public and the Congress to do away with existing programs. Bowen also used the time to hone the proposal and reach out to some untraditional supporters. Bowen's greatest help would come from congressional Democrats and liberal-oriented interest groups representing the elderly. His biggest headaches came from administration colleagues and Reagan's conservative supporters.

After Reagan requested the study, Bowen named a pair of task forces. An external group included two members of Congress, health group leaders, and consumer organizations. An internal HHS group was split into three parts: One would study acute care coverage for the elderly, another would look into long-term nursing home care for the elderly, and a third would examine the needs of working-age Americans faced with catastrophic medical bills. The external group, chaired by James Balog, vice chairman of the Wall Street firm, Drexel Burnham Lambert, was more for show than for substance. Nearly all of the members were supportive of Bowen's ideas and the product of their work was a foregone conclusion: They supported a government role in providing catastrophic insurance for the elderly.

The internal task forces were also more show than substance. Bowen did not intend to back off from the basic premise of his plan as presented in the *FAH Review* back in November. What he needed to do was refine the plan to knock out any objectionable features without losing the core of his proposal.

Clearly, the biggest problem Bowen faced was the size of his proposed monthly premium. The $12 estimate included in his article was designed to cover costs that would be incurred in 1985; with the one-year delay Reagan ordered, the program wouldn't go into effect until at least 1986. The new estimate approached $14 monthly, or $168 per year. For most retired Americans that was a manageable amount; but for the millions of Medicare beneficiaries living in poverty, $168 might as well have been $1680—it simply wasn't possible. Bowen had to scale back his proposal to lower that premium to a politically feasible amount.

After the initial flurry of opposition from health insurers, the opponents to Bowen's plan lay low. Perhaps they believed that the problem was over when Reagan agreed to hold off Bowen for a year. But insurers weren't Bowen's only problem. In fact, their opposition served a useful purpose for Bowen because their motives were so clearly financially based. By opposing the Bowen plan, the insurers looked like a classical special interest group out to protect their pocketbooks.

Bowen's real problems would come from the conservative wing of the Republican party. Having risen to prominence with Reagan's 1980 election, the right wing had been frustrated by its inability to get Reagan to concentrate on its agenda. Now it seemed that the administration was moving in the opposite direction.

The first salvo came from the conservative Heritage Foundation. Until 1980, the group was relatively unknown; but with the new President one of its biggest fans, Heritage became a hot prospect. Its *Mandate for Leadership* report in 1980 laid the groundwork for some of the administration's policy initiatives in Reagan's first term. A similar effort in 1985 for the President's second term drew little attention. Many of the best minds in Heritage had been recruited into the administration; the foundation was suffering from brain drain. To replace those it lost, Heritage had brought in some of the administration officials who had fallen by the wayside. One of those was Peter Ferrara, a Washington attorney who had briefly served in the White House Office of Domestic Policy.

In April 1986, Heritage published a diatribe against the Bowen plan written by Ferrara. In it Ferrara called Bowen's proposal "another expansion of the welfare state based on an outdated 1960s policy mindset." Ferrara said the Bowen plan—which he called the idea of "some HHS staffers"—would "drive the private insurers out of the business, replacing them with [a] public program." Bowen's plan was based on "faulty assumptions" that only a few elderly Americans would need the catastrophic coverage Bowen offered. Ferrara predicted Medicare catastrophic coverage would result in "physicians, hospitals, and patients [being] far more inclined to opt for more prolonged care in many instances where it is not strictly necessary." Guaranteed coverage, he added, would "induce the development of new and highly expensive medical technologies and techniques," leading to higher medical costs.

The plan must never get to Congress, Ferrara argued. "Congressional liberals and elderly groups" would expand it to include expensive long-term care. Pulling out all stops, Ferrara said Bowen's plan would lead to new calls for national health insurance and a "massive increase in Medicare." In conclusion, Ferrara said Bowen's plan ran counter to Reagan's "basic policy goals: to reduce government spending and interference in the private sector."

To those in Washington familiar with the workings of Medicare and federal health policy, Ferrara's charges were hollow and, in some cases, just downright silly. But the substance of what Ferrara had written had little to do with the impact his words had on the development of a catastrophic insurance policy in the Reagan administration. Despite its decline, the Heritage Foundation imprimatur lent Ferrara's words some force; his former position on the White House staff, although short-lived, added some weight.

Bowen was not pleased with Ferrara's accusations but was determined to remain above the fray. Burke was not so inclined. During nearly twenty years in the federal bureaucracy, Burke had a reputation as a man who "shot from the lip." Now Bowen's right-hand man, Burke hadn't learned to curb those impulses. Allies said to let Ferrara talk; he'd soon show how little he knew about health policy. Instead, Burke fired back at Ferrara and shot Bowen in the foot. Burke broke a cardinal Washington rule: Never turn a one-day story into a two-day story. By responding, Burke brought Ferrara's article to the attention of those who might have missed it.

Ferrara, who would later go to work for the Medigap insurers, wasn't the last voice raised against Bowen in 1986. In September, the U.S. Chamber of Commerce picked up Ferrara's arguments. The public accusations Heritage and the Chamber of Commerce hurled at Bowen were the first sign that the health secretary's attempts to convince the President to back him would not be easy. The basic tenet of their opposition—federalization versus privatization—would become the core issue for the opposition that would arise in the Reagan Cabinet.

By the time the Chamber of Commerce launched its broadside, Bowen was putting the finishing touches to his refined catastrophic plan. In November, he took it before Reagan's Domestic Policy Council (DPC). The DPC was created at the beginning of Reagan's second term. Its chairman was Attorney General Edwin Meese. In Reagan's first term, Meese had served as White House counselor and as the President's link to his conservative supporters. When he moved to the Justice Department in 1985, Meese wanted to keep a handle on domestic policy development; the DPC was the perfect answer. The council was made up of several members of Reagan's Cabinet whose departments dealt with domestic issues. It would meet sporadically to debate major policy proposals and present recommendations to the President.

When Bowen presented his proposal to the DPC in November, there was surprisingly little reaction. As he finished his presentation, Bowen asked if it would be all right if he released the plan to the public at a press conference the next day. In what proved to be an astounding miscalculation of Bowen's ability to garner public support, Meese agreed.

Bowen's decision to "go public" with his proposals was a stroke of genius. Once the plan was a matter of public knowledge, the White House was forced to deal with it. It could not be ignored and swept under the rug. If Bowen were to be rejected, that would be a public event, one that would be an embarrassment to the administration and a slap to a well-respected and well-liked Cabinet secretary.

On November 20, Bowen stepped before a phalanx of television cameras to lay out his proposal to the President. The centerpiece was a new Medicare catastrophic insurance policy for acute illnesses. Much like the original Bowen-Burke proposal, Bowen's new plan called for an annual limit on the elderly's out-of-pocket spending on covered Medicare services. The limit would be set at $2000 in 1987 and would grow each year to keep up with medical cost inflation. Limits on hospitalization coverage would be eliminated along with the copayments charged for stays over sixty days. The elderly would be asked to pay a maximum of about $1000 per year for hospital care and $1000 for physician services. To cover the costs of that protection, Bowen asked the elderly to pay a monthly premium of $4.92, or $59 yearly. The premium would cover the entire cost of the benefit; there would be no additional cost to the government or to the Medicare Trust Fund.

Bowen also offered some ideas for dealing with the costs of long-term nursing home care and the catastrophic medical bills of working Americans. Unlike his Medicare proposals, these other plans would require no increased direct federal spending. For nursing home care, for example, Bowen suggested that the government create IMAs that would allow working Americans to put up to $1000 a year in a tax-free account to be used in later years to pay for nursing home care. Bowen also proposed that the government offer a $100 annual tax credit to Americans over age 55 who purchased long-term care insurance. He also wanted to extend the same preferable tax treatment to the reserves of long-term care insurance companies.

Bowen's catastrophic baby arrived about one month early and the wily health secretary had a reason for the premature delivery. In 1985, Bowen's attempt to convince Reagan to back him failed because of a lack of time before the President was to deliver his State of the Union address. This time around, Bowen was determined not to run out of time. There were two months left before Reagan would journey to Capitol Hill for his 1986 State of the Union. Bowen planned to make the most of that time; so did his opponents.

Now that the Bowen plan was out, it was open season for its

opponents. The DPC was to have its first meeting after Bowen's presentation on December 3. Insurance industry lobbyists began briefing council members on the flaws in Bowen's logic. Some members were not very receptive. Labor Secretary William Brock, for example, was an early Bowen ally. The two had known each other back in the days when Bowen was chairman of the Republican Governors' Conference and Brock was chairman of the Republican National Committee. Bowen had backed Brock on a civil rights fight with Meese; now Brock returned the favor. Another supporter was Defense Secretary Caspar Weinberger, not one who many would expect to support expansion of a domestic program. But Weinberger had served as one of Nixon's health secretaries and felt an allegiance to Bowen. Just as Weinberger believed the defense secretary should make defense policy, he thought the health secretary should make health policy.

The leadership of the Cabinet conservatives' opposition to Bowen was left to Beryl Sprinkel, chairman of the President's Council of Economic Advisers. Until 1987, his role in administration health policymaking was either nonexistent or one of the best kept secrets in Washington. By 1987, however, Reagan's Cabinet was running quite low on health policy experts. Stockman's departure in 1985 left a big hole at OMB, one that was not nearly filled by his successor James Miller. Miller's very able deputy, Deborah Steelman, tried to frame the opposition to Bowen but with Miller presenting her case it was a difficult undertaking. In the White House, Reagan lost his health policy adviser, William Roper, when Roper joined Bowen's team at HHS as Health Care Financing administrator; no replacement was ever named. Bowen was the beneficiary of this vacuum.

Sprinkel worked closely with the Heritage Foundation and the Chamber of Commerce to come up with an alternative to the Bowen plan. The internal administration argument by this time had stretched beyond its original deadline—Reagan's 1987 State of the Union address. As a result, the President was forced to make a promise to send the Congress a plan at some later date. Bowen had hoped the deadline would have pulled the rug out from under the opposition; now, with the due date past, he feared the plan might lose its momentum. He called on his allies in Congress to keep the pressure on the White House. Indiana's two Republican senators—Dan Quayle and Richard Lugar—and Massachusetts Congressman Silvio Conte urged Reagan to make a decision before the issue was lost to the Democrats.

Sprinkel was given one last chance to convince Reagan to reject Bowen. At the next Domestic Policy Council meeting with the President, Sprinkel laid out his alternative. Rather than providing direct Medicare coverage of catastrophic medical bills, Sprinkel suggested the government give each elderly person a government voucher that could be used to purchase private catastrophic insurance. In that way, Sprinkel argued, the private insurance industry would not only be retained but strengthened. And, it fit in perfectly with Reagan's privatization effort.

Next, it was Bowen's turn to talk. The HHS secretary had already briefed the President on the specifics of his plan in mid-December. At that meeting, Bowen had gone for Reagan's heartstrings, recounting the battle his first wife had undergone with cancer and adding some other case histories researched by HHS. Now it was time to go for Sprinkel's throat. The mild-mannered Bowen often fooled his political adversaries with his low-key style and country doctor image, much as the President had lulled his own opponents with his genial storyteller exterior. But like Reagan, beneath Bowen's surface was a hardened political soul. Bowen knew this was his last chance. He approached a large tripod with a white paper pad on it and took out a black magic marker. First, Bowen again went through his own plan, drawing a straight line from the government to the beneficiary to show how the catastrophic benefits would be paid. Then he outlined the Sprinkel voucher option in which the money would go from the government to the beneficiary, who would then turn it over to the insurance company, which would then pay the providers. Off to the side, Bowen drew several circles representing the federal regulators who would have to watch over a voucher system to make sure the government's money was being spent wisely. By the time Bowen was done, the pad was covered with black lines, circles, and arrows. And when he was done, so was Sprinkel. Nothing could get to the President more than an example of too much government bureaucracy.

On February 12, Reagan announced that he had decided to endorse the Bowen plan and would send it to Congress. In announcing his support, Reagan said: "I am asking Congress to help give Americans that last full measure of security, to provide a health insurance plan that fights the fear of catastrophic illness. For too long, many of our senior citizens have been faced with making an intolerable choice—a choice between bankruptcy and death."

* * *

While Bowen was battling his administration colleagues, his plan was gaining favor on Capitol Hill with the newly elected Democratic leadership in the Senate and House. The 1986 election had ended six years of Republican rule in the Senate. New committee chairmen like Lloyd Bentsen of Texas at Finance and Ted Kennedy of Massachusetts at Human Resources were strongly backing Bowen and promising quick action. In fact, while Reagan dawdled over Bowen's plan, Kennedy introduced it word-for-word in the Senate. In the House, the chairman of the Ways and Means health subcommittee, Pete Stark, was an enthusiastic supporter of the catastrophic notion; in fact, he had been pushing a similar plan the past two years with no success and little publicity.

Bowen's Democratic supporters on Capitol Hill were a mix of old- and new-breed politicians. Kennedy had long been a fixture on the national political scene as well as in the health policy picture. Beginning in the early 1970s, Kennedy had gone well beyond his early image as "Jack and Bobby Kennedy's younger brother" to one of a savvy politician and a very good senator. During the decade he had chaired the Senate's health subcommittee Kennedy helped to push the issue of national health insurance to the top of the Democratic party's domestic policy agenda. His record also was filled with accomplishments in the health arena, including creation of government support for medical students and other health professionals in training, expanded government efforts to fight preventable diseases, and efforts to press the medical profession to address the ethical questions that arose in the modern age.

Kennedy had taken Reagan's 1980 election victory hard. Coming on the heels of his own disastrous challenge of Carter in the Democratic primaries, the victory of a leader of the conservative movement that made Kennedy its symbol of evil was almost too much to take. Add to that the fact that the Democrats' defeat in the congressional election stripped him of the chairmanship of the Senate Judiciary Committee and of the Senate's health subcommittee. For six years, Kennedy watched Utah Republican Orrin Hatch chair the Human Resources Committee that he and his two brothers had sat on throughout the 1950s, 1960s, and 1970s. Kennedy would prove to be a formidable "ranking minority member" of the committee, often taking control as Hatch botched the leadership challenge (see Chapter 3). With the 1986 election returning him to power, Kennedy was anxious to reassert his health policy leadership role.

But the politics of the 1980s had changed the focus of federal health policymaking away from the public health jurisdiction of Kennedy's Human Resources Committee to the health care financing jurisdiction of the Finance Committee. At Finance the new chairman was Texas Democrat Lloyd Bentsen. This was Bentsen's first crack at congressional leadership. In the sixteen years since his 1970 election to the Senate, Bentsen had built a reputation as an economic conservative with a heart. He briefly rose to national attention with a run for the 1976 Democratic presidential nomination but quickly faded from view. In 1987, as he took over the Senate's most powerful committee; more than just the "eyes of Texas" were upon him. Despite Kennedy's posturing, catastrophic insurance would be Bentsen's baby. Early in the year, the two men met for a private discussion in Bentsen's office. Bentsen made it clear that he wanted Kennedy to keep his hands off the catastrophic insurance bill. He did not want to see a repeat of the fights of the 1970s, when Long's attempts went for naught because of Kennedy's meddling. Kennedy agreed to be supportive of Bentsen and not seek jurisdiction over the bill.

In the House, the fight over catastrophic insurance would shine a spotlight on Stark, perhaps one of the more eccentric members of the House leadership. Congress has had its share of odd characters over the years—and still has quite a few today—but most have played minor roles and remained on the sidelines, providing the public and the press with entertainment but little else. Stark was an exception. Before coming to Congress, Stark had already made a name for himself as the president of an Oakland, California savings and loan by placing a giant peace symbol on the bank's roof to attract the accounts of the Oakland–San Francisco–Berkeley "hippies." Once in Washington, Stark quit the banking business but kept his quirks. His banking experience and close ties with the California delegation leader, Representative Philip Burton, helped him gain a spot on the Ways and Means Committee. Stark proved to be a hard worker who got results, a good recipe for advancement on the results-oriented committee.

By the time Chicago's Dan Rostenkowski took over the panel in 1981, Stark was one of the senior members of the panel and a close ally of the new chairman. During Reagan's first term, Stark chaired the important Subcommittee on Select Revenues, which handled major tax bills. He helped Rostenkowski frame the Democratic response to Reagan's tax cut bills. In 1985, several of the Ways and Means subcommittee chairmen were ready to change jobs. In a game of musical chairs, Stark wound up heading the health subcommittee, replacing Andrew Jacobs, Jr.

During his first two years at the helm, Stark proved to be a colorful chairman. In 1985 he angered the American Medical Association by labeling its leaders "troglodytes living in the nineteenth century." Stark's animosity toward the AMA was the natural by-product of the fact that the American Medical Political Action Committee (AMPAC) had consistently contributed to the campaigns of his opponents. In the 1986 election, AMPAC outdid itself, spending nearly $250,000 to promote Stark's unknown opponent. Stark won with nearly 70 percent of the vote, and returned to Washington in 1987, stronger than ever.

In 1987, Stark and Bentsen would lead the congressional effort to take Bowen's plan, improve it, and push it toward enactment. Despite its allure, the Bowen plan contained several problems. First, the out-of-pocket spending cap would only affect those services already covered by Medicare. Bills paid by the elderly for such uncovered services as outpatient prescription drugs, dental care, and eyeglasses would not count. Neither would the bills charged by doctors who refused to accept Medicare's fee and chose to bill the patient for the rest. In 1985, it was estimated the elderly spent about $8 billion on prescription drugs and another $3 billion on doctors' bills that exceeded Medicare's allowance. Dental care cost the elderly $3.8 billion. None of those costs would be covered under the Bowen plan.

The Medicare restructuring proposal advanced by Bowen and Reagan would do little to help the elderly with nursing home costs. Two types of nursing home stays are common in the lives of many elderly Americans. For many, a stay in an acute care hospital is followed by additional care in a skilled nursing facility (SNF); for those who are in need of still more care, it is on to an intermediate care facility (ICF). Those who are well enough to go home but still need care can rely on home health care services. Medicare coverage of SNF care was limited to 100 days yearly, but elderly people who needed more than twenty days of care had to pay a stiff daily coinsurance that in many areas of the country exceeded the cost of a day of care. Home health care coverage was limited to 100 visits per year, with a limit of thirty days per illness.

Medicare paid for very little long-term nursing home care; most elderly Americans who needed such care either paid for it themselves—quickly depleting even the best lifetime savings— or turned to Medicaid. To get Medicaid coverage, however, a senior citizen had to exhaust all savings and most assets. For many, such humiliation was worse than the illness that sent them to the nursing home in the first place.

Bowen's idea of setting up IMAs had been referred by Reagan

to his Treasury Department, where it would remain through the rest of the year. Perhaps the biggest problem with Bowen's proposal was its plan to finance the coverage via a monthly premium—originally estimated at $4.92; later revised upward to $6—charged to all beneficiaries, which clearly would be regressive. The low-income elderly could barely afford the premiums and deductibles they paid for basic Medicare benefits; the extra charge Bowen proposed could make things worse, not better, for them. At the same time, the upper-income elderly, who could well afford to pay more, would get a cut-rate insurance benefit.

Bentsen and Stark were determined to improve on Bowen's plan by making its financing progressive and by expanding on the post-acute care coverage of SNF and home health care. Neither man felt it was possible to address long-term care and neither was particularly interested in confronting the controversial area of drug coverage.

Stark would be the first ahead of the pack, and he wouldn't work alone. His partner would be Republican Congressman Bill Gradison of Ohio. Where Stark was flash and color, Gradison was subtlety and substance. Stark led with his heart, Gradison with his head. Each knew the other's strengths and weaknesses; together they were quite a combination. By teaming up, Stark and Gradison would appeal both to the liberal Democrats in the House and the mainstream Republicans. Gradison was a respected member of the House who previously had served in the executive branch in the Department of Health, Education, and Welfare.

Stark and Gradison were disturbed by the regressive nature of Bowen's financing mechanism. They saw in the catastrophic bill a chance for a breakthrough in Medicare reform that could pave the way for future changes in the program. The fact that its benefits are available to all Americans over age 65 gave Medicare universal support. On the other hand, Medicaid, the health benefits program for the poor, had been labeled a "welfare program for a select few, paid for by the working many." As a result, lawmakers were very leery of changing the basic entitlement nature of Medicare. When the Reagan administration made noises about applying a "means test" to Medicare benefits—that is, cutting off benefits to any senior with income above a certain level—legislators of both parties issued loud condemnations.

While a means test for eligibility was out of the question—and probably will be for some time—Stark and Gradison tapped a receptive lode when they suggested applying an income test to the premium that Congress would charge for the new catastrophic illness coverage. Rather than charging every elderly American the same premium, they suggested financing the entire benefit by requiring taxpaying seniors—about 40 percent of the thirty-one million total—to pay a tax on the actuarial value of Medicare benefits (about $1800 in 1986). The tax revenue gained would go to pay for catastrophic coverage for all beneficiaries, and it would cost 60 percent of the elderly absolutely nothing.

To address the shortcomings in Medicare's post-acute care benefit, Stark and Gradison proposed extending SNF coverage to 150 days and applying a much smaller coinsurance to the first seven days of care. Medicare's home health benefit also would be extended, to forty-two consecutive days instead of twenty-one.

Their plan also set a slightly lower spending cap than Bowen suggested; instead of $2000 yearly, Stark-Gradison proposed two separate caps. For Part A coverage of hospital stays, they would limit cost-sharing to a single deductible each year; Bowen's plan would allow two. Medicare's Part A deductible had been set to rise each year to cover the cost of an average day of care; it is paid for the first day of hospital care in each spell of illness. (A beneficiary would not pay a second deductible, for example, if he were readmitted to the hospital for further treatment related to the same illness but would pay twice if the second hospitalization was for an unrelated illness.) For the first seventeen years of Medicare, the deductible had climbed steadily along with health care inflation. Beginning in 1984, when Medicare switched to a prospective payment system for hospitals (see Chapter 7), the number of days per hospitalization began to drop even as fixed payments forced the average cost per day upward. But that increase had no effect on government spending, because the new payment system paid a flat fee no matter how long the stay. It did, however, bite hard into the income of the elderly. The Part A deductible shot up from $304 in 1983 to $356 in 1984, $400 in 1985, and $492 in 1986. Policymakers ignored the discrepancy in the program as long as the public seemed not to notice, and the Medicare program was collecting some easy new money. In 1986, however, the deductible was set to jump a whopping $80 to $572, on January 1, 1987. This time, Congress wasn't willing to let the elderly continue to pay this ridiculous price. It capped the 1987 deductible at $520 and changed the formula so that future increases would more accurately follow inflation, but the damage had been done. The Part A deductible was now a big hindrance to some elderly who needed hospital care. Many weren't able to pay it; some didn't go to the hospital, others left the provider to foot the bill. Stark and Gradison wanted to limit the damage by holding the number of deductibles to one each year. Out-of-pocket spending for Part B services would be held to about $1200 per year for an annual cap of about $1750.

Stark and Gradison introduced their plan at the end of April, and quickly pushed for consideration by the Ways and Means health subcommittee. After three days of closed door debate and votes, the panel approved the proposal. But there was an early sign of trouble for the financing alternative Stark and Gradison had proposed; it cleared the subcommittee but by a six to five vote. The authors knew they had to come up with a new formula before the full committee took up the matter.

When Ways and Means took up the Stark-Gradison plan, the authors had an alternative financing method in mind. Rather than taxing the actuarial value of the Medicare benefit, they proposed to charge a surtax on all taxpaying retirees of up to $580 per person to bring in most of the necessary revenues to pay for the benefit. After a couple of years, the rest of the elderly would pay a small monthly premium of $2.60 to help finance the benefit. The new proposal was acceptable to a majority of the Ways and Means Committee and was approved.

The passage of the Stark-Gradison plan hit another hitch in March. Lobbyists for America's elderly liked the revisions the two congressmen had made in the Bowen plan—in fact, they helped draft some of them—but still wanted more. The American Association of Retired Persons (AARP) had, by 1987, become the leading voice for the elderly, eclipsing the more liberal National Council of Senior Citizens. In earlier years, AARP tended to represent the better-off elderly, while the council led the way for the poorer senior citizens. In the 1970s and 1980s, AARP's membership had broadened and so had its lobbying focus.

In 1987, AARP leaders were in a quandary. They were excited by the prospect of passage of a Medicare catastrophic insurance bill and were willing to ask their members to foot the bill through higher premiums, but they also knew the benefits would accrue to a very few of the elderly who were faced by catastrophic acute care costs. They worried that once the elderly began paying the premiums and saw little tangible results, they would balk. AARP knew it had to expand the legislation further, so that a new benefit could help a majority of the elderly. That benefit was outpatient prescription drugs.

The first week of March, AARP Executive Director Cy Brickfield, Council President William Hutton, and congressmen Henry Waxman and Claude Pepper held a press conference in the U.S. Capitol to call for prescription drug coverage, expansion of home health care coverage, and protection for the low-income elderly. Stark and Gradison had already granted their requests on home health and the poor, but were not willing to go for the drug coverage. Stark said the costs of such a program were too uncertain, and he was unwilling to take on that task while trying to push through his progressive financing scheme.

As it would turn out, Stark didn't have much to say about the matter; AARP leaders went to Speaker of the House Jim Wright of Texas to press their case. Wright, who had just replaced the retired Tip O'Neill as Speaker, was worried about his reputation as more conservative than his predecessor. He promised AARP he would deliver the drug benefit and ordered Ways and Means Chairman Rostenkowski to carry out that promise.

Wright's commitment to a drug benefit scrambled Stark and Gradison's carefully laid plans, but an order from the Speaker and the chairman of the Ways and Means Committee is law in the House of Representatives. Stark went to work designing a drug benefit that would provide coverage to elderly people with very high drug bills. Like the overall catastrophic benefit, the drug coverage would have to be paid for by the elderly. Stark decided to offer coverage of drug costs above $700 per year and require the elderly to pay 20 percent of each prescription that fell above the limit. To finance the new benefit, Stark proposed to raise the surtax on the taxpaying elderly.

Stark and Gradison had one last hurdle to cross before they could take the package to the House floor. The House Commerce Committee had exercised its right to claim jurisdiction over the bill. Under Waxman's leadership, it added a more liberal drug benefit—a $500 annual deductible and no coinsurance—as well as a limited respite care benefit and a requirement that states pick up all of the Medicare cost-sharing for Medicaid-eligible elderly. Most of Waxman's additions were acceptable to Stark, but a month of negotiation was needed to iron out the differences on drugs. The final product: a $500 annual deductible and a 20 percent coinsurance on each prescription.

As the Stark-Gradison bill neared floor consideration, the White House, which had been fairly quiet until now, began complaining about the modifications made in the Bowen plan. But the administration had waited too long to voice its objections, and a Republican alternative plan was shot down on the House floor. The Stark-Gradison bill was then approved on July 22, by a margin of 302 to 127.

Meanwhile, over in the Senate, Bentsen had been busy putting together his own version of catastrophic insurance. It was quite similar to the Stark-Gradison model but had more streamlined features. Bentsen, too, would limit beneficiaries to about $1750 per year in out-of-pocket spending for covered Medicare services. Bentsen offered 150 days of SNF coverage with a small coinsurance charge for the first seven days, and would extend home health coverage to as many as forty-five consecutive days.

To finance the new benefit, Bentsen wanted to charge all beneficiaries an extra $4 monthly and the taxpaying elderly would pay an 8 percent surtax on taxes above $150 per year, up to a maximum of $800 per person. The Bentsen bill breezed through the Finance Committee at the end of May with no nay votes. Bentsen did not include a prescription drug benefit in his plan, but, like Stark, he was forced to promise to add such a plan when the bill reached the Senate floor. Bentsen asked his health subcommittee chairman, Maine Democrat George Mitchell, to draft such a plan.

With House passage at the end of July, Bentsen was ready to move his bill to the Senate floor for a vote. Things looked good for enactment of a final bill by Labor Day. Mitchell and Republican senators John Chafee of Rhode Island and John Heinz of Pennsylvania, teamed up with Democrat Tom Daschle of South Dakota, had worked out a deal on drug coverage calling for a three-year phase-in of the benefit, which would pay 80 percent of drug costs above $600 per year.

As the Senate prepared for an August vote, drug makers began to get nervous. The Pharmaceutical Manufacturers Association (PMA), representing most of the big name-brand drug makers, had successfully lobbied to change the House drug benefit to limit some of the controls that would have been placed on its members. But as the Senate got ready to vote on the Mitchell amendment, the PMA pulled out its big guns. Drug makers went to the Republican leadership of the Senate, and asked for a delay in the vote until after the upcoming August congressional recess. Don't rush into these things, the PMA argued. Senate Republicans, unhappy with the way things were going, agreed to stall and kept Bentsen from bringing his bill to the floor before the recess.

During their month-long absence from Washington, lawmakers were pelted with a $3.5 million lobbying campaign by PMA and its members. Elderly citizens received a mailing from PMA warning that the drug benefit would be expensive and help only a few seniors. The result was an outpouring of letters to congressional offices opposing or questioning the wisdom of a new drug benefit. The PMA showed no shame; it even told the elderly that they would be paying for costly AIDS drugs for victims of that epidemic. Illinois Senator Paul Simon received nearly 600 letters of opposition in August, nearly ten times the number he had received on the subject of catastrophic insurance all year.

The PMA would not prove to have enough clout to stop the catastrophic bill or the Mitchell amendment, but its lobbying campaign slowed the Senate bill dramatically. That delay enabled the administration to collect its thoughts and begin pressing the Senate for changes in the Bentsen bill before it reached the Senate floor. Bentsen, recognizing that the President still had something to say about the bill even though Democrats controlled Congress, agreed to open discussions with the White House about its concerns.

It was too late to push Congress back to the Bowen plan, but the White House hoped to force the Senate to curb its bill so that the final product would be closer to Bowen than to Stark-Gradison. White House officials asked Bentsen to move his cap up from $1750 to the $2000 Bowen had proposed. They also wanted him to link the annual increase in that cap to the rise in Medicare spending; the House bill limited the rise to the annual increase in the Consumer Price Index. The White House argued that if the cap weren't tied to costs it would lead to an explosion of costs. Finally, the White House wanted Bentsen to phase in the drug benefit over four years instead of three and to include some specific cost containment methods.

Bentsen, anxious to get his bill off the mark, agreed to compromise with the White House on most issues. He would up his cap from $1750 to $1850 and would agree to a complex formula that would raise the cap each year so that the same proportion of elderly qualified for the benefit. He and Mitchell agreed to the four-year phase-in for drug coverage but stuck to the $600 annual deductible. With those changes made, the modified Bentsen bill sailed to Senate passage, eighty-six to eleven.

The three-month delay in Senate action was costly to Medicare beneficiaries. By the time the Senate had voted, there was precious little time left in 1987 to complete a House-Senate negotiating session. Instead, legislators put off final action until early 1988 and, in effect, decided to delay the start of the program until 1989. But in May 1988 House-Senate negotiators pinned down a final bill and sent it to Reagan for his signature.

Enactment of the catastrophic insurance benefit marked a turning point in federal health policymaking. While the budget cutting mania of the 1980s did not end, lawmakers could actually point to a concrete advance for the nation's elderly. At the same time, the introduction of progressive financing for the benefit opened a door that many believe future Congresses will use to broaden the base of financial support for Medicare and lighten the load on the estimated 3.3 million elderly Americans living in poverty. For Bowen, the accomplishment ensured that his tenure at HHS would be one that will be remembered.

12

AIDS

With all of the developments in health care during the Reagan years, what will most probably be remembered longest is an issue that no policymaker could have anticipated—a national epidemic known as AIDS, or acquired immune deficiency syndrome. The arrival of AIDS on the scene nearly coincided with Reagan's arrival in Washington. The epidemic would encompass Reagan's two terms in office; by the time he would leave Washington, no end would be in sight.

1981

As the epidemic began, few in Washington, in fact, few people around the country, were aware of the issue. The first public attention began in June, after the publication of a scientific report in the *Center for Disease Control Morbidity and Mortality Weekly Report.* The *MMWR,* as the report is known, arrives on the desks of many health care professionals and reporters each Thursday. The June 5, 1981, issue contained a seemingly innocuous report on page two by Dr. Michael Gottlieb, entitled *"Pneumocystis* Pneumonia in Homosexual Men in Los Angeles." Gottlieb charted five cases of a usually rare form of pneumonia, all of which were found in gay men living in the Los Angeles area. *Pneumocystis* was not a disease normally found in young men; it was more often found in people with a depressed immune system—cancer patients on chemotherapy, for example. The fact that Gottlieb had found these five unusual cases caught the attention of the medical research community but went right by the eyes of most policymakers in Washington and health reporters around the country.

As 1981 went on, the toll of AIDS cases began to mount. Early patterns showed that nearly 80 percent of cases were among homosexual men. Many of the other cases were among intravenous drug abusers and recent Haitian refugees to the United States. Most of the early cases of AIDS were in New York City, Los Angeles, and San Francisco, each with a fairly substantial gay population. The gay connection led many in government and the press to label AIDS the "gay plague." (In fact, in the earliest days of the epidemic, AIDS was formally known as Gay-Related Immune Deficiency, or GRID. For the sake of continuity, throughout this chapter, the disease will be called AIDS.)

For most of 1981, AIDS would remain a private torment for the growing number of Americans who were affected by this mysterious new plague. In the gay community and in places like New York and San Francisco, worried whispers turned to concerned conversations. By the end of 1981, when Reagan sent his 1982 budget to Congress, the number of AIDS cases had risen to 271, yet he asked for no money to trace AIDS or to pursue its cause.

1982

In the summer of 1982 Congress would first begin to look into AIDS. Once again, it would be Los Angeles Congressman Henry Waxman, chairman of the House Commerce health subcommittee, who would lead the congressional action. This time Waxman had more reason than usual to be prodding the Reagan administration to act on a health issue: Waxman's congressional district was home to one of Los Angeles' largest gay communities. In April, Waxman held a one-day hearing at the Los Angeles Gay and Lesbian Community Services Center. Because the hearing was held in Los Angeles, it would be several days before word of the proceedings would get back to Washington.

Waxman pulled no punches at this first hearing. In his statement opening the hearing, Waxman noted that AIDS was attacking a population that was already one of the most stigmatized in the nation—gay men. "There is no doubt in my mind that, if the same disease had appeared among Americans of Norwegian descent, or among tennis players, rather than gay males, the responses of both the government and the medical community would have been different." Waxman paraded a string of administration health experts before his audience and grilled them on the status of the government's efforts to track and solve the mystery of AIDS.

Waxman was preaching to the converted. The predominantly gay audience certainly agreed that the government should be doing more, and so did the career government health officials testifying that day. But those officials remained silent about their feelings. Dr. James Curran, who headed the CDC's AIDS task force, reported that his agency had redirected funds from other programs to pay for the early work in tracking AIDS. Waxman pressed for details of CDC's budget requests for AIDS work; Curran said there were none.

Curran was telling the truth; one year into the epidemic, CDC had made no plans to budget for its AIDS work. Rather than ask for money from the Congress, the administration continued to assert that it could handle the AIDS work within its current budget. The reasons behind the government's delay lay in many of the conflicts going on in the Reagan administration at the time.

* * *

First, like many of the public health agencies in the government after Reagan was elected, the CDC was in the midst of "damage control" efforts. Reagan's first budget proposed to slash CDC funding from $327 million to $161 million. Congress rejected some of those cuts in 1981 but in 1982, CDC officials weren't about to rock the boat by asking for money to track a gay disease.

The fact that AIDS was thought of as a gay disease was the second factor working against a strong government effort. Waxman was right when he said the population affected by AIDS was stigmatized. The gay community had made great progress in the 1970s in overcoming societal prejudice, but its success angered its opponents in the religious right. With a new president in office, thanks to the support of those fundamentalists, gay rights activists, much like the public health officials in government, were in retreat. Many of the top officials of the Reagan administration were at best indifferent and at worst antagonistic to the gay community; others thought a negative stance was necessary to win favor with those in power. Verbal "gay bashing" was in; new government efforts to prevent disease were out.

A third factor was the administration's antipathy to the Washington bureaucracy. Reagan had been elected, in part, because of his opposition to the Washington establishment; he and his supporters believed that most people who worked for the government worked against the interests of the people.

The Public Health Service (PHS), the agency responsible for coordinating the government's AIDS response, was considered a particular problem area. The PHS had long been a semi-independent agency; no matter what party was in power, the PHS went its own way. Officials working in the agency often had stronger allegiances to the programs and constituencies they served than to the political appointees who were their bosses for the next four or eight years. Most figured, and correctly so, that the politicians would come and go, but the programs and the people they served would still be around when the next president took office. The new Reagan regime viewed PHS as a den of liberal Democrats, determined to fight the President tooth and nail. In 1981, PHS had been hit hard by staff reductions; in 1982, more positions were lost as the block grants approved by Congress got under way. During the course of the Reagan years, the overall HHS staff would shrink from more than 150,000 job slots to less than 120,000. Many of the cuts were in the PHS.

Those bureaucrats who survived Reagan's staff cuts were kept at arm's length. Many were transferred away from the programs that they had been working in under Carter. By moving the bureaucrats, the administration hoped to cut the cord between them and the constituencies they served. People found themselves working on programs in which they had little or no experience. On the surface, such moves would seem absurd: Why assign people to programs if they didn't have the knowledge and skills to run them well? Because the Reagan administration didn't want the programs run well; well run programs cost money. Poorly run programs became easier targets for budget cuts or termination. Besides, if they kept moving people around, no one would be in one place long enough to detect whether the budget cuts were doing harm.

When it came to AIDS, the administration's distrust of the established bureaucracy at PHS would exact a horrible price. When CDC officials began pleading for money to track AIDS in 1981 and 1982, their requests were viewed in Washington as an attempt to end-run the budget cuts Reagan was exacting on Capitol Hill. In the view of those running the government, AIDS was being used by liberals at CDC to continue the federal bureaucracy. Some even went so far as to doubt that AIDS even existed.

With the combination of government antipathy to federal solutions to health problems, the homophobia exhibited by many of the administration's leaders, and the distrust for the career health officials at the PHS, it was no wonder that the administration's response to AIDS was so miserable. That isn't to say that all of the administration political appointees responded poorly to AIDS. A handful of officials merit praise for their attempts— usually unsuccessful—to prod the administration to action. Most notable was Reagan's first assistant secretary for health, Dr. Edward Brandt. Recruited from the University of Texas Southwestern Medical School, Brandt was the government's top health official and was responsible for managing the huge PHS bureaucracy. Brandt was a Reagan loyalist, journeying to Capitol Hill to press for enactment of the block grants and for cuts in many of the programs he administered. But Brandt seemed uncomfortable with his role in dismantling programs. Like most people who come to Washington to serve their government, Brandt wanted to leave his mark. What kind of mark would budget cuts leave? But Brandt's discomfort would pale in comparison to the frustration he would feel as he tried to press the case for more AIDS funding within the administration.

* * *

Waxman's hearing had little effect on the government's response to AIDS in 1982. The administration still refused to ask Congress for any money specifically aimed at AIDS. The CDC continued to make do by shifting money from other programs. Later in the year, Waxman teamed up with his California colleague, Edward Roybal, and the chairman of the House Appropriations health subcommittee, Representative William Natcher of Kentucky, to gain $2 million in appropriations for CDC to continue its surveillance of AIDS; that was the first money Congress directly appropriated for AIDS.

But while Waxman, Roybal, and Natcher were able to get the ball rolling on CDC's AIDS effort, concern began to rise about the lack of any response to AIDS by the National Institutes of Health (NIH), the government's giant biomedical research complex in Bethesda, Maryland. With AIDS in its second year, and building toward epidemic size, NIH could not identify a single research grant or project aimed at AIDS.

* * *

The NIH represents the best and the worst of the government's health care network. Built by Congress in the 1950s and 1960s, under the leadership of former senators Warren Magnuson of Washington and Lister Hill of Alabama, NIH had been responsible for some of the major medical breakthroughs of the late twentieth century. Through its intramural research program and its vast extramural grant program, NIH money was behind almost every major research project. By the 1980s, NIH had gained the moniker, "the crown jewels" of the Public Health Service.

The luster of NIH meant little to the budgeteers in the Reagan administration. By the time Reagan took office, the government was spending nearly $3.5 billion on NIH and paying for more than 5000 new extramural grants every year. While those figures meant success to many in the medical community, they meant excess to the officials in Reagan's budget office. In Reagan's first budget, Stockman and Schweiker spent nearly two months fighting over NIH funding. Stockman wanted to cut Carter's budget request of $3.8 billion; Schweiker wanted it maintained. During his tenure in Congress, Schweiker had held the senior Republican position on the Senate Appropriations health subcommittee. There he had helped Magnuson push the NIH spending total upward and took pride in the accomplishments that money had created. Now Stockman wanted to reverse that progress. In the end—after taking his case all the way to Reagan—Schweiker prevailed; Reagan asked Congress for $3.76 billion for NIH in the FY82 budget. In a year in which almost every federal health program absorbed deep cuts in funding, NIH came away clean.

Schweiker and Stockman would rerun their NIH budget brouhaha in 1982 and 1983. In 1982, Schweiker won again; in 1983, Stockman prevailed and Schweiker quit. His replacement, Margaret Heckler, cared little for budget fights with Stockman. In her eyes, Schweiker had paid with his job; she wanted to keep hers. Beginning in 1984 and extending to the end of the Reagan era, the administration would consistently ask Congress to pare back the NIH budget; lawmakers would continue to ignore those requests and would increase the NIH budget to more than $7 billion by the time Reagan left office.

The NIH also benefited from an unusual amount of independence from political influence. On paper, the NIH was under the control of one director; under Reagan that would be Dr. James Wyngaarden. But in reality the institutes that made up the NIH were individual kingdoms run by powerful rulers. In fact, several of the major institutes—those in charge of research into cancer, heart and lung disease, and blood disorders—reported directly to the Congress without going through Wyngaarden's office. That independence would prove useful during the AIDS epidemic, as institute directors took their case for more funds to Capitol Hill, not to OMB. But that same independence made it difficult for leaders of Congress to get an accounting of what was being done with those billions of dollars being spent each year.

* * *

In 1982, Waxman began to press NIH directors to show him what was being done on AIDS. At first, Waxman and his aide, Tim Westmoreland, ran into a brick wall. The NIH officials were reluctant to share information with their benefactors on Capitol Hill. The irony did not escape Waxman; as he fought the administration on NIH's behalf for more money, its leaders refused to cooperate with his investigation into the administration's response to AIDS. Waxman and Westmoreland would soon find out the reason behind that recalcitrance. Nothing was being done at NIH on AIDS. Not a single grant had been awarded for an AIDS research contract nearly two years after the government began tracing the beginning of this epidemic. Waxman was apoplectic: He hauled the leaders of NIH before his subcommittee and demanded some answers. Mysteriously, when those officials reached Waxman's hearing room, they had a list of AIDS research projects funded by NIH. Waxman and Westmoreland weren't about to be fooled; it was quickly apparent that these "AIDS projects" were really unrelated investigations into immune deficiency and other disorders. The point remained: In late 1982, NIH still had not funded a single AIDS grant.

As 1982 ended, CDC reported the number of AIDS cases had risen to 1292, with 1047 deaths.

1983

Waxman began to turn up the heat in 1983; now he had a new ally. In the Senate, the chairman of the Appropriations health subcommittee, Senator Harrison "Jack" Schmitt of New Mexico, had been defeated in his bid for a second term. Schmitt had been disinterested in the AIDS issue during his two years in charge of the subcommittee. The ex-astronaut had, in fact, shown little interest in most of the health programs before him. Early in his tenure, Schmitt confused and astounded the witnesses and audience at a subcommittee hearing by asking NIH officials what was being spent to determine the effectiveness of copper bracelets in fighting arthritis. The laughter in the room faded as the audience and witnesses realized the new chairman was serious. Following his defeat in 1982, a liberal Republican, Senator Lowell Weicker of Connecticut, took over as chairman. Weicker, Waxman, and Natcher would combine in the next year to kick-start the government's AIDS effort.

In 1983, for the first time, the Reagan administration would ask Congress to appropriate money to track AIDS and to research its causes. In his fiscal 1984 budget, the President asked for $39.8 million for AIDS. Proponents of more AIDS funding—led by National Gay Task Force lobbyist Jeff Levi—called Reagan's request "too small," but privately were glad to see the administration was finally coming around. As long as Reagan requested some money for AIDS, they figured they could convince Congress to up the ante.

At HHS, Brandt continued to press his case for more AIDS spending and a greater focus on the epidemic by the administration. Brandt also was disappointed; Schweiker's resignation in February forestalled a promotion for Brandt to HHS under secretary, the number two post in the department. Schweiker planned to press for his nomination to the post after the incumbent, David Swoap, resigned to return to California. Such a move would have given AIDS and the rest of Brandt's agenda a powerful base and a more visible leader. But Schweiker's resignation cut that short. The White House instead promoted Social Security administrator Jack Svahn, another alumnus of Reagan's California government, to serve as under secretary in the Heckler regime at HHS. Svahn had no interest in AIDS. At PHS, Brandt decided he too would soon leave government, but Schweiker and Heckler persuaded him to stay on during the transition. That interim period would stretch into nearly two years, until Brandt finally did quit in December 1984.

As the new secretary, Heckler took a much more active interest in the epidemic and provided the administration with a visible leader on the issue. Schweiker had left much of the AIDS work to Brandt and his colleagues at PHS but had given them little of the political support that was needed to get the government's AIDS response in gear. Schweiker's administrative style emphasized delegation; he ran HHS much like he had run his Senate office. Heckler delegated very little, preferring a "hands-on" management approach; the result was a secretary spread too thin and little authority in lower ranks to move on a question. Heckler gave AIDS a higher profile with her declaration that the issue was her department's "number one priority." Unfortunately, her actions never matched her rhetoric. Waxman would ruefully remark: "If that's how she treats her number one priority, I'd hate to be number two."

Brandt was heartened by the new attention being paid to AIDS by Heckler and others in the administration. When the new secretary asked him to provide her with a memo outlining budget needs for the AIDS fight, Brandt set about the task eagerly. By mid-1983, PHS determined it needed another $12 million in fiscal 1984 to handle the growing AIDS problem. By this time, more than 1500 cases of AIDS had been reported to the CDC; nearly half those people were already dead. Brandt delivered his memo to Heckler and awaited her action; it never came. Heckler ran into a brick wall at OMB where Stockman would not hear of any requests for supplemental appropriations. Heckler was told to "reprogram" from other programs within her existing budget. She passed that message on to a crestfallen Brandt.

Stockman's refusal to grant Brandt's request began a new pattern in the government's reaction to the AIDS epidemic. Quietly, Brandt instructed his staff to leak his memo asking for $12 million in new AIDS money to Waxman and Natcher in time for its consideration as part of the FY83 supplemental appropriation. That done, Congress voted the $12 million Brandt wanted. Time and again in years to come, Brandt and his successors would use this underground railroad to get the message to the Hill that more money was needed for AIDS. But each time PHS succeeded, OMB grew angrier.

* * *

While the Reaganauts in Washington were fighting over when to start a government response to AIDS, a remarkable thing was going on in cities like New York and Los Angeles, where AIDS was a fact of life. The gay community, which had struggled in vain to interest its largely silent masses in a fight for civil rights, now came to life to fight the death that was cutting down its members. Beginning with New York's Gay Men's Health Crisis (GMHC), spreading to San Francisco's Kaposi Sarcoma Foundation, and later to Los Angeles' LA Cares and AIDS Project LA, the gay community was doing for itself what the government was refusing to do. Social services for the hundreds—later thousands—of victims of AIDS were being provided by hundreds—later thousands—of volunteers from the gay community. Community members cared for people with AIDS, did their shopping, washed their laundry, and, most importantly, listened to their fears and calmed their minds. These same groups fought, mainly at the local level, for a greater government response.

Back in Washington, the National Gay Task Force's Levi was also fighting a lonely battle for a federal response. Levi had some early allies on Capitol Hill—chiefly Waxman and Ted Weiss, who represented New York's Greenwich Village—but he knew that to win in Congress he had to broaden his base from these two able congressmen who were so closely allied with the gay communities in their districts. Unlike some of his colleagues in the gay political movement, Levi believed he could reach out to nontraditional supporters when it came to AIDS; more importantly, he knew he had to if his efforts were to succeed. Throughout 1982 and 1983, Levi became a fixture in the offices of congressional health committees and the Public Health Service. He got no help in those early days from the health lobbying giants like the American Medical Association and the American Public Health Association. They had other concerns; chiefly protecting their programs and their turf. In an age of constant budget battles to retain existing programs, the health lobbying industry looked away from AIDS until it became unavoidable in 1985 and beyond. But without Levi's early work, many of those later efforts would have been that much harder.

* * *

Remarkably, by 1983, scientists knew little more about AIDS than they did in 1981. They suspected that the disease was sexually transmitted, chiefly because of its prevalence in gay men. If it were a sexually transmitted disease, then it was likely that a virus was the cause. But others argued that if a virus were the culprit, AIDS would not have been as contained as it had been so far.

Waxman's hectoring of NIH officials had its effect. Beginning in 1983, NIH began to treat AIDS as a serious matter. Money was freed up for extramural researchers and NIH's own team of scientists began to work on the disease themselves. The work of the CDC with its meager budget was now supplemented by the NIH and its munificent money pile. The NIH scientists went about their work assuming that AIDS was a viral disease transmitted by sex.

But sex could not be the only means of transmission. Even from the earliest days of AIDS, an inordinate number of cases had appeared in the small hemophiliac population. Evidence seemed to point to a blood-borne disease. In the 1970s, U.S. researchers had made great strides in helping hemophiliacs live safer and far more comfortable lives. Development of Factor-VIII treatments for hemophiliacs controlled the bleeding that had so often spelled death in the past. But Factor VIII was a by-product of donated blood, each lot drawn from more than 5000 individual donors.

In early 1983, the blood link to AIDS became stronger, as the CDC reported the first two cases of AIDS that seemed to have been the result of blood transfusions. The blood connection would prove to be the first turning point in the fight against AIDS. No longer was AIDS a problem for "those people," it now was considered a threat to all Americans. Each year an estimated ten million people received a blood transfusion; each of those people was now considered at risk.

The blood connection woke up a lot of the Reagan administration officials who were hoping AIDS would just go away. Again, it would fall to Brandt to come up with a government response. While the U.S. blood supply is a private business—run mainly by the American Red Cross and the American Association of Blood Banks—the federal Food and Drug Administration (FDA) was responsible for regulating their actions. And Brandt was responsible for the FDA.

On March 4, 1983, Brandt announced what he called "interim measures" to prevent the transmission of AIDS. He called them "prudent and temporary measures that should reduce the risk of acquiring and transmitting AIDS." Sexual contact should be avoided with persons known or suspected to have AIDS. Members of high-risk groups—gays and drug users—should "be aware that multiple sexual partners increase the probability of developing AIDS." This advice mirrored much of what the gay community had been telling its members for more than a year.

As for the blood connection, Brandt had this advice: "Members of groups at increased risk for AIDS should refrain from donating plasma and/or blood. This recommendation includes all individuals belonging to such groups, even though many individuals may be at little risk of AIDS." The health chief instructed blood banks to inform potential blood donors of this new policy.

The reaction to Brandt's blood policy was quick and angry. Waxman criticized the recommendations in a press release dated March 3, the day before Brandt released his plan. As per an agreement reached earlier in the year, Brandt had consulted with Waxman before making his recommendations public. Waxman called Brandt's plan "an overreaction to the facts of AIDS and blood." Instead of screening donors, Waxman argued, blood banks should screen blood. He suggested testing all blood donations for the presence of antibodies to the hepatitis B virus (hepatitis and AIDS had several common traits, and some researchers believed such a screen would be a good proxy for a test for AIDS virus antibodies). Levi and other gay political leaders joined Waxman in condemning Brandt's policy, but really had no alternative to offer.

The existence of the blood connection and the uproar that

resulted from Brandt's interim policy created greater impetus in the government to find the cause of AIDS. The threat that AIDS could break out of its original risk groups to the general population made AIDS a national health issue. The government stepped up its efforts to identify the cause of AIDS. If the cause could be found, there might be a better way to prevent its transmission. The NIH stepped up its efforts, including the involvement of National Cancer Institute researcher Dr. Robert Gallo, whose earlier work on leukemia was widely praised.

As 1983 drew to a close, CDC said the AIDS case total had risen by 2833 to 4125; 3553 Americans had died of AIDS since 1981.

1984

Gallo followed his hunch that the AIDS virus was related to the leukemia virus he had identified earlier in his career. At the same time, French researchers were following another path to the virus. The work of the French and American researchers would take nearly two years. Their paths would later collide in a series of angry accusations and lawsuits.

At NIH, Gallo and his research team at the National Cancer Institute worked feverishly to identify the cause of AIDS. Gallo and his team had decided that the AIDS virus was a new type of leukemia virus; they called it the human T-cell leukemia virus (HTLV-III). By April, they felt ready to present their findings. Most scientific findings are presented in medical journals or at medical conferences. But 1984 was, after all, an election year in which the incumbent president was seeking a second term. Over at HHS, Margaret Heckler was looking for ways to polish the administration's image on social issues like AIDS. Since the revelation of the AIDS blood connection in 1983, the public's interest in AIDS had grown dramatically. So too had the criticism of the White House for its lackadaisical response. Heckler was determined to change that. She decided that Gallo's news was too important to wait for the *New England Journal of Medicine* or the *Journal of the American Medical Association*; she wanted a national press conference.

On April 23, 1984, Gallo, Brandt, and Heckler stepped before a bank of microphones and a roomful of reporters and television cameras to announce Gallo's findings. As was her custom, Heckler blew the announcement way out of proportion. The news was, indeed, a major breakthrough in the fight against AIDS, but to hear Heckler tell it, Gallo had just cured the epidemic and the American public could stop worrying about it.

"Today, I am proud to announce that the arrow of funds, medical personnel, research, and experimentation which the Department of Health and Human Services and its allies around the world have aimed and fired at the disease AIDS has hit the target. Only two or three rings away from the bull's-eye." Heckler went on to summarize Gallo's findings and make some amazing promises, promises the health officials on the stage with her knew the government could not keep. Heckler said a blood test for AIDS had been developed and would be ready for use "within about six months." In reality, only the concept of the test was developed (and would be patented that day), and use of the test was just over one year away. Heckler said the Gallo discovery "will enable us to develop a vaccine to prevent AIDS. We hope to have such a vaccine ready for testing in about two years." No such hope had been held out by Gallo or other government scientists; they certainly had said nothing about having a vaccine ready to test in two years. In reality, vaccine testing would not begin until late 1987. Heckler didn't seem to care that her statement was inaccurate. Heckler had a hot story that put her department in a good light just eight months before her President's reelection; a few facts weren't going to stand in her way.

The announcement that the government had found the cause of AIDS also meant that Americans could begin to prevent the transmission of the virus. Since the virus was borne in blood or semen, then sexually active people must avoid sharing those fluids. Use of condoms during sex had been advocated by gay community leaders since 1982. Now those warnings took on a new urgency, as gay men realized they no longer had to be passive pawns in the AIDS rampage. Levi sought help from the government to begin a massive public education effort to spread the word about AIDS prevention; they got no response. The CDC officials were 100 percent behind Levi's plan, but political leaders at HHS were too concerned about the reaction of their conservative colleagues to touch the education issue. A clear sign of the internal administration conservative backlash on AIDS came in mid-1984 when Ed Brandt accepted the invitation of the National Gay Task Force to present an award to the Blood Sister Project of San Diego, a group of lesbians who had recruited their sisters to donate blood in place of gay males. On the eve of the dinner, Brandt backed out, claiming a scheduling conflict. The reality was that Brandt was ordered to cancel his appearance after conservative Reagan supporters got word of his plans to dine with homosexuals.

Government officials were caught in a difficult position in 1983. The need to educate the public and alert them to the dangers of AIDS carried with it a distinct risk of panicking that same public and producing an overreaction and backlash against those hit first—gay men. Even gay leaders worried that if the public became too concerned about AIDS, the panic would overwhelm their lobbying efforts in Washington and force policymakers to make unwise decisions. Discrimination against gays in housing and education was already beginning to be based on a fear of AIDS; the prospect of a gay quarantine was not that far off the table. Rather than balancing those concerns, however, the administration chose to ignore the education issue. The small amount of money appropriated by Congress in 1984 to start an education program was channeled to the U.S. Conference of Mayors; the administration wanted no part of direct distribution of government funds to the gay groups that were willing to help educate their community.

The administration's decision to delay an education program stands as its greatest failure in the AIDS epidemic. While an earlier start on AIDS research might have produced quicker results, many of the Americans who would develop AIDS in the 1980s had been infected in the 1970s before anyone knew what AIDS was. How many cases of AIDS and AIDS-related deaths could have been prevented if the government had launched an education effort in 1983 will never be known.

* * *

Meanwhile, the PHS was in the midst of another budget rewrite. Following Gallo's announcement, Brandt ordered his agencies to reconsider their funding needs. With a virus identified, more money would have to go into development of a blood test. Those agencies came back to Brandt with a list of new projects that they believed should begin as soon as possible. The bottom line was an additional $20.1 million in fiscal 1984 and an increase in the projected FY85 budget of $35.8 million. The total request of $55.9 million was approved by Brandt on May 25 and sent on to Heckler for her approval.

But the same secretary who worked so hard to make political hay out of the Gallo findings was not anxious to cross swords with the White House budget office. Brandt's memo sat on Heckler's desk for two months. In July, a copy of Brandt's memo was leaked to the press. Stories of Heckler's delay embarrassed the administration, but not enough to free the money. Again, Brandt was told to find the money elsewhere by cutting back on other programs. Congress was not willing to approve such a shift in funds; instead, the new money Brandt wanted was approved near year's end as part of the FY85 HHS appropriations bill. Shortly thereafter, exhausted from nearly four years of budget battling, Brandt resigned his post and left government to become chancellor of the University of Maryland in Baltimore.

At the end of 1984, the number of reported AIDS cases was up to 9846; 8216 people had died of AIDS.

1985

The administration's squeamishness to the contrary, 1985 would be the year of AIDS education. Despite the HHS refusal to request any AIDS education money, Congress included funds within the $33.3 million it appropriated for fiscal 1985 for AIDS work at CDC. Growing public awareness was encouraging to government officials involved with AIDS, but public knowledge remained murky.

In February, Waxman and his allies got new ammunition in their battle for more AIDS money. The congressional Office of Technology Assessment (OTA), an independent panel created by Congress to advise it on the increasingly complex scientific and medical questions facing Americans, issued a highly critical report on the administration's AIDS efforts. While the report praised the PHS for its work to "build a foundation" of AIDS data, OTA said the agency had been forced to operate with "insufficient resources." The administration had paid little attention to AIDS treatments, public education, and prevention, OTA said. The Office of Technology Assessment predicted that the AIDS toll would rise to more than 40,000 by 1986, a projection that would prove to be uncannily accurate.

Within a month of the OTA report, the PHS began yet another reevaluation of its AIDS funding needs. This time the protagonist was acting Assistant Secretary for Health Dr. James Mason. Mason had take Brandt's place until Heckler and the White House could agree on a permanent replacement. His full-time job was running CDC, so Mason was quite familiar with the AIDS epidemic. Like Brandt, Mason would be an unexpected hero in the AIDS fight. Before taking the CDC post in November 1983, Mason had been director of the department of public health for the state of Utah. He had been recommended for the CDC post by conservative Utah Republican Senator Orrin Hatch. At the time of his appointment, public health community members worried that Mason would be too conservative for the job. When Waxman called Mason before his subcommittee in February to respond to the OTA charges, Mason could only provide vague defenses of the administration's efforts. Embarrassed and angry, Mason returned to his office to order the funding evaluation.

While the Reagan budget makers were dragging their feet, HHS scientists continued to press ahead with the resources provided by Congress. On March 4, the Food and Drug Adminis tration licensed the first blood test to determine the presence of antibodies to the HTLV-III virus. Development of the test had taken about a year—twice as long as Heckler had promised at Gallo's 1984 press conference. But late or not, the test would alleviate one of the PHS' major AIDS concerns: By testing all blood donations, the United States could feel comfortable that the blood supply was protected from the AIDS virus. Fear of widespread contamination of the blood supply eased.

But the licensing of the antibody test also caused problems. While it was designed to screen blood donations, the test also could give an indication of a person's exposure to the AIDS virus. In effect, the test could be used to screen people as well as blood. Health and life insurance companies, already worried about the future cost of AIDS to their bulging reserves, saw the test as a way to limit their financial exposure. Gay men, who were living in almost constant fear that a head cold or case of the flu was actually the first sign of an AIDS-related opportunistic infection, saw the test as a way to either confirm their fears or allay them. But the blood test wasn't perfect; while the number of false negative tests would later prove to be small, in 1985, blood banks feared that a rush by members of AIDS risk groups to donate blood to determine antibody status would result in more bad blood slipping through the gaps.

Blood bankers and PHS scientists agreed that alternative testing sites were needed to allow people who wanted to know their antibody status to get the test without endangering the blood supply. The PHS asked for $10.4 million to finance the creation of these testing clinics. But again, the budget makers balked; they said PHS could have the money, but it had to take it away from other health programs—a phenomenon that was dubbed "robbing Peter to pay Peter." Cooler heads prevailed on Capitol Hill, and the $10.4 million in new money was appropriated and spent. By the time the blood test was ready for use, the testing sites were ready to open.

In July, Mason's AIDS funding reevaluation was completed and he asked Heckler to boost the AIDS budget by $40 million, to $126 million. Heckler didn't make the same mistake she made with Brandt's request in 1984; she approved all the money Mason requested. The House voted a $190 million AIDS budget in September, but by the time the Senate took up the HHS funding bill, Mason had upped his request to $196 million. Weicker ran with Mason's request and the Senate approved a $200 million AIDS budget.

In the midst of the congressional budget one-upmanship, Reagan made his first public comments on AIDS. The President had been criticized strongly for his failure to use his skills as the "great communicator" to address AIDS. In one way, the criticism, particularly that from the press, was unfair. The same reporters who noted Reagan's silence failed to take the opportunity Reagan's rare press conferences afforded them to ask the President about AIDS. Finally, in September, as school board officials in Indiana were battling with the question of admitting a student diagnosed with AIDS, Reagan was asked his opinion. Reagan's rambling answer indicated that the President wasn't quite ready to talk about AIDS. He defended the administration's AIDS budget as "something of a vital contribution" and claimed the government had spent "over a half a billion dollars" on AIDS since 1981. "AIDS," Reagan said, "is one of the top priorities with us. There is no question about the seriousness of this." As to the question of schools, Reagan punted, saying he could see "both sides of the issue."

Despite the cryptic nature of the President's comments, many hoped Reagan's remarks marked a new positive phase in the administration response to the epidemic; they would not. Many believed the President had begun to pay more attention to AIDS after he and the world learned of the diagnosis of movie actor Rock Hudson. Hudson's somewhat involuntary decision to reveal his diagnosis to the world's press had galvanized public opinion. The actor's long career had made him a familiar name and face to millions of people around the world. Pictures of the ailing Hudson brought home to many of those people the devastation of AIDS. By mid-1985 many Americans knew, or knew of, someone who had been diagnosed as having, or had died of, AIDS; but for the vast majority of Americans, Hudson was the first time AIDS touched home. The President and First Lady Nancy Reagan weren't immune to the impact of Hudson's plight. Both had known Hudson during their Hollywood days; in fact, the actor had been a guest at a White House dinner just a few months before his diagnosis became public knowledge.

Hudson's diagnosis also touched off another round of public response to AIDS. Again, the attention was useful to those pressing for a government response but troubling to many of those same people who were trying to avoid public panic; AIDS leaped back to the front page of newspapers and magazines and to the lead story on nightly newscasts. There is little doubt that the attention also made it easier for Congress to up the ante on AIDS funding. For fiscal 1986, Congress appropriated $233.8 million, more than double the FY85 total.

In October, the PHS issued a sobering report on the status of AIDS and its future, saying it was "unlikely an AIDS vaccine or treatment" would be developed in the next five years. As a result, PHS said, it would launch a education and information program to alert the public to the nature of the disease and ways to prevent its spread. If everything worked the way PHS wanted, the spread of AIDS could be reduced by 1990 and eliminated by 2000. On Capitol Hill, Waxman's aide, Tim Westmoreland, was astounded. His boss had been pushing for an AIDS education program for two years, to no avail. The small amount of money that Congress appropriated over the administration's objections had been handed over to the mayors. Now, PHS was saying education was the answer to the AIDS epidemic. At the time, 14,000 Americans had been diagnosed with AIDS; PHS predicted that number would double in 1986.

But while Mason was announcing that his agency wanted to move ahead on education, CDC was holding up funds that were supposed to go to four education projects in New York, Los Angeles, and Pittsburgh because of concerns about the explicit nature of the material to be used. The projects were aimed at the gay community, to help teach ways to prevent transmission of the AIDS virus by encouraging "safer sex" practices among gay men. But CDC was worried that federal funding of such projects would seem to be "endorsing the gay lifestyle." To prevent any offense to local communities, CDC instructed the four applicants—the University of Pittsburgh, the University of California at Los Angeles, Memorial Sloan-Kettering Cancer Center, and AIDS Project LA—to create a "program review panel" to clear the material with state and local health officials. The panels would review and approve any written or audiovisual materials, pictorials, questionnaires, or survey instruments. On the one hand, CDC was announcing that education was the way to curb the spread of AIDS; on the other, it didn't want to offend any moral sensibilities.

As 1985 ended, CDC said AIDS cases totaled 20,070—nearly double the total at the end of 1984—and 15,908 people were dead of AIDS-related illnesses.

1986

Despite the CDC moralizing on AIDS education, 1985 had ended on an up note for proponents of a greater government response to the AIDS crisis. Reagan's public comments were seen as a sign that the administration was taking AIDS more seriously; the White House lodged no protests against the increases voted by Congress in AIDS funding. Observers hoped the AIDS fight had turned a corner and that they could look forward to a period of cooperation between the White House and Capitol Hill.

Those hopes were dashed when the administration announced its proposed fiscal 1987 AIDS budget. Not only was the administration not asking for a significant increase in AIDS funding, as many believed was necessary, but the White House was asking Congress to cut AIDS funding from $224 million in FY86 to $213 million in FY87. At the same time, Reagan also asked Congress to rescind $41 million of that FY86 total, including money added to open more AIDS testing clinics, expand an AIDS information telephone hotline, and test alternative ways to care for AIDS patients at a lower cost.

When HHS Secretary Otis Bowen walked out to announce the administration's new AIDS budget, the roomful of reporters was ready to do battle. How could the administration propose to cut AIDS funds and still call it "public health priority number one," Bowen was asked. Didn't this just affirm what all of the administration critics had been saying about the lack of an adequate government response? Bowen hemmed, hawed, and left. His abrupt departure didn't end the questions; but his budget aides could do no better and the press conference was quickly ended. The controversy had just begun.

Remarkably, administration officials seemed baffled by the press and public reaction to the proposed AIDS budget cut. After all, they pointed out, the reduction was small and dealt only with programs that it did not deem necessary. Those officials seemed to miss the symbolism behind a proposal to cut funds for an epidemic that had, by now, caught the full attention of the nation.

But budget day also included a small surprise for the health community. President Reagan made his first trip to HHS since taking office in 1981, and announced that he had asked U.S. Surgeon General Dr. C. Everett Koop to prepare a comprehensive report on the AIDS epidemic. Reagan said AIDS was "one of our highest public health priorities."

Reagan's announcement sent AIDS lobbyists into a tailspin. Before 1986, Koop had played virtually no role in the government's response to AIDS. In his post as Surgeon General, he was the number two official in the Public Health Service, but he and Brandt had never seen eye to eye and the assistant secretary had kept the AIDS issue to himself. With Brandt out of the way, and with little else to do in the mostly ceremonial surgeon general's job, Koop had been angling for months for a greater role in the AIDS fight. Neither Heckler nor Mason responded to Koop's requests for something to do; the White House, however, did.

* * *

While the Surgeon General had a fairly low profile in 1986 when Reagan asked him to take on the AIDS issue, Koop's arrival in

Washington in 1981 had been anything but quiet. His selection by the White House was seen by many as a payoff by the new administration to its fundamentalist conservative supporters in the antiabortion movement. Koop was a force in that movement, lending the credibility he had earned as one of the nation's leading pediatric surgeons to the cause. He had appeared at rallies, in films, and in print, preaching against abortion on demand in the United States. Just before getting the nod for the Surgeon General post, Koop had completed work on a book entitled *Whatever Happened to the Human Race?*, in which he expounded his belief that abortion was a step toward euthanasia, in which Americans would cast off unwanted babies, senior citizens, and handicapped children. Koop's nomination was one of several choices made by the White House, sending a message that it would not be business as usual in Washington under President Reagan.

Normally, a new President gets a lot of leeway in the appointment of his first team; Reagan was certainly no exception. With the new Republican majority in the Senate, Reagan had little trouble pushing through such controversial nominees as Interior Secretary James Watt and Secretary of State Alexander Haig. Few thought there would a problem with Koop's nomination. The chairman of the Senate Human Resources Committee, Utah's Orrin Hatch, was a fan of Koop's and promised his full support to get Koop confirmed.

But there was one small hitch in those plans. The White House had neglected to check the rules regarding service in the Public Health Service corps. The Surgeon General is the chief of the corps and must abide by those rules. While Congress had eliminated most of the mandatory retirement rules in effect for federal government employees, it had neglected to repeal the rule that limited membership in the corps to people under age 62; Koop was 64. Before he could be confirmed, both houses of Congress had to approve a bill to raise or eliminate the retirement age limit.

The technicality that caught Koop allowed congressional Democrats more of a say on his nomination. While only the Senate would have to vote on the nomination, the House would have its say on the rule change. Democrats still controlled the House in 1981, and they were determined to make things as difficult as possible for Koop. In March, North Carolina Republican Senator Jesse Helms slipped an amendment through the Senate eliminating the retirement requirement. But Waxman and Michigan Congressman John Dingell blocked House action on the matter. Waxman's subcommittee scheduled a hearing and called Koop to testify; the White House refused to allow him to appear, arguing that Koop was a private citizen and no expert on mandatory retirement. Waxman was merely using the excuse of the age limit to haul Koop before Congress to question him about his views; that was the Senate's job, the White House said. But the refusal to send Koop to testify angered Waxman and stiffened his resolve to hold up the nomination.

Waxman, with support from the American Public Health Association, argued that Koop lacked the public health experience needed to serve as Surgeon General. He wanted to add such requirements to the statute governing the post. Hatch and the White House refused; the ensuing stalemate would last until the end of the summer of 1981. Waxman and Hatch cut a deal on the issue as part of the budget negotiations and added language eliminating the mandatory retirement rule but requiring future Surgeons General to have public health qualifications. The new law was written in such a way that Koop could serve, but allowed Waxman to make his point. In November, Koop's nomination was approved by the Senate.

* * *

After his tumultuous arrival on the Washington scene, the new Surgeon General lay low. His boss, Brandt, gave him a few odds and ends to handle but, for the most part, cut him out of the policymaking loop at HHS; Koop made the Surgeon General's familiar calls for Americans to quit smoking. But in 1986, his mission would change.

Koop took Reagan's charge to prepare an AIDS report very

seriously. He set out to write a comprehensive study of the epidemic and offer Americans some solid advice on ways to avoid getting the deadly illness. He called in leaders from the public health community—including many of those who had so strongly opposed him nomination in 1981—the religious community, and the gay community.

National Gay Task Force chief Jeff Levi went into his meeting with Koop warily; Koop's past condemnations of homosexuality made Levi worry that he was in for a lambasting. The Koop report, he feared, could be a giant step backward in the gay community's fight for greater government response to the AIDS epidemic. But Levi emerged from his meeting with a very different impression of the Surgeon General. Koop had asked pointed questions; it was clear he knew a lot about the subject. The questions he asked were very encouraging; the two men seemed to be on the same wavelength on the critical issue of AIDS prevention and public education. Could it be that this conservative pariah would actually be an AIDS savior?

Others who met with Koop came away similarly impressed. Koop seemed headed in the right direction. The next worry was what the White House would do when it saw Koop's report. Too many times in the past, the White House and its budget office had stepped in to quash AIDS policies drafted by health specialists at HHS. Would Koop suffer the same fate?

Surgeon General Koop had an advantage that his public health colleagues didn't; he did not have to clear his reports through any higher official. He fended off requests by HHS and White House officials for a glimpse at early drafts of his report. Koop knew if the White House got drift of the direction his report was taking, there would be political pressure exerted on him to change his mind. But Koop did share his drafts with the public health and gay community leaders with whom he had consulted. They were amazed. The report contained a frank discussion of AIDS, how it was transmitted, and, more importantly, how it wasn't. Koop minced no words: AIDS was not a casually transmitted disease. To spread the virus, people had to exchange blood or semen. Anal intercourse and shared needles were the two most dangerous modes of transmission. To halt the spread, Koop said, sexually active people should use condoms. But prevention must go beyond sexually active adults. Koop said children should be educated about AIDS, beginning in grade school; safe sexual practices, including condom use, should be taught in these sex education classes.

Levi was elated. Koop was saying just what he and his organization had been saying since 1982. If Koop could succeed in making his report public, Levi felt the war on AIDS could truly begin.

In October, Koop stepped before a phalanx of television cameras and announced the findings of his report. On the same day, he had sent the final copy of the report to the White House and to the printers. There would be no turning back. The man who "looked like Lincoln and sounded like Moses" had become the new de facto leader in the fight against AIDS.

* * *

While Koop was at work on his report, PHS officials were once again reevaluating the administration's AIDS budget. By now, Mason had tired of the job of acting assistant secretary for health and had returned to Atlanta to run CDC full time. His replacement as acting assistant secretary was Dr. Donald Ian Macdonald, the director of the Alcohol, Drug Abuse, and Mental Health Administration. Macdonald's estimate was that the $213 million Reagan had asked for AIDS was $100 million short. Again, the administration's budget officials would go through the motions of studying Macdonald's request before telling him to find the money elsewhere; but by now, Congress was used to this charade and took Macdonald's advice to heart. The final FY86 AIDS budget was set at $410 million, nearly double the FY85 total.

* * *

Congress' decision to double the AIDS budget may have been aided by Koop's report and Macdonald's budget recommendation, but the driving force may have been the report of a group of scientists who gathered at the Coolfont Conference Center in Berkeley Springs, West Virginia from June 4 to 6. The meeting was kept very quiet until a week later, when Macdonald and CDC's Walter Dowdle, who had been named HHS' first AIDS policy coordinator, held a press conference in Washington. To date, Macdonald noted, there had been 21,000 AIDS cases reported in the United States with more than 11,000 deaths. To get a handle on things to come, HHS had asked its team of experts to predict the course of the epidemic over the following five years. Its prediction, Macdonald said, was "staggering." By 1991, the Coolfont conference predicted, there would be a cumulative total of 270,000 cases of AIDS in the United States and 179,000 deaths. In 1991 alone, 74,000 Americans would be diagnosed with AIDS and 54,000 would die. The United States would spend anywhere from $8 billion to $16 billion in treating AIDS in 1991.

Macdonald said the government would step up its efforts to track the gestation period of the AIDS virus in the human body, determine why some infected people developed AIDS and others didn't, find out why some people with AIDS developed one opportunistic disease while others developed a different malady. Expanded efforts would be made to develop drugs to treat AIDS patients. Vaccine research also would be expanded, with the hope that the government could begin testing a vaccine on humans by 1988. In the meantime, Macdonald said, "our most effective tool for the next few years will continue to be the traditional public health infectious disease control measures." Again, he promised to expand government efforts to educate the populace on ways to prevent AIDS viral infection. Finally, Macdonald said, he was recommending creation of a "national commission" made up of people from the government, the private sector, medicine, and other fields "to look at anticipated needs and resource availability and to make recommendations on how all sectors of our society can handle this major crisis."

The Coolfont report was a splash of cold water in the faces of those who thought America had made progress in its fight against AIDS. News reports quickly pointed out that the PHS projections for 1991 meant more Americans would die of AIDS by that year than had been killed in the decade of fighting in the jungles of Vietnam.

At the end of 1986, AIDS cases totaled 35,587; deaths were up to 24,654.

1987

It may have taken six years, but by 1987, the Reagan administration seemed to catch on to the fact that AIDS was serious business. When the President submitted his fiscal 1988 budget in February, there was no proposal to cut the AIDS funding; in fact, Reagan proposed a record $534 million budget for AIDS research and education, up $124 million from FY87. Included was $121 million for public education, another record. The turnaround on AIDS funding was due mostly to the influence of Bowen. His arrival at HHS in late 1985 came too late to have much impact on the FY87 budget and the horrendous decision to propose a funding cut; by the time the FY88 budget was written, Bowen and his team had been firmly ensconced in Washington.

While Bowen was successful in turning the White House around on AIDS funding, he would have a harder time getting his way on AIDS education. Koop may have hoodwinked the White House by issuing his AIDS report without prior editing or censorship, but the violent reaction from the conservative wing of the Republican party had Reagan's advisers on red alert. They would have their say in the formulation of the government's AIDS education effort. Koop may have favored a direct education campaign aimed at school-age children, but he would have to fight tooth and nail to get his way.

Koop's biggest antagonist on AIDS education would be William Bennett, Reagan's second secretary of Education, who had taken office in 1985 at the beginning of Reagan's second term. Unlike Bowen and Koop, who had no plans for future government posts or careers after their terms in Reagan's service ended, Bennett in 1987 had his sights set on higher office; he was, in one insider's words, "résumé writing." Bennett blasted Koop and Bowen in private Cabinet council meetings and in public speeches and interviews. American children should not be taught about safe sex and condom use, Bennett argued, but should be told to "just say no" to sex. Abstinence was the key.

Koop and Bennett squared off at a January 21 Cabinet council meeting. Both presented their cases to the gathered administration leaders. But the Koop-Bennett feud wouldn't end there. The education secretary would continue to snipe at the Surgeon General whenever Koop spoke out on his education views. Both men had huge egos. To Koop, Bennett was interfering with health matters. To Bennett, Koop was treading on his turf.

On February 11, the council decided. According to a memo prepared by Attorney General Meese, President Reagan had approved five principles on AIDS education:

> Despite intensive research efforts, prevention is the only effective AIDS control strategy at present. Thus, there should be an aggressive federal effort in AIDS education.
>
> The scope and content of the school portion of this AIDS education effort should be locally determined, and should be consistent with parental values.
>
> The federal role should focus on developing and conveying accurate health information on AIDS to educators and others, not mandating a specific school curriculum on this subject, and trusting the American people to use this information in a manner appropriate to their community's needs.
>
> Any health information developed by the federal government that will be used for education should encourage responsible sexual behavior—based on fidelity, commitment, and maturity, placing sexuality within the context of marriage.
>
> Any health information provided by the federal government that might be used in schools should teach that children should not engage in sex, and should be used with the consent and involvement of parents.

So, Koop got the go-ahead to spend federal funds for a school-based AIDS education program and Bennett got his way on content. The White House said that AIDS education should be "grounded in the moral and cultural values of our diverse national communities." In other words, educate but don't proselytize.

The AIDS education program wouldn't be the only topic of dispute among administration officials. Growing use of the AIDS blood test to determine whether people were infected led the administration into a new battleground. Again, the fight would pit Bowen and Koop against Bennett and his former under secretary, Gary Bauer, who was now on the White House staff. Bennett and Bauer began pressing the President to support mandatory AIDS testing of people considered high risks for AIDS infection—gays, drug addicts, and their sex partners. Such testing was the only way to identify who was infected and encourage them to stop spreading the AIDS virus. Koop and Bowen argued that mandatory testing would drive the infected underground. If persons who believed they might be infected knew they would be tested if they went to a clinic or hospital, they would avoid those services.

To build its case, the CDC held a two-day conference to get the opinions of public health experts on AIDS testing. The deck, as they say, was stacked. Public health experts had been decrying use of the AIDS blood test to identify virus carriers since the test was licensed in 1985. When the meeting in Atlanta was held in February, the conclusion was nearly unanimous: no mandatory AIDS testing. Instead, participants favored voluntary testing coupled with extensive counseling of those who were tested. Test records had to be kept confidential, and people who tested positive had to be protected from discrimination, the conference said.

The testing question would become a topic of debate in the Cabinet council, pitting the usual opponents. Both sides made their arguments but no decision was reached. The council seemed at a standstill, but a decision had to be made in time for Reagan's first public speech on AIDS. The President had accepted the invitation of a former Hollywood colleague, actress Elizabeth Taylor, to speak at a Washington dinner being held by the American Foundation for AIDS Research (AmFAR). Taylor had become active in the organization in 1984 and stepped up her involvement after her longtime friend, Rock Hudson, was diagnosed with AIDS in 1985.

Once the President had accepted Taylor's invitation, the White House staff knew it had to come up with something for him to say. The ensuing argument was termed a "bloody battle" by one of the participants. When all was said and done, the White House had a policy and the President had a speech. In it, he announced his support for mandatory testing of federal prisoners and immigrants to the United States. States, he said, also should require testing of their prisoners. Next, the President coined a new term in the testing game. He said he favored "routine testing" of people treated at drug abuse clinics, VD clinics, and at hospitals. Finally, Reagan said he favored routine testing of marriage license applicants.

Reagan's new position on AIDS testing was greeted with boos by some in the AmFAR audience and by gays picketing the dinner outside. State health officials, for the most part, ignored the President's call. But later in the year, the federal government issued rules requiring testing in federal prisons and of all immigrants to the United States.

While the White House was fighting over AIDS education and testing, there were some positive developments. In September 1986, the government had given its permission to drug maker Burroughs Wellcome to begin testing a new AIDS treatment drug on a small group of AIDS patients. Azidothymidine (AZT) was the first drug licensed for AIDS treatment; in 1987 that test was dropped and the drug was approved for wider use. But optimism met reality when Burroughs announced that the price for AZT would amount to nearly $10,000 per year per patient. Many health insurance policies excluded coverage of experimental drugs; others didn't cover outpatient drugs like AZT.

In Washington, Jeff Levi worked with Waxman aide Tim Westmoreland to put together a plan to give states money to help defray the AZT bills for poor AIDS patients. Waxman and Senator Lowell Weicker on the Senate's Appropriations health subcommittee, pushed through an emergency $30 million to pay for AZT.

The money provided an important link that allowed people who were receiving AZT for free during the test period to stay on the drug now that they had to pay for it. By the time 1987 was over, forty-six states had voted to pay for AZT through their Medicaid programs (the four that did not were Florida, Texas, Alabama, and Arkansas).

The administration's family feud over AIDS policy led the White House to try to defuse some of the AIDS issues. On May 4, Reagan announced that he would create a national commission to advise him on AIDS issues. Reagan was only one step ahead of Congress. Senator Robert Dole of Kansas and Congressman Roy Rowland of Georgia were pushing legislation to create a commission on Congress' terms. To make sure that he would control the membership, the White House staff convinced Reagan to move first.

The announcement that Reagan would name an AIDS commission didn't halt the administration fighting. Bennett's alter ego, Bauer, saw the commission as his chance to make some headlines. He told reporters that the panel would not include a gay representative. His comments stirred up more conflict just as the White House was trying to cool the AIDS issue. In June, Reagan named Dr. Eugene Mayberry, Mayo Clinic chief executive officer, to chair the commission but put off naming the other members. Mayberry embarrassed the White House by telling reporters he knew "very little" about AIDS.

Meanwhile the many sides of the AIDS dispute were lobbying the White House for a representative on the commission. Public outcry convinced the White House to ignore Bauer's braying and name New York geneticist and Gay Men's Health Crisis official Dr. Frank Lilly, as the panel's gay member. To offset Lilly, the White House also named Cardinal John O'Connor of New York. Appointees who raised eyebrows included a sexual therapist from San Diego, the president of Amway, the publisher of the *Saturday Evening Post,* and an Illinois state legislator who favored mandatory AIDS testing of marriage license applicants and was closely aligned with conservative gadfly Phyllis Schlafly. The membership list drew laughter from most of the public and groans from Capitol Hill. The panel got off to a very slow start, hampered by infighting and a lack of staff. In September, the White House ordered Mayberry to fire his staff director; in October, Mayberry and vice chairman Woody Myers quit. By that point the commission was in shambles and could only improve. The White House rejected conservative counsel to replace Mayberry and Myers with right-wing activists. With two middle-of-the-road replacements on board and under the forceful leadership of retired Navy Admiral James Watkins, the panel became a more respectable force.

By the end of the year, Congress was ready again to double the AIDS budget. A total of $951 million was appropriated for AIDS research and education. AIDS cases now were up to 53,798, and 30,153 Americans were dead of AIDS-related illnesses.

1988

As Reagan entered his final year in office, the turnaround on AIDS seemed complete. Bowen continued to press for higher budgets, and the White House agreed to request a record $1.3 billion. By the time Reagan's request went to Capitol Hill, 54,233 Americans had been diagnosed with AIDS, and 30,355 of them were dead.

* * *

The Reagan administration's AIDS legacy will probably never recover from the self-inflicted damage incurred from 1981 to 1986. Budget-driven policymakers left the country with short-sighted policies. But Congress—with the help of government scientists and political appointees who were willing to stick their necks out—overcame those shortcomings and provided the leadership on AIDS that the White House lacked. But Waxman provided the best summary of the administration's place in the history books on AIDS when he spoke at an August 10, 1986 meeting of the American Bar Association. "The Reagan administration, for all its sweeping change and sudden shifts in politics, will not be remembered for its Space Shield, its secret wars, or its tax plans. [It] will be remembered for its failure to deal with AIDS. We will remember the President as showing less foresight with more information than any leader since Herbert Hoover or Neville Chamberlain.''

Index

AARP (American Association of Retired Persons), 197
Abortion issue, 125–139
Acquired immune deficiency syndrome (AIDS), 2, 68, 203–237
(*See also* AIDS *entries*)
ACR (adjusted community rate), 167–168
Adjusted community rate (ACR), 167–168
Adolescent Family Life Act, 53
AFDC (Aid to Families with Dependent Children), 20
Aid to Families with Dependent Children (AFDC), 20
AIDS (acquired immune deficiency syndrome) 2, 68, 203–237
AIDS testing, 233–234
AMA (American Medical Association) 90–92, 100
American Association of Retired Persons (AARP), 197
American Foundation for AIDS Research (AmFAR), 233
American Hospital Association, 100
American Medical Association (AMA), 90–92, 100
American Medical Political Action Committee (AMPAC), 192–193
AmFAR (American Foundation for AIDS Research), 233
AMPAC (American Medical Political Action Committee), 192–193

Ancillary services, 107
Antiabortion movement, 125–139
Azidothymidine (AZT), 234–235
AZT (Azidothymidine), 234–235

"Baby Doe" infants, 130–136
Baker, Howard, 10, 18–19, 49–50, 124
Baker, James, III, 63
Balanced budget, 6
Balog, James, 183
Baucus, Max, 146
Bauer, Gary, 233, 235
Bennett, William, 231–233
Bentsen, Lloyd, 190–194, 198–200
Biles, Brian, 143–144
Block grants, 40–55
Blood transfusions, 214–215
Boll Weevils, 31
Bowen, Elizabeth, 71
Bowen, Otis, 8, 70–73, 137–139, 152, 169, 178–190, 201, 224–225, 231–233
Brandt, Edward, 35, 207–208, 211–212, 215–219
Brickfield, Cy, 197
Brock, William, 188
Bromberg, Michael, 101, 107–108
Broyhill, James, 32
Budget, balanced, 6
Budget deficits, 106
Budget government, 1–2
Burke, Sheila, 108–110, 160

239

Burke, Thomas, 71–72, 180–181, 185
Burton, Philip, 192
Bush, George, 6, 142
Byrd, Harry, Sr., 91–93, 179

Cabinet government, 7–8
Califano, Joseph, 99–100
Carter, Jimmy, 99–102, 125
Catastrophic insurance, 73, 177–201
CBO (Congressional Budget Office), 114
CDC (Centers for Disease Control), 203, 205–208, 223–224
Centers for Disease Control (CDC), 203, 205–208, 223–224
Certificates of need (CON), 143
Chafee, John, 199
Chandler, Rod, 135
CHAP (Child Health Assurance Program), 22, 34
"Chastity bill," 53
CHC (Community Health Centers) program, 38–39, 51–52
Child Health Assurance Program (CHAP), 22, 34
Child support enforcement, 69
Childhood Immunization program, 38
Clark, Dick, 125
Cogan, John, 162–163
COLA (cost of living adjustment), 98
Commerce committee, 80
Community Health Centers (CHC) program, 38–39, 51–42
CON (certificates of need), 143
Congressional Budget Office (CBO), 114
Constantine, Jay, 156, 160
Conte, Silvio, 64, 189
Coolfont report, 230
Cost containment, 5
Cost of living adjustment (COLA), 98
Cranston, Alan, 136
Curran, James, 205

Dannemeyer, William, 48
Daschle, Tom, 199
Davis, Carolyne, 152, 162–163, 165, 167, 168
Del Real, Juan, 168
Denton, Jeremiah, 53, 135–136

Diagnosis-related groups (DRGs), 112–113, 115–121
Dingell, John, 152, 227
"Doe, Baby," infants, 130–136
Dole, Elizabeth, 63
Dole, Robert, 10, 18–19, 59, 81–82, 85, 108, 110, 116, 118, 160
Domenici, Pete, 10, 18–19, 50
Domestic Policy Council (DPC), 186, 188
Dowdle, Walter, 230
DPC (Domestic Policy Council), 186, 188
DRGs (diagnosis-related groups), 112–113, 115–121
Durenberger, David, 118, 145–147

Eisenhower, Dwight, 91
Eldercare, 92–93
Elderly, 90

Factor VIII, 214
Falwell, Jerry, 123
Family Planning program, 39–40, 128–130
FDA (Food and Drug Administration), 215
Federal spending, 1–2
Ferrara, Peter, 184–186
50-50 rule, 167
Flemming, Arthur, 91
Food and Drug Administration (FDA), 215
Ford, Gerald, 58
Frank, Barney, 62–63
Fundamentalists, 123–124

Gallo, Robert, 216–218
Gasper, JoAnn, 137–138
Gay Men's Health Crisis (GMHC), 213
Gephardt, Richard, 101–102, 160
Gesell, Gerhard, 132
Ginsburg, Paul, 117
GMHC (Gay Men's Health Crisis), 213
Gold Plus Plan, 166–167
Gottlieb, Michael, 203–204
Gradison, Bill, 160, 194–198
Gramm, Phil, 24, 31
Gray, Robert, 182
Gunter, Bill, 171, 175
Gypsy Moths, 31–32

Index

Haddow, Alice, 68
Haddow, C. McClain ("Mac"), 66–69, 168, 169
Harris, Patricia, 148
Hatch, Orrin, 43–47, 54–55, 127, 130, 136, 191, 226
Hawkins, Paula, 165
HCFA (Health Care Financing Administration), 119, 164–176
Health care deregulation, 141–153
Health Care Financing Adminstration (HCFA), 119, 164–176
Health care prices, 105
Health care spending, 3
Health, Education, and Welfare Department (HEW), 91
Health and Human Services Department (HHS), 8, 161–163
Health Incentives Reform package, 14
Health insurance, 77–78
  catastrophic, 73, 177–201
  Medigap, 158, 181–182
Health maintenance organizations (HMOs), 156, 159–166
Health policy, 1
Health Systems Agency (HSA), 143, 144
Heckler, John, 65, 66
Heckler, Margaret, 8, 62–70, 115, 129, 161–162, 168, 169, 209, 211–212, 216–217, 221–222
Heinz, John, 149, 160, 199
Helms, Jesse, 126–127, 130, 227
Heritage Foundation, 12, 184, 185
HEW (Health, Education, and Welfare) Department, 91
HMOs (health maintenance organizations), 156, 159–166
Hospital Insurance Trust Fund, Medicare, 112–114
Hospitalization coverage, 94
Hospitals, 2–3
  closing of, 120–121
HSA (Health Systems Agency), 143, 144
Hudson, Rock, 222–223, 234
Human Resources Committee, 43–44
Human T-cell leukemia virus (HTLV-III), 216, 221
Humana Inc., 173–175

Humphrey, Gordon, 45, 139
Hutton, William, 197
Hyde, Henry, 125–127

ICFs (intermediate care facilities), 151, 193
IMAs (Individual Medical Accounts), 180, 193
IMC (International Medical Centers Inc.), 163–176
Individual Medical Accounts (IMAs), 180, 193
Inflation, 75
Institute of Medicine (IOM), 149–152
Insurance, health (see Health Insurance)
Intermediate care facilities (ICFs), 151, 193
International Medical Centers Inc. (IMC), 163–176

Javits, Jacob, 44, 45
Johnson, Lyndon, 89–93
Jones, Jim, 24

Katz, Sidney, 150
Kemp, Jack, 5, 137–138
Kennedy, Edward ("Ted"), 43–47, 53, 85, 87, 130, 179–180, 190–192
Kennedy, John, 90, 91
Kennedy, Robert, 39
Kern, John, 109
Kerr, Robert, 92
Kidney dialysis program, 97, 99
Kirkpatrick, Jeanne, 62
Koop, C. Everett, 132–134, 225–229, 231–233
Kusserow, Richard, 136

Latta, Delbert, 24, 31
Levi, Jeff, 211, 213–214, 218, 228–229, 234
Lilly, Frank, 235
Lobbying, 42
Long, Russell, 22, 95, 179
Luce, Bryan, 163
Lugar, Richard, 189

McCormack, John, 93
Macdonald, Donald Ian, 229–230

McIntyre, Thomas, 125
Madigan, Edward, 20, 29–30, 47, 83–84
Mason, James, 220–223
Mayberry, Eugene, 235–236
"Means test," 195
Mecklenburg, Marjory, 138
Medicaid, 8–9, 13, 17–35, 92
Medicaid cap, 25, 28–34
Medicare, 9, 14, 78
  cuts in, 106–114
  state of chaos in, 89–103
Medicare Economic Index (MEI), 98
Medicare Hospital Insurance Trust Fund, 112–114
Medigap insurance, 158, 181–182
Meese, Edwin, 186, 232
MEI (Medicare Economic Index), 98
Mental Health Systems Act, 54
Mica, Dan, 171–172
Michel, Bob, 19
Miller, James, 8, 152, 188
Mills, Wilbur, 91–92
Mitchell, George, 152, 199, 200
MMWR (Morbidity and Mortality Weekly Report), 203
Morbidity and Mortality Weekly Report (MMWR), 203
Mortality statistics, 2
Myers, Woody, 236

Natcher, William, 208
National Council of Senior Citizens, 197
National Institutes of Health (NIH), 208–211
Nelson, Karen, 25
Newhall, David, 60, 65
Newman, Donald, 72
NIH (National Institutes of Health), 208–211
Nixon, Richard, 58, 94–95
Nofziger, Lyn, 168
Nursing home regulations, 147–153

Oakar, Mary Rose, 149
O'Connor, John, 235
Office of Management and Budget (OMB), 5, 7–8

Office of Technology Assessment (OTA), 220
OMB (Office of Management and Budget), 5, 7–8
Omnibus-bill approach, 10–11
O'Neill, Thomas ("Tip"), Jr., 10, 76–77, 115, 197
OTA (Office of Technology Assessment), 220

PACs (political action committees), 27–28
Peer Review Organizations (PROs), 146–147
Pepper, Claude, 115, 149, 164, 165, 169
Pharmaceutical Manufacturers Association (PMA), 199–200
PHP (prepaid health plans), 159
PHS (Public Health Service), 206–207
Pickle, J. J. ("Jake"), 118
Planned Parenthood Federation, 137, 138
PMA (Pharmaceutical Manufacturers Association), 199–200
Political action committees (PACs), 27–28
Poverty, 20
Prepaid Health Plans (PHP), 159
Preyer, Richardson, 26–28
Professional Standards Review Organizations (PSROs) program, 99, 142, 144–147
PROs (Peer Review Organizations), 146–147
Pryor, David, 149
PSROs (Professional Standards Review Organizations) program, 99, 142, 144–147
Public Health Service (PHS), 206–207
Pursell, Carl, 165

Quayle, Dan, 85, 189

Ratchford, William, 149
Reagan, Ronald, 1, 4, 6–8, 40–42, 57–60, 93, 102–103, 105–106, 123–124, 131, 141–142, 145, 159, 178, 222, 234
Recarey, Miguel, Jr., 163–175
Regan, Donald, 69–70
Ribicoff, Abraham, 179
Right-to-life movement, 125–139

Index

Rockefeller, Nelson, 59
Roe v. Wade, 125–128
Rogers, Paul, 100–101
Roosevelt, Franklin, 90
Roper, William, 152, 169–175, 188
Rostenkowski, Dan, 79–81, 100–101, 116, 118, 192, 197
Rowland, Roy, 235
Roy, Bill, 144
Roybal, Edward, 208
Rubin, Robert, 11, 60

Schmitt, Harrison ("Jack"), 210–211
Schneider, Andreas, 25
Schweiker, Richard, 8, 11, 44–45, 57–62, 65, 111–119, 128–129, 148–149, 152, 209, 211–212
Sears, John, 58–59, 165, 168
Section 223 limits, 107–111
SHPDA (Statewide Health Planning and Development Agency) programs, 143
Siguler, George, 65
Simon, Paul, 200
Skilled nursing facilities (SNFs), 151, 193, 194
SNFs (skilled nursing facilities), 151, 193, 194
"Social safety net," 106
Social Security trust fund, 114
Spending, federal, 1–2
  for health care, 3
Sprinkel, Beryl, 188–189
Squeal rule, 129
SSI (Supplemental Security Income), 21
Stafford, Robert, 44–46
Stark, Pete, 169, 171–172, 190, 192–198
Statewide Health Planning and Development Agency (SHPDA) programs, 143

Steelman, Deborah, 188
Stockman, David, 5–11, 22–25, 29–32, 47–49, 61–62, 81–85, 101, 105–109, 145, 152, 162–163, 209, 212
Supplemental Security Income (SSI), 21
Svahn, Jack, 64–66, 211
Swoap, David, 211

Talmadge, Herman, 109
Tax cap, 83
Tax Equity and Fiscal Responsibility Act (TEFRA), 111, 112
Taylor, Elizabeth, 233–234
TEFRA (Tax Equity and Fiscal Responsibility Act), 111, 112
Truman, Harry, 90–91

UAW (United Auto Workers), 83
Unemployment rate, 75–76
United Auto Workers (UAW), 83

Venereal disease (VD), 41
Voluntary effort (VE), 101–102
Voting records, 10
Voucher program, 155–176

Watkins, James, 236
Waxman, Henry, 15–16, 25–34, 42–43, 79–81, 100–101, 130, 135, 143–144, 159–161, 197–198, 204–205, 208, 210, 211, 213–215, 220, 227, 234, 236–237
Ways and Means Committee, 80
Weicker, Lowell, 139, 211
Weinberger, Caspar, 188
Weiss, Ted, 213
Westmoreland, Tim, 210, 223
Windom, Robert, 138
Winston, David, 11–13, 60–61
Wright, Jim, 197–198
Wyngaarden, James, 209

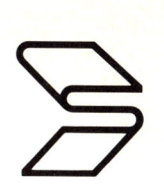

Ref.
DK
17
.L46

The Soviet Union
Figures - Facts - Data

Die Sowjetunion
Zahlen - Fakten - Daten

Edited by / Herausgegeben von
Borys Lewytzkyj

Distributed by
GALE RESEARCH COMPANY
Book Tower
Detroit, Michigan 48226

K·G·Saur
München·New York·London·Paris 1979

K. G. Saur Verlag KG
Pössenbacherstr. 2b, 8000 München 71
Federal Republic of Germany
Tel. (089) 79 89 01
Telex 5212067 saur d

ISBN 3-598-07040-3

K. G. Saur Publishing, Inc.
175 Fifth Avenue
New York, N.Y. 10010, U.S.A.
Tel. (212) 477-2500
Telex 0023/238386 kgspur

ISBN 0-89664-010-8

CIP-Kurztitelaufnahme der Deutschen Bibliothek

The Soviet Union : figures, facts, data =
Die Sowjetunion / ed. by Borys Lewytzkyj.
— München, New York, London, Paris: Saur,
1979.
   ISBN 3-598-07040-3 (München)
   ISBN 0-89664-010-8 (New York)

NE: Lewytzkyj, Borys [Hrsg.]; PT

Library of Congress Cataloging in Publication Data

Lewytzkyj, Borys.
   Die Sowjetunion, Zahlen - Fakten - Daten = The Soviet Union, figures - facts - data.

   English and German.
   1. Russia. I. Title. II. Title: The Soviet Union, figures - facts - data.
DK17.L46   947.085   79-11237
ISBN 0-89664-010-8

© 1979 by K. G. Saur Verlag KG, München
Printed in the Federal Republic of Germany
by grafik + druck GmbH & Co., München
Bound by Thomas-Buchbinderei GmbH, Augsburg

CONTENTS

Preface VII

Systematic Index XI

List of Diagrams XXXI

Introduction: The Political System of the USSR... XXXIII

Figures, Facts, Data 1

INHALT

Vorwort IX

Systematische Übersicht XXI

Verzeichnis der Graphischen Darstellungen XXXI

Einführung: Das Politische System der UdSSR XXXV

Zahlen, Fakten, Daten 1

Note for English users: geographical and proper names as well as headlines and technical terms were transliterated from the Russian according to the international German transliteration system (whereby the diacritical sign ˇ had to be rendered ^ for technical reasons), i.e.:

$$ts = c$$
$$ch = \hat{c}$$
$$kh = ch$$
$$i = i$$

etc.

Examples: Ashkhabad = Aŝchabad
Chrushchev = Chruŝchev
Chekhov = Čechov
Arkhangelsk = Archangelsk
Sovetskaia entsiklopediia = Sovjetskaja enciklopedija
Zhitomir = Žitomir
Chita = Čita
Soiuz = Sojuz

PREFACE

For the first time ever in western documentation this work attempts to give an insight into all aspects of the Soviet state and Soviet society by using an encyclopedic approach (names, figures and other data are presented in tabular form). The information contained ranges from details about size of territories, population, structure of administration, party and state apparat, national economy, science and education to information about public organizations and various other instructive details. The data is presented in three languages (English, German and Russian), with Russian included only as an aid to prevent any misinterpretation.

This volume offers quick and comprehensive information to institutions, government agencies, libraries and to specialists in a wide range of fields and is a valuable aid to individuals engaged in politics, science, business and trade, to students, and last but not least, to the interested general public. At the same time, editors, journalists and publishers will find this handbook a clearly arranged and easy-to-use reference tool.

The information on the national economy was taken from official Soviet sources and does not always entirely satisfy western readers and users. It should be pointed out in this context that an increasing readiness to release information did not set in until the beginning of the sixties. The first statistical collection, "Narodnoe Khozjaistvo", was published by the Central Statistical Administration in 1956. Meanwhile, more detailed and comprehensive works are published annually, but unfortunately those relating to the economy of the union republics are not regularly published by the Central Statistical Administrations of these republics. At the beginning of every year, the daily papers publish a report describing how the plan was fulfilled in the preceding year in the USSR as a whole as well as in the republics. This type of information was also processed for the present volume. It should be kept in mind that in the Soviet Union statistics and surveys are prepared for a select group of specialists and high-ranking functionaries which are not accessible in the West but sometimes appear in the studies of a number of Soviet specialists.

The criteria and methods applied in Soviet statistics posed a special problem. Very often they differ considerably from the standard figures generally used in the West, and frequently the reckoning methods and criteria used are not elaborated. The size of the country alone made standardized and centralized data collecting and surveying difficult in the past. Electronic data processing has improved the situation significantly, though it has remained impossible to this day to guarantee the accuracy of information received from the lower-echelon organizations. Factories, kolkhozes and sovkhozes still tend to embellish their records by giving them a "face lifting" according to the traditional practice of "pripiski" (attribution).

VII

The most irritating factor in all state surveys - including areas not connected with the national economy - is the ideological tenet that the function of statistics is to "prove" the ever-increasing productivity resulting from the construction of socialism. This is criticized by many Soviet economists and statisticians too. At the beginning of the sixties, when discussion was still relatively liberal, hard and open criticism of these built-in errors was also expressed. An analysis attributed to A. Aganbegian, the famous economist, said bluntly: "Several statistical findings which were published by the Central Statistical Administration prove to be downright absurd." One must admit, however, that with increasing modernization of statistical methods and tools, some improvement has been achieved.

The greater part of the material used here comes from the archives of the author, especially the information on persons and institutions. It is the result of decades of research and study of the Soviet newspapers, journals, encyclopedias, lexica and other relevant publications. In this work the author was aided by an experienced researcher. Among the literature published within the last years, a number of publications on special subject groups which reflect the somewhat improved methods applied in Soviet statistics deserve special mention.

Numerous w e s t e r n studies also cover various aspects and fields of Soviet life in detail. Among those, the publications by the U.S. Department of Commerce, Industry and Trade (Administration Bureau of East-West Trade) and those of the Joint Economic Committee, in particular "Soviet Economic Prospects for the Seventies", all of them being accessible to the public, are of special value. A number of publications attempt to render a comprehensive picture of developments in the Soviet Union. The (German) Federal Institute for East-European and International Studies in Cologne publishes an annual report entitled "The Soviet Union 19--. Domestic policy, economy, foreign policy - Analysis and review", containing carefully edited information on the subjects named in the title for the year in question.

A new edition of the present volume is scheduled for 1980/81. By then the figures for the results of the Tenth Five-Year Plan (1976-80) as well as the target goals for the Eleventh Five-Year Plan (1981-85) will be available. Furthermore, the XXVI. Party Congress of the CPSU as well as the Party Congresses of the union republics will have taken place, very likely resulting in considerable change in personnel within the top leadership and an accelerated influx of the younger generation, a trend which is already noticeable. And perhaps most important of all: the information on the census which is to take place in 1979 will be available for the next edition.

Munich, 1978   Borys Lewytzkyj

VORWORT

Mit der vorliegenden Arbeit wird erstmals in der westlichen Literatur versucht, in enzyklopädischer Art durch Namen und Daten, in Tabellen geordnet, Einblick in alle Bereiche des sowjetischen Systems und der sowjetischen Gesellschaft zu geben. Die Informationen reichen von Gebietsgröße, Bevölkerungszahl, Verwaltungsgliederung, Partei- und Staatsapparaten, Wirtschaft, Wissenschaft und Erziehung bis hin zu gesellschaftlichen Organisationen und verschiedenen wissenswerten Einzelinformationen. Das Werk ist dreisprachig (Englisch, Deutsch, Russisch), wobei Russisch nur als Hilfsmittel gedacht ist, um jegliche Mißverständnisse auszuschließen.

Diese Arbeit soll eine rasche und umfassende Information bieten für Institute, Behörden, Bibliotheken, Fachleute der verschiedensten Richtungen, Persönlichkeiten aus Politik, Wirtschaft, Wissenschaft und Handel, aber last not least auch für Studenten sowie für eine interessierte Öffentlichkeit. Zugleich dient dieser Band als übersichtliches und leicht zu handhabendes Nachschlagwerk für Redakteure, Journalisten und Verlage.

Bei den Angaben für die Wirtschaft werden offizielle Daten aus sowjetischen Quellen wiedergegeben. Sie können westliche Leser und Benutzer des Werkes nicht immer vollständig befriedigen. In diesem Zusammenhang sei daran erinnert, daß eine allmählich wachsende Informationsfreudigkeit erst seit den sechziger Jahren zu beobachten ist. Der erste statistische Sammelband "Narodnoe chozjaistvo SSSR" wurde 1956 von der Statistischen Zentralverwaltung der UdSSR herausgebracht. Inzwischen werden jährlich umfangreichere Sammelbände veröffentlicht, leider erscheinen jedoch die von den Statistischen Zentralverwaltungen der jeweiligen Republiken herausgegebenen Sammelbände über die Volkswirtschaft der Republiken nicht regelmäßig. Zu Beginn eines jeden Jahres wird ein Bericht über die Planerfüllung im vorangegangenen Jahr in der gesamten UdSSR wie in den Unionsrepubliken in Tageszeitungen veröffentlicht. Auch diese Daten wurden für die vorliegende Arbeit ausgewertet. Hierbei ist zu beachten, daß in der Sowjetunion für einen engen Expertenkreis bzw. für verantwortliche Funktionäre Statistiken und Übersichten erstellt werden, die im Westen nicht zugänglich sind, die jedoch manchmal in Studien einiger sowjetischer Fachleute auftauchen.

Eine besondere Schwierigkeit lag in den von der sowjetischen Statistik verwendeten Kriterien und Methoden. Sie weichen sehr oft stark von den üblichen westlichen Erfassungsgrößen ab, sie bedienen sich häufig nicht explizierter Zählungsmethoden und -kriterien. Allein die Größe des Landes hat lange Zeit eine einheitliche und zentralisierte Datenerfassung erschwert. Hier hat die EDV inzwischen erhebliche Verbesserungen gebracht. Bis heute gelang es allerdings nicht, die Zuverlässigkeit der von unten nach oben gelangenden Informationen zu gewährleisten. Betriebe, Kolchosen und Sowchosen neigen nach wie vor dazu, ihre eigenen Leistungen aufzuwerten, also nach oben zu "korrigieren" - nach der traditionellen Unsitte der "pripiski" (Zuschreibungen).

Als wesentlichster Störfaktor aller statistischen Erhebungen – auch außerhalb der Wirtschaft – erweist sich die ideologische Verpflichtung, die Statistik habe die kontinuierliche Zunahme der Errungenschaften beim Aufbau des Sozialismus "nachzuweisen". Damit sind auch zahlreiche sowjetische Wirtschaftler und Statistiker unzufrieden. Zu Beginn der sechziger Jahre, als noch ein relativ breiter Diskussionsspielraum bestand, gab es auch harte, offene Kritiken an diesen "immanenten" Fehlerquellen. Eine Analyse, die dem bekannten Ökonomen A. Aganbegian zugeschrieben wird, formulierte schonungslos: "Mehrere statistische Angaben, die von der Statistischen Zentralverwaltung publiziert wurden, erweisen sich beim Versuch, sie zu analysieren, als schlichtweg absurd". Man muß allerdings anerkennen, daß bei der Modernisierung der statistischen Verfahren und der zuständigen statistischen Apparate und Institute einige Erfolge erzielt werden konnten.

Das Gros der hier vorgelegten Angaben stammt aus dem Archiv des Verfassers, das gilt vor allem für die Informationen über Personen und Institutionen. Sie sind das Ergebnis jahrzehntelanger Forschungstätigkeit auf der Grundlage der Auswertung sowjetischer Zeitungen, Zeitschriften, Enzyklopädien, Lexika und anderer einschlägiger Veröffentlichungen, unterstützt durch eine erfahrene Fachkraft. Unter den in den letzten Jahren erschienenen Informationsquellen sind hier Sammelbände nach Fachgebieten hervorzuheben, in denen sich auch etwas verbesserte Methoden der sowjetischen Statistik spiegeln.

Viele w e s t l i c h e Studien befassen sich auch mit einer eingehenden Darstellung verschiedener Einzelaspekte bzw. Einzelbereiche des sowjetischen Lebens. Von besonderem Wert sind dabei die öffentlich zugänglichen Publikationen, die vom U.S. Department of Commerce, Industry and Trade, Administration Bureau of East-West Trade, herausgegeben werden, sowie die Publikationen des Joint Economic Committee, insbesondere "Soviet Economic Prospects for the Seventies". In einigen Publikationen wurde auch versucht, eine Gesamtdarstellung der sowjetischen Entwicklung zu leisten. Das Bundesinstitut für ostwissenschaftliche und internationale Fragen in Köln (Bundesrepublik Deutschland) veröffentlicht als Jahresbericht einen Band "Sowjetunion 19.. (Jahreszahl). Innenpolitik, Wirtschaft, Aussenpolitik – Analyse und Bilanz", der kritisch aufbereitete Informationen aus den im Titel genannten Bereichen für das genannte Jahr bietet.

In den Jahren 1980/81 soll eine Neuauflage der vorliegenden Arbeit erscheinen. Bis dahin werden Zahlen über die Erfüllung des X. Fünfjahrplanes (1976-80) bekannt sein, desgleichen die Planziele des XI. Fünfjahrplanes (1981-85). In diesen Zeitraum fallen dann auch der XXVI. Parteitag der KPdSU und Parteitage in den Unionsrepubliken, die mit Sicherheit erhebliche personelle Veränderungen in den Führungsgremien bringen werden, gekennzeichnet vor allem durch einen sich bereits heute beschleunigenden Generationswechsel. Und vielleicht das Wichtigste: die Unterlagen über die Volkszählung von 1979 werden zur Verfügung stehen.

München, 1978   Borys Lewytzkyj

SYSTEMATIC INDEX

1.	**Administrative-territorial survey**	
1.1	Union Republics	1
1.2	Union Republics (Territory and Capitals)	4
1.3	Autonomous Republics	5
1.4	Autonomous Regions, National Krais, Oblasts, Raions, and Village Soviets in the Union Republics	6
1.5	Cities, Urban-Type Settlements and Raions in the Cities	6
2.	**Population**	
2.1	Population 1897-1977	7
2.2	Population of the USSR and the Union Republics	8
2.2.1	Urban	9
2.2.2	Rural	9
2.3	Population of the Union Republics	10
2.4	Population of the Economic Raions, Autonomous Republics and Oblasts	12
2.5	Cities with more than 50,000 inhabitants	24
2.6	Increase in population	33
2.7	Cities and Urban-type Settlements by Population	34
2.8	Male and Female	35
2.9	Population by Sex	36
2.9.1	Urban population	37
2.9.2	Rural population	38
2.10	Distribution of Population by Sex and Age	40
2.10.1	Urban population	40
2.10.2	Rural population	42
2.11	Peoples of the Soviet Union	46
2.11.1	Principal Nationalities of the Union Republics	46
2.11.2	Peoples of the Soviet Union by Ethnic-Linguistic Groups	47
2.11.3	National Composition of Population	51
2.11.4	Nationalities represented among the Population of the USSR and the Union Republics	54
3.	**Communist Party of the Soviet Union**	
3.1	Party Congresses	57
3.2	Number of Members 1917-1975	59
3.3	Politburo CC CPSU	62
3.3.1	Secretariat CC CPSU	75
3.4	Social Composition of the CPSU	83
3.4.1	Social Composition	83
3.4.2	Communist Party Members by Profession	83
3.5	Level of Education of Communist Party Members	84
3.5.1	Level of Education of Communist Party Members (in thous.)	84
3.5.2	Level of Education of Communist Party Members (in percent)	85
3.5.3	Number of Communist Party Members with Academic Degree	85
3.6	Women in the CPSU	86
3.7	National Composition of the CPSU	87
3.7.1	Nationalities represented in the CPSU	87
3.7.2	National Composition as of 1/1/1976	88
3.8	Primary Party Organizations	89
3.8.1	Network of Primary Organizations	89
3.8.2	Primary Party Organizations by Percentage of Communist Party Members	90
3.8.3	Communist Party Members by Field of Economic Activity	90

XI

3.8.4	Structure of the Primary Party Organizations	91
3.9	Elected Leading Party Organizations	95
3.9.1	CC CPSU	95
3.9.2	Politburo CC CPSU	95
3.9.3	Secretariat CC CPSU	97
3.9.4	Network of Leading Party Organizations	98
3.9.5	Elected Leading Party Organizations of the Union Republics	98
3.10	Nominated Party Apparatus	109
3.10.1	CPSU CC Apparatus under the Direction of the CC Secretariat	109
3.10.2	CC Apparatus of CPs of the Union Republics	110
3.10.3	Nominated Apparatus of the Local Party Organizations	112
4.	**State Structure**	
4.1	Soviet State Organs	114
4.2.1	Number of the Soviets of the People's Deputies	117
4.2.2	Chairmen of the USSR Supreme Soviet Presidium	117
4.2.3	Number of the Elected Deputies of the USSR Supreme Soviet	118
4.2.4	USSR Supreme Soviet	118
4.2.5	Composition of the Deputies of the USSR Supreme Soviet	120
4.3	USSR Council of Ministers	122
4.3.1	Chairmen of the USSR Council of Ministers	122
4.3.2	Composition of the USSR Council of Ministers	123
4.3.3	USSR Ministry of Foreign Affairs	127
4.3.4	USSR Ministry of Defense	133
4.4	Supreme Soviets and Councils of Ministers of the Union Rep.	139
4.4.1	RSFSR	139
4.4.2	Ukrainskaja SSR	141
4.4.3	Belorusskaja SSR	144
4.4.4	Uzbekskaja SSR	146
4.4.5	Kazachskaja SSR	149
4.4.6	Gruzinskaja SSR	151
4.4.7	Azerbajdžanskaja SSR	154
4.4.8	Litovskaja SSR	156
4.4.9	Moldavskaja SSR	158
4.4.10	Latvijskaja SSR	161
4.4.11	Kirgizskaja SSR	163
4.4.12	Tadžikskaja SSR	165
4.4.13	Armjanskaja SSR	167
4.4.14	Turkmenskaja SSR	169
4.4.15	Estonskaja SSR	172
5.	**Economy**	
5.1	Industry	174
5.1.1	Output of the most important Industrial Branches	174
5.1.2	Electric Power	192
5.1.2.1	Capacity of Electric Power Stations and Output of Electric Power	192
5.1.2.2	Consumption of Electric Power	193
5.1.2.3	Energetic Capacity and Consumption of Electric Power by the most important Industrial Branches	194
5.1.2.4	Power Capacity of the Power Stations in the USSR	195
5.1.2.5	Electric Power Output per capita	195
5.1.2.6	Electric Power Output in the Union Republics	196
5.1.3	Iron and Steel Industry	197
5.1.3.1	Output of Pig Iron Steel, Finished Rolled Steel and Steel Tubes	197
5.1.3.2	Output of Iron and Manganese Ore (Commercial Type)	198
5.1.3.3	Pig Iron Output in the Union Republics	198
5.1.3.4	Steel Output in the Union Republics	199

5.1.3.5	Production of Finished Rolled Steel in the Union Republics	199
5.1.4	Fuel Industry	200
5.1.4.1	Fuel Output by Types	200
5.1.4.2	Coal Output by Types	201
5.1.4.3	Coal Output in the Union Republics	202
5.1.4.4	Mineral Oil Output (incl.Gas Condensate) in the Union Rep.	202
5.1.4.5	Natural Gas Output in the Union Republics	203
5.1.5	Machine Building and Metal Working Industry	204
5.1.5.1	Output of Equipment for Various Branches of the Industry	204
5.1.5.2	Output of Instruments, Means of Automation, and Computers	206
5.1.5.3	Production of Chemical Equipment	207
5.1.5.4	Production of Material-Handling Equipment	208
5.1.5.5	Output of Production Equipment for the Light, Food and Printing Industries and for Trade and Catering Enterprises	209
5.1.5.6	Output of Sanitary Engineering Equipment	213
5.1.5.7	Output of Agricultural Machines	214
5.1.5.8	Output of Tractors by Types	216
5.1.6	Chemical Industry	217
5.1.6.1	Output of Mineral Fertilizers by Types	217
5.1.6.2	Output of Mineral Fertilizers in the Union Republics	218
5.1.6.3	Output of Synthetic Resins and Plastics	218
5.1.6.4	Output of Chemical Fibres and Yarns	219
5.1.6.5	Output of Tires by Types	220
5.1.7	Forestry, Wood Working and Cellulose-Paper Industry	221
5.1.7.1	Timber Logging	221
5.1.7.2	Exploitation of Densely Wooded Regions	221
5.1.7.3	Output of Sawed Timber and Plywood	223
5.1.7.4	Output of Sawed Timber in the Union Republics	223
5.1.7.5	Timber Logging in the Union Republics	224
5.1.7.6	Output of Cellulose, Newsprint, and Cardboard	226
5.1.7.7	Output of Newsprint in the Union Republics	226
5.1.8	Construction Materials Industry	227
5.1.8.1	Output of Cement by Types, in 1975	227
5.1.8.2	Output of Cement in the Union Republics	227
5.1.8.3	Output of Various Types of Precast Concrete Structures and Components	228
5.1.8.4	Output of Wall Construction Materials	229
5.1.8.5	Output of Roofing Materials	230
5.1.8.6	Output of Linoleum	230
5.1.9	Light Industry	231
5.1.9.1	Output of the most important Products of the Light Industry	231
5.1.9.2	Output of Cotton Fabrics in the Union Republics	233
5.1.9.3	Output of Woolen Fabrics in the Union Republics	233
5.1.9.4	Output of Linen Fabrics in the Union Republics	234
5.1.9.5	Output of Silk Fabrics in the Union Republics	234
5.1.9.6	Output of Cotton Fibres in the Union Republics	234
5.1.9.7	Output of Raw Silk in the Union Republics	235
5.1.9.8	Output of Hosiery and Socks in the Union Republics	235
5.1.9.9	Output of Linen Hosiery in the Union Republics	236
5.1.9.10	Output of Outer Hosiery in the Union Republics	236
5.1.9.11	Output of Woven Fabrics and Hosiery containing Synthetic Fibres	237
5.1.10	Food Industry	238
5.1.10.1	Output of the most important Products of the Food Industry	238
5.1.10.2	Production of Castor and Refined Sugar	239
5.1.10.3	Production of Castor Sugar by Union Republics	239
5.1.10.4	Meat Production by Types	240
5.1.10.5	Meat Production by Union Republics	240
5.1.10.6	Production of Animal Fats by Union Republics	241
5.1.10.7	Production of Vegetable Fats by Union Republics	241

Index

5.1.10.8	Production of Canned Goods by Types	242
5.2	Agriculture	243
5.2.1	Gross Agricultural Output by Union Republics	243
5.2.1.1	Agricultural Output - Output of Livestock Products	244
5.2.2	Output of Agricultural Products	245
5.2.3	Yield of Agricultural Crops	247
5.2.4	Share of Total Production of Agricultural Raw Products of State Farms, Collective Farms and Other State-owned Enterprises	248
5.2.5	Production of Marketable Goods in Agriculture	250
5.2.6	Share of Total Marketable Production of the Co-operative Agriculture of State and Collective Farms and Other State-owned Enterprises (in percent)	251
5.2.7	Gross Yield of Grain Crops by Union Republics	253
5.2.8	Gross Yield of Winter and Summer Wheat by Union Republics	253
5.2.9	Gross Yield of Winter and Summer Rye by Union Republics	254
5.2.10	Gross Yield of Maize (Ripe) by Union Republics	254
5.2.11	Gross Yield of Millet by Union Republics	254
5.2.12	Gross Yield of Buckwheat by Union Republics	255
5.2.13	Gross Yield of Rice by Union Republics	255
5.2.14	Gross Yield of Legumes by Union Republics	255
5.2.15	Gross Yield of Sugar-Beet (for Factory Processing) by Union Republics	256
5.2.16	Gross Yield of Flax Fibre by Union Republics	256
5.2.17	Gross Yield of Sunflower Seeds by Union Republics	256
5.2.18	Gross Yield of Potatoes by Union Republics	256
5.2.19	Gross Yield of Vegetables by Union Republics	257
5.2.20	Gross Yield of Grapes by Union Republics	257
5.2.21	Gross Yield of Fruit and Berries by Union Republics	258
5.2.22	Sowing Area of Grain by Union Republics	258
5.2.23	Sowing Area of Winter Wheat by Union Republics	259
5.2.24	Sowing Area of Summer Wheat by Union Republics	259
5.2.25	Total Sowing Area of Winter and Summer Rye by Union Republics	260
5.2.26	Sowing Area of Maize (Ripe) by Union Republics	260
5.2.27	Sowing Area of Millet by Union Republics	260
5.2.28	Sowing Area of Buckwheat by Union Republics	260
5.2.29	Sowing Area of Rice by Union Republics	261
5.2.30	Sowing Area of Legumes by Union Republics	261
5.2.31	Total Sowing Area of Industrial Crops by Union Republics	261
5.2.32	Sowing Area of Cotton by Union Republics	262
5.2.33	Sowing Area of Sugar-Beet by Union Republics	262
5.2.34	Sowing Area of Long-Fibre Flax by Union Republics	262
5.2.35	Sowing Area of Sunflower Seeds by Union Republics	263
5.2.36	Sowing Area of Potatoes by Union Republics	263
5.2.37	Sowing Area of Vegetables by Union Republics	263
5.2.38	Sowing Area of Fodder Crops by Union Republics	264
5.2.39	Sowing Area of Seasonal and Perennial Grass incl. Winter Sowing for Green Fodder by Union Republics	264
5.2.40	Area of Irrigated Ground in Collective and State Farms and Other State Enterprises by Union Republics	265
5.2.41	Sowing Area of Agricultural Crops on Irrigated Ground in Collective and State Farms and other State Enterprises by Union Republics	266
5.2.42	Fruit-Growing and Viticulture	267
5.2.43	Area of Viticulture of all Growing Phases by Union Republics	265
5.2.44	Area of Viticulture at Fruit-Bearing State by Union Republics	268
5.2.45	Sowing Area of Tea by Union Republics	268
5.2.46	Livestock Breeding	269
5.2.46.1	Livestock	269

Index

5.2.46.2	Dairy Cattle and Livestock in Individual Agricultural Enterprises	270
5.2.46.3	Beef Cattle by Union Republics	272
5.2.46.4	Dairy Cattle by Union Republics	272
5.2.46.5	Pigs by Union Republics	273
5.2.46.6	Sheep and Goats by Union Republics	273
5.2.46.7	Sheep by Union Republics	274
5.2.46.8	Poultry by Union Republics	274
5.2.46.9	Basic Livestock Products	275
5.2.46.10	Basic Livestock Products by Union Republics	277
5.2.46.11	Meat Production by Union Republics	278
5.2.46.12	Milk Production by Union Republics	278
5.2.46.13	Egg Production by Union Republics	279
5.2.46.14	Wool Production by Union Republics	279
5.2.47	Collective Farms	280
5.2.47.1	Basic Indicators of Collective Farm Development	280
5.2.47.2	Breakdown of Collective Farms by Amount of Gross Income per 100 Hectares Arable Land	283
5.2.47.3	Breakdown of Collective Farms by Number of Households	284
5.2.47.4	Breakdown of Collective Farms by Livestock	285
5.2.47.5	Basic Indicators of Collective Farm Development by Union Rep.	286
5.2.48	State Farms	288
5.2.48.1	Number of State Farms	288
5.2.48.2	Basic Indicators on State Farm Development	289
5.2.48.3	Number of State Farms by Union Republics	291
5.2.49	State Purchases of Agricultural Products	292
5.2.49.1	State Purchases of Basic Agricultural Products from the Collective and State Farms and other State Agricultural Enterprises	292
5.2.49.2	State Purchases of Agricultural Products	293
5.2.49.3	State Purchases of Staple Agricultural Products	295
5.2.49.4	State Purchases of Grain Crops by Union Republics	296
5.2.49.5	State Purchases of Wheat by Union Republics	297
5.2.49.6	State Purchases of Rye by Union Republics	297
5.2.49.7	State Purchases of Sugar-Beet by Union Republics	297
5.2.49.8	State Purchases of Flax Fibres by Union Republics	298
5.2.49.9	State Purchases of Sunflower Seeds by Union Republics	298
5.2.49.10	State Purchases of Potatoes by Union Republics	298
5.2.49.11	State Purchases of Vegetables by Union Republics	299
5.2.49.12	State Purchases of Fruits and Berries by Union Republics	299
5.2.49.13	State Purchases of Grapes by Union Republics	299
5.2.49.14	Gross Yield (Purchases) of Raw Tea by Union Republics	300
5.2.49.15	State Purchases of Basic Livestock Products in Individual Agricultural Enterprises	300
5.2.49.16	State Purchases of Cattle and Poultry by Union Republics (live weight)	301
5.2.49.17	State Purchases of Cattle and Poultry by Union Republics (slaughter weight)	302
5.2.49.18	State Purchases of Milk and Dairy Products by Union Republics	302
5.2.49.19	State Purchases of Eggs by Union Republics	303
5.2.49.20	State Purchases of Wool by Union Republics	303
5.2.50	Supply of Tractors, Lorries and Agricultural Machines to Agriculture	304
5.2.51	Number of Tractors in Agriculture by Union Republics	305
5.2.52	Number of Grain Harvesters in Agriculture by Union Republics	306
5.2.53	Supply of Mineral Fertilizers to Agriculture	307
5.2.54	Cadres in Agriculture	308
5.2.54.1	Average Annual Number of Persons engaged at Collective and State Farms, Subsidiary and Other Agricultural Prod.Enterpr.	308

XV

Index

5.2.54.2	Average Annual Number of all Collective Farmers participating in Work on Collective Farms, by Union Republics	309
5.2.54.3	Number of Specialists with Higher and Specialized Secondary Education Engaged at Collective and State Farms, Subsidiary and Other Agricultural Production Enterprises	310
5.2.54.4	Number of Specialists with Higher and Specialized Secondary Education Engaged at Collective and State Farms, Subsidiary and Other Agricultural Production Enterprises, by Union Rep.	311
5.2.54.5	Number of Leading Cadres on Collective Farms by Jobs and Union Republics	312
5.2.54.6	Number of Leading Cadres on State Farms by Jobs and Union Rep.	313
5.2.54.7	Number of Mechanist-Cadres at Collective and State Farms	314
5.2.54.8	Number of Mechanist-Cadres at Collective and State Farms by Union Republics	315
5.3	Transport and Communications	316
5.3.1	Freight Transport by All Types of Public Transport Facilities	316
5.3.2	Passenger Transport by All Types of Public Transport	317
5.3.3	Railway Transport	318
5.3.3.1	Length of Railway Network from the Ministry of Railways	318
5.3.3.2	Length of Railway Network from the Ministry of Railways by Union Republics	319
5.3.3.3	Passenger Traffic by Railway	319
5.3.4	Marine Transport	320
5.3.4.1	Basic Indicators of Marine Transport from the Ministry of the High-Sea Fleet	320
5.3.5	Inland Water Transport	321
5.3.5.1	Basic Indicators on Public Inland Waterway Transport	321
5.3.5.2	Freight Carried and Passenger Traffic in Public Inland Water Transport, by Union Republics	323
5.3.6	Pipeline	324
5.3.6.1	Pipeline for Petroleum and Petroleum Products	324
5.3.6.2	Gas Lines	324
5.3.7	Motor Transport	325
5.3.7.1	Basic Indicators for Freight Transport	325
5.3.7.2	Length of Motor Roads with Hard Pavement	325
5.3.7.3	Length of Motor Roads by Union Republics	326
5.3.7.4	Passenger Bus Transport in the Public Transportation System, by Union Republics	328
5.3.7.5	Municipal Passenger Transport with Buses of the Public Transport System	328
5.3.7.6	Suburban Passenger Transport with Buses of the Public Transport System	329
5.3.7.7	Utilization of Passenger Taxis in the Public Transp.System	329
5.3.8	Municipal Electrified Passenger Transportation	330
5.3.8.1	Development of Municipal Electrified Passenger Transportation	330
5.3.8.2	Passenger Transport on Subways by Union Republics	331
5.3.8.3	Length of Public Transportation Routes by Union Republics	332
5.3.8.4	Movable Stock of the Municipal Electrified Passenger Transport System by Union Republics	333
5.3.9	Air Traffic	334
5.3.9.1	Basic Indicators on Air Traffic from the Ministry of Civil Aviation	334
5.3.9.2	Basic Indicators on Air Traffic on an International Basis	335
5.3.10	Communications	336
5.3.10.1	Basic Indicators on Communication Development	336
5.3.10.2	Number of Post, Telegraph and Telephone Offices by Union Rep.	338
5.3.10.3	Number of Radio Receivers (Radio Sets, TV Sets and Rediffusion Loudspeakers) by Union Republics	339
5.4	Capital Construction	340
5.4.1	Commissioned Fixed Assets	340

5.4.2	Productive Capacities Commissioned by Expanding and Reconstructing Existing and Building New Enterprises	341
5.4.3	Investments by the State and Collective Farms in Agriculture	345
5.4.4	Structure of Investments in Fixed Assets	347
5.4.5	Number of Plants, Building and Other Projects which were Constructed, are Being Constructed or Are Planned with the Technical Aid of the USSR since 1945	348
5.4.6	Number of Enterprises, Buildings and Other Projects which were Constructed, Are Being Constructed or are planned in Foreign Countries with the Technical Aid of the USSR since 1945	349
5.5	Foreign Trade	351
5.5.1	Foreign Trade Turnover	351
5.5.2	Foreign Trade by Country Groups	352
5.5.3	Foreign Trade by Countries	353
5.5.4	Export Structure	364
5.5.5	Import Structure	365
5.5.6	Share of the Most Important Products in Export	366
5.5.7	Foreign Trade Organizations	369
6.	Labour	
6.1	Share of the Working-Age Population Based on Total Population	392
6.2	Educational Level of the Working-Age Population	396
6.3	Educational Level of the Population of the USSR by Professions	408
6.4	Average Annual Number of Workers and Employees by Branches of the National Economy	412
6.5	Average Annual Number of Workers and Employees in the National Economy	414
6.6	Percentage of Females in Relation to Total Number of Workers and Employees by Branches of the National Economy	415
6.7	Percentage of Females in Relation to Total Number of Workers and Employees by Union Republics	417
6.8	Percentage of Females in Relation to Average Annual Number of all Collective Farmers having Participated in the Work at Collective Farms, by Union Republics	417
6.9	Number of Female Specialists with Higher and Specialized Secondary Education, Engaged in the National Economy	418
6.10	Number of Woman Doctors in all Special Branches	418
6.11	Percentage of Workers and Employees of 55 Years of Age and Older by Branches of the National Economy	419
7.	Social Structure	
7.1	Breakdown of the Population of the USSR and the Union Republics by Social Groups	420
7.2	Breakdown of Gainfully Employed Population of the USSR and the Union Republics by Social Groups	426
7.3	Breakdown of the Population of the USSR and the Union Republics by Means of Income	432
7.4	Breakdown of the Population of the USSR and the Union Republics by Means of Income and Social Groups	437
7.5	Social Structure of the Population of the Union Republics 1939	449
7.6	Social Structure of the Population of the Union Republics 1959	450
8.	Science	
8.1	Academy of Sciences of the USSR, Academies of Sciences of the Union Republics and Branch Academies	451
8.2	Scientific Centers of the Academy of Sciences	453
8.3	Personnel Composition of the Academy of Sciences of the USSR	456
8.3.1	USSR Branch Academies	478
8.3.2	Academies of Sciences of the Union Republics	479
8.4	List of Institutes	480
8.5	Number of Persons Working in the Scientific Field	494
8.5.1	Number of Persons Engaged in the Scientific Field by Nationality	495
8.5.2	Number of Persons Engaged in the Scientific Field by Union Rep.	495

Index

8.5.3	Number of Females Engaged in the Scientific Field, by Union Rep.	496
8.5.4	Number of Aspirants	497
8.5.5	Number of Aspirants by Union Republics	498
8.5.6	Number of Female Aspirants	499
8.5.7	Breakdown of Aspirants by Nationalities and Ethnic Groups	500
8.6	Scientific and Technical Information	502

9. Education

9.1	Number of Pupils and Students by Types of Education	505
9.2	General Educational Day Schools by Union Republics	506
9.3	Graduates from General Educational Schools of All Types, by Union Republics	513
9.4	Percentage of Females in Relation to Total Number of Teachers at General Educational Day Schools	515
9.5	Number of Teachers at General Educational Day Schools by Jobs, Education and Duration of Their Pedagogical Occupation	516
9.6	Number of Teachers of the Upper Forms at General Educational Day Schools by Subjects and Education	521
9.7	General Educational Evening (Shift) Schools in the Union Republics	522
9.8	Permanent Preparatory Educational Establishments in the Union Rep.	524
9.9	Number of Other Educational Institutions of the USSR Ministry of Education	527
9.10	Music, Art and Ballet Schools of the USSR Ministry of Culture in the Union Republics	528

10. Printing and Publishing

10.1	Publication of Books and Brochures in the Languages of the USSR and Foreign Languages in 1976	529
10.2	Books and Booklets in Russian and in Other Languages of USSR Peoples	534
10.3	Book Production by Subjects	534
10.4	Publication of Literature (Books and Brochures) Divided by Subjects for the Year 1976	538
10.5	Publication of Books and Brochures Divided by Subjects for the Year 1976	544
10.6	Publication of Books and Brochures by Subjects	548
10.7	Publication of Periodicals and Serialized Literature (without Newspapers)	551
10.8	Publication of Periodicals and Serials (without Newspapers) in the Languages of the Main Nationalities of the USSR for 1976	553
10.9	Publication of Periodicals and Serials (without newspapers) by Subjects for the Year 1976	554
10.10	Publication of Periodicals and Serials (without Newspapers) by Destination for the Year 1976	557
10.11	Publication of Newspapers by Types	559
10.12	Publication of Newspapers in the Languages of the Nationalities of the USSR and Foreign Languages in 1976	561

11. Standard of Living, Social Security

11.1	Income of the Population	562
11.1.1	Growth of the Real Income of the Population	562
11.1.2	Average Monthly Wages and Salaries of Workers and Employees in the National Economy	562
11.1.3	Average Monthly Wages and Salaries of Workers and Employees by Branches of the National Economy	563
11.1.4	Growth of the Monthly Wages and Salaries of Workers & Employees	565
11.1.5	Average Monthly Wage and Salary in the National Economy and in Branches with Highest and Lowest Wage and Salary Bracket	565
11.1.6	Correlation Between Average and Minimum Wage and Salary	565
11.1.7	Growth of Pay of Kolkhoz Workers	566
11.1.8	Share of Income from Private Farming of Total Income of Industrial and Kolkhoz Workers	566

11.1.9	Allowances and Benefits for the Population out of the Public Consumer Funds	567
11.1.10	Growth of Allowances and Benefits for the Population out of the Public Consumer Funds	568
11.2	Housing Construction	569
11.2.1	Number of Newly Built Apartment Houses	569
11.2.2	Municipal Housing Fund	570
11.2.3	Housing Funds of the Capitals of the Union Republics	571
11.3	Retail Trade	571
11.3.1	Retail Stores and Sales Floor Space of State and Cooperative Organizations in the Union Republics	571
11.3.2	Communal Catering Organizations and Number of Available Places in the Union Republics	572
11.3.3	Self-Service Shops	573
11.3.4	Growth in Trade Turnover and Retail Outlets	574
11.3.5	Provision of City and Rural Population with Durable Consumer and Household Goods	575
11.4	Health	576
11.4.1	Basic Indicators of the Development of Health Services	576
11.4.2	Number of Doctors of All Special Branches by Union Republics	579
11.4.3	Number of Woman Doctors of All Special Branches	580
11.4.4	Number of Medical Facilities for Ambulant Treatment	580
11.4.5	Growth in Number of Hospitals and Hospital Beds	581

12. Public Organizations

12.1	List of Leading Public Organizations	582
12.2	Trade Unions	584
12.2.1	Number of Trade Union Members at USSR Trade Union Congresses	584
12.2.2	Chairmen of the All-Union Central Council of Trade Unions	585
12.2.3	All-Union Central Council of Trade Unions	585
12.2.4	CCs of the Branch Trade Unions	585
12.2.5	Trade Union Councils of the Union Republics	587
12.2.6	Societies and Organizations Working under the Guidance of Trade Unions	588
12.3	All-Union Leninist Young Communist League	588
12.3.1	Number of Members at Komsomol Congresses	588
12.3.2	CC of USSR Komsomol	590
12.3.3	CCs of the Komsomol of the Union Republics	591
12.3.4	Number of CPSU Members and Candidates within the Komsomol	591
12.3.5	All-Union Pioneers Organization	592
12.4	Number of Members of some Voluntary All-Union Societies	592
12.5	Additional Information on Some Public Organizations	593

13. Religion

13.1	Council for Religious Affairs at the USSR Council of Ministers	596
13.2	General Data	596
13.3	The Russian Orthodox Church	597
13.4	The Georgian Orthodox Church	599
13.5	The Armenian Gregorian Church	599
13.6	The Old Believers	599
13.7	Islam	599
13.8	The Roman Catholic Church	600
13.9	The Evangelical Lutheran Church	600
13.10	The Evangelical Christians-Baptists	600
13.11	Judaism	600
13.12	Buddhism	601
13.13	Other Denominations	601
13.14	Most Important Illegal Churches and Sects	601

Index

14. Miscellaneous Information
14.1	Soviet Anthem	603
14.2	Territorial Expansion after the Second World War	604
14.3	The Boundaries of the USSR	604
14.4	The Highest Mountains	605
14.5	Volcanoes	605
14.6	The Principal Rivers	605
14.7	The Biggest Lakes	606
14.8	The Principal Peninsulas	607
14.9	Economy	607
14.9.1	Official Exchange Rate of the Ruble (March 1978)	607
14.9.2	Five-Year Plans	609
14.9.3	Wheat Imports	609
14.9.4	Mineral Oil and Mineral Oil Products Exports	609
14.9.5	Natural Gas Export	610
14.9.6	Share of Agricultural Production of Private Subsidiary Enterprises	610
14.10	Other Organizations and Institutions of CPSU CC	611
14.11	Press Agencies	611
14.12	USSR Orders	
14.13	Some Cultural Institutions	613
14.13.1	Libraries	613
14.13.2	Public Libraries in the Union Republics	613
14.13.3	Number of Theatres in the Union Republics	613
14.13.4	Circuses	614
14.13.5	Number of Museums in the Union Republics	614

SYSTEMATISCHE INHALTSÜBERSICHT

1.	**Administrativ-territoriale Zusammensetzung**	
1.1	Unionsrepubliken	1
1.2	Unionsrepubliken (Territorium und Hauptstädte)	4
1.3	Autonome Republiken	5
1.4	Autonome Gebiete, nationale Kreise, Krajs, Oblast, Rayons und Dorfsowjets in den Unionsrepubliken	6
1.5	Städte, städtische Siedlungen und Rayons in den Städten	6
2.	**Bevölkerung**	
2.1	Bevölkerung 1897-1977	7
2.2	Bevölkerung der UdSSR und der Unionsrepubliken	8
2.2.1	Stadtbevölkerung	9
2.2.2	Landbevölkerung	9
2.3	Bevölkerung der Unionsrepubliken	10
2.4	Bevölkerung der Wirtschaftsrayons, Autonomen Republiken, Krai und Oblasti	12
2.5	Städte mit über 50.000 Einwohnern	24
2.6	Bevölkerungszuwachs	33
2.7	Städte und städtische Siedlungen nach Einwohnerzahl	34
2.8	Männer und Frauen	35
2.9	Bevölkerung nach Geschlechtern	36
2.9.1	Stadtbevölkerung	37
2.9.2	Landbevölkerung	38
2.10	Verteilung der Bevölkerung nach Geschlecht und Alter	40
2.10.1	Stadtbevölkerung	40
2.10.2	Landbevölkerung	42
2.11	Völker der Sowjetunion	46
2.11.1	Hauptnationen der Unionsrepubliken	46
2.11.2	Völker der Sowjetunion nach ethnisch-linguistischen Gruppen	47
2.11.3	Nationale Zusammensetzung der Bevölkerung	51
2.11.4	Anteil der Hauptnationen an der Bevölkerung der UdSSR und den Unionsrepubliken	54
3.	**Kommunistische Partei der Sowjetunion**	
3.1	Parteitage	57
3.2	Mitgliederzahlen 1917-1975	59
3.3	Politbüro ZK KPdSU	62
3.3.1	Sekretariat ZK KPdSU	75
3.4	Soziale Zusammensetzung der KPdSU	83
3.4.1	Soziale Zusammensetzung	83
3.4.2	Zusammensetzung der Angestellten-Kommunisten nach Berufen	83
3.5	Bildungsstand der Kommunisten	84
3.5.1	Bildungsstand der Kommunisten (in Tausend)	84
3.5.2	Bildungsstand der Kommunisten (in Prozent)	85
3.5.3	Zahl der Kommunisten mit Akademischem Grad	85
3.6	Frauen in der KPdSU	86
3.7	Nationale Zusammensetzung der KPdSU	87
3.7.1	Anteil der Hauptnationen	87
3.7.2	Nationale Zusammensetzung nach dem 1.1.1976	88
3.8	Grundorganisationen der Partei	89
3.8.1	Netz der Grundorganisationen	89
3.8.2	Grundorganisationen der Partei nach Anteil der Kommunisten	90
3.8.3	Verteilung der Kommunisten nach Wirtschaftszweigen	90

Inhaltsübersicht

3.8.4	Struktur der Grundorganisationen der Partei	91
3.9	Gewählte leitende Organe der Partei	95
3.9.1	ZK der KPdSU	95
3.9.2	Politbüro ZK KPdSU	95
3.9.3	Sekretariat ZK KPdSU	97
3.9.4	Netz der leitenden Parteiorgane	98
3.9.5	Gewählte leitende Organe der Partei der Unionsrepubliken	98
3.10	Ernannter Parteiapparat	109
3.10.1	Apparat des ZK der KPdSU unter der Leitung des ZK-Sekretar.	109
3.10.2	Apparate der ZKs der KPs der Unionsrepubliken	110
3.10.3	Ernannter Apparat der lokalen Parteiorganisationen	112
4.	Staatsordnung	
4.1	Sowjetische Staatsorgane	114
4.2.1	Zahl der Sowjets der Volksdeputierten	117
4.2.2	Vorsitzende des Präsidiums des Obersten Sowjets der UdSSR	117
4.2.3	Zahl der gewählten Deputierten des Obersten Sowjets d.UdSSR	118
4.2.4	Oberster Sowjet der UdSSR	118
4.2.5	Zusammensetzung der Deputierten des Obersten Sowjets d.UdSSR	120
4.3	Ministerrat der UdSSR	122
4.3.1	Vorsitzende des Ministerrates der UdSSR	122
4.3.2	Zusammensetzung des Ministerrates der UdSSR	123
4.3.3	Außenministerium der UdSSR	127
4.3.4	Verteidigungsministerium der UdSSR	133
4.4	Oberste Sowjets und Ministerräte der Unionsrepubliken	139
4.4.1	RSFSR	139
4.4.2	Ukrainskaja SSR	141
4.4.3	Belorusskaja SSR	144
4.4.4	Uzbekskaja SSR	146
4.4.5	Kazachskaja SSR	149
4.4.6	Gruzinskaja SSR	151
4.4.7	Azerbajdžanskaja SSR	154
4.4.8	Litovskaja SSR	156
4.4.9	Moldavskaja SSR	158
4.4.10	Latvijskaja SSR	161
4.4.11	Kirgizskaja SSR	163
4.4.12	Tadžikskaja SSR	165
4.4.13	Armjanskaja SSR	167
4.4.14	Turkmenskaja SSR	169
4.4.15	Estonskaja SSR	172
5.	Wirtschaft	
5.1	Industrie	174
5.1.1	Produktion der wichtigsten Industriezweige	174
5.1.2	Elektroenergie	192
5.1.2.1	Kapazität der Elektrizitätswerke und Elektroenergieerzeugung	192
5.1.2.2	Verbrauch an Elektroenergie	193
5.1.2.3	Energetische Kapazitäten und Verbrauch an Elektroenergie nach den wichtigsten Industriezweigen	194
5.1.2.4	Energetische Kapazitäten in den Kraftwerken der UdSSR	195
5.1.2.5	Elektroenergieerzeugung pro Kopf der Bevölkerung	195
5.1.2.6	Elektroenergieerzeugung in den Unionsrepubliken	196
5.1.3	Eisen- und Stahlindustrie	197
5.1.3.1	Produktion von Roheisen, Stahl, Eisen- und Stahlwalzgut und Stahlrohren	197
5.1.3.2	Gewinnung von Eisen- und Manganerz (Handelsware)	198
5.1.3.3	Roheisengewinnung in den Unionsrepubliken	198
5.1.3.4	Stahlgewinnung in den Unionsrepubliken	199

5.1.3.5	Produktion von fertigem Eisen- und Stahlwalzgut in den Unionsrepubliken	199
5.1.4	Brennstoffindustrie	200
5.1.4.1	Brennstoffgewinnung nach Arten	200
5.1.4.2	Kohlegewinnung nach Arten	201
5.1.4.3	Kohlegewinnung in den Unionsrepubliken	202
5.1.4.4	Erdölgewinnung (mit Gaskondensat) in den Unionsrepubliken	202
5.1.4.5	Gasgewinnung in den Unionsrepubliken	203
5.1.5	Maschinenbau und metallbearbeitende Industrie	204
5.1.5.1	Produktion von Ausrüstungen für verschiedene Industriezweige	204
5.1.5.2	Produktion von Geräten, Automatisationsmitteln und EDV	206
5.1.5.3	Produktion von chemischen Ausrüstungen	207
5.1.5.4	Produktion von Hebe- und Transportausrüstungen	208
5.1.5.5	Produktion von technologischen Ausrüstungen für die Leicht-, Nahrungsmittel- und polygraphische Industrie und für Betriebe des Handels und der öffentlichen Ernährung	209
5.1.5.6	Produktion von sanitär-technischen Ausrüstungen	213
5.1.5.7	Produktion von Landwirtschaftsmaschinen	214
5.1.5.8	Produktion von Traktoren nach Arten	216
5.1.6	Chemische Industrie	217
5.1.6.1	Produktion von Mineraldünger nach Arten	217
5.1.6.2	Produktion von Mineraldünger in den Unionsrepubliken	218
5.1.6.3	Produktion von synthetischen Harzen und Kunststoffen	218
5.1.6.4	Produktion von chemischen Fasern	219
5.1.6.5	Produktion von Kraftfahrzeug- und Fahrraddecken	220
5.1.7	Forst-, holzbearbeitende und Zellulose-Papier-Industrie	221
5.1.7.1	Nutzholzeinschlag	221
5.1.7.2	Erschließung der waldreichen Regionen	221
5.1.7.3	Produktion von Schnittholz und Furnierplatten	223
5.1.7.4	Produktion von Schnittholz in den Unionsrepubliken	223
5.1.7.5	Holzeinschlag in den Unionsrepubliken	224
5.1.7.6	Produktion von Zellulose, Papier und Karton	226
5.1.7.7	Papiererzeugung in den Unionsrepubliken	226
5.1.8	Baustoffindustrie	227
5.1.8.1	Zementerzeugung nach Sorten im Jahre 1975	227
5.1.8.2	Zementerzeugung in den Unionsrepubliken	227
5.1.8.3	Produktion einzelner Arten von montierbaren Stahlbetonkonstruktionen und Details	228
5.1.8.4	Produktion von Baustoffen nach Arten	229
5.1.8.5	Produktion von Bedachungsmaterialien	230
5.1.8.6	Produktion von Linoleum	230
5.1.9	Leichtindustrie	231
5.1.9.1	Produktion der wichtigsten Erzeugnisse der Leichtindustrie	231
5.1.9.2	Produktion von Baumwollgeweben nach Unionsrepubliken	233
5.1.9.3	Produktion von Wollgeweben nach Unionsrepubliken	233
5.1.9.4	Produktion von Leinengeweben nach Unionsrepubliken	234
5.1.9.5	Produktion von Seidengeweben nach Unionsrepubliken	234
5.1.9.6	Produktion von Baumwollfasern nach Unionsrepubliken	234
5.1.9.7	Produktion von Rohseide nach Unionsrepubliken	235
5.1.9.8	Produktion von Strumpf-Socken-Erzeugnissen n.Unionsrepubliken	235
5.1.9.9	Produktion von Wäschetrikotagen nach Unionsrepubliken	236
5.1.9.10	Produktion von Obertrikotagen nach Unionsrepubliken	236
5.1.9.11	Produktion von Geweben und Trikotagenerzeugnissen unter Verwendung von chemischen Fasern	237
5.1.10	Nahrungsmittelindustrie	238
5.1.10.1	Produktion der wichtigsten Erzeugnisse der Nahrungsmittelindustrie	238
5.1.10.2	Produktion von Streuzucker und Raffinade	239
5.1.10.3	Produktion von Streuzucker in den Unionsrepubliken	239

Inhaltsübersicht

5.1.10.4	Fleischproduktion nach Arten	240
5.1.10.5	Fleischproduktion nach Unionsrepubliken	240
5.1.10.6	Produktion von tierischen Fetten nach Unionsrepubliken	241
5.1.10.7	Produktion von pflanzlichen Fetten nach Unionsrepubliken	241
5.1.10.8	Konservenproduktion nach Arten	242
5.2	Landwirtschaft	243
5.2.1	Bruttoproduktion der Landwirtschaft nach Unionsrepubliken	243
5.2.1.1	Produktion von Getreide u.Feldfrüchten - Viehwirtschaft	244
5.2.2	Erzeugung der landwirtschaftlichen Produkte	245
5.2.3	Bruttoernteertrag der landwirtschaftlichen Kulturen	247
5.2.4	Anteil der Produktion landwirtschaftlicher Grunderzeugnisse der Kolchosen,Sowchosen und anderen staatlichen landwirtschaftlichen Betrieben an der Gesamtproduktion	248
5.2.5	Marktproduktion der Landwirtschaft	250
5.2.6	Anteil der Warenproduktion der gesellschaftlichen Landwirtschaft der Kolchosen,Sowchosen und anderen staatlichen Wirtschaft an der gemeinsamen Warenproduktion	251
5.2.7	Bruttoernteertrag an Getreide nach Unionsrepubliken	253
5.2.8	Bruttoernteertrag an Winter-u.Sommerweizen n.Unionsrepubliken	253
5.2.9	Bruttoernteertrag an Winter-u.Sommerroggen n.Unionsrepubliken	254
5.2.10	Bruttoernteertrag an Körnermais nach Unionsrepubliken	254
5.2.11	Bruttoernteertrag an Hirse nach Unionsrepubliken	254
5.2.12	Bruttoernteertrag an Buchweizen nach Unionsrepubliken	255
5.2.13	Bruttoernteertrag an Reis nach Unionsrepubliken	255
5.2.14	Bruttoernteertrag an Hülsenfrüchten nach Unionsrepubliken	255
5.2.15	Bruttoernteertrag an Zuckerrüben nach Unionsrepubliken	256
5.2.16	Bruttoernteertrag an Flachsfaser nach Unionsrepubliken	256
5.2.17	Bruttoernteertrag an Sonnenblumensamen nach Unionsrepubliken	256
5.2.18	Bruttoernteertrag an Kartoffeln nach Unionsrepubliken	256
5.2.19	Bruttoernteertrag an Gemüse nach Unionsrepubliken	257
5.2.20	Bruttoernteertrag an Weintrauben nach Unionsrepubliken	257
5.2.21	Bruttoernteertrag an Obst und Beerenobst nach Unionsrepubliken	258
5.2.22	Getreideanbaufläche nach Unionsrepubliken	258
5.2.23	Winterweizenanbaufläche nach Unionsrepubliken	259
5.2.24	Sommerweizenanbaufläche nach Unionsrepubliken	259
5.2.25	Gesamtanbaufläche an Winter- und Sommerroggen n.Unionsrep.	260
5.2.26	Anbaufläche an Körnermais nach Unionsrepubliken	260
5.2.27	Hirseanbaufläche nach Unionsrepubliken	260
5.2.28	Anbaufläche an Buchweizen nach Unionsrepubliken	260
5.2.29	Reisanbaufläche nach Unionsrepubliken	261
5.2.30	Anbaufläche an Hülsenfrüchten nach Unionsrepubliken	261
5.2.31	Gesamtanbaufläche an technischen Kulturen n.Unionsrepubliken	261
5.2.32	Baumwollanbaufläche nach Unionsrepubliken	262
5.2.33	Anbaufläche an Zuckerrüben nach Unionsrepubliken	262
5.2.34	Anbaufläche an Faserlein nach Unionsrepubliken	262
5.2.35	Anbaufläche an Sonnenblumensamen nach Unionsrepubliken	263
5.2.36	Kartoffelanbaufläche nach Unionsrepubliken	263
5.2.37	Gemüseanbaufläche nach Unionsrepubliken	263
5.2.38	Anbaufläche an Viehfutter nach Unionsrepubliken	264
5.2.39	Anbaufläche an mehr- und einjährigen Gräsern einschl. Winteraussaat für Grünfutter nach Unionsrepubliken	264
5.2.40	Bewässerte Bodenfläche in Kolchosen, Sowchosen und anderen staatlichen Wirtschaften nach Unionsrepubliken	265
5.2.41	Anbaufläche an landwirtschaftl.Kulturen auf dem bewässerten Boden in Kolchosen,Sowchosen u.a.staatl.Wirtschaften nach Unionsrepubliken	266
5.2.42	Obst- und Weinbau	267
5.2.43	Weinbaufläche aller Wachstumsphasen nach Unionsrepubliken	265

Inhaltsübersicht

5.2.44	Weinbaufläche im fruchttragenden Stadium n.Unionsrepubliken	268
5.2.45	Teeanbaufläche nach Unionsrepubliken	268
5.2.46	Viehwirtschaft	269
5.2.46.1	Viehbestand	269
5.2.46.2	Nutzviehbestand in den einzelnen landwirtschaftl.Betrieben	270
5.2.46.3	Rinderbestand nach Unionsrepubliken	272
5.2.46.4	Kühebestand nach Unionsrepubliken	272
5.2.46.5	Schweinebestand nach Unionsrepubliken	273
5.2.46.6	Schaf- und Ziegenbestand nach Unionsrepubliken	273
5.2.46.7	Schafbestand nach Unionsrepubliken	274
5.2.46.8	Geflügelbestand nach Unionsrepubliken	274
5.2.46.9	Grunderzeugnisse der Viehwirtschaft	275
5.2.46.10	Grunderzeugnisse der Viehwirtschaft nach Unionsrepubliken	277
5.2.46.11	Fleischerzeugung nach Unionsrepubliken	278
5.2.46.12	Milcherzeugung nach Unionsrepubliken	278
5.2.46.13	Eierproduktion nach Unionsrepubliken	279
5.2.46.14	Erzeugung von Wolle nach Unionsrepubliken	279
5.2.47	Kolchosen	280
5.2.47.1	Hauptkennziffern der Entwicklung der Kolchosen	280
5.2.47.2	Gliederung der Kolchosen nach Höhe des Bruttoeinkommens pro 100 ha Ackerland	283
5.2.47.3	Gliederung der Kolchosen nach Anzahl der Höfe	284
5.2.47.4	Gliederung der Kolchosen nach Viehbestand	285
5.2.47.5	Hauptkennziffern der Entwicklung der Kolchosen nach Unionsrepubliken	286
5.2.48	Sowchosen	288
5.2.48.1	Anzahl der Sowchosen	288
5.2.48.2	Grundkennziffern der Entwicklung der Sowchosen	289
5.2.48.3	Anzahl der Sowchosen nach Unionsrepubliken	291
5.2.49	Staatliche Aufkäufe von landwirtschaftlichen Erzeugnissen	292
5.2.49.1	Anteil der Aufkäufe der landwirtschaftl.Grunderzeugnisse in den Kolchosen, Sowchosen und anderen staatlichen Betrieben an den gesamten staatlichen Aufkäufen	292
5.2.49.2	Staatl.Aufkäufe von landwirtschaftl.Erzeugnissen	293
5.2.49.3	Staatl.Aufkäufe von Grunderzeugnissen der Landwirtschaft	295
5.2.49.4	Staatl.Aufkäufe an Getreidekulturen nach Unionsrepubliken	296
5.2.49.5	Staatl.Aufkäufe an Weizen nach Unionsrepubliken	297
5.2.49.6	Staatl.Aufkäufe an Roggen nach Unionsrepubliken	297
5.2.49.7	Staatl.Aufkäufe an Zuckerrüben nach Unionsrepubliken	297
5.2.49.8	Staatl.Aufkäufe an Flachsfasern nach Unionsrepubliken	298
5.2.49.9	Staatl.Aufkäufe an Sonnenblumensamen nach Unionsrepubliken	298
5.2.49.10	Staatl.Aufkäufe an Kartoffeln nach Unionsrepubliken	298
5.2.49.11	Staatl.Aufkäufe an Gemüse nach Unionsrepubliken	299
5.2.49.12	Staatl.Aufkäufe an Obst und Beeren nach Unionsrepubliken	299
5.2.49.13	Staatl.Aufkäufe von Weintrauben nach Unionsrepubliken	299
5.2.49.14	Bruttoernteertrag (Aufkäufe) an Sortenteeblättern nach Unionsrepubliken	300
5.2.49.15	Staatl.Aufkäufe von Grunderzeugnissen der Viehwirtschaft	300
5.2.49.16	Staatl.Aufkäufe von Vieh und Geflügel nach Unionsrepubliken (Lebendgewicht)	301
5.2.49.17	Staatl.Aufkäufe von Vieh und Geflügel nach Unionsrepubliken (umgerechnet auf Schlachtgewicht)	302
5.2.49.18	Staatl.Aufkäufe von Milch u.Milchprodukten n.Unionsrep.	302
5.2.49.19	Staatl.Aufkäufe von Eiern nach Unionsrepubliken	303
5.2.49.20	Staatl.Aufkäufe von Wolle nach Unionsrepubliken	303
5.2.50	Belieferung der Landwirtschaft mit Traktoren, Lastkraftwagen und Landmaschinen	304
5.2.51	Traktorenpark in der Landwirtschaft nach Unionsrepubliken	305
5.2.52	Mähdrescherpark in der Landwirtschaft nach Unionsrepubliken	306

Inhaltsübersicht

5.2.53	Belieferung der Landwirtschaft mit mineralischen Düngemitteln	307
5.2.54	Kader in der Landwirtschaft	308
5.2.54.1	Jahresdurchschnittszahl der Beschäftigten in Kolchosen, Sowchosen,Neben-u.anderen landwirtschaftl.Produktionsbetr.	308
5.2.54.2	Jahresdurchschnittszahl aller Kolchosbauern, die sich an der Arbeit der Kolchosen beteiligen, nach Unionsrepubliken	309
5.2.54.3	Anzahl der Spezialisten mit Hochschul-u.mittl.Fachschulbildung, die in Kolchosen,Sowchosen,Neben- u.anderen landwirtschaftl.Produktionsbetrieben beschäftigt sind	310
5.2.54.4	Anzahl der Spezialisten mit Hoch-u.mittl.Fachschulbildung, die in Kolchosen,Sowchosen,Neben-u.anderen landwirtschaftl. Produktionsbetrieben beschäftigt sind,nach Unionsrepubliken	311
5.2.54.5	Anzahl der leitenden Kader der Kolchosen nach ihren Posten, nach Unionsrepubliken	312
5.2.54.6	Anzahl der leitenden Kader der Sowchosen nach ihren Posten, nach Unionsrepubliken	313
5.2.54.7	Anzahl der Mechanisatoren-Kader in Kolchosen u.Sowchosen	314
5.2.54.8	Anzahl der Mechanisatoren-Kader in Kolchosen u.Sowchosen nach Unionsrepubliken	315
5.3	Transport-, Post- und Fernmeldewesen	316
5.3.1	Gütertransportleistung aller Transportzweige des öffentlichen Verkehrs	316
5.3.2	Personenbeförderungsleistung aller Transportzweige des öffentlichen Verkehrs	317
5.3.3	Eisenbahntransport	318
5.3.3.1	Länge des benutzten Eisenbahnnetzes des Ministeriums für Verkehrswesen	318
5.3.3.2	Länge des benutzten Eisenbahnnetzes des Ministeriums für Verkehrswesen nach Unionsrepubliken	319
5.3.3.3	Personenbeförderung per Bahn	319
5.3.4	Seetransport	320
5.3.4.1	Grundkennziffern des Seetransports des Ministeriums für Hochseeschiffahrt	320
5.3.5	Binnenwassertransport	321
5.3.5.1	Grundkennziffern des öffentlichen Binnenwassertransports	321
5.3.5.2	Gütertransport und Personenbeförderung im öffentlichen Binnenwassertransport, nach Unionsrepubliken	323
5.3.6	Rohrfernleitungen	324
5.3.6.1	Rohrfernleitungen für Erdöl und Erdölprodukte	324
5.3.7	Kraftverkehr	325
5.3.7.1	Grundkennziffern des volkswirtschaftl.Kraftverkehrs	325
5.3.7.2	Länge der Autostraßen mit harter Decke	325
5.3.7.3	Länge der Autostraßen nach Unionsrepubliken	326
5.3.7.4	Personenbeförderung mit Autobussen der öffentlichen Verkehrsmittel, nach Unionsrepubliken	328
5.3.7.5	Städtische Personenbeförderung mit Autobussen der öffentlichen Verkehrsmittel	328
5.3.7.6	Vorort-Personenbeförderung mit Autobussen der öffentlichen Verkehrsmittel	329
5.3.7.7	Nutzung der Personentaxi d.öffentl.Verkehrsmittel	329
5.3.8	Städtische elektrifizierte Personenverkehrsmittel	330
5.3.8.1	Entwicklung der städtischen elektrifzierten Personenverkehrsmittel	330
5.3.8.2	Passagierbeförderung in U-Bahnen nach Unionsrepubliken	331
5.3.8.3	Länge der benutzten Verkehrswege nach Unionsrepubliken	332
5.3.8.4	Beweglicher Bestand der städtischen elektrifizierten Verkehrsmittel nach Unionsrepubliken	333
5.3.9	Luftverkehr	334
5.3.9.1	Grundkennziffern des Luftverkehrs des Ministeriums für zivile Luftfahrt	334

Inhaltsübersicht

5.3.9.2	Grundkennziffern des Luftverkehrs auf internationaler Ebene	335
5.3.10	Post- und Fernmeldewesen	336
5.3.10.1	Grundkennziffern der Entwicklung des Post-u.Fernmeldewesens	336
5.3.10.2	Anzahl der Post-, Telegraphen-u.Telephonämter n.Unionsrep.	338
5.3.10.3	Anzahl der Funkempfangsanschlüsse(Rundfunkgeräte, Fernsehgeräte u.drahtfunkleitstellen) nach Unionsrepubliken	339
5.4	Investitionsbau	340
5.4.1	Inanspruchnahme der Grundfonds	341
5.4.2	Anteil der Produktionskapazitäten durch Erweiterung und Rekonstruktion von bestehenden und Bau von neuen Betrieben	341
5.4.3	Investitionen des Staates u.d.Kolchosen i.d.Landwirtschaft	345
5.4.4	Struktur der Investitionen	347
5.4.5	Anzahl der Betriebe,Bauten u.a.Objekte, die seit 1945 mit techn. Hilfe der UdSSR im Ausland gebaut wurden, sich im Bau befinden oder gebaut werden sollen	348
5.4.6	Anzahl der Betriebe,Bauten u.a.Objekte, die seit 1945 mit techn. Hilfe der UdSSR im Ausland gebaut wurden, sich im Bau befinden oder gebaut werden sollen, nach Wirtschaftszweigen	349
5.5	Außenwirtschaftliche Beziehungen	351
5.5.1	Außenhandelsumsatz	351
5.5.2	Außenhandel nach Ländergruppen	352
5.5.3	Außenhandelsumsatz nach Ländern	353
5.5.4	Struktur des Exports	364
5.5.5	Struktur des Imports	365
5.5.6	Anteil der wichtigsten Güter am Export	366
5.5.7	Außenhandelsorganisationen	369
6.	Arbeitsreserven	
6.1	Anteil der Bevölkerung im arbeitsfähigen Alter an der Gesamtbevölkerung	392
6.2	Bildungsstand der Bevölkerung im arbeitsfähigen Alter	396
6.3	Bildungsstand der Bevölkerung der UdSSR nach Berufen	408
6.4	Jahresdurchschnittszahl der Arbeiter und Angestellten nach Volkswirtschaftsbereichen	412
6.5	Jahresdurchschnittszahl der Arbeiter und Angestellten in der Volkswirtschaft	414
6.6	Prozentualer Anteil der Frauen an der Gesamtzahl der Arbeiter und Angestellten nach Volkswirtschaftszweigen	415
6.7	Prozentualer Anteil der Frauen an der Gesamtzahl der Arbeiter und Angestellten nach Unionsrepubliken	417
6.8	Prozentualer Anteil der Frauen a.d.Jahresdurchschnittszahl aller Kolchosbauern,die sich an Arbeiten in den Kolchosen beteiligt haben, nach Unionsrepubliken	417
6.9	Zahl der in der Volkswirtschaft beschäftigten Frauen-Spezialisten mit Hochschul- und mittlerer Fachschulbildung	418
6.10	Zahl der Ärztinnen aller Fachrichtungen	418
6.11	Prozentualer Anteil von Arbeitern und Angestellten, die 55 Jahre alt und älter sind, nach Volkswirtschaftszweigen	419
7.	Soziale Struktur	
7.1	Aufteilung der Bevölkerung der UdSSR und der Unionsrepubliken nach gesellschaftlichen Gruppen	420
7.2	Aufteilung der beschäftigten Bevölkerung der UdSSR und der Unionsrepubliken nach gesellschaftlichen Gruppen	426
7.3	Aufteilung der Bevölkerung der UdSSR und der Unionsrepubliken nach Einkommensquellen	432
7.4	Aufteilung der Bevölkerung der UdSSR und der Unionsrepubliken nach Einkommensquellen und gesellschaftlichen Gruppen	437
7.5	Soziale Struktur der Bevölkerung der Unionsrepubliken 1939	449
7.6	Soziale Struktur der Bevölkerung der Unionsrepubliken 1959	450

XXVII

Inhaltsübersicht

8. Wissenschaft

8.1	Akademie der Wissenschaften der UdSSR, Akademien der Wissenschaften der Unionsrepubliken und Branchenakademien	451
8.2	Wissenschaftliche Zentren der Akademie der Wissenschaften	453
8.3	Personelle Zusammensetzung der Akademie d.Wissenschaften d.UdSSR	456
8.3.1	Zweigakademien der UdSSR	478
8.3.2	Akademien der Wissenschaften der Unionsrepubliken	479
8.4	Verzeichnis der Institute	480
8.5	Zahl der im wissenschaftl.Bereich tätigen Personen	494
8.5.1	Zahl der im wissenschaftl.Bereich tätigen Personen nach Nationalität	495
8.5.2	Zahl der im wissenschaftl.Bereich tätigen Personen nach Unionsrepubliken	495
8.5.3	Zahl der im wissenschaftl.Bereich tätigen Frauen nach Unionsrepubliken	496
8.5.4	Zahl der Aspiranten	497
8.5.5	Zahl der Aspiranten nach Unionsrepubliken	498
8.5.6	Zahl der Frauen-Aspiranten	499
8.5.7	Aufteilung der Aspiranten nach Nationalität bzw. ethnischer Abstammung	500
8.6	Wissenschaftlich-technische Information	502

9. Bildungswesen

9.1	Zahl der Schüler und Studenten nach Schularten	505
9.2	Allgemeinbildende Tagesschulen nach Unionsrepubliken	506
9.3	Absolventen aus den allgemeinbildenden Schulen aller Arten nach Unionsrepubliken	513
9.4	Anteil der Frauen an der Gesamtzahl der Lehrer der allgemeinbildenden Tagesschulen	515
9.5	Zahl der Lehrer an allgemeinbildenden Tagesschulen nach Posten, Bildung und Dauer ihrer pädagogischen Tätigkeit	516
9.6	Zahl der Lehrer der oberen Klassen der allgemeinbildenden Tagesschulen nach Fächern und Bildung	521
9.7	Allgemeinbildende Abend(Schicht-)schulen i.d.Unionsrepubliken	522
9.8	Ständige Vorschuleinrichtungen in den Unionsrepubliken	524
9.9	Zahl der außerschulischen Einrichtungen des Ministeriums für Volksbildung der UdSSR	527
9.10	Musik-, Kunst- und Ballettschulen des Kulturministeriums der UdSSR in den Unionsrepubliken	528

10. Druck- und Verlagswesen

10.1	Publikation von Büchern und Broschüren in den Sprachen der Völker der UdSSR und der Völker des Auslands im Jahre 1976	529
10.1.1	in den Unionsrepubliken	532
10.2	Bücher u.Broschüren in russischer Sprache und in Sprachen anderer Völker der UdSSR	534
10.3	Buchproduktion in thematischer Aufteilung	534
10.4	Publikation von Literatur (Bücher und Broschüren) in thematischer Aufteilung im Jahre 1976	538
10.5	Publikation von Büchern und Broschüren in thematischer Aufteilung im Jahre 1976	544
10.6	Publikation von Büchern und Broschüren nach Zielbestimmung	548
10.7	Publikation von periodischen und Fortsetzungspublikationen (ohne Zeitungen)	551
10.8	Publikation von periodischen und Fortsetzungspublikationen (ohne Zeitungen) in den Sprachen der Hauptnationen der UdSSR im Jahre 1976	553
10.9	Publikation von periodischen und Fortsetzungspublikationen (ohne Zeitungen) in thematischer Aufteilung im Jahre 1976	554

10.10	Publikation von periodischen und Fortsetzungspublikationen (ohne Zeitungen) nach Zielbestimmung im Jahre 1976	557
10.11	Publikation von Zeitungen nach Typen	559
10.12	Publikation von Zeitungen in den Sprachen der Völker der UdSSR und des Auslands im Jahre 1976	561

11. Lebensstandard, Sozialfürsorge

11.1	Einkommen der Bevölkerung	562
11.1.1	Wachstum des Realeinkommens der Bevölkerung	562
11.1.2	Durchschnittl.Monatslohn d.Arbeiter u.Angestellten in der Volkswirtschaft	562
11.1.3	Durchschnittl.Monatslohn d.Arbeiter u.Angestellten nach Volkswirtschaftszweigen	563
11.1.4	Wachstum des durchschnittl.Monatslohnes d.Arbeiter u.Angest.	565
11.1.5	Durchschnittl.Monatslohn in der Volkswirtschaft und in den Zweigen mit höchster und niedrigster Lohnstufe	565
11.1.6	Verhältnis zwischen Durchschnitts- und Minimallohn	565
11.1.7	Wachstum der Entlohnung der Kolchosbauern	566
11.1.8	Anteil des Einkommens aus privaten Nebenwirtschaften am Einkommen der Industriearbeiter und Kolchosbauern	566
11.1.9	Zahlungen und Leistungen für die Bevölkerung aus den öffentlichen Bedarfsfonds	567
11.1.10	Wachstum der Zahlungen und Leistungen für die Bevölkerung aus den öffentlichen Bedarfsfonds	568
11.2	Wohnungsbau	569
11.2.1	Fertiggestellte Wohnhäuser	569
11.2.2	Städtischer Wohnungsfonds	570
11.2.3	Wohnungsfonds der Hauptstädte der Unionsrepubliken	571
11.3	Einzelhandel	571
11.3.1	Einzelhandelsbetriebe u.Verkaufsfläche der Läden der staatl. u.genossenschaftl.Organisationen in den Unionsrepubliken	571
11.3.2	Betriebe der Gemeinschaftsverpflegung und Zahl der dort vorhandenen Plätze in den Unionsrepubliken	572
11.3.3	Selbstbedienungsläden	573
11.3.4	Wachstum des Warenumsatzes u.d.Handelsnetzes im Einzelhandel	574
11.3.5	Versorgung der Stadt-u.Landbevölkerung mit langlebigen Kultur- und Haushaltsgütern	575
11.4	Gesundheitswesen	576
11.4.1	Grundkennziffern der Entwicklung des Gesundheitswesens	576
11.4.2	Zahl der Ärzte aller Fachrichtungen nach Unionsrepubliken	579
11.4.3	Zahl der Ärztinnen aller Fachrichtungen	580
11.4.4	Zahl der medizinischen Einrichtungen für ambulant-poliklinische ärztliche Betreuung	580
11.4.5	Wachstum des Netzes der Krankenanstalten u.d.Bettenkontingents	581

12. Gesellschaftliche Organisationen

12.1	Verzeichnis der wichtigsten gesellschaftlichen Organisationen	582
12.2	Gewerkschaften	584
12.2.1	Zahl der Gewerkschaftsmitglieder zu Gewerkschaftskongressen der UdSSR	584
12.2.2	Vorsitzende des Unionszentralrates der Gewerkschaften	585
12.2.3	Unionszentralrat der Gewerkschaften	585
12.2.4	ZKs der Branchengewerkschaften	585
12.2.5	Gewerkschaftsräte der Unionsrepubliken	587
12.2.6	Unter der Leitung der Gewerkschaften tätige Gesellschaften und Organisationen	588
12.3	Leninscher Kommunistischer Jugendverband - Komsomol	588
12.3.1	Zahl der Mitglieder zu Komsomolkongressen	588
12.3.2	ZK des Komsomol der UdSSR	590
12.3.3	ZKs des Komsomol der Unionsrepubliken	591

Inhaltsübersicht

12.3.4	Zahl der im Komsomol tätigen Mitglieder u.Kandidaten d.KPdSU	591
12.3.5	Unionspionierorganisation	592
12.4	Mitgliederzahl einiger freiwilliger Unionsgesellschaften	592
12.5	Zusätzliche Informationen über einige gesellschaftliche Organisationen	593

13. Religion

13.1	Rat für Religiöse Angelegenheiten beim Ministerrat der UdSSR	596
13.2	Allgemeine Daten	596
13.3	Die Russisch-Orthodoxe Kirche	597
13.4	Die Georgische Orthodoxe Kirche	599
13.5	Die Armenisch-Gregorianische Kirche	599
13.6	Die Altgläubigen	599
13.7	Moslems	599
13.8	Die Römisch-Katholische Kirche	600
13.9	Die Evangelisch-Lutherische Kirche	600
13.10	Die Christlich-Evangelischen Baptisten	600
13.11	Mosaische Glaubensgemeinschaften	600
13.12	Buddhismus	601
13.13	Andere Konfessionen	601
13.14	Wichtigste illegale Kirchen und Sekten	601

14. Diverses

14.1	Hymne der Sowjetunion	603
14.2	Territoriale Ausdehnung nach dem Zweiten Weltkrieg	604
14.3	Die Staatsgrenze der UdSSR	604
14.4	Die höchsten Bodenerhebungen	605
14.5	Vulkane	605
14.6	Die wichtigsten Flüsse	605
14.7	Die größten Seen	606
14.8	Die wichtigsten Inseln	607
14.9	Wirtschaft	607
14.9.1	Offizieller Rubelkurs (März 1978)	607
14.9.2	Fünfjahrpläne	609
14.9.3	Weizenimporte	609
14.9.4	Export von Erdöl und Erdölprodukten	609
14.9.5	Export von Erdgas	610
14.9.6	Anteil der privaten Nebenwirtschaftn an der landwirtschaftlichen Produktion	610
14.10	Weitere Organisationen und Institutionen des ZK der KPdSU	611
14.11	Presseagenturen	611
14.12	Orden der UdSSR	611
14.13	Einige kulturelle Institutionen	613
14.13.1	Bibliotheken	613
14.13.2	Öffentliche Bibliotheken in den Unionsrepubliken	613
14.13.3	Zahl der Theater in den Unionsrepubliken	613
14.13.4	Zirkusse	614
14.13.5	Zahl der Museen in den Unionsrepubliken	614

LIST OF DIAGRAMS

National State Structure of the USSR	3
Age-Sex-Pyramid 1926	44
Age Sex-Pyramid 1970	45
Communist Party of the Soviet Union	56
CPSU Central Committee	61
Primary Organization with less than 50 Communist Party Members	92
Primary Organization with Party Committee	93
Primary Organization with the Rights of a Rayon Committee	94
Main Political Directorate of the Soviet Army	108
Soviets of the USSR People's Deputies	116
General Assembly of the Academy of Sciences of the USSR	455
Scheme of the State System of Scientific-Technical Information	501
Congress of the USSR Trade Unions	589

VERZEICHNIS DER GRAPHISCHEN DARSTELLUNGEN

National-staatlicher Aufbau der UdSSR	3
Alter-Geschlecht-Pyramide 1926	44
Alter-Geschlecht-Pyramide 1970	45
Kommunistische Partei der Sowjetunion	56
Zentralkomitee der KPdSU	61
Grundorganisation mit weniger als 50 Kommunisten	92
Grundorganisation mit Parteikomitee	93
Grundorganisation mit Parteikomitee mit den Rechten eines Raykoms	94
Politische Hauptverwaltung der Armee und Seekriegsflotte der UdSSR	108
Sowjets der Volksdeputierten der UdSSR	116
Generalversammlung der Akademie der Wissenschaften der UdSSR	455
Schema des staatlichen Systems der wissenschaftlich-technischen Information	501
Kongreß der Gewerkschaften der UdSSR	589

INTRODUCTION: THE POLITICAL SYSTEM OF THE USSR

The political system embraces all interdependent parts - the state apparat as well as all organizations and institutions - which are active within this system.

The CPSU is described as the "guiding force" of the whole system, i.e. it guides (rukovodit) all parts of the system, determines (opredeljajet) and directs (napravljajet) all its activities.

All decisions of the Party, the Central Committee of the CPSU and of the union republics are meant as directives for the activities of the state apparat, the institutions and organizations of the whole society. Every Five-Year Plan is drafted by the Central Committee (first) and then ratified by the state agencies. In legislature too the Party is the sole determining force, i.e. it initiates laws or amends or corrects bills before submitting them to the Supreme Soviet of the USSR for voting. The total Party operates through its elected party administration (s.p.95) and the nominated apparat (s.p.109).

The implementation of Party and Government decisions is the responsibility of the basic Party organizations in all organizations and institutions (in the Supreme Soviet of the USSR and of the republics it is the party groups, the same goes for the Councils of the People's Deputies on all levels, the trade unions and other public organizations).

One of the Party's most important tools of power is its c a d r e   p o l i c y , guaranteeing the Party a monopoly on the appointment (nomination) of important posts, and this within the Party as well as in   a l l   a r e a s   o u t s i d e   t h e   P a r t y . For this cadre policy the following principles are applied: "r e c o m e n d a c i j a" (recommendation) means that the next-highest Party agency "recommends" those eligible for the election to leading Party posts; in the sphere outside the Party it is the Party organizations which "recommend" those persons to be nominated (appointed) to leading posts in   a l l   areas (except ministries and the Armed Forces); "n o m e n - c l a t u r a" (nomenclature) is the second system with which a list of posts (especially in the economic and administrative sector) is drafted which are to be filled exclusively by the Party even in cases where various regulations stipulate that the nomination (appointment) of these posts is the responsibility of administrative agencies or individuals; "k o m p l e k t i - r o v a n i e" (completion) describes a system guaranteeing the composition of an entire apparat with persons - including non-Party affiliated persons - who suit the Party (scientific councils, for example, or Councils of the People's Deputies).

The Party organizations are empowered to control the administration (except the ministries and the Armed Forces) as far as the implementation of Party and Government decisions on the local (primary) level is concerned; it has the right to formulate suggestions for improvement and recommend changes in personnel.

The Party has a monopoly on the whole field of "ideological work" which encompasses education, literature and the arts, mass communications media, all cultural institutions and **agitation** work.

In addition there are a number of other mechanisms which were developed outside the legislature but which were recognized by all organizations and institutions, with which the Party tries to secure its supremacy which is permanently "to be perfected" and to further strengthen and expand its function as a guiding and inspiring force of the whole society.

THE POLITICAL SYSTEM OF THE USSR – DAS POLITISCHE SYSTEM DER UdSSR

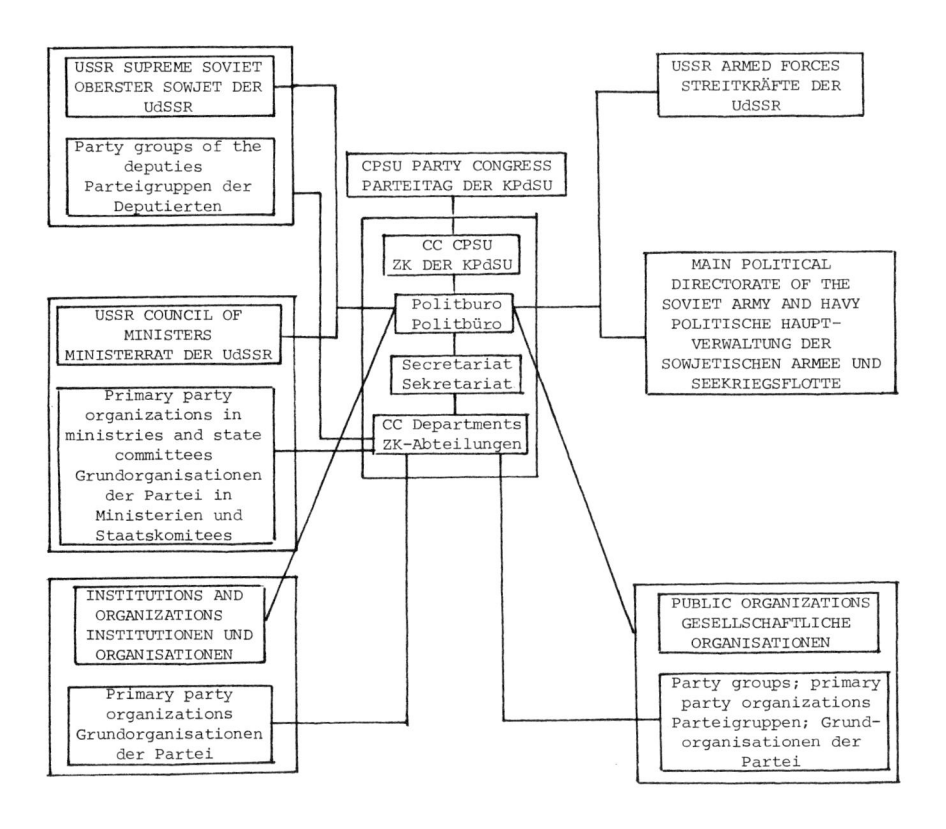

```
┌─────────────────────┐                                           ┌─────────────────────┐
│ USSR SUPREME SOVIET │                                           │  USSR ARMED FORCES  │
│  OBERSTER SOWJET    │                                           │   STREITKRÄFTE DER  │
│      DER UdSSR      │                                           │        UdSSR        │
├─────────────────────┤      ┌────────────────────┐               └─────────────────────┘
│ Party groups of the │      │ CPSU PARTY CONGRESS│
│      deputies       │      │ PARTEITAG DER KPdSU│
│  Parteigruppen der  │      └────────────────────┘
│     Deputierten     │      ┌────────────────────┐
└─────────────────────┘      │      CC CPSU       │
                             │   ZK DER KPdSU     │               ┌─────────────────────┐
                             ├────────────────────┤               │   MAIN POLITICAL    │
┌─────────────────────┐      │     Politburo      │               │  DIRECTORATE OF THE │
│  USSR COUNCIL OF    │      │     Politbüro      │               │ SOVIET ARMY AND NAVY│
│     MINISTERS       │      ├────────────────────┤               │  POLITISCHE HAUPT-  │
│ MINISTERRAT DER UdSSR│     │    Secretariat     │               │   VERWALTUNG DER    │
├─────────────────────┤      │    Sekretariat     │               │ SOWJETISCHEN ARMEE  │
│   Primary party     │      ├────────────────────┤               │ UND SEEKRIEGSFLOTTE │
│  organizations in   │      │   CC Departments   │               └─────────────────────┘
│ ministries and state│      │   ZK-Abteilungen   │
│     committees      │      └────────────────────┘
│  Grundorganisationen│
│   der Partei in     │
│   Ministerien und   │
│    Staatskomitees   │
└─────────────────────┘
┌─────────────────────┐                                           ┌─────────────────────┐
│   INSTITUTIONS AND  │                                           │ PUBLIC ORGANIZATIONS│
│    ORGANIZATIONS    │                                           │   GESELLSCHAFTLICHE │
│  INSTITUTIONEN UND  │                                           │    ORGANISATIONEN   │
│    ORGANISATIONEN   │                                           ├─────────────────────┤
├─────────────────────┤                                           │ Party groups; primary│
│   Primary party     │                                           │ party organizations │
│   organizations     │                                           │ Parteigruppen; Grund-│
│ Grundorganisationen │                                           │  organisationen der │
│     der Partei      │                                           │       Partei        │
└─────────────────────┘                                           └─────────────────────┘
```

Article 6 of the Soviet constitution of 1977 reads: "The leading and guiding forces of Soviet society and the nucleus of its political system, of all state organizations and public organizations, is the Communist Party of the Soviet Union. The CPSU exists for the people and serves the people."
Die sowjetische Verfassung von 1977 sagt in Artikel 6: "Die führende und lenkende Kraft der sowjetischen Gesellschaft, der Kern ihres politischen Systems, der staatlichen Organe und gesellschaftlichen Organisationen ist die Kommunistische Partei der Sowjetunion. Die KPdSU ist für das Volk da und dient dem Volk."

EINFÜHRUNG: DAS POLITISCHE SYSTEM DER UdSSR

Dem politischen System gehören alle voneinander abhängigen Teile - Staatsapparate ebenso wie alle Organisationen und Institutionen - an und wirken darin zusammen. Als "leitender Kern" des gesamten Systems wird die KPdSU beschrieben, sie leitet (rukovodit) alle Teile des Systems, bestimmt (opredeljajet) und steuert (napravljajet) deren gesamte Tätigkeit.

Alle Beschlüsse der Partei, der ZKs der KPdSU wie der Parteien der Unionsrepubliken, haben den Charakter von Direktiven für die Tätigkeit aller Staatsapparate, Institutionen und Organisationen der gesamten Gesellschaft. Alle Fünfjahrpläne werden zunächst vom ZK beschlossen und anschließend von den Staatsapparaten bestätigt. Die Partei ist auch im Bereich der Legislative die alleinbestimmende Kraft, indem sie als Initiatorin von Gesetzen auftritt, gegebenenfalls Gesetzesvorlagen ergänzt und korrigiert und sie erst dann dem Obersten Sowjet der UdSSR zur Abstimmung vorlegt. Für die totale Parteileitung sind gewählte Leitungsorgane der Partei (s.S.95) und der ernannte Apparat (s.S.109) zuständig.

Die Realisierung der Partei- und Regierungsbeschlüsse übernehmen in allen Organisationen und Institutionen die Grundorganisationen der Partei (in den Obersten Sowjets der UdSSR und der Unionsrepubliken sind es Parteigruppen, das gleiche gilt für die Räte der Volksdeputierten auf allen Ebenen, die Gewerkschaften und andere gesellschaftliche Organisationen).

Eines der wichtigsten Machtinstrumente der Partei ist die K a d e r p o l i t i k . Sie garantiert dem Parteiapparat das Monopol auf die Besetzung aller wichtigen Posten, und zwar sowohl innerhalb der Partei wie i n   a l l e n   B e r e i c h e n a u ß e r h a l b   d e r   P a r t e i . Für die Kaderpolitik bedient sie sich folgender Mechanismen: "r e k o m e n d a - c i j a" (Empfehlung) bedeutet, daß die nächsthöhere Parteiinstanz bei der Wahl der leitenden Parteiorgane die für Führungsposten zu Wählenden "empfiehlt"; im außerparteilichen Bereich sind es die Parteiorganisationen, die die Personen "empfehlen", die in   a l l e n   Bereichen für führende Posten nominiert werden (Ausnahme: Ministerien und Streitkräfte); "n o m e n k l a t u r a" (Nomenklatur) ist ein zweites "System", mit dessen Hilfe eine Liste von Posten erstellt wird, insbesondere in Wirtschaft und Verwaltung, die ausschließlich durch die Partei zu besetzen sind, selbst dann, wenn verschiedene Bestimmungen und Verordnungen ausdrücklich die personelle Besetzung in die Kompetenz von Behörden oder Einzelpersonen stellen; "k o m p l e k t i r o v a n i e" (Komplettierung) ist ein System, das die Zusammensetzung eines ganzen Apparates mit solchen Personen - darunter auch Parteilosen - garantiert, die der Partei genehm sind (z.B. Wissenschaftliche Räte oder Räte der Volksdeputierten).

Die Parteiorganisationen haben das Recht, die Tätigkeit der Verwaltung (Ausnahme: Ministerien und Streitkräfte) daraufhin zu kontrollieren, ob durch sie die Beschlüsse von Partei und Regierung vor Ort realisiert wurden; sie sind berechtigt, Verbesserungsvorschläge auszuarbeiten und notfalls personelle Veränderungen vorzuschlagen.

Die Partei hat das Monopol auf dem gesamten Gebiet der "ideologischen Arbeit", zu dem Bildung, Literatur und Kunst, Massenmedien, alle kulturellen Institutionen und Agitationsarbeit gehören.

Hinzu kommen verschiedene andere, außerhalb der Legislative entstandene, aber von allen Organisationen und Institutionen anerkannte Mechanismen, mit deren Hilfe die Partei versucht, ihre stets zu "vervollkommnende" Herrschaft zu sichern, ihre Funktion als leitende und inspirierende Kraft der gesamten Gesellschaft immer weiter zu festigen und auszubauen.

1. ADMINISTRATIVE-TERRITORIAL SURVEY
ADMINISTRATIV-TERRITORIALE ZUSAMMENSETZUNG
NACIONAL'NO-GOSUDARSTVENNOE DELENIE

1.1 UNION REPUBLICS - UNIONSREPUBLIKEN - SOJUZNYE RESPUBLIKI

Sojuz Sovetskich Socialistiĉeskich respublik, SSSR, Sojuz SSR;
 Sovetskij Sojuz
Union of Soviet Socialist Republics, U.S.S.R.; Soviet Union
Union der Sozialistischen Sowjetrepubliken, UdSSR; Sowjetunion

Rossijskaja Sovetskaja Federativnaja Socialistiĉeskaja respublika;
 RSFSR
Russian Soviet Federative Socialist Republic; RSFSR
Russische Sozialistische Föderative Sowjetrepublik; Rußland

Ukrainskaja Sovetskaja Socialistiĉeskaja respublika, Ukrainskaja SSR,
 USSR; Ukraina
Ukrainian Soviet Socialist Republic; Ukraine
Ukrainische Sozialistische Sowjetrepublik; Ukraine

Belorusskaja Sovetskaja Socialistiĉeskaja respublika, Belorusskaja
 SSR, BSSR; Belorussija
Belorussian Soviet Socialist Republic; Belorussia
Belorussische Sozialistische Sowjetrepublik; Belorußland

Uzbekskaja Sovetskaja Socialistiĉeskaja respublika, Uzbekskaja SSR,
 UZBSSR; Uzbekistan
Uzbek Soviet Socialist Republic; Uzbekistan
Usbekische Sozialistische Sowjetrepublik; Usbekistan

Kazachskaja Sovetskaja Socialistiĉeskaja respublika, Kazachskaja
 SSR, KAZSSR; Kazachstan
Kazakh Soviet Socialist Republic; Kazakhstan
Kasachische Sozialistische Sowjetrepublik; Kasachstan

Gruzinskaja Sovetskaja Socialistiĉeskaja respublika, Gruzinskaja
 SSR, GRUZSSR; Gruzija
Georgian Soviet Socialist Republic; Georgia
Grusinische Sozialistische Sowjetrepublik; Grusien, Grusinien

Azerbajdžanskaja Sovetskaja Socialistiĉeskaja respublika,
 Azerbajdžanskaja SSR, AZERBSSR; Azerbajdžan
Azerbaidzhan Soviet Socialist Republic; Azerbaidzhan
Aserbaidschanische Sozialistische Sowjetrepublik; Aserbaidschan

1.1 Administrative-territorial survey
Administrativ-territoriale Zusammensetzung

Latvijskaja Sovetskaja Socialističeskaja respublika, Latvijskaja
SSR, LATVSSR; Latvija
Latvian Soviet Socialist Republic; Latvia
Lettische Sozialistische Sowjetrepublik; Lettland

Kirgizskaja Sovetskaja Socialističeskaja respublika, Kirgizskaja
SSR, KIRGSSR; Kirgizija
Kirghiz Soviet Socialist Republic; Kirghizia
Kirgisische Sozialistische Sowjetrepublik; Kirgisien

Tadžikskaja Sovetskaja Socialističeskaja respublika, Tadžikskaja
SSR, TADŽSSR; Tadžikistan
Tadzhik Soviet Socialist Republic; Tadzhikistan
Tadschikische Sozialistische Sowjetrepublik; Tadschikistan

Armjanskaja Sovetskaja Socialističeskaja respublika, Armjanskaja
SSR, ARMSSR; Armenija
Armenian Soviet Socialist Republic; Armenia
Armenische Sozialistische Sowjetrepublik; Armenien

Turkmenskaja Sovetskaja Socialističeskaja respublika, Turkmenskaja
SSR, TURKMSSR; Turkmenija, Turkmenistan
Turkmen Soviet Socialist Republic; Turkmenistan
Turkmenische Sozialistische Sowjetrepublik; Turkmenien

Estonskaja Sovetskaja Socialističeskaja respublika, Estonskaja SSR,
ESTSSR; Estonija
Estonian Soviet Socialist Republic; Estonia
Estnische Sozialistische Sowjetrepublik; Estland

Litovskaja Sovetskaja Socialističeskaja respublika, Litovskaja SSR,
LITSSR; Litva
Lithuanian Soviet Socialist Republic; Lithuania
Litauische Sozialistische Sowjetrepublik; Litauen

Moldavskaja Sovetskaja Socialističeskaja respublika, Moldavskaja
SSR, MOLDSSR; Moldavija
Moldavian Soviet Socialist Republic; Moldavia
Moldauische Sozialistische Sowjetrepublik; Moldau

Administrative-territorial survey
Administrativ-territoriale Zusammensetzung

NATIONAL STATE STRUCTURE OF THE USSR
NATIONAL-STAATLICHER AUFBAU DER UdSSR
NACIONAL'NO-GOSUDARSTVENNOE USTROJSTVO SSSR

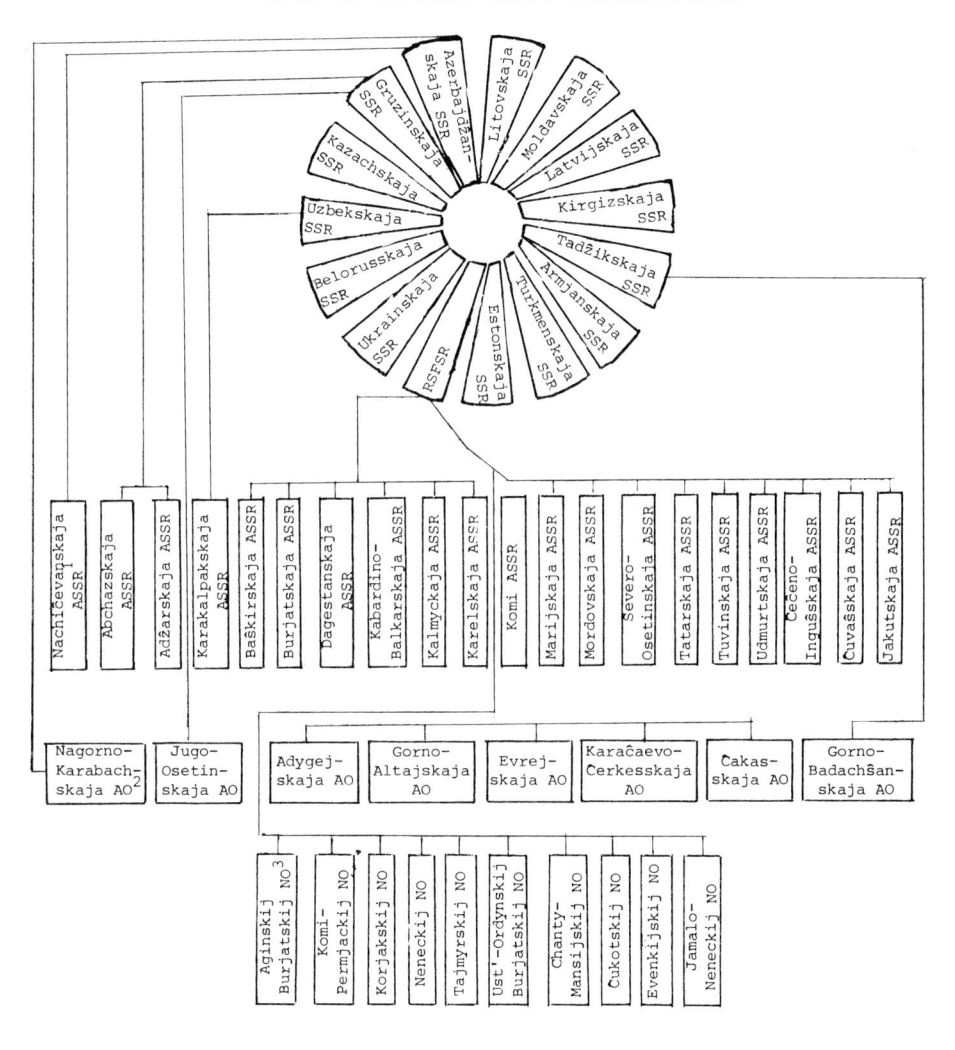

Union Republics (radial diagram):
- Azerbajdžanskaja SSR
- Gruzinskaja SSR
- Kazachskaja SSR
- Uzbekskaja SSR
- Belorusskaja SSR
- Ukrainskaja SSR
- RSFSR
- Estonskaja SSR
- Turkmenskaja SSR
- Armjanskaja SSR
- Tadžikskaja SSR
- Kirgizskaja SSR
- Latvijskaja SSR
- Moldavskaja SSR
- Litovskaja SSR

ASSR:
- Nachičevanskaja ASSR
- Abchazskaja ASSR
- Adžarskaja ASSR
- Karakalpakskaja ASSR
- Baškirskaja ASSR
- Burjatskaja ASSR
- Dagestanskaja ASSR
- Kabardino-Balkarskaja ASSR
- Kalmyckaja ASSR
- Karelskaja ASSR
- Komi ASSR
- Marijskaja ASSR
- Mordovskaja ASSR
- Severo-Osetinskaja ASSR
- Tatarskaja ASSR
- Tuvinskaja ASSR
- Udmurtskaja ASSR
- Čečeno-Ingušskaja ASSR
- Čuvašskaja ASSR
- Jakutskaja ASSR

AO:
- Nagorno-Karabachskaja AO[2]
- Jugo-Osetinskaja AO
- Adygejskaja AO
- Gorno-Altajskaja AO
- Evrejskaja AO
- Karačaevo-Čerkesskaja AO
- Čakasskaja AO
- Gorno-Badachšanskaja AO

NO:
- Aginskij Burjatskij NO[3]
- Komi-Permjackij NO
- Korjakskij NO
- Neneckij NO
- Tajmyrskij NO
- Ust'-Ordynskij Burjatskij NO
- Chanty-Mansijskij NO
- Čukotskij NO
- Evenkijskij NO
- Jamalo-Neneckij NO

---

1 ASSR — Avtonomnaja respublika — Autonomous Republic — Autonome Republik

2 AO   — Avtonomnaja oblast' — Autonomous Oblast — Autonomes Gebiet

3 NO   — Nacional'nyj okrug — National Okrug — Nationaler Kreis

1.2 Administrative-territorial survey
Administrativ-territoriale Zusammensetzung

1.2 UNION REPUBLICS (TERRITORY AND CAPITALS)
UNIONSREPUBLIKEN (TERRITORIUM UND HAUPTSTÄDTE)
SOJUZNYE RESPUBLIKI (PLOČSAD' I STOLICY)

	Territory Territorium ploščad' ('000 sq km) (1000 km^2)	Capitals Hauptstädte stolicy	Date of Foundation Gründungs- datum Data obrazo- vanija	Date of Entry into the USSR Datum des Eintritts in die UdSSR Data vchoždenija v SSSR
RSFSR	17,075.4	Moskva	7.11.1917	30.12.1922
Ukrainskaja SSR	603.7	Kiev	25.12.1917	30.12.1922
Belorusskaja SSR	207.6	Minsk	1. 1.1919	30.12.1922
Uzbekskaja SSR	447.4	Taškent	27.10.1924	27.10.1924
Kazachskaja SSR	2,717.3	Alma-Ata	5.12.1936	5.12.1936
Gruzinskaja SSR	69.7	Tbilisi	25. 2.1921	30.12.1922 +)
Azerbajdžanskaja SSR	86.6	Baku	28. 4.1920	30.12.1922 +)
Litovskaja SSR	65.2	Vilnius	21. 7.1940	3. 8.1940
Moldavskaja SSR	33.7	Kišinev	2. 8.1940	2. 8.1940
Latvijskaja SSR	63.7	Riga	21. 7.1940	5. 8.1940
Kirgizskaja SSR	198.5	Frunze	5.12.1936	5.12.1936
Tadžikskaja SSR	143.1	Dušanbe	16.10.1929	5.12.1929
Armjanskaja SSR	29.8	Erevan	29.11.1920	30.12.1922 +)
Turkmenskaja SSR	488.1	Aschabad	27.10.1924	27.10.1924
Estonskaja SSR	45.1	Tallin	21. 7.1940	6. 8.1940

+) as a member of the Transcaucasian Federation
+) als Mitglied der Transkaukasischen Föderation
+) v sostave Zakavkazskoj Federacii

4

Administrative-territorial survey
Administrativ-territoriale Zusammensetzung 1.3

1.3 AUTONOMOUS REPUBLICS - AUTONOME REPUBLIKEN - AVTONOMNYE RESPUBLIKI

	Territory Territorium ploŝĉad' ('000 sq.km) (1000 km²)	Capital Hauptstadt stolicy	Date of Foundation Gründungs- datum data obra- zovanija
RSFSR			
Baŝkirskaja ASSR	143.6	Ufa	23. 3.1919
Burjatskaja ASSR	351.3	Ulan-Ude	30. 5.1923
Dagestanskaja ASSR	50.3	Machaĉkala	20. 1.1921
Kabardino-Balkarskaja ASSR	12.5	Nal'ĉik	5.12.1936
Kalmyckaja ASSR	75.9	Elista	20.10.1935
Karelskaja ASSR	172.4	Petrozavodsk	25. 7.1923
Komi ASSR	415.9	Syktyvkar	5.12.1936
Marijskaja ASSR	23.2	Joŝkar-Ola	5.12.1936
Mordovskaja ASSR	26.2	Saransk	20.12.1934
Severo-Osetinskaja ASSR	8.0	Ordžonikidze	5.12.1936
Tatarskaja ASSR	68.0	Kazan'	27. 5.1920
Tuvinskaja ASSR	170.5	Kyzyl	10.10.1961
Udmurtskaja ASSR	42.1	Iževsk	28.12.1934
Ĉeĉeno-Inguŝskaja ASSR	19.3	Groznyj	5.12.1936
Ĉuvaŝskaja ASSR	18.3	Ĉeboksary	21. 4.1925
Jakutskaja ASSR	3,103.2	Jakutsk	27. 4.1922
Uzbekskaja SSR			
Karakalpakskaja ASSR	165.6	Nukus	20. 3.1932
Gruzinskaja SSR			
Abchazskaja ASSR	8.6	Suchumi	4. 3.1921
Adžarskaja ASSR	3.0	Batumi	16. 7.1921
Azerbajdžanskaja SSR			
Nachiĉevanskaja ASSR	5.5	Nachiĉevan'	9. 2.1924

1.4 AUTONOMOUS REGIONS, NATIONAL KRAIS, OBLASTS, RAIONS, AND
VILLAGE SOVIETS IN THE UNION REPUBLICS (as of Jan.1, 1977)
AUTONOME GEBIETE, NATIONALE KREISE, KRAJS, OBLAST, RAYONS UND
DORFSOWJETS IN DEN UNIONSREPUBLIKEN (zum 1.1.1977)
AVTONOMNYE OBLASTI, NACIONAL'NYE OKRUGA, KRAJA, OBLASTI,
RAJONY I SEL'SOVETY V SOJUZNYCH RESPUBLIKACH (1.1.1977)

Union Republics Unionsrepubliken Sojuznye respubliki	Autonomous Oblasts Autonome Oblast Avtonomnye Oblasti	Krais Krajs Kraja	Oblasts Oblast Oblasti	National Krais Nationale Kreise Nacional'- nye okruga	Raions(without cities) Rayons(ohne Städte) Rajony(bez gorodskich)	Village Soviets Dorfsowjets Sel'skie sovety
SSSR	8	6	120	10	3,117	41,249
RSFSR	5	6	49	10	1,783	22,710
Ukrainskaja SSR	-	-	25	-	477	8,542
Belorusskaja SSR	-	-	6	-	117	1,512
Uzbekskaja SSR	-	-	11	-	134	977
Kazachskaja SSR	-	-	19	-	210	2,174
Gruzinskaja SSR	1	-	-	-	65	923
Azerbajdžanskaja SSR	1	-	-	-	61	1,051
Litovskaja SSR	-	-	-	-	44	594
Moldavskaja SSR	-	-	-	-	34	712
Latvijskaja SSR	-	-	-	-	26	507
Kirgizskaja SSR	-	-	3	-	34	362
Tadžikskaja SSR	1	-	2	-	41	293
Armjanskaja SSR	-	-	-	-	36	469
Turkmenskaja SSR	-	-	5	-	40	229
Estonskaja SSR	-	-	-	-	15	194

1.5 CITIES, URBAN-TYPE SETTLEMENTS AND RAIONS IN THE CITIES
STÄDTE, STÄDTISCHE SIEDLUNGEN UND RAYONS IN DEN STÄDTEN
GORODA, POSELKI GORODSKOGO TIPA I RAJONY V GORODACH
(as of Jan.1, 1977 - zum 1.1.1977)

	Cities Städte Goroda Total Insg. Vsego	Urban-type settlements[1] Städtische Siedlungen[1] Poselki gorodskogo tipa	Raions in the Cities Rayons in den Städten Rajony v gorodach
SSSR	2,040	3,784	572
RSFSR	995	2,015	344
Ukrainskaja SSR	398	896	115
Belorusskaja SSR	96	109	16
Uzbekskaja SSR	82	84	12
Kazachskaja SSR	82	189	29
Gruzinskaja SSR	51	62	8
Azerbajdžanskaja SSR	60	125	10
Litovskaja SSR	92	20	7
Moldavskaja SSR	21	37	3
Latvijskaja SSR	56	36	6
Kirgizskaja SSR	17	32	4
Tadžikskaja SSR	18	47	4
Armjanskaja SSR	24	33	7
Turkmenskaja SSR	15	73	3
Estonskaja SSR	33	26	4

[1] Urban-type settlements: all suburbs lying outside the city limits - workers' settlements with more than 3,000 inhabitants, health resorts with more than 2,000 inhabitants, vacation colonies - Städtische Siedlungen: alle Vororte, die außerhalb der Stadtgrenze liegen - Arbeitersiedlungen mit über 3.000 Einwohnern, Kurorte mit über 2.000 Einwohnern, Feriensiedlungen

Population 2.1
Bevölkerung

2. POPULATION — BEVÖLKERUNG — NASELENIE

2.1 POPULATION - BEVÖLKERUNG - NASELENIE 1897 - 1977

Year Jahr Gody	Number Gesamtzahl<čislennost' in Mill.	urban Stadt gorod- skoge	rural Land sel'- skoge	Percent of total urban in % zur Gesamtbevölkerung Stadt % ko vsemu naseleniju gorodskoe	rural Land sel'skoe
1897	124,6	18,4	106,2	15	85
1913	159,2	28,5	130,7	18	82
1940	194,1	63,1	131,0	33	67
1951	181,6	73,0	108,6	40	60
1956	197,9	88,2	109,7	45	55
1959	208,8	100,0	108,8	48	52
1961	216,3	107,9	108,4	50	50
1966	232,2	123,7	108,5	53	47
1967	234,8	126,9	107,9	54	46
1968	237,2	129,8	107,4	55	45
1969	239,5	132,9	106,6	55	45
1970	241,7	136,0	105,7	56	44
1971	243,9	139,0	104,9	57	43
1972	246,3	142,5	103,8	58	42
1973	248,6	146,1	102,5	59	41
1974	250,9	149,6	101,3	60	40
1975	253,3	153,1	100,1	60	40
1976	255,5	156,6	98,9	61	39
1977	257,8	159,6	98,2	62	38
1978	260,0				

2.2 Population
Bevölkerung

2.2 POPULATION OF USSR AND THE UNION REPUBLICS
BEVÖLKERUNG DER UdSSR UND DER UNIONSREPUBLIKEN
NASELENIE SSSR I SOJUZNYCH RESPUBLIK

CENSUS - VOLKSZÄHLUNG - PEREPIS' NASELENIJA 1939, 1959, 1970

	Total - Gesamtbevölkerung - vse naselenie		
	1939	1959	1970
SSSR	190,677,890	208,826,650	241,720,134
RSFSR	108,377,210	117,534,306	130,079,210
Ukrainskaja SSR	40,468,848	41,869,046	47,126,517
Belorusskaja SSR	8,912,218	8,055,714	9,002,338
Uzbekskaja SSR	6,346,928	8,119,103	11,799,429
Kazachskaja SSR	6,081,361	9,294,741	13,008,726
Gruzinskaja SSR	3,540,023	4,044,045	4,686,358
Azerbajdžanskaja SSR	3,205,150	3,697,717	5,117,081
Litovskaja SSR	2,880,000	2,711,445	3,128,236
Moldavskaja SSR	2,452,023	2,884,477	3,568,873
Latvijskaja SSR	1,884,756	2,093,458	2,364,127
Kirgizskaja SSR	1,458,213	2,065,837	2,932,805
Tadžikskaja SSR	1,484,922	1,980,547	2,899,602
Armjanskaja SSR	1,282,338	1,763,048	2,491,873
Turkmenskaja SSR	1,251,883	1,516,375	2,158,880
Estonskaja SSR	1,052,017	1,196,791	1,356,079

Population 2.2.1
Bevölkerung 2.2.2

2.2.1 URBAN - STADTBEVÖLKERUNG - GORODSKOE NASELENIE

	1939 Total Insg. vsego	%	1959 Total Insg. vsego	%	1970 Total Insg. vsego	%
SSSR	60,409,216	32	99,977,695	48	135,991,514	56
RSFSR	36,295,552	33	61,611,074	52	80,981,143	62
Ukrainskaja SSR	13,568,999	34	19,147,419	46	25,688,560	55
Belorusskaja SSR	1,854,817	21	2,480,505	31	3,907,783	43
Uzbekskaja SSR	1,469,847	23	2,728,580	34	4,321,603	37
Kazachskaja SSR	1,689,450	28	4,067,224	44	6,538,652	50
Gruzinskaja SSR	1,066,226	30	1,712,897	42	2,239,738	48
Azerbajdžanskaja SSR	1,156,798	36	1,767,270	48	2,564,551	50
Litovskaja SSR	658,900	23	1,045,965	39	1,571,737	50
Moldavskaja SSR	328,581	13	642,244	22	1,130,048	32
Latvijskaja SSR	662,669	35	1,173,976	56	1,476,602	62
Kirgizskaja SSR	270,086	19	696,207	34	1,097,498	37
Tadžikskaja SSR	249,301	17	646,178	33	1,076,700	37
Armjanskaja SSR	366,447	29	881,844	50	1,481,532	59
Turkmenskaja SSR	416,264	33	700,797	46	1,034,199	48
Estonskaja SSR	355,279	34	675,515	56	881,168	65

2.2.2 RURAL - LANDBEVÖLKERUNG - SEL'SKOE NASELENIE

	1939 Total Insg. vsego	%	1959 Total Insg. vsego	%	1970 Total Insg. vsego	%
SSSR	130,268,674	68	108,848,955	52	105,728,620	44
RSFSR	72,081,658	67	55,923,232	48	49,098,067	38
Ukrainskaja SSR	26,899,849	66	22,721,627	54	21,437,957	45
Belorusskaja SSR	7,057,401	79	5,575,209	69	5,094,555	57
Uzbekskaja SSR	4,877,081	77	5,390,523	66	7,477,826	63
Kazachskaja SSR	4,391,911	72	5,227,517	56	6,470,074	50
Gruzinskaja SSR	2,473,797	70	2,331,148	58	2,446,620	52
Azerbajdžanskaja SSR	2,048,352	64	1,930,447	52	2,552,530	50
Litovskaja SSR	2,221,100	77	1,665,480	61	1,556,499	50
Moldavskaja SSR	2,123,442	87	2,242,233	78	2,438,825	68
Latvijskaja SSR	1,222,087	65	919,482	44	887,525	38
Kirgizskaja SSR	1,188,127	81	1,369,630	66	1,835,307	63
Tadžikskaja SSR	1,235,621	83	1,334,369	67	1,822,902	63
Armjanskaja SSR	915,891	71	881,204	50	1,010,341	41
Turkmenskaja SSR	835,619	67	815,578	54	1,124,681	52
Estonskaja SSR	696,738	66	521,276	44	474,911	35

2.3 Population / Bevölkerung

2.3 POPULATION OF UNION REPUBLICS - BEVÖLKERUNG DER ('000)

	1897	1920	1926	1939	1951
SSSR	124,649	136,810	147,028	190,678	181,603
A urban Stadtbevölkerung gorodskoe naselenie	18,436	20,885	26,314	60,409	73,005
B rural Landbevölkerung sel'skoe naselenie	106,213	115,925	120,714	130,269	108,598
1. RSFSR	67,473	88,247	92,735	108,377	102,945
A	9,894	12,553	16,455	36,296	45,901
B	57,579	75,694	76,280	72,081	57,044
2. Ukrainskaja SSR	28,445	26,400	29,515	40,469	37,223
A	4,320	5,110	5,673	13,569	13,447
B	24,125	21,290	23,842	26,900	23,776
3. Belorusskaja SSR	6,673	4,359	4,986	8,912	7,781
A	899	740	848	1,855	1,726
B	5,774	3,619	4,138	7,057	6,055
4. Uzbekskaja SSR	3,948	4,470	4,621	6,347	6,434
A	743	807	1,012	1,470	1,975
B	3,205	3,663	3,609	4,877	4,459
5. Kazachskaja SSR	4,333	5,400	6,025	6,082	6,813
A	303	380	519	1,690	2,675
B	4,030	5,020	5,506	4,392	4,138
6. Gruzinskaja SSR	1,894	2,408	2,677	3,540	3,560
A	359	481	594	1,066	1,291
B	1,535	1,927	2,083	2,474	2,269
7. Azerbajdžanskaja SSR	1,807	1,952	2,314	3,205	2,933
A	305	406	650	1,157	1,320
B	1,502	1,546	1,664	2,048	1,613
8. Litovskaja SSR	2,536	...	...	2,880	2,561
A	355	...	...	659	792
B	2,181	...	...	2,221	1,769
9. Moldavskaja SSR	1,615	2,331	2,421	2,452	2,392
A	251	48	31	328	418
B	1,364	185	211	2,124	1,974
10. Latvijskaja SSR	1,929	...	...	1,885	1,954
A	542	...	...	663	917
B	1,387	...	...	1,222	1,037
11. Kirgizskaja SSR	663	860	1,002	1,458	1,764
A	63	93	122	270	503
B	600	767	880	1,188	1,261
12. Tadžikskaja SSR	810	924	1,032	1,485	1,554
A	69	58	106	249	424
B	741	866	926	1,236	1,130
13. Armjanskaja SSR	798	720	881	1,282	1,360
A	97	122	167	366	599
B	701	598	714	916	761
14. Turkmenskaja SSR	750	837	998	1,252	1,225
A	79	87	137	416	469
B	671	750	861	836	756
15. Estonskaja SSR	975	...	...	1,052	1,104
A	157	...	...	355	548
B	818	...	...	697	556

Population 2.3
Bevölkerung

UNIONSREPUBLIKEN - NASELENIJE SOJUZNYCH RESPUBLIK
(1000)

1956	1959	1961	1966	1970	1974	1976	
197,902	208,827	216,286	232,243	241,720	250,869	255,524	
88,171	99,978	107,883	123,720	135,991	149,589	156,590	A
109,731	108,849	108,403	108,523	105,729	101,280	98,934	B
112,266	117,534	120,766	127,189	130,079	132,913	134,650	1.
55,392	61,611	66,098	74,698	80,981	88,231	92,101	A
56,874	55,923	54,668	52,491	49,098	44,682	42,549	B
39,742	41,869	43,097	45,548	47,126	48,521	49,075	2.
16,038	19,147	20,647	23,358	25,688	28,195	29,341	A
23,704	22,722	22,450	22,190	21,438	20,326	19,734	B
7,850	8,056	8,233	8,656	9,002	9,268	9,371	3.
2,115	2,481	2,745	3,337	3,908	4,549	4,868	A
5,735	5,575	5,488	5,319	5,094	4,719	4,503	B
7,341	8,119	8,722	10,399	11,800	13,289	14,079	4.
2,382	2,729	3,036	3,704	4,322	5,030	5,484	A
4,959	5,390	5,686	6,695	7,478	8,259	8,595	B
8,283	9,295	10,236	12,047	13.009	13,928	14,337	5.
3,368	4,067	4,590	5,702	6,538	7,348	7,706	A
4,915	5,228	5,646	6,345	6,471	6,580	6,631	B
3,876	4,044	4,190	4,505	4,686	4,878	4,954	6.
1,549	1,713	1,803	2,073	2,240	2,398	2,507	A
2,327	2,331	2,387	2,432	2,446	2,480	2,447	B
3,375	3,698	3,973	4,640	5,117	5,514	5,689	7.
1,617	1,767	1,946	2,300	2,564	2,821	2,943	A
1,758	1,931	2,027	2,340	2,553	2,693	2,746	B
2,644	2,711	2,802	2,989	3,128	3,262	3,315	8.
928	1,046	1,127	1,343	1,571	1,796	1,903	A
1,716	1,665	1,675	1,646	1,557	1,466	1,412	B
2,652	2,885	3,039	3,367	3,569	3,764	3,850	9.
534	643	725	949	1,130	1,332	1,433	A
2,118	2,242	2,314	2,418	2,439	2,432	2,417	B
2,020	2,093	2,144	2,279	2,364	2,454	2,497	10.
1,056	1,174	1,226	1,374	1,477	1,584	1,650	A
964	919	918	905	887	870	847	B
1,920	2,066	2,214	2,615	2,933	3,219	3,368	11.
611	696	760	965	1,098	1,228	1,312	A
1,309	1,370	1,454	1,650	1,835	1,991	2,056	B
1,808	1,981	2,120	2,556	2,900	3,283	3,486	12.
577	646	720	921	1,077	1,242	1,300	A
1,231	1,335	1,400	1,635	1,823	2,041	2,186	B
1,592	1,763	1,905	2,239	2,492	2,728	2,834	13.
755	882	988	1,258	1,482	1,699	1,806	A
837	881	917	981	1,010	1,029	1,028	B
1,371	1,516	1,623	1,917	2,159	2,430	2,581	14.
609	700	763	924	1,034	1,182	1,254	A
762	816	860	993	1,125	1,248	1,327	B
1,162	1,197	1,222	1,297	1,356	1,418	1,438	15.
640	676	709	814	881	954	982	A
522	521	513	483	475	464	456	B

2.4 Population / Bevölkerung

2.4 POPULATION OF THE ECONOMIC RAIONS, AUTONOMOUS
BEVÖLKERUNG DER WIRTSCHAFTSRAYONS, AUTONOMEN
NASELENIE EKONOMIČESKICH RAJONOV, AVTONOMNYCH
(1000)

	1926 Total Insg. vsego	1926 urban Stadt gorodskoe	1926 rural Land sel'skoe	1939 Total Insg. vsego	1939 urban Stadt gorodskoe	1939 rural Land sel'skoe
SSSR	147,028	26,314	120,714	190,678	60,409	130,269
RSFSR	92,735	16,455	76,280	108,377	36,296	72,081
1. Severo-Zapadnyj rajon	8,538	2,491	6,047	11,174	5,366	5,808
Archangel'skaja oblast'	861	114	747	1,109	435	674
Neneckij nacional'nyj okrug	14	--	14	46	14	32
Vologodskaja oblast'	1,728	156	1,572	1,601	288	1,313
g. Leningrad[1]	1,737	1,737	---	3,401	3,401	---
Leningradskaja oblast'	923	142	781	1,279	375	904
Murmanskaja oblast'	32	17	15	291	245	46
Novgorodskaja oblast'	1,092	133	959	1,153	243	910
Pskovskaja oblast'	1,678	128	1,550	1,551	100	1,451
Karel'skaja ASSR	261	54	207	469	150	319
Komi ASSR	226	10	216	320	29	291
2. Central'nyj rajon	22,472	5,183	17,289	26,595	10,934	15,661
Brjanskaja oblast'	1,709	265	1,444	1,802	450	1,352
Vladimirskaja oblast'	1,211	262	949	1,344	494	850
Ivanovskaja oblast'	1,064	330	734	1,385	727	658
Kalininskaja oblast'	2,667	325	2,342	2,487	609	1,878
Kalužskaja oblast'	1,324	138	1,186	1,183	235	948
Kostromskaja oblast'	1,081	128	953	1,077	239	838
g. Moskva[1]	2,080	2,080	---	4,542	4,542	---
Moskovskaja oblast'	2,608	630	1,978	4,256	1,686	2,570
Orlovskaja oblast'	1,537	146	1,391	1,286	162	1,124
Rjazanskaja oblast'	2,079	163	1,916	1,925	204	1,721
Smolenskaja oblast'	2,166	216	1,950	1,980	363	1,617
Tul'skaja oblast'	1,523	221	1,302	1,726	616	1,110
Jaroslavskaja oblast'	1,423	279	1,144	1,602	607	995
3. Volgo-Vjatskij rajon	7,602	699	6,903	8,695	1,778	6,917
Gor'kovskaja oblast'	2,754	444	2,310	3,565	1,143	2,422
Kirovskaja oblast'	2,209	142	2,067	2,284	346	1,938
Marijskaja ASSR	489	20	469	581	76	505
Mordovskaja ASSR	1,259	48	1,211	1,187	82	1,105
Čuvašskaja ASSR	891	45	846	1,078	131	947
4. Central'no-Černozemnyj rajon	9,542	900	8,642	9,153	1,293	7,860
Belgorodskaja oblast'	1,677	118	1,559	1,440	95	1,345
Voronežskaja oblast'	2,525	277	2,248	2,709	553	2,156
Kurskaja oblast'	1,846	161	1,685	1,773	182	1,591
Lipeckaja oblast'	1,478	128	1,350	1,353	185	1,168
Tambovskaja oblast'	2,016	216	1,800	1,878	278	1,600

[1] Including urban-type settlements under the jurisdiction of the City Soviet
[1] Einschl. der dem Stadtsowjet unterstellten Siedlungen städtischen Typs
[1] i gorodskie poselenija, podčinennye gorsovetu

Population 2.4
Bevölkerung

REPUBLICS, KRAIS AND OBLASTS
REPUBLIKEN, KRAI UND OBLASTI
RESPUBLIK, KRAEV I OBLASTEJ
(1000)

	1959			1970			1974		
Total Insg. vsego	urban Stadt gorod- skoe	rural Land sel' skoe	Total Insg. vsego	urban Stadt gorod- skoe	rural Land sel' skoe	Total Insg. vsego	urban Stadt gorod- skoe	rural Land sel' skoe	
208,827	99,978	108,849	241,720	135,991	105,729	250,869	149,589	101,280	
117,534	61,611	55,923	130,079	80,981	49,098	132,913	88,231	44,682	
10,865	7,023	3,842	12,157	8,913	3,244	12,611	9,658	2,953	1.
1,267	666	601	1,401	921	480	1,421	993	428	
37	17	20	39	21	18	39	22	17	
1,309	453	856	1,296	616	680	1,283	690	593	
3,340	3,340	---	3,987	3,987	---	4,243	4,243	---	
1,226	609	617	1,399	834	565	1,471	911	560	
568	523	45	799	708	91	881	782	99	
736	281	455	722	386	336	718	424	294	
953	258	695	875	373	502	860	421	439	
651	409	242	713	490	223	722	533	189	
815	484	331	965	598	367	1,012	661	351	
25,718	15,287	10,431	27,652	19,703	7,949	28,136	21,128	7,008	2.
1,550	540	1,010	1,582	750	832	1,540	819	721	
1,405	796	609	1,511	1,023	488	1,537	1,099	438	
1,320	876	444	1,339	1,010	329	1,323	1,037	286	
1,805	786	1,019	1,717	976	741	1,693	1,049	644	
938	350	588	995	516	479	986	563	423	
921	366	555	871	465	405	814	494	320	
6,044	6,044	---	7,077	7,077	---	7,528	7,528	---	
4,906	2,755	2,151	5,759	3,957	1,802	6,015	4,275	1,740	
929	221	708	931	362	569	897	424	473	
1,445	433	1,012	1,412	665	747	1,375	733	642	
1,141	366	775	1,106	529	577	1,090	593	497	
1,918	1,160	758	1,952	1,392	560	1,938	1,471	467	
1,396	814	582	1,400	981	419	1,400	1,043	357	
8,252	3,216	5,036	8,348	4,412	3,936	8,271	4,790	3,481	3.
3,618	1,882	1,736	3,683	2,378	1,305	3,656	2,526	1,130	
1,886	704	1,182	1,727	944	783	1,666	1,012	654	
648	183	465	685	280	405	690	329	361	
1,002	184	818	1,029	373	656	1,002	415	587	
1,098	263	835	1,224	437	787	1,257	508	749	
7,769	2,117	5,652	7,998	3,214	4,784	7,823	3,635	4,188	4.
1,226	240	986	1,261	444	817	1,257	547	710	
2,369	821	1,548	2,527	1,151	1,376	2,498	1,259	1,239	
1,483	303	1,180	1,474	486	988	1,423	581	842	
1,142	345	797	1,224	542	682	1,215	605	610	
1,549	408	1,141	1,512	591	921	1,430	643	787	

2.4 Population
Bevölkerung

	1926			1939		
	Total Insg. vsego	urban Stadt gorodskoe	rural Land sel' skoe	Total Insg. vsego	urban Stadt gorodskoe	rural Land sel' skoe
5. Povolžskij rajon	14,876	2,075	12,801	15,456	3,938	11,518
Astrachanskaja oblast'	615	207	408	683	294	389
Volgogradskaja oblast'	1,724	280	1,444	1,775	613	1,162
Kujbyševskaja oblast'	1,454	262	1,192	1,644	577	1,067
Penzenskaja oblast'	1,997	220	1,777	1,648	285	1,363
Saratovskaja oblast'	2,541	470	2,071	2,273	788	1,485
Ul'janovskaja oblast'	1,276	126	1,150	1,183	196	987
Baškirskaja ASSR	2,546	229	2,317	3,157	541	2,616
Kalmyckaja ASSR	135	---	135	179	30	149
Tatarskaja ASSR	2,588	281	2,307	2,914	614	2,300
6. Severo-Kavkazskij rajon	9,135	1,740	7,395	10,332	3,077	7,255
Krasnodarskij kraj	3,196	553	2,643	3,167	784	2,383
of which-darunter- v tom čisle: Adygejskaja avtonomnaja oblast'	262	53	209	278	56	222
Stavropol'skij kraj	1,695	247	1,448	1,764	351	1,413
of which-darunter- v tom čisle: Karačaevo-Čerkesskaja avtonomnaja oblast'	178	19	159	251	39	212
Rostovskaja oblast'	2,450	643	1,807	2,893	1,264	1,629
Dagestanskaja ASSR	744	85	659	1,023	220	803
Kabardino-Balkarskaja ASSR	224	16	208	350	85	265
Severo-Osetinskaja ASSR	287	94	193	408	174	234
Čečeno-Ingušskaja ASSR	539	102	437	727	199	528
7. Ural'skij rajon	8,261	1,599	6,662	10,298	4,213	6,085
Kurganskaja oblast'	1,236	62	1,174	976	97	879
Orenburgskaja oblast'	1,498	213	1,285	1,675	380	1,295
Permskaja oblast'	1,734	317	1,417	2,084	827	1,257
of which-darunter- v tom čisle: Komi-Permjackij nacional'nyj okrug	171	---	171	169	14	155
Sverdlovskaja oblast'	1,716	557	1,159	2,611	1,555	1,056
Čeljabinskaja oblast'	1,052	322	730	1,729	1,034	695
Udmurtskaja ASSR	1,025	128	897	1,223	320	903
8. Zapadno-Sibirskij rajon	7,432	877	6,555	8,927	2,581	6,346
Altajskij kraj	2,586	199	2,387	2,387	411	1,976
of which-darunter- v tom čisle: Gorno-Altajskaja avtonomnaja oblast'	107	6	101	162	24	138
Kemerovskaja oblast'	798	120	678	1,654	910	744
Novosibirskaja oblast'	1,588	171	1,417	1,862	582	1,280
Omskaja oblast'	1,122	193	929	1,390	330	1,060
Tomskaja oblast'	395	94	301	643	172	471
Tjumenskaja oblast'	943	100	843	991	176	815
of which-darunter- v tom čisle: Chanty-Mansijskij nacional'nyj okrug	39	3	36	93	8	85
Jamalo-Neneckij nacional'nyj okrug	19	---	19	48	13	35

Population
Bevölkerung 2.4

	1959			1970			1974		
Total Insg. vsego	urban Stadt gorod- skoe	rural Land sel' skoe	Total Insg. vsego	urban Stadt gorod- skoe	rural Land sel' skoe	Total Insg. vsego	urban Stadt gorod- skoe	rural Land sel' skoe	
15,975	7,348	8,627	18,374	10,482	7,892	18,845	11,695	7,150	5.
702	365	337	868	526	342	899	577	322	
1,854	1,008	846	2,323	1,523	800	2,399	1,660	739	
2,256	1,397	859	2,751	1,970	781	2,956	2,247	709	
1,508	500	1,008	1,536	679	857	1,504	741	763	
2,163	1,164	999	2,454	1,598	856	2,495	1,732	763	
1,117	404	713	1,225	641	584	1,230	722	508	
3,340	1,281	2,059	3,818	1,839	1,979	3,825	2,027	1,798	
185	39	146	268	92	176	269	107	162	
2,850	1,190	1,660	3,131	1,614	1,517	3,268	1,882	1,386	
11,601	4,961	6,640	14,281	7,106	7,175	14,899	7,849	7,050	6.
3,756	1,462	2,294	4,510	2,121	2,389	4,666	2,308	2,358	
324	105	219	385	152	233	400	180	220	
1,889	587	1,302	2,306	980	1,326	2,400	1,118	1,282	
285	66	219	345	113	232	356	124	232	
3,312	1,899	1,413	3,831	2,420	1,411	3,967	2,633	1,334	
1,063	315	748	1,429	505	924	1,521	566	955	
420	166	254	588	280	308	634	354	280	
451	238	213	552	356	196	582	389	193	
710	294	416	1,065	444	621	1,129	481	648	
14,184	8,863	5,321	15,185	10,440	4,745	15,233	11,047	4,186	7.
999	328	671	1,085	464	621	1,065	511	554	
1,832	827	1,005	2,050	1,088	962	2,057	1,189	868	
2,991	1,765	1,226	3,023	2,031	992	2,974	2,122	852	
236	34	202	212	40	172	188	40	148	
4,045	3,074	971	4,320	3,485	835	4,356	3,639	717	
2,979	2,275	704	3,289	2,563	726	3,345	2,688	657	
1,338	594	744	1,418	809	609	1,436	898	538	
11,252	5,724	5,528	12,109	7,431	4,678	12,291	8,071	4,220	8.
2,682	882	1,800	2,670	1,228	1,442	2,638	1,336	1,302	
157	30	127	168	40	128	165	45	120	
2,786	2,149	637	2,918	2,401	517	2,910	2,467	443	
2,299	1,275	1,024	2,505	1,638	867	2,531	1,755	776	
1,645	711	934	1,824	1,008	816	1,858	1,134	724	
747	360	387	786	466	320	818	525	293	
1,093	347	746	1,406	690	716	1,536	854	682	
124	33	91	271	170	101	362	249	113	
62	22	40	80	34	46	109	58	51	

2.4 Population
Bevölkerung

	1926			1939		
	Total Insg. vsego	urban Stadt gorod- skoe	rural Land sel' skoe	Total Insg. vsego	urban Stadt gorod- skoe	rural Land sel' skoe
9. Vostočno-Sibirskij rajon	3,305	523	2,782	4,771	1,731	3,040
Krasnojarskij kraj	1,426	167	1,259	1,959	585	1,374
of which - darunter - v tom čisle:						
Chakasskaja avtonomnaja oblast'	121	6	115	276	111	165
Tajmyrskij(Dolgano-Nenec- kij)nacional'nyj okrug	7	---	7	15	---	15
Evenkijskij nacional'nyj okrug	5	---	5	10	2	8
Irkutskaja oblast'	861	186	675	1,303	581	722
of which - darunter - v tom čisle:						
Ust'-Ordynskij Burjatskij nacional'nyj okrug	119	---	119	131	---	131
Čitinskaja oblast'	629	120	509	963	398	565
of which-darunter-v tom čisle: Aginskij Burjatskij nacional'nyj okrug	34	---	34	36	---	36
Burjatskaja ASSR	389	50	339	546	167	379
Tuvinskaja ASSR	...	...	...	...	...	...
10. Dal'nevostočnyj rajon	1,572	368	1,204	2,976	1,385	1,591
Primorskij kraj	637	173	464	888	452	436
Chabarovskij kraj	183	69	114	658	416	242
of which-darunter-v tom čisle: Evrejskaja avto- nomnaja oblast'	36	9	27	109	72	37
Amurskaja oblast'	414	106	308	634	289	345
Kamčatskaja oblast'	19	2	17	109	35	74
of which-darunter-v tom čisle: Korjakskij nacional' nyj okrug	10	---	10	23	---	23
Magadanskaja oblast'	20	---	20	173	31	142
of which-darunter-v tom čisle: Čukotskij nacional' nyj okrug	13	---	13	21	3	18
Sachalinskaja oblast'	12	3	9	100	50	50
Jakutskaja ASSR	287	15	272	414	112	302
Ukrainskaja SSR	29,515	5,673	23,842	40,469	13,569	26,900
11. Donecko-Pridneprovskij rajon	13,735	2,727	11,008	15,942	7,651	8,291
Vorošilovgradskaja oblast'	1,322	286	1,036	1,837	1,209	628
Dnepropetrovskaja oblast'	1,790	396	1,394	2,273	1,206	1,067
Doneckaja oblast'	1,645	648	997	3,104	2,421	683
Zaporožskaja oblast'	1,108	129	979	1,389	546	843

Population 2.4
Bevölkerung

	1959			1970			1974		
Total Insg. vsego	urban Stadt gorodskoe	rural Land sel'	Total Insg. vsego	urban Stadt gorodskoe	rural Land sel'	Total Insg. vsego	urban Stadt gorodskoe	rural Land sel'	
6,473	3,413	3,060	7,463	4,612	2,851	7,733	5,101	2,632	9.
2,615	1,296	1,319	2,962	1,831	1,131	3,041	2,006	1,035	
411	222	189	446	266	180	471	300	171	
33	20	13	38	23	15	42	26	16	
11	2	9	13	4	9	14	5	9	
1,977	1,227	750	2,313	1,673	640	2,411	1,827	584	
146	20	126	146	25	121	140	27	113	
1,036	564	472	1,145	658	487	1,192	730	462	
46	---	46	66	14	52	68	18	50	
673	276	397	812	363	449	841	440	401	
172	50	122	231	87	144	248	98	150	
4,834	3,265	1,569	5,780	4,132	1,648	6,300	4,674	1,626	10.
1,381	928	453	1,721	1,254	467	1,872	1,410	462	
1,142	848	294	1,346	1,047	299	1,451	1,150	301	
163	117	46	172	118	54	184	127	57	
718	429	289	793	490	303	849	552	297	
221	141	80	288	219	69	334	276	58	
28	6	22	31	10	21	33	13	20	
236	191	45	353	264	89	411	312	99	
47	27	20	101	70	31	118	85	33	
649	489	160	615	483	132	647	530	117	
487	239	248	664	375	289	736	444	292	
41,869	19,147	22,722	47,126	25,688	21,438	48,521	28,195	20,326	
17,766	11,248	6,518	20,057	14,107	5,950	20,620	15,081	5,539	11.
2,452	1,944	508	2,751	2,271	480	2,802	2,355	447	
2,705	1,899	806	3,343	2,549	794	3,505	2,760	745	
4,263	3,656	607	4,892	4,276	616	5,061	4,481	580	
1,464	829	635	1,775	1,167	608	1,861	1,288	573	

2.4 Population / Bevölkerung

	1926			1939		
	Total Insg. vsego	urban Stadt gorodskoe	rural Land sel' skoe	Total Insg. vsego	urban Stadt gorodskoe	rural Land sel' skoe
Kirovogradskaja oblast'	1,522	165	1,357	1,222	225	997
Poltavskaja oblast'	2,199	273	1,926	1,890	381	1,509
Sumskaja oblast'	1,824	236	1,588	1,673	319	1,354
Charkovskaja oblast'	2,325	594	1,731	2,554	1,344	1,210
12. Jugo-Zapadnyj rajon	12,115	1,864	10,251	19,664	4,133	15,531
Vinnickaja oblast'	2,434	273	2,161	2,268	271	1,997
Volynskaja oblast'	...	...	...	1,034	169	865
Žitomirskaja oblast'	1,760	286	1,474	1,692	347	1,345
Zakarpatskaja oblast'	...	...	...	...	...	...
Ivano-Frankovskaja oblast'	...	...	...	1,282	294	988
g. Kiev	514	514	---	851	851	---
Kievskaja oblast'	1,931	170	1,761	1,716	209	1,507
L'vovskaja oblast'	...	...	...	2,457	779	1,678
Rovenskaja oblast'	...	...	...	1,052	139	913
Ternopol'skaja oblast'	...	...	...	1,413	204	1,209
Chmel'nickaja oblast'	1,788	203	1,585	1,732	204	1,528
Čerkasskaja oblast'	1,825	192	1,633	1,556	218	1,338
Černigovskaja oblast'	1,863	226	1,637	1,799	282	1,517
Černovickaja oblast'	...	...	...	812	166	646
13. Južnyj rajon	3,665	1,082	2,583	4,863	1,785	3,078
Krymskaja oblast'	712	330	382	1,124	586	538
Nikolaevskaja oblast'	940	168	772	917	248	669
Odesskaja oblast'	1,277	484	793	2,079	784	1,295
Chersonskaja oblast'	736	100	636	743	167	576
14. Pribaltijskij rajon	...	...	...	5,817	1,677	4,140
Litovskaja SSR	...	...	...	2,880	659	2,221
15. g. Vil'njus	...	...	...	215	215	---
Latvijskaja SSR	...	...	...	1,885	663	1,222
g. Riga	...	...	...	348	348	---
Estonskaja SSR	...	...	...	1,052	355	697
16. g. Tallin	...	...	...	160	160	---
Kaliningradskaja oblast'	...	...	...	...	...	...
Zakavkazskij rajon	5,872	1,411	4,461	8,027	2,589	5,438
Gruzinskaja SSR	2,677	594	2,083	3,540	1,066	2,474
17. g. Tbilisi	294	294	---	519	519	---
Abchazskaja ASSR	212	32	180	312	88	224
Adžarskaja ASSR	132	50	82	200	76	124
Jugo-Osetinskaja avtonomnaja oblast'	87	6	81	106	14	92
Azerbajdžanskaja SSR	2,314	650	1,664	3,205	1,157	2,048
18. g. Baku[1]	453	453	---	773	773	---
Nachičevanskaja ASSR	105	15	90	127	23	104
Nagorno-Karabachskaja avtonomnaja oblast'	125	8	117	151	16	135

1 Including urban-type settlements under the jurisdiction of the City Soviet
1 Einschl. der dem Stadtsowjet unterstellten Siedlungen städtischen Typs
1 i gorodskie poselenija, podčinennye gorsovetu

Population 2.4
Bevölkerung

	1959			1970			1974		
Total Insg. vsego	urban Stadt gorod- skoe	rural Land sel' skoe	Total Insg. vsego	urban Stadt gorod- skoe	rural Land sel' skoe	Total Insg. vsego	urban Stadt gorod- skoe	rural Land sel' skoe	
1,250	380	870	1,259	552	707	1,266	599	667	
1,627	484	1,143	1,706	679	1,027	1,730	794	936	
1,486	482	1,004	1,505	655	850	1,465	690	775	
2,519	1,574	945	2,826	1,958	868	2,930	2,114	816	
19,028	5,434	13,594	20,689	7,940	12,749	21,158	9,032	12,126	12.
2,132	363	1,769	2,132	542	1,590	2,104	639	1,465	
893	231	662	974	313	661	1,002	357	645	
1,606	417	1,189	1,626	568	1,058	1,589	629	960	
920	265	655	1,057	314	743	1,112	381	731	
1,095	250	845	1,249	384	865	1,295	432	863	
1,110	1,110	---	1,632	1,632	---	1,887	1,887	---	
1,717	438	1,279	1,834	655	1,179	1,863	755	1,108	
2,111	821	1,290	2,429	1,149	1,280	2,501	1,254	1,247	
921	157	764	1,048	288	760	1,084	337	747	
1,086	180	906	1,153	269	884	1,173	310	863	
1,606	305	1,301	1,615	431	1,184	1,602	497	1,105	
1,484	341	1,143	1,535	563	972	1,553	640	913	
1,573	353	1,220	1,560	540	1,020	1,524	606	918	
774	203	571	845	292	553	869	308	561	
5,075	2,465	2,610	6,380	3,641	2,739	6,743	4,082	2,661	13.
1,201	775	426	1,813	1,146	667	1,982	1,299	683	
1,012	401	611	1,148	605	543	1,189	690	499	
2,038	957	1,081	2,389	1,335	1,054	2,491	1,470	1,021	
824	332	492	1,030	555	475	1,081	623	458	
6,612	3,290	3,322	7,580	4,465	3,115	7,905	4,917	2,988	14.
2,711	1,046	1,665	3,128	1,571	1,557	3,262	1,796	1,466	
236	236	---	372	372	---	420	420	---	15.
2,093	1,174	919	2,364	1,477	887	2,454	1,584	870	
580	580	---	732	732	---	776	776	---	
1,197	676	521	1,356	881	475	1,418	954	464	
282	282	---	363	363	---	392	392	---	16.
611	394	217	732	536	196	771	583	188	
9,505	4,362	5,143	12,295	6,286	6,009	13,120	6,918	6,202	
4,044	1,713	2,331	4,686	2,240	2,446	4,878	2,398	2,480	
703	703	---	889	889	---	984	984	---	17.
405	150	255	487	215	272	497	224	273	
245	111	134	310	137	173	334	150	184	
97	24	73	99	36	63	103	39	64	
3,698	1,767	1,931	5,117	2,564	2,553	5,514	2,821	2,693	
968	968	---	1,266	1,266	---	1,359	1,359	---	18.
141	38	103	202	50	152	219	54	165	
131	27	104	150	57	93	154	61	93	

2.4 Population / Bevölkerung

	1926			1939		
	Total Insg. vsego	urban Stadt gorodskoe	rural Land sel' skoe	Total Insg. vsego	urban Stadt gorodskoe	rural Land sel' skoe
Armjanskaja SSR	881	167	714	1,282	366	916
19. g. Erevan	65	65	---	204	204	---
Sredneaziatskij rajon	7,653	1,377	6,276	10,542	2,405	8,137
Uzbekskaja SSR	4,621	1,012	3,609	6,347	1,470	4,877
20. Andižanskaja oblast'	483	90	393	653	96	557
Bucharskaja oblast'	477	64	413	481	83	398
Džizakskaja oblast'	129	14	115	177	10	167
Kaškadar'inskaja oblast'	343	39	304	460	41	419
Namanganskaja oblast'	400	107	293	521	103	418
Samarkandskaja oblast'	628	150	478	844	182	662
Surchandar'inskaja oblast'	203	17	186	315	17	298
Syrdar'inskaja oblast'	97	3	94	157	16	141
g. Taškent	314	314	---	556	556	---
Taškentskaja oblast'	325	24	301	605	96	509
Ferganskaja oblast'	597	144	453	779	175	604
Chorezmskaja oblast'	294	29	265	323	37	286
Karakalpakskaja ASSR	331	17	314	476	58	418
Kirgizskaja SSR	1,002	122	880	1,458	270	1,188
21. g. Frunze	37	37	---	93	93	---
Issyk-Kul'skaja oblast'	134	13	121	174	27	147
Narynskaja oblast'	102	2	100	124	4	120
Ošskaja oblast'	477	55	422	675	107	568
Tadžikskaja SSR	1,032	106	926	1,485	249	1,236
22. g. Dušanbe	6	6	---	83	83	---
Kuljabskaja oblast'	233	4	229	226	11	215
Leninabadskaja oblast'	364	91	273	513	121	392
Gorno-Badachšanskaja avtonomnaja oblast'	56	1	55	72	4	68
Turkmenskaja SSR	998	137	861	1,252	416	836
23. g. Aschabad	52	52	---	127	127	---
Aschabadskaja oblast'	170	5	165	191	25	166
Krasnovodskaja oblast'	81	23	58	128	80	48
Maryjskaja oblast'	242	29	213	290	74	216
Tašauzskaja oblast'	128	4	124	249	24	225
Čardžouskaja oblast'	325	24	301	266	85	181
Kazachstanskij rajon						
Kazachskaja SSR	6,025	519	5,506	6,082	1,690	4,392
24. Aktjubinskij oblast'	365	34	331	338	89	249
g. Alma-Ata	44	44	---	222	222	---
Alma-Atinskaja oblast'	384	3	381	308	19	289
Vostočno-Kazachstanskaja oblast'	452	37	415	537	134	403

Population 2.4
Bevölkerung

	1959			1970			1974	
Total Insg. vsego	urban Stadt gorod- skoe	rural Land sel' skoe	Total Insg. vsego	urban Stadt gorod- skoe	rural Land sel' skoe	Total Insg. vsego	urban Stadt gorod- skoe	rural Land sel' skoe
1,763	882	881	2,492	1,482	1,010	2,728	1,699	1,029
493	493	---	767	767	---	870	870	---
13,682	4,771	8,911	19,792	7,531	12,261	22,221	8,682	13,539
8,119	2,729	5,390	11,800	4,322	7,478	13,289	5,030	8,259
768	174	594	1,059	255	804	1,193	311	982
574	130	444	934	292	642	1,068	347	721
218	26	192	341	39	302	396	76	320
508	67	441	801	132	669	907	159	748
594	155	439	847	242	605	963	301	662
953	288	665	1,363	387	976	1,527	457	1,070
422	65	357	662	106	556	751	128	623
245	66	179	341	100	241	394	117	277
927	927	---	1,385	1,385	---	1,552	1,552	---
1,080	327	753	1,479	592	887	1,623	677	946
939	301	638	1,332	440	892	1,510	499	1,011
381	64	317	554	103	451	625	119	506
510	139	371	702	249	453	780	287	493
2,066	696	1,370	2,933	1,098	1,835	3,219	1,228	1,991
220	220	---	431	431	---	474	474	---
234	60	174	312	89	223	337	102	235
135	27	108	186	28	158	209	34	175
869	278	591	1,233	381	852	1,377	435	942
1,981	646	1,335	2,900	1,077	1,823	3,283	1,242	2,041
227	227	---	374	374	---	422	422	---
255	43	212	368	99	269	418	113	305
666	247	419	938	354	584	1,061	404	657
73	8	65	98	12	86	110	14	96
1,516	700	816	2,159	1,034	1,125	2,430	1,182	1,248
170	170	---	253	253	---	280	280	---
185	53	132	294	86	208	334	107	227
192	154	38	259	210	49	283	232	51
351	121	230	482	160	322	549	182	367
295	71	224	411	119	292	460	140	320
321	129	192	457	203	254	521	238	283
9,295	4,067	5,228	13,009	6,538	6,471	13,928	7,348	6,580
401	174	227	551	248	303	592	272	320
456	456	---	730	730	---	813	813	---
468	37	431	712	131	581	791	156	635
735	394	341	845	485	360	861	508	353

19.

20.

21.

22.

23.

24.

21

2.4 Population / Bevölkerung

	1926 Total Insg. vsego	1926 urban Stadt gorodskoe	1926 rural Land sel' skoe	1939 Total Insg. vsego	1939 urban Stadt gorodskoe	1939 rural Land sel' skoe
Gur'evskaja oblast'	238	16	222	245	83	162
Džambulskaja oblast'	347	30	317	354	94	260
Džezkazganskaja oblast'	77	--	77	108	61	47
Karagandinskaja oblast'	203	5	198	295	174	121
Kzyl-Ordinskaja oblast'	319	42	277	328	95	233
Kokčetavskaja oblast'	321	11	310	330	50	280
Kustanajskaja oblast'	436	27	409	339	49	290
Mangyšlakskaja oblast'	45	2	43	42	10	32
Pavlodarskaja oblast'	322	18	304	222	34	188
Severo-Kazachstanskaja oblast'	334	47	287	371	92	279
Semipalatinskaja oblast'	462	61	401	409	154	255
Taldy-Kurganskaja oblast'	299	16	283	269	55	214
Turgajskaja oblast'	107	--	107	79	--	79
Ural'skaja oblast'	416	44	372	380	68	312
Celinogradskaja oblast'	324	20	304	269	40	229
Čimkentskaja oblast'	530	62	468	637	167	470
Belorusskij rajon Belorusskaja SSR	4,986	848	4,138	8,912	1,855	7,057
25. Brestskaja oblast'	...	...	...	1,209	203	1,006
Vitebskaja oblast'	1,281	219	1,062	1,702	374	1,328
Gomel'skaja oblast'	1,320	207	1,113	1,529	324	1,205
Grodnenskaja oblast'	...	...	...	1,239	201	1,038
g. Minsk	132	132	---	237	237	---
Minskaja oblast'	1,001	104	897	1,599	199	1,400
Mogilevskaja oblast'	1,252	186	1,066	1,397	317	1,080
Moldavskaja SSR	242	31	211	2,452	328	2,124
26. g. Kišinev	...	...	...	112	112	---

[1] Including urban-type settlements under the jurisdiction of the City Soviet
[1] Einschl. der dem Stadtsowjet unterstellten Siedlungen städtischen Typs
[1] i gorodskie poselenija, podčinennye gorsovetu

Population 2.4
Bevölkerung

	1959			1970			1974		
Total Insg. vsego	urban Stadt gorod- skoe	rural Land sel' skoe	Total Insg. vsego	urban Stadt gorod- skoe	rural Land sel' skoe	Total Insg. vsego	urban Stadt gorod- skoe	rural Land sel' skoe	
252	146	106	336	194	142	362	214	148	
560	202	358	794	320	474	870	377	493	
279	217	62	411	313	98	441	343	98	
740	580	160	1,141	946	195	1,223	1,044	179	
327	152	175	492	269	223	529	300	229	
492	123	369	589	178	411	598	195	403	
654	184	470	889	367	522	921	417	504	
36	16	20	164	136	28	218	190	28	
455	132	323	698	340	358	750	402	348	
469	156	313	556	212	344	551	228	323	
516	224	292	714	317	397	744	354	390	
485	166	319	610	237	373	655	264	391	
127	14	113	222	58	164	249	74	175	
381	113	268	513	158	355	547	193	354	
555	248	307	755	399	356	797	447	350	
907	333	574	1,287	500	787	1,416	557	859	
8,056	2,481	5,575	9,002	3,908	5,094	9,268	4,549	4,719	
1,182	284	898	1,295	451	844	1,324	528	796	25.
1,276	410	866	1,370	623	747	1,391	715	676	
1,364	389	975	1,533	616	917	1,560	718	842	
1,077	251	826	1,120	369	751	1,132	420	712	
509	509	---	917	917	---	1,095	1,095	---	
1,471	273	1,198	1,540	410	1,130	1,527	462	1,065	
1,177	365	812	1,227	522	705	1,239	611	628	
2,885	643	2,242	3,569	1,130	2,439	3,764	1,332	2,432	
216	216	---	356	356	---	432	432	---	26.

23

2.5 Population
    Bevölkerung

2.5 CITIES WITH MORE THAN 50,000 INHABITANTS
    STÄDTE MIT ÜBER 50.000 EINWOHNERN
    GORODA S NASELENIEM SVYŠE 50 TYS. ČELOVEK

(1000)

	1926	1939	1959	1970	1974	1976	1977
Abakan	3	37	56	90	112	120	123
Azov	18	25	40	59	68	73	75
Aktjubinsk	21	49	97	150	170	179	184
Alapaevsk	12	25	47	52	52	52	52
Aleksandrija	19	20	49	69	75	78	79
Aleksandrov	13	28	37	50	55	57	58
Aleksin	4	22	46	61	64	65	66
Alma-Ata	44	222	456	730	813	851	871
Almalyk	--	--	40	81	91	95	97
Almetevsk	--	--	49	87	97	102	104
Anadyr	--	2	2.7	7.7	9.7	--	--
Angarsk	--	--	135	203	224	231	233
Angren	--	--	56	76	84	99	102
Andižan	73	85	131	188	210	220	224
Anžero-Sudžensk	30	69	116	106	103	104	105
Antracit	7	36	56	55	58	59	60
Apatity	--	4	15	46	53	56	58
Arzamas	15	26	42	67	79	85	89
Armavir	75	84	111	145	155	158	158
Arsenev	--	11	26	47	56	58	60
Artem	4	35	55	61	67	69	70
Artemovsk (Oblast Doneck)	38	58	63	82	89	91	91
Archangelsk	77	251	258	343	369	383	391
Asbest	8	30	63	76	79	80	80
Astrachan	184	259	305	410	445	458	466
Ačinsk	18	32	50	97	109	114	117
Ašchabad	52	127	170	253	280	297	302
Baku	453	773	968	1,266	1,359	1,406	1,435
+)	453	544	643	852	913	943	961
Balakovo	19	23	36	103	123	135	140
Balašicha	8	29	58	92	101	106	108
Balašov	27	48	64	83	88	90	91
Balchaš	--	33	53	76	80	78	79
Baranoviči	...	27	58	101	115	123	126
Barnaul	74	148	303	439	488	514	522
Batajsk	23	48	52	85	96	100	102
Batumi	48	70	82	101	111	117	118
Bekabad	--	8	41	58	60	61	63
Belaja Cerkov'	43	47	71	109	128	137	141
Belgorod	31	34	72	151	198	219	227
Belovo	1	43	100	108	110	111	112
Belogorsk (Oblast Amur)	8	34	49	57	62	64	65
Beloreck	20	41	59	67	70	72	72
Belcy	...	30	66	101	115	121	123

+) not including urban-type settlements under the jurisdiction of the City Soviet
+) ohne dem Stadtsowjet unterstellte Siedlungen städtischen Typs
+) v tom čisle bez gorodskich poselenij, podčinennych gorsovetu

Population 2.5
Bevölkerung

	1926	1939	1959	1970	1974	1976	1977
Bendery	...	31	43	72	89	97	100
Berdičev	56	62	53	71	77	80	80
Berdsk	--	11	29	53	60	63	64
Berdjansk	26	52	65	100	113	117	119
Berezniki	7	51	106	146	161	172	176
Bijsk	46	80	146	186	203	209	212
Birobidžan	--	30	41	56	62	65	67
Blagoveščensk (Oblast Amur)	61	58	94	128	157	171	177
Bobrujsk	51	84	98	138	170	185	192
Bor	10	25	43	55	59	62	62
Borisov	26	49	59	84	95	102	106
Borisoglebsk	40	53	54	64	67	69	69
Boroviči	19	41	49	55	57	58	59
Bratsk	--	--	43	155	184	195	203
Brest	...	41	74	122	150	162	167
Brjanka	14	56	78	71	69	68	67
Brjansk	86	174	207	318	358	375	385
Buguruslan	18	21	42	49	51	53	53
Bugulma	14	25	61	72	78	81	82
Buzuluk	25	42	55	67	72	75	76
Buchara	47	50	69	112	133	144	147
Velikije Luki	21	35	59	85	98	101	103
Vilnius	...	215	236	372	420	447	458
Vinnica	58	93	122	212	264	288	297
Vitebsk	99	167	148	231	265	279	286
Vičuga	25	47	52	53	52	52	52
Vjazma	--	34	32	44	--	50	51
Vladivostok	108	206	291	441	495	526	536
Vladimir	40	67	154	234	263	278	284
Volgograd	151	445	591	818	885	918	931
Volžsk	--	19	33	43	--	53	54
Volžskij	--	--	67	142	178	195	203
Vologda	58	95	139	178	205	219	224
Volsk	35	56	62	69	71	72	72
Vorkuta	--	--	83	90	93	96	96
Voronež	122	344	447	660	729	764	779
Vorošilovgrad	73	215	275	383	423	439	445
Voskresensk	4	29	45	67	71	73	74
Votkinsk	19	39	60	74	80	86	88
Vyborg	...	...	51	65	69	71	72
Vyšnij Voloček	32	64	66	74	76	75	75
Gatčina	19	38	37	63	70	73	74
Georgievsk	--	32	35	44	--	50	51
Georgiu-Dej	7	25	38	49	51	52	52
Glazov	7	16	59	68	75	79	82
Gomel	86	139	168	272	324	349	360
Gori	11	20	35	48	52	54	54
Gorlovka	41	189	308	335	341	342	342
Gorkij	222	644	941	1,170	1,260	1,305	1,319
Grodno	...	49	73	132	161	176	182
Groznyj	97	172	250	341	369	381	387
Gubkin	--	--	21	54	63	67	68
Gukovo	--	9	53	65	69	70	71
Gurev	12	41	79	114	125	131	134
Gus'-Chrustalnyj	18	40	54	65	67	69	70

2.5 Population
Bevölkerung

	1926	1939	1959	1970	1974	1976	1977
Daugaupils	...	52	65	100	109	112	114
Derbent	23	34	47	57	63	66	69
Džalal-Abad	10	15	31	44	50	53	54
Džambul	25	64	113	187	228	246	252
Džezkazgan	--	3	32	62	74	82	85
Dzeržinsk (Oblast Gorkij)	9	103	164	221	235	245	248
Dimitrov	6	27	51	52	55	57	58
Dimitrovgrad	18	32	51	81	92	97	99
Dneprodzeržinsk	34	148	194	227	242	248	251
Dnepropetrovsk	237	528	661	862	941	976	995
Dolgoprudnyj	--	8	25	53	59	63	64
Doneck	174	474	708	879	934	967	984
Drogobyč	...	37	42	56	63	66	68
Družkovka	13	32	43	53	59	60	61
Dubna	--	10	33	44	--	50	51
Dušanbe	6	83	227	374	422	448	460
Evpatorija	24	47	57	79	88	92	94
Egorevsk	30	56	59	67	71	71	71
Ejsk	36	45	55	64	69	71	71
Elgava	...	32	36	55	61	64	65
Elec	43	51	78	101	108	112	113
Enakievo	--	109	117	115	--	114	114
Erevan	65	204	493	767	870	928	956
Essentuki	7	16	48	65	70	73	74
Efremov	10	27	29	48	52	53	53
Ždanov	63	222	284	417	451	467	474
Železnogorsk	--	--	2	31	--	57	60
Železnodorožnyj	1	17	40	57	64	69	72
Želtye Vody	--	7	32	40	--	51	52
Žitomir	77	95	106	161	209	229	236
Žukovskij	--	11	42	74	82	85	87
Zagorsk	21	45	74	92	98	100	101
Zaporože	54	289	449	658	729	760	772
Zelenograd	--	--	--	89	112	121	125
Zelenodolsk	3	30	60	77	83	86	86
Zima	--	28	39	42	--	50	51
Zlatoust	48	99	161	180	188	195	197
Zyrjanovsk	3	16	54	56	54	54	55
Ivanovo	111	285	335	420	447	458	461
Ivano-Frankovsk	...	65	66	105	128	139	142
Iževsk	63	176	285	422	489	522	534
Izmail	...	24	48	70	75	78	79
Izjum	23	35	38	52	56	58	58
Inta	--	--	45	50	51	51	52
Irbit	12	26	45	49	51	52	52
Irkutsk	108	250	366	451	497	519	532
Iskitim	--	14	34	45	53	57	59
Išim	14	31	48	56	61	62	63
Išimbaj	--	22	47	54	56	57	58
Joškar-Ola	4	27	89	166	195	210	216
Kadievka[1]	27	96	123	137	140	141	141
Kazan	179	406	667	869	931	958	970
Kalinin	108	216	261	345	383	395	401
Kaliningrad (Oblast Kaliningrad)	...	...	204	297	331	345	353
Kaliningrad (Oblast Moskau)	--	44	72	106	114	119	121

[1] as of Feb.15,1978 - ab 15.2.78: Stachanov

Population 2.5
Bevölkerung

	1926	1939	1959	1970	1974	1976	1977
Kaluga	52	89	134	211	240	255	262
Kaluš	...	14	13	41	51	55	57
Kamenec-Podolskij	30	35	40	57	71	77	79
Kamensk-Uralskij	5	51	141	169	178	185	187
Kamensk-Šachtinskij	17	43	58	68	73	75	76
Kamyŝin	18	24	57	97	103	108	109
Kansk	19	42	74	95	96	97	98
Karaganda	--	154	383	523	559	570	576
Karŝi	15	23	33	71	84	91	95
Kaunas	...	152	219	305	337	352	359
Kemerovo	22	137	289	385	425	446	454
Kentau	--	3	37	55	58	60	61
Kerĉ	36	104	98	128	145	152	154
Kzyl-Orda	23	47	66	122	135	143	148
Kiev	514	851	1,110	1,632	1,887	2,013	2,079
Kimry	19	35	41	53	58	59	59
Kinešma	34	75	85	96	98	100	101
Kirov	62	144	252	333	364	376	381
Kirovabad	57	99	136	190	203	211	216
Kirovakan	9	18	49	107	123	130	133
Kirovograd	71	103	132	189	211	224	228
Kirovo-Čepeck	--	--	29	51	57	62	64
Kiselevsk	--	44	128	127	125	125	124
Kislovodsk	26	51	78	90	94	97	98
Kišinev	...	112	216	356	432	471	489
Klajpeda	...	...	90	140	160	169	173
Klimovsk	--	11	29	43	--	52	52
Klin	9	28	53	81	86	88	89
Klincy	22	40	42	58	63	66	66
Kovrov	27	67	99	123	132	138	140
Kokand	69	85	105	133	147	152	155
Kokĉetav	11	19	53	81	91	97	98
Kolomna	35	87	118	136	141	144	145
Kolomyja	--	38	31	41	--	50	51
Kolpino	17	38	35	70	95	102	104
Kommunarsk	16	55	98	123	127	129	129
Komsomolsk-na-Amure	--	71	177	218	234	246	252
Konotop	33	46	54	68	73	76	77
Konstantinovka	25	96	89	105	109	111	111
Kopejsk	9	60	162	156	156	157	157
Kcĉkino	--	12	81	71	69	67	66
Korosten'	12	31	38	56	58	61	62
Kostroma	74	121	172	223	240	247	250
Kotlas	4	27	53	56	59	62	63
Kochtla-Jarve	--	--	56	68	71	71	72
Kramatorsk	12	94	115	150	162	167	171
Krasnoarmejsk (Oblast Doneck)	11	30	48	55	57	59	59
Krasnovodsk	10	21	39	49	53	54	55
Krasnogorsk (Oblast Moskau)	--	18	35	63	68	71	72
Krasnodar	153	193	313	464	519	543	552
Krasnokamsk	--	30	55	55	56	57	58
Krasnoturinsk	6	10	62	59	58	59	60
Krasnojarsk	72	190	412	648	728	758	769
Krasnyj Luĉ	13	59	94	103	104	105	105
Kremenĉug	--	90	93	166	171	202	206
Krivoj Rog	33	192	401	573	620	634	641

27

2.5 Population / Bevölkerung

	1926	1939	1959	1970	1974	1976	1977
Kropotkin	31	42	54	68	72	73	74
Kstovo	--	--	24	48	53	55	56
Kuzneck	30	38	57	84	91	94	96
Kujbyšev	176	390	806	1,045	1,140	1,186	1,204
Kumečtau	--	--	31	44	--	52	54
Kungur	21	36	65	74	79	82	83
Kurgan	28	53	146	244	278	257	304
Kursk	82	120	205	284	338	363	373
Kustanaj	25	34	86	124	143	151	154
Kutaisi	48	78	128	161	169	177	182
Kyzyl	...	10	34	52	60	57	59
Labinsk	29	---	42	50	55	57	57
Leninabad	37	46	77	103	116	121	123
Leninakan	42	68	108	165	180	188	192
Leningrad	1,737	3,401	3,340	3,987	4,243	4,372	4,425
+)	1,619	3,119	3,003	3,550	3,786	3,911	3,963
Leninogorsk (Oblast Ost-Kasachstan)	9	50	74	72	70	69	69
Leninogorsk (Tatarskaja ASSR)	--	--	39	47	--	51	52
Leninsk-Kuzneckij	20	83	132	128	130	131	131
Lida	...	33	29	48	52	55	56
Liepaja	...	53	71	93	98	103	104
Lipeck	21	67	157	289	339	363	375
Lisičansk	35	85	104	118	120	123	123
Luck	...	39	56	94	115	128	133
Lvov	...	340	411	553	605	629	612
Lysva	27	51	73	73	74	75	76
Ljubercy	10	48	95	139	151	154	156
Magadan	--	27	62	92	105	112	116
Magnitogorsk	--	146	311	364	384	393	398
Majkop	53	56	82	110	124	127	128
Makeevka	--	270	407	429	--	437	437
Margilan	44	46	68	95	108	113	115
Mary	22	37	48	62	70	70	72
Machačkala	34	87	119	186	214	231	239
Meždurečensk	---	--	55	82	88	89	91
Melitopol	25	76	95	137	149	155	157
Miass	20	38	98	131	141	145	146
Mingečaur	--	--	20	43	--	52	54
Minsk	132	237	509	917	1,095	1,189	1,231
Mineralnye Vody	18	31	40	55	60	62	64
Michajlovka	13	18	35	50	55	57	58
Mičurinsk	50	72	81	94	99	101	102
Mogilev	50	99	122	202	244	264	275
Mozyr	10	17	26	49	61	69	72
Molodečno	...	7	26	50	60	64	66

+) not including urban-type settlements under the jurisdiction of the City Soviet
+) ohne dem Stadtsowjet unterstellte Siedlungen städtischen Typs
+) v tom čisle bez gorodskich poselenij, podčinennych gorsovetu

Population 2.5
Bevölkerung

	1926	1939	1959	1970	1974	1976	1977
Moskva	2,080	4,542	6,044	7,077	7,528	7,734	7,819
+)	2,079	4,537	6,009	6,942	7,368	7,563	7,644
Mukačevo	...	...	46	57	65	69	71
Murmansk	9	119	222	309	347	369	374
Murom	23	40	72	99	107	111	112
Mytišči	17	60	99	119	127	133	136
Naberežnye Čelny	4	9	16	38	163	225	253
Navoi	4	3	10	61	77	85	87
Nalčik	13	48	88	146	182	195	199
Namangan	74	80	123	175	202	217	224
Narva	...	20	27	58	68	71	72
Naro-Fominsk	16	32	35	49	53	54	54
Nachodka	--	--	64	104	121	127	129
Nebit-Dag	--	4	33	56	62	65	67
Nevinnomyssk	--	--	40	85	95	100	101
Nežin	38	39	46	56	63	68	70
Neftekamsk	--	--	--	46	57	62	63
Nižnekamsk	--	--	--	49	84	112	120
Nižnevartovsk	--	--	--	16	--	63	76
Nižnij Tagil	39	160	338	378	390	396	399
Nikolaev	105	184	251	362	412	436	447
Nikopol	14	58	83	125	137	143	146
Novgorod	33	40	61	128	158	172	179
Novoaltajsk	--	9	34	49	51	52	53
Novokuzneck	4	166	382	499	519	530	537
Novokujbyševsk	--	--	63	104	111	113	114
Novomoskovsk (Oblast Dnepropetrovsk)	17	37	44	61	66	68	70
Novomoskovsk (Oblast Tula)	1	76	107	134	143	146	147
Novopolock	--	--	--	40	56	62	65
Novorossijsk	68	95	93	133	143	150	153
Novosibirsk	120	404	885	1,161	1,243	1,286	1,304
Novotroick	--	3	54	83	91	95	96
Novočeboksarsk	--	--	--	39	58	69	74
Novočerkassk	62	81	123	162	178	183	184
Novošachtinsk	7	48	104	102	101	101	101
Noginsk	38	81	93	104	108	111	112
Norilsk	--	14	118	135	156	168	173
Nukus	--	10	39	74	88	96	100
Obninsk	--	--	16	49	61	66	69
Odessa	418	599	664	892	981	1,023	1,039
Odincovo	3	13	20	67	72	78	80
Oktjabrskij	--	--	65	77	80	86	88
Omsk	162	289	581	821	935	1,002	1,026
Ordžonikidze	78	131	164	236	265	276	281
Orel	76	111	150	232	265	282	289
Orenburg	123	172	267	344	400	435	446
Orechovo-Zuevo	63	99	108	120	125	128	130
Orsk	14	66	176	225	237	243	244
Orša	22	54	64	101	111	114	116
Osinniki	--	25	67	62	60	60	60
Oš	31	33	65	120	143	155	161
Pavlovo	16	32	48	63	67	68	68
Pavlovskij Posad	21	43	55	66	68	69	69

+) not including urban-type settlements under the jurisdiction of the City Soviet
+) ohne dem Stadtsowjet unterstellte Siedlungen städtischen Typs
+) v tom čisle bez gorodskich poselenij, podčinennych gorsovetu

2.5 Population / Bevölkerung

	1926	1939	1959	1970	1974	1976	1977
Pavlograd	21	40	46	80	94	97	100
Pavlodar	18	29	90	187	228	247	258
Panevežis	...	27	41	73	88	94	97
Penza	92	160	255	374	414	436	443
Pervomajsk (Oblast Nikolaev)	32	33	44	59	69	73	75
Pervouralsk	9	44	90	117	122	125	126
Perm	121	306	629	850	920	957	972
Petrozavodsk	27	70	135	184	203	216	220
Petrodvorec	12	44	39	60	63	64	65
Petropavlovsk	47	92	131	173	188	196	199
Petropavlovsk-Kamĉatskij	2	35	86	154	187	202	207
Pinsk	..	30	42	62	77	84	87
Podolsk	20	72	129	169	183	191	193
Polevskoj	11	25	47	58	60	62	64
Polock	26	30	44	64	73	75	76
Poltava	91	128	143	220	254	270	274
Poti	13	25	42	46	51	54	54
Prževalsk	13	21	33	42	48	50	51
Priluki	29	37	44	57	63	66	66
Prokopevsk	11	107	282	274	269	267	267
Pskov	43	60	81	127	146	155	167
Puŝkin	25	56	46	79	82	86	86
Puŝkino (Oblast (Moskau)	4	21	30	48	57	62	65
Pjatigorsk	41	62	70	93	100	103	105
Ramenskoe	14	28	46	61	69	72	73
Revda	10	32	55	59	60	61	61
Reutov	7	15	24	50	56	58	59
Reĉica	17	30	31	48	55	59	60
Ržev	33	54	49	61	66	68	69
Riga	...	348	580	732	776	806	816
Romny	--	26	36	48	--	51	51
Rovenki	13	36	57	61	62	62	62
Rovno	...	43	56	116	147	162	167
Roslavl	26	41	37	49	54	55	55
Rostov-na-Donu	308	510	600	789	867	907	921
Rubežnoe	5	22	35	58	66	67	68
Rubcovsk	16	38	111	145	163	171	173
Rudnyj	--	--	33	96	105	108	108
Rustavi	--	--	62	98	117	127	131
Rybinsk	60	144	182	218	230	236	237
Rjazan	51	95	214	350	405	432	442
Salavat	--	--	61	114	126	130	131
Salsk	7	11	35	50	55	57	57
Samarkand	105	136	196	267	293	304	312
Saransk	15	41	91	191	223	241	248
Saran	--	5	40	49	52	54	55
Sarapul	25	42	69	97	102	107	108
Saratov	220	372	579	757	820	848	856
Safonovo	--	4	32	46	51	53	53
Sverdlovsk	140	423	779	1,025	1,122	1,171	1,187
Sverdlovsk (Oblast Vorošilovgrad)	3	37	62	68	69	71	72
Svetlogorsk (Oblast Gomel)	--	--	6	40	51	56	57
Svobodnyj	10	44	56	63	68	70	72

Population 2.5
Bevölkerung

	1926	1939	1959	1970	1974	1976	1977
Sevastopol	--	109	142˙	229	259	290	283
Severodvinsk	--	21	79	145	166	180	188
Severodoneck	--	5	33	90	104	109	111
Semipalatinsk	57	110	156	236	265	277	282
Serov	33	65	98	101	100	100	101
Serpuchov	56	91	106	124	130	131	132
Simferopol	82	143	186	249	275	286	291
Slavjansk	29	81	99	124	133	137	138
Slavjansk-na-Kubani	--	--	39	52	55	56	57
Smela	28	34	45	55	58	60	60
Smolensk	79	157	147	211	242	258	264
Snežnoe	5	44	69	64	65	64	63
Soligorsk	--	--	--	38	--	54	57
Solikamsk	6	38	83	89	93	95	97
Solncevo	--	--	--	41	--	51	51
Soĉi	13	71	127	224	244	251	255
Spassk-Dalnij	--	23	40	45	--	52	52
Stavropol	59	85	141	198	226	239	245
Staryj Oskol	20	11	27	52	66	80	92
Sterlitamak	25	39	112	185	205	210	211
Stryj	...	34	36	48	54	56	57
Stupino	--	19	40	59	62	64	64
Sumgait	--	6	51	124	152	168	174
Sumy	44	64	98	159	189	199	203
Surgut	1	--	6	34	53	67	74
Suchumi	22	44	65	102	112	118	120
Syzran	50	83	148	173	181	185	187
Syktyvkar	5	24	69	125	148	157	161
Taganrog	86	189	202	254	272	282	285
Taldy-Kurgan	--	--	41	61	76	82	84
Tallin	...	160	282	363	392	408	415
Tambov	72	106	172	230	252	262	265
Tartu	...	57	74	90	96	99	100
Taŝauz	4	15	38	63	75	81	84
Taŝkent	314	556	927	1,385	1,552	1,643	1,689
Tbilisi	294	519	703	889	984	1,030	1,042
Temirtau	--	5	77	166	192	200	202
Termez	10	13	28	45	52	55	57
Ternopol	...	50	52	85	112	127	133
Tiraspol	19	38	63	105	126	137	142
Tichoreck	19	37	50	60	62	63	63
Tichvin	--	16	18	34	--	52	54
Tobolsk	--	32	36	49	--	51	53
Tokmak (Kirgizskaja SSR)	16	19	29	42	50	54	56
Togliatti	6	--	72	251	403	463	479
Tomsk	92	145	249	338	386	413	423
Torez	2	49	92	93	95	96	96
Troick	30	47	76	85	90	92	92
Tuapse	12	30	37	51	58	61	63
Tula	155	285	351	462	494	506	510
Tulun	6	28	42	49	51	51	51
Turkestan	22	36	38	54	57	60	61
Tjumen	50	79	150	269	312	335	347
Užgorod	...	30	47	65	72	77	85
Uzlovaja	3	18	54	62	64	64	64
Ulan-Ude	29	126	174	254	287	302	308
Uljanovsk	66	98	206	351	410	436	447
Uman	44	44	45	63	75	79	81

2.5 Population
Bevölkerung

	1926	1939	1959	1970	1974	1976	1977
Uralsk	36	67	99	134	149	157	162
Urgenč	5	22	44	76	87	91	94
Usolje-Sibirskoe	8	20	48	87	96	100	101
Ussurijsk	35	72	104	128	142	145	147
Ust-Kamenogorsk	14	20	150	230	252	262	267
Ufa	99	258	547	771	871	923	942
Uchta	--	3	36	63	75	78	77
Feodosija	29	45	46	65	71	75	77
Fergana	14	36	72	111	124	132	135
Frunze	37	93	220	431	474	498	511
Chabarovsk	52	207	323	436	488	513	524
Charcyzsk	5	14	34	51	55	59	60
Charkov	417	840	953	1,223	1,330	1,385	1,405
Chasavjurt	7	23	34	54	60	64	66
Cherson	59	97	158	261	299	315	324
Chimki	3	23	48	87	97	103	106
Chmelnickij	32	37	62	113	144	161	167
Celinograd	13	31	99	180	209	217	222
Čajkovskij	--	--	13	48	60	63	64
Čapaevsk	14	58	83	86	86	87	87
Čardžou	14	51	66	96	104	110	113
Čeboksary	9	31	104	216	251	278	292
Čeljabinsk	59	273	689	875	947	989	1,007
Červonograd	...	...	12	44	51	52	53
Čeremchovo	14	56	122	99	91	88	87
Čerepovec	22	32	92	188	223	238	246
Čerkassy	40	52	85	158	204	221	229
Čerkessk	19	29	42	67	78	82	85
Černigov	35	69	90	159	205	225	233
Černovcy	...	106	152	187	199	209	214
Černogorsk	1	17	51	60	66	69	70
Čimkent	21	74	153	247	284	296	303
Čirčik	--	15	66	107	121	128	131
Čistopol	18	32	52	60	64	66	67
Čita	64	121	172	241	275	290	294
Čusovoj	18	43	61	58	58	58	59
Šadrinsk	19	31	52	73	79	81	82
Šachtersk (Oblast Doneck)	--	29	65	65	70	72	73
Šachtinsk	--	--	7	40	--	51	52
Šachty	49	135	196	205	217	222	223
Ševčenko	--	--	--	59	89	104	111
Šostka	9	29	39	64	65	64	64
Šuja	34	58	65	69	70	72	72
Šjauljaj	...	31	60	93	107	112	115
Ščekino	--	11	46	61	70	71	72
Ščelkovo	12	27	58	78	86	89	91
Ekibastuz	--	--	25	44	51	54	55
Elektrostal	--	43	97	123	130	134	135
Elista	--	17	23	50	59	62	63
Engels	34	69	91	130	148	159	163
Južno-Sachalinsk	...	...	86	106	124	131	134
Jurga	--	--	47	62	69	73	75
Jurmala	...	13	38	54	57	59	59
Jakutsk	11	53	74	108	133	143	149
Jalta	29	33	44	62	73	76	77
Jangijul	4	16	45	55	59	60	62
Jaroslavl	116	309	407	517	558	577	584

2.6
INCREASE IN POPULATION - BEVÖLKERUNGSZUWACHS - PRIROST NASELENIJA
(in percent - in Prozent - v procentach)

Year Jahr Gody	Urban Stadt Gorod- skoe	Rural Land Sel' skoe	Absolute Increase or Decrease Absoluter Zuwachs bzw. Abnahme Absoljutnyj prirost ili ubyl'	
			Urban Stadt Gorod- skoe	Rural Land Sel'- skoe
1950	69,4	109,1	3,6	- 0,5
1951	73,0	108,6	3,8	- 0,6
1952	76,8	108,0	3,4	- 0,2
1953	80,2	107,8	3,4	- 0,4
1954	83,6	107,4	2,7	+ 0,7
1955	86,3	108,1	1,9	+ 1,6
1956	88,2	109,7	3,2	+ 0,3
1957	91,4	110,0	4,2	- 0,7
1958	95,6	109,3	4,4	- 0,5
1959	100,0	108,8	3,6	- 0,0
1960	103,6	108,8	4,3	- 0,4
1961	107,9	108,4	3,3	+ 0,4
1962	111,2	108,8	3,2	+ 0,3
1963	114,4	109,1	3,3	- 0,1
1964	117,7	109,0	3,0	- 0,1
1965	120,7	108,9	3,0	- 0,4
1966	123,7	108,5	3,2	- 0,6
1967	126,9	107,9	2,9	- 0,5
1968	129,8	107,4	3,1	- 0,8
1969	132,9	106,6	3,0	- 0,9
1970	135,9	105,7	3,1	- 0,8
1971	139,0	104,9	3,5	- 1,1
1972	142,5	103,8	3,6	- 1,3
1973	146,1	102,5	3,8	- 1,3
1974	149,6	101,3	3,5	- 1,2
1975	153,1	100,2	3,5	- 1,0
1976	156,6	98,9	3,5	- 1,3
1977	160,8	98,1	3,5	- 1,3

2.7 Population
Bevölkerung

2.7 CITIES AND URBAN-TYPE SETTLEMENTS BY POPULATION
STÄDTE UND STÄDTISCHE SIEDLUNGEN NACH EINWOHNERZAHL
GORODA I POSELKI GORODSKOGO TIPA PO ČISLU ŽITELEJ

	Number of urban-type settlements Anzahl städtischer Siedlungen Cislo gorodskich poselenij				Population Einwohnerzahl Cislo žitelej (1000)			
	1926	1959	1970	1974	1926	1959	1970	1974
Total urban settlements Gesamte städtische Siedlungen Vse gorodskie poselenia	1,925	4,619	5,505	5,699	26,316	99,978	135,991	149,589
- 3,000	748	843	1,118	1,115	1,207	1,610	2,052	2,040
3,000 - 5,000	320	904	1,028	1,040	1,256	3,597	4,098	4,097
5,000 - 10,000	378	1,296	1,430	1,502	2,688	9,214	10,070	10,611
10,000 - 20,000	253	798	919	973	3,523	11,150	12,722	13,588
20,000 - 50,000	135	474	600	618	3,983	14,828	18,469	19,096
50,000 - 100,000	60	156	189	213	4,109	10,990	13,055	14,718
100,000 - 500,000	28	123	188	203	5,397	24,426	38,239	43,713
500,000 and above und mehr i bolee	3	25	33	35	4,153	24,163	37,286	41,726
Cities-Städte-goroda	709	1,679	1,935	1,999	21,696	82,941	116,267	128,692
- 3,000	51	90	78	71	106	191	156	138
3,000 - 5,000	90	115	90	76	361	460	364	303
5,000 - 10,000	168	283	255	264	1,208	2,123	1,954	1,989
10,000 - 20,000	182	443	546	564	2,574	6,507	7,911	8,242
20,000 - 50,000	127	444	556	573	3,788	14,081	17,302	17,863
50,000 - 100,000	60	156	189	213	4,109	10,990	13,055	14,718
100,000 - 500,000	28	123	188	203	5,397	24,426	38,239	43,713
500,000 and above und mehr i bolee	3	25	33	35	4,153	24,163	37,286	41,726
Urban-type settlements Siedlungen städtischen Typs Poselki gorodskogo tipa	1,216	2,940	3,570	3,700	4,620	17,037	19,724	20,897
- 3,000	697	753	1,040	1,044	1,101	1,419	1,896	1,902
3,000 - 5,000	230	789	938	964	895	3,137	3,734	3,794
5,000 - 10,000	210	1,013	1,175	1,238	1,480	7,091	8,116	8,622
10,000 - 20,000	71	355	373	409	949	4,643	4,811	5,346
20,000 and above und mehr i bolee	8	30	44	45	195	747	1,167	1,233

Population 2.8
Bevölkerung

2.8
MALE AND FEMALE - MÄNNER UND FRAUEN - MUŽČINY I ŽENŠČINY

Year Jahr Gody	Total population Gesamtbevölkerung Vse naselenie (mill.)	male Männer mužčiny	female Frauen ženščiny	male Männer mužčiny	female Frauen ženščiny
				(%)	
1897	124,6	62,0	62,6	49,8	50,2
1913	159,2	79,1	80,1	49,7	50,3
1920	136,8	65,3	71,5	47,7	52,3
1922	136,1	65,0	71,1	47,7	52,3
1926	147,0	71,0	76,0	48,3	51,7
1939	190,7	91,4	99,3	47,9	52,1
1950	178,5	78,4	100,1	43,9	56,1
1951	181,6	79,9	101,7	44,0	56,0
1952	184,8	81,5	103,3	44,1	55,9
1953	188,0	83,3	104,7	44,3	55,7
1954	191,0	84,8	106,2	44,4	55,6
1955	194,4	86,5	107,9	44,5	55,5
1956	197,9	88,5	109,4	44,7	55,3
1957	201,4	90,2	111,2	44,8	55,2
1958	204,9	92,0	112,9	44,9	55,1
1959	208,8	94,0	114,8	45,0	55,0
1960	212,4	95,9	116,5	45,2	54,8
1961	216,3	97,9	118,4	45,3	54,7
1962	220,0	99,9	120,1	45,4	54,6
1963	223,5	101,7	121,8	45,5	54,5
1964	226,7	103,4	123,3	45,6	54,4
1965	229,6	104,9	124,7	45,7	54,3
1966	232,2	106,3	125,9	45,8	54,2
1967	234,8	107,7	127,1	45,9	54,1
1968	237,2	108,9	128,3	45,9	54,1
1969	239,5	110,1	129,4	46,0	54,0
1970	241,7	111,4	130,3	46,1	53,9
1971	243,9	112,5	131,4	46,1	53,9
1972	246,3	113,8	132,5	46,2	53,8
1973	248,6	115,0	133,6	46,3	53,7
1974	250,9	116,2	134,7	46,3	53,7
1975	253,3	117,5	135,8	46,4	53,6
1976	255,5	118,7	136,8	46,4	53,6

2.9 Population
Bevölkerung

2.9 POPULATION BY SEX - BEVÖLKERUNG NACH GESCHLECHTERN - NASELENIE PO POLU

1939, 1959, 1970 (Census-Volkszählungen-Perepis'naselenija)

2.9 Total population
Gesamtbevölkerung

Vse naselenie	1939	1959	1970
SSSR	190,677,890	208,826,650	241,720,134
A. male -Männer-mužčiny	91,404,452	94,050,303	111,399,377
B. female -Frauen-ženščiny	99,273,438	114,776,347	130,320,757
RSFSR	108,377,210	117,534,306	130,079,210
A.	51,100,972	52,424,832	59,324,787
B.	57,276,238	65,109,474	70,754,423
Ukrainskaja SSR	40,468,848	41,869,046	47,126,517
A.	19,362,060	18,575,382	21,305,320
B.	21,106,788	23,293,664	25,821,197
Belorusskaja SSR	8,912,218	8,055,714	9,002,338
A.	4,316,755	3,581,485	4,137,816
B.	4,595,463	4,474,229	4,864,522
Uzbekskaja SSR	6,346,928	8,119,103	11,799,429
A.	3,278,175	3,897,342	5,743,956
B.	3,068,753	4,221,761	6,055,473
Kazachskaja SSR	6,081,361	9,294,741	13,008,726
A.	3,161,954	4,414,699	6,262,721
B.	2,919,407	4,880,042	6,746,005
Gruzinskaja SSR	3,540,023	4,044,045	4,686,358
A.	1,764,967	1,865,345	2,202,580
B.	1,775,056	2,178,700	2,483,778
Azerbajdžanskaja SSR	3,205,150	3,697,717	5,117,081
A.	1,642,612	1,756,561	2,483,035
B.	1,562,538	1,941,156	2,634,046
Litovskaja SSR	2,880,000	2,711,445	3,128,236
A.	1,381,300	1,244,678	1,467,950
B.	1,498,700	1,466,767	1,660,286
Moldavskaja SSR	2,452,023	2,884,477	3,568,873
A.	1,214,489	1,333,794	1,662,275
B.	1,237,534	1,550,683	1,906,598
Latvijskaja SSR	1,884,756	2,093,458	2,364,127
A.	886,181	919,008	1,080,616
B.	998,575	1,174,450	1,283,511
Kirgizskaja SSR	1,458,213	2,065,837	2,932,805
A.	742,169	974,620	1,401,557
B.	716,044	1,091,217	1,531,248
Tadžikskaja SSR	1,484,922	1,980,547	2,899,602
A.	769,674	964,728	1,426,255
B.	715,248	1,015,819	1,473,347

Population 2.9
Bevölkerung 2.9.1

	1939	1959	1970
Armjanskaja SSR	1,282,338	1,763,048	2,491,873
A.	648,614	842,406	1,217,163
B.	633,724	920,642	1,274,710
Turkmenskaja SSR	1,251,883	1,516,375	2,158,880
A.	645,280	730,333	1,063,151
B.	606,603	786,042	1,095,729
Estonskaja SSR	1,052,017	1,196,791	1,356,079
A.	489,250	525,090	620,195
B.	562,767	671,701	735,884

2.9.1 Urban population
Stadtbevölkerung

Gorodskoe naselenie	1939	1959	1970
SSSR	60,409,216	99,977,695	135,991,514
A.	28,920,615	45,208,278	63,026,095
B.	31,488,601	54,769,417	72,965,419
RSFSR	36,295,552	61,611,074	80,981,143
A.	17,202,121	27,652,664	37,137,193
B.	19,093,431	33,958,410	43,843,950
Ukrainskaja SSR	13,568,999	19,147,419	25,688,560
A.	6,462,266	8,664,550	11,881,383
B.	7,106,733	10,482,869	13,807,177
Belorusskaja SSR	1,854,817	2,480,505	3,907,783
A.	896,618	1,105,079	1,835,603
B.	958,199	1,375,426	2,072,180
Uzbekskaja SSR	1,469,847	2,728,580	4,321,603
A.	756,134	1,284,590	2,089,086
B.	713,713	1,443,990	2,232,517
Kazachskaja SSR	1,689,450	4,067,224	6,538,652
A.	876,882	1,922,760	3,151,725
B.	812,568	2,144,464	3,386,927
Gruzinskaja SSR	1,066,226	1,712,897	2,239,738
A.	521,425	779,420	1,046,903
B.	544,801	933,477	1,192,835
Azerbajdžanskaja SSR	1,156,798	1,767,270	2,564,551
A.	580,669	836,017	1,254,991
B.	576,129	931,253	1,309,560
Litovskaja SSR	658,900	1,045,965	1,571,737
A.	325,500	472,738	741,258
B.	333,400	573,227	830,479
Moldavskaja SSR	328,581	642,244	1,130,048
A.	160,841	293,768	529,339
B.	167,740	348,476	600,709
Latvijskaja SSR	662,669	1,173,976	1,476,602
A.	303,397	508,815	675,437
B.	359,272	665,161	801,165

2.9.1 Population
2.9.2 Bevölkerung

	1939	1959	1970
Kirgizskaja SSR	270,086	696,207	1,097,498
A.	142,716	326,442	515,622
B.	127,370	369,765	581,876
Tadžikskaja SSR	249,301	646,178	1,076,700
A.	133,424	308,021	527,776
B.	115,877	338,157	548,924
Armjanskaja SSR	366,447	881,844	1,481,532
A.	186,287	422,307	725,022
B.	180,160	459,537	756,510
Turkmenskaja SSR	416,264	700,797	1,034,199
A.	215,873	335,199	512,621
B.	200,391	365,598	521,578
Estonskaja SSR	355,279	675,515	881,168
A.	156,462	295,908	402,136
B.	198,817	379,607	479,032

2.9.2 Rural population
Landbevölkerung

Sel'skoe naselenie	1939	1959	1970
SSSR	130,268,674	108,848,955	105,728,620
A.	62,483,837	48,842,025	48,373,282
B.	67,784,837	60,006,930	57,355,338
RSFSR	72,081,658	55,923,232	49,098,067
A.	33,898,851	24,772,168	22,187,594
B.	38,182,807	31,151,064	26,910,473
Ukrainskaja SSR	26,899,849	22,721,627	21,437,957
A.	12,899,794	9,910,832	9,423,937
B.	14,000,055	12,810,795	12,014,020
Belorusskaja SSR	7,057,401	5,575,209	5,094,555
A.	3,420,137	2,476,406	2,302,213
B.	3,637,264	3,098,803	2,792,342
Uzbekskaja SSR	4,877,081	5,390,523	7,477,826
A.	2,522,041	2,612,752	3,654,870
B.	2,355,040	2,777,771	3,822,956
Kazachskaja SSR	4,391,911	5,227,517	6,470,074
A.	2,285,072	2,491,939	3,110,996
B.	2,106,839	2,735,578	3,359,078
Gruzinskaja SSR	2,473,797	2,331,148	2,446,620
A.	1,243,542	1,085,925	1,155,677
B.	1,230,255	1,245,223	1,290,943
Azerbajdžanskaja SSR	2,048,352	1,930,447	2,552,530
A.	1,061,943	920,544	1,228,044
B.	986,409	1,009,903	1,324,486
Litovskaja SSR	2,221,100	1,665,480	1,556,499
A.	1,055,800	771,940	726,692
B.	1,165,300	893,540	829,807

Population 2.9.2
Bevölkerung

	1939	1959	1970
Moldavskaja SSR	2,123,442	2,242,233	2,438,825
A.	1,053,648	1,040,026	1,132,936
B.	1,069,794	1,202,207	1,305,889
Latvijskaja SSR	1,222,087	919,482	887,525
A.	582,784	410,193	405,179
B.	639,303	509,289	482,346
Kirgizskaja SSR	1,188,127	1,369,630	1,835,307
A.	599,453	648,178	885,935
B.	588,674	721,452	949,372
Tadžikskaja SSR	1,235,621	1,334,369	1,822,902
A.	636,250	656,707	898,479
B.	599,371	677,662	924,423
Armjanskaja SSR	915,891	881,204	1,010,341
A.	462,327	420,099	492,141
B.	453,564	461,105	518,200
Turkmenskaja SSR	835,619	815,578	1,124,681
A.	429,407	395,134	550,530
B.	406,212	420,444	574,151
Estonskaja SSR	696,738	521,276	474,911
A.	332,788	229,182	218,059
B.	363,950	292,094	256,852

2.10 Population
2.10.1 Bevölkerung

DISTRIBUTION OF POPULATION BY SEX AND AGE-VERTEILUNG DER BEVÖLKERUNG

2.10 Total population
Gesamtbevölkerung
Vse naselenie

	1959 total zusammen oba pola	male (m.) Männer(M.) mužčiny(m.)	female (f.) Frauen (F.) ženščiny(ž.)
Total - Insg. - vsego	208,826,650	94,050,303	114,776,347
0 - 4 years-Jahre-let	24,433,215	12,405,396	11,927,819
5 - 9	22,029,147	11,202,904	10,826,243
10 - 14	15,337,202	7,807,678	7,529,524
15 - 19	16,471,448	8,258,809	8,212,639
20 - 24	20,343,028	10,055,978	10,287,050
25 - 29	18,190,129	8,916,969	9,273,160
30 - 34	18,998,899	8,611,011	10,387,888
35 - 39	11,590,509	4,528,340	7,062,169
40 - 44	10,408,095	3,998,239	6,409,856
45 - 49	12,263,494	4,705,764	7,557,730
50 - 54	10,446,734	4,010,114	6,436,620
55 - 59	8,698,854	2,905,486	5,793,368
60 - 69	11,736,245	4,098,922	7,637,323
70 - 79	6,168,022	2,020,519	4,147,503
80 - 89	1,578,473	464,794	1,113,679
90 - 99	203,086	49,940	153,146
100 and older - und älter - i starše	21,708	5,432	16,276
Age not indicated-Alter nicht angegeben-Vozrast ne ukazan	8,362	4,008	4,354
Gainfully employed population Bevölkerung im arbeitsfähigen Alter Naselenie v trudosposobnom vozraste (m.,M. 16-59, f.,F.,ž. 16-54)	119,821,618	55,076,204	64,745,414

2.10.1 Urban population
Stadtbevölkerung
Gorodskoe naselenie

Total - Insg. - vsego	99,977,695	45,208,278	54,769,417
0 - 4 years-Jahre-let	10,161,001	5,186,946	4,974,055
5 - 9	9,534,431	4,848,497	4,685,934
10 - 14	7,001,362	3,540,864	3,460,498
15 - 19	8,056,716	3,978,033	4,078,683
20 - 24	10,891,855	5,294,947	5,596,908
25 - 29	9,504,857	4,693,941	4,810,916
30 - 34	10,269,278	4,701,605	5,567,673
35 - 39	6,039,259	2,352,370	3,686,889
40 - 44	5,513,994	2,219,355	3,294,639
45 - 49	6,221,233	2,518,349	3,702,884

Population 2.10
Bevölkerung 2.10.1

NACH GESCHLECHT UND ALTER-RASPREDELENIE NASELENIJA PO POLU I VOZRASTU

			1970 % in relation to % Verhältnis zu % k			per 1,000 inhabitants auf 1.000 Einwohner na 1000 žitelej			
1970			1959			1959		1970	
total zusammen oba pola	m. M. m.	f. F. ž.	total zusammen oba pola	m. M. m.	f. F. ž.	m. M. m.	f. F. ž.	m. M. m.	f. F. ž.
241,720,134	111,399,377	130,320,757	+ 16	+ 18	+ 14	450	550	461	539
20,509,889	10,434,611	10,075,278	- 16	- 16	- 16	510	490	509	491
24,475,707	12,474,721	12,000,986	+ 11	+ 11	+ 11	509	491	510	490
24,988,366	12,730,029	12,258,337	+ 63	+ 63	+ 63	509	491	509	491
21,999,236	11,225,249	10,773,987	+ 34	+ 36	+ 31	501	499	510	490
17,105,210	8,626,904	8,478,306	- 16	- 14	- 18	494	506	504	496
13,770,411	6,813,420	6,956,991	- 24	- 24	- 25	490	510	495	505
21,144,685	10,408,341	10,736,344	+ 11	+ 21	+ 3	453	547	492	508
16,593,854	8,139,761	8,454,093	+ 43	+ 80	+ 20	391	609	491	509
19,003,071	8,758,628	10,244,443	+ 83	+119	+ 60	384	616	461	539
12,255,572	4,743,540	7,512,032	--	+ 1	- 1	384	616	387	613
9,077,740	3,429,835	5,647,905	- 13	- 14	- 12	384	616	378	622
12,013,176	4,273,019	7,740,157	+ 38	+ 47	+ 34	334	666	356	644
17,595,299	5,922,428	11,672,871	+ 50	+ 44	+ 53	349	651	337	663
8,024,761	2,505,750	5,519,011	+ 30	+ 24	+ 33	328	672	312	688
2,597,266	711,842	1,885,424	+ 65	+ 53	+ 69	294	706	274	726
277,799	66,664	211,135	+ 37	+ 33	+ 38	246	754	240	760
19,304	4,252	15,052	- 11	- 22	- 8	250	750	220	780
268,788	130,383	138,405							
130,486,541	64,003,489	66,483,052	+ 9	+ 16	+ 3	460	540	490	510
135,991,514	63,026,095	72,965,419	+ 36	+ 39	+ 33	452	548	463	537
9,866,019	5,029,626	4,836,393	- 3	- 3	- 3	510	490	510	490
11,699,893	5,972,123	5,727,770	+ 23	+ 23	+ 22	509	491	510	490
12,120,124	6,172,929	5,947,195	+ 73	+ 74	+ 72	506	494	509	491
13,723,142	6,924,741	6,798,401	+ 70	+ 74	+ 67	494	506	505	495
11,910,115	5,981,465	5,928,650	+ 9	+ 13	+ 6	486	514	502	498
8,821,452	4,407,079	4,414,373	- 7	- 6	- 8	494	506	500	500
13,409,641	6,599,988	6,809,653	+ 31	+ 40	+ 22	458	542	492	508
9,772,862	4,791,556	4,981,306	+ 62	+104	+ 35	390	610	490	510
11,423,242	5,339,814	6,083,428	+107	+141	+ 85	402	598	467	533
7,102,885	2,751,857	4,351,028	+ 14	+ 9	+ 18	405	595	387	613

2.10.1 Population
2.10.2 Bevölkerung

	1959		
	total zusammen oba pola	m. M. m.	f. F. ž.
50 - 54 years-Jahre-let	5,094,463	2,003,762	3,090,701
55 - 59	3,896,021	1,358,958	2,537,063
60 - 69	4,873,355	1,669,587	3,203,768
70 - 79	2,323,923	693,570	1,630,353
80 - 89	534,551	133,674	400,877
90 - 99	53,863	11,259	42,604
100 and older- und älter - i starše	4,436	912	3,524
Age not indicated-Alter nicht angegeben-Vozrast ne ukazan	3,097	1,649	1,448
Gainfully employed population Bevölkerung im arbeitsfähigen Alter Naselenie v trudosposobnom vozraste (m.,M.16-59,f.,F.,ž.16-54)	62,187,956	28,744,501	33,443,455

2.10.2 Rural population
Landbevölkerung
Sel'skoe naselenie

Total - Insg. - vsego	108,848,955	48,842,025	60,006,930
0 - 4 years-Jahre-let	14,172,214	7,218,450	6,953,764
5 - 9	12,494,716	6,354,407	6,140,309
10 - 14	8,335,840	4,266,814	4,069,026
15 - 19	8,414,732	4,280,776	4,133,956
20 - 24	9,451,173	4,761,031	4,690,142
25 - 29	8,685,272	4,223,028	4,462,244
30 - 34	8,729,621	3,909,406	4,820,215
35 - 39	5,551,250	2,175,970	3,375,280
40 - 44	4,894,101	1,778,884	3,115,217
45 - 49	6,042,261	2,187,415	3,854,846
50 - 54	5,352,271	2,006,352	3,345,919
55 - 59	4,802,833	1,546,528	3,256,305
60 - 69	6,862,890	2,429,335	4,433,555
70 - 79	3,844,099	1,326,949	2,517,150
80 - 89	1,043,922	331,120	712,802
90 - 99	149,223	38,681	110,542
100 and older - und älter - i starše	17,272	4,520	12,752
Age not indicated-Alter nicht angegeben-Vozrast ne ukazan	5,265	2,359	2,906
Gainfully employed population Bevölkerung im arbeitsfähigen Alter Naselenie v trudosposobnom vozraste (m.,M.16-59,f.,F.,ž.16-54)	57,633,662	26,331,703	31,301,959

Population 2.10.1
Bevölkerung 2.10.2

			1970 % in relation to % Verhältnis zu			per 1,000 inhabitants auf 1.000 Einwohner na 1000 žitelej			
	1970		% k	1959		1959		1970	
total	m.	f.	total	m.	f.	m.	f.	m.	f.
zusammen	M.	F.	zusammen	M.	F.	M.	F.	M.	F.
oba pola	m.	ž.	oba pola	m.	ž.	m.	ž.	m.	ž.
5,295,610	2,076,603	3,219,007	+ 4	+ 4	+ 4	393	607	392	608
6,607,335	2,473,908	4,133,427	+ 70	+ 82	+ 63	349	651	374	626
9,044,334	3,026,044	6,018,290	+ 86	+ 81	+ 88	343	657	335	665
3,834,642	1,112,470	2,722,172	+ 65	+ 60	+ 67	298	702	290	710
1,112,570	275,197	837,373	+108	+106	+109	250	750	247	753
104,476	21,505	82,971	+ 94	+ 91	+ 95	209	791	206	794
5,368	955	4,413	+ 21	+ 5	+ 25	206	794	178	822
137,804	68,235	69,569							
81,363,923	40,034,653	41,329,270	+ 31	+ 39	+ 24	462	538	492	508
105,728,620	48,373,282	57,355,338	- 3	- 1	- 4	449	551	458	542
10,643,870	5,404,985	5,238,885	- 25	- 25	- 25	509	491	508	492
12,775,814	6,502,598	6,273,216	+ 2	+ 2	+ 2	509	491	509	491
12,868,242	6,557,100	6,311,142	+ 54	+ 54	+ 55	512	488	510	490
8,276,094	4,300,508	3,975,586	- 2	0	- 4	509	491	520	480
5,195,095	2,645439	2,549,656	- 45	- 44	- 46	504	496	509	491
4,948,959	2,406,341	2,542,618	- 43	- 43	- 43	486	514	486	514
7,735,044	3,808,353	3,926,691	- 11	- 3	- 19	448	552	492	508
6,820,992	3,348,205	3,472,787	+ 23	+ 54	+ 3	392	608	491	509
7,579,829	3,418,814	4,161,015	+ 55	+ 92	+ 34	363	637	451	549
5,152,687	1,991,683	3,161,004	- 15	- 9	- 18	362	638	387	613
3,782,130	1,353,232	2,428,898	- 29	- 33	- 27	375	625	358	642
5,405,841	1,799,111	3,606,730	+ 13	+ 16	+ 11	322	678	333	667
8,550,965	2,896,384	5,654,581	+ 25	+ 19	+ 28	354	646	339	661
4,190,119	1,393,280	2,796,839	+ 9	+ 5	+ 11	345	655	333	667
1,484,696	436,645	1,048,051	+ 42	+ 32	+ 47	317	683	294	706
173,323	45,159	128,164	+ 16	+ 17	+ 16	259	741	261	739
13,936	3,297	10,639	- 19	- 27	- 17	262	738	237	763
130,984	62,148	68,836							
49,122,618	23,968,836	25,153,782	- 15	- 9	- 20	457	543	488	512

2. Population
   Bevölkerung

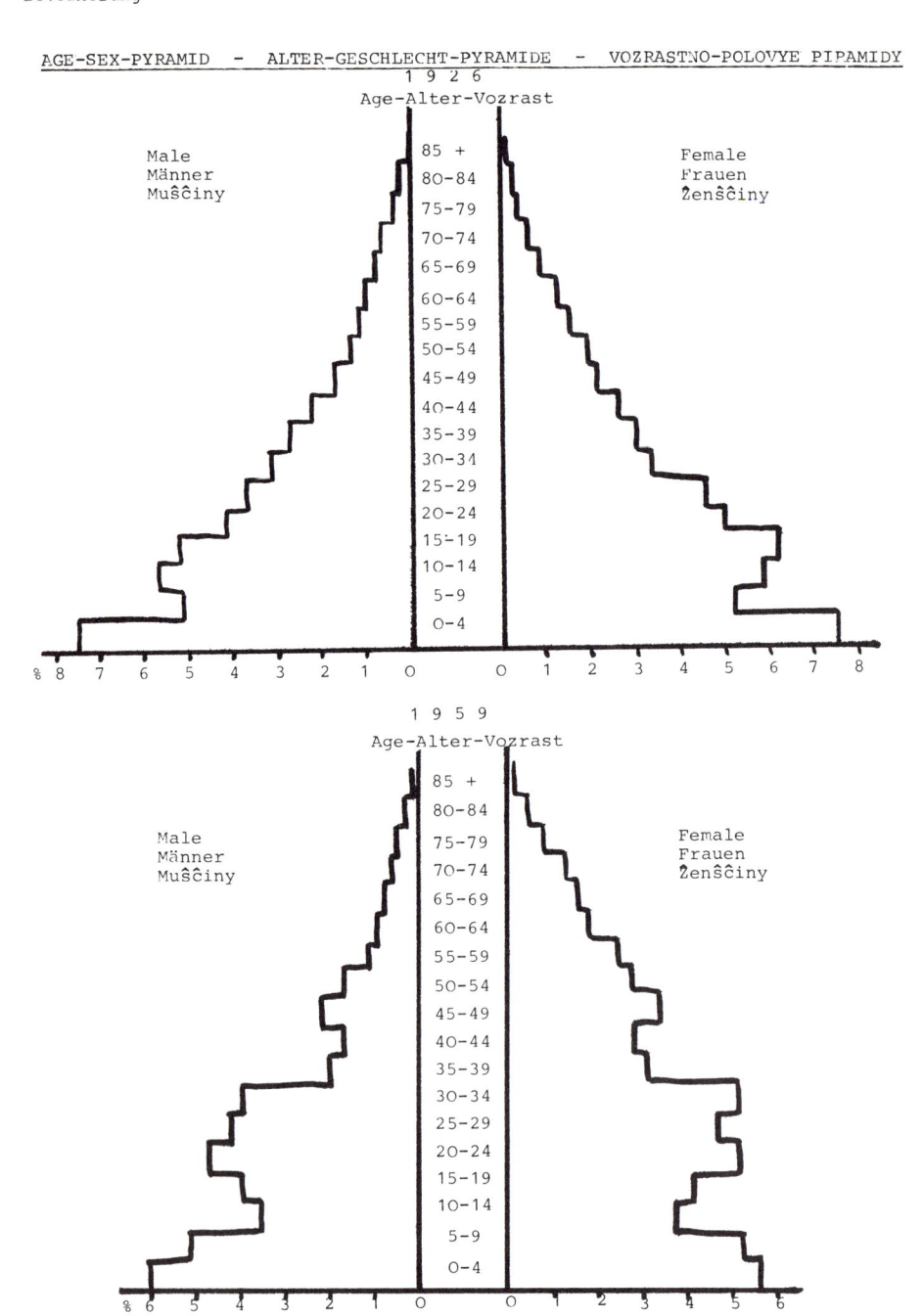

AGE-SEX-PYRAMID - ALTER-GESCHLECHT-PYRAMIDE - VOZRASTNO-POLOVYE PIPAMIDY

1 9 2 6
Age-Alter-Vozrast

Male / Männer / Mušĉiny

Female / Frauen / Ženšĉiny

85 +
80-84
75-79
70-74
65-69
60-64
55-59
50-54
45-49
40-44
35-39
30-34
25-29
20-24
15-19
10-14
5-9
0-4

1 9 5 9
Age-Alter-Vozrast

Male / Männer / Mušĉiny

Female / Frauen / Ženšĉiny

85 +
80-84
75-79
70-74
65-69
60-64
55-59
50-54
45-49
40-44
35-39
30-34
25-29
20-24
15-19
10-14
5-9
0-4

Population
Bevölkerung

AGE-SEX-PYRAMID - ALTER-GESCHLECHT-PYRAMIDE - VOZRASTNO-POLOVYE PIRAMIDY

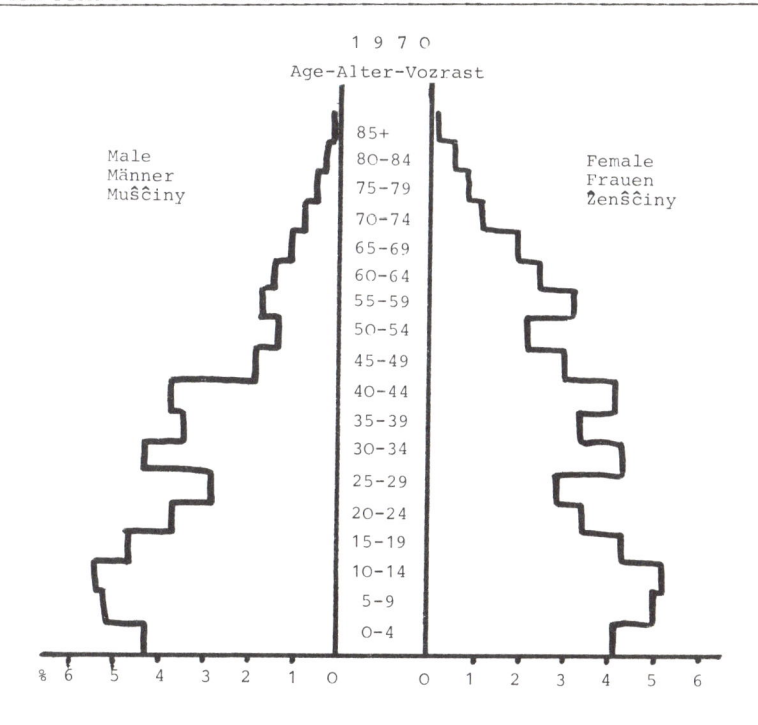

1 9 7 0
Age-Alter-Vozrast

Male	85+	Female
Männer	80-84	Frauen
Muŝĉiny	75-79	Ženŝĉiny
	70-74	
	65-69	
	60-64	
	55-59	
	50-54	
	45-49	
	40-44	
	35-39	
	30-34	
	25-29	
	20-24	
	15-19	
	10-14	
	5-9	
	0-4	

% 6 5 4 3 2 1 0   0 1 2 3 4 5 6

2.11 Population
2.11.1 Bevölkerung

2.11 PEOPLES OF THE SOVIET UNION
VÖLKER DER SOWJETUNION
NARODY SSSR

2.11.1 PRINCIPAL NATIONALITIES OF THE UNION PEPUBLICS
HAUPTNATIONEN DER UNIONSREPUBLIKEN
GLAVNYE NACII SOJUZNYCH RESPUBLIK

English	Deutsch	Po russki	Self-Designation Selbstbezeichnung Samonazvanie
Russians	Russen	Russkie	Russkie
Ukrainians	Ukrainer	Ukraincy	Ukrainci
Belorussians	Belorussen	Belorusy	Belarusy
Uzbeks	Usbeken	Uzbeki	Ozbeklar
Kazakhs	Kasachen	Kazachi	Kazakdar
Georgians	Georgier	Gruziny	Kartveli
Azerbaidzhans	Aserbaidschaner	Azerbajdžan$_{cy}$	Azerbajĝan
Lithuanians	Litauer	Litovcy	Lietuvi
Moldavians	Moldauer	Moldavane	Moldoven'
Latvians	Letten	Latyŝi	Latvieŝi
Kirghiz	Kirgisen	Kirgizy	Kirghizdar
Tadzhiks	Tadschiken	Tadžiki	Todžik
Armenians	Armenier	Armjane	Chaj
Turkmens	Turkmenier	Turkmeny	Türkmenlar
Estonians	Esten	Estoncy	Eesti(-Rahvas)

Population / Bevölkerung 2.11.2

2.11.2 PEOPLES OF THE SOVIET UNION BY ETHNIC-LINGUISTIC GROUPS
VÖLKER DER SOWJETUNION NACH ETHNISCH-LINGUISTISCHEN GRUPPEN
NARODY SSSR PO ETNIČESKO-LINGVISTIČESKIM GRUPPAM

English	Deutsch	Po russki	Self-Designation / Selbstbezeichnung / Samozvanie
Slavic group	Slawische Gruppe	Slavjanskaja gruppa	
Russians	Russen	Russkie	Russkie
Ukrainians	Ukrainer	Ukraincy	Ukrainci
Belorussians	Belorussen	Belorusy	Belarusy
Poles	Polen	Poljaki	Polacy
Bulgarians	Bulgaren	Bolgary	Bolgary
Lithuanian-Latvian group	Lettisch-litauische Gruppe	Letto-litovskaja gruppa	
Lithuanians	Litauer	Litovcy	Lietuvi
Latvians	Letten	Latyši	Latvieši
Germanic group	Germanische Gruppe	Germanskaja gruppa	
Germans	Deutsche	Nemcy	Deutsche
Romance group	Romanische Gruppe	Romanskaja gruppa	
Moldavians	Moldauer	Moldavane	Moldoven'
Albanian group	Albanische Gruppe	Albanskaja gruppa	
Albanians	Albaner	Albancy (Arnauty)	Škipetary
Greek group	Griechische Gruppe	Grečeskaja gruppa	
Greeks (south russ.)	Griechen (südruss.)	Greki (južno-russkie)	Elliny
Iranian group	Iranische Gruppe	Iranskaja gruppa	
Tadshiks	Tadschiken	Tadžiki	Todžik
Baluchi	Beludschen	Beludži	Baluč
Djemshids	Dschemschiden	Džemšidy	Džamšid (či)
Central Asiatic Jews	Mittelasiatische Juden	Evrei sredne-aziatskie	Ivri, Jachudi
Ossetians	Osetinen	Osetiny	Iron, Digor
Talysh	Talyschen	Talyši	Tolyšon
Kurds	Kurden	Kurdy	Kurmandž
Tats	Taten	Taty	Taty
Mountain Jews	Bergjuden	Gorskie Evrei	Dag(h) Čufut
Indian group	Indische Gruppe	Indijskaja gruppa	
Gipsy	Zigeuner	Cygane, Cygany	Roma, Lom, Dom, Mazang, Džugi, Ljuli
Armenian group	Armenische Gruppe	Armjanskaja gruppa	
Armenians	Armenier	Armjane	Chaj
Southern Caucasians	Kartveli-Gruppe (Südkaukasische)	Kartvelijskaja (Južno-karkazskaja) gruppa	
Georgians	Georgier	Gruziny	Kartveli

47

2.11.2 Population / Bevölkerung

English	Deutsch	Po russki	Self-Designation Selbstbezeichnung Samozvanie
Adigai-Abkhazian (Northwestern Caucasian) group	Adygeisch-Abchasische (Nordwestkaukasische) Gruppe	Adygejsko-Abchazskaja (severo-zapadnaja Kavkazskaja) gruppa	
Abkhazians	Abchasen	Abchazy	Apsua
Adegeys	Adygen	Adygejcy	Adyge
Kabardians	Kabardiner	Kabardincy	Kabardej, Adyge
Circassians	Tscherkessen	Čerkesy	Čerkes, Adyge
Abazins	Abasiner	Abaziny	Abaza
Chechen-Dagestan (Northeastern Caucasian) group	Tschetscheno-Dagestanische (Nordostkaukasische) Gruppe	Čečeno-Dagestanskaja (severo-vostočnaja Kavkazskaja) gruppa	
Chechens	Tschetschen	Čečency	Nachče
Inghushs	Inguschen	Inguŝi	Galga
Avarks	Awaren	Avarcy	Avaral
Laks	Laken	Laki	Lak (kuču)
Dargins	Darginer	Dargincy	Dargante
Tabasarans	Tabasaranen	Tabasarany	Tabasaran
Lesgians	Lesgier	Lezginy	Lezgijar
Apuls	Agulen	Aguly	Aguly
Rutuls	Rutulen	Rutulcy	Rutul
Tsakhurs	Zachuren	Cachury	Cachur
Chinalugs	Chinaluger	Chinalugi	Kettiturdur
Semitic group	Semitische Gruppe	Semitskaja gruppa	
Jewish	Juden	Evrei	Idn
Central Asian Arabs	Mittelasiatische Araber	Araby sredneaziatskie	
Ajsors	Ajsoren	Ajsory	Osurai
Finnish group	Finnische Gruppe	Finskaja gruppa	
Estonians	Esten	Estoncy	Eesti (-Rahvas)
Livs	Liven	Livy	Liivi
Karelians	Karelier	Karely	Kar'jalajne (Karjalaiset)
Izhors	Ingrier (Ischoren)	Ižorcy (Ižora)	Ingry, Inkerikot
Finns	Finnen	Finny	Suomi, Suomalaiset
Vepsy	Wepsen	Vepsy	Vepsy, Čichari
Saams	Saamen (Loparen)	Saamy	Saam(i)
Komi	Komi	Komi	Komi(-Mort)
Komi and Permyaks	Komi-Permjaken	Komi-Permjaki	Komi(-Mort) Komi-Otir
Udmurts	Udmurten	Udmurty	Udmurty
Mari (Cheremis)	Mari (Scheremissen)	Marijcy	Mari
Mordvinians	Mordwinen	Mordva, Mordviny, Mordovcy	Mokŝa, Erzja, Mokŝerzja

Population
Bevölkerung 2.11.2

English	Deutsch	Po russki	Self-Designation Selbstbezeichnung Samozvanie
	Ugrische Gruppe	Ugorskaja gruppa	
Khanty	Chanten	Chanty	Chanti, Chante, Chantych
Mansi	Mansen (Wogulen)	Mansi	Man'si
Samoyedic group	Samojedische Gruppe	Samodijskaja gruppa	
Nenets	Nenzen	Nency	Neneče
Ents	Enzen	Ency	Madu, Pe-baj
Nganasans	Nganassanen	Nganasany	Nja
Selkups	Selkupen	Sel'kupy	Sel'kup, Šel'kup, Čumyl'kup, Sjussekum, Šeŝkum
Turkish group	Türkische Gruppe	Tjurskaja gruppa	
Chuvash	Tschuwaschen	Čuvaŝi	Čuvaŝlar
Tatars	Tataren	Tatary	Tatarlar
Bashkirs	Baschkiren	Baŝkiry	Baŝkirdlar
Nogais	Nogaier	Nogajcy	Noghailar
Kumuks	Kumyken	Kumyki	Kumuklar
Karachays	Karatschaier	Karačaevcy	Karačaylar
Balkars	Balkaren	Balkarcy	Balkarlar
Kazakhs	Kasachen	Kazachi	Kazakdar
Karakalpaks	Karakalpaken	Karakalpaki	Karakalpakdar
Kirgiz	Kirgisen	Kirgizy	Kirghizdar
Altays	Altaier	Altajcy	Altaylilar
Shors	Schoren	Šorcy	Šorlar
Khakas	Chakassen	Chakasy	Hakazdar
Tuvins	Tuwiner	Tuvincy	Tuva'dar
Yakuts	Jakuten	Jakuty	Jakutlar (Sacha)
Tofalars	Topaer	Tofalary	Tofalar
Dolgans	Dolghanen	Dolgany	Dolghanlar
Uyghurs	Ujguren	Ujgury	Uyghurlar
Uzbeks	Usbeken	Uzbeki	Ozbeklär
Turkmens	Turkmenen	Turkmeny	Türkmenler
Aserbaidzhani	Aserbajdschaner	Azerbajdžancy	Azarîlar, Azerbajĝanli
Gagauz	Gagausen	Gaugauzy	Gagauzlar
Karaims	Karaimer	Karaimy	Karaimlar
Mongolian group	Mongolische Gruppe	Mongol'skaja gruppa	
Buryats	Burjaten	Burjaty	Burjat
Kalmyks	Kalmücken	Kalmyki	Kalmyk, Kalmük
Sart-Kalmaks	Sart-Kalmaken	Sart-Kalmaki	Sart
Tungus-Manchurian group	Tungusisch-Mandschurische Gruppe	Tunguso-Mančžurskaja gruppa	
Evenks	Ewenken	Evenki	Evenki
Negidals	Negidalen	Negidal'cy	Elkenbee
Evens	Ewenen	Eveny	Even, Mene, Oroč-Orač, Turgechal
Nanajs	Nanai	Nanajcy	Nanaj, Nani
Ulchis	Ultscha	Ul'či	Ul'či, Ol'či
Oroks	Oroken	Oroki	Ul'ta
Udegeys	Ude(he)	Udechejcy	Ude(he)
Orochis	Orotschen	Oroči	Oroči, Nani

49

2.11.2 Population / Bevölkerung

English	Deutsch	Po russki	Self-Designation Selbstbezeichnung Samozvanie
Paleoasiatic Peoples	Paläoasiatische Völker	Paleoaziatskie narody	
Chukchi	Tschuktschen	Čukči	Čaucu, Čavču, Luoravetlany
Koryaks	Korjaken	Korjaki	Čavčyv, Nymyl'yn
Itelmens	Itelmenen	Itel'meny	Itel'men
Jukagiry	Jukagiren	Jukagiry	Odul
Nivchis	Niwchi (Giljaken)	Nivchi	Nivchi
Eskimo-group	Eskimo-Gruppe	Eskimosskaja gruppa	
Eskimos	Eskimo	Eskimosy	Jupigyt, Nivokagmit, Ukazigmit etc.
Aleuts	Aleuten	Aleuty	Aleuty, Sasignan, Unangany
Ketskaya group	Ketische Gruppe	Ketskaja gruppa	
Kety	Keten	Kety	Ket
Aynskaya group	Ainu-Gruppe	Ajnskaja gruppa	
Ayny	Ainu	Ajny	Ajno, Ajnu
Chinese-Tibetan group	Chinesisch-Tibetanische Gruppe	Kitajskaja gruppa	
Dungans	Dunganen	Dungane	Huei-dsu
Chinese	Chinesen	Kitajcy	Chan'
Korean group	Koreanische Gruppe	Korejskaja gruppa	
Koreans	Koreaner	Korejcy	Čosen-Saram

50

Population 2.11.3
Bevölkerung

2.11.3 NATIONAL COMPOSITION OF POPULATION
NATIONALE ZUSAMMENSETZUNG DER BEVÖLKERUNG
NACIONAL'NYJ SOSTAV NASELENIJA

	A Total Gesamtzahl Vsego (1000)		B of which - davon - iz nich speak their mother tongue bekennen sich zur Muttersprache sčitajut rodnym jazyk svojej nacii (%)		C of which - davon - iz nich speak another language spoken in the USSR beherrschen eine andere Sprache der Völker der UdSSR svobodno vladejut vtorym jazykom narodov SSSR 1970; %)	
	1959	1970	1959	1970	Russian russisch russkim	others andere drugimi
Total population Gesamtbevölkerung Vse naselenie	208,827	241,720	94.3	93.9	17.3	4.2
Russkie	114,114	129,015	99.8	99.8	0.1	3.0
Ukraincy	37,253	40,753	87.7	85.7	36.3	6.0
Uzbeki	6,015	9,195	98.4	98.6	14.5	3.3
Belorusy	7,913	9,052	84.2	80.6	49.0	7.3
Tatary	4,968	5,931	92.1	89.2	62.5	5.3
Kazachi	3,622	5,299	98.4	98.0	41.8	1.8
Azerbajdžancy	2,940	4,380	97.6	98.2	16.6	2.5
Armjane	2,787	3,559	89.9	91.4	30.1	6.0
Gruziny	2,692	3,245	98.6	98.4	21.3	1.0
Moldavane	2,214	2,698	95.2	95.0	36.1	3.6
Litovcy	2,326	2,665	97.8	97.9	35.9	1.9
Evrei	2,268	2,151	21.5	17.7	16.3	28.8
Tadžiki	1,397	2,136	98.1	98.5	15.4	12.0
Nemcy	1,620	1,846	75.0	66.8	59.6	1.1
Čuvaši	1,470	1,694	90.8	86.9	58.4	5.5
Turkmeny	1,002	1,525	98.9	98.9	15.4	1.3
Kirgizy	969	1,452	98.7	98.8	19.1	3.3
Latyši	1,400	1,430	95.1	95.2	45.2	2.4
Nationalitis of Dagestan Nationalitäten Dagestans Narodnosti Dagestana of which - davon - iz nich:	945	1,365	96.2	96.5	41.7	8.9
Avarcy	270	396	97.2	97.2	37.8	5.7
Lezginy	223	324	92.7	93.9	31.6	22.3
Dargincy	158	231	98.6	98.4	43.0	2.8
Kumyki	135	189	98.0	98.4	57.4	1.2
Lakcy	64	86	95.8	95.6	56.0	3.5
Tabasarany	35	55	99.2	98.9	31.9	10.2
Nogajcy	39	52	90.0	89.8	68.5	1.1
Rutul'cy	6.7	12	99.9	98.9	30.7	18.8
Cachury	7.3	11	99.2	96.5	12.2	43.5
Aguly	6.7	8.8	99.4	99.4	39.8	9.6

2.11.3 Population / Bevölkerung

	A 1959	A 1970	B 1959	B 1970	C Russian russisch russkim	C others andere drugimi
Mordva	1,285	1,263	78.1	77.8	65.7	8.1
Baŝkiry	989	1,240	61.9	66.2	53.3	2.6
Poljaki	1,380	1,167	45.2	32.5	37.0	12.7
Estoncy	989	1,007	95.2	95.5	29.0	2.0
Udmurty	625	704	89.1	82.6	63.3	6.9
Čečency	419	613	98.8	98.7	66.7	1.0
Marijcy	504	599	95.1	91.2	62.4	6.2
Osetiny	413	488	89.1	88.6	58.6	10.7
Komi i Komi-Permjaki	431	475	88.7	83.7	64.8	5.2
of which - davon - iz nich:						
Komi	287	322	89.3	82.7	63.1	5.4
Komi-Permjaki	144	153	87.6	85.8	68.5	4.6
Korejcy	314	357	79.3	68.6	50.3	1.7
Bolgary	324	351	79.4	73.1	58.8	7.9
Greki	309	337	41.5	39.3	35.4	14.5
Burjaty	253	315	94.9	92.6	66.7	2.7
Jakuty	233	296	97.6	96.3	41.7	1.1
Kabardincy	204	280	97.9	98.0	71.4	0.8
Karakalpaki	173	236	95.0	96.6	10.4	3.6
Cygane	132	175	59.3	70.8	53.0	16.4
Ujgury	95	173	85.0	88.5	35.6	9.5
Vengry	155	166	97.2	96.6	25.8	9.8
Inguŝi	106	158	97.9	97.4	71.2	0.9
Gagauzy	124	157	94.0	93.6	63.3	8.6
People of North, Sibiria and Far East Völkerschaften des Nordens, Sibiriens u.des Fernen Ostens Narodnosti Severa, Sibiri i Dal'nego Vostoka	129	151	75.7	67.4	52.5	7.1
of which - davon - iz nich:						
Nency	23	29	84.7	83.4	55.1	3.3
Evenki	24	25	54.9	51.3	54.9	7.5
Chanty	19	21	77.0	68.9	48.1	7.3
Čukči	12	14	93.9	82.6	58.7	4.8
Eveny	9.1	12	81.4	56.0	46.4	17.6
Nanajcy	8.0	10	86.3	69.1	58.0	9.4
Mansi	6.45	7.7	59.2	52.4	38.6	5.4
Korjaki	6.3	7.5	90.5	81.1	64.3	5.5
Dolgany	3.9	4.9	93.9	89.8	61.9	3.2
Nivchi	3.7	4.4	76.3	49.5	43.8	5.6
Sel'kupy	3.8	4.3	50.6	51.1	40.8	8.6
Ul'či	2.1	2.4	84.9	60.8	56.8	7.0
Saamy	1.8	1.9	69.9	56.2	52.9	9.3
Udegejcy	1.4	1.5	73.7	55.1	46.0	10.1
Itel'meny	1.1	1.3	36.0	35.7	32.5	4.3
Kety	1.0	1.2	77.1	74.9	59.1	2.0
Oroči	0.8	1.1	68.4	48.6	44.4	6.6
Nganasany	0.75	1.0	93.4	75.4	40.0	15.7

Population 2.11.3
Bevölkerung

	A		B		C	
	1959	1970	1959	1970	Russian russisch russkim	others andere drugimi
Jukagiry	0.4	0.6	52.5	46.8	29.1	32.8
Negidal'cy[1]	...	0.5	...	53.3	45.1	6.0
Karely	167	146	71.3	63.0	59.1	15.1
Tuvincy	100	139	99.1	98.7	38.9	0.4
Kalmyki	106	137	91.0	91.7	81.1	1.5
Rumyny	106	119	83.3	63.9	28.5	16.3
Karačaevcy	81	113	96.8	98.1	67.6	1.2
Adygejcy	80	100	96.8	96.5	67.9	1.4
Kurdy	59	89	89.9	87.6	19.9	36.2
Finny	93	85	59.5	51.0	47.0	8.5
Abchazy	65	83	95.0	95.9	59.2	2.8
Chakasy	57	67	86.0	83.7	65.5	3.4
Balkarcy	42	60	97.0	97.2	71.5	2.5
Altajcy	45	56	88.5	87.2	54.9	3.2
Čerkesy	30	40	89.7	92.0	70.0	2.5
Dungane	22	39	95.1	94.3	48.0	5.7
Irancy (Persy)	21	28	44.7	36.9	33.9	12.7
Abaziny	20	25	94.8	96.1	69.5	6.1
Assirijcy	22	24	64.3	64.5	46.2	14.7
Čechi	25	21	49.0	42.9	35.6	21.4
Taty	11	17	70.9	72.6	57.7	15.3
Šorcy	15	16	83.7	73.5	59.8	5.9
Beludži	7.8	13	94.9	98.1	2.9	40.4
Slovaki	15	12	61.2	52.0	39.3	31.3
Vepsy	16	8.3	46.1	34.3	32.8	16.4
Udiny	3.7	5.9	92.6	93.5	36.4	32.6
Chalcha-mongoly	1.8	5.2	86.6	92.9	54.4	1.6
Karaimy	5.7	4.6	13.9	12.8	11.3	21.4
Albancy	5.3	4.4	79.0	56.7	47.4	7.0
Afgancy	1.9	4.2	71.8	70.7	26.7	31.9
French-Franzosen- Francuzy	1.0	2.5	56.4	75.1	19.6	17.7
People of India and Pakistan Völker Indiens und Pakistans Narody Indii i Pakistana	0.4	1.9	84.4	87.7	47.8	2.2
Eskimosy	1.1	1.3	84.0	60.0	50.5	3.4
Ižorcy	1.1	0.8	34.7	26.6	24.5	32.0
Tofy	0.6	0.6	89.1	56.3	48.7	4.5
Aleuty	0.4	0.4	22.3	21.8	18.8	1.8
Others-andere-drugie	97	152	69.1	81.3	33.9	19.0

[1] 1959 recorded under Evenks - 1959 unter Ewenken erfaßt -
1959 g. negidal'cy učityvalis' v sostave evenkov

53

2.11.4 Population
Bevölkerung

2.11.4 NATIONALITIES REPRESENTED AMONG THE POPULATION
ANTEIL DER HAUPTNATIONEN AN DER BEVÖLKERUNG
GLAVNYE NACII V NASELENII
1970 - %

	Total population Gesamtbevölkerung Vse naselenie	Russkie	Ukraincy	Belorusy	Uzbeki	Kazachi	Gruziny	Azerbajdžancy
SSSR	100,0	53,4	16,9	3,7	3,8	2,2	1,3	1,8
RSFSR	100,0	82,8	2,6	0,7	---	0,4	0,1	0,1
Ukrainskaja SSR	100,0	19,4	74,9	0,8	---	---	---	---
Belorusskaja SSR	100,0	10,4	2,1	81,0	---	---	---	---
Uzbekskaja SSR	100,0	12,5	0,9	---	65,5	4,0	---	---
Kazachskaja SSR	100,0	42,4	7,2	1,5	1,7	32,6	---	---
Gruzinskaja SSR	100,0	8,5	1,1	---	---	---	66,8	4,6
Azerbajdžanskaja SSR	100,0	10,0	---	---	---	---	---	73,8
Litovskaja SSR	100,0	8,6	0,8	1,5	---	---	---	---
Moldavskaja SSR	100,0	11,6	14,2	---	---	---	---	---
Latvijskaja SSR	100,0	29,8	2,3	4,0	---	---	---	---
Kirgizskaja SSR	100,0	29,2	4,1	---	11,3	0,8	---	---
Tadžikskaja SSR	100,0	11,9	1,1	---	23,0	0,3	---	---
Armjanskaja SSR	100,0	2,7	---	---	---	---	---	5,9
Turkmenskaja SSR	100,0	14,5	1,6	---	8,3	3,2	---	---
Estonskaja SSR	100,0	24,7	2,1	1,4	---	---	---	---

Population 2.11.4
Bevölkerung

OF THE USSR AND THE UNION REPUBLICS
DER UdSSR UND DEN UNIONSREPUBLIKEN
SSSR I SOJUZNYCH RESPUBLIK
1970 - %

v tom čisle

Litovcy	Moldavane	Latyši	Kirgizy	Tadžiki	Armjane	Turkmeny	Estoncy	Tatary	Evrei	Other nationalities / Andere Nationali-täten / Drugie nacional-nosti
1,1	1,2	0,6	0,6	0,9	1,5	0,6	0,4	2,4	0,9	6,7
---	0,1	---	---	---	0,2	---	---	3,7	0,6	8,7
---	0,6	---	---	---	---	---	---	---	1,6	2,7
---	---	---	---	---	---	---	---	---	1,6	4,9
---	---	---	0,9	3,8	---	0,6	---	4,9	0,9	6,0
---	---	---	---	---	---	---	---	2,2	---	12,4
---	---	---	---	---	9,7	---	---	---	1,2	8,1
---	---	---	---	---	9,4	---	---	---	---	6,8
80,1	---	---	---	---	---	---	---	---	0,8	8,2
---	64,6	---	---	---	---	---	---	---	2,7	6,9
1,7	---	56,8	---	---	---	---	---	---	1,6	3,8
---	---	---	43,8	0,7	---	---	---	2,4	---	7,7
---	---	---	1,2	56,2	---	0,4	---	2,4	0,5	3,0
---	---	---	---	---	88,6	---	---	---	---	2,8
---	---	---	---	---	1,1	65,6	---	1,7	---	4,0
---	---	---	---	---	---	---	68,2	---	0,4	3,2

55

Communist Party of the Soviet Union
Kommunistische Partei der Sowjetunion

COMMUNIST PARTY OF THE SOVIET UNION
KOMMUNISTISCHE PARTEI DER SOWJETUNION
KOMMUNISTIČESKAJA PARTIJA SOVETSKOGO SOJUZA

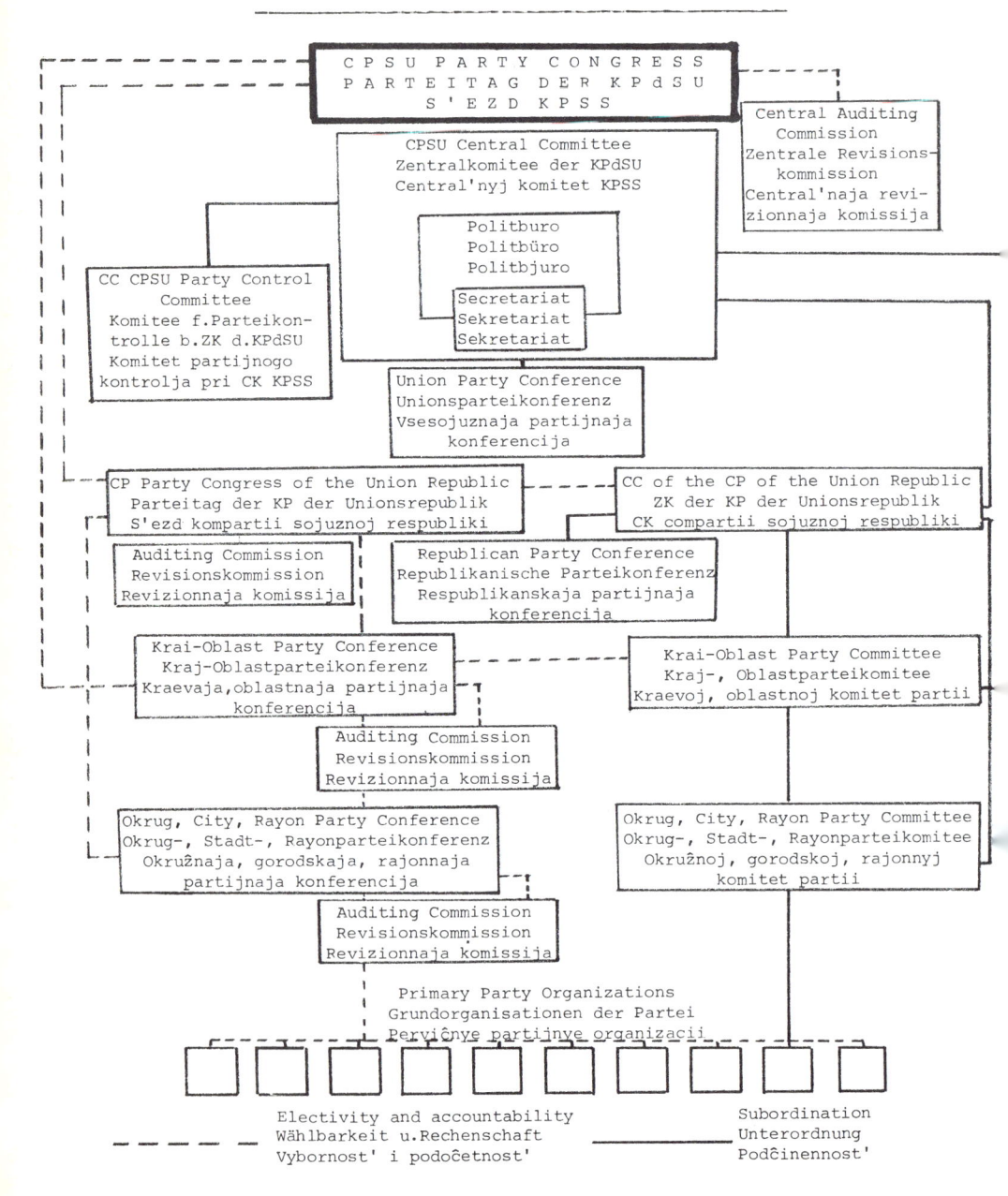

```
┌─────────────────────────────────────┐
│   CPSU  PARTY  CONGRESS             │
│   PARTEITAG  DER  KPdSU             │
│         S'EZD  KPSS                 │
└─────────────────────────────────────┘
```

Central Auditing Commission
Zentrale Revisionskommission
Central'naja revizionnaja komissija

CPSU Central Committee
Zentralkomitee der KPdSU
Central'nyj komitet KPSS

- Politburo / Politbüro / Politbjuro
- Secretariat / Sekretariat / Sekretariat

CC CPSU Party Control Committee
Komitee f. Parteikontrolle b. ZK d. KPdSU
Komitet partijnogo kontrolja pri CK KPSS

Union Party Conference
Unionsparteikonferenz
Vsesojuznaja partijnaja konferencija

CP Party Congress of the Union Republic
Parteitag der KP der Unionsrepublik
S'ezd kompartii sojuznoj respubliki

CC of the CP of the Union Republic
ZK der KP der Unionsrepublik
CK compartii sojuznoj respubliki

Auditing Commission
Revisionskommission
Revizionnaja komissija

Republican Party Conference
Republikanische Parteikonferenz
Respublikanskaja partijnaja konferencija

Krai-Oblast Party Conference
Kraj-Oblastparteikonferenz
Kraevaja, oblastnaja partijnaja konferencija

Krai-Oblast Party Committee
Kraj-, Oblastparteikomitee
Kraevoj, oblastnoj komitet partii

Auditing Commission
Revisionskommission
Revizionnaja komissija

Okrug, City, Rayon Party Conference
Okrug-, Stadt-, Rayonparteikonferenz
Okružnaja, gorodskaja, rajonnaja partijnaja konferencija

Okrug, City, Rayon Party Committee
Okrug-, Stadt-, Rayonparteikomitee
Okružnoj, gorodskoj, rajonnyj komitet partii

Auditing Commission
Revisionskommission
Revizionnaja komissija

Primary Party Organizations
Grundorganisationen der Partei
Pervičnye partijnye organizacii

--- Electivity and accountability / Wählbarkeit u. Rechenschaft / Vybornost' i podočetnost'

——— Subordination / Unterordnung / Podčinennost'

Communist Party of the Soviet Union
Kommunistische Partei der Sowjetunion 3.1

3. COMMUNIST PARTY OF THE SOVIET UNION
KOMMUNISTISCHE PARTEI DER SOWJETUNION
KOMMUNISTIČESKAJA PARTIJA SOVETSKOGO SOJUZA

3.1 PARTY CONGRESSES - PARTEITAGE - S'EZDY PARTII

		Delegates-Delegierte-Delegaty Total Insg. Vsego	of which-davon-iz nich with deciding vote mit entscheidender Stimme s reš.golosom	in an advisory capacity mit beratender Stimme s sovešč. golosom
		A	B	C
1.	RSDRP [1] 1.-3. (13.-15.) 3.1898 Minsk	9	9	-
2.	RSDRP 17.(30.)7.- 10.(23.)8.1903 Bruxelles-London	57	43	14
3.	RSDRP 12.-27.4.(25.4.- 10.5.)1905 London	38	24	14
4.	(Ob'edinitel'nyj) RSDRP 10.-25.4.(23.4.- 8.5.)1906 Stockholm	134	112	22
5.	(Londonskij) RSDRP 30.4.-19.5. (13.5.-1.6.)1907 London	342	303	39
6.	RSDRP(b) [2] 26.7.-3.8. (8.-16.8.)1917 Petrograd	267	157	110
7.	(ekstrennyj) RKP(b) [3] 6.-8.3.1918 Petrograd	106	47	59
8.	RKP(b) 18.-23.3.1919 Moskva	403	301	102
9.	RKP(b) 29.3.-5.4.1920 Moskva	716	554	162

[1] 1898-1917 RSDRP
   Social Democratic Workers' Party of Russia
   Sozialdemokratische Arbeiterpartei Rußlands
   Rossijskaja Social-Demokratičeskaja rabočaja partija

[2] 1917-1918 RSDRP(b)
   Social Democratic Workers' Party of Russia (Bolshevik)
   Sozialdemokratische Arbeiterpartei (Bolschewiki) Rußlands
   Rossijskaja Social-Demokratičeskaja rabočaja partija (bol'ševikov)

[3] 1918-1925 RKP(b)
   Communist Party of Russia (Bolshevik)
   Kommunistische Partei (Bolschewiki) Rußlands
   Rossijskaja Kommunisticheskaja partija (bol'ševikov)

3.1 Communist Party of the Soviet Union
Kommunistische Partei der Sowjetunion

			A	B	C
10.	RKP(b) 8.-16.3.1921	Moskva	990	694	296
11.	RKP(b) 27.3.-2.4.1922	Moskva	687	522	165
12.	RKP(b) 17.-25.4.1923	Moskva	825	408	417
13.	RKP(b) 23.-31.5.1924	Moskva	1,164	748	416
14.	VKP(b)[4] 18.-31.12.1925	Moskva	1,306	665	641
15.	VKP(b) 2.-19.12.1927	Moskva	1,669	898	771
16.	VKP(b) 26.6.-13.7.1930	Moskva	2,159	1,268	891
17.	VKP(b) 26.1.-10.2.1934	Moskva	1,961	1,225	736
18.	VKP(b) 10.-21.3.1939	Moskva	2,035	1,569	466
19.	KPSS[5] 5.-14.10.1952	Moskva	1,359	1,192	167
20.	KPSS 14.-25.2.1956	Moskva	1,430	1,349	81
21.	(Vneočerednoj) KPSS 27.1.-25.2.1959	Moskva	1,367	1,261	106
22.	KPSS 17.-31.10.1961	Moskva	4,799	4,394	405
23.	KPSS 29.3.-8.4.1966	Moskva	4,942	4,619	323
24.	KPSS 30.3.-9.4.1971	Moskva	4,963	4,740	223
25.	KPSS 24.2.-5.3.1976	Moskva	4,998	--	--

---

[4] 1925-1952 VKP(b)
   Communist Party of the Soviet Union (Bolshevik)
   Kommunistische Partei der Sowjetunion (Bolschewiki)
   Vsesojuznaja Kommunističeskaja partija (bol'ševikov)

[5] seit 1952 KPSS
   Communist Party of the Soviet Union
   Kommunistische Partei der Sowjetunion
   Kommunističeskaja partija Sovetskogo Sojuza

Communist Party of the Soviet Union
Kommunistische Partei der Sowjetunion 3.2

3.2 NUMBER OF MEMBERS - MITGLIEDERZAHLEN - ČISLENNYJ SOSTAV
1 9 1 7 - 1 9 7 5

	Members Mitglieder Členy	Candidates Kandidaten Kandidaty	Total Insgesamt Vsego
1917 (1. 3.)	24,000	--	24,000
1917 (1.10.)	350,000	--	350,000
1918 (1. 3.)	390,000	--	390,000
1919 (1. 3.)	350,000	--	350,000
1920 (1. 3.)	611,978	--	611,978
1921 (1. 3.)	732,521	--	732,521
1922 (1. 1.)[1]	410,430	117,924	528,354
1923	381,400	117,700	499,100
1924	350,000	122,000	472,000
1925	440,365	361,439	801,804
1926	639,652	440,162	1,079,814
1927	786,288	426,217	1,212,505
1928	914,307	391,547	1,305,854
1929	1,090,508	444,854	1,535,362
1930	1,184,651	493,259	1,677,910
1931	1,369,406	842,819	2,212,225
1932	1,769,773	1,347,477	3,117,250
1933	2,203,951	1,351,387	3,555,338
1934	1,826,756	874,252	2,701,008
1935	1,659,104	699,610	2,358,714
1936	1,489,907	586,935	2,076,842
1937	1,453,828	527,869	1,981,697
1938	1,405,879	514,123	1,920,002
1939	1,514,181	792,792	2,306,973
1940	1,982,743	1,417,232	3,399,975
1941	2,490,479	1,381,986	3,872,465
1942	2,155,336	908,540	3,063,876
1943	2,451,511	1,403,190	3,854,701
1944	3,126,627	1,791,934	4,918,561
1945	3,965,530	1,794,839	5,760,369

[1] as of 1921: 1.1. - ab 1921: zum 1.1. - s 1921 na 1.1.

3.2 Communist Party of the Soviet Union
Kommunistische Partei der Sowjetunion

	Members Mitglieder Členy	Candidates Kandidaten Kandidaty	Total Insgesamt Vsego
1946	4,127,689	1,383,173	5,510,862
1947	4,774,886	1,277,015	6,051,901
1948	5,181,199	1,209,082	6,390,281
1949	5,334,811	1,017,761	6,352,572
1950	5,510,787	829,396	6,340,183
1951	5,658,577	804,398	6,462,975
1952	5,853,200	854,339	6,707,539
1953	6,067,027	830,197	6,897,224
1954	6,402,284	462,579	6,864,863
1955	6,610,238	346,867	6,957,105
1956	6,767,644	405,877	7,173,521
1957	7,001,114	493,459	7,494,573
1958	7,296,559	546,637	7,843,196
1959	7,622,356	616,775	8,239,131
1960	8,017,249	691,418	8,708,667
1961	8,472,396	803,430	9,275,826
1962	9,051,934	839,134	9,891,068
1963	9,581,149	806,047	10,387,196
1964	10,182,916	839,453	11,022,369
1965	10,811,443	946,726	11,758,169
1966	11,548,287	809,021	12,357,308
1967	12,135,103	549,030	12,684,133
1968	12,484,836	695,389	13,180,225
1969	12,958,303	681,588	13,639,891
1970	13,395,253	616,531	14,011,784
1971	13,745,980	626,583	14,372,563
1972	14,109,432	521,857	14,631,289
1973	14,330,525	490,506	14,821,031
1974	14,493,524	532,391	15,025,915
1975	14,719,062	575,741	15,294,803
1976	15,029,562	602,329	15,638,891
1977 (July 1 - 1.7.)	15,545,097	658,349	16,203,446

Communist Party of the Soviet Union
Kommunistische Partei der Sowjetunion 3.

C P S U   C E N T R A L   C O M M I T T E E
Z E N T R A L K O M I T E E   D E R   K P d S U
EXECUTIVE AND ADMINISTRATIVE APPARATUS [1]
EXEKUTIVE UND VERWALTUNGSAPPARAT
(1. 1. 1979)

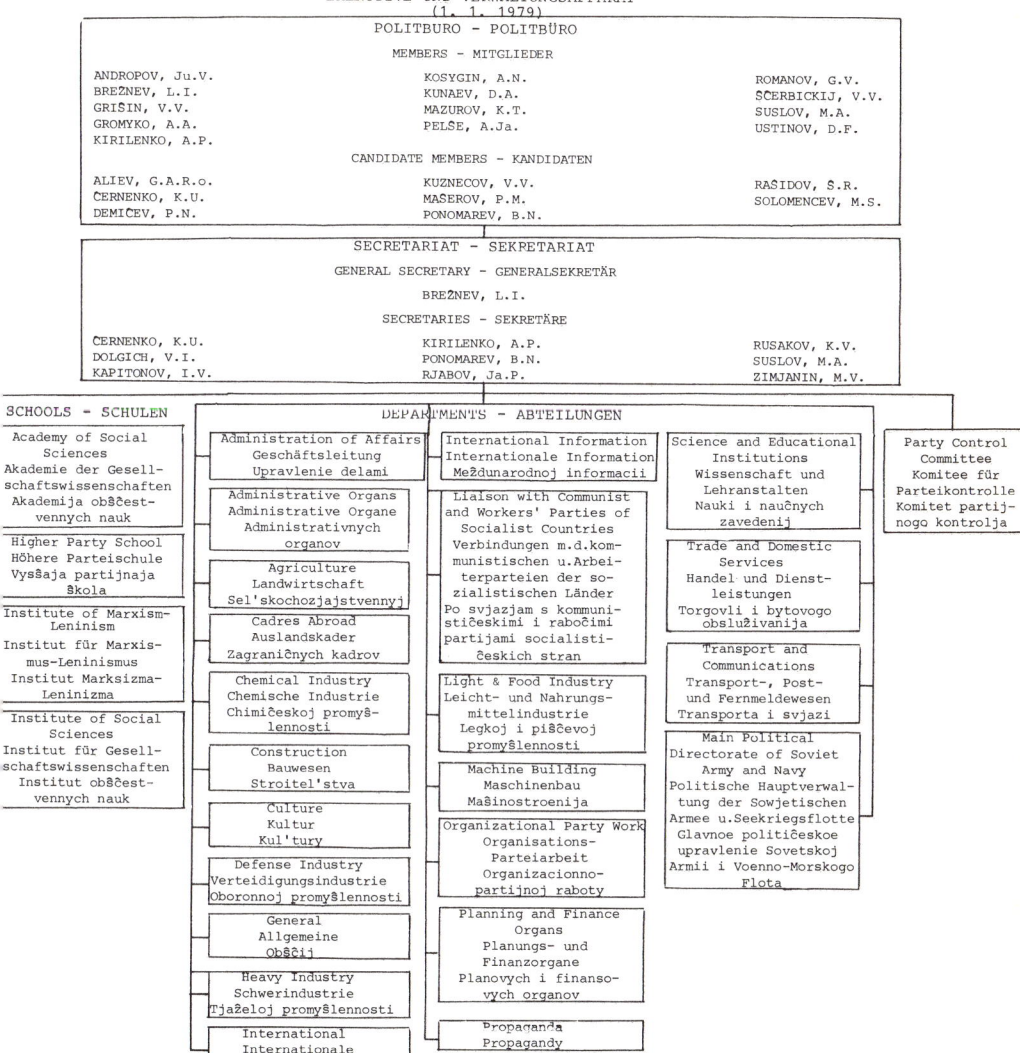

POLITBURO - POLITBÜRO

MEMBERS - MITGLIEDER

ANDROPOV, Ju.V.	KOSYGIN, A.N.	ROMANOV, G.V.
BREŽNEV, L.I.	KUNAEV, D.A.	ŠČERBICKIJ, V.V.
GRIŠIN, V.V.	MAZUROV, K.T.	SUSLOV, M.A.
GROMYKO, A.A.	PELŠE, A.Ja.	USTINOV, D.F.
KIRILENKO, A.P.		

CANDIDATE MEMBERS - KANDIDATEN

ALIEV, G.A.R.o.	KUZNECOV, V.V.	RAŠIDOV, Š.R.
ČERNENKO, K.U.	MAŠEROV, P.M.	SOLOMENCEV, M.S.
DEMIČEV, P.N.	PONOMAREV, B.N.	

SECRETARIAT - SEKRETARIAT

GENERAL SECRETARY - GENERALSEKRETÄR
BREŽNEV, L.I.

SECRETARIES - SEKRETÄRE

ČERNENKO, K.U.	KIRILENKO, A.P.	RUSAKOV, K.V.
DOLGICH, V.I.	PONOMAREV, B.N.	SUSLOV, M.A.
KAPITONOV, I.V.	RJABOV, Ja.P.	ZIMJANIN, M.V.

SCHOOLS - SCHULEN

- Academy of Social Sciences
  Akademie der Gesellschaftswissenschaften
  Akademija obščestvennych nauk
- Higher Party School
  Höhere Parteischule
  Vysšaja partijnaja škola
- Institute of Marxism-Leninism
  Institut für Marxismus-Leninismus
  Institut Marksizma-Leninizma
- Institute of Social Sciences
  Institut für Gesellschaftswissenschaften
  Institut obščestvennych nauk

DEPARTMENTS - ABTEILUNGEN

- Administration of Affairs
  Geschäftsleitung
  Upravlenie delami
- Administrative Organs
  Administrative Organe
  Administrativnych organov
- Agriculture
  Landwirtschaft
  Sel'skochozjajstvennyj
- Cadres Abroad
  Auslandskader
  Zagraničnych kadrov
- Chemical Industry
  Chemische Industrie
  Chimičeskoj promyšlennosti
- Construction
  Bauwesen
  Stroitel'stva
- Culture
  Kultur
  Kul'tury
- Defense Industry
  Verteidigungsindustrie
  Oboronnoj promyšlennosti
- General
  Allgemeine
  Obščij
- Heavy Industry
  Schwerindustrie
  Tjaželoj promyšlennosti
- International
  Internationale
  Meždunarodnyj
- International Information
  Internationale Information
  Meždunarodnoj informacii
- Liaison with Communist and Workers' Parties of Socialist Countries
  Verbindungen m.d.kommunistischen u.Arbeiterparteien der sozialistischen Länder
  Po svjazjam s kommunističeskimi i raboči mi partijami socialističeskich stran
- Light & Food Industry
  Leicht- und Nahrungsmittelindustrie
  Legkoj i piščevoj promyšlennosti
- Machine Building
  Maschinenbau
  Mašinostroenija
- Organizational Party Work
  Organisationsparteiarbeit
  Organizacionnopartijnoj raboty
- Planning and Finance Organs
  Planungs- und Finanzorgane
  Planovych i finansovych organov
- Propaganda
  Propagandy
- Science and Educational Institutions
  Wissenschaft und Lehranstalten
  Nauki i naučnych zavedenij
- Trade and Domestic Services
  Handel und Dienstleistungen
  Torgovli i bytovogo obsluživanija
- Transport and Communications
  Transport-, Postund Fernmeldewesen
  Transporta i svjazi
- Main Political Directorate of Soviet Army and Navy
  Politische Hauptverwaltung der Sowjetischen Armee u.Seekriegsflotte
  Glavnoe političeskoe upravlenie Sovetskoj Armii i Voenno-Morskogo Flota
- Party Control Committee
  Komitee für Parteikontrolle
  Komitet partijnogo kontrolja

Besides there are following schools of the CC of the CPSU -
Außerdem bestehen beim ZK der KPdSU folgende Schulen:

Institute of Scientific Atheism of the Academy of Social Sciences - Institut für wissenschaftlichen Atheismus -
   Institut naučnogo ateizma Akademii obščestvennych nauk;
Higher Party School for Correspondence Courses - Höhere Parteischule für Fernstudium - Zaočnaja vysšaja partijnaja škola;
Institute for Further Education of the Leading Party and Soviet Cadre of the Higher Party School -
   Institut für die Erhöhung der Qualifikation der leitenden Partei- und Sowjetkader der Höheren Parteischule -
   Institut povyšenija kvalifikacii rukovodjaščich partijnych i sovetskich kadrov Vysšej partijnoj školy.

[1] also see page - siehe auch Seite 95 ff.

3.3 Communist Party of the Soviet Union
Kommunistische Partei der Sowjetunion

3.3 POLITBURO CC CPSU - POLITBÜRO ZK KPdSU - POLITBJURO CK KPSS
(1952-66 Presidium - Präsidium - Prezidium)

	Members Mitglieder Členy			Candidate members Kandidaten Kandidaty		
	Name Name Familija	Date of birth/death Geburts-/ Sterbedat. data rožd./ smerti	Party affiliation Parteizugehörigkeit Partijnyj staž	Name Name Familija	Date of birth/death Geburts-/ Sterbedat. data rožd./ smerti	Party affiliation Parteizugehörigkeit Partijnyj staž
	A	B	C	A	B	C
Zasedanie[1] CK RSDRP(b) 10.(23.)10. 1917	LENIN, V.I. BUBNOV, A.S. ZINOVEV, G.E.	1870-1924[5] 1883-1940[3] 1883-1936[3]	1893 1903 1901-27 1928-32 1933-34			
	KAMENEV, L.B.	1883-1936[3]	1901-27 1928-32 1933-34			
	SOKOLNIKOV, G.Ja. STALIN, J.V. TROCKIJ, L.D.	1888-1939[5] 1879-1953 1879-1940[4]	1905-36 1898 1917-27			
Plenum CK RKP(b) 25.3.1919	KAMENEV, L.B. KRESTINSKIJ, N.N. LENIN, V.I. STALIN, J.V. TROCKIJ, L.D.	1883-1938[3]	1903	BUCHARIN, N.I. ZINOVEV, G.E. KALININ, M.I.	1888-1938[3] 1875-1946	1906 1898
Plenum CK RKP(b) 5.4.1920	KAMENEV, L.B. KRESTINSKIJ, N.N. LENIN, V.I. STALIN, J.V. TROCKIJ, L.D.			BUCHARIN, N.I. ZINOVEV, G.E. KALININ, M.I.		

1 Meeting - Tagung - Zasedanie
2 Joint Plenum - Vereinigtes Plenum - Ob'edinennyj plenum
3 liquidated - liquidiert - likvidirovan
4 murdered - ermordet - ubit
5 died in arrest - in Haft gestorben - umer v tjurme
6 suicide - Selbstmord - samoubijstvo
7 Joint Session of the Plenum of the CC CPSU, of the Council of Ministers of the USSR, of the Presidium of the Supreme Soviet of the USSR -
Gemeinsame Tagung des Plenums des ZK der KPdSU, des Ministerrates der UdSSR, des Präsidiums des Obersten Sowjets der UdSSR -
Sovmestnoe zasedanie plenuma CK KPSS, Soveta Ministrov SSSR, Prezidiuma Verchovnogo Soveta SSSR

Communist Party of the Soviet Union
Kommunistische Partei der Sowjetunion   3.3

	Members Mitglieder Členy			Candidate members Kandidaten Kandidaty		
	A	B	C	A	B	C
Plenum CK RKP(b) 16.3.1921	KAMENEV, L.B. ZINOVEV, G.E. LENIN, V.I. STALIN, J.V. TROCKIJ, L.D.			BUCHARIN, N.I. KALININ, M.I. MOLOTOV, V.M.*	1890	1906
Plenum CK RKP(b) 3.4.1922	ZINOVEV, G.E. KAMENEV, L.B. LENIN, V.I. STALIN, J.V. TROCKIJ, L.D.			BUCHARIN, N.I. KALININ, M.I. MOLOTOV, V.M.		
Plenum CK RKP(b) 26.4.1923	ZINOVEV, G.E. KAMENEV, L.B. LENIN, V.I. RYKOV, A.I. STALIN, J.V. TOMSKIJ, M.P. TROCKIJ, L.D.	1881-1938[3] 1880-1936[6]	1899 1904	BUCHARIN, N.I. KALININ, M.I. MOLOTOV, V.M. RUDZUTAK, Ja.E.	1887-1938[3]	1905
Plenum CK RKP(b) 2.6.1924	BUCHARIN, N.I. ZINOVEV, G.E. KAMENEV, L.B. RYKOV, A.I. STALIN, I.V. TOMSKIJ, M.P. TROCKIJ, L.D.			DZERŽINSKIJ, F.E. KALININ, M.I. MOLOTOV, V.M. RUDZUTAK, Ja.E. SOKOLNIKOV, G.Ja. FRUNZE, M.V.	1877-1926 1885-1925	1895 1904
Plenum CK VKP(b) 1.1.1926	BUCHARIN, N.I. VOROŠILOV, K.E. ZINOVEV, G.E. KALININ, M.I. MOLOTOV, V.M. RYKOV, A.I. STALIN, J.V. TOMSKIJ, M.P. TROCKIJ, L.D.	1881-1969	1903	DZERŽINSKIJ, F.E. KAMENEV, L.B. PETROVSKIJ, G.I. RUDZUTAK, Ja.E. UGLANOV, N.A.	1878-1958 1886-1940[5]	1897 1907-32 1932-36
Plenum CK VKP(b) 14.-23.7.1926	BUCHARIN, N.I. VOROŠILOV, K.E. KALININ, M.I. MOLOTOV, V.M. RUDZUTAK, Ja.E. RYKOV, A.I. STALIN, J.V. TOMSKIJ, M.P. TROCKIJ, L.D.			ANDREEV, A.A. KAGANOVIČ, L.M.* KAMENEV, L.B. KIROV, S.M. MIKOJAN, A.I. ORDŽONIKIDZE, G.K. PETROVSKIJ, G.I. UGLANOV, N.A.	1895-1971 1893 1886-1934[4] 1895 1886-1937[6]	1914 1911 1904 1915 1903
Ob'edinennyj[2] plenum CK CKK VKP(b) 23.10.1926	BUCHARIN, N.I. VOROŠILOV, K.E. KALININ, M.I. MOLOTOV, V.M. RUDZUTAK, Ja.E. RYKOV, A.I. STALIN, J.V. TOMSKIJ, M.P.			ANDREEV, A.A. KAGANOVIČ, L.M. KIROV, S.M. MIKOJAN, A.I. ORDŽONIKIDZE, G.K. PETROVSKIJ, G.I. UGLANOV, N.A.		

* 1957 relieved from all party and government posts for "forming group hostiled to party" - 1957 wegen "Bildung einer parteifeindlichen Gruppe" aller Partei-u.Staatsämter enthoben

63

3.3 Communist Party of the Soviet Union
Kommunistische Partei der Sowjetunion

	Members Mitglieder Členy			Candidate members Kandidaten Kandidaty		
	A	B	C	A	B	C
Ob'edinnenyj plenum CK i CCK VKP(b) 3.11.1926	BUCHARIN, N.I. VOROŠILOV, K.E. KALININ, M.I. MOLOTOV, V.M. RUDZUTAK, Ja.E. RYKOV, A.I. STALIN, J.V. TOMSKIJ, M.P.			ANDREEV, A.A. KAGANOVIČ, L.M. KIROV, S.M. MIKOJAN, A.I. PETROVSKIJ, G.I. UGLANOV, N.A. ČUBAR, V.Ja.	1891-1939[3]	1907
Plenum CK VKP(b) 19.12.1927	BUCHARIN, N.I. VOROŠILOV, K.E. KALININ, M.I. KUIBYŠEV, V.V. MOLOTOV, V.M. RYKOV, A.I. RUDZUTAK, Ja.E. STALIN, J.V. TOMSKIJ, M.P.	1888-1935[4]	1904	ANDREEV, A.A. KAGANOVIČ, L.M. KIROV, S.M. KOSIOR, S.V. MIKOJAN, A.I. PETROVSKIJ, G.I. UGLANOV, N.A. ČUBAR, V.Ja.	1889-1939[3]	1907
Plenum CK VKP(b) 29.4.1929	BUCHARIN, N.I. VOROŠILOV, K.E. KALININ, M.I. KUIBYŠEV, V.V. MOLOTOV, V.M. RYKOV, A.I. RUDZUTAK, Ja.E. STALIN, J.V. TOMSKIJ, M.P.			ANDREEV, A.A. BAUMAN, K.Ja. KAGANOVIČ, L.M. KIROV, S.M. KOSIOR, S.V. MIKOJAN, A.I. PETROVSKIJ, G.I. ČUBAR, V.Ja.	1892-1937[3]	1907
Plenum CK VKP(b) 21.6.1929	BUCHARIN, N.I. VOROŠILOV, K.E. KALININ, M.I. KUIBYŠEV, V.V. MOLOTOV, V.M. RYKOV, A.I. RUDZUTAK, Ja.E. STALIN, J.V. TOMSKIJ, M.P.			ANDREEV, A.A. BAUMAN, K.Ja. KAGANOVIČ, L.M. KIROV, S.M. KOSIOR, S.V. MIKOJAN, A.I. PETROVSKIJ, G.I. SYRCOV, S.I. ČUBAR, V.Ja.	1893-1938[3]	1913
Plenum CK VKP(b) 10.-17.11.1929	VOROŠILOV, K.E. KALININ, M.I. KUIBYŠEV, V.V. MOLOTOV, V.M. RYKOV, A.I. RUDZUTAK, Ja.E. STALIN, J.V. TOMSKIJ, M.P.			ANDREEV, A.A. BAUMAN, K.Ja. KAGANOVIČ, L.M. KIROV, S.M. KOSIOR, S.V. MIKOJAN, A.I. PETROVSKIJ, G.I. SYRCOV, S.I. ČUBAR, V.Ja.		
Plenum CK VKP(b) 13.7.1930	VOROŠILOV, K.E. KAGANOVIČ, L.M. KALININ, M.I. KIROV, S.M. KOSIOR, S.V. KUIBYŠEV, V.V. MOLOTOV, V.M. RUDZUTAK, Ja.E. RYKOV, A.I. STALIN, J.V.			ANDREEV, A.A. MIKOJAN, A.I. PETROVSKIJ, G.I. SYRCOV, S.I. ČUBAR, V.Ja.		

Communist Party of the Soviet Union
Kommunistische Partei der Sowjetunion 3.3

	Members Mitglieder Členy			Candidate members Kandidaten Kandidaty		
	A	B	C	A	B	C
Ob'edinnenyj plenum CK i CKK VKP(b) 17.-21.12.1930	VOROŠILOV, K.E. KAGANOVIČ, L.M. KALININ, M.I. KIROV, S.M. KOSIOR, S.V. KUIBYŠEV, V.V. MOLOTOV, V.M. ORDŽONIKIDZE, G.K. RUDZUTAK, Ja.E. STALIN, J.V.			MIKOJAN, A.I. PETROVSKIJ, G.I. SYRCOV, S.I. ČUBAR, V.Ja.		
Plenum CK VKP(b) 10.2.1934	ANDREEV, A.A. VOROŠILOV, K.E. KAGANOVIČ, L.M. KALININ, M.I. KIROV, S.M. KOSIOR, S.V. KUIBYŠEV, V.V. MOLOTOV, V.M. ORDŽONIKIDZE, G.K. STALIN, J.V.			MIKOJAN, A.I. PETROVSKIJ, G.I. POSTYŠEV, P.P. RUDZUTAK, Ja.E. ČUBAR, V.Ja.	1887-1940[3]	1904
Plenum CK VKP(b) 1.2.1935	ANDREEV, A.A. VOROŠILOV, K.E. KAGANOVIČ, L.M. KALININ, M.I. KIROV, S.M. KOSIOR, S.V. KUIBYŠEV, V.V. MIKOJAN, A.I. MOLOTOV, V.M. ORDŽONIKIDZE, G.K. STALIN, J.V.			ŽDANOV, A.A. PETROVSKIJ, G.I. POSTYŠEV, P.P. RUDZUTAK, Ja.E. ČUBAR, V.Ja. EICHE, R.I.	1896-1948 1890-1940[3]	1915 1905
Plenum CK VKP(b) 11.-12.10.1937	ANDREEV, A.A. VOROŠILOV, K.E. KAGANOVIČ, L.M. KALININ, M.I. KIROV, S.M. KOSIOR, S.V. KUIBYŠEV, V.V. MIKOJAN, A.I. MOLOTOV, V.M. ORDŽONIKIDZE, G.K. STALIN, J.V.			EŽOV, N.I. ŽDANOV, A.A. PETROVSKIJ, G.I. POSTYŠEV, P.P. RUDZUTAK, Ja.E. ČUBAR, V.Ja. EICHE, R.I.	1901-1938[3]	1917
Plenum CK VKP(b) Jan. 1938	ANDREEV, A.A. VOROŠILOV, K.E. KAGANOVIČ, L.M. KALININ, M.I. KIROV, S.M. KOSIOR, S.V. KUIBYŠEV, V.V. MIKOJAN, A.I. MOLOTOV, V.M. ORDŽONIKIDZE, G.K. STALIN, J.V.			ŽDANOV, A.A. PETROVSKIJ, G.I. RUDZUTAK, Ja.E. CHRUŠČEV, N.S.* ČUBAR, V.Ja. EICHE, R.I.	1894-1971	1918

* 1938-1939 and 1939-Oct.1964: member - 1938-1939 und 1939-Okt.1964: Mitglied

3.3 Communist Party of the Soviet Union
Kommunistische Partei der Sowjetunion

	Members Mitglieder Členy			Candidate members Kandidaten Kandidaty		
	A	B	C	A	B	C
Plenum CK VKP(b) 22.3.1939	ANDREEV, A.A. VOROŠILOV, K.E. ŽDANOV, A.A. KAGANOVIČ, L.M. KALININ, M.I. MIKOJAN, A.I. MOLOTOV, V.M. STALIN, J.V. CHRUŠČEV, N.S.			BERIJA, L.P. ŠVERNIK, N.M.	1899-1953[3] 1888-1970	1917 1905
Plenum CK VKP(b) Feb. 1941	ANDREEV, A.A. VOROŠILOV, K.E. ŽDANOV, A.A. KAGANOVIČ, L.M. KALININ, M.I. MIKOJAN, A.I. MOLOTOV, V.M. STALIN, J.V. CHRUŠČEV, N.S.			BERIJA, L.P. VOZNESENSKIJ, N.A. MALENKOV, G.M.[*] ŠVERNIK, N.M. ŠČERBAKOV, A.S.	1903-1950[3] 1902 1901-1945	1919 1920 1918
Plenum CK VKP(b) March-März 1946	ANDREEV, A.A. BERIJA, L.P. VOROŠILOV, K.E. ŽDANOV, A.A. KAGANOVIČ, L.M. KALININ, M.I. MALENKOV, G.M. MIKOJAN, A.I. MOLOTOV, V.M. STALIN, J.V. CHRUŠČEV, N.S.			BULGANIN, N.A.[**] VOZNESENSKIJ,N.A. KOSYGIN, A.N. ŠVERNIK, N.M. ŠČERBAKOV, A.S.	1895-1975 1904	1917 1927
Plenum CK VKP(b) Feb. 1948	ANDREEV, A.A. BERIJA, L.P. BULGANIN, N.A. VOROŠILOV, K.E. ŽDANOV, A.A. KAGANOVIČ, L.M. KOSYGIN, A.N. MALENKOV, G.M. MIKOJAN, A.I. MOLOTOV, V.M. STALIN, J.V. CHRUŠČEV, N.S.			VOZNESENSKIJ,N.A. ŠVERNIK, N.M. ŠČERBAKOV, A.S.		
Plenum CK KPSS 16.10.1952	ANDRIANOV, V.M. ARISTOV, A.B. BERIJA, L.P. BULGANIN, N.A. VOROŠILOV, K.E. IGNATEV, S.D. KAGANOVIČ, L.M. KOROTČENKO,D.S. KUZNECOV, V.V.	1902 1903 1903 1894-1969 1901	1926 1921 1924 1918 1927	BREŽNEV, L.I. VYŠINSKIJ,A.Ja. ZVEREV, A.G. IGNATOV, N.G. KABANOV, I.G. KOSYGIN, A.N. PATOLIČEV, N.S. PEGOV, N.M. PUZANOV, A.M.	1906 1883-1954 1900-1969 1901-1966 1898-1972 1908 1905 1906	1931 1920 1919 1924 1917 1928 1930 1925

[*] 1957 relieved from all party and government posts for "forming group hostiled to party 1957 wegen "Bildung einer parteifeindlichen Gruppe" aller Partei-u.Staatsämter enthob

[**] 1958 expelled from Politburo - 1958 aus dem Politbüro ausgeschlossen

Communist Party of the Soviet Union
Kommunistische Partei der Sowjetunion 3.3

	Members Mitglieder Členy			Candidate members Kandidaten Kandidaty		
	A	B	C	A	B	C
	KUUSINEN, O.V.	1881-1964	1905	TEVOSJAN, I.F.	1902-1958	1918
	MALENKOV, G.M.			JUDIN, P.F.	1899-1968	1928
	MALYŠEV, V.A.	1902-1957	1926			
	MELNIKOV, L.G.	1906	1928			
	MIKOJAN, A.I.					
	MICHAJLOV, N.A.	1906	1930			
	MOLOTOV, V.M.					
	PERVUCHIN, M.G.	1904-1978	1919			
	PONOMARENKO,P.K.	1902	1925			
	SABUROV, M.Z.	1900*	1920			
	STALIN, J.V.					
	SUSLOV, M.A.	1902	1921			
	CHRUŠČEV, N.S.					
	ČESNOKOV, D.I.	--	1939			
	ŠVERNIK, N.M.					
	ŠKIRJATOV, M.F.	1883-1954	1906			
Sovmestnoe zase- danie plenuma CK KPSS,Soveta Mi- nistrov SSSR, Prezidiuma Ver- chovnogo Soveta SSSR⁷ March-März 1953	BERIJA, L.P. BULGANIN, N.A. VOROŠILOV, K.E. KAGANOVIČ, L.M. MALENKOV, G.M. MIKOJAN, A.I. MOLOTOV, V.M. PERVUCHIN, M.G. SABUROV, M.Z. CHRUŠČEV, N.S.			BAGIROV, M.D. MELNIKOV, L.G. PONOMARENKO, P.K. ŠVERNIK, N.M.	1896-1956³	1917
Plenum CK KPSS July-Juli 1953	BULGANIN, N.A. VOROŠILOV, K.E. KAGANOVIČ, L.M. MALENKOV, G.M. MIKOJAN, A.I. MOLOTOV, V.M. PERVUCHIN, M.G. SABUROV, M.Z. CHRUŠČEV, N.S.			MELNIKOV, L.G. PONOMARENKO, P.K. ŠVERNIK, N.M.		
Plenum CK KPSS 4.-12.7.1955	BULGANIN, N.A. VOROŠILOV, K.E. KAGANOVIČ, L.M. KIRIČENKO, A.I.** MALENKOV, G.M. MIKOJAN, A.I. MOLOTOV, V.M. PERVUCHIN, M.G. SABUROV, M.Z. SUSLOV, M.A. CHRUŠČEV, N.S.	1908	1930	MELNIKOV, L.G. PONOMARENKO, P.K. ŠVERNIK, N.M.		
Plenum CK KPSS 27.2.1956	BULGANIN, N.A. VOROŠILOV, K.E. KAGANOVIČ, L.M. KIRIČENKO, A.I.			BREŽNEV, L.I. ŽUKOV, G.K. MUCHITDINOV, N.A. ***	1896-1974 1917	1919 1942

* 1957 relieved from all party and government posts for "forming group hostiled to party"
  1957 wegen "Bildung einer parteifeindlichen Gruppe" aller Partei-u.Staatsämter enthoben
** until May - bis Mai 1960
*** 1956-57; 1957-Nov.1961 Member-Mitglied

67

3.3 Communist Party of the Soviet Union
Kommunistische Partei der Sowjetunion

	Members Mitglieder Členy			Candidate members Kandidaten Kandidaty		
	A	B	C	A	B	C
	MALENKOV, G.M. MIKOJAN, A.I. MOLOTOV, V.M. PERVUCHIN, M.G. SABUROV, M.Z. SUSLOV, M.A. CHRUŠČEV, N.S.			FURCEVA, E.A. ŠVERNIK, N.M. ŠEPILOV, D.T.*	1910-1974 1905	1930 1926
Plenum CK KPSS 13.-14.2.1957	BULGANIN, N.A. VOROŠILOV, K.E. KAGANOVIČ, L.M. KIRIČENKO, A.I. MALENKOV, G.M. MIKOJAN, A.I. MOLOTOV, V.M. PERVUCHIN, M.G. SABUROV, M.Z. SUSLOV, M.A. CHRUŠČEV, N.S.			BREŽNEV, L.I. ŽUKOV, G.K. KOZLOV, F.R. MUCHITDINOV, N.A. FURCEVA, E.A. ŠVERNIK, N.M. ŠEPILOV, D.T.	1908-1965	1926
Plenum CK KPSS 22.-29.6.1957	ARISTOV, A.B. BELJAEV, N.I. BREŽNEV, L.I. BULGANIN, N.A. VOROŠILOV, K.E. ŽUKOV, G.K. IGNATOV, N.G. KIRIČENKO, A.I. KOZLOV, F.R. KUUSINEN, O.V. MIKOJAN, A.I. SUSLOV, M.A. FURCEVA, E.A. CHRUŠČEV, N.S. ŠVERNIK, N.M.	1903-1966	1921	KALNBERZIN, Ja.E. KIRILENKO, A.P. KOROTČENKO, D.S. KOSYGIN, A.N. MAZUROV, K.T. MŽAVANADZE, V.P.** MUCHITDINOV, N.A. PERVUCHIN, M.G. POSPELOV, P.N.	1893 1906 1914 1902 1898	1917 1931 1940 1927 1916
Plenum CK KPSS Oct.-Okt.1957	ARISTOV, A.B. BELJAEV, N.I. BREŽNEV, L.I. BULGANIN, N.A. VOROŠILOV, K.E. IGNATOV, N.G. KIRIČENKO, A.I. KOZLOV, F.R. KUUSINEN, O.V. MIKOJAN, A.I. SUSLOV, M.A. FURCEVA, E.A. CHRUŠČEV, N.S. ŠVERNIK, N.M.			KALNBERZIN, Ja.E. KIRILENKO, A.P. KOROTČENKO, D.S. KOSYGIN, A.N. MAZUROV, K.T. MŽAVANADZE, V.P. MUCHITDINOV, N.A. PERVUCHIN, M.G. POSPELOV, P.N.		

* 1957 expelled from CC CPSU for "forming group opposing the party" -
  1957 wegen "Bildung einer antiparteilichen Gruppe" aus dem ZK der KPdSU ausgeschlossen
** until December - bis Dezember 1972

Communist Party of the Soviet Union
Kommunistische Partei der Sowjetunion 3.3

	Members Mitglieder Členy			Candidate members Kandidaten Kandidaty		
	A	B	C	A	B	C
Plenum CK KPSS 16.-17.12.1957	ARISTOV, A.B. BELJAEV, N.I. BREŽNEV, L.I. BULGANIN, N.A. VOROŠILOV, K.E. IGNATOV, N.G. KIRIČENKO, A.I. KOZLOV, F.R. KUUSINEN, O.V. MIKOJAN, A.I. MUCHITDINOV, N.A. SUSLOV, M.A. FURCEVA, E.A. CHRUŠČEV, N.S. ŠVERNIK, N.M.			KALNBERZIN, Ja.E. KIRILENKO, A.P. KOROTČENKO, D.S. KOSYGIN, A.N. MAZUROV, K.T. MŽAVANADZE, V.P. PERVUCHIN, M.G. POSPELOV, P.N.		
Plenum CK KPSS 17.-18.6.1958	ARISTOV, A.B. BELJAEV, N.I. BREŽNEV, L.I. BULGANIN, N.A. VOROŠILOV, K.E. IGNATOV, N.G. KIRIČENKO, A.I. KOZLOV, F.R. KUUSINEN, O.V. MIKOJAN, A.I. MUCHITDINOV, N.A. SUSLOV, M.A. FURCEVA, E.A. CHRUŠČEV, N.S. ŠVERNIK, N.M.			KALNBERZIN, Ja.E. KIRILENKO, A.P. KOROTČENKO, D.S. KOSYGIN, A.N. MAZUROV, K.T. MŽAVANADZE, V.P. PERVUCHIN, M.G. PODGORNYJ, N.V.* POLJANSKIJ, D.S. POSPELOV, P.N.	1903 1917	1930 1939
Plenum CK KPSS 5.9.1958	ARISTOV, A.B. BELJAEV, N.I. BREŽNEV, L.I. VOROŠILOV, K.E. IGNATOV, N.G. KIRIČENKO, A.I. KOZLOV, F.R. KUUSINEN, O.V. MIKOJAN, A.I. MUCHITDINOV, N.A. SUSLOV, M.A. FURCEVA, E.A. CHRUŠČEV, N.S. ŠVERNIK, N.M.			KALNBERZIN, Ja.E. KIRILENKO, A.P. KOROTČENKO, D.S. KOSYGIN, A.N. MAZUROV, K.T. MŽAVANADZE, V.P. PERVUCHIN, M.G. PODGORNYJ, N.V. POLJANSKIJ, D.S. POSPELOV, P.N.		
Plenum CK KPSS 4.5.1960	ARISTOV, A.B. BREŽNEV, L.I. VOROŠILOV, K.E. IGNATOV, N.G. KOSYGIN, A.N. KOZLOV, F.R. KUUSINEN, O.V. MIKOJAN, A.I. MUCHITDINOV, N.A.			KALNBERZIN, Ja.E. KIRILENKO, A.P. KOROTČENKO, D.S. MAZUROV, K.T. MŽAVANADZE, V.P. PERVUCHIN, M.G. POSPELOV, P.N.		

* 1958-1960 and 1960-May 1977: Member - 1958-1960 und 1960-Mai 1977: Mitglied

3.3 Communist Party of the Soviet Union
Kommunistische Partei der Sowjetunion

	Members Mitglieder Členy A	B	C	Candidate members Kandidaten Kandidaty A	B	C
	PODGORNYJ, N.V. POLJANSKIJ, D.S. SUSLOV, M.A. FURCEVA, E.A. CHRUŠČEV, N.S. ŠVERNIK, N.M.					
Plenum CK KPSS 13.-16.7.1960	ARISTOV, A.B. BREŽNEV, L.I. IGNATOV, N.G. KOSYGIN, A.N. KOZLOV, F.R. KUUSINEN, O.V. MIKOJAN, A.I. MUCHITDINOV, N.A. PODGORNYJ, N.V. POLJANSKIJ, D.S. SUSLOV, M.A. FURCEVA, E.A. CHRUŠČEV, N.S. ŠVERNIK, N.M.			KALNBERZIN, Ja.E. KIRILENKO, A.P. KOROTČENKO, D.S. MAZUROV, K.T. MŽAVANADZE, V.P. PERVUCHIN, M.G. POSPELOV, P.N.		
Plenum CK KPSS 10.-18.1.1961	ARISTOV, A.B. BREŽNEV, L.I. IGNATOV, N.G. KOSYGIN, A.N. KOZLOV, F.R. KUUSINEN, O.V. MIKOJAN, A.I. MUCHITDINOV, N.A. PODGORNYJ, N.V. POLJANSKIJ, D.S. SUSLOV, M.A. FURCEVA, E.A. CHRUŠČEV, N.S. ŠVERNIK, N.M.			VORONOV, G.I. GRIŠIN, V.V. KALNBERZIN, Ja.E. KIRILENKO, A.P. KOROTČENKO, D.S. MAZUROV, K.T. MŽAVANADZE, V.P. PERVUCHIN, M.G. POSPELOV, P.N.	1910 1914	1931 1939
Plenum CK KPSS 31.10.1961	BREŽNEV, L.I. VORONOV, G.I. KOZLOV, F.R. KOSYGIN, A.N. KUUSINEN, O.V. MIKOJAN, A.I. PODGORNYJ, N.V. POLJANSKIJ, D.S. SUSLOV, M.A. CHRUŠČEV, N.S. ŠVERNIK, N.M.			GRIŠIN, V.V. RAŠIDOV, Š.R. MAZUROV, K.T. MŽAVANADZE, V.P. ŠČERBICKIJ, V.V.	1917 1918	1939 1941
Plenum CK KPSS 26.4.1962	BREŽNEV, L.I. VORONOV, G.I. KIRILENKO, A.P. KOZLOV, F.R. KOSYGIN, A.N. KUUSINEN, O.V. MIKOJAN, A.I.			GRIŠIN, V.V. RAŠIDOV, Š.R. MAZUROV, K.T. MŽAVANADZE, V.P. ŠČERBICKIJ, V.V.		

Communist Party of the Soviet Union
Kommunistische Partei der Sowjetunion   3.3

| | Members Mitglieder Členy | | | Candidate members Kandidaten Kandidaty | | |
	A	B	C	A	B	C
	PODGORNYJ, N.V. POLJANSKIJ, D.S. SUSLOV, M.A. CHRUŠČEV, N.S. ŠVERNIK, N.M.					
Plenum CK KPSS 23.11.1962	BREŽNEV, L.I. VORONOV, G.I. KIRILENKO, A.P. KOZLOV, F.R. KOSYGIN, A.N. KUUSINEN, O.V. MIKOJAN, A.I. PODGORNYJ, N.V. POLJANSKIJ, D.S. SUSLOV, M.A. CHRUŠČEV, N.S. ŠVERNIK, N.M.			GRIŠIN, V.V. EFREMOV, L.N. RAŠIDOV, Š.R. MAZUROV, K.T. MŽAVANADZE, V.P. ŠČERBICKIJ, V.V.	1912	1941
Plenum CK KPSS 13.12.1963	BREŽNEV, L.I. VORONOV, G.I. KIRILENKO, A.P. KOZLOV, F.R. KOSYGIN, A.N. KUUSINEN, O.V. MIKOJAN, A.I. PODGORNYJ, N.V. POLJANSKIJ, D.S. SUSLOV, M.A. CHRUŠČEV, N.S. ŠVERNIK, N.M.			GRIŠIN, V.V. EFREMOV, L.N. MAZUROV, K.T. MŽAVANADZE, V.P. RAŠIDOV, Š.R. ŠELEST, P.E.*	1908	1928
Plenum CK KPSS 15.10.1964	BREŽNEV, L.I. VORONOV, G.I. KIRILENKO, A.P. KOZLOV, F.R. KOSYGIN, A.N. MIKOJAN, A.I. PODGORNYJ, N.V. POLJANSKIJ, D.S. SUSLOV, M.A. ŠVERNIK, N.M.			GRIŠIN, V.V. EFREMOV, L.N. MAZUROV, K.T. MŽAVANADZE, V.P. RAŠIDOV, Š.R. ŠELEST, P.E.		
Plenum CK KPSS 16.11.1964	BREŽNEV, L.I. VORONOV, G.I. KIRILENKO, A.P. KOSYGIN, A.N. MIKOJAN, A.I. PODGORNYJ, N.V. POLJANSKIJ, D.S. SUSLOV, M.A. ŠELEPIN, A.N. ŠELEST, P.E. ŠVERNIK, N.M.	1918	1940	GRIŠIN, V.V. DEMIČEV, P.N. EFREMOV, L.N. MAZUROV, K.T. MŽAVANADZE, V.P. RAŠIDOV, Š.R.	1918	1939

* 1963-1964 and 1964-April 1973: Member - Mitglied

71

3.3 Communist Party of the Soviet Union
Kommunistische Partei der Sowjetunion

	Members Mitglieder Členy			Candidate Members Kandidaten Kandidaty		
	A	B	C	A	B	C
Plenum CK KPSS 26.3.1965	BREŽNEV, L.I. VORONOV, G.I. KIRILENKO, A.P. KOSYGIN, A.N. MAZUROV, K.T. MIKOJAN, A.I. PODGORNYJ, N.V. POLJANSKIJ, D.S. SUSLOV, M.A. ŠELEPIN, A.N. ŠELEST, P.E. ŠVERNIK, N.M.			GRIŠIN, V.V. DEMIČEV, P.N. EFREMOV, L.N. MŽAVANADZE, V.P. RAŠIDOV, Š.R. USTINOV, D.F.	1908	1927
Plenum CK KPSS 6.12.1965	BREŽNEV, L.I. VORONOV, G.I. KIRILENKO, A.P. KOSYGIN, A.N. MAZUROV, K.T. MIKOJAN, A.I. PODGORNYJ, N.V. POLJANSKIJ, D.S. SUSLOV, M.A. ŠELEPIN, A.N. ŠELEST, P.E. ŠVERNIK, N.M.			GRIŠIN, V.V. DEMIČEV, P.N. EFREMOV, L.N. MŽAVANADZE, V.P. RAŠIDOV, Š.R. ŠČERBICKIJ, V.V. USTINOV, D.F.		
Plenum CK KPSS 8.4.1966	BREŽNEV, L.I. VORONOV, G.I. KIRILENKO, A.P. KOSYGIN, A.N. MAZUROV, K.T. PELŠE, A.Ja. PODGORNYJ, N.V. POLJANSKIJ, D.S. SUSLOV, M.A. ŠELEPIN, A.N. ŠELEST, P.E.	1899	1915	GRIŠIN, V.V. DEMIČEV, P.N. KUNAEV, D.A. MAŠEROV, P.M. MŽAVANADZE, V.P. RAŠIDOV, Š.R. USTINOV, D.F. ŠČERBICKIJ, V.V.	1912 1918	1939 1943
Plenum CK KPSS 21.6.1967	BREŽNEV, L.I. VORONOV, G.I. KIRILENKO, A.P. KOSYGIN, A.N. MAZUROV, K.T. PELŠE, A.Ja. PODGORNYJ, N.V. POLJANSKIJ, D.S. SUSLOV, M.A. ŠELEPIN, A.N. ŠELEST, P.E.			ANDROPOV, Ju.V. GRIŠIN, V.V. DEMIČEV, P.N. KUNAEV, D.A. MAŠEROV, P.M. MŽAVANADZE, V.P. RAŠIDOV, Š.R. USTINOV, D.F. ŠČERBICKIJ, V.V.	1914	1939
Plenum CK KPSS 9.4.1971	BREŽNEV, L.I. VORONOV, G.I. GRIŠIN, V.V. KIRILENKO, A.P. KOSYGIN, A.N.			ANDROPOV, Ju.V. DEMIČEV, P.N. MAŠEROV, P.M. MŽAVANADZE, V.P. RAŠIDOV, Š.R.		

Communist Party of the Soviet Union
Kommunistische Partei der Sowjetunion 3.3

	Members Mitglieder Členy			Candidate Members Kandidaten Kandidaty		
	A	B	C	A	B	C
	KULAKOV, F.D. KUNAEV, D.A. MAZUROV, K.T. PELŠE, A.Ja. PODGORNYJ, N.V. POLJANSKIJ, D.S. SUSLOV, M.A. ŠELEPIN, A.N. ŠELEST, P.E. ŠČERBICKIJ, V.V.	1918-1978	1940	USTINOV, D.F.		
Plenum CK KPSS 22.-23.11.1971	BREŽNEV, L.I. VORONOV, G.I. GRIŠIN, V.V. KIRILENKO, A.P. KOSYGIN, A.N. KULAKOV, F.D. KUNAEV, D.A. MAZUROV, K.T. PELŠE, A.Ja. PODGORNYJ, N.V. POLJANSKIJ, D.S. SUSLOV, M.A. ŠELEPIN, A.N. ŠELEST, P.E. ŠČERBICKIJ, V.V.			ANDROPOV, Ju.V. DEMIČEV, P.N. MAŠEROV, P.M. MŽAVANADZE, V.P. RAŠIDOV, Š.R. SOLOMENCEV, M.S. USTINOV, D.F.	1913	1940
Plenum CK KPSS 19.5.1972	BREŽNEV, L.I. VORONOV, G.I. GRIŠIN, V.V. KIRILENKO, A.P. KOSYGIN, A.N. KULAKOV, F.D. KUNAEV, D.A. MAZUROV, K.T. PELŠE, A.Ja. PODGORNYJ, N.V. POLJANSKIJ, D.S. SUSLOV, M.A. ŠELEPIN, A.N. ŠELEST, P.E. ŠČERBICKIJ, V.V.			ANDROPOV, Ju.V. DEMIČEV, P.N. MAŠEROV, P.M. MŽAVANADZE, V.P. PONOMAREV, B.N. RAŠIDOV, Š.R. SOLOMENCEV, M.S. USTINOV, D.F.	1905	1919
Plenum CK KPSS 18.12.1972	BREŽNEV, L.I. VORONOV, G.I. GRIŠIN, V.V. KIRILENKO, A.P. KOSYGIN, A.N. KULAKOV, F.D. KUNAEV, D.A. MAZUROV, K.T. PELŠE, A.Ja. PODGORNYJ, N.V. POLJANSKIJ, D.S. SUSLOV, M.A. ŠELEPIN, A.N. ŠELEST, P.E. ŠČERBICKIJ, V.V.			ANDROPOV, Ju.V. DEMIČEV, P.N. MAŠEROV, P.M. PONOMAREV, B.N. RAŠIDOV, Š.R. SOLOMENCEV, M.S. USTINOV, D.F.		

3.3 Communist Party of the Soviet Union
Kommunistische Partei der Sowjetunion

	Members Mitglieder Členy			Candidate members Kandidaten Kandidaty		
	A	B	C	A	B	C
Plenum CK KPSS 26.-27.4.1973	ANDROPOV, Ju.V. BREŽNEV, L.I. GREČKO, A.A. GRIŠIN, V.V. GROMYKO, A.A. KIRILENKO, A.P. KOSYGIN, A.N. KULAKOV, F.D. KUNAEV, D.A. MAZUROV, K.T. PELŠE, A.Ja. PODGORNYJ, N.V. POLJANSKIJ, D.S. SUSLOV, M.A. ŠELEPIN, A.N. ŠČERBICKIJ, V.V.	1903-1976 1909	1928 1931	DEMIČEV, P.N. MAŠEROV, P.M. PONOMAREV, B.N. ROMANOV, G.V. RAŠIDOV, Š.R. SOLOMENCEV, M.S. USTINOV, D.F.	1923	1944
Plenum CK KPSS 16.4.1975	ANDROPOV, Ju.V. BREŽNEV, L.I. GREČKO, A.A. GRIŠIN, V.V. GROMYKO, A.A. KIRILENKO, A.P. KOSYGIN, A.N. KULAKOV, F.D.	KUNAEV, D.A. MAZUROV, K.T. PELŠE, A.Ja. PODGORNYJ, N.V. POLJANSKIJ, D.S. SUSLOV, M.A. ŠČERBICKIJ, V.V.		DEMIČEV, P.N. MAŠEROV, P.M. PONOMAREV, B.N. RAŠIDOV, Š.R. ROMANOV, G.V. SOLOMENCEV, M.S. USTINOV, D.F.		
Plenum CK KPSS 24.2.-4.3.1976	ANDROPOV, Ju.V. BREŽNEV, L.I. GREČKO, A.A. GRIŠIN, V.V. GROMYKO, A.A. KIRILENKO, A.P. KOSYGIN, A.N. KULAKOV, F.D.	KUNAEV, D.A. MAZUROV, K.T. PELŠE, A.Ja. PODGORNYJ, N.V. ROMANOV, G.V. SUSLOV, M.A. ŠČERBICKIJ, V.V. USTINOV, D.F.		ALIEV, G.A.R. DEMIČEV, P.N. MAŠEROV, P.M. PONOMAREV, B.N. RAŠIDOV, Š.R. SOLOMENCEV, M.S.	1923	1945
Plenum CK KPSS 24.5.1977	ANDROPOV, Ju.V. BREŽNEV, L.I. GRIŠIN, V.V. GROMYKO, A.A. KIRILENKO, A.P. KOSYGIN, A.N. KULAKOV, F.D.	KUNAEV, D.A. MAZUROV, K.T. PELŠE, A.Ja. ROMANOV, G.V. SUSLOV, M.A. ŠČERBICKIJ, V.V. USTINOV, D.F.		ALIEV, G.A.R.o. DEMIČEV, P.N. MAŠEROV, P.M. PONOMAREV, B.N. RAŠIDOV, Š.R. SOLOMENCEV, M.S.		
Plenum CK KPSS 3.10.1977	ANDROPOV, Ju.V. BREŽNEV, L.I. GRIŠIN, V.V. GROMYKO, A.A. KIRILENKO, A.P. KOSYGIN, A.N. KULAKOV, F.D.	KUNAEV, D.A. MAZUROV, K.T. PELŠE, A.Ja. ROMANOV, G.V. SUSLOV, M.A. ŠČERBICKIJ, V.V. USTINOV, D.F.		ALIEV, G.A.R.o. ČERNENKO, K.U. DEMIČEV, P.N. KUZNECOV, V.V. MAŠEROV, P.M. PONOMAREV, B.N. RAŠIDOV, Š.R. SOLOMENCEV, M.S.		

Communist Party of the Soviet Union
Kommunistische Partei der Sowjetunion 3.3.1

3.3.1
SECRETARIAT CC CPSU — SEKRETARIAT ZK KPdSU — SEKRETARIAT CK KPSS

	Name Name Familija A	Date of birth/death Geburts-/ Sterbedat. data rożd./ smerti B	Party affiliation Partei- zugehö- rigkeit Partij- nyj staż C
Plenum CK RKP(b) 25.3.1919	STASOVA, E.D.	1873-1966	1898
Plenum CK RKP(b) 29.11.1919	STASOVA, E.D. KRESTINSKIJ, N.N.	1883-1938[3]	1903
Plenum CK RKP(b) 5.4.1920	KRESTINSKIJ, N.N. PREOBRAŻENSKIJ, E.A. SEREBRJAKOV, L.P.	1886-1938[3] 1890-1937[3]	1903 1905-27 1930-36
Plenum CK RKP(b) 16.3.1921	MOLOTOV, V.M. MICHAJLOV, V.M. JAROSLAVSKIJ, E.M.	1890 1894-1937 1878-1943	1906 1915 1898
Plenum CK RKP(b) 10.4.1922	STALIN, J.V.[8] KUIBYŠEV, V.V. MOLOTOV, V.M.	1879-1953 1888-1935[4]	1898 1904
Plenum CK RKP(b) 26.4.1923	STALIN, J.V.[8] MOLOTOV, V.M. RUDZUTAK, Ja.E.	1887-1938[3]	1905
Plenum CK RKP(b) 2.6.1924	STALIN, J.V.[8] ANDREEV, A.A. ZELENSKIJ, I.A. KAGANOVIČ, L.M. MOLOTOV, V.M.	1895-1971 1890-1938[3] 1893	1914 1906 1911
Plenum CK VKP(b) 1.1.1926	STALIN, J.V.[8] EVDOKIMOV, G.E. KOSIOR, S.V. MOLOTOV, V.M. UGLANOV, N.A. ARTJUCHINA, A.V.[10] BUBNOV, A.S.[10]	1884-1936[3] 1889-1939[3] 1886-1940[5] 1889-1969[5] 1883-1940[5]	1903-27 1928-34 1907 1907-32 1932-36 1910 1903
Plenum CK VKP(b) 19.12.1927	STALIN, J.V.[8] KOSIOR, S.V. KUBJAK, N.A. MOLOTOV, V.M. UGLANOV, N.A. ARTJUCHINA, A.A.[10] BUBNOV, A.S.[10] MOSKVIN, I.M.[10]	1881-1942[5]	1898

[8] Secretary General – Generalsekretär – General'nyj sekretar'
[9] First Secretary – Erster Sekretär – Pervyj sekretar'
[10] Candidate to Secretariate – Kandidat zum Sekretariat – Kandidat sekretariata

3.3.1 Communist Party of the Soviet Union
Kommunistische Partei der Sowjetunion

	A	B	C
Plenum CK VKP(b) 6.-11.4.1928	STALIN, J.V.[8] KOSIOR, S.V. KUBJAK, N.A. MOLOTOV, V.M. UGLANOV, N.A. ARTJUCHINA, A.V.[10] BAUMAN, K.Ja.[10] BUBNOV, A.S.[10] MOSKVIN, I.M.[10]	1892-1937	1907
Plenum CK VKP(b) 4.-12.7.1928	STALIN, J.V.[8] KAGANOVIČ, L.M. KUBJAK, N.A. MOLOTOV, V.M. UGLANOV, N.A. ARTJUCHINA, A.V.[10] BAUMAN, K.Ja.[10] BUBNOV, A.S.[10] MOSKVIN, I.M.[10]		
Plenum CK VKP(b) 29.4.1929	STALIN, J.V.[8] BAUMAN, K.Ja. KAGANOVIČ, L.M. KUBJAK, N.A. MOLOTOV, V.M. ARTJUCHINA, A.V.[10] BUBNOV, A.S.[10] MOSKVIN, I.M.[10]		
Plenum CK VKP(b) 13.7.1930	STALIN, J.V.[8] BAUMAN, K.Ja. KAGANOVIČ, L.M. MOLOTOV, V.M. POSTYŠEV, P.P. MOSKVIN, I.M. ŠVERNIK, N.M.	1887-1940[3] 1888-1970	1904 1905
Plenum CK VKP(b) 10.2.1934	STALIN, J.V.[8] ŽDANOV, A.A. KAGANOVIČ, L.M. KIROV, S.M.	1896-1948 1886-1934[4]	1915 1904
Plenum CK VKP(b) 1.2.1935	STALIN, J.V.[8] EŽOV, N.I. ŽDANOV, A.A. KAGANOVIČ, L.M.	1901-1938[3]	1917
Plenum CK VKP(b) 22.3.1939	STALIN, J.V.[8] ANDREEV, A.A. ŽDANOV, A.A. MALENKOV, G.M.	1902	1920
Plenum CK VKP(b) May-Mai 1941	STALIN, J.V.[8] ANDREEV, A.A. ŽDANOV, A.A. MALENKOV, G.M. ŠČERBAKOV, A.S.	1901-1945	1918

Communist Party of the Soviet Union
Kommunistische Partei der Sowjetunion 3.3.1

	A	B	C
Plenum CK VKP(b) March-März 1946	STALIN, J.V.[8] ŽDANOV, A.A. KUZNECOV, A.A. MALENKOV, G.M. POPOV, G.M.	1905-1949[3] 1906-1968	1925 1926
Plenum CK VKP(b) May-Mai 1946	STALIN, J.V.[8] ŽDANOV, A.A. KUZNECOV, A.A. MALENKOV, G.M. PATOLIČEV, N.S. POPOV, G.M.	1908	1928
Plenum CK VKP(b) May-Mai 1947	STALIN, J.V.[8] ŽDANOV, A.A. KUZNECOV, A.A. MALENKOV, G.M. POPOV, G.M. SUSLOV, M.A.	1902	1921
Plenum CK VKP(b) Oct.-Okt. 1948	STALIN, J.V.[8] KUZNECOV, A.A. MALENKOV, G.M. PONOMARENKO, P.K. POPOV, G.M. SUSLOV, M.A.	1902	
Plenum CK VKP(b) Feb. 1949	STALIN, J.V.[8] MALENKOV, G.M. PONOMARENKO, P.K. POPOV, G.M. SUSLOV, M.A.		
Plenum CK VKP(b) Dec.-Dez. 1949	STALIN, J.V.[8] MALENKOV, G.M. PONOMARENKO, P.K. POPOV, G.M. SUSLOV, M.A. CHRUŠČEV, N.S.*	1894-1971	1918
Plenum CK KPSS 16.10.1952	STALIN, J.V.[8] ARISTOV, A.B. BREŽNEV, L.I. IGNATOV, N.G. MALENKOV, G.M. MICHAJLOV, N.A. PEGOV, N.M. PONOMARENKO, P.K. SUSLOV, M.A. CHRUŠČEV, N.S.	1903 1906 1901-1966 1906 1905	1921 1931 1924 1930 1930
Plenum CK KPSS 14.3.1953	IGNATEV, S.D. POSPELOV, P.N. SUSLOV, M.A. CHRUŠČEV, N.S. ŠATALIN, N.N.	1903 1898 --	1924 1916 1925
Plenum CK KPSS 6.4.1953	POSPELOV, P.N. SUSLOV, M.A. CHRUŠČEV, N.S. ŠATALIN, N.N.		

* 1949-1953; 1953-Oct./Okt.1964: First Secretary-Erster Sekretär

3.3.1 Communist Party of the Soviet Union
Kommunistische Partei der Sowjetunion

	A	B	C
Plenum CK KPSS Sept. 1953	CHRUŠČEV, N.S.[9] POSPELOV, P.N. SUSLOV, M.A. ŠATALIN, N.N.		
Plenum CK KPSS 4.-12.7.1955	CHRUŠČEV, N.S.[9] ARISTOV, A.B. BELJAEV, N.I. POSPELOV, P.N. SUSLOV, M.A. ŠATALIN, N.N. ŠEPILOV, D.T.	1906-1966 1905	1921 1926
Plenum CK KPSS 27.2.1956	CHRUŠČEV, N.S.[9] ARISTOV, A.B. BELJAEV, N.I. BREŽNEV, L.I. POSPELOV, P.N. SUSLOV, M.A. FURCEVA, E.A. ŠEPILOV, D.T.	1910-1974	1930
Plenum CK KPSS 20.-24.12.1956	CHRUŠČEV, N.S.[9] ARISTOV, A.B. BELJAEV, N.I. BREŽNEV, L.I. POSPELOV, P.N. SUSLOV, M.A. FURCEVA, E.A.		
Plenum CK KPSS 13.-14.2.1957	CHRUŠČEV, N.S.[9] ARISTOV, A.B. BELJAEV, N.I. BREŽNEV, L.I. POSPELOV, P.N. SUSLOV, M.A. FURCEVA, E.A. ŠEPILOV, D.T.		
Plenum CK KPSS 29.6.1957	CHRUŠČEV, N.S.[9] ARISTOV, A.B. BELJAEV, N.I. BREŽNEV, L.I. KUUSINEN, O.V. POSPELOV, P.N. SUSLOV, M.A. FURCEVA, E.A.	1881-1964	1905
Plenum CK KPSS 16.-17.12.1957	CHRUŠČEV, N.S.[9] ARISTOV, A.B. BELJAEV, N.I. BREŽNEV, L.I. IGNATOV, N.G. KIRIČENKO, A.I.[*] KUUSINEN, O.V. MUCHITDINOV, N.A.[**] POSPELOV, P.N. SUSLOV, M.A. FURCEVA, E.A.	1908 1917	1930 1942

[*] until May - bis Mai 1960
[**] until - bis November 1961

Communist Party of the Soviet Union
Kommunistische Partei der Sowjetunion 3.3.1

	A	B	C
Plenum CK KPSS 12.11.1958	CHRUŠČEV, N.S.[9] ARISTOV, A.B. BREŽNEV, L.I. IGNATOV, N.G. KIRIČENKO, A.I. KUUSINEN, O.V. MUCHITDINOV, N.A. POSPELOV, P.N. SUSLOV, M.A. FURCEVA, E.A.		
Plenum CK KPSS 4.5.1960	CHRUŠČEV, N.S.[9] BREŽNEV, L.I. KOZLOV, F.R. KUUSINEN, O.V. MUCHITDINOV, N.A. SUSLOV, M.A.	1908-1965	1926
Plenum CK KPSS 12.-16.7.1960	CHRUŠČEV, N.S.[9] KOZLOV, F.R. KUUSINEN, O.V. MUCHITDINOV, N.A. SUSLOV, N.A.		
Plenum CK KPSS 31.10.1961	CHRUŠČEV, N.S.[9] DEMIČEV, P.N. ILIČEV, L.F. KOZLOV, F.R. KUUSINEN, O.V. PONOMAREV, B.N. SPIRIDONOV, I.V. SUSLOV, M.A. ŠELEPIN, A.N.	1918 1906 1905 1905 1918	1939 1924 1919 1928 1940
Plenum CK KPSS April 1962	CHRUŠČEV, N.S.[9] DEMIČEV, P.N. ILIČEV, L.F. KOZLOV, F.R. KUUSINEN, O.V. PONOMAREV, B.N. SUSLOV, M.A. ŠELEPIN, A.N.		
Plenum CK KPSS 19.-23.11.1962	CHRUŠČEV, N.S.[9] ANDROPOV, Ju.V. DEMIČEV, P.N. ILIČEV, L.F. KOZLOV, F.R. KUUSINEN, O.V. POLJAKOV, V.I. PONOMAREV, B.N. RUDAKOV, A.P. SUSLOV, M.A. TITOV, V.N. ŠELEPIN, A.N.	 1914 1913 1910-1966 1907	 1939 1939 1931 1938
Plenum CK KPSS 18.-22.6.1963	CHRUŠČEV, N.S.[9] ANDROPOV, Ju.V. BREŽNEV, L.I. DEMIČEV, P.N. ILIČEV, L.F.		

3.3.1 Communist Party of the Soviet Union
Kommunistische Partei der Sowjetunion

	A	B	C
	KOZLOV, F.R. KUUSINEN, O.V. PODGORNYJ, N.V. * POLJAKOV, V.I. PONOMAREV, B.N. RUDAKOV, A.P. SUSLOV, M.A. TITOV, V.N. ŠELEPIN, A.N.	1903	1930
Plenum CK KPSS 14.10.1964	BREŽNEV, L.I.[9] ANDROPOV, Ju.V. DEMIČEV, P.N. ILIČEV, L.F. KOZLOV, F.R. PODGORNYJ, N.V. POLJAKOV, V.I. PONOMAREV, B.N. RUDAKOV, A.P. SUSLOV, M.A. TITOV, V.N. ŠELEPIN, A.N.		
Plenum CK KPSS 16.11.1964	BREŽNEV, L.I.[9] ANDROPOV, Ju.V. DEMIČEV, P.N. ILIČEV, L.F. PODGORNYJ, N.V. PONOMAREV, B.N. RUDAKOV, A.P. SUSLOV, M.A. TITOV, V.N. ŠELEPIN, A.N.		
Plenum CK KPSS 26.3.1965	BREŽNEV, L.I.[9] ANDROPOV, Ju.V. DEMIČEV, P.N. PODGORNYJ, N.V. PONOMAREV, B.N. RUDAKOV, A.P. SUSLOV, M.A. TITOV, V.N. USTINOV, D.F.** ŠELEPIN, A.N.	1908	1927
Plenum CK KPSS 29.9.1965	BREŽNEV, L.I.[9] ANDROPOV, Ju.V. DEMIČEV, P.N. KULAKOV, F.D. PODGORNYJ, N.V. PONOMAREV, B.N. RUDAKOV, A.P. SUSLOV, M.A. USTINOV, D.F. ŠELEPIN, A.N.	1918	1940

* until - bis April 1966
** as of April 30, 1976: USSR Minister of Defense -
   ab 30.4.1976: Verteidigungsminister der UdSSR

Communist Party of the Soviet Union
Kommunistische Partei der Sowjetunion 3.3.1

	A	B	C
Plenum CK KPSS 8.4.1966	BREŽNEV, L.I.[8] ANDROPOV, Ju.V. DEMIČEV, P.N. KAPITONOV, I.V. KIRILENKO, A.P. KULAKOV, F.D. PONOMAREV, B.N. RUDAKOV, A.P. SUSLOV, M.A. USTINOV, D.F. ŠELEPIN, A.N.	1906	1931
Plenum CK KPSS 12.-13.12.1966	BREŽNEV, L.I.[8] ANDROPOV, Ju.V. DEMIČEV, P.N. KAPITONOV, I.V. KIRILENKO, A.P. KULAKOV, F.D. PONOMAREV, B.N. SOLOMENCEV, M.S. SUSLOV, M.A. USTINOV, D.F. ŠELEPIN, A.N.	1913	1940
Plenum CK KPSS 20.-21.6.1967	BREŽNEV, L.I.[8] DEMIČEV, P.N. KAPITONOV, I.V. KIRILENKO, A.P. KULAKOV, F.D. PONOMAREV, B.N. SOLOMENCEV, M.S. SUSLOV, M.A. USTINOV, D.F. ŠELEPIN, A.N.		
Plenum CK KPSS 26.9.1967	BREŽNEV, L.I.[8] DEMIČEV, P.N. KAPITONOV, I.V. KIRILENKO, A.P. KULAKOV, F.D. PONOMAREV, B.N. SOLOMENCEV, M.S. SUSLOV, M.A. USTINOV, D.F.		
Plenum CK KPSS 10.4.1968	BREŽNEV, L.I.[8] DEMIČEV, P.N. KAPITONOV, I.V. KATUŠEV, K.F.* KIRILENKO, A.P. KULAKOV, F.D. PONOMAREV, B.N. SOLOMENCEV, M.S. SUSLOV, M.A. USTINOV, D.F.	1927	1952

* until May - bis Mai 1977

3.3.1 Communist Party of the Soviet Union
Kommunistische Partei der Sowjetunion

	A	B	C	A	B	C
Plenum CK KPSS 9.4.1971	BREŽNEV, L.I.[8] DEMIČEV, P.N. KAPITONOV, I.V. KATUŠEV, K.F. KIRILENKO, A.P.			KULAKOV, F.D. PONOMAREV, B.N. SOLOMENCEV, M.S. SUSLOV, M.A. USTINOV, D.F.		
Plenum CK KPSS 22.-23.11.1971	BREŽNEV, L.I.[8] DEMIČEV, P.N. KAPITONOV, I.V. KATUŠEV, K.F. KIRILENKO, A.P.			KULAKOV, F.D. PONOMAREV, B.N. SUSLOV, M.A. USTINOV, D.F.		
Plenum CK KPSS 18.12.1972	BREŽNEV, L.I.[8] DEMIČEV, P.N. DOLGICH, V.I. KAPITONOV, I.V. KATUŠEV, K.F.	1924	1942	KIRILENKO, A.P. KULAKOV, F.D. PONOMAREV, B.N. SUSLOV, M.A. USTINOV, D.F.		
Plenum CK KPSS 16.12.1974	BREŽNEV, L.I.[8] DOLGICH, V.I. KAPITONOV, I.V. KATUŠEV, K.F. KIRILENKO, A.P.			KULAKOV, F.D. PONOMAREV, B.N. SUSLOV, M.A. USTINOV, D.F.		
Plenum CK KPSS 24.2.-4.3.1976	BREŽNEV, L.I.[8] DOLGICH, V.I. ZIMJANIN, M.V. KAPITONOV, I.V. KATUŠEV, K.F. KIRILENKO, A.P.	1914	1939	KULAKOV, F.D. PONOMAREV, B.N. SUSLOV, M.A. USTINOV, D.F. ČERNENKO, K.U.	1911	1931
Plenum CK KPSS 25.-26.10.1976	BREŽNEV, L.I.[8] DOLGICH, V.I. ZIMJANIN, M.V. KAPITONOV, I.V. KATUŠEV, K.F. KIRILENKO, A.P.			KULAKOV, F.D. PONOMAREV, B.N. RJABOV, Ja.P. SUSLOV, M.A. ČERNENKO, K.U.		
Plenum CK KPSS 24.5.1977	BREŽNEV, L.I.[8] DOLGICH, V.I. ZIMJANIN, M.V. KAPITONOV, I.V. KIRILENKO, A.P. KULAKOV, F.D.			PONOMAREV, B.N. RJABOV, Ja.P. RUSAKOV, K.V. SUSLOV, M.A. ČERNENKO, K.U.		

Communist Party of the Soviet Union 3.4.1
Kommunistische Partei der Sowjetunion 3.4.2

3.4 SOCIAL COMPOSITION OF CPSU
SOZIALE ZUSAMMENSETZUNG DER KPdSU
SOCIAL'NYJ SOSTAV KPSS

3.4.1 SOCIAL COMPOSITION - SOZIALE ZUSAMMENSETZUNG - SOCIAL'NYJ SOSTAV
(Mill. & %)

	1971 Mill.	%	1973 Mill.	%	1974 Mill.	%	1975 Mill.	%	1977 Mill.	%
Workers Arbeiter Rabočie	5,76	40,1	6,04	40,7	6,16	41,0	6,35	41,3	6,7	42,0
Kolkhoznik Kolchosbauern kolchozniki	2,17	15,1	2,17	14,7	2,16	14,4	2,17	14,1	2,18	13,9
Employees Angestellte služaščie	6,44	44,8	6,61	44,6	6,70	44,6	6,85	44,6	7,0	44,4

3.4.2 COMMUNIST PARTY MEMBERS BY PROFESSION
ZUSAMMENSETZUNG DER ANGESTELLTEN-KOMMUNISTEN NACH BERUFEN
SOSTAV KOMMUNISTOV-SLUŽAŠČICH PO RODU ZANJATIJ

	1956	1961	1972	1976
Total - Insgesamt - vsego	100	100	100	100
of which - davon - iz nich				
Directors of organizations, institutions, enterprises, construction, projects, sovkhoz and their structural subdivisions Leiter der Organisationen, Institutionen, Betriebe, Bauten, Sowchosen und ihrer strukturellen Unterteilungen rukovoditeli organizacij, učreždenij, predprijatij, stroek, sovchozov i ich strukturnych podrazdelenij	14,0	10,4	8,5	8,9
Engineering, technical and agricultural specialists Ingenieur-technische Kader, Spezialisten der Landwirtschaft inženerno-techničeskich rabotnikov, specialistov sel'skogo chozjajstva	18,2	26,4	38,5	40,0

83

3.4.2 Communist Party of the Soviet Union
3.5.1 Kommunistische Partei der Sowjetunion

3.4.2

	1956	1961	1972	1976
Scientists, teachers, doctors, writers and artists Wissenschaftler, Lehrer, Ärzte, Literatur- und Kunstschaffende naučnych rabotnikov, učitelej, vračej, dejatelej literatury i iskusstva	18,9	21,3	24,0	24,2

3.5 LEVEL OF EDUCATION OF COMMUNIST PARTY MEMBERS
BILDUNGSSTAND DER KOMMUNISTEN
SOSTAV KOMMUNISTOV PO OBRAZOVANIJU

3.5.1 LEVEL OF EDUCATION OF COMMUNIST PARTY MEMBERS (in thousands)
BILDUNGSSTAND DER KOMMUNISTEN (in Tausenden)
SOSTAV KOMMUNISTOV PO OBRAZOVANIJU (tysjač)

	1971	1976	1977
Members and candidates of the CPSU - total Mitglieder und Kandidaten der KPdSU - insg. Vsego členov i kandidatov v členy KPSS	14,373	15,639	15,994
of which with - davon mit - iz nich imejut obrazovanie: completed college or university education - abgeschlossener Hochschulbildung - vysšee	2,820	3,808	4,009
not completed college or university education - nicht abgeschlossener Hochschulbildung - nezakončennoe vysšee	338	383	380
intermediate school education - mittlerer Schulbildung - srednee	4,933	6,022	6,268
not completed intermediate school education - nicht abgeschlossener mittl.Schulbildung - nepolnoe srednee	3,573	3,175	3,154
elementary school education - Grundschulbildung - načal'noe	2,709	2,251	2,182

Communist Party of the Soviet Union 3.5.2
Kommunistische Partei der Sowjetunion 3.5.3

3.5.2 LEVEL OF EDUCATION OF COMMUNIST PARTY MEMBERS (in percent)
BILDUNGSSTAND DER KOMMUNISTEN (in Prozenten)
SOSTAV KOMMUNISTOV PO OBRAZOVANIJU (v procentach)

Year Jahr Gody	compl.college or university educ. abgeschl. Hochschulbildung vysšee	not compl.coll. or univ.educ. nicht abgeschl. Hochschulbild. nezakončennoe vysšee	elementary school educ. mittlere Schulbildung srednee	not compl.inter-med.school educ. nicht abgeschl. mittl.Schulbild. nepolnoe srednee	elementary school ed. Grundschulbildung načal'noe	no elem. school ed. keine Grundschulbild. bez nač.
1927	0.8	--	9.1	--	63.0	27.1
1941	6.2	1.9	15.1	16.6	45.2	15.0
1952	8.9	2.8	22.2	27.6	31.4	7.1
1956	11.2	3.6	22.2	29.6	28.4	5.0
1961	13.2	3.0	26.2	28.6	25.8	3.2
1966	15.7	2.5	30.9	27.5	23.4	--
1971	19.6	2.4	34.3	24.9	18.8	--
1972	20.5	2.3	35.0	24.1	18.1	--
1976	24.3	2.5	38.5	20.3	14.4	--
1977	25.1	2.4	39.2	19.7	13.6	--

3.5.3 NUMBER OF COMMUNIST PARTY MEMBERS WITH ACADEMIC DEGREE
ZAHL DER KOMMUNISTEN MIT AKADEMISCHEM GRAD
ČISLO KOMMUNISTOV IMEJUŠČICH UČENUJU STEPEN'

Year Jahr Gody	Doctors of Science[1] Doktoren der Wissenschaften[1] doktora nauk	Candidates of Science[1] Kandidaten der Wissenschaften[1] kandidaty nauk
1950	2,144	14,463
1952	2,767	18,370
1956	3,840	34,513
1961	5,211	47,343
1966	7,488	69,320
1971	12,978	110,131
1972	14,656	120,840
1976	21,511	168,547

[1] The titles "Doctor of Science" and "Candidate of Science" cannot be compared to degrees earned in Western countries. Both are full academic degrees, attainable in all fields of study. The title "Candidate" precedes that of "Doctor". -

Die beiden akademischen Titel "Doktor der Wissenschaften" und "Kandidat der Wissenschaften" sind mit akademischen Graden in westlichen Ländern nicht zu vergleichen. Beide sind volle akademische Titel, die in allen Studienfächern verliehen werden. Der Grad "Kandidat" ist eine Vorstufe zum "Doktor".

3.6 Communist Party of the Soviet Union
Kommunistische Partei der Sowjetunion

3.6 WOMEN IN THE CPSU - FRAUEN IN DER KPdSU - ŽENŠČINY V KPSS

Year Jahr Gody	Total Insg. Vsego	As a percentage of total Communist Party Members In % zur Gesamtzahl der Kommunisten v % k obščemu čislu kommunistov
1920	45,297	7.5
1925	76,804	9.6
1927	148,306	12.2
1930	219,338	13.1
1934	395,763	14.7
1939	333,821	14.5
1941	575,853	14.9
1946	1,033,115	18.7
1952	1,276,560	19.0
1956	1,414,456	19.7
1962	1,942,080	19.6
1966	2,548,901	20.6
1971	3,195,556	22.2
1972	3,311,281	22.6
1973	3,442,029	23.0
1974	3,518,086	23.6
1975	3,657,231	23.8
1976	3,793,859	24.3
1977	3,947,616	24.7

Communist Party of the Soviet Union
Kommunistische Partei der Sowjetunion 3.7.1

3.7 NATIONAL COMPOSITION OF THE CPSU
NATIONALE ZUSAMMENSETZUNG DER KPdSU
NACIONAL'NYJ SOSTAV KPSS

3.7.1　　　　NATIONALITIES PEPPESENTED IN THE CPSU
　　　　　　　ANTEIL DER HAUPTNATIONEN
　　　　　　　ČISLO KOMMUNISTOV GLAVNYCH NACIJ

	1967 Total Insg. vsego	%	1973 Total Insg. vsego	%	1977 Total Insg. vsego	%
Russkie	7,846,292	61.8	9,025,363	60.9	9,679,129	60.5
Ukraincy	1,983,090	15.6	2,369,200	16.5	2,561,818	16.0
Belorusy	424,360	3.3	521,544	3.5	580,833	3.6
Uzbeki	219,381	1.7	291,550	2.0	333,907	2.1
Kazachi	199,196	1.6	254,667	1.7	292,936	1.8
Gruziny	209,196	1.6	246,214	1.7	265,625	1.7
Azerbaidžancy	162,181	1.3	212,122	1.4	241,677	1.5
Litovcy	71,316	0.6	96,558	0.7	110,934	0.7
Moldavane	46,562	0.4	59,434	0.4	72,331	0.5
Latyŝi	49,559	0.4	61,755	0.4	66,402	0.4
Kirgizy	39,053	0.3	46,049	0.3	51,112	0.3
Tadžiki	46,593	0.4	58,668	0.4	65,477	0.4
Armjane	200,605	1.6	225,132	1.5	239,460	1.5
Turkmeny	35,781	0.3	44,218	0.3	50,269	0.3
Estoncy	37,705	0.3	46,424	0.3	50,984	0.3
Total-Insg.-vsego	11,570,870	91.2	13,558,898	92.5	15,994,476	91.6

3.7.2 Communist Party of the Soviet Union
Kommunistische Partei der Sowjetunion

3.7.2 NATIONAL COMPOSITION AS OF 1.1.1976
NATIONALE ZUSAMMENSETZUNG ZUM 1.1.1976
NACIONAL'NYJ SOSTAV NA 1.1.1976

	Total Insg. vsego	%
Total - Insg. - vsego	15,638,891	100.0
Russkie	9,481,536	60.6
Ukraincy	2,505,378	16.0
Belorusy	563,408	3.6
Uzbeki	321,458	2.1
Kazachi	282,471	1.8
Gruziny	259,520	1.7
Azerbaidžancy	232,223	1.5
Litovcy	106,967	0.7
Moldavane	67,707	0.4
Latyŝi	65,116	0.4
Kirgizy	49,542	0.3
Tadžiki	63,611	0.4
Armjane	234,253	1.5
Turkmeny	48,021	0.3
Estoncy	49,739	0.3
Abchazy	5,274	0.03
Avarcy	19,387	0.1
Adygejcy	5,975	0.04
Altajcy	3,317	0.02
Balkarcy	3,893	0.02
Baŝkiry	55,122	0.4
Burjaty	20,476	0.1
Dargincy	8,408	0.1
Evrei	294,774	1.9
Inguŝi	2,763	0.02
Kabardincy	15,608	0.1
Kalmyki	6,411	0.04
Karakalpaki	9,072	0.1
Karačaevcy	5,191	0.03
Karely	10,284	0.1
Komi	24,986	0.2
Kumyki	8,909	0.1
Lakcy	6,681	0.04
Lezginy	19,716	0.1
Marijcy	21,171	0.1
Mordviny	73,464	0.5
Osetiny	36,758	0.2
Tatary	300,714	1.9
Tuvincy	6,584	0.04
Udmurty	31,666	0.2
Chakasy	2,489	0.02
Čerkesy	2,858	0.02
Čečency	12,959	0.1
Čuvaŝi	83,109	0.5
Jakuty	15,910	1.2
others-andere-drugie nacional'nosti	194,012	1.2

3.8 PRIMARY PARTY ORGANIZATIONS
GRUNDORGANISATIONEN DER PARTEI
PERVIČNYE ORGANIZACII PARTII

3.8.1 NETWORK OF PRIMARY ORGANIZATIONS - NETZ DER GRUNDORGANISATIONEN - SET' PERVIČNYCH PARTIJNYCH ORGANIZACIJ

	1. 1. 1971 Total Insg. vsego	%	1. 1. 1976 Total Insg. vsego	%
Total - Insg. - vsego	369,695	100.0	390,387	100,0
of which-darunter-iz nich:				
Industry, transport, post and telecommunications and construction work Industrie-,Transport-,Post-und Fernmeldewesen und Baubetriebe predprijatij promyšlennosti, transporta, svjazi i stroitelstv	95,375	25.8	101,472	26.0
Sovkhoz - Sowchosen - sovchozov	16,972	4.6	18,941	4.9
Kolkhoz - Kolchosen - kolchozov	33,644	9.1	29,081	7.4
Enterprises for trade and provision of foodstuffs Betriebe des Handels und der öffentlichen Lebensmittelversorgung predprijatij torgovli i obščestvennogo pitanija	14,848	4.0	14,488	3.7
Schools-Lehranstalten-učebnych zavedenij	61,881	16.7	67,446	17.3
Scientific institutions-wissenschaftliche Institutionen-naučnych učreždenij	5,148	1.4	6,018	1.5
Cultural and educational institutions (theatre,clubs,museums,cultural centers,etc.) Kulturelle und Bildungsanstalten (Theater, Klubs, Museen, Kulturparks u.a.) kul'turno-prosvetitel'nych i zrelišcnych učreždenij (teatry, kluby, muzei, parki kul'tury i.t.d.)	5,169	1.4	5,280	1.4
Public health institutions (hospitals, sanatoriums,outpatient medical centers,etc.) Kuranstalten (Krankenhäuser, Sanatorien, Polykliniken u.a.) lečebnych učreždenij (bol'nicy, sanatorii, polikliniki i.t.d.)	15,341	4.1	16,147	4.1
Institutions, organizations, economic institutes (from central to rayon) Institutionen, Organisationen, Wirtschaftsorgane (zentrale bis Rayons) učreždenij, organizacij i chozorganov (ot central'nych do rajonnych vključitel'no)	59,809	16.2	65,060	16.7
Rural, territorial and property management Ländliche, territoriale und Hausverwaltungen sel'skich territorialnych, pri domoupravlenijach i pročich vidov	61,508	16.7	66,454	17.0

3.8.2 Communist Party of the Soviet Union
3.8.3 Kommunistische Partei der Sowjetunion

3.8.2

PRIMARY PARTY ORGANIZATIONS BY PERCENTAGE OF COMMUNIST PARTY MEMBERS
GRUNDORGANISATIONEN DER PARTEI NACH ANTEIL DER KOMMUNISTEN
PERVIČNYE PARTIJNYE ORGANIZACII PO ČISLU KOMMUNISTOV

	1946	1957	1961	1966	1972	1977
- 15	63.0	57.5	43.7	40.0	40.2	40.4
15 - 49	29.7	36.4	43.8	43.3	42.0	40.9
50 - 100	5.4	4.2	8.1	10.7	11.6	12.1
above-über-svyše 100	1.9	1.9	4.4	6.0	6.2	6.6

3.8.3

COMMUNIST PARTY MEMBERS BY FIELD OF ECONOMIC ACTIVITY (in percentages)
VERTEILUNG DER KOMMUNISTEN NACH WIRTSCHAFTSZWEIGEN (in Prozenten)
RASSTANOVKA KOMMUNISTOV PO OTRASLJAM NARODNOGO CHOZJAJSTVA
(v procentach)

	1.1.1971	1.1.1976
Total - insg. - vsego	100.0	100.0
of which - davon - iz nich:		
in the manufacturing industry		
in den materiellen Produktionszweigen on		
v otrasljach material'nogo proizvodstva	73.4	73.0
of which - darunter - v tom čisle:		
in industry, construction work, transport, post and telecommunications		
in Industrie, Bauwesen, Transport-, Post- und Fernmeldewesen		
v promyšlennosti, stroitel'stve, na transporte i v svjazi	46.4	47.0
in agriculture		
in der Landwirtschaft		
v sel'skom chozjajstve	21.5	20.5
of which - davon - iz nich:		
in Sovkhoz - in Sowchosen - v sovchozach	8.2	8.0
in Kolkhoz - in Kolchosen - v kolchozach	11.7	10.8
Trade, provision of foodstuffs, procurement, material-technical supply and other productive branches		
Handel, öffentl. Lebensmittelversorgung, Beschaffungen, materiell-techn. Versorgung u.a. Produktionszweige		
v torgovle, obščestvennom pitanii, zagotovkach, material'-no-techničeskom snabženii i pročich otrasljach material'nogo proizvodstva	5.5	5.5
in science, education, public services		
in den nicht-materiellen Produktionszweigen		
v neproizvodstvennych otrasljach	26.6	27.0
of which - darunter - v tom čisle:		
Science - Wissenschaft - v nauke	4.0	4.3

Communist Party of the Soviet Union 3.8.3
Kommunistische Partei der Sowjetunion 3.8.4

	1.1.1971	1.1.1976
Elementary schools, colleges and universities, public health, culture and art Volksbildung, Hochschulen, Gesundheitswesen, Kultur und Kunst v prosveščenii, vysšich učebnych zavedenijach, zdravoochranenii, kul'ture i iskusstve	12.5	12.4
in leading state and economic agencies, in the party apparat and social organizations In den Organen der Staats-und Wirtschaftsleitung, im Apparat der Partei- und gesellschaftlichen Organisationen v organach gosudarstvennogo i chozjajstvennogo upravlenija, v apparate partijnych i obščestvennych organizacij	8.6	8.6
in housing, communal administration and public services In Wohnungs- und Kommunalwirtschaft und in Dienstleistungsbetrieben v žiliščnom, kommunal'nom chozjajstve i v bytovom obsluživanii	1.5	1.7

3.8.4 STRUCTURE OF THE PRIMARY PARTY ORGANIZATIONS
STRUKTUR DER GRUNDORGANISATIONEN DER PARTEI
STRUKTURA PERVIČNYCH PARTIJNYCH ORGANIZACIJ

	1.1.1971	1.1.1976
Primary party organizations with party committees Grundorganisationen der Partei mit Parteikomitees Pervičnych partorganizacij, imejuščich partkomy	31,219	35,951
party committees with the rights of rayon party committees darunter Parteikomitees mit den Rechten eines Rayonparteikomitees v tom čisle partkomov, imejuščich prava rajkoma partii	610	783
Secondary party organizations Parteiorganisationen der Betriebsabteilungen Cechovych partorganizacij	352,871	400,388
with the rights of a primary party organization davon mit den Rechten einer Grundorganisation der Partei iz nich s pravami pervičnych partorganizacij	235,660	274,454
Secondary party organizations with party committees Parteiorganisationen der Betriebsabteilungen mit Parteikomitee Cechovych partorganizacij, imejuščich partkomy	415	955
Party groups - Parteigruppen - Partijnych grupp	443,233	528,894
Party committees at main railway junctions Knotenpunktparteikomitees im Eisenbahntransport Uzlovych partkomov na železnodorožnom transporte	124	179

Communist Party of the Soviet Union
Kommunistische Partei der Sowjetunion

PRIMARY ORGANIZATION WITH LESS THAN 50 COMMUNIST PARTY MEMBERS
GRUNDORGANISATION MIT WENIGER ALS 50 KOMMUNISTEN
PERVIČNAJA ORGANIZACIJA NASČITYVAJUŠČAJA MENEE 50 KOMMUNISTOV

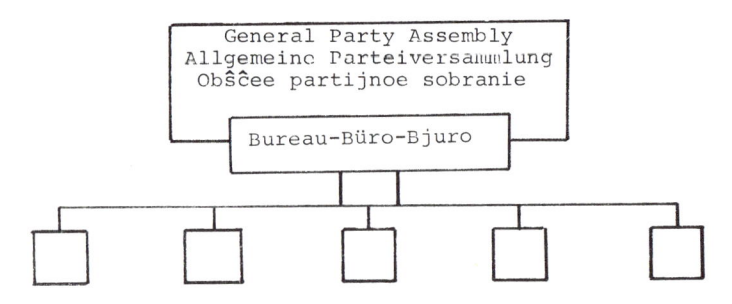

```
          ┌─────────────────────────────────┐
          │    General Party Assembly       │
          │  Allgemeine Parteiversammlung   │
          │    Obšĉee partijnoe sobranie    │
          │  ┌───────────────────────────┐  │
          └──┤   Bureau-Büro-Bjuro       ├──┘
             └───────────────────────────┘
                          │
        ┌────────┬────────┼────────┬────────┐
      ┌─┴─┐    ┌─┴─┐    ┌─┴─┐    ┌─┴─┐
      │   │    │   │    │   │    │   │
      └───┘    └───┘    └───┘    └───┘
```

Party groups in the brigades and other production groups
Parteigruppen in den Brigaden und anderen Produktionsgruppen
Partijnye gruppy po brigadam i drugim proizvodstvennym gruppy

PRIMARY ORGANIZATION WITH MORE THAN 50 COMMUNIST PARTY MEMBERS
GRUNDORGANISATION MIT MEHR ALS 50 KOMMUNISTEN
PERVIČNAJA ORGANIZACIJA NASČITYVAJUŠČAJA SVYŠE 50 KOMMUNISTOV

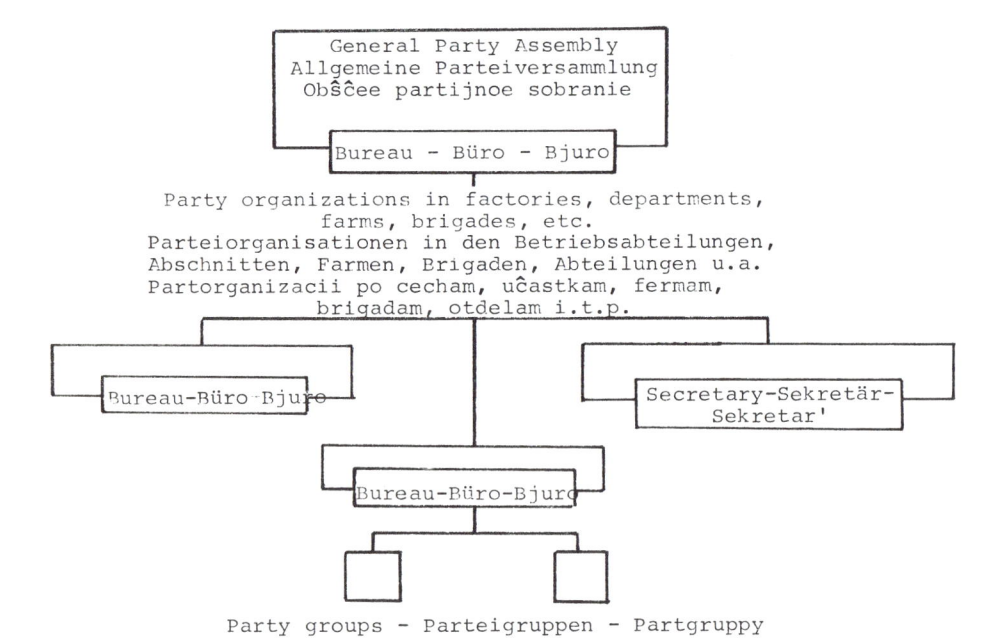

```
          ┌─────────────────────────────────┐
          │    General Party Assembly       │
          │  Allgemeine Parteiversammlung   │
          │    Obšĉee partijnoe sobranie    │
          │  ┌───────────────────────────┐  │
          └──┤   Bureau - Büro - Bjuro   ├──┘
             └───────────────────────────┘
```

Party organizations in factories, departments,
farms, brigades, etc.
Parteiorganisationen in den Betriebsabteilungen,
Abschnitten, Farmen, Brigaden, Abteilungen u.a.
Partorganizacii po cecham, učastkam, fermam,
brigadam, otdelam i.t.p.

```
  ┌──────────────────────┐         ┌──────────────────────────┐
  │  Bureau-Büro-Bjuro   │         │  Secretary-Sekretär-     │
  └──────────────────────┘         │        Sekretar'         │
                                   └──────────────────────────┘
              ┌──────────────────────┐
              │  Bureau-Büro-Bjuro   │
              └──────────────────────┘
                    ┌────┐   ┌────┐
                    │    │   │    │
                    └────┘   └────┘
```

Party groups - Parteigruppen - Partgruppy

92

Communist Party of the Soviet Union
Kommunistische Partei der Sowjetunion

PRIMARY ORGANIZATION WITH PARTY COMMITTEE
GRUNDORGANISATION MIT PARTEIKOMITEE
PERVIČNAJA ORGANIZACIJA IMEJUŠČAJA PARTIJNYJ KOMITET

General Party Assembly (Conference)
Allgemeine Parteiversammlung (Konferenz)
Obščee partijnoe sobranie (Konferencija)

Party Committee
Parteikomitee
Partijnyj komitet

Party organizations in factories, departments,
farms, brigades etc.
Parteiorganisationen in den Betriebsabteilungen,
Abschnitten, Farmen, Bri- gaden, Abteilungen u.a.
Partorganizacii po cecham , učastkam, fermam,
brigadam, otdelam i.t.p.

Bureau
Büro
Bjuro

Bureau
Büro
Bjuro

Bureau
Büro
Bjuro

Party groups
Parteigruppen
Partgruppy

Party groups
Parteigruppen
Partgruppy

Secretary
Sekretär
Sekretar'

Secretary
Sekretär
Sekretar'

Secretary
Sekretär
Sekretar'

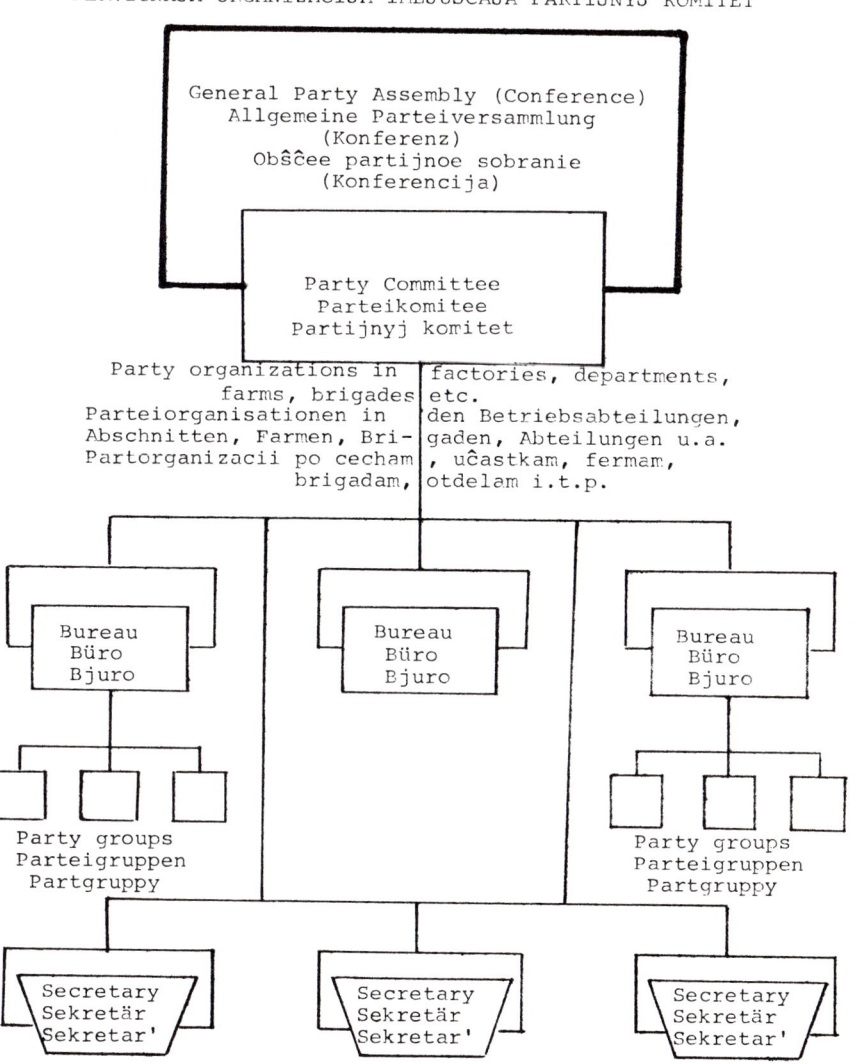

Communist Party of the Soviet Union
Kommunistische Partei der Sowjetunion

PRIMARY ORGANIZATION WITH THE RIGHTS OF A RAYON COMMITTEE[1]
GRUNDORGANISATION MIT PARTEIKOMITEE MIT DEN RECHTEN EINES RAYKOMS[1]
PERVIČNAJA ORGANIZACIJA IMEJUŠČAJA PARTIJNYJ KOMITET S PRAVAMI RAJKOMA PARTII[1]

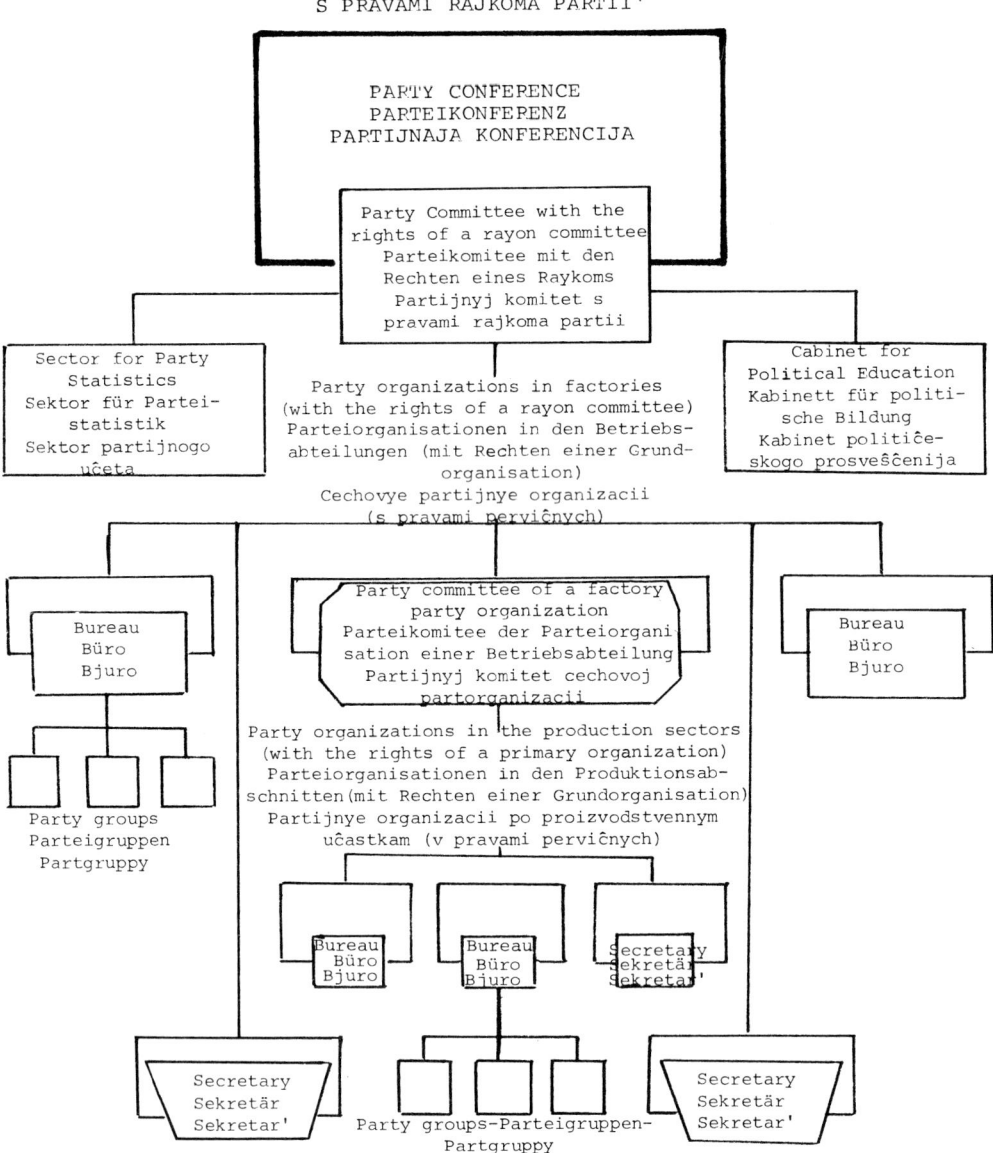

PARTY CONFERENCE
PARTEIKONFERENZ
PARTIJNAJA KONFERENCIJA

Party Committee with the rights of a rayon committee
Parteikomitee mit den Rechten eines Raykoms
Partijnyj komitet s pravami rajkoma partii

Sector for Party Statistics
Sektor für Parteistatistik
Sektor partijnogo učeta

Party organizations in factories (with the rights of a rayon committee)
Parteiorganisationen in den Betriebsabteilungen (mit Rechten einer Grundorganisation)
Cechovye partijnye organizacii (s pravami pervičnych)

Cabinet for Political Education
Kabinett für politische Bildung
Kabinet političeskogo prosveščenija

Bureau / Büro / Bjuro

Party committee of a factory party organization
Parteikomitee der Parteiorganisation einer Betriebsabteilung
Partijnyj komitet cechovoj partorganizacii

Bureau / Büro / Bjuro

Party groups
Parteigruppen
Partgruppy

Party organizations in the production sectors (with the rights of a primary organization)
Parteiorganisationen in den Produktionsabschnitten (mit Rechten einer Grundorganisation)
Partijnye organizacii po proizvodstvennym učastkam (v pravami pervičnych)

Bureau / Büro / Bjuro

Bureau / Büro / Bjuro

Secretary / Sekretär / Sekretar'

Secretary / Sekretär / Sekretar'

Party groups-Parteigruppen-Partgruppy

Secretary / Sekretär / Sekretar'

---

1 In charge of admission to membership in the CPSU, personal background files of members and candidate members and personal affairs of Communists -
in den Fragen der Aufnahme in die KPdSU, Führung der Personalakten der Mitglieder u. Kandidaten d.Partei u.Untersuchung der persönlichen Angelegenheiten der Kommunisten -
po voprosam priema v KPSS, vedenija učeta členov i kandidatov partii i rassmotrenija personal'nych del kommunistov

Communist Party of the Soviet Union 3.9.1
Kommunistische Partei der Sowjetunion 3.9.2

3.9 ELECTED LEADING PARTY ORGANIZATIONS
GEWÄHLTE LEITENDE ORGANE DER PARTEI
VYBORNYE RUKOVODJAŠČIE ORGANY PARTII

3.9.1 CC CPSU - ZK der KPdSU - CK KPSS [+)]

Members Mitglieder Členy	- 287
Candidate Members Kandidaten Kandidaty	- 139

3.9.2 POLITBURO CC CPSU - POLITBÜRO ZK KPdSU - POLITBJURO CK KPSS

Name Familija	Date of Birth Geburtsdatum Data rožd.	Party Affiliation Parteizugehörigkeit Partijnyj staž	Further positions Weitere Positionen Drugie dolžnosti
A	B	C	D
Members - Mitglieder - Členy			
ANDROPOV, Ju.V.	1914	1939	Chairman, Committee for State Security of the USSR - Vorsitzender d.Komitees f.Staatssicherheit der UdSSR
BREŽNEV, L.I.	1906	1931	Secretary General, CC CPSU; Chairman, Presidium of USSR Supreme Soviet - Generalsekretär d.ZK d.KPdSU; Vorsitzender d.Präsidiums d.Obersten Sowjets d.UdSSR
GRIŠIN, V.V.	1914	1939	First City Secretary, CPSU Moscow - Erster Stadtsekretär d.KPdSU in Moskau
GROMYKO, A.A.	1909	1931	Minister of Foreign Affairs of the USSR- Außenminister der UdSSR
KIRILENKO, A.P.	1906	1931	Secretary, CC CPSU - Sekretär des ZK der KPdSU
KOSYGIN, A.N.	1904	1927	Chairman, USSR Council of Ministers - Vorsitzender d.Ministerrates d.UdSSR

+) Elected at the XXV.CPSU Party Congress in March 1976. 13 members died prior to Sept. 1978, 8 candidate members were promoted to members -
Gewählt auf dem XXV.Parteitag der KPdSU im März 1976. Bis Sept. 1978 sind 13 Mitglieder gestorben, 8 Kandidaten sind zu Mitgliedern aufgestiegen.

3.9.2 Communist Party of the Soviet Union
Kommunistische Partei der Sowjetunion

A	B	C	D
KULAKOV, F.D.[1]	1918	1940	Secretary, CC CPSU; Chief, CC CPSU Department of Agriculture - Sekretär d.ZK d.KPdSU; Leiter d. Landwirtschaftsabteilung b.ZK d.KPdSU
KUNAEV, D.A.	1912	1939	First Secretary, CC CP of Kazakhstan- Erster Sekretär d.ZK d.KP Kasachstans
MAZUROV, K.T.	1914	1940	First vice-chairman, USSR Council of Ministers - Erster stellv.Vorsitzender d.Ministerrates der UdSSR
PELŠE, A.Ja.	1899	1915	Chairman, CC CPSU Committee for Party Control - Vorsitzender d.Komitees f.Parteikontrolle b.ZK d.KPdSU
ROMANOV, G.V.	1923	1944	First Obkom Secretary of the CPSU in Leningrad - Erster Obkomsekretär d.KPdSU in Leningrad
ŠCERBICKIJ, V.V.	1918	1941	First Secretary, CC CP of the Ukraine- Erster Sekretär d.ZK d.KP d.Ukraine
SUSLOV, M.A.	1902	1921	Secretary, CC CPSU - Sekretär d.ZK d.KPdSU
USTINOV, D.F.	1908	1927	USSR Minister of Defense - Verteidigungsminister der UdSSR

Candidate Members - Kandidaten - Kandidaty

ALIEV, G.A.R.o.	1923	1945	First Secretary, CC CP of Azerbaijan - Erster Sekretär d.ZK d.KP Aserbaidschans
ČERNENKO, K.U.	1911	1931	Secretary, CC CPSU; Chief, CC CPSU General Department - Sekretär d.ZK d.KPdSU; Leiter der Allgemeinen Abteilung b.ZK d.KPdSU
DEMIČEV, P.N.	1918	1939	USSR Minister of Culture - Kulturminister der UdSSR
KUZNECOV, V.V.	1901	1927	First Vice-Chairman, Presidium of USSR Supreme Soviet - Erster stellv.Vorsitzender d.Präsidiums d.Obersten Sowjets d.UdSSR
MAŠEROV, P.M.	1918	1943	First Secretary, CC CP of Belorussia - Erster Sekretär d.ZK d.KP Belorußlands
PONOMAREV, B.N.	1905	1919	Secretary, CC CPSU; Chief, CC CPSU International Department - Sekretär d.ZK d.KPdSU; Leiter d.Internationalen Abteilung b.ZK d.KPdSU
RAŠIDOV, Š.R.	1917	1939	First Secretary, CC CP of Uzbekistan - Erster Sekretär d.ZK d.KP Usbekistans
SOLOMENCEV, M.S.	1913	1940	Chairman, RSFSR Council of Ministers - Vorsitzender d.Ministerrates d.RSFSR

[1] died on July 17, 1978 - am 17.7.78 gestorben

Communist Party of the Soviet Union
Kommunistische Partei der Sowjetunion 3.9.3

3.9.3

SECRETARIAT CC CPSU - SEKRETARIAT ZK KPdSU - SEKRETARIAT CK KPSS

Name Familija	Date of Birth Geburtsdatum Data rožd.	Party Affiliation Parteizuge- hörigkeit Partijnyj staž	Further positions Weitere Positionen Drugie dolžnosti
Secretary General - Generalsekretär - General'nyj sekretar'			
BREŽNEV, L.I.	1906	1931	
Secretaries - Sekretäre - Sekretari			
ČERNENKO, K.U.	1911	1931	
DOLGICH, V.I.	1924	1942	Secretary; Chief, CC CPSU Department for Heavy Industry - Sekretär; Leiter d.Abteilung f. Schwerindustrie b.ZK d.KPdSU
KAPITONOV, I.V.	1915	1939	Secretary; Chief, CC CPSU Department for Organizational Party Work - Sekretär; Leiter d.Abteilung für Organisations-Parteiarbeit beim ZK d.KPdSU
KIRILENKO, A.P.	1906	1931	
KULAKOV, F.D.[1]	1918	1940	
PONOMAREV, B.N.	1905	1919	
RJABOV, Ja.P.	1928	1954	Secretary, Armament Industry - Sekretär für Rüstungsindustrie
RUSAKOV, K.V.	1909	1943	Secretary; Chief, CC CPSU Department for Liaison with Communist & Workers' Parties of the Socialist Countries - Sekretär; Leiter d.Abteilung f.Verbindungen m.kommunistischen u.Arbeiterparteien d.sozialistischen Länder b.ZK d.KPdSU
SUSLOV, M.A.	1902	1921	
ZIMJANIN, M.V.	1914	1939	Secretary, Ideological Section - Sekretär für den ideologischen Bereich

[1] died on July 17, 1978 - am 17.7.78 gestorben

3.9.4 Communist Party of the Soviet Union
3.9.5 Kommunistische Partei der Sowjetunion

3.9.4 NETWORK OF LEADING PARTY ORGANISATIONS
NETZ DER LEITENDEN PARTEIORGANE
SET'RUKOVODJAŠČICH PARTIJNYCH ORGANOV

	1922	1926	1930	1934	1939	1952	1956	1961	1966	1971	1972	1977
CC of CPs of the Union Republics - ZK der KPs der Unionsrepubliken CK kompartij sojuznych respublik	6	7	8	8	10	15	15	14	14	14	14	14
Krajkom	1	4	9	12	6	6	6	7	6	6	6	6
Obkom	17	37	37	58	104	156	148	135	133	142	142	149
Gubkom	75	40	--	--	--	--	--	--	--	--	--	--
Okružkom	--	114	228	20	29	23	10	10	10	10	10	10
Ukom	759	442	26	--	--	--	--	--	--	--	--	--
Gorkom		..	..	132	-23	531	554	596	739	760	763	832
Raykom gorodskoj	517	..	..	93	345	490	485	341	410	448	448	594
Raykom sel'skoj		1,530	3,012	2,466	3,492	4,373	4,248	3,231	2,519	2,810	2,813	2,870

3.9.5 ELECTED LEADING PARTY ORGANIZATIONS OF THE UNION REPUBLICS
GEWÄHLTE LEITENDE ORGANE DER PARTEI DER UNIONSREPUBLIKEN
VYBORNYE RUKOVODJAŠČIE ORGANY PARTII SOJUZNYCH RESPUBLIK

RSFSR [1]

CPSU City Committees - Gorkoms der KPdSU - Gorkomy KPSS [2]

| Leningrad | -- | Moskva | - GRIŠIN, V.V. |

CPSU Krai Committees - Krajkomitees der KPdSU - Krajkomy KPSS

Altai	- AKSENOV, N.F.	Krasnojarsk	- FEDIRKO, P.S.
Chabarovsk	- ČERNYJ, A.K.	Primore	- LOMAKIN, V.P.
Krasnodar	- MEDUNOV, S.F.	Stavropol	- GORBAČEV, M.S.

---

1 No party of its own - the party organizations in the RSFSR are subordinate to the CC of the CPSU -
Keine eigene Partei - die Parteiorganisationen auf dem Gebiet der RSFSR sind direkt dem ZK der KPdSU untergeordnet

2 For all Krai-,Oblast- and Gorkoms the First Secretaries are listed -
Bei allen Krai-,Oblast-und Gorkoms werden die Ersten Sekretäre angeführt

Communist Party of the Soviet Union
Kommunistische Partei der Sowjetunion 3.9.5

CPSU Oblast Committees - Oblastkomitees der KPdSU - Obkomy KPSS

Adygejskaja avto-		Kostroma	- BALANDIN, Ju.N.
nomnaja oblast'	- BERSEGOV, N.A.	Kuibyšev	- ORLOV, V.P.
Amur	- AVRAMENKO, S.S.	Kurgan	- KNJAZEV, F.K.
Archangelsk	- POPOV, B.V.	Kursk	- GUDKOV, A.F.
Astrachan	- BORODIN, L.A.	Leningrad	- ROMANOV, G.V.
Baškirskaja ASSR	- SAKIROV, M.Z.	Lipeck	- PAVLOV, G.P.
Belgorod	- TRUNOV, M.P.	Magadan	- SAJDUROV, S.A.
Brjansk	- SIZENKO, E.I.	Mari ASSR	- NIKONOV, V.P.
Čečeno-Ingušskaja		Mordovskaja ASSR	- BEREZIN, A.I.
ASSR	- VLASOV, A.V.	Moskva	- KONOTOP, V.I.
Čeljabinsk	- VOROPOAEV, M.G.	Murmansk	- PTICYN, V.N.
Chakasskaja avto-		Novgorod	- ANTONOV, N.A.
nomnaja oblast'	- KRYLOV, A.I.	Novosibirsk	- GORJAČEV, F.S.
Čita	- MATAFONOV, M.I.	Omsk	- MANJAKIN, S.I.
Čuvašskaja ASSR	- PROKOPEV, I.P.	Orel	- MEŠKOV, F.S.
Burjatskaja ASSR	- MODOGOEV, A.U.	Orenburg	- KOVALENKO, A.V.
Dagestanskaja ASSR	- UMACHANOV, M.-S.I.	Penza	- ERMIN, L.B.
Evrejskaja avto-		Perm	- KONOPLEV, B.V.
nomnaja oblast'	- ŠAPIRO, L.B.	Pskov	- RYBAKOV, A.M.
Gorkij	- CHRISTORADNOV,Ju.N.	Rjazan	- PRIEZZEV, N.S.
Gorno-Altajskaja		Rostov	- BONDARENKO, I.A.
avtonomnaja oblast'	- LAZEBNYJ, N.S.	Sachalin	- LEONOV, P.A.
Ivanovo	- KLJUEV, V.G.	Saratov	- GUSEV, V.K.
Irkutsk	- BANNIKOV, N.V.	Severo-Osetinskaja	
Jakutskaja ASSR	- ČIRJAEV, G.I.	ASSR	- KABALOEV, B.E.
Jaroslavl	- LOŠČENKOV, F.I.	Smolensk	- KLIMENKO, I.E.
Kabardino-Balkar-		Sverdlovsk	- ELCIN, B.N.
skaja ASSR	- MALBACHOV, T.K.	Tambov	- CHOMJAKOV, A.A.
Kalinin	- KORYTKOV, N.G.	Tatarskaja ASSR	- TABEEV, F.A.
Kaliningrad	- KONOVALOV, N.S.	Tjumen	- BOGOMJAKOV, G.P.
Kalmyckaja ASSR	- GORODOVIKOV, B.B.	Tomsk	- LIGAČEV, E.K.
Kaluga	- KANDRENKOV, A.A.	Tula	- JUNAK, I.Ch.
Kamčatka	- KAČIN, D.I.	Tuvinskaja ASSR	- ŠIRŠIN, G.Č.
Karačaevo-Čerkesskaja		Udmurtskaja ASSR	- MARISOV, V.K.
avtonomnaja oblast'	- MURACHOVSKIJ, V.S.	Uljanovsk	- KUZNECOV, I.M.
Karelskaja ASSR	- SEN'KIN, I.I.	Vladimir	- PONOMAREV, M.A.
Kemerovo	- GORŠKOV, L.A.	Volgograd	- KULIČENKO, L.S.
Kirov	- BESPALOV, I.P.	Vologda	- DRYGIN, A.S.
Komi ASSR	- MOROZOV, I.P.	Voronež	- IGNATOV, V.N.

Ukrainskaja SSR

Politburo - Politbüro - Politbjuro

Members-Mitglieder-Členy

    BORISENKO, N.M.   SOKOLOV, I.Z.
    BOTVIN, A.P.   SOLOGUB, V.A.
    FEDORČUK, V.V.   TITARENKO, A.A.
    LJAŠKO, A.P.   VAŠČENKO, G.I.
    POGREBNJAK, P.L.   VATČENKO, A.F.
    ŠČERBICKIJ, V.V.

Candidate Members-Kandidaten-Kandidaty

    DOBRIK, V.F.   MALANČUK, V.Ju.
    GERASIMOV, I.A.   POGREBNJAK, Ja.P.
    KAČURA, B.V.

3.9.5 Communist Party of the Soviet Union
Kommunistische Partei der Sowjetunion

Secretariat - Sekretariat

| First Secretary
Erster Sekretär
Pervyj Sekretar' | - ŠČERBICKIJ, V.V. | Second Secretary
Zweiter Sekretär
Vtoroj Sekretar' | - SOKOLOV, I.Z. |

Secretaries
Sekretäre
Sekretari
- BORISENKO, N.M.
- MALANČUK, V.Ju.
- POGREBNJAK, Ja.P.
- TITARENKO, A.A.

CPU City Committee - Gorkom der KPU - Gorkom KPU, Kiev

BOTVIN, A.P.

CPU Oblast Committees - Oblastkomitees der KPU - Obkomy KPU

Čerkassy	- LUTAK, I.K.	Nikolaev	- VASLJAEV, V.A.
Černigov	- UMANEC, N.V.	Odessa	- KIRIČENKO, N.K.
Černovcy	- DIKUSAROV, V.G.	Poltava	- MORGUN, F.T.
Charkov	- SACHNJUK, I.I.	Rovno	- PANASENKO, T.I.
Cherson	- MOZGOVOJ, I.A.	Sumy	- GRINCOV, I.G.
Chmelnickij	- LISOVYJ, T.G.	Ternopol	- JARKOVOJ, I.M.
Dnepropetrovsk	- KAČALOVSKIJ, E.V.	Vinnica	- TARATUTA, V.N.
Doneck	- KAČURA, B.V.	Volynskaja oblast'	
Ivano-Frankovsk	- BEZRUK, P.F.	(Luck)	- KORŽ, M.P.
Kiev	- CYBUL'KO, V.M.	Vorošilovgrad	- GONČARENKO, B.T.
Kirovograd	- KOBYLČAK, M.M.	Zakarpatskaja oblast'	
Krim	- MAKARENKO, V.S.	(Užgorod)	- ILNICKIJ, Ju.V.
Lvov	- DOBRIK, V.F.	Zaporože	- VSEVOLOŽSKIJ, M.N.
		Žitomir	- KAVUN, V.M.

Belorusskaja SSR

Buro - Büro - Bjuro

Members-Mitglieder-Členy

AKSENOV, A.N. MICKEVIČ, V.F.
GVOZDEV, V.A. MIKULIČ, V.A.
JAKUŠEV, I.F. NIKULKIN, Ja.P.
KISELEV, T.Ja. POLOZOV, N.N.
KOLOKOLOV, Ju.B. POLJAKOV, I.E.
KUZMIN, A.T. ŠEVELUCHA, V.S.
LAGIR, M.I. FIRISANOV, L.S.
MAŠEROV, P.M. ZAJCEV, M.M.

Candidate Members-Kandidaten-Kandidaty

LOBANOK, V.E. SNEŽKOVA, N.L.
PLATONOV, K.M.

Secretariat - Sekretariat

| First Secretary
Erster Sekretär
Pervyj sekretar' | - MAŠEROV, P.M. | Second Secretary
Zweiter Sekretär
Vtoroj Sekretar' | - AKSENOV, A.N. |

Secretaries
Sekretäre
Sekretari
- KOLOKOLOV, Ju.B.
  KUZMIN, A.T.
  ŠEVELUCHA, V.S.
  FIRISANOV, L.S.

Communist Party of the Soviet Union
Kommunistische Partei der Sowjetunion 3.9.5

CPB City Committee - Gorkom der KPB - Gorkom KPB, Minsk

LEPEŠKIN, V.A.

CPB Oblast Committees - Oblastkomitees der KPB - Obkomy KPB

Brest	- SOKOLOV, E.E.	Minsk	- MIKULIČ, V.A.
Gomel	- GVOZDEV, V.A.	Mogilev	- PRIŠČEPČIK, V.V.
Grodno	- KLECKOV, L.G.	Vitebsk	- ŠABAŠOV, S.M.

UZBEKSKAJA SSR

Buro - Büro - Bjuro

Members-Mitglieder-Členy

ANISIMKIN, I.G.   MATČANOV, N.M.
BELONOŽKO, S.E.   MUSACHANOV, M.M.
CHODŽAEV, A.A.   OSETROV, T.N.
CHUDAJBERDYEV, N.D.   RAŠIDOV, Š.R.
GREKOV, L.I.   SALIMOV, A.U.
KURBANOV, Ju.R.

Candidate Members-Kandidaten-Kandidaty

KAMALOV, K.   ORLOV, G.M.
MACHMUDOV, H.   SULTANOVA, S.U.
NORDMAN, E.B.

Secretariat - Sekretariat

First Secretary   Second Secretary
Erster Sekretär   - RAŠIDOV, Š.R.   Zweiter Sekretär - GREKOV, L.I.
Pervyj Sekretar'   Vtoroj Sekretar'

Secretaries   - ANISIMKIN, I.G.
Sekretäre   - KURBANOV, Ju.R.
Sekretari   - SALIMOV, A.U.

CPU City Committee - Gorkom der KPU - Gorkom KPU, Taškent

CHODŽAEV, A.A.

CPU Oblast Committees - Oblastkomitees der KPU - Obkomy KPU

Andižan	- USMANCHODŽAEV, I.B.	Kaška-Darja	- GAIPOV, R.G.
Buchara	- KARIMOV, A.	Namangan	- KAMALOV, M.
Chorezm	- CHUDAJBERGENOV, M.Ch.	Samarkand	- RACHIMOV, B.R.
Džizak	- BAJMIROV, T.B.	Surchan-Darja	- KARIMOV, A.
Fergana	- SAMSUDINOV, F.S.	Syr-Darja	- CHAJDUROV, V.A.
Kara-Kalpaken ASSR	- KAMALOV, K.	Taškent	- MUSACHANOV, M.M.

KAZACHSKAJA SSR

Buro - Büro - Bjuro

Members-Mitglieder-Členy

AŠIMOV, B.A.
ASKAROV, A.A.   KUNAEV, D.A.
IMAŠEV, S.N.   MIROŠKIN, O.S.
KLIMOV, A.I.   NIJAZBEKOV, S.B.
KORKIN, A.I.   SMIRNOV, S.A.
KOSPANOV, S.K.

101

3.9.5 Communist Party of the Soviet Union
Kommunistische Partei der Sowjetunion

Candidate Members-Kandidaten-Kandidaty

MUKAŠEV, S.M.
ŠEVČENKO, V.T.
SLAŽNEV, I.G.

Secretariat - Sekretariat

First Secretary
Erster Sekretär   - KUNAEV, D.A.
Pervyj Sekretar'

Second Secretary
Zweiter Sekretär   - KORKIN, A.G.
Vtoroj Sekretar'

Secretaries   - IMAŠEV, S.N.
Sekretäre   - KLIMOV, A.I.
Sekretari   - KOSPANOV, S.K.
                - MIROŠKIN, O.S.

CPK City Committee - Gorkom der KPK - Gorkom KPK, Alma-Ata

ERPILOV, P.I.

CPK Oblast Committees - Oblastkomitees der KPK - Obkomy KPK

Aktjubinsk	- LIVENCOV, V.A.	Pavlodar	- ISAEV, B.V.
Alma-Ata	- AUCHADIEV, K.M.	Semipalatinsk	- RAMAZANOV, A.G.
Celinograd	- MOROZOV, N.E.	Severo-Kazachstan-	
Čimkent	- ASKAROV, A.	skaja oblast'	
Džambul	- BEKTURGANOV,Ch.Š.	(Petropavlovsk)	- DEMIDENKO, V.P.
Džezkazgan	- LOSEV, K.S.	Taldy-Kurgan	- KUSAINOV, S.K.
Gurev	- MUKAŠEV, S.M.	Turgajskaja oblast'	
Karaganda	- AKULINCEV, V.K.	(Arkalyk)	- AUELBEKOV, E.N.
Kokčetav	- KUANYŠEV, O.S.	Uralsk	- IKSANOV, M.B.
Kzyl-Orda	- ABDUKARIMOV, I.A.	Vostočno-Kazachstan-	
Kustanai	- BORODIN, A.M.	skaja oblast'	
Mangyšlakskaja ob-		(Ust'-Kamenogorsk)	- PROTOZANOV, A.K.
last'(Ševčenko)	- AŠIMBAEV, T.A.		

GRUZINSKAJA SSR

Buro - Büro - Bjuro

Members-Mitglieder-Členy

ČCHEIDZE, Z.A.   MENTEŠAŠVILI, T.N.
GILAŠVILI, P.G.   PATARIDZE, Z.A.
INAURI, A.N.   PATIAŠVILI, D.I.
KIKNADZE, Š.D.   ŠEVARDNADZE, E.A.
KOLBIN, G.V.   SIRADZE, V.M.
KULIŠEV, O.F.

Candidate Members-Kandidaten-Kandidaty

ČERKEZIJA, O.E.   MOSAŠVILI, T.I.
CHABEIŠVILI, S.E.   SARTAVA, Ž.K.
ČITANAVA, N.A.

Secretariat - Sekretariat

First Secretary
Erster Sekretär   - ŠEVARDNADZE, E.A.
Pervyj Sekretar'

Second Secretary
Zweiter Sekretär   - KOLBIN, G.V.
Vtoroj Sekretar'

Secretaries   - ČCHEIDZE, Z.A.
Sekretäre   - PATIAŠVILI, D.I.
Sekretari   - SIRADZE, V.M.

Communist Party of the Soviet Union
Kommunistische Partei der Sowjetunion

CPG City Committee - Gorkom der KPG - Gorkom KPG, Tbilisi

MENTEŠAŠVILI, T.N.

CPG Oblast Committees - Oblastkomitees der KPG - Obkomy KPG

Abchazskaja ASSR   - ADLEJBA, B.V.
Adžarskaja ASSR   - PAPUNIDZE, V.R.
Jugo-Osetinskaja avtonom-
naja oblast'   - SANAKOEV, F.S.

AZERBAJDŽANSKAJA SSR

Buro - Büro - Bjuro

Members-Mitglieder-Členy

ALIEV, G.A.R.o.	KERIMOV, A.G.
BAGIROV, K.M.	KONSTANTINOV, A.U.
CHALILOV, K.A.	KRASILNIKOV, V.S.
IBRAGIMOV, G.Ch.	PUGAČEV, Ju.N.
IBRAGIMOV, I.A.	SEIDOV, G.N.

Candidate Members-Kandidaten-Kandidaty

ASKEROV, I.N.   GUSEJNOVA, Z.I.
EFENDIEV, G.S.   KEVORKOV, B.S.

Secretariat - Sekretariat

First Secretary
Erster Sekretär   - ALIEV, G.A.R.o.
Pervyj Sekretar'

Second Secretary
Zweiter Sekretär   - PUGAČEV, Ju.N.
Vtoroj Sekretar'

Secretaries   - IBRAGIMOV, G.Ch.
Sekretäre   - MAMEDZADE, R.C.
Sekretari   - SEIDOV, G.N.

CPA City Committee - Gorkom der KPA - Gorkom KPA, Baku

KERIMOV, A.G.

CPA Oblast Committees - Oblastkomitees der KPA - Obkomy KPA

Nagorno-Karabachskaja avtonomnaja
oblast'   - KEVORKOV, B.S.
Nachičevanskaja ASSR   - RAGIMOV, K.N.

LITOVSKAJA SSR

Buro - Büro - Bjuro

Members-Mitglieder-Členy

BARAUSKAS, A.B.	KAJRIS, K.K.
BARKAUSKAS, A.S.	MANJUŠIS, Ju.A.
BRAZAUSKAS, A.M.	SAKALAUSKAS, V.V.
CHARAZOV, V.I.	ŠEPETIS, L.K.
FERENSAS, A.A.	SONGAJLA, R.-B.I.
GRIŠKJAVIČJUS, P.P.	

3.9.5 Communist Party of the Soviet Union
Kommunistische Partei der Sowjetunion

Candidate Members-Kandidaten-Kandidaty

           ASTRAUSKAS, V.S.   MIKUČJAUSKAS, V.K.
           BALTRUNAS, V.   PETKJAVIČJUS, Ju.Ju.

Secretariat - Sekretariat

First Secretary		Second Secretary	
Erster Sekretär	- GRIŠKJAVIČJUS, P.P.	Zweiter Sekretär	- CHARAZOV, V.I.
Pervyj Sekretar'		Vtoroj Sekretar'	

           Secretaries   - BRAZAUSKAS, A.M.
           Sekretäre   - ŠEPETIS, L.K.
           Sekretari   - SONGAJLA, R.-B.I.

CPL City Committee - Gorkom der KPL - Gorkom KPL, Vilna

           SAKALAUSKAS, V.V.

MOLDAVSKAJA SSR

Buro - Büro - Bjuro

Members-Mitglieder-Členy

           BODJUL, I.I.
           GROSSU, S.K.   MERENIŠČEV, N.V.
           EREMEJ, G.I.   PETRIK, P.P.
           ILJAŠENKO, K.P.   SAVOČKO, B.N.
           KALENIK, E.P.   VORONIN, P.V.
           KALIN, I.P.

Candidate Members-Kandidaten-Kandidaty

           DYGAJ, G.G.   ZAJČENKO, N.M.
           RAGOZIN, A.P.

Secretariat - Sekretariat

First Secretary		Second Secretary	
Erster Sekretär	- BODJUL, I.I.	Zweiter Sekretär	- MERENIŠČEV, N.V.
Pervyj Sekretar'		Vtoroj Sekretar'	

           Secretaries   - KALENIK, E.P.
           Sekretäre   - KALIN, I.P.
           Sekretari   - SAVOČKO, B.N.

CPM City Committee - Gorkom der KPM - Gorkom KPM, Kišinev

           KIKTENKO, V.K.

LATVIJSKAJA SSR

Buro - Büro - Bjuro

Members-Mitglieder-Členy

           ANDERSON, I.A.   PETERSON, E.K.
           AUŠKAP, E.Ja.   RUBEN, Ju.Ja.
           BEMAN, E.K.   STRAUTMANIS, P.Ja.
           ČEMM, V.A.   STRELKOV, I.K.
           MAJOROV, A.M.   VERRO, R.O.
                                         VOSS, A.E.

Communist Party of the Soviet Union
Kommunistische Partei der Sowjetunion 3.9.5

Candidate Members-Kandidaten-Kandidaty

    AVDJUKEVIČ, L.I.   ZITMANIS, A.K.
    VAGRIS, Ja.Ja.

Secretariat - Sekretariat

First Secretary		Second Secretary
Erster Sekretär	- VOSS, A.E.	Zweiter Sekretär - STRELKOV, I.K.
Pervyj Sekretar'		Vtoroj Sekretar'

    Secretaries   - ANDERSON, I.A.
    Sekretäre   - AUŠKAP, E.Ja.
    Sekretari   - ČEMM, V.A.

CPL City Committee - Gorkom der KPL - Gorkom KPL, Riga

    VAGRIS, Ja.Ja.

KIRGIZSKAJA SSR

Buro - Büro - Bjuro

Members-Mitglieder-Členy

CHODOS, P.M.	MINIČ, N.G.
FOMIČENKO, K.E.	MOLDOBAEV, K.
IBRAIMOV, S.	NAUMOV, P.I.
KULATOV, T.	SUJUMBAEV, A.S.
KULMATOV, K.	USUBALIEV, T.
MASALIEV, A.M.	

Candidate Members-Kandidaten-Kandidaty

    ABAKIROV, E.   BEGMATOVA, S.
                      KABANOV, M.F.

Secretariat - Sekretariat

First Secretary		Second Secretary
Erster Sekretär	- USUBALIEV, T.	Zweiter Sekretär - FOMIČENKO, K.E.
Pervyj Sekretar'		Vtoroj Sekretar'

    Secretaries   - KULMATOV, K.K.
    Sekretäre   - MASALIEV, A.M.
    Sekretari   - NAUMOV, P.I.

CPK City Committee - Gorkom der KPK - Gorkom KPK, Frunze

    MOLDOBAEV, K.M.

CPK Oblast Committees - Oblastkomitees der KPK - Obkomy KPK

    Issyk-Kulskaja oblast'
    (Prževalsk)   - DUJŠEEV, A.
    Naryn   - SAVITACHUNOV, A.
    Oš   - KOŠOEV, T.Ch.

TADŽIKSKAJA SSR

Buro - Büro - Bjuro

Members-Mitglieder-Členy

BABAEV, M.B.	NABIEV, R.
BOBOSADYKOVA, G.B.	PERVENCEV, E.I.
CHOLOV, M.	POLUKAROV, Ju.I.
DADABAEV, A.	RACHIMOVA, I.R.
DEDOV, I.F.	RASULOV, D.R.
KARMYŠEV, L.K.	

3.9.5 Communist Party of the Soviet Union
Kommunistische Partei der Sowjetunion

Candidate Members-Kandidaten-Kandidaty

CHAJDAROV, A.Ch.   USMANOV, U.G.
NOVIČKOV, V.E.

Secretariat - Sekretariat

First Secretary
Erster Sekretär - RASULOV, D.R.
Pervyj Sekretar'

Second Secretary
Zweiter Sekretär - POLUKAROV, Ju.I.
Vtoroj Sekretar'

Secretaries   - BABAEV, M.B.
Sekretäre   - DADABAEV, A.D.
Sekretari   - RACHIMOVA, I.R.

CPT City Committee - Gorkom der KPT - Gorkom KPT, Dušanbe

BOBOSADYKOVA, G.B.

CPT Oblast Committees - Oblastkomitees der KPT - Obkomy KPT

Gorno-Badachšanskaja avto-
nomnaja oblast' (Chorog) - DAVLJATKADAMOV, Ch.
Kuljab   - CHISAMUTDINOV, A.B.
Kurgan-Tjube   - PALLAEV, G.
Leninabad   - CHODŽIEV, R.

ARMJANSKAJA SSR

Buro - Büro - Bjuro

Members-Mitglieder-Členy

ANISIMOV, P.P.   NERSESJAN, L.N.
ARZUMANJAN, R.A.   POSTNIKOV, S.I.
DALLAKJAN, K.L.   SARKISJAN, F.T.
DEMIRČJAN, K.S.   SARKISOV, B.E.
GALUMJAN, V.B.   VOSKANJAN, G.M.
MARTIROSJAN, G.A.

Candidate Members-Kandidaten-Kandidaty

ARZUMANJAN, M.B.   MURADJAN, M.O.
ASCATRJAN, E.T.   SAAKJAN, L.G.
KOTANDŽJAN, G.S.

Secretariat - Sekretariat

First Secretary
Erster Sekretär - DEMIRČJAN, K.S.
Pervyj Sekretar'

Second Secretary
Zweiter Sekretär - ANISIMOV, P.P.
Vtoroj Sekretar'

Secretaries   - DALLAKJAN, K.L.
Sekretäre   - GALUMJAN, V.B.
Sekretari   - VOSKANJAN, G.M.

CPA City Committee - Gorkom der KPA - Gorkom KPA, Erevan

NERSESJAN, L.N.

Communist Party of the Soviet Union
Kommunistische Partei der Sowjetunion 3.9.5

TURKMENSKAJA SSR

Buro - Büro - Bjuro

Members-Mitglieder-Členy

ANNAORAZOV, P.A.	KLYČEV, A.-M.
BURASNIKOV, B.F.	MAKARKIN, N.V.
DOLGOV, P.S.	MOLLAEVA, M.
GAPUROV, M.	PEREUDIN, V.M.
JASKULIEV, B.Ja.	ŠMIDT, M.G.
KARRYEV, Č.S.	

Candidate Members-Kandidaten-Kandidaty

| ČARYEV, M.A. | KISELEV, Ja.P. |
| DURDYEV, A.A. | |

Secretariat - Sekretariat

First Secretary   Second Secretary
Erster Sekretär - GAPUROV, M.   Zweiter Sekretär - PEREUDIN, V.M.
Pervyj Sekretar'   Vtoroj Sekretar'

Secretaries   - DOLGOV, P.S.
Sekretäre   - KARRYEV, Č.S.
Sekretari   - MOLLAEVA, M.

CPT City Committee - Gorkom der KPT - Gorkom KPT, Ašchabad

DURDYEV, A.A.

CPT Oblast Committees - Oblastkomitees der KPT - Obkomy KPT

Ašchabad   - ANNAORAZOV, P.A.   Mary   - AKGAEV, A.
Čardžou   - ČARYEV, B.   Tašauz   - ATAEV, B.
Krasnovodsk - MITRIN, E.T.

ESTONSKAJA SSR

Buro - Büro - Bjuro

Members-Mitglieder-Členy

JUHANSON, N.O.	RJUJTEL, A.
KEBIN, I.G.	TYNURIST, E.G.
KLAUSON, V.I.	KIAO, V.A.
LEBEDEV, K.V.	VAJNO, K.G.
LENCMAN, L.N.	VJALJAS, V.I.
MERIMAA, O.O.	

Candidate Members-Kandidaten-Kandidaty

| | ŠISOV, L.D. |
| PORK, A.P. | ZARUBIN, L.K. |

Secretariat - Sekretariat

First Secretary   Second Secretary
Erster Sekretär - VAJNO, K.G.   Zweiter Sekretär - LEBEDEV, K.V.
Pervyj Sekretar'   Vtoroj Sekretar'

Secretaries   - RJUJTEL, A.
Sekretäre   - KIAO, V.A.
Sekretari   - VJALJAS, V.I.

CPE City Committee - Gorkom der KPE - Gorkom KPE, Tallin

JUHANSON, N.O.

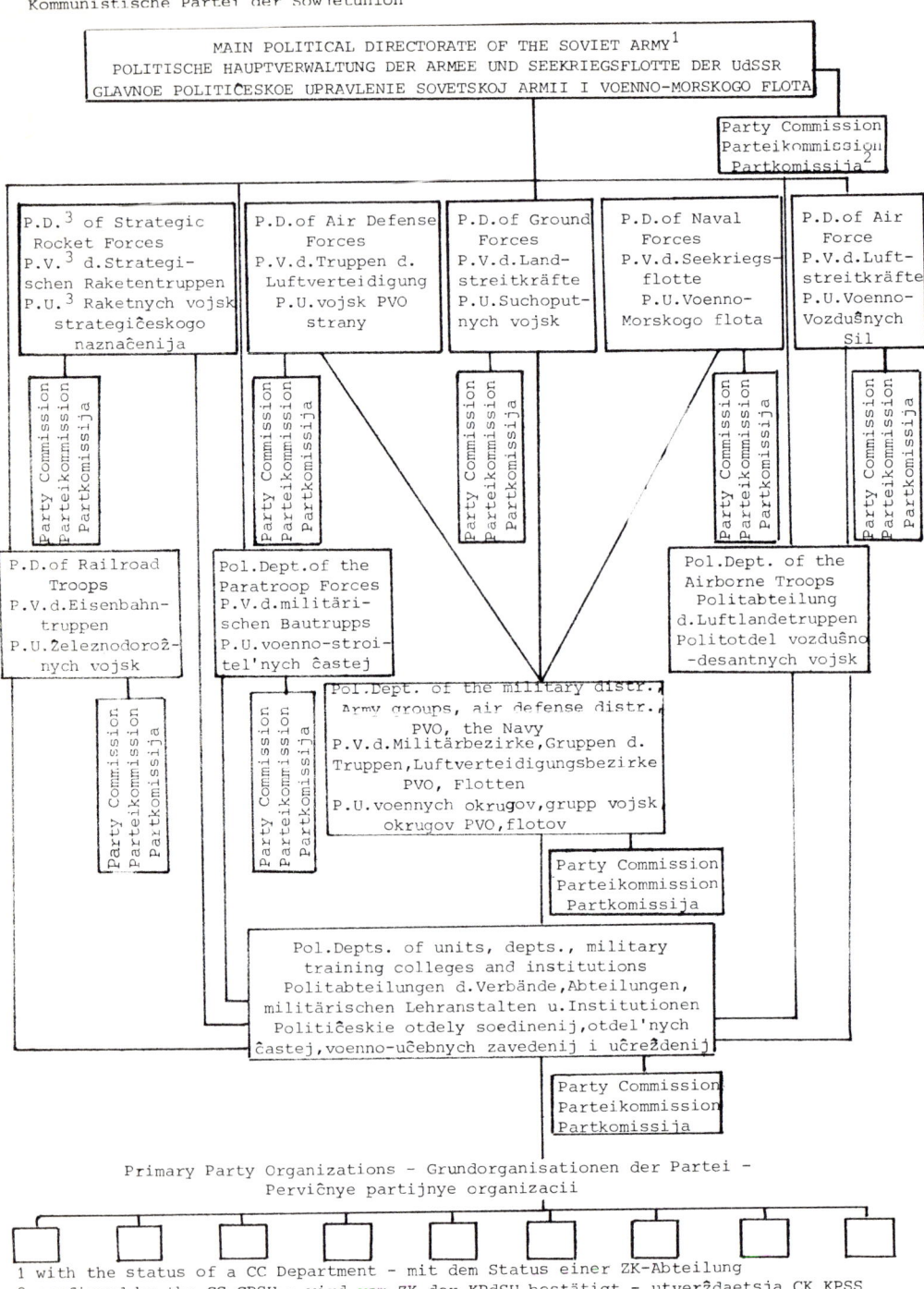

Communist Party of the Soviet Union
Kommunistische Partei der Sowjetunion

MAIN POLITICAL DIRECTORATE OF THE SOVIET ARMY[1]
POLITISCHE HAUPTVERWALTUNG DER ARMEE UND SEEKRIEGSFLOTTE DER UdSSR
GLAVNOE POLITIČESKOE UPRAVLENIE SOVETSKOJ ARMII I VOENNO-MORSKOGO FLOTA

Party Commission
Parteikommission
Partkomissija[2]

P.D.[3] of Strategic Rocket Forces
P.V.[3] d.Strategischen Raketentruppen
P.U.[3] Raketnych vojsk strategičeskogo naznačenija

P.D. of Air Defense Forces
P.V.d.Truppen d. Luftverteidigung
P.U.vojsk PVO strany

P.D. of Ground Forces
P.V.d.Landstreitkräfte
P.U.Suchoputnych vojsk

P.D. of Naval Forces
P.V.d.Seekriegsflotte
P.U.Voenno-Morskogo flota

P.D. of Air Force
P.V.d.Luftstreitkräfte
P.U.Voenno-Vozdušnych Sil

Party Commission / Parteikommission / Partkomissija (for each)

P.D. of Railroad Troops
P.V.d.Eisenbahntruppen
P.U.Železnodorožnych vojsk

Pol.Dept. of the Paratroop Forces
P.V.d.militärischen Bautrupps
P.U.voenno-stroitel'nych častej

Pol.Dept. of the Airborne Troops
Politabteilung d.Luftlandetruppen
Politotdel vozdušno-desantnych vojsk

Party Commission / Parteikommission / Partkomissija

Pol.Dept. of the military distr., Army groups, air defense distr., PVO, the Navy
P.V.d.Militärbezirke,Gruppen d. Truppen,Luftverteidigungsbezirke PVO, Flotten
P.U.voennych okrugov,grupp vojsk, okrugov PVO,flotov

Party Commission
Parteikommission
Partkomissija

Pol.Depts. of units, depts., military training colleges and institutions
Politabteilungen d.Verbände,Abteilungen, militärischen Lehranstalten u.Institutionen
Političeskie otdely soedinenij,otdel'nych častej,voenno-učebnych zavedenij i učreždenij

Party Commission
Parteikommission
Partkomissija

Primary Party Organizations - Grundorganisationen der Partei - Pervičnye partijnye organizacii

---

1 with the status of a CC Department - mit dem Status einer ZK-Abteilung
2 confirmed by the CC CPSU - wird vom ZK der KPdSU bestätigt - utverždaetsja CK KPSS
3 P.D.: Political Directora -P.V.: Politische Verwaltung-P.U.: Političeskoe upravlenie

Communist Party of the Soviet Union
Kommunistische Partei der Sowjetunion   3.10.1

3.10 NOMINATED PARTY APPARATUS
ERNANNTER PARTEIAPPARAT
NAZNAČENNYJ PARTIINYI APPARAT

3.10.1 CPSU CC APPARATUS UNDER THE DIRECTION OF THE CC SECRETARIAT
APPARAT DES ZK DER KPdSU UNTER DER LEITUNG DES ZK-SEKRETARIATS
APPARAT CK KPSS POD RUKOVODSTVOM SEKRETARIATA CK

Departments	Abteilungen	Otdely	Chief-Leiter
General	Allgemeine Abteilung	Obščij otdel	ČERNENKO, K.U.
Organizational Party Work	Organisations- Parteiarbeit	Organizacionno-par- tijnoj raboty	KAPITONOV, I.V.
Administrative Organs	Administrative Organe	Administrativnych organov	SAVINKIN, N.I.
Defense Industry	Verteidigungs- industrie	Oboronnoj promyš- lennosti	SERBIN, I.D.
Heavy Industry	Schwerindustrie	Tjaželoj promyšlenn.	DOLGICH, V.I.
Machine Building	Maschinenbau	Mašinostroenija	FROLOV, V.S.
Chemical Industry	Chemische Industrie	Chimičeskoj promyšlenn.	LISTOV, V.V.
Construction	Bauwesen	Stroitel'stva	DMITRIEV, I.N.
Light & Food Industry	Leicht-u.Nahrungs- mittelindustrie	Legkoj i piščevoj promyšlennosti	MOCALIN, F.I.
Agriculture	Landwirtschaft	Sel'skochozjajstvennyj otdel	KARLOV, V.A.
Transport and Communications	Transport-, Post- u.Fernmeldewesen	Transporty i svjazi	SIMONOV, K.S.
Trade and Domestic Services	Handel und Dienst- leistungen	Torgovli i bytovogo obsluživanija	KABKOV, Ja.I.
Planning and Finance Organs	Planungs- u.Finanz- organe	Planovych i finanso- vych organov	GOSTEV, B.I.
Political Main Admi- nistration of the Soviet Army and Maritime Fleet	Politische Hauptver- waltung d.Sowjeti- schen Armee und Seekriegsflotte	Glavnoe Upravlenie Sovetskoj Armii i Voenno-Morskogo Flota	EPIŠEV, A.A.
Science & Educational Institutions	Wissenschaft und Lehranstalten	Nauki i učebnych zavedenij	TRAPEZNIKOV, S.P.
Propaganda	Propaganda	Propagandy	TJAŽELNIKOV, E.M.
Culture	Kultur	Kul'tury	ŠAURO, V.F.
International	Internationale Abteil.	Mežmdunarodnyj otdel	PONOMAREV, B.N.
Liaison with Commu- nist & Workers' Par- ties of the Socia- list Countries	Verbindungen m.d.kom- munistischen u.Arbei- terparteien d.sozia- listischen Länder	Po svjazjam s kommuni- stičeskimi i rabočimi partijami socialisti- českich stran	RUSAKOV, K.V.
Cadres Abroad	Auslandskader	Zagraničnych kadrov	PEGOV, N.M.
International Information	Internationale Information	Mežmdunarodnoj informacii	ZAMJATIN, L.M.
Administration of Affairs	Geschäftsleitung	Upravlenie delami	PAVLOV, G.S.

3.10.2 Communist Party of the Soviet Union
Kommunistische Partei der Sowjetunion

3.10.2 CC APPARATUS OF CPs OF THE UNION REPUBLICS
APPARATE DER ZKs DER KPs DER UNIONSREPUBLIKEN
APPARATY CK KP SOJUZNYCH RESPUBLIK

Department - Abteilung	Ukrainskaja SSR	Belorusskaja SSR	Uzbekskaja SSR	Kazachskaja SSR	Gruzinskaja SSR	Azerbajdžanskaja SSR	Litovskaja SSR	Moldavskaja SSR	Latvijskaja SSR	Kirgizskaja SSR	Tadžikskaja SSR	Armjanskaja SSR	Turkmenskaja SSR	Estonskaja SSR
Administration of Affairs - Geschäftsleitung - Upravlenie delami	x	x	x	x	x	x	x	x	x	x	x	x	x	x
Administrative Organs - Administrative Organe - Otdel administrativnych organ.	x	x	x	x	x	x	x	x	x	x	x	x	x	x
General - Allgemeine Abteilung - Obščij otdel	x	x	x	x	x	x	x	x	x	x	x	x	x	x
Construction & Municipal Services - Bauwesen und städtische Wirtschaft - Otdel stroitel'stva i gorodskogo chozjajstva	x	x	x	x	x	x	x	x	x	x	x	x	x	x
Chemical Industry - Chemische Industrie - Chimičeskoj promyšlennosti	x													
Chemical & Light Industry - Chemische u.Leichtindustrie - Otdel chimičeskoj i legkoj promyšlennosti		x												
Chemical & Petroleum Industry - Chemische u.Erdölindustrie - Otdel chimičeskoj i neftjanoj promyšlennosti						x								
Petroleum & Chemical Industry - Erdöl-u.chemische Industrie - Otdel neftjanoj i chimičeskoj promyšlennosti													x	
Trade & Domestic Services - Handel u. Dienstleistungen - Otdel torgovli i bytovogo obsluživanija	x	x			x		x		x					x
Trade, Planning & Finance Organs - Handel, Planungs-u.Finanzorgane - Otdel torgovli,planovych i finansovych organov			x	x	x	x			x			x	x	
Industry & Transport - Industrie u. Transport - Promyšlenno-transportnyj otdel						x		x	x	x	x		x	x	x
Culture - Kultur - Otdel kul'tury	x	x	x	x	x	x	x	x	x	x	x	x	x	x
Information & liaison w.foreign countr. - Information u.Verbindungen m.d.Ausland-Otdel informacii i zarubežnych svjazej	x	x					x			x				
Agriculture - Landwirtschaft - Sel'skochozjajstvennyj otdel	x	x	x	x	x	x		x	x	x	x	x	x	x
Agriculture & Food Industry - Landwirtschaft u.Nahrungsmittelindustrie - Otdel sel'skogo chozjajstva i piščevoj promyšlennosti							x							

110

Communist Party of the Soviet Union
Kommunistische Partei der Sowjetunion 3.10.2

Department - Abteilung	Ukrainskaja SSR	Belorusskaja SSR	Uzbekskaja SSR	Kazachskaja SSR	Gruzinskaja SSR	Azerbajdžanskaja SSR	Litovskaja SSR	Moldavskaja SSR	Latvijskaja SSR	Kirgizskaja SSR	Tadžikskaja SSR	Armjanskaja SSR	Turkmenskaja SSR	Estonskaja SSR
Light & Food Industry - Leicht-u.Nahrungsmittelindustrie - Otdel legkoj i piščevoj promyšlennosti	x		x	x	x	x	x		x	x	x	x	x	x
Machine Building - Maschinenbau - Otdel mašinostroenija	x	x												
Food Industry - Nahrungsmittelindustrie- Otdel piščevoj promyšlennosti			x											
Organizational Party Work - Organisations-Parteiarbeit - Otdel organizacionno-partijnoj raboty	x	x	x	x	x	x	x	x	x	x	x	x	x	x
Planning & Finance Organs - Planungs- u.Finanzorgane - Otdel planovo-finansovych organov	x							x						
Propaganda & Agitation - Propaganda u. Agitation - Otdel propagandy i agitacii	x	x	x	x	x	x	x	x	x	x	x	x	x	x
Heavy Industry - Schwerindustrie - Otdel tjaželoj promyšlennosti	x		x											
Heavy Industry & Machine Building - Schwerindustrie u.Maschinenbau - Otdel tjaželoj promyšlennosti i mašinostroenija			x											
Heavy Industry & Transport - Schwerindustrie u.Transport - Otdel tjaželoj promyšlennosti i transporta		x												
Transport & Communications - Transport, Post-u.Fernmeldewesen - Otdel transporta i svjazi	x	x	x	x										
Liaison w.foreign countr.-Verbindungen m.d.Ausland-Otdel zarubežnych svjazej		x		x	x	x	x		x					x
Water resources - Wasserwirtschaft - Otdel vodnogo chozjajstva			x											
Water resources & Rural Construction - Wasserwirtschaft und Landbauwesen - Otdel vodnogo chozjajstva i sel'skogo stroitel'stva						x						x	x	
Science & Educational - Wissenschaft u.Lehranstalten - Otdel nauki i učebnych zavedenij	x	x	x	x	x	x	x	x	x	x	x	x	x	x

111

3.10.3 Communist Party of the Soviet Union
Kommunistische Partei der Sowjetunion

NOMINATED APPARATUS OF THE LOCAL PARTY ORGANISATIONS
ERNANNTER APPARAT DER LOKALEN PARTEIORGANISATIONEN
NAZNAČENNYJ APPARAT MESTNYCH PARTIJNYCH ORGANIZACIJ

Departments - Abteilungen - Otdely

Krai, Oblast Committees - Kraj-,Oblastkomitees - Kraevoj, oblastnoj komitet[1]

General	Allgemeine Abteilung	Obščij otdel
Organizational Party Work	Organisations-Parteiarbeit	Organizacionno-partijnoj raboty
Propaganda & Agitation	Propaganda u.Agitation	Propagandy i agitacii
Industry & Transport	Industrie u.Transport	Promyšlenno-transportnyj
Light & Food Industry	Leicht- u.Nahrungsmittelindustrie	Legkoj i piščevoj promyšlennosti
Construction	Bauwesen	Stroitel'stva
Agriculture	Landwirtschaft	Sel'skochozjajstvennyj
Administrative, Trade & Finance Organs	Administrative, Handelsu.Finanzorgane	Administrativnych i torgovofinansovych organov
Finances & Economics	Finanzen u.Wirtschaft	Finansovo-chozjajstvennyj
Science & Educational Institutions	Wissenschaft u.Lehranstalten	Nauki i učebnych zavedenij
Party Commission	Parteikommission	Partijnaja komissija

City Committees - Stadtkomitees - Gorodskoj komitet[2]

General	Allgemeine Abteilung	Obščij otdel
Organisation	Organisation	Organizacionnyj
Industry & Transport	Industrie u.Transport	Promyšlenno-transportnyj
Propaganda & Agitation	Propaganda u.Agitation	Propagandy i agitacii
Cabinet for Political Education	Kabinett für politische Bildung	Kabinet političeskogo prosveščenija
Sector for Party Statistics	Sektor f.Parteistatistik	Sektor partijnogo učeta
Extrabudgetary departments and commissions	Außeretatmäßige Abteilungen u.Kommissionen	Vneštatnye otdely i komissii

District Committees - Kreiskomitees - Okružnoj komitet[3]

General	Allgemeine Abteilung	Obščij otdel
Organisation	Organisation	Organizacionnyj
Industry & Transport	Industrie u.Transport	Promyšlenno-transportnyj

---

1 headed by the bureau and secretariat of the krai or oblast committees - geleitet von Büro und Sekretariat des Kraj- oder Oblastkomitees
2 headed by the bureau of the city committee - geleitet vom Büro des Stadtkomitees
3 headed by the bureau of the district committee - geleitet vom Büro des Kreiskomitees

Communist Party of the Soviet Union
Kommunistische Partei der Sowjetunion 3.10.3

Agriculture	Landwirtschaft	Sel'skochozjajstvennyj
Propaganda & Agitation	Propaganda u.Agitation	Propagandy i agitacii
Extrabudgetary departments and commissions	Außeretatmäßige Abteilungen u.Kommissionen	Vneštatnye otdely i komissii

Rayon Committees - Rayonkomitees - Rajonnyj komitet[4]

General	Allgemeine Abteilung	Obščij otdel
Organisation	Organisation	Organizacionnyj
Propaganda & Agitation	Propaganda u.Agitation	Propagandy i agitacii
Cabinet for Political Education	Kabinett f.politische Bildung	Kabinet političeskogo prosveščenija
Sector for Party Statistics	Sektor f.Parteistatistik	Sektor partijnogo učeta
Extrabudgetary departments and commissions	Außeretatmäßige Abteilungen u.Kommissionen	Vneštatnye otdely i komissii

---
[4] headed by the bureau of the rayon committee - geleitet vom Büro des Rayonkomitees

4.1 State Structur / Staatsordnung

4. STATE STRUCTURE
STAATSORDNUNG
GOSUDARSTVENNOE USTROJSTVO

4.1 SOVIET STATE ORGANS
SOWJETISCHE STAATSORGANE
ORGANY SOVETSKOGO GOSUDARSTVA

STATE POWER ORGANS - ORGANE DER STAATSMACHT - ORGANY GOSUDARSTVENNOJ VLASTI

Supreme-Oberste-Vysšie:

USSR Supreme Soviet	Oberster Sowjet der UdSSR	Verchovnyj Sovet SSSR
Supreme Soviet Presidium	Präsidium d.Obersten Sowjets	Prezidium Verchovnogo Soveta SSSR
Supreme Soviets of the Union Republics	Oberste Sowjets der Unionsrepubliken	Verchovnye Sovety sojuznych respublik
Supreme Soviet Presidiums Union Republics	Präsidien der Obersten Sowjets d.Unionsrepubliken	Prezidiumy Verchovnych Sovetov sojuznych respublik
Supreme Soviets of the Autonomous Republics	Oberste Sowjets der Autonomen Republiken	Verchovnye Sovety avtonomnych respublik
Supreme Soviet Presidiums of the Autonomous Republics	Präsidien d.Obersten Sowjets d.Autonomen Republiken	Prezidiumy Verchovnych Sovetov avtonomnych respublik

Local-Lokale-Mestnye

Soviets of the people's deputies:	Sowjets d.Volksdeputierten:	Sovety narodnych deputatov:
of the krai,oblast,autonomous districts,rajons, cities,villages and settlements	der Kraj,Oblast,autonomen Oblast,Nationalkreise, Rayons,Städte,Dörfer u. Siedlungen	Kraevye,oblastnye,avtonomnych okrugov,rajonnye,gorodskie,sel'skie,poselkovye nych okrugov,rajonnye,go-

STATE ADMINISTRATION ORGANS - ORGANE DER STAATSVERWALTUNG - ORGANY GOSUDARSTVENNOGO UPRAVLENIJA

Supreme-Oberste-Vysšie:

USSR Council of Ministers	Ministerrat der UdSSR	Sovet Ministrov SSSR
Councils of Ministers of the Union Republics	Ministerräte der Unionsrepubliken	Sovety Ministrov sojuznych respublik
Councils of Ministers of the Autonomous Republics	Ministerräte d.Autonomen Republiken	Sovety Ministrov avtonomnych respublik

Central-Zentrale-Central'nye

USSR Ministries	Ministerien der UdSSR	Ministerstva SSSR
USSR Authorities	Behörden der UdSSR	Vedomstva SSSR

State Structure 4.1
Staatsordnung

Ministries of the Union Republics	Ministerien der Unionsrepubliken	Ministerstva sojuznych respublik
Authorities of the Union Republics	Behörden der Unionsrepubliken	Vedomstva sojuznych respublik
Ministries of the Autonomous Republics	Ministerien der Autonomen Republiken	Ministerstva avtonomnych respublik
Authorities of the Autonomous Republics	Behörden der Autonomen Republiken	Vedomstva avtonomnych respublik

Local-Lokale-Mestnye:

Local Soviets' Executive Committees of the people's deputies	Exekutivkomitees der lokalen Sowjets der Volksdeputierten	Ispolnitel'nye komitety mestnych Sovetov narodnych deputatov
Departments & Administration of the Local Soviets' Executive Committees of the people's deputies	Abteilungen u.Verwaltungen der Exekutivkomitees der lokalen Sowjets der Volksdeputierten	Otdely i upravlenija ispolnitel'nych komitetov mestnych Sovetov narodnych deputatov

JUDICIAL ORGANS - JUSTIZORGANE - ORGANY PRAVOSUDIJA

USSR courts	Gerichte der UdSSR	Sudy SSSR
USSR Supreme Court	Oberster Gerichtshof der UdSSR	Verchovnye Sudy SSSR
Court-martials	Kriegsgerichte	Voennye tribunaly
Courts of the Union Republics	Gerichte d.Unionsrepubliken	Sudy sojuznych respublik
Supreme Courts of the Union and Autonomous Republics	Oberste Gerichtshöfe der Unions-u.Autonomen Republiken	Verchovnye Sudy sojuznych i avtonomnych respublik
Krai & District Courts	Kraj-u.Gebietsgerichte	Kraevye, oblastnye sudy
Courts of the Autonomous Oblast & National Districts	Gerichte d.Autonomen Oblast u.Nationalkreise	Sudy avtonomnych oblastej i nacional'nych okrugov
	Rayon-u.Stadtvolksgerichte	Rajonnye, gorodskie narodnye sudy

ORGANS FOR THE ADMINISTRATION OF THE LAW
ORGANE ZUR ÜBERWACHUNG DER RECHTSORDNUNG
ORGANY NADZORA ZA ZAKONNOSTJU

Public Prosecutor's Office	Organe d.Staatsanwaltschaft	Organy prokuratury
Attorney-General of the USSR	Generalstaatsanwalt d.UdSSR	General'nyj prokuror SSSR
District Attorney of the Union's Republics	Staatsanwälte der Unionsrepubliken	Prokurory sojuznych respublik
District Attorneys of the Autonomous Republics	Staatsanwälte der Autonomen Republiken	Prokurory avtonomnych respublik
District Attorneys of the Krai,Oblast, and autonomous Oblast	Staatsanwälte d.Kraj,Oblast u.autonomen Oblast	Prokurory kraev, oblastej i avtonomnych oblastej
District Attorneys of the National Districts	Staatsanwälte d.Nationalen Kreise	Prokurory nacional'nych okrugov
District Attorneys of the Rayons and Cities	Staatsanwälte der Rayons und Städte	Prokurory rajonov i gorodov

4. State Structure
Staatsordnung

4.2 SOVIETS OF THE USSR PEOPLE'S DEPUTIES
SOWJETS DER VOLKSDEPUTIERTEN DER UdSSR
SOVETY NARODNYCH DEPUTATOV SSSR

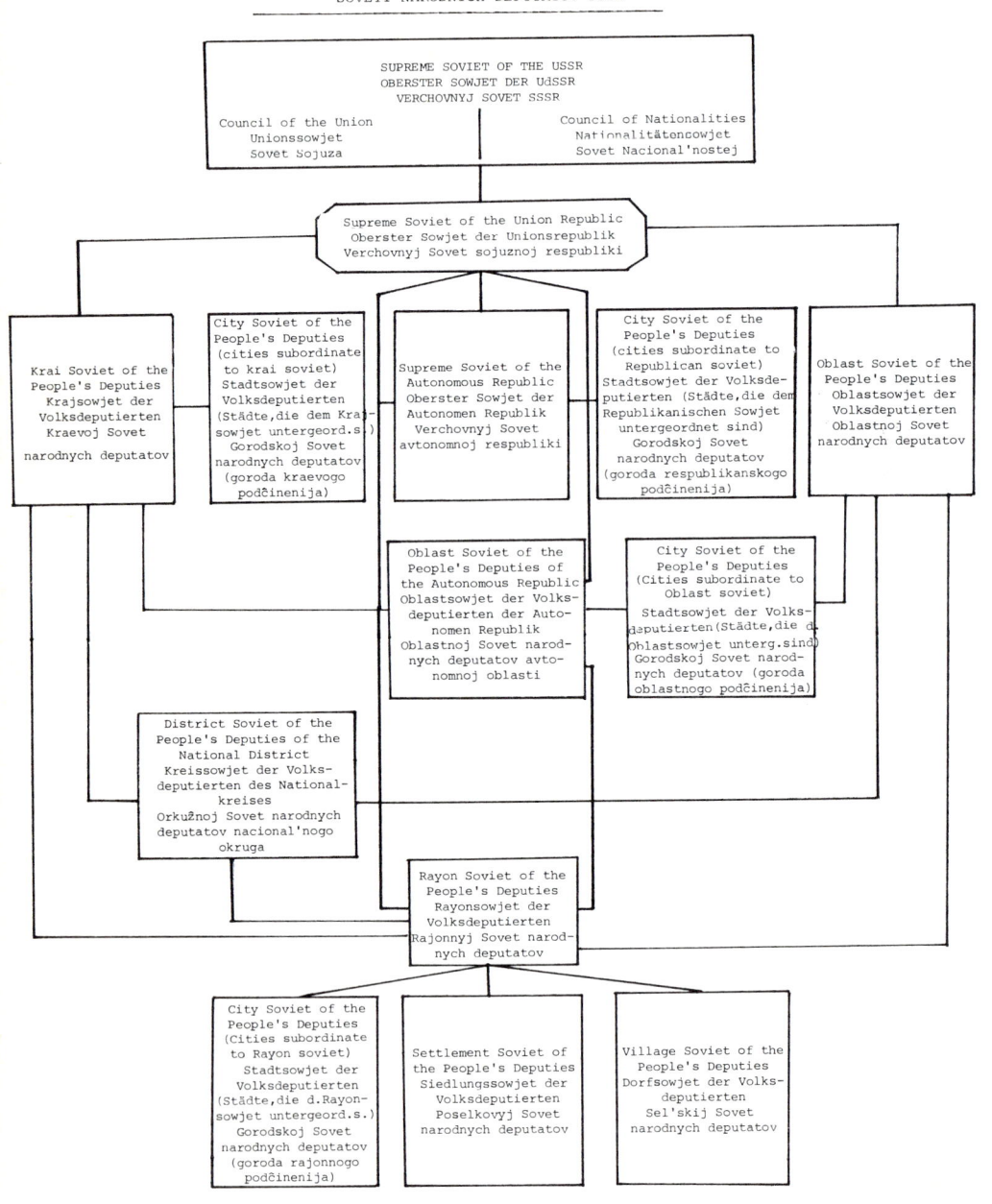

SUPREME SOVIET OF THE USSR
OBERSTER SOWJET DER UdSSR
VERCHOVNYJ SOVET SSSR

- Council of the Union / Unionssowjet / Sovet Sojuza
- Council of Nationalities / Nationalitätensowjet / Sovet Nacional'nostej

Supreme Soviet of the Union Republic
Oberster Sowjet der Unionsrepublik
Verchovnyj Sovet sojuznoj respubliki

- Krai Soviet of the People's Deputies / Krajsowjet der Volksdeputierten / Kraevoj Sovet narodnych deputatov

- City Soviet of the People's Deputies (cities subordinate to krai soviet) / Stadtsowjet der Volksdeputierten (Städte, die dem Kraisowjet untergeord.s.) / Gorodskoj Sovet narodnych deputatov (goroda kraevogo podčinenija)

- Supreme Soviet of the Autonomous Republic / Oberster Sowjet der Autonomen Republik / Verchovnyj Sovet avtonomnoj respubliki

- City Soviet of the People's Deputies (cities subordinate to Republican soviet) / Stadtsowjet der Volksdeputierten (Städte, die dem Republikanischen Sowjet untergeordnet sind) / Gorodskoj Sovet narodnych deputatov (goroda respublikanskogo podčinenija)

- Oblast Soviet of the People's Deputies / Oblastsowjet der Volksdeputierten / Oblastnoj Sovet narodnych deputatov

- Oblast Soviet of the People's Deputies of the Autonomous Republic / Oblastsowjet der Volksdeputierten der Autonomen Republik / Oblastnoj Sovet narodnych deputatov avtonomnoj oblasti

- City Soviet of the People's Deputies (Cities subordinate to Oblast soviet) / Stadtsowjet der Volksdeputierten (Städte, die d. Oblastsowjet unterg.sind) / Gorodskoj Sovet narodnych deputatov (goroda oblastnogo podčinenija)

- District Soviet of the People's Deputies of the National District / Kreissowjet der Volksdeputierten des Nationalkreises / Okružnoj Sovet narodnych deputatov nacional'nogo okruga

- Rayon Soviet of the People's Deputies / Rayonsowjet der Volksdeputierten / Rajonnyj Sovet narodnych deputatov

- City Soviet of the People's Deputies (Cities subordinate to Rayon soviet) / Stadtsowjet der Volksdeputierten (Städte, die d. Rayonsowjet untergeord.s.) / Gorodskoj Sovet narodnych deputatov (goroda rajonnogo podčinenija)

- Settlement Soviet of the People's Deputies / Siedlungssowjet der Volksdeputierten / Poselkovyj Sovet narodnych deputatov

- Village Soviet of the People's Deputies / Dorfsowjet der Volksdeputierten / Sel'skij Sovet narodnych deputatov

State Structure 4.2.1
Staatsordnung 4.2.2

4.2.1 NUMBER OF THE SOVIETS OF THE PEOPLE'S DEPUTIES
ZAHL DER SOWJETS DER VOLKSDEPUTIERTEN
KOLIČESTVO SOVETOV NARODNYCH DEPUTATOV
(15.6.1975)

USSR Supreme Soviet - Oberster Sowjet der UdSSR - Verchovnyj Sovet SSSR	1
Supreme Soviets of the Union Republics - Oberste Sowjets der Unionsrepubliken - Verchovnye Sovety sojuznych respublik	15
Supreme Soviets of the Autonomous Republics - Oberste Sowjets der Autonomen Republiken - Verchovnye Sovety avtonomnych respublik	20
Krai Soviets - Krajsowjets - Kraevye Sovety	6
Oblast Soviets - Oblastsowjets - Oblastnye Sovety	120
Oblast Soviets of the Autonomous Districts - Oblastsowjets der Autonomen Gebiete - Oblastnye Sovety avtonomnych oblastej	8
District Soviets - Kreissowjets - Okružnye Sovety	10
Rayon Soviets - Rayonsowjets - Rajonnye Sovety	3,003
City Soviets - Stadtsowjets - Gorodskie Sovety	2,006
Rayon Soviets in the Cities - Rayonsowjets in den Städten - Rajonnye Sovety v gorodach	558
Settlement Soviets - Siedlungssowjets - Poselkovye Sovety	3,598
Village Soviets - Dorfsowjets - Sel'skie Sovety	41,128

4.2.2 CHAIRMEN OF THE USSR SUPREME SOVIET PRESIDIUM[1]
VORSITZENDE DES PRÄSIDIUMS DES OBERSTEN SOWJETS DER UdSSR
PREDSEDATELI PREZIDIUMA VERCHOVNOGO SOVETA SSSR

KALININ, M.I.	1922-1946	ŠVERNIK, N.M.	1946-1953
PETROVSKIJ, G.I.	1922-1938	VOROŠILOV, K.E.	1953-1960
ČERVJAKOV, A.G.	1922-1937	BREŽNEV, L.I.	1960-1964
NARIMANOV, N.N.	1922-1925	MIKOJAN, A.I.	1964-1965
AJTAKOV, N.	1925-1937	PODGORNYJ, N.V.	1965-1977
CHODŽAEV, F.A.	1925-1937	BREŽNEV, L.I.	1977-
MAKSUM, N.	1931-1934		
MUSABEKOV, G.M.	1925-1937		
RACHIMBAEV, A.R.	1934-1937		

---

[1] 1922-1938 USSR Central Executive Committee - Zentrales Exekutivkomitee der UdSSR - Central'nyj Ispolnitel'nyj Komitet SSSR (CIK) - with several chairmen - mit mehreren Vorsitzenden

4.2.3 State Structure
4.2.4 Staatsordnung

4.2.3 NUMBER OF THE ELECTED DEPUTIES OF THE USSR SUPREME SOVIET
ZAHL DER GEWÄHLTEN DEPUTIERTEN DES OBERSTEN SOWJETS DER UdSSR
ČISLO VYBRANNYCH DEPUTATOV VERCHOVNOGO SOVETA SSSR

Election Day Wahltag Data vyborov	Legislative Periods Legislaturperioden Sozyvy	Number of Deputies Zahl der Deputierten Čislo deputatov
12.12.1937	1.	1,143
10. 2.1946	2.	1,339
12. 3.1950	3.	1,316
14. 3.1954	4.	1,347
16. 3.1958	5.	1,378
18. 3.1962	6.	1,443
12. 6.1966	7.	1,517
14. 6.1970	8.	1,517
16. 6.1974	9.	1,517

4.2.4 USSR SUPREME SOVIET
OBERSTER SOWJET DER UdSSR
VERCHOVNYJ SOVET SSSR

Presidium-Präsidium-Prezidium

Chairman-Vorsitzender-
Predsedatel'   - BREŽNEV, L.I.

First Deputy Chairman-Erster
Stellvertreter-Pervyj Zamestitel   - KUZNECOV, V.V.

| Deputy Chairmen -
Stellvertreter -
Zamestiteli | JASNOV, M.A.
VATČENKO, A.F.
POLJAKOV, I.E.
MATČANOV, N.M.
NIJAZBEKOV, S.B. | GILAŠVILI, P.V.
CHALILOV, K.A.
BARKAUSKAS, A.S.
ILJAŠENKO, K.F.
STRAUTMANIS, P.Ja. | KULATOV, T.
CHOLOV, M.
SARKISOV, B.E.
KLYČEV, A.-M. |

Secretary-Sekretär-Sekretar'   - GEORGADZE, M.P.

| Presidium members -
Mitglieder des
Präsidiums -
Členy prezidiuma | CECEGOV, S.S.
FEDOROV, E.K.
GAMZATOV, R.G.
GITALOV, A.V.
GRIŠIN, V.V.
KONOTOP, V.I.
KUNAEV, D.A.
MAŠEROV, P.M. | NIKOLAEVA-
TEREŠKOVA, V.V.
NOVOSELOVA, N.A.
PASTUCHOV, B.N.
PUCHOVA, Z.P.
RAŠIDOV, S.R.
ROMANOV, G.V. | ŠAKIROV, M.Z.
ŠČERBICKIJ, V.V.
ŠIBAEV, A.I.
SMIRNOV, G.N.
TABEEV, F.A.
TYNEL, L.G.
ZLOBIN, N.A. |

Soviet of the Union-Unionssowjet-Sovet Sojuza

Chairman-Vorsitzender-
Predsedatel'   - ŠITIKOV, A.P.

| Deputy Chairmen - Stellvertreter -
Zamestiteli | ALIEV, G.A.
DAVIDČIK, A.L. | DŽUMAEV, A.
PATON, B.E. |

State Structure 4.2.4
Staatsordnung

Standing Commissions-Ständige Kommissionen-Postojannye Komissii

Credentials Commission - Mandatskommission - Mandatnaja komissija	- BEKTURGANOV, Ch.Š.
Legislative Proposals Commission - Kommission f.Gesetzentwürfe - Komissija zakonodatel'nych predloženij	- KAPITONOV, I.V.
Planning and Budget Commission - Plan-u.Budgetkommission - Planovo-bjudžetnaja komissija	- VAŠČENKO, G.I.
Foreign Affairs Commission - Kommission für auswärtige Angelegenheiten - Komissija po inostrannym delam	- SUSLOV, M.A.
Youth Affairs Commission - Kommission für Jugendfragen - Komissija po delam molodeži	- GORBAČEV, M.S.
Industrial Commission - Kommission für Industrie - Komissija po promyšlennosti	- RJABOV, Ja.P.
Transport and Communications Commission - Kommission f. Transport,Post-u.Fernmeldewesen - Komissija po transportu i svjazi	- KLIMENKO, I.E.
Construction and Construction Materials Industry Commission - Kommission f.Bauwesen u.Baustoffindustrie - Komissija po stroitel'stvu i promyšlennosti stroitel' nych materialov	- LOMAKIN, V.P.
Agriculture Commission - Kommission für Landwirtschaft - Komissija po sel'skomu chozjajstvu	- KAVUN, V.M.
Consumer Goods Commission - Kommission für Konsumgüter - Komissija po tovaram narodnogo potreblenija	- ORLOV, V.P.
Health and Social Security Commission - Kommission für Gesundheitswesen u.Sozialfürsorge - Komissija po zdravoochraneniju i social'nomu obespečeniju	- BLOCHINA, I.N.
Education, Science and Culture Commission - Kommission f.Volksbildung,Wissenschaft u.Kultur - Komissija po narodnomu obrazovaniju, nauke i kul'ture	- VOSS, A.E.
Trade, Consumer Services and Municipal Economy Commission - Kommission f.Handel,Dienstleistungen u.Kommunalwirtschaft - Komissija po torgovle, bytovomu obsluživaniju i kommunal'nomu chozjajstvu	- KONOPLEV, B.V.
Commission for Women's Working and Living Conditions, Maternity and Child Care - Kommission f.Arbeits-u. Lebensbedingungen der Frauen, f.Mutter-u.Kindschutz - Komissija po voprosam truda i byta ženščin, ochrany materinstva i detstva	- KULIEVA, Z.T.k.
Nature Conservation Commission - Kommission f.Naturschutz - Komissija po ochrane prirody	- UMACHANOV, M.S.

Soviet of Nationalities-Nationalitätensowjet-Sovet Nacional'nostej

Chairman-Vorsitzender-
Predsedatel'   - RUBEN, V.P.

| Deputy Chairmen - Stellvertreter - Zamestiteli | TAŠPULATOVA, D. TICHONOV, N.S. | ZAJČENKO, N.M. ŽAKSYBEKOV, S.Š. |

Standing Commissions-Ständige Kommissionen-Postojannye Komissii

Credentials Commission - Mandatskommission - Mandatnaja komissija	- ŠEVARDNADZE, E.A.
Legislative Proposals Commission - Kommission f.Gesetzentwürfe - Komissija zakonodatel'nych predloženij	- KEBIN, I.O.
Planning and Budget Commission - Plan-u.Budgetkommission - Planovo-bjudžetnaja komissija	- MASLENNIKOV, N.I.

119

4.2.4 State Structure
4.2.5 Staatsordnung

Foreign Affairs Commission - Kommission für auswärtige Angelegenheiten - Komissija po inostrannym delam	- PONOMAREV, B.N.
Youth Affairs Commission - Kommission f.Jugendfragen - Komissija po delam molodeži	- ASKAROV, A.
Industrial Commission - Kommission für Industrie - Komissija po promyšlennosti	- KAJRIS, K.K.
Transport and Communications Commission - Kommission f. Transport,Post-u.Fernmeldewesen - Komissija po transportu i svjazi	- MARTIROSJAN, G.A.
Construction and Construction Materials Industry Commission - Kommission f.Bauwesen u.Baustoffindustrie - Komissija po stroitel'stvu i promyšlennosti stroitel'- nych materialov	- KALAŠNIKOV, A.M.
Agriculture Commission - Kommission für Landwirtschaft - Komissija po sel'skomu chozjajstvu	- KARLOV, V.A.
Consumer Goods Commission - Kommission für Konsumgüter - Komissija po tovaram narodnogo potreblenija	- SMIRNOV, A.A.
Health and Social Security Commission - Kommission für Gesundheitswesen u.Sozialfürsorge - Komissija po zdravoochraneniju i social'nomu obespečeniju	- TIMAKOV, V.D.
Education, Science & Culture Commission - Kommission f.Volksbildung, Wissenschaft u.Kultur - Komissija po narodnomu obrazovaniju, nauke i kul'ture	- FEDOSEEV, P.N.
Trade, Consumer Services and Municipal Economy Commission - Kommission f.Handel, Dienstleistungen u.Kommunalwirtschaft - Komissija po torgovle, bytovomu obsluživaniju i kommunal'nomu chozjajstvu	- OSETROV, T.N.
Commission for Women's Working and Living Conditions, Maternity and Child Care - Kommission f.Arbeits-u.Lebensbedingungen der Frauen, f.Mutter-u.Kindschutz - Komissija po voprosam truda i byta ženščin, ochrany materinstva i detstva	- LYKOVA, L.P.
Nature Conservation Commission - Kommission für Naturschutz - Komissija po ochrane prirody	- GRIDASOV, D.M.

4.2.5 COMPOSITION OF THE DEPUTIES OF THE USSR SUPREME SOVIET
ZUSAMMENSETZUNG DER DEPUTIERTEN DES OBERSTEN SOWJETS DER UdSSR
SOSTAV DEPUTATOV VERCHOVNOGO SOVETA SSSR

	elected-gewählt					
	June-Juni 1966		June-Juni 1970		June-Juni 1974	
		%		%		%
Total of Deputies - Gesamtzahl d. Deputierten - Vsego deputatov	1,517	100	1,517	100	1,517	100
of which - davon - iz nich: firstly elected - erstmals gewählt - izbrany vpervye	992	65.4	846	55.8	846	55.8
males - Männer - mužčin	1,092	72.0	1,054	69.5	1,042	68.7
females - Frauen - ženščin	425	28.0	463	30.5	475	31.3
CPSU members and candidate members- Mitglieder u.Kandidaten der KPdSU - Členov i kandidatov v členy KPSS.	1,141	75.8	1,096	72.3	1,096	72.2
Non-party members - Parteilose - Bespartijnych	376	24.2	421	27.7	421	27.8

State Structure 4.2.5
Staatsordnung

	June-Juni 1966 %	elected-gewählt June-Juni 1970 %	June-Juni 1974 %
by professions-nach Berufen- po rodu zanjatij:			
Workers - Arbeiter - Raboçich	404 26.6	481 31.7	498 32.8
Kolkhozniks-Kolchosbauern-Kolchoznikov	294 19.4	282 18.6	271 17.9
Directors of enterprises and specialists of all political economy branches- Leiter d.Betriebe u.Spezialisten aller Volkswirtschaftszweige - Rukovoditelej predprijatij i specialistov vsech otraslej narodnogo chozjajstva	91 6.0	73 4.8	-- --
Party, Soviet, Labor Union and Komsomol functionaries - Partei-,Sowjet-,Gewerkschafts-u. Komsomolfunktionäre - Rabotnikov partijnych,sovetskich,profsojuznych i komsomol'skich organov	518 34.1	478 31.5	-- --
Scientists, writers, artists and employees of public instruction and Public Health - Wissenschaftler,Kultur-,Literatur-u. Kunstschaffende u.Beschäftigte d. Volksbildung u.d.Gesundheitswesens - Rabotniki nauki,kultury,literatury i iskusstva,prosveščenija i zdravoochranenija	154 10.2	146 9.6	-- --
Military-Militärs-Voennoslužaščich	56 3.7	57 3.8	-- --
by education-nach Ausbildung- po obrazovaniju:			
university-Hochschule-vysšee	761 50.2	734 48.4	803 53.0
not completed university-nicht abgeschl.Hochschule-nezakončennoe vysšee	47 3.1	46 3.0	
intermediate school-Mittelschule- srednee	275 18.1	448 29.5	698 46.0
not completed intermediate school - nicht abgeschl. Mittelschule - nepolnoe srednee	344 22.7	252 16.6	
elementary school-Grundschule-načal'noe	90 5.9	37 2.5	16 1.0
by age - nach Alter - po vozrastu:			
- 30 years-Jahre-let	182 12.0	281 18.5	279 18.4
31 - 40	434 28.6	349 23.0	-- --
41 - 50	420 27.7	386 25.5	-- --
51 - 60	386 25.4	329 21.7	-- --
above - über - starše 60	95 6.3	172 11.3	-- --

4.3 USSR COUNCIL OF MINISTERS
MINISTERRAT DER UdSSR
SOVET MINISTROV SSSR

Presidium-Präsidium-Prezidija

  Chairman-Vorsitzender-Predsedatel'
  First Deputy Chairman-Erster Stellv.Vorsitzender-Pervyj
    zamestitel'predsedatelja
  Deputy Chairmen-Stellv.Vorsitzende-Zamestiteli predsedatelja

  All-Union Ministries-Unionsministerien-Vsesojuznye ministerstva

  Union Republic Ministries-Unionsrepublikanische Ministerien-Sojuznorespublikanskie ministerstva

  State Committees-Staatskomitees-Gosudarstvennye komitety

  Other Agencies-Andere Verwaltungen-drugie upravlenija

  Chairmen of the Republic Councils of Ministers-Vorsitzende der Republikanischen Ministerräte-Predsedateli respublikanskich Sovetov Ministrov

  Agencies of the Council of Ministers without Ministerial Status - Verwaltungen des Ministerrates ohne Ministerialstatus - Upravlenija Soveta Ministrov bez statusa Ministerstva

4.3.1 CHAIRMEN OF THE USSR COUNCIL OF MINISTERS[1]
VORSITZENDE DES MINISTERRATES DER UdSSR
PREDSEDATELI SOVETA MINISTROV SSSR

LENIN, V.I.	1917-1923 (RSFSR)
	1923-1924
RYKOV, A.I.	1924-1930
MOLOTOV, V.M.	1930-1941
STALIN, J.V.	1941-1953
MALENKOV, G.M.	1953-1955
BULGANIN, N.A.	1955-1958
CHRUŠČEV, N.S.	1958-1964
KOSYGIN, A.N.	1964-

---

[1] until 1946 Council of the People's Commissars of the USSR
bis 1946 Rat der Volkskommissare der UdSSR -
Sovet Narodnych Komissarov SSSR

State Structure 4.3.2
Staatsordnung

4.3.2 COMPOSITION OF THE USSR COUNCIL OF MINISTERS - ZUSAMMENSETZUNG DES
MINISTERRATES DER UdSSR - SOSTAV SOVETA MINISTROV SSSR
(as of September 1, 1978 - zum 1. September 1978)

Chairman-Vorsitzender-Predsedatel' — KOSYGIN, A.N.

First Deputy Chairmen-Erste Stellvertreter-Pervye zamestiteli — MAZUROV, K.T.
TICHONOV, N.A.

Deputy Chairmen-Stellvertreter- — ARCHIPOV, I.V.   MARTYNOV, N.V.
Zamestiteli   BAJBAKOV, N.K.   NOVIKOV, I.T.
                                   DYMŠIC, V.E.   NOVIKOV, V.N.
                                   KATUŠEV, K.F.   NURIEV, Z.N.
                                   KIRILLIN, V.A.   SMIRNOV, L.V.

All-Union Ministries of - Unionsministerien für - Obščesojuznye Ministerstva:

Automotive Industry-Automobilindustrie-avtomobil'noj promyšlennosti
Moskva, K-265, Kuzneckij Most, 21/5 — POLJAKOV, V.N.[1]

Aviation Industry-Luftfahrtindustrie-aviacionnoj promyšlennosti
Moskva, Ulanskij Pereulok, 16 — KAZAKOV, V.A.

Chemical Industry-chemische Industrie-chimičeskoj promyšlennosti
Moskva, Centr, Ulica Kirova, 20 — KOSTANDOV, L.A.

Chemical and Petroleum Machine Building-chemischen u.Erdöl-
maschinenbau-chimičeskogo i neftjanogo mašinostroenija
Moskva, I-110, Bezbožnyj Pereulok, 25 — BRECHOV, K.I.

Civil Aviation-zivile Luftfahrt-graždanskoj aviacii
Moskva, A-167, Leningradskij Prospekt, 37 — BUGAEV, B.P.

Communications Equipment Industry-Kommunikationsmittel-
industrie-promyšlennosti sredstv svjazi — PERVYŠIN, E.K.

Construction of Petroleum and Gas Industry Enterprises -
Bau von Betrieben der Erdöl- und Gasindustrie -
stroitel'stva predprijatij neftjanoj i gazovoj promyšlennosti — ŠČERBINA, B.E.

Construction, Road and Municipal Machine Building -
Bau-, Straßenbaumaschinen und kommunalen Maschinenpark -
stroitel'nogo, dorožnogo i kommunal'nogo mašinostroenija
Moskva, K-12, Malyj Čerkasskij Pereulok, 1/3 — NOVOSELOV, E.S.

Defense - Verteidigung - oborony
Moskva, Z-35, Nabereznaja Morisa Toreza, 34 — USTINOV, D.F.

Defense Industry-Verteidigungsindustrie-oboronnoj promyšlennosti- ZVEREV, S.A.

Electrical Equipment Industry-elektrotechnische Industrie-
elektrotechničeskoj promyšlennosti
Moskva, D-242, Bol'šaja Gruzinskaja Ulica, 12 — ANTONOV, A.K.

Electronics Industry-Elektronenindustrie-elektronnoj promyšlennosti
Moskva, K-74, Kitajskij Pereulok, 7 — ŠOKIN, A.I.

Foreign Trade-Außenhandel-vnešnej torgovli
Moskva, G-200, Smolenskaja-Sennaja Ploščad', 32/34 — PATOLIČEV, N.S.

Gas Industry-Gasindustrie-gazovoj promyšlennosti
Moskva, Centr, Ulica Kirova, 13 — ORUDŽEV, S.A.

General Machine Building-allgemeinen Maschinenbau-
obščego mašinostroenija — AFANASEV, S.A.

Heavy and Transport Machine Building-schweren und Transport-
maschinenbau-tjažëlogo i transportnogo mašinostroenija
Moskva, Centr, Ulica Bogdana Chmel'nickogo, 12 — ŽIGALIN, V.F.

---
1 Minister-Ministr

123

4.3.2 State Structure
Staatsordnung

Instrument Making, Automation Equipment and Control Systems -
Gerätebau, elektronische Geräte und Steuerungssysteme -
priborostroenija, sredsts avtomatizacii i sistem upravlenija
Moskva, K-9, Ulica Ogareva, 5 — RUDNEV, K.N.

Machine Building-Maschinenbau-mašinostroenija — BACHIREV, V.V.

Machine Building for Animal Husbandry and Fodder Production -
Maschinenbau f.Viehwirtschaft u.Futterproduktion -
mašinostroenija dlja životnovodstva i kormoproizvodstva
Moskva, Prospekt Kalinina, 27 — BELJAK, K.N.

Machine Building for Light and Food Industry and Household
Appliances-Maschinenbau f.Leicht-u.Nahrungsmittelindustrie
u.Herstellung v.Haushaltsgeräten-mašinostroenija dlja legkoj
i piščevoj promyšlennosti i bytovych priborov
Moskva, D-22, Presnenskij Val, 17 — PUDKOV, I.I.

Machine Tool and Tool Building Industry-Werkzeugmaschinen-
u.Instrumentenbau-stankostroitel'noj i instrumental'noj
promyšlennosti
Moskva, K-50, Ulica Gor'kogo 20 — KOSTOUSOV, A.I.

Maritime Fleet-Hochseeschiffahrt-morskogo flota
Moskva, K-25, Ulica Ždanova, 1/4 — GUŽENKO, T.B.

Medical Industry-medizinische Industrie-medicinskoj promyšlennosti
Moskva, K-12, Čerkasskij Pereulok, 15 — MELNIČENKO, A.K.

Medium Machine Building-mittleren Maschinenbau-srednego
mašinostroenija — SLAVSKIJ, E.P.

Petroleum Industry-Erdölindustrie-neftjanoj promyšlennosti
Moskva, Ž-35, Nabereżnaja Morisa Toreza, 26/1 — MALCEV, N.A.

Power Machine Building-Generatoren und Turbinenbau -
energetičeskogo mašinostroenija — KROTOV, V.V.

Pulp and Paper Industry-Zellulose-u.Papierindustrie-
cellulozno-bumažnoj promyšlennosti
Moskva, K-45, Bol'šoj Kisel'nyj Pereulok, 13/15 — GALANŠIN, K.I.

Radio Industry-Radioindustrie-radiopromyšlennosti
Moskva, K-74, Kitajskij Pereulok, 7 — PLEŠAKOV, P.S.

Railways-Verkehrswesen-putej soobščenija
Moskva, B-174, Novaja Bastmannaja Ulica, 2 — PAVLOVSKIJ, I.G.

Shipbuilding Industry-Schiffsbauindustrie-sudostroitel'noj
promyšlennosti
Moskva, D-242, Sadovaja-Kudrinskaja Ulica, 11/13 — EGOROV, M.V.

Tractor and Agricultural Machine Building-Traktoren-u.Land-
maschinenbau-traktornogo i sel'skochozjajstvennogo mašinostroen.
Moskva, K-265, Kuzneckij Most, 21/5 — SINICYN, I.F.

Transport Construction-Transportbauwesen-transportnogo stroitel'stva
Moskva, B-217, Sadovaja-Spasskaja Ulica, 21 — SOSNOV, I.D.

Union Republic Ministries of - Unionsrepublikanische Ministerien für - Sojuzno-
respublikanskie Ministerstva:

Agriculture-Landwirtschaft-sel'skogo chozjajstva
Moskva, I-139, Orlikov Pereulok, 1/11 — MESJAC, V.K.

Coal Industry-Kohlenindustrie-ugol'noj promyšlennosti
Moskva, K-45, Kisel'nyj Pereulok, 13/5 — BRATČENKO, B.F.

State Structure 4.3.2
Staatsordnung

Communications-Post-u.Fernmeldewesen-svjazi
Moskva, K-9, Ulica Gor'kogo, 7 — TALYZIN, N.V.

Construction-Bauwesen-stroitel'stva
Moskva, V-311, Pervaja Ulica Stroitelej, 8, Korpus 2 — KARAVAEV, G.A.

Construction of Heavy Industry Enterprises-Bau v.Betrieben d.
Schwerindustrie-stroitel'stva predprijatij tjaželoj industrii
Moskva, D-242, Sadovaja-Kudrinskaja Ulica, 11/13 — GOLDIN, N.V.

Construction Materials Industry-Baustoffindustrie-
promyšlennosti stroitel'nych materialov
Moskva, K-9, Prospekt Chudožestvennogo Teatra, 2 — GRIŠMANOV, I.A.

Culture-Kultur-kul'tury
Moskva, K-12, Ulica Kuibyševa, 10 — DEMIČEV, P.N.

Education-Volksbildung-prosveščenija
Moskva, B-174, Žabolovka, 49 — PROKOFEV, M.A.

Ferrous Metallurgy-Eisenhüttenindustrie-černoj metallurgii
Moskva, K-74, Ploščad' Nogina, 2/5 — KAZANEC, I.P.

Finance-Finanzen-finansov
Moskva, K-97, Ulica Kuibyševa, 9 — GARBUZOV, V.F.

Fish Industry-Fischereiwirtschaft-rybnogo chozjajstva
Moskva, K-45, Roždestvenskij Bul'var, 12 — IŠKOV, A.A.

Food Industry-Nahrungsmittelindustrie-piščevoj promyšlennosti
Moskva, K-265, Kuzneckij Most, 21/5 — LEIN, V.P.

Foreign Affairs-auswärtige Angelegenheiten-inostrannych del
Moskva, G-200, Smolenskaja-Sennaja Ploščad, 32-34 — GROMYKO, A.A.

Geology-Geologie-geologii
Moskva, D-242, Bol'šaja Gruzinskaja Ulica, 4/6 — KOZLOVSKIJ, E.A.

Health-Gesundheitswesen-zdravoochranenija
Moskva, K-51, Rachmanovskij Pereulok, 3 — PETROVSKIJ, B.V.

Higher and Secondary Specialized Education-Hochschul-u.
mittlere Fachschulbildung-vysšego-srednego special'nogo
Moskva, K-31, Ulica Ždanova, 11 — ELJUTIN, V.P.

Industrial Construction-Industriebauwesen-promyšlennogo stroitel'stva
Moskva, K-25, Prospekt Mazksa, 4 — TOKAREV, A.M.

Installation and Special Construction Work-Montage-u.Spezial-
bauarbeiten-montažnych i special'nych stroitel'nych rabot
Moskva, K-379, Bol'šaja Sadovaja Ulica, 8-a — BAKIN, B.V.

Internal Affairs-innere Angelegenheiten-vnutrennich del
Moskva, K-9, Ulica Ogareva, 6 — ŠČELOKOV, N.A.

Justice-Justiz-justicii
Moskva, G-260, Ulica Vorovskogo, 15 — TEREBILOV, V.I.

Land Reclamation and Water Resources-Melioration u.Wasser-
wirtschaft-melioracii i vodnogo chozjajstva
Moskva, I-139, Orlikov Pereulok, 1/11 — ALEKSEEVSKIJ, E.E.

Light Industry-Leichtindustrie-legkoj promyšlennosti
Moskva, C-19, Prospekt Marksa, 11/1 — TARASOV, N.N.

Meat and Dairy Industry-Fleisch-u.Milchindustrie-
mjasnoj i moločnoj promyšlennosti
Moskva, B-140, Verchnjaja Krasnosel'skaja Ulica, 15 — ANTONOV, S.F.

4.3.2 State Structure
Staatsordnung

Nonferrous Metallurgy - Buntmetallurgie - cvetnoj metallurgii
Moskva, K-74, Ploščad' Nogina, 2/5 — LOMAKO, P.F.

Petroleum Refining and Petrochemical Industry - erdölverarbeitende Industrie und Petrochemie - neftepererabatyvajuš-
čej i neftechimičeskoj promyšlennosti — FEDOROV, V.S.

Power and Electrification - Energiewirtschaft und Elektri-
fizierung - energetiki i elektrifikacii — NEPOROŽNIJ, P.S.
Moskva, K-74, Kitajskij Pereulok, 7

Procurement - Beschaffungen - zagotovok
Moskva, Christoprudnyj Bul'var, 12-A — ZOLOTUCHIN, G.S.

Rural Construction - Landbauwesen - sel'skogo stroitel'stva
Moskva, K-25, Prospekt Marksa, 4, Pervoe Stroenie — CHITROV, S.D.

Timber and Wood Processing Industry - Holz-u.holzbearbeitende
Industrie - lesnoj i derevoobrabatyvajuščej promyšlennosti
Moskva, G-19, Ulica Gricevec, 2/16 — TIMOFEEV, N.V.

Trade - Handel - torgovli
Moskva, K-12, Ulica Razina, 26-28 — STRUEV, A.I.

All-Union State Comitees of the USSR -   Chairman/Chief
Unions-Staatskomitees der UdSSR -   Vorsitzender/Leiter
Obščesojuznye Gosudarstvennye Komitety SSSR: Predsedatel'/Načalnik

for Science and Technology - für Wissenschaft u.Technik -
po nauke i technike
Moskva, Centr, Ulica Gor'kogo, 11 — KIRILLIN, V.A.[1]

for Inventions and Discoveries - für Erfindungen und
Entdeckungen - po delam izobretenij i otkrytij
Moskva, Centr, Malyj Čerkasskij Pereulok, 2/6 — MAKSAREV, Ju.E.[2]

for Standards - für Normen - standartov
Moskva, M-49, Leninskij Prospekt, 9 — BOJCOV, V.V.

for Foreign Economic Relations - für Wirtschaftsbeziehungen
mit dem Ausland - po vnešnim ekonomičeskim svjazjam
Moskva, V-324, Ovčinnikovskaja Naberežnaja, 18/1 — SKAČKOV, S.A.

for Hydrometeorology and Environment Control -
für Hydrometeorologie und Kontrolle der Umwelt -
po gidrometeorologii i kontrolju prirodnoj sredy — IZRAEL, Ju.A.

for Material Reserves - für materielle Reserven -
po material'nym rezervam — KOKAREV, A.A.

Union Republic State Committees of the USSR -
Unionsrepublikanische Staatskomitees der UdSSR -
Sojuzno-respublikanskie Gosudarstvennye Komitety SSSR:

State Planning Committee - Staatliches Plankomitee -
Gosudarstvennyj Planovyj komitet - GOSPLAN
Moskva, Centr, Prospekt Marksa, 12 — BAJBAKOV, N.K.[1]

for Construction Affairs - für Bauwesen -
po delam stroitel'stva - GOSSTROJ
Moskva, K-25, Prospekt Marksa, 4 — NOVIKOV, I.T.[1]

for Material and Technical Supply - für materiell-technische
Versorgung - po material'no-techničeskomu snabženiju
Moskva, I-139, Pervyj Djakovskij Pereulok, 4 — MARTYNOV, N.V.

---
[1] at the same time Deputy Chairman of the Council of Ministers -
gleichzeitig stellv.Vorsitzender des Ministerrates
[2] until August 9, 1978 - bis 9.8.1978

State Structure 4.3.2
Staatsordnung 4.3.3

for Labor and Social Questions - für Arbeit und soziale
Fragen - po trudu i social'nym voprosam
Moskva, Centr, Ploščad' Kuibyševa, 1 — LOMONOSOV, V.G.

for Prices - für Preispolitik - cen
Moskva, Ž-72, Bersenevskaja Naberežnaja, 20 — GLUŠKOV, N.T.

for Vocational and Technical Education - für berufstechnische
Ausbildung - po professional'no-techničeskomu obrazovaniju
Moskva, K-12, Sadovaja-Sucharevskaja Ulica, 16 — BULGAKOV, A.A.

for Television and Radio Broadcasting - für Fernseh-und Rundfunkwesen - po televideoniju i radioveščaniju
Moskva, Ž-326, Pjatnickaja Ulica, 25 — LAPIN, S.G.

for Cinematography - für Filmwesen - po kinematografii
Moskva, K-9, Malyj Gnezdnikovskij Pereulok, 7 — ERMAŠ, F.T.

for Publishing Houses, Printing Plants and the Book Trade -
für Verlagswesen, Polygraphie und Buchhandel -
po delam izdatel'stv, poligrafii i knižnoj torgovli
Moskva, K-51, Petrovka, 26 — STUKALIN, B.I.

for Forestry - für Forstwirtschaft - lesnogo chozjajstva
Moskva, M-162, Chavsko-Šabolovskij Pereulok, 4-A — VOROBEV, G.I.

for State Security of the USSR - für Staatssicherheit der
UdSSR - Komitet gosudarstvennoj bezopasnosti SSSR
Moskva, Centr, Ulica Dzeržinskogo, 2 — ANDROPOV, Ju.V.

for Production-Technological Supply in Agriculture -
für produktionstechnische Versorgung der Landwirtschaft -
po proizvodstvenno-techničeskomu obespečeniju sel'skogo choz-
Moskva, I-139, Orlikov Pereulok, 1/11   jajstva — EŽEVSKIJ, A.A.

Committee for People's Control - Komitee für Volkskontrolle -
Komitet narodnogo kontrolja
Moskva, K-132, Ulica Kuibyševa, 21 — ŠKOLNIKOV, A.M.

USSR State Bank - Staatsbank der UdSSR - Gosbank SSSR
Moskva, K-16, Neglinnaja Ulica, 12 — ALCHIMOV, V.S.

Central Statistical Administration - Statistische Zentralverwaltung - Central'noe statističeskoe upravlenie
Moskva, K-430, Ulica Kirova, 39 — VOLODARSKIJ, L.M.

Head - Geschäftsführer - upravljajuščij delami — SMIRTJUKOV, M.S.

4.3.3 USSR MINISTRY OF FOREIGN AFFAIRS
AUSSENMINISTERIUM DER UdSSR
MINISTERSTVO INOSTRANNYCH DEL SSSR

Minister - Ministr — GROMYKO, A.A.

First Deputy Ministers - Erste stellv. Minister -
Pervyj zamestitel'ministra — KORNIENKO, G.M.
MALCEV, V.F.

Deputy Ministers - Stellv. Minister -
Zamestiteli Ministra — FIRJUBIN, N.P.   MALIK, Ja.A.
ILIČEV, L.F.   SEMENOV, V.S.
KOVALEV, A.G.   ZEMSKOV, I.M.
KOZYREV, S.P.

4.3.3 State Structure / Staatsordnung

Secretary General-Generalsekretär-General'nyj sekretar'			- EŽOV, I.M.
Collegium Members –	BONDARENKO, A.P.	KAPICA, M.S.	SEMENOV, V.S.
Mitglieder des Kollegiums –	CHLESTOV, O.N.	KORNIENKO, G.M.	SUDARIKOV, N.G.
Členy kollegii	DUBININ, Ju.V.	KOVALEV, A.G.	SUSLOV, V.P.
	EŽOV, I.M.	KOZYREV, S.P.	SYTENKO, M.D.
	FIRJUBIN, N.P.	MALIK, Ja.A.	TITOV, F.E.
	GROMYKO, A.A.	RODIONOV, N.N.	VORONCOV, Ju.M.
	ILIČEV, L.F.		ZEMSKOV, I.N.
	ISRAELJAN, V.L.		

Apparatus of the Ministry – Apparat des Ministeriums – Apparat Ministerstva

Administration of Affairs-Geschäftsleitung-Upravlenie delami — - DUČKOV, B.I.

Administration for Foreign Policy Planning –
Verwaltung für Planung der außenpolitischen Maßnahmen –
Upravlenie po planirovaniju vnešnepolitičeskich meroprijatij — - KOVALEV, A.G.

Administration for General International Problems –
Verwaltung für allgemeine internationale Probleme –
Upravlenie po obščim meždunarodnym problemam — - ADAMIŠIN, A.L.

Department for Cultural Relations with Foreign Countries –
Abteilung für kulturelle Verbindungen mit dem Ausland –
Otdel po kul'turnym svjazjam s zarubežnymi stranami — --

Protocol Department – Protokollabteilung – Protokol'nyj otdel — - NIKIFOROV, D.S.

Press Department – Presseabteilung – Otdel pečati — - SOFINSKIJ, V.N.

Information Department – Informationsabteilung –
Otdel informacii — - MAKSUDOV, L.M.

International Organizations Department – Abteilung für Internationale Organisationen – Otdel meždunarodnych organizacij — - ISRAELJAN, V.L.

International Economic Organizations Department –
Abteilung für internationale Wirtschaftsorganisationen –
Otdel meždunarodnych ekonomičeskich organizacij — - NESTERENKO, A.E.

Treaty and Legal Department – Vertrags-u.Rechtsabteilung –
Dogovorno-pravovyj otdel — - CHLESTOV, O.N.

Tenth Department (responsible for diplomatic couriers) –
Zehnte Abteilung (zuständig für diplomatischen Kurierdienst) –
Desjatyj otdel (vedaet kur'erskoj služboj) — - ŽEREBČOV, N.S.

Consular Administration – Konsularverwaltung –
Konsul'skoe upravlenie — - IPPOLITOV, I.I.

Archives Administration – Historisch-Diplomatische Archiv-
Verwaltung – Istoriko-diplomatičeskoe upravlenie — - TICHVINSKIJ, S.L.

Currency & Finance Administration – Valuta-u.Finanzverwaltung-
Valjutno-finansovoe upravlenie — - RJABIN, V.A.

Administration for Servicing the Diplomatic Corps –
Verwaltung für die Betreuung des diplomatischen Korps –
Upravlenie po obsluživaniju diplomatičeskogo korpusa — - KUZNECOV, V.N.

Bureau of Translations – Übersetzungsbüro – Bjuro perevodov — - PASTOEV, V.V.

Moscow State Institute of International Relations –
Moskauer Staatliches Institut für Internationale Beziehungen –
Moskovskij gosudarstvennyj institut meždunarodnych otnošenij — - LEBEDEV, N.I.
(Rektor)

State Structure 4.3.3
Staatsordnung

Higher Diplomatic School - Höhere Diplomatische Schule -   - POPOV, V.I.
Vysšaja diplomatičeskaja škola   (Rektor)

Higher Courses in Foreign Languages - Höhere Kurse für
Fremdsprachen - Vysšie kursy inostrannych jazykov   - LIFANOV, N.M.

First African Department - Erste Afrikanische Abteilung -
Pervyj Afrikanskij otdel   - SVEDOV, A.A.
(Algeria,Central African Empire,Chad,Libya,Mali,
Mauritania,Morocco,Senegal,Tunisia,Upper Volta -
Algerien,Libyen,Mauretanien,Mali,Marokko,Obervolta,
Senegal,Tschad,Tunesien,Zentralafrikanisches Kaiserreich)

Second African Department - Zweite Afrikanische Abteilung -
Vtoroj Afrikanskij otdel   - LICHAČEV, V.A.
(all countries south of the Sahara not belonging to the
First or Third Department - alle Länder südlich der
Sahara,die nicht zur Ersten oder Dritten Abteilung gehören)

Third African Department - Dritte Afrikanische Abteilung -
Tretij Afrikanskij otdel   - USTINOV, V.A.
(Burundi,Ethiopia,Kenya,Malawi,Mauritius,Rwanda,
Zambia,Somalia,Tanzania,Uganda -
Äthiopien,Burundi,Kenia,Mauritius,Malawi,Ruanda,Sambia,
Somalia,Tansania,Uganda)

First European Department - Erste Europäische Abteilung -
Pervyj Evropejskij otdel   - DUBININ, Ju.V.
(Belgium,France,Italy,Luxemburg,Netherlands,Portugal,
Switzerland - Belgien,Frankreich,Italien,Luxemburg,
Niederlande,Portugal,Schweiz)

Second European Department - Zweite Europäische Abteilung -
Vtoroj Evropejskij otdel   - SUSLOV, V.P.
(Australia,Great Britain,Ireland,Canada,New Zealand -
Australien,Großbritannien,Irland,Kanada,Neuseeland)

Third European Department - Dritte Europäische Abteilung -
Tretij Evropejskij otdel   - BONDARENKO, A.P.
(Germany,Austria - Deutschland,Österreich)

Fourth European Department - Vierte Europäische Abteilung -
Četvertyj Evropejskij otdel   - DEEV, M.M.
(Czechoslovakia,Poland - Polen,Tschechoslowakei)

Fifth European Department - Fünfte Europäische Abteilung -
Pjatyj Evropejskij otdel   - GRUBJAKOV, V.F.
(Albania,Bulgaria,Cyprus,Greece,Hungary,Romania,Yugoslavia -
Albanien,Bulgarien,Griechenland,Jugoslawien,Rumänien,Ungarn,Zypern)

First Far Eastern Department - Erste Fernost-Abteilung -
Pervyj Dal'nevostočnyj otdel   - KAPICA, M.S.
(China,Korea,Mongolia - China,Korea,Mongolei)

Second Far Eastern Department - Zweite Fernost-Abteilung -
Vtoroj Dal'nevostočnyj otdel   - SOLOVEV, N.N.
(Indonesia,Japan,Philippines - Indonesien,Japan,Philippinen)

Latin American Department - Lateinamerikanische Abteilung -
Otdel stran Latinskoj Ameriki   - ALEKSEEV, N.B.

Middle Eastern Department - Abteilung für den Mittleren Osten-
Otdel stran Srednego Vostoka   - BOLDYREV, V.K.
(Afghanistan,Iran,Turkey- Türkei)

Near Eastern Department - Nahost-Abteilung -
Otdel stran Bližnego Vostoka   - SYTENKO, M.D.

4.3.3 State Structure
Staatsordnung

(Egypt,Irak,Israel,Jordan,Kuwait,Lebanon,Saudi-Arabia,Syria,
Sudan,Yemen Arab Republic,People's Democratic Republic of Yemen –
Ägypten,Irak,Israel,Arabische Republik Jemen,Volksdemokratische
Republik Jemen,Jordanien,Kuweit,Libanon,Saudi-Arabien,Sudan,Syrien)

Scandinavian Department – Abteilung für Skandinavische Länder –
Otdel skandinavskich stran   – SOBOLEV, V.M.
(Denmark,Finland,Iceland,Norway,Sweden – Dänemark,
Finnland,Island,Norwegen,Schweden)

South Asian Department – Abteilung für Südasien –
Otdel Južnoj Azii   – SUDARIKOV, N.G.
(Bangladesh,Burma,India,Nepal,Pakistan,Sri Lanka –
Bangladesch,Birma,Indien,Nepal,Pakistan,Sri Lanka)

Southeast Asian Department – Abteilung für Südostasien –
Otdel Jugo-Vostočnoj Azii   –   --
(Cambodia,Laos,Malaysia,Singapore,Thailand,Vietnam –
Kambodscha,Laos,Malaysia,Singapur,Thailand,Vietnam)

United States of America Department – US-Abteilung – Otdel SŠA – KORNIENKO, G.M.

Ambassadors for Special Assignments – Sonderbotschafter – Posly po osobym poručenijam

                BELOCHVOSTIKOV, N.D.   PODCEROB, B.F.
                CARAPKIN, S.K.   STRIGANOV, S.R.
                KOLOSOVSKIJ, I.K.   ZORIN, V.A.
                MENDELEVIČ, L.I.

Ambassadors – Botschafter – Posly

Afghanistan   – PUZANOV, A.M.
Algeria – Algerien   – RYKOV, V.N.
Angola   – LOGINOV, V.P.
Argentina – Argentinien   – STRIGANOV, S.R.
Australia   – BASOV, A.V.
                                                 (Also ambassador to Fiji –
                                                 glz.Botschafter in Fidschi)

Austria – Österreich   – EFREMOV, M.T.
Bangladesh – Bangladesch   – STEPANOV, V.P.
Belgium – Belgien   – ROMANOVSKIJ, S.K.
Benin   – ILIN, I.S.
Bolivia – Bolivien   – KAZANCEV, B.A.
Botswana – Botsuana   – PETROV, M.N.
Brazil – Brasilien   – ŽUKOV, D.A.
Bulgaria – Bulgarien   – BAZOVSKIJ, V.N.
Burma – Birma   – GRUZINOV, S.S.
Burundi   – POŽIDAEV, D.P.
Cameroon – Kamerun   – TIKUNOV, V.S.
Canada – Kanada   – JAKOVLEV, A.N.
Cape Verde Islands – Kapverdische Inseln   – SEMENOV, V.M.
                                                 (Also ambassador to Guinea-Bissau –
                                                 glz.Botschafter in Guinea-Bissau)

Central African Empire –
Zentralafrikanisches Kaiserreich   – NAUMOV, A.F.
Chad – Tschad   – MARČUK, I.I.
China   – ŠČERBAKOV, I.S.
Colombia – Kolumbien   – ROMANOV, L.M.
                                                 (Also ambassador to Surinam –
                                                 glz.Botschafter in Suriname)

Comores   – STARCEV, A.K.
                                                 (Also Ambassador to Seychelles –
                                                 glz.Botschafter auf den Seychellen)

Congo – Kongo   – KUZNECOV, S.A.

State Structure 4.3.3
Staatsordnung

Costa Rica	- ZELENOV, D.A.
Cuba - Kuba	- TOLUBEEV, N.P.
Cyprus - Zypern	- ASTAVIN, S.T.
Czechoslovakia - Tschechoslowakei	- MACKEVIČ, V.V.
Denmark - Dänemark	- EGORYČEV, N.G.
Ecuador	- ŠLJAPNIKOV, H.E.
Egypt - Ägypten	- POLJAKOV,V.P.
Eqatorial Guinea - Äquatorial-Guinea	- BELOUS, N.A.
Ethiopia - Äthiopien	- RATANOV, A.P.
Fiji - Fidschi	- BASOV, A.V.
	(Also ambassador to Australia - glz.Botschafter in Australien)
Finland - Finnland	- STEPANOV, V.S.
France - Frankreich	- ČERVONENKO, S.V.
Gabon - Gabun	- FILATOV, V.G.
Gambia	- TER-GAZARJANC, G.A.
Germany, Federal Republic of - Deutsche Bundesrepublik	- FALIN, V.M.
German Democratic Republic - DDR	- ABRASIMOV, P.A.
Ghana	- BERNOV, Ju.V.
Greece - Griechenland	- UDALCOV, I.I.
Guinea	- MININ, V.I.
Guinea-Bissau	- SEMENOV, V.M.
	(Also ambassador to Cape Verde Islands - glz.Botschafter a.d.Kapverdischen Inseln
Guyana - Guayana	- KOTENEV, V.V.
Hungary - Ungarn	- PAVLOV, V.Ja.
Iceland - Island	- FARAFONOV, G.N.
India - Indien	- VORONCOV, Ju.M.
Indonesia - Indonesien	- ŠPED'KO, I.F.
Iran	- VINOGRADOV, V.M.
Iraq - Irak	- BAPKOVSKIJ, A.A.
Ireland - Irland	- KAPLIN, A.S.
Italy - Italien	- RYŽOV, N.S.
Jamaica - Jamaika	- MUSIN, D.P.
Japan	- POLJANSKIJ, D.S.
Jordan - Jordanien	- NIŠANOV, R.N.
Kenya - Kenia	- MIROŠNIČENKO, B.P.
Korea, Democratic People's Republic of - Koreanische Volksdemokratische Republik	- KRIULIN, G.A.
Kuwait - Kuweit	- SIKAČEV, N.N.
Laos	- PODOLSKIJ, M.G.
Lebanon - Libanon	- SOLDATOV, A.A.
Liberia	- ULANOV, A.A.
Libya - Libyen	- ANISIMOV, A.V.
Luxembourg - Luxemburg	- KOSAREV, E.A.
Madagascar - Madagaskar	- ALEKSEEV, A.I.
Malaysia	- KULIK, B.T.
Maldives - Malediven	- PASJUTIN, A.S.
	(Also ambassador to Sri Lanka - glz.Botschafter in Sri Lanka)
Mali	- FAZYLOV, M.S.
Malta	- LUNKOV, N.M.
	(Also ambassador to the United Kingdom - glz.Botschafter in Großbritannien)
Mauritania - Mauretanien	- STARCEV, V.I.

4.3.3 State Structure / Staatsordnung

Mauritius	- SAFRONOV, I.I.
Mexico - Mexiko	- VOLSKIJ, Ju.I.
Mongolia - Mongolei	- SMIRNOV, A.I.
Morocco - Marokko	- NERSESOV, E.V.
Mozambique - Mosambik	- EVSJUKOV, P.N.
Nepal	- UDUMJAN, K.B.
Netherlands - Niederlande	- ROMANOV, A.Jo.
New Zealand - Neuseeland	- SELJANINOV, O.P. (Also ambassador to the Kingdom of Tonga - glz.Botschafter im Königreich Tonga)
Niger	- KUDAŠKIN, V.N.
Nigeria	- SNEGIREV, V.V.
Norway - Norwegen	- KIRIČENKO, Ju.A.
Pakistan	- ASIMOV, S.A.
Peru	- KUZMIN, L.F.
Philippines - Philippinen	- MICHAJLOV, V.V.
Poland - Polen	- ARISTOV, B.I.
Portugal	- KALININ, A.I.
Romania - Rumänien	- DROZDENKO, V.I.
Rwanda - Ruanda	- RYKOV, G.V.
Sao Tome and Principe - Sao Tome und Principe	- DJAKONOV, D.A.
Senegal	- TER-GAZARJANC, G.A. (Also ambassador to Gambia - glz.Botschafter in Gambia)
Seychelles - Seschellen	- STARCEV, A.K. (Also ambassador to Comores - glz.Botschafter in Comores)
Sierra Leone	- FILIPPOV, I.F.
Singapore - Singapur	- RAZDUCHOV, Ju.I.
Somalia	- SAMSONOV, G.E.
Spain - Spanien	- BOGOMOLOV, S.A.
Sri Lanka	- PASJUTIN, A.S. (Also ambassador to the Maldives - glz.Botschafter in Malediven)
Sudan	- FEDOTOV, F.N.
Surinam - Suriname	- ROMANOV, L.M. (Also Ambassador to Colombia - glz.Botschafter in Kolumbien)
Sweden - Schweden	- JAKOVLEV, M.D.
Switzerland - Schweiz	- LAVROV, V.S.
Syria - Syrien	- ČERNJAKOV, Ju.N.
Tanzania - Tansania	- SLIPČENKO, S.A.
Thailand	- KUZNECOV, Ju.I.
Togo	- ILJUCHIN, I.A.
Tonga	- SELJANINOV, O.P. (Also ambassador to New Zealand - glz.Botschafter in Neuseeland)
Trinidad and Tobago	- KAZIMIROV, V.N. (Also ambassador to Venezuela - glz.Botschafter in Venezuela)
Tunisia - Tunesien	- KOLOKOLOV, B.L.
Turkey - Türkei	- RODIONOV, A.A.
Uganda	- MUSIJKO, E.V.
United Kingdom - Großbritannien	- LUNKOV, N.M. (Also ambassador to Malta - glz.Botschafter auf Malta)

State Structure 4.3.3
Staatsordnung 4.3.4

United States of America - USA — DOBRYNIN, A.F.
Upper Volta - Obervolta — KAZANSKIJ, A.N.
Uruguay — LEBEDEV, Ju.V.
Venezuela — KAZIMIROV, V.N.
 (Also ambassador to Trinidad and Tobago-
 glz.Botschafter in Trinidad und Tobago)
Vietnam — ČAPLIN, B.N.
Yemen Arab Republic - Jemen (Arabische
 Republik) — KORNEV, V.I.
Yemen, People's Democratic Republic of -
 Jemen (Volksdemokratische Republik) — KABOŠKIN, V.F.
Yugoslavia - Jugoslawien — RODIONOV, N.N.
Zaire — LAVROV, I.M.
Zambia - Sambia — SOLODOVNIKOV, V.G.

4.3.4   USSR MINISTRY OF DEFENSE
VERTEIDIGUNGSMINISTERIUM DER UdSSR
MINISTERSTVO OBORONY SSSR

Minister - Ministr — USTINOV, D.F.
 Marshal of the Soviet Union -
 Marschall der Sowjetunion

First Deputy Ministers - — KULIKOV, V.G.
Erste stellv. Minister - Marshal of the Soviet Union -
Pervye zamestiteli ministra Marschall der Sowjetunion
 OGARKOV, N.V.
  Marshal of the Soviet Union -
  Marschall der Sowjetunion
 SOKOLOV, L.S.
  Marshal of the Soviet Union -
  Marschall der Sowjetunion

Deputy Ministers -
Stellv. Minister -
Zamestiteli ministra — ALEKSEEV, N.N.
  Colonel-General - Generaloberst
 ALTUNIN, A.T.
  Colonel-General - Generaloberst
 BATICKIJ, P.F.
  Marshal of the Soviet Union -
  Marschall der Sowjetunion
 GORŠKOV, S.G.
  Naval Admiral of the Soviet Union -
  Flottenadmiral der Sowjetunion
 KURKOTKIN, S.K.
  Army General - Armeegeneral
 KUTACHOV, P.S.
  Captain Marshal of the Air Force -
  Hauptmarschall der Luftwaffe
 MOSKALENKO, K.S.
  Marshal of the Soviet Union -
  Marschall der Sowjetunion
 PAVLOVSKIJ, I.G.
  Army General - Armeegeneral
 TOLUBKO, V.F.
  Army General - Armeegeneral

133

4.3.4 State Structure / Staatsordnung

General Staff of the USSR Armed Forces -
Generalstab der Streitkräfte der UdSSR -
General'nyj Stab Vooružennych Sil SSSR
    Chief - Chef - Načal'nik   - OGARKOV, N.V.
                                                       Marshal of the Soviet Union
                                                       Marschall der Sowjetunion

    Chief, Political Department - Chef der Polit-
    abteilung - Načal'nik politotdela   --

Main Political Directorate of the Soviet Army and Navy -
Politische Hauptverwaltung der Sowjetischen Armee und
Seekriegsflotte -
Glavnoe političeskoe upravlenie Sovetskoj Armii i
Voenno-Morskogo Flota
    Chief - Chef - Načal'nik   - EPIŠEV, A.A.
                                                       Army General - Armeegeneral

Supreme Forces Command - Oberkommando der Waffen-
gattungen - Glavnokomandovanija zodov vojsk

    Air Defense Forces - Truppen der Luftverteidigung
    des Landes - Vojska Protivovozdušnoj oborony strany -
    PVO
        Commander-in-Chief - Oberkommandierender -
        Glavnokomandujuščij   - BATICKIJ, P.F.
                                                        Marshal of the Soviet Union
                                                          Marschall der Sowjetunion

        Chief, Political Directorate/Member,
        Military Council - Chef der Politischen
        Verwaltung, Mitglied des Militärrates -
        Načal'nik Političeskogo upravlenija,
        člen Voennogo soveta   - BOBYLEV, S.
                                                       Colonel-General - Generaloberst

    Air Force - Luftstreitkräfte -
    Voenno-Vozdušnye Sily SSSR
        Commander-in-Chief - Oberkommandierender   - KUTACHOV, P.S.
                                                                 Captain Marshal of the Air
                                                                 Force - Hauptmarschall
                                                                 der Luftwaffe

        Chief, Political Directorate/Member,
        Military Council - Chef der Politischen   - MOROZ, I.
        Verwaltung, Mitglied des Militärrates   Colonel-General - Generaloberst

    Ground Forces - Landstreitkräfte -
    Suchoputnye vojska SSSR
        Commander-in-Chief - Oberkommandierender   - PAVLOVSKIJ, I.G.
                                                                 Army General - Armeegeneral
        Chief, Political Directorate/Member,
        Military Council - Chef der Politischen   - VASJAGIN, S.
        Verwaltung, Mitglied des Militärrates   Army General - Armeegeneral

    Naval Forces - Seekriegsflotte -
    Voenno-Morskoj flot SSSR
        Commander-in-Chief - Oberkommandierender   - GORŠKOV, S.G.
                                                                 Naval Admiral of the Soviet
                                                                 Union - Flottenadmiral der
                                                                 Sowjetunion

        Chief, Political Directorate/Member,
        Military Council - Chef der Politischen   - GRIŠANOV, V.M.
        Verwaltung, Mitglied des Militärrates   Naval Admiral - Flottenadmiral

State Structure 4.3.4
Staatsordnung

Strategic Rocket Forces - Strategische Raketentruppen - Raketnye vojska strategičeskogo naznačenija
    Commander-in-Chief - Oberkommandierender — TOLUBKO, V.F.
        Army General - Armeegeneral

    Chief, Political Directorate/Member,
    Military Council - Chef der Politischen — GORČAKOV, P.A.
    Verwaltung, Mitglied des Militärrates   Colonel-General - Generaloberst

Joint Armed Forces of Warsaw Pact Nations - Vereinte Streitkräfte der Teilnehmerstaaten des Warschauer Paktes - Ob'edinennye Vooružennye Sily gosudarstv učastnikov Waršavskogo Dogovora
    Commander-in-Chief - Oberkommandierender — KULIKOV, V.G.
        Marshal of the Soviet Union - Marschall der Sowjetunion

    Chief of Staff - Chef des Stabes - Načal'nik Štaba — GRIBKOV, A.I.
        Army General - Armeegeneral

Groups of Forces - Gruppen der Truppen - Gruppy vojsk

    Central Group of Forces - Zentralgruppe der Truppen - Central'naja Gruppa vojsk (CSSR)
        Commander-Kommandierender-Komandujuščij — TENIŠČEV, I.
        Colonel-General - Generaloberst

        Chief, Political Directorate/Member,
        Military Council - Chef der Politischen — MAKSIMOV, K.
        Verwaltung, Mitglied des Militärrates   Lieutenant-General - Generalleutnant

    Group of Soviet Forces in Germany - Gruppe der Sowjetischen Streitkräfte in Deutschland - Gruppa Sovetskich vojsk v Germanii (DDR)
        Commander-in-Chief - Oberkommandierender — IVANOVSKIJ, E.F.
        Army General - Armeegeneral

        Chief, Political Directorate/Member,
        Military Council - Chef der Politischen — MEDNIKOV, I.S.
        Verwaltung, Mitglied des Militärrates   Colonel-General - Generaloberst

    Northern Group of Forces - Nordgruppe der Truppen - Severnaja Gruppa vojsk (Poland-Polen)
        Commander - Kommandierender — KULIŠEV, O.
        Colonel-General - Generaloberst

        Chief, Political Directorate/Member,
        Military Council - Chef der Politischen — DANILOV, V.A.
        Verwaltung, Mitglied des Militärrates   Lieutenant-General - Generalleutnant

    Southern Group of Forces - Südgruppe der Truppen - Južnaja Gruppa vojsk (Hungary-Ungarn)
        Commander - Kommandierender — KRIVDA, F.
        Colonel-General - Generaloberst

        Chief, Political Directorate/Member,
        Military Council - Chef der Politischen — --
        Verwaltung, Mitglied des Militärrates

4.3.4 State Structure
Staatsordnung

Military Districts - Militärbezirke - Voennye okruga

Baltic Military District - Militärbezirk Baltikum -
Pribaltijskij voennyj okrug
   Commander - Kommandierender — - MAJOROV, A.M.
                                                 Army General - Armeegeneral
   Chief, Political Directorate/Member,
   Military Council - Chef der Politischen — - GUBIN, I.
   Verwaltung, Mitglied des Militärrates   Lieutenant-General -
Belorussian Military District - Militärbezirk   Generalleutnant
Belorußland - Belorusskij voennyj okrug
   Commander - Kommandierender — - ZAJCEV, M.M.
                                                 Lieutenant-General of the
                                               Tank Forces - Generalleut-
                                               nant der Panzertruppen
   Chief, Political Directorate/Member,
   Military Council - Chef der Politischen — - DEBALJUK, A.
   Verwaltung, Mitglied des Militärrates   Colonel-General -
                                               Generaloberst
Carpathian Military District - Militärbezirk
Karpaten - Prikarpatskij voennyj okrug
   Commander - Kommandierender — - VARENNIKOV, V.I.
                                               Army-General - Armeegeneral
   Chief, Political Directorate/Member,
   Military Council - Chef der Politischen — - ŠEVKUN, N.
   Verwaltung, Mitglied des Militärrates   Lieutenant-General -
Central Asian Military District - Militärbezirk   Generalleutnant
Mittelasien - Sredneaziatskij voennyj okrug
   Commander - Kommandierender — - LUŠEV, P.G.
                                               Colonel-General - Generaloberst
   Chief, Political Directorate/Member,
   Military Council - Chef der Politischen — - POPKOV, M.
   Verwaltung, Mitglied des Militärrates   Lieutenant-General -
                                               Generalleutnant
Far East Military District - Militärbezirk
Fernost - Dal'nevostočnyj voennyj okrug
   Commander - Kommandierender — - TRETJAK, I.
                                               Army General - Armeegeneral
   Chief, Political Directorate/Member,
   Military Council - Chef der Politischen — - DRUŽININ, M.
   Verwaltung, Mitglied des Militärrates   Lieutenant-General -
Kiev, Military District - Militärbezirk Kiev -   Generalleutnant
Kievskij voennyj okrug
   Commander - Kommandierender — - GERASIMOV, I.A.
                                               Army General - Armeegeneral
   Chief, Political Directorate/Member,
   Military Council - Chef der Politischen — - DEMENTEV, V.
   Verwaltung, Mitglied des Militärrates   Lieutenant-General -
                                               Generalleutnant
Leningrad Military District - Militärbezirk
Leningrad - Leningradskij voennyj okrug
   Commander - Kommandierender — - SOROKIN, M.
                                               Colonel-General-Generaloberst
   Chief, Political Directorate/Member,
   Military Council - Chef der Politischen — - NOVIKOV, V.
   Verwaltung, Mitglied des Militärrates   Lieutenant-General -
                                               Generalleutnant

State Structure 4.3.4
Staatsordnung

Moscow Military District - Militärbezirk Moskau -
Moskovskij voennyj okrug
    Commander - Kommandierender   - GOVOROV, V.L.
        Army General - Armeegeneral
    Chief, Political Directorate/Member,
    Military Council - Chef der Politischen - GRUŠEVOJ, K.
    Verwaltung, Mitglied des Militärrates   Colonel-General - Generaloberst
North Caukasus Military District - Militärbezirk
Nordkaukasus - Severokavkazskij voennyj okrug
    Commander - Kommandierender   - BELIKOV, V.
        Colonel-General - Generaloberst
    Chief, Political Directorate/Member,
    Military Council - Chef der Politischen
    Verwaltung, Mitglied des Militärrates   - KOSTENKO, N.
        Lieutenant-General -
Odessa Military District - Militärbezirk Odessa -   Generalleutnant
Odesskij voennyj okrug
    Commander - Kommandierender   - VOLOŠIN, I.
        Colonel-General-Generaloberst
    Chief, Political Directorate/Member,
    Military Council - Chef der Politischen
    Verwaltung, Mitglied des Militärrates   --

Siberian Military District - Militärbezirk Sibirien -
Sibirskij voennyj okrug
    Commander - Kommandierender   - CHOMULO, M.G.
        Colonel-General - Generaloberst
    Chief, Political Directorate/Member,
    Military Council - Chef der Politischen - LYKOV, I.
    Verwaltung, Mitglied des Militärrates   Lieutenant-General -
        Generalleutnant
Transbaikal Military District - Militärbezirk
Transbaikal - Zabajkal'skij voennyj okrug
    Commander - Kommandierender   - BELIK, P.A.
    Chief, Political Directorate/Member,   Colonel-General - Generaloberst
    Military Council - Chef der Politischen
    Verwaltung, Mitglied des Militärrates   - LIZIČEV, A.
        Lieutenant-General -
Transcaucasus Military District - Militärbezirk   Generalleutnant
Transkaukasus - Zakavkazskij voennyj okrug
    Commander - Kommandierender   - KULIŠEV, O.V.
        Colonel-General - Generaloberst
    Chief, Political Directorate/Member,
    Military Council - Chef der Politischen - OVERČUK, A.M.
    Verwaltung, Mitglied des Militärrates   Major-General - Generalmajor
Turkestan Military District - Militärbezirk
Turkestan - Turkestanskij voennyj okrug
    Commander - Kommandierender   - BELONOŽKO, S.
        Lieutenant-General -
        Generalleutnant
    Chief, Political Directorate/Member,
    Military Council - Chef der Politischen - RODIN, V.
    Verwaltung, Mitglied des Militärrates   Major-General - Generalmajor
Ural Military District - Militärbezirk Ural -
Ural'skij voennyj okrug
    Commander - Kommandierender   - SILČENKO, N.K.
        Lieutenant-General -
        Generalleutnant
    Chief, Political Directorate/Member,
    Military Council - Chef der Politischen - SAMOJLENKO, V.
    Verwaltung, Mitglied des Militärrates   Lieutenant-General -
        Generalleutnant

4.3.4 State Structure
Staatsordnung

Volga Military District - Militärbezirk Wolga -
Privolžskij voennyj okrug
   Commander - Kommandierender   - --
   Chief, Political Directorate/Member,
   Military Council - Chef der Politischen - UTKIN, B.
   Verwaltung, Mitglied des Militärrates   Major-General - Generalmajor

Air Defense Districts - Luftverteidigungsbezirke -
Okruga protivovozdušnoj oborony - PVO

  Baku Air Defense District -
  Luftverteidigungsbezirk Baku -
  Bakinskij okrug protivovozdušnoj oborony
    Commander - Kommandierender   - KONSTANTINOV, A.U.
                                                     Colonel-General of the airforce-
    Chief, Political Directorate/Member,   Generaloberst der Luftwaffe
    Military Council - Chef der Politischen
    Verwaltung, Mitglied des Militärrates   - SVIRIDOV, I.
                                                       Major-General - Generalmajor
  Moscow Air Defense District -
  Luftverteidigungsbezirk Moskau -
  Moskovskij okrug protivovozdušnoj oborony
    Commander - Kommandierender   - BOČKOV, B.V.
                                                       Colonel-General-Generaloberst

    Chief, Political Directorate/Member,
    Military Council - Chef der Politischen - PONOMAREV, V.
    Verwaltung, Mitglied des Militärrates   Lieutenant-General of the air
                                                       force - Generalleutnant der
                                                       Luftwaffe

Fleets - Flotten - Floty
  Baltic Fleet - Baltische Flotte - Baltijskij Flot
    Commander - Kommandierender   - MICHAJLIN, V.V.
                                                       Admiral
    Chief, Political Directorate/Member,
    Military Council - Chef der Politischen
    Verwaltung, Mitglied des Militärrates   --
  Black Sea Fleet - Schwarzmeerflotte - Černomorskij Flot
    Commander - Kommandierender   - CHOVRIN, N.I.
    Chief, Political Directorate/Member,   Admiral
    Military Council - Chef der Politischen
    Verwaltung, Mitglied des Militärrates   --
  Northern Fleet - Nordmeerflotte - Severnyj Flot
    Commander - Kommandierender   - ČERNAVIN, V.N.
                                                       Vice-admiral - Vizeadmiral
    Chief, Political Directorate/Member,
    Military Council - Chef der Politischen - PADORIN, Ju.
    Verwaltung, Mitglied des Militärrates   Rear-admiral - Konteradmiral
  Pacific Fleet - Pazifikflotte - Tichookeanskij Flot
    Commander - Kommandierender   - MASLOV, V.P.
                                                     Admiral
    Chief, Political Directorate/Member,
    Military Council - Chef der Politischen --
    Verwaltung, Mitglied des Militärrates

State Structure 4.4.1
Staatsordnung

4.4 SUPREME SOVIETS AND COUNCILS OF MINISTERS OF THE UNION'S REPUBLICS
OBERSTE SOWJETS UND MINISTERRÄTE DER UNIONSREPUBLIKEN
VERCHOVNYE SOVETY I SOVETY MINISTROV SOJUZNYCH RESPUBLIK

4.4.1 RSFSR

Supreme Soviet of the RSFSR - Oberster Sowjet der RSFSR - Verchovnyj Sovet RSFSR

Presidium-Präsidium-Prezidija

Chairman-Vorsitzender-Predsedatel'	- JASNOV, M.A.	
Deputy Chairmen-stellv.Vorsitzende-Zamestiteli predsedatelja	- KOLČINA, O.P.	ASTAJKIN, I.P.
	SULTANOV, F.V.	BASIEV, O.A.
	SEMENOV, B.S.	BATYEV, S.G.
	ŠAMCHALOV, Š.M.	DOLČANMAA, B.-K.Š.
	GETTUEV, M.I.	SYSOEV, P.P.
	NAMSINOV, I.E.	BOKOV, Ch.Ch.
	PROKKONEN, P.S.	ISLJUKOV, S.M.
	PANEV, Z.V.	OVČINNIKOVA, A.Ja.
	ALMAKAEV, P.A.	
Secretary-Sekretär-Sekretar'	- NEŠKOV, Ch.P.	
Presidium members-Mitglieder des Präsidiums-Členy prezidiuma	- BABIN, S.D.	KORŽEV-ČUVELEV, G.M.
	BOGATYREV, N.G.	LALETINA, M.F.
	DEMENTEVA, R.F.	MALKOV, N.I.
	DEMIDOVA, A.I.	SILINA, A.I.
	FILATOV, V.A.	SOLOVEV, Ju.F.
	ILIČEV, L.A.	TICHOMIROVA, L.A.
	KIRILENKO, A.P.	VETLICKIJ, V.F.
Chairman of the Supreme Soviet - Vorsitzender des Obersten Sowjets - Predsedatel' Verchovnogo Soveta	- KOTELNIKOV, V.A.	
Deputies-Stellvertreter-Zamestiteli	- AMOSOVA, E.G.	LEVIN, G.M.
	BONDAREV, Ju.V.	MAMAEVA, T.N.
	EFIMOV, S.V.	UGUŽAKOV, V.A.
	GOROVOJ, N.I.	VOROBEV, B.M.

Council of Ministers of the RSFSR - Ministerrat der RSFSR - Sovet Ministrov RSFSR

Chairman-Vorsitzender-Predsedatel'	- SOLOMENCEV, M.S.	
First Deputies-Erste Stellvertreter-Pervyj Zamestiteli	- VASILEV, N.F.	VOROTNIKOV, V.I.
Deputies-Stellvertreter-Zamestiteli	- ALEKSANKIN, A.V.	KAZAKOV, V.I.
	DEMČENKO, V.A.	KOČEMASOV, V.I.
	KALAŠNIKOV, A.M.	LYKOVA, L.P.
	KARPOVA, E.F.	MASLENNIKOV, N.I.

4.4.1 State Structure
Staatsordnung

Union Republican Ministries of – Unionsrepublikanische Ministerien für – Sojuzno-respublikanskie Ministerstva:

Agriculture – Landwirtschaft – sel'skogo chozjajstva	– FLORENTEV, L.Ja.
Construction Materials Industry – Baustoffindustrie – promyšlennosti stroitel'nych materialov	– MARAKOV, G.N.
Culture – Kultur – kul'tury	– MELENTEV, Ju.S.
Education – Volksbildung – prosveščenija	– DANILOV, A.I.
Finance – Finanzen – finansov	– BOBROVNIKOV, A.A.
Fish Industry – Fischereiwirtschaft – rybnogo chozjajstva	– VANJAEV, N.A.
Food Industry – Nahrungsmittelindustrie – piščevoj promyšlennosti	– KLEMENČUK, A.P.
Foreign Affairs – auswärtige Angelegenheiten – inostrannych del	– TITOV, F.E.
Forestry – Forstwirtschaft – lesnogo chozjajstva	– ZVEREV, A.I.
Geology – Geologie – geologii	– ROVNIN, L.I.
Health – Gesundheitswesen – zdravoochranenija	– TROFIMOV, V.V.
Higher and Secondary Specialized Education – Hochschul-u.mittl. Fachschulbildung – vysšego i srednego special'nogo obrazovanija	– OBRAZOCV, I.F.
Justice – Justiz – justicii	– BLINOV, V.M.
Land Reclamation and Water Resources – Melioration u.Wasserwirtschaft – melioracii i vodnogo chozjajstva	– KORNEV, K.S.
Light Industry – Leichtindustrie – legkoj promyšlennosti	– KONDRATKOV, E.F.
Meat and Dairy Industry – Fleisch-u.Milchindustrie – mjasnoj i moločnoj promyšlennosti	– KONARYGIN, V.S.
Procurement – Beschaffungen – zagotovok	– MERKULOV, P.I.
Rural Construction – Landbauwesen – sel'skogo stroitel'stva	– MALCEV, N.S.
Textile Industry – Textilindustrie – tekstil'noj promyšlennosti	– PARAMONOV, A.M.
Trade – Handel – torgovli	– ŠIMANSKIJ, V.P.

Republican Ministries of – Republikanische Ministerien für – Respublikanskie Ministerstva:

Construction and Utilization of Roads – Bau und Nutzung der Autobahnen – stroitel'stva i ekspluatacii avtomobil'nych dorog	– NIKOLAEV, A.A.
Consumer Services – Dienstleistungen – bytovogo obsluživanija naselenija	– DUDENKOV, I.G.
Domestic Construction – zivilen Wohnungsbau – žiliščno-graždanskogo stroitel'stva	– GLADYREVSKIJ, A.V.
Fuel Industry – Brennstoffindustrie – toplivnoj promyšlennosti	– PANKRATOV, Ju.A.
Housing and Municipal Services – Wohnungs-u.Kommunalwirtschaft-žiliščno-kommunal'nogo chozjajstva	– BUTUSOV, S.M.
Inland Water Transport – Binnenschiffahrt – rečnogo flota	– BAGROV, L.V.
Local Industry – lokale Industrie – mestnoj promyšlennosti	– USPENSKIJ, V.K.
Motor Transport – Kraftverkehr – avtomobil'nogo transporta	– TRUBICYN, E.G.
Social Security – Sozialfürsorge – social'nogo obespečenija	– KOMAROVA, D.P.

Chairman/Chief
Vorsitzender/Leiter
Predsedatel'Načalnik

State Planning Committee – Staatl. Plankomitee – Gosudarstvennyj Planovyj komitet – GOSPLAN	– MASLENNIKOV, N.I.[1]

1 also Deputy Chairman of the Council of Ministers – glz.stellv.Vorsitzender des Ministerrates

State Structure 4.4.1
Staatsordnung 4.4.2

Committee for People's Control - Komitee für Volkskontrolle -
Komitet narodnogo kontrolja — - KONNOV, V.F.
State Committee for Construction Affairs - Staatskomitee für
Bauwesen - Gosudarstvennyj komitet po delam stroitel'stva — - BASILOV, D.P.
State Committee for Labor - Staatskomitee für Arbeit -
Gosudarstvennyj komitet po trudu — - SOZYKIN, A.G.
State Committee for Vocational and Technical Education -
Staatskomitee für berufstechnische Ausbildung - Gosudarstvennyj
komitet po professional'no-techničeskomu obrazovaniju — - KAMAEV, G.L.
State Committee for Cinematography - Staatskomitee f.Filmwesen -
Gosudarstvennyj komitet po kinematografii — - FILIPPOV, A.G.
State Committee for Publishing Houses, Printing Plants and the
Book Trade - Staatskomitee für Verlagswesen, Polygraphie und
Buchhandel - Gosudarstvennyj komitet po delam izdatel'stv,
poligrafii i knižnoj torgovli — - SVIRIDOV, N.V.
State Committee for Prices - Staatskomitee für Preispolitik -
Gosudarstvennyj komitet cen — - FROLOV, K.I.
State Committee for Production-Technological Supply in
Agriculture - Staatskomitee für produktionstechnische Versor-
gung der Landwirtschaft - Gosudarstvennyj komitet po proiz-
vodstvenno-techničeskom obespečeniju sel'skogo chozjajstva — - BOSENKO, N.V.
Central Statistical Administration - Zentrale Statistische
Verwaltung - Central'noe statističeskoe upravlenie — - DRJUČIN, A.P.

4.4.2 Ukrainskaja SSR

Supreme Soviet of the Ukrainian SSR - Oberster Sowjet der
Ukrainischen SSR - Verchovnyj Sovet Ukrainskoj SSSR

Presidium-Präsidium-Prezidija

Chairman-Vorsitzender-Predsedatel'   - VATČENKO, A.F.

First Deputy Chairman -
  Erster stellv.Vorsitzender -
  Pervyj zamestitel'predsedatelja   - ŠEVČENKO, V.S.

Deputy Chairmen-stellv.Vorsitzende -
  Zamestiteli predsedatelja   - ČEMODUROV, T.N.   ŠČERBINA, V.P.

Secretary-Sekretär-Sekretar'   - KOLOTUCHA, Ja.Ja.

Presidium members-Mitglieder des
  Präsidiums-Členy prezidiuma   - BABIČ, Ju.P.   POVEDA, G.A.
                                  EREMENKO, A.A.   POCHODIN, V.P.
                                  ERŠOV, I.D.   RADZIEVSKIJ, I.I.
                                  GRINCOV, I.G.   RYŽUK, M.M.
                                  JUPKO, L.D.   ŠČERBICKIJ, V.V.
                                  KAČURA, B.V.   SOLOGUB, V.A.
                                  KORNIENKO, A.I.   TELIŠEVSKIJ, T.D.
                                  LEGUNOV, G.A.   TKAČENKO, I.G.
                                  LUTAK, I.K.   ZAJKOVSKAJA, T.A.
                                  PATON, B.E.   SOKOLOV, I.Z.

Chairman of the Supreme Soviet -
  Vorsitzender des Obersten Sowjets -
  Predsedatel' Verchovnogo Soveta   - BILYJ, M.U.

Deputies-Stellvertreter-Zamestiteli   - GAVRILOVA, T.A.   MIŠČENKO, N.V.
                                        KAČALOVSKIJ, E.V.   PUDENKO, G.I.

141

4.4.2 State Structure
Staatsordnung

Council of Ministers of the Ukrainian SSR - Ministerrat der Ukrainischen SSR - Sovet Ministrov Ukrainskoj SSR

Chairman-Vorsitzender-Predsedatel'	- LJAŠKO, A.P.	
First Deputies-Erste Stellvertreter-Pervyj Zamestiteli	- POGREBNJAK, P.L.	VAŠČENKO, G.I.
Deputies-Stellvertreter-Zamestiteli	- BURMISTROV, A.A. ESYPENKO, P.E. KOČEVYCH, I.P. ROZENKO, P.Ja.	SEMIČASTNYJ, V.E. STEPANENKO, I.D. ORLIK, M.A.

Union Republican Ministries of - Unionsrepublikanische Ministerien für - Sojuzno-respublikanskie Ministerstva:

Agriculture - Landwirtschaft - sel'skogo chozjajstva	- CHORUNŽIJ, M.V.
Coal Industry - Kohlenindustrie - ugol'noj promyšlennosti	- KOLESOV, O.A.
Communications - Post-u.Fernmeldewesen - svjazi	- SINČENKO, G.Z.
Construction of Heavy Industries Enterprises - Bau v.Betrieben d.Schwerindustrie - stroitel'stva predprijatij tjaželoj industrii	- LUBENEC, G.K.
Construction Materials Industry - Baustoffindustrie - promyšlennosti stroitel'nych materialov	- BAKLANOV, G.M.
Culture - Kultur - kul'tury	- BEZKLUBENKO, S.D.
Education - Volksbildung - prosveščenija	- MARINIČ, A.M.
Ferrous Metallurgy - Eisenhüttenindustrie - černoj metallurgii	- KULIKOV, Ja.P.
Finance - Finanzen - finansov	- BARANOVSKIJ, A.M.
Food Industry - Nahrungsmittelindustrie - piščevoj promyšlennosti	- SANOV, N.M.
Foreign Affairs - auswärtige Angelegenheiten - inostrannych del	- ŠEVEL, G.G.
Forestry - Forstwirtschaft - lesnogo chozjajstva	- LUKJANOV, B.N.
Geology - Geologie - geologii	- ŠPAK, P.F.
Health - Gesundheitswesen - zdravoochranenija	- ROMANENKO, A.E.
Higher and Secondary Specialized Education - Hochschul-u.mittl. Fachschulbildung - vysšego i srednego special'nogo obrazovanija	- EFIMENKO, G.G.
Industrial Construction - Industriebauwesen - promyšlennogo stroitel'stva	- AREŠKOVIČ, V.D.
Installation and Special Construction Work - Montage-u.Spezialbauarbeiten - montažnych i special'nych stroitel'nych rabot	- BAGRATUNI, G.R.
Internal Affairs - innere Angelegenheiten - vnutrennich del	- GOLOVČENKO, I.Ch.
Justice - Justiz - justicii	- ZAJČUK, V.I.
Land Reclamation and Water Resources - Melioration u.Wasserwirtschaft - melioracii i vodnogo chozjajstva	- GARKUŠA, N.A.
Light Industry - Leichtindustrie - legkoj promyšlennosti	- KASJANENKO, O.Ja.
Meat and Dairy Industry - Fleisch-u.Milchindustrie - mjasnoj i moločnoj promyšlennosti	- SENNIKOV, A.A.
Power and Electrification - Energiewirtschaft u.Elektrifizierungenergetiki i elektrifikacii	- MAKUCHIN, A.N.
Procurement - Beschaffungen - zagotovok	- ŠMATOLJAN, I.I.
Rural Construction - Landbauwesen - sel'skogo stroitel'stva	- KOTOV, Ju.B.
State Farms - Sowchose - sovchozov	- KOLOMIEC, Ju.P.

State Structure 4.4.2
Staatsordnung

Timber and Wood Processing Industry - Holz- u.holzbearbeitende
Industrie - lesnoj i derevoobrabatyvajuščej promyšlennosti — GRUNJANSKIJ, I.I.
Trade - Handel - torgovli — STARUNSKIJ, V.G.

Republican Ministries of - Republikanische Ministerien für - Respublikanskie Ministerstva:

Construction and Utilization of Roads - Bau und Nutzung der
Autobahnen - stroitel'stva i ekspluatacii avtomobil'nych dorog — ŠULGIN, N.P.
Consumer Services - Dienstleistungen - bytovogo
obsluživanija naselenija — ŠPAKOVSKIJ, L.K.
Housing and Municipal Services - Wohnungs-u.Kommunalwirtschaft -
žilisčno-kommunal'nogo chozjajstva — PLOSČENKO, V.D.
Local Industry - lokale Industrie - mestnoj promyšlennosti — GAEVSKIJ, Ju.F.
Motor Transport - Kraftverkehr - avtomobil'nogo transporta — GOLOVČENKO, F.D.
Social Security - Sozialfürsorge - social'nogo obespečenija — FEDOROV, A.F.

Chairman/Chief
Vorsitzender/Leiter
Predsedatel'Načalnik

State Planning Committee - Staatl. Plankomitee -
Gosudarstvennyj Planovyj komitet - GOSPLAN — ROZENKO, P.Ja.[1]
State Committee for Construction Affairs - Staatskomitee für
Bauwesen - Gosudarstvennyj komitet po delam stroitel'stva — ZLOBIN, G.K.
Committee for People's Control - Komitee für Volkskontrolle -
Komitet narodnogo kontrolja — KUCEVOL, V.S.
State Committee for Prices - Staatskomitee für Preispolitik -
Gosudarstvennyj komitet cen — ŠAMBORSKIJ, V.K.
State Committee for Cinematography - Staatskomitee f.Filmwesen -
Gosudarstvennyj komitet po kinematografii — BOLŠAK, V.G.
State Committee for Vocational and Technical Education -
Staatskomitee für berufstechnische Ausbildung - Gosudarstvennyj
komitet po professional'no-techničeskomu obrazovaniju — KOVALČUK, N.M.
State Committee for Publishing Houses, Printing Plants and the
Book Trade - Staatskomitee für Verlagswesen, Polygraphie und
Buchhandel - Gosudarstvennyj komitet po delam izdatel'stv,
poligrafii i knižnoj torgovli — PAŠČENKO, A.Ja.
State Committee for Labor - Staatskomitee für Arbeit -
Gosudarstvennyj komitet po trudu — PANTELEEV, N.A.
State Committee for Television and Radio Broadcasting -
Staatskomitee für Fernseh- und Rundfunkwesen -
Gosudarstvennyj komitet po televideniju i radioveščaniju — IVANENKO, B.V.
State Committee for the Protection of Nature - Staatskomitee
für Naturschutz - Gosudarstvennyj komitet po ochrane prirody — PROCENKO, D.Jo.
State Committee for the Supervision of Labor Safety in
Industry and Mining - Staatskomitee f.d.Überwachung
d.Arbeitssicherheit i.d.Industrie u.f.Bergwerksaufsicht -
Gosudarstvennyj komitet po nadzoru za bezopasnym vedeniem
rabot v promyšlennosti i gornomu nadzoru — DEGTJAREV, V.I.

State Committee for Materials and Technical Supply -
Staatskomitee für materiell-technische Versorgung -
Gosudarstvennyj komitet po material'no-techničeskomu snabženiju — MOSTOVOJ, P.I.
Committee for State Security - Komitee für Staatssicherheit -
Komitet gosudarstvennoj bezopasnosti — FEDORČUK, V.V.
State Committee for Production-Technological Supply in
Agriculture - Staatskomitee für produktionstechnische Ver-
sorgung der Landwirtschaft - Gosudarstvennyj komitet po proiz-
vodstvenno-techničeskom obespečeniju sel'skogo chozjajstva — MOMOTENKO, N.P.

---

[1] also Deputy Chairman of the Council of Ministers -
glz.stellv.Vorsitzender des Ministerrates

4.4.2 State Structure
4.4.3 Staatsordnung

Main Administration of Horticulture, Wine-growing and Wine
Industry - Hauptverwaltung für Gartenbau, Weinanbau und
Weinindustrie - Glavnoe upravlenie po sadovodstvu, vino-
gradarstvu i vinodel'noj promyšlennosti — LYSENKO, V.G.
Main Administration of the Petroleum Refining and Petro-
chemical Industry - Hauptverwaltung für erdölverarbeitende
Industrie und Petrochemie - Glavnoe upravlenie po nefteperera-
batyvajuščej i neftechimičeskoj promyšlennosti — LISNIČIJ, G.E.
Central Statistical Administration - Statistische Zentral-
verwaltung - Central'noe statističeskoe upravlenie — TROJAN, A.I.

4.4.3 Belorusskaja SSR

Supreme Soviet of the Belorussian SSR - Oberster Sowjet der Belorussischen SSR - Verchovnyj Sovet Belorusskoj SSR

Presidium-Präsidium-Prezidija

Chairman-Vorsitzender-Predsedatel'	- POLJAKOV, I.E.	
Deputy Chairmen-stellv.Vorsitzende-Zamestiteli predsedatelja	- BYČKOVSKAJA, Z.M.	LOBANOK, V.E.
Secretary-Sekretär-Sekretar'	- ČAGINA, E.P.	
Presidium members-Mitglieder des Präsidiums-Členy prezidiuma	- AKSENOV, A.N.	MAŠEROV, P.M.
	CEKUNOVA, R.S.	MATJUŠEVSKIJ, K.V.
	CHUSAINOV, Ju.M.	RUBIS, P.E.
	DEBALJUK, A.V.	SALENIK, K.P.
	KABJAK, S.T.	SUCHIJ, N.A.
	KOVALEV, M.V.	TJABUT, D.V.
	MACHNAČ, A.S.	ŽURBILO, L.N.
	MASLAKOV, A.V.	
Chairman of the Supreme Soviet - Vorsitzender des Obersten Sowjets - Predsedatel'Verchovnogo Soveta	- ŠAMJAKIN, I.P.	
Deputies-Stellvertreter-Zamestiteli	- CAGELNIK, A.K.	PASAMANOVA, E.N.
	GORBAČ, F.S.	STAROVOJTOV, V.K.

Council of Ministers of the Belorussian SSR - Ministerrat der Belorussischen SSR - Sovet Ministrov Belorusskoj SSR

Chairman-Vorsitzender-Predsedatel'	- KISELEV, T.Ja.	
First Deputy-Erster Stellvertreter-Pervyj Zamestitel'	- MICKEVIČ, V.F.	
Deputies-Stellvertreter-Zamestiteli	- CHITRUN, L.I.	GVOZDEV, V.A.
	DANILOV, D.A.	KOLOKOLOV, Ju.B.
	GLAZKOV, I.M.	PILOTOVIČ, S.A.
		SNEŽKOVA, N.L.

Union Republican Ministries of - Unionsrepublikanische Ministerien für - Sojuzno-respublikanskie Ministerstva:

Agriculture - Landwirtschaft - sel'skogo chozjajstva	- KOZLOV, V.A.
Communications - Post-u.Fernmeldewesen - svjazi	- AFANASEV, P.V.
Construction Materials Industry - Baustoffindustrie - promyšlennosti stroitel'nych materialov	- TARASOV, M.P.

144

State Structure 4.4.3
Staatsordnung

Culture - Kultur - kul'tury	- MICHNEVIČ, Ju.M.
Education - Volksbildung - prosveščenija	- MINKEVIČ, M.G.
Finance - Finanzen - finansov	- SATILO, B.J.
Food Industry - Nahrungsmittelindustrie - piščevoj promyšlennosti	- EREJ, A.I.
Foreign Affairs - auswärtige Angelegenheiten - inostrannych del	- GURINOVIČ, A.E.
Forestry - Forstwirtschaft - lesnogo chozjajstva	- MOISEENKO, S.T.
Health - Gesundheitswesen - zdravoochranenija	- SAVČENKO, N.E.
Higher and Secondary Specialized Education - Hochschul-u.mittl. Fachschulbildung - vysšego i srednego special'nogo obrazovanija	- MEŠKOV, N.M.
Industrial Construction - Industriebauwesen - promyšlennogo stroitel'stva	- ARCHIPEC, N.T.
Installation and Special Construction Work - Montage-u.Spezialbauarbeiten - montažnych i special'nych stroitel'nych rabot	- ANTONOVIČ, Jo.A.
Internal Affairs - innere Angelegenheiten - vnutrennich del	- KLIMOVSKOJ, A.A.
Justice - Justiz - justicii	- ZDANOVIČ, A.A.
Land Reclamation and Water Resources - Melioration und Wasserwirtschaft - melioracii i vodnogo chozjajstva	- PAVLJUČUK, V.Jo.
Light Industry - Leichtindustrie - legkoj promyšlennosti	- NAGIBOVIČ, L.N.
Meat and Dairy Industry - Fleisch-u.Milchindustrie - mjasnoj i moločnoj promyšlennosti	- BAVRIN, V.I.
Procurement - Beschaffungen - zagotovok	- KALITKO, A.Ja.
Rural Construction - Landbauwesen - sel'skogo stroitel'stva	- DANILENKO, V.D.
Timber and Wood Processing Industry - Holz-u.holzbearbeitende Industrie - lesnoj i derevoobrabatyvajuščej promyšlennosti	- KIJKOV, A.Ja.
Trade - Handel - torgovli	- MOLOČKO, N.P.
Republican Ministries of - Republikanische Ministerien für - Respublikanskie Ministerstva:	
Construction and Utilization of Highways - Bau u.Nutzung der Autobahnen - stroitel'stva i ekspluatacii avtomobil'nych dorog	- ŠARAPOV, V.I.
Consumer Services - Dienstleistungen - bytovogo obsluživanija naselenija	- GRIB, A.L.
Fuel Industry - Brennstoffindustrie - toplivnoj promyšlennosti	- FILIPPOV, G.A.
Housing and Municipal Services - Wohnungs-u.Kommunalwirtschaft - žilišcno-kommunal'nogo chozjajstva	- BEZLJUDOV, A.Jo.
Local Industry - lokale Industrie - mestnoj promyšlennosti	- RUSAKOV, L.V.
Motor Transport - Kraftverkehr - avtomobil'nogo transporta	- ANDREEV, A.E.
Social Security - Sozialfürsorge - social'nogo obespečenija	- LUZGIN, V.I.
	Chairman/Chief Vorsitzender/Leiter Predsedatel'/Načalnik
State Planning Committee - Staatl. Plankomitee - Gosudarstvennyj Planovyj komitet - GOSPLAN	- GVOZDEV, V.A.[1]
State Committee for Construction Affairs - Staatskomitee für Bauwesen - Gosudarstvennyj komitet po delam stroitel'stva	- KOROL, V.A.
Committee for People's Control - Komitee für Volkskontrolle - Komitet narodnogo kontrolja	- LAGIR, M.I.
State Committee for Labor - Staatskomitee für Arbeit - Gosudarstvennyj komitet po trudu	- ROMMA, F.D.

[1] also Deputy Chairman of the Council of Ministers - glz.stellv.Vorsitzender des Ministerrates

4.4.3 State Structure
4.4.4 Staatsordnung

State Committee for Television and Radio Broadcasting - Staatskomitee für Fernseh- und Rundfunkwesen - Gosudarstvennyj komitet po televideniju i radioveŝč niju	- PUCILEV, S.M.
State Committee for Cinematography - Staatskomitee für Filmwesen - Gosudarstvennyj komitet po kinematografii	- MATVEEV, V.V.
State Committee for Prices - Staatskomitee für Preispolitik - Gosudarstvennyj komitet cen	- ŽDANKO, G.S.
State Committee for Publishing Houses, Printing Plants and the Book Trade - Staatskomitee für Verlagswesen, Polygraphie und Buchhandel - Gosudarstvennyj komitet po delam izdatelstv, poligrafii i knižnoj torgovli	- DELEC, M.I.
State Committee for Vocational and Technical Education - Staatskomitee für berufstechnische Ausbildung - Gosudarstvennyj komitet po professional'no-techničeskomu obrazovaniju	- MAKSIMOV, L.G.
State Committee for the Protection of Nature - Staatskomitee für Naturschutz - Gosudarstvennyj komitet po ochrane prirody	- VORONCOV, A.I.
State Committee for Materials and Technical Supply - Staatskomitee für materiell-technische Versorgung - Gosudarstvennyj komitet po material'no-techničeskogo snabženija	- NEGERIŠ, E.F.
Committee for State Security - Komitee für Staatssicherheit - Komitet gosudarstvennoj bezopasnosti	- NIKULKIN, Ja.P.
State Committee for Production-Technological Supply in Agriculture - Staatskomitee für produktionstechnische Versorgung der Landwirtschaft - Gosudarstvennyj komotet po proizvodstvenno-techničeskom obespečeniju sel'skogo chozjajstva	- POŽARSKIJ, B.M.
Central Statistical Administration - Statistische Zentralverwaltung - Central'noe statističeskoe upravlenie	- ČERVANEV, D.L.
Main Administration for Gasification - Hauptverwaltung für Gasifizierung - Glavnoe upravlenie gazifikacii	- CAJKA, E.M.

4.4.4 Uzbekskaja SSR

Supreme Soviet of the Uzbek SSR - Oberster Sowjet der Usbekischen SSR - Verchovnyj Sovet Uzbekskoj SSR

Presidium-Präsidium-Prezidija

Chairman-Vorsitzender-Predsedatel'	- MATČANOV, N.M.	
Deputy Chairmen-stellv.Vorsitzende-Zamestiteli predsedatelja	- ABDALIN, A.S.	EŠIMBETOV, D.
Secretary-Sekretär-Sekretar'	- PULATOVA, Ch.M.	
Presidium members-Mitglieder des Präsidiums-Členy prezidiuma	- ACHUNBABAEV, K.Ju. ATAKUZIEV, R. CHVAN, M.-G.G. GAFURŽANOV, E.G. JUSUPOV, P.Ju. KADYROV, A.M. KARAMATOVA, M. KAZIMOV, V.A.	MACHMUDOVA, N.M. MUCHSINOVA, T.K. MUJDINOV, M. RAŠIDOV, S.R. ŠEVELEV, P.F. SIVEC, V.N. USMANCHODŽAEV, I.B. VLADIMIROVA, A.M.
Chairman of the Supreme Soviet - Vorsitzender des Obersten Sowjets - Predsedatel'Verchovnogo Soveta	MACHMUDOVA, T. - SIRAŽDUNOV, S.Ch.	
Deputies-Stellvertreter-Zamestiteli	- CHALMATOV, I. CHALMURATOV, P.	ISRAILOVA, Z. NOVOSELOV, V.D.

State Structure 4.4.4
Staatsordnung

Council of Ministers of the Uzbek SSR - Ministerrat der Usbekischen SSR - Sovet Ministrov Uzbekskoj SSR

Chairman-Vorsitzender-Predsedatel'	- CHUDAJBERDYEV, N.D.
First Deputy-Erster Stellvertreter-Pervyj Zamestitel'	- OSETROV, T.N.
Deputies-Stellvertreter-Zamestiteli	- ABDULLAEVA, R.Ch. MAMARASULOV, S.
	ACHMEDOV, K.A. MUCHORTOV, M.D.
	CHODŽAEV, A.R. TURSUNOV, M.T.

Union Republican Ministries of - Unionsrepublikanische Ministerien für - Sojuzno-respublikanskie Ministerstva:

Agriculture - Landwirtschaft - sel'skogo chozjajstva	- URKINBAEV, A.A.
Communications - Post-u.Fernmeldewesen - svjazi	- TOCHTAEV, T.M.
Construction - Bauwesen - stroitel'stva	- OMEROV, S.A.
Cotton Cleaning Industry - Baumwollreinigungsindustrie - chlopkoočistitel'noj promyšlennosti	- USMANOV, V.
Construction Materials Industry - Baustoffindustrie - promyšlennosti stroitel'nych materialov	- MIRZABEKOV, B.G.
Culture - Kultur - kul'tury	- NADŽIMOV, G.
Education - Volksbildung - prosveščenija	- ŠERMUCHAMEDOV, S.
Finance - Finanzen - finansov	- MURATCHODŽAEV, V.M.
Food Industry - Nahrungsmittelindustrie - piščevoj promyšlennosti	- SADYKOV, V.
Foreign Affairs - auswärtige Angelegenheiten - inostrannych del	- TURSUNOV, M.T.[1]
Forestry - Forstwirtschaft - lesnogo mozjajstva	- TAIROV, S.M.
Geology - Geologie - geologii	- TULJAGANOV, Ch.T.
Health - Gesundheitswesen - zdravoochranenija	- ZAIROV, K.S.
Higher and Secondary Specialized Education - Hochschul-u.mittl. Fachschulbildung - vysšego i srednego special'nogo obrazovanija	- ABDURACHMANOV, G.
Installation and Special Construction Work - Montage-u.Spezialbauarbeiten - montažnych i special'nych stroitel'nych rabot	- BORODAVKO, I.K.
Internal Affairs - innere Angelegenheiten - vnutrennich del	- JACHJAEV, Ch.Ch.
Justice - Justiz - justicii	- VASIKOVA, M.S.
Land Reclamation and Water Resources - Melioration und Wasserwirtschaft - melioracii i vodnogo chozjajstva	- DŽURABEKOV, I.Ch.
Light Industry - Leichtindustrie - legkoj promyšlennosti	- KURBANOV, M.Ch.
Meat and Dairy Industry - Fleisch-und Milchindustrie - mjasnoj i moločnoj promyšlennosti	- MAMADŽANOV, Ju.
Power and Electrification - Energiewirtschaft und Elektrifizierung - energetiki i elektrifikacii	- CHAMIDOV, A.Ch.
Procurement - Beschaffungen - zagotovok	- AŠURALIEV, R.
Rural Construction - Landbauwesen - sel'skogo stroitel'stva	- NASYROV, Ch.M.
Trade - Handel - torgovli	- JUSUPOV, G.G.
Furniture and Wood Processing Industry - Möbel-und holzbearbeitende Industrie - mebel'noj i derevoobrabatyvajuščej promyšlennosti	- UMAROV, A.Ch.

Republican Ministries of - Republikanische Ministerien für - Respublikanskie Ministerstva:

Construction and Utilization of Roads - Bau und Nutzung der Autobahnen - stroitel'stva i ekspluatacii avtomobil'nych dorog	- KAJUMOV, A.K.

---

[1] also Deputy Chairman of the Council of Ministers - glz.stellv.Vorsitzender des Ministerrates

4.4.4 State Structure / Staatsordnung

Consumer Services – Dienstleistungen – bytovogo obsluživanija naselenija	– BRODOVA, A.I.
Municipal Services – Kommunalwirtschaft – kommunal'nogo chozjajstva	– ILJUCHIN, A.M.
Local Industry – lokale Industrie – mestnoj promyšlennosti	– NASREDDINOV, G.
Motor Transport – Kraftverkehr – avtomobil'nogo transporta	– GAVRILOV, A.F.
Social Security – Sozialfürsorge – social'nogo obespečenija	– SADYKOVA, V.S.

Chairman/Chief
Vorsitzender/Leiter
Predsedatel'/Načalnik

State Planning Committee – Staatliches Plankomitee – Gosudarstvennyj Planovyj komitet – GOSPLAN	– ACHMEDOV, K.A.[1]
State Committee for Construction Affairs – Staatskomitee für Bauwesen – Gosudarstvennyj komitet po delam stroitel'stva	– SKREBNEV, V.S.
Committee for People's Control – Komitee für Volkskontrolle – Komitet narodnogo kontrolja	– MACHMUDOV, N.
State Committee for Labor – Staatskomitee für Arbeit – Gosudarstvennyj komitet po trudu	– MURTAZAEV, K.
State Committee for Vocational and Technical Education – Staatskomitee für berufstechnische Ausbildung – Gosudarstvennyj komitet po professional'no-techničeskomu obrazovaniju	– KAJUMOV, P.
State Committee for Cinematography – Staatskomitee für Filmwesen – Gosudarstvennyj komitet po kinematografii	– ABDULLAEV, A.
State Committee for Fishery – Staatskomitee für Fischereiwirtschaft – Gosudarstvennyj komitet po rybnomu chozjajstvu	– MACHMUDOV, A.
State Committee for Publishing Houses, Printing Plants and the Book Trade – Staatskomitee für Verlagswesen, Polygraphie und Buchhandel – Gosudarstvennyj komitet po delam izdatel'stv, poligrafii i knižnoj torgovli	– ESENBAEV, Z.I.
State Committee on Prices – Staatskomitee für Preispolitik – Gosudarstvennyj komitet cen	– TADŽIEV, N.
State Committee for Television and Radio Broadcasting – Staatskomitee für Fernseh- und Rundfunkwesen – Gosudarstvennyj komitet po televideniju i radioveščaniju	– IBRAGIMOV, U.Ja.
Committee for State Security – Komitee für Staatssicherheit – Komitet gosudarstvennoj bezopasnosti	– MELKUMOV, L.N.
State Committee for Production-Technological Supply in Agriculture – Staatskomitee für produktionstechnische Versorgung der Landwirtschaft – Gosudarstvennyj komitet po proizvodstvenno-techničeskom obespečeniju sel'skogo chozjajstva	– SAFAROV, R.
State Committee for Gasification – Staatskomitee für Gasifizierung – Gosudarstvennyj komitet po gazifikacii	– ATADŽANOV, A.R.
Main Administration of Materials and Technical Supply – Hauptverwaltung für materiell-technische Versorgung – Glavnoe upravlenie material'no-techničeskogo snabženija	– ŠARIPOV, T.Ja.
Main Administration for Construction in Tashkent City – Hauptverwaltung für Bauwesen in der Stadt Taškent – Glavnoe upravlenie po stroitel'stvu v gorode Taškente	– NABIEV, T.
State-Cooperative Administration for Construction on Collective Farms – Staatliche Genossenschaftsvereinigung für Bauwesen in den Kolchosen – Gosudarstvenno-kooperativnoe ob'edinenie po stroitel'stvu v kolchozach "Uzkolchozstroj"	– AŠUROV, I.
Agrarian-Industrial Association for the Production, Procurement, Industrial Processing and Wholesale of Potatoes, Vegetables, Melons, Fruits and Grapes – Agrar-industrielle Vereinigung	

---
[1] Also Deputy Chairman of the Council of Ministers – glz.Stellv.Vorsitzender des Ministerrates

State Structure 4.4.4
Staatsordnung   4.4.5

für Produktion, Beschaffung, industrielle Verarbeitung und Engros-
Verkauf von Kartoffeln, Gemüse, Melonen, Obst und Weintrauben -
Agrarno-promyšlennoe ob'edinenie po proizvodstvu, zagotovkam,
promyšlennoj pererabotke i optovoj realizacii kartofelja,
ovoščej, bachčevych kul'tur, fruktov i vinograda
"Uzplodovošč"   - ALIMOV, A.A.
Central Statistical Administration - Statistische Zentral-
verwaltung - Central'noe statističeskoe upravlenie   - MACHMUDOV, S.M.

4.4.5 Kazachskaja SSR

Supreme Soviet of the Kazakh SSR - Oberster Sowjet der Kasachischen SSR - Verchovnyj Sovet Kazachskoj SSR

Presidium-Präsidium-Prezidija

Chairman-Vorsitzender-Predsedatel'   - NIJAZBEKOV, S.B.

Deputy Chairman-stellv.Vorsitzender-
 Zamestitel' predsedatelja   - --

Secretary-Sekretärin-Sekretar'   - ABAEVA, N.B.

Presidium members-Mitglieder des
 Präsidiums-Členy prezidiuma   - ALIMŽANOV, A.T.   KORKIN, A.G.
                                             BELALOV, I.M.   KULBAEVA, Ch.
                                             BORISOVA, L.A.   KUNAEV, D.A.
                                             EFREMOV, V.V.   MAKUŠEV, V.V.
                                             PLOTNIKOV, A.P.   MYRZAŠEV, R.
                                             GUKASOV, E.Ch.   ŠARF, I.I.
                                             IKSANOV, M.B.   TITENKOVA, G.N.
                                             ISMAGANBETOV, S.M.   TURGUMBAEV, K.S.
                                             IZDIKULOVA, R.
Chairman of the Supreme Soviet -
Vorsitzender des Obersten Sowjets -
Predsedatel'Verchovnogo Soveta   - IMAŠEV, S.N.

Deputies-Stellvertreter-Zamestiteli   - PODOJNIKOVA, N.I.   SARSENOVA, D.Ž.
                                             POCELUEV-SNEGIN, D.F.

Council of Ministers of the Kazakh SSR - Ministerrat der Kasachischen SSR - Sovet Ministrov Kasachskoj SSR

Chairman-Vorsitzender-Predsedatel'   - AŠIMOV, B.

First Deputies-Erste Stellvertreter-
 Pervye Zamestiteli   --   SMIRNOV, S.A.

Deputies-Stellvertreter-Zamestiteli   - BAŠMAKOV, E.F.   TAKEŽANOV, S.T.
                                             DŽIENBAEV, S.S.   ŽANYBEKOV, Š.
                                             KUBAŠEV, S.

Union Republican Ministries of - Unionsrepublikanische Ministerien für -
Sojuzno-respublikanskie Ministerstva:

Agriculture - Landwirtschaft - sel'skogo chozjajstva   - MOTORIKO, M.G.

Communications - Post-u.Fernmeldewesen - svjazi   - ELIBAEV, A.A.

Construction of Heavy Industry Enterprises - Bau von Betrieben
 der Schwerindustrie - stroitel'stva predprijatij tjaželoj
 promyšlennosti   - OL'KOV, N.P.
Culture - Kultur - kul'tury   - ERKIMBEKOV, Ž.

Education - Volksbildung - prosveščenija   - BALACHMETOV, K.B.

149

4.4.5 State Structure / Staatsordnung

Finance – Finanzen – finansov	– BAJSEITOV, R.S.
Fish Industry – Fischereiwirtschaft – rybnogo chozjajstva	– UTEGALIEV, I.M.
Food Industry – Nahrungsmittelindustrie – piščevoj promyšlennosti	-ZARICKIJ, E.E.
Foreign Affairs – auswärtige Angelegenheiten – inostrannych del	– BAZARBAEV, M.
Forestry – Forstwirtschaft – lesnogo chozjajstva	– ZAJCEV, A.M.
Geology – Geologie – geologii	– CAKABAEV, S.F.
Health – Gesundheitswesen – zdravoochranenija	– SARMANOV, T.S.
Higher and Secondary Specialized Education – Hochschul-und mittlere Fachschulbildung – vysšego i srednego special'nogo obrazovanija	– KATAEV, T.
Installation and Special Construction Work – Montage- und Spezialbauarbeiten – po montažnym i special'nym stroitel'nym rabotam	– ERŽANOV, B.M.
Internal Affairs – innere Angelegenheiten – vnutrennich del	– ESBULATOV, M.
Justice – Justiz – justicii	– DŽUSUPOV, B.
Land Reclamation and Water Economy – Melioration und Wasserwirtschaft – melioracii i vodnogo chozjajstva	– TYNYBAEV, A.A.
Light Industry – Leichtindustrie – legkoj promyšlennosti	– IBRAGIMOV, V.G.
Meat and Dairy Industry – Fleisch-und Milchindustrie – mjasnoj i moloČnoj promyšlennosti	– ALYBAEV, A.A.
Nonferrous Metallurgy – Buntmetallurgie – cvetnoj metallurgii	– GREBENJUK, V.A.
Power and Electrification – Energiewirtschaft und Elektrifizierung – energetiki i elektrifikacii	– BATUROV, T.I.
Procurement – Beschaffungen – zagotovok	– DAIROV, M.D.
Rural Construction – Landbauwesen – sel'skogo stroitel'stva	– MUSIN, K.N.
Timber and Wood Processing Industry – Holz- und holzbearbeitende Industrie – lesnoj i derevoobrabatyvajuščej promyšlennosti	– ALDERBAEV, M.
Trade – Handel – torgovli	– IVANOV, M.S.
Construction Materials Industry – Baustoffindustrie – promyšlennosti stroitel'nych materialov	– TREBUCHIN, F.V.

Republican Ministries of – Republikanische Ministerien für – Respublikanskie Ministerstva:

Consumer Services – Dienstleistungen – bytovogo obsluživanija naselenija	– KONAKBAEV, K.D.
Local Industry – lokale Industrie – mestnoj promyšlennosti	– MUCHAMED-RACHIMOV, T.G.
Motor Highways – Landstraßen – šossejnych dorog	– GONČAROV, L.B.
Motor Transport – Kraftverkehr – avtomobil'nogo transporta	– KADYRBAEV, V.K.
Municipal Services – Kommunalwirtschaft – kommunal'nogo chozjajstva	– ČERNYŠOV, A.I.
Social Security – Sozialfürsorge – social'nogo obespečenija	– OMAROVA, Z.S.

Chairman/Chief
Vorsitzender/Leiter
Predsedatel'/Načalnik

State Planning Committee – Staatl. Plankomitee – Gosudarstvennyj Planovyj komitet – GOSPLAN	– TAKEŽANOV, S.T.[1]
State Committee for Construction Affairs – Staatskomitee für Bauwesen – Gosudarstvennyj komitet po delam stroitel'stva	– BEKTEMISOV, A.I.

1 Also Deputy Chairman of the Council of Ministers – glz.stellv.Vorsitzender des Ministerrates

State Structure 4.4.5
Staatsordnung 4.4.6

Committee for People's Control - Komitee für Volkskontrolle -
Komitet narodnogo kontrolja   - KANCELJARISTOV, P.S.
State Committee for Publishing Houses, Printing Plants and the
Book Trade - Staatskomitee für Verlagswesen, Polygraphie und
Buchhandel - Gosudarstvennyj komitet po delam izdatel'stv,
poligrafii i knižnoj torgovli   - ELEUKENOV, Š.R.
State Committee for Labor - Staatskomitee für Arbeit -
Gosudarstvennyj komitet po trudu   - KASYMKANOV, A.K.
State Committee for Cinematography - Staatskomitee für
Filmwesen - Gosudarstvennyj komitet po kinematografii   - GALIMŽANOVA, L.G.
State Committee for the Supervision of Labor Safety in
Industry and Mining - Staatskomitee f.d.Überwachung
d.Arbeitssicherheit i.d.Industrie u.f.Bergwerksaufsicht -
Gosudarstvennyj komitet po nadzoru za bezopasnym vedeniem
rabot v promyšlennosti i gornomu nadzoru   · GALIMŽANOV, K.G.
State Committee for Vocational and Technical Education -
Staatskomitee für berufstechnische Ausbildung -
Gosudarstvennyj komitet po professional'no-techničeskomu
obrazovaniju   - ISABEKOV, A.
State Committee for Television and Radio Broadcasting -
Staatskomitee für Fernseh- und Rundfunkwesen -
Gosudarstvennyj komitet po televideniju i radioveščeniju   - CHASENOV, Ch.
State Committee on Prices - Staatskomitee für Preispolitik -
Gosudarstvennyj komitet cen   - NAKIPOV, Š.K.
Committee for State Security - Komitee für Staatssicherheit -
Komitet gosudarstvennoj bezopasnosti   - ŠEVČENKO, V.T.
Main Administration for Material and Technical Supply -
Hauptverwaltung für materiell-technische Versorgung -
Glavnoe upravlenie po material'no-techničeskom snabženiju   - TANKIBAEV, Ž.A.
State Committee for Production-Technological Supply in
Agriculture - Staatskomitee für produktionstechnische Versor-
gung der Landwirtschaft - Gosudarstvennyj komitet po proiz-
vodstvenno-techničeskom obespečeniju sel'skogo chozjajstva   - EGOROV, A.M.
Central Statistical Administration - Statistische Zentral-
verwaltung - Central'noe statističeskoe upravlenie   - TROCENKO, Z.P.

4.4.6 Gruzinskaja SSR

Supreme Soviet of the Georgian SSR - Oberster Sowjet der Georgischen
SSR - Verchovnyj Sovet Gruzinskoj SSR

Presidium-Präsidium-Prezidija

Chairman-Vorsitzender-Predsedatel'   - GILAŠVILI, P.G.

Deputy Chairmen-stellv.Vorsitzende-
Zamestiteli predsedatelja   - DIASAMIDZE, D.D.   ŠINKUBA, B.V.

Secretary-Sekretärin-Sekretar'   - LAŠKARAŠVILI, T.V.

Presidium members-Mitglieder des
Präsidiums-Členy prezidiuma   - CIKLAURI, A.N.   MARDANOV, G.I.
                                             DVALIŠVILI, D.N.   MEZVRIŠVILI, M.A.
                                             DŽAVACHIŠVILI, G.D.   SARTAVA, Ž.K.
                                             GAPRINDAŠVILI, C.D.   ŠEVARDNADZE, E.A.
                                             KARKARAŠVILI, Š.V.   TODUA, I.T.
                                             KOČOJAN, V.A.   ZURABAŠVILI, A.D.
                                             LOBŽANIDZE, B.F.   KVAČADZE, Z.A.

151

4.4.6 State Structure
Staatsordnung

Chairman of the Supreme Soviet – Vorsitzender des Obersten Sowjets – Predsedatel'Verchovnogo Soveta	– ABAŠIDZE, I.V.	
Deputies-Stellvertreter-Zamestiteli	– GURGENIDZE, N.V. KABULOVA, T.Š.	KARBA, O.N. VASADZE, Z.O.

Council of Ministers of the Georgian SSR – Ministerrat der Georgischen SSR – Sovet Ministrov Gruzinskoj SSR

Chairman-Vorsitzender-Predsedatel'	– PATARIDZE, Z.A.	
First Deputy-Erster Stellvertreter- Pervyj Zamestitel'	– KIKNADZE, Š.D.	
Deputies-Stellvertreter-Zamestiteli	– ČERKEZIJA, O.E. DŽAPARIDZE, E.M. GELDIAŠVILI, Z.V.	KEDIŠVILI, Ju.I. VADAČKORIJA, V.I.

Union Republican Ministries of – Unionsrepublikanische Ministerien für –
Sojuzno-respublikanskie Ministerstva:

Agriculture – Landwirtschaft – sel'skogo chozjajstva	– ČITANAVA, N.A.
Communications – Post-u.Fernmeldewesen – svjazi	– KOBACHIDZE, V.I.
Construction – Bauwesen – stroitel'stva	– MEDZMARIAŠVILI, N.A.
Construction Materials Industry – Baustoffindustrie – promyšlennosti stroitel'nych materialov	– LOLAŠVILI, O.I.
Culture – Kultur – kul'tury	– TAKTAKIŠVILI, O.V.
Education – Volksbildung – prošvešćenija	– KINKLADZE, O.D.
Finance – Finanzen – finansov	– ANANIAŠVILI, P.A.
Food Industry – Nahrungsmittelindustrie – piščevoj promyšl.	– KONCELIDZE, R.Ch.
Foreign Affairs – auswärtige Angelegenheiten – inostranych del	– KIKNADZE, Š.D.[1]
Forestry – Forstwirtschaft – lesnogo chozjajstva	– CALAGANIDZE, S.I.
Health – Gesundheitswesen – zdravoochranenija	– LEŽAVA, G.G.
Higher and Secondary Specialized Education – Hochschul-u.mittl. Fachschulbildung – vysšego i srednego special'nogo obrazovanija	–DŽIBLADZE, G.N.
Internal Affairs – innere Angelegenheiten – vnutrennich del	– KETILADZE, K.E.
Justice – Justiz – justicii	– SUČANAŠVILI, A.A.
Land Reclamation and Water Resources – Melioration u.Wasser- wirtschaft – melioracii i vodnogo chozjajstva	– GADELIJA, G.B.
Light Industry – Leichtindustrie – legkoj promyšlennosti	– GAMCEMLIDZE, G.P.
Meat and Dairy Industry – Fleisch-u.Milchindustrie – mjasnoj i moločnoj promyšlennosti	–
Procurement – Beschaffungen – zagotovok	– ČANUKVADZE, Š.I.
Rural Construction – Landbauwesen – sel'skogo stroitel'stva	– CHARATIŠVILI, Jo.A.
Timber and Woodworking Industry – Holz-u.holzbearbeitende Industrie – lesnoj i derevoobrabatyvajuščej promyšlennosti	– TITBERIDZE, Š.A.
Trade – Handel – torgovli	– MEGRELIŠVILI, M.A.

Republican Ministries of – Republikanische Ministerien für – Respublikanskie
Ministerstva:

Consumer Services – Dienstleistungen – bytovogo obsluživanija naselenija	– SOBOLEV, V.A.
Highways – Autobahnen – avtomobil'nych dorog	– ROBITAŠVILI, G.V.
Motor Transport – Kraftverkehr – avtomobil'nogo transporta	– DAVITAŠVILI, T.N.

1 Also Deputy Chairman of the Council of Ministers
glz.stellv.Vorsitzender des Ministerrates

State Structure 4.4.6
Staatsordnung

Housing and Municipal Services - Wohnungs-u.Kommunalwirt-
  schaft - Žiliščno-kommunal'nogo chozjajstva — VAŠADZE, N.G.
Local Industry - lokale Industrie - mestnoj promyšlennosti — MAGRADZE, M.K.
Social Security - Sozialfürsorge - social'nogo obespečenija — GARDABCHADZE, K.K.

                                                                                         Chairman/Chief
                                                                                         Vorsitzender/Leiter
                                                                                         Predsedatel'/Načalnik

State Planning Committee - Staatl. Plankomitee -
  Gosudarstvennyj Planovyj komitet - GOSPLAN — DŽAPARIDZE, E.M.[1]
State Committee for Construction Affairs - Staatskomitee für
  Bauwesen - Gosudarstvennyj komitet po delam stroitel'stva — MIZIANAŠVILI, G.Z.
Committee for People's Control - Komitee für Volkskontrolle -
  Komitet narodnogo kontrolja — MELKADZE, O.V.
State Committee for Science and Technology - Staatskomitee
  für Wissenschaft und Technik - Gosudarstvennyj komitet po
  nauke i technike — GVERDCITELI, I.G.
State Committee for Television and Broadcasting - Staats-
  komitee für Fernseh-u.Rundfunkwesen - Gosudarstvennyj
  komitet po televideniju i radioveščaniju — ENUKIDZE, G.N.
State Committee for Vocational and Technical Education -
  Staatskomitee f.berufstechnische Ausbildung - Gosudarstvennyj
  komitet po professional'no-techničeskomu obrazovaniju — ŠEVARDNADZE, I.A.
State Committee for Publishing Houses, Printing Plants and the
  Book Trade - Staatskomitee für Verlagswesen, Polygraphie und
  Buchhandel - Gosudarstvennyj komitet po delam izdatel'stv,
  poligrafii i knižnoj torgovli — ČIKVAIDZE, A.D.
State Committee for the Protection of Nature - Staatskomitee
  für Naturschutz - Gosudarstvennyj komitet po ochrane prirody — KAČARAVA, V.Ja.
State Committee for Cinematography - Staatskomitee für Film-
  wesen - Gosudarstvennyj komitet po kinematografii — DVALIŠVILI, A.A.
State Committee for Labor - Staatskomitee für Arbeit -
  Gosudarstvennyj komitet po trudu — DŽAPARIDZE, R.A.
State Committee for the Supervision of Labor Safety in
  Industry and Mining - Staatskomitee f.d.Überwachung
  d.Arbeitssicherheit i.d.Industrie u.f.Bergwerksaufsicht -
  Gosudarstvennyj komitet po nadzoru za bezopasnym vedeniem
  rabot v promyšlennosti i gornomu nadzoru — GAMCHARAŠVILI, A.G.
State Committee for Prices - Staatskomitee für Preispolitik -
  Gosudarstvennyj komitet cen — CIMAKURIDZE, K.S.
Committee for State Security - Komitee für Staatssicherheit -
  Komitet gosudarstvennoj bezopasnosti — INAURI, A.N.
State Committee for Production-Technological Supply in
  Agriculture - Staatskomitee für produktionstechnische Versor-
  gung der Landwirtschaft - Gosudarstvennyj komitet po proiz-
  vodstvenno-techničeskom obespečeniju sel'skogo chozjajstva — SARIŠVILI, D.E.
State Committee for Material and Technical Supply -
  Staatskomitee für materiell-technische Versorgung -
  Gosudarstvennyj komitet po material'no-techničeskogo snabžen. — BUADZE, A.I.
Main Administration of the Gas Industry - Hauptverwaltung
  für Gasifizierung - Glavnoe upravlenie po gazifikacii — --
Main Administration for Installation and Specialized
  Construction Work - Hauptverwaltung für Montage-u.Spezial-
  bauarbeiten - Glavnoe upravlenie montažnych i special'nych
  stroitel'nych rabot — BUCHRAŠVILI, Š.E.
Main Administration for the Industrial Construction - Hauptverwaltung für Investitionsbau - Glavnoe upravlenie
  kapital'nogo stroitel'stva — ZATUAŠVILI, B.A.
Central Statistical Administration - Statistische Zentralverwaltung - Central'noe statističeskoe upravlenie — BASARIJA, R.V.

---
[1] Also Deputy Chairman of the Council of Ministers
  glz.stellv.Vorsitzender des Ministerrates

153

4.4.7 State Structure
Staatsordnung

4.4.7 Azerbajdžanskaja SSR

Supreme Soviet of the Azerbaijan SSR - Oberster Sowjet der
Aserbaidschanischen SSR - Verchovnyj Sovet Azerbajdžanskoj SSR

Presidium-Präsidium-Prezidija

Chairman-Vorsitzender-Predsedatel'	- CHALILOV, K.A.o.	
Deputy Chairmen-stellv.Vorsitzende- Zamestiteli predsedatelja	- ALIEVA, S.A.k.	ASLANOV, A.A.
Secretary-Sekretärin-Sekretar'	- ABILOVA, G.A.k.	
Presidium members-Mitglieder des Präsidiums-Členy prezidiuma	- ACHMEDOVA, T.R. ALIEV, G.A.R.o. ALIEV, N.A. KIRILJUK, V.K. DADAŠEV, M.M.o. GADŽIEV, B.A.o. GRIGORJAN, S.A. GUSEJNOV, A.N.o.	GUSEJNOVA, F.R.k. ISMAILOV, V.A.o. KULIEV, I.B.o. MAMEDOV, I.A.o. NIKITIN, N.V. SULEJMANOV, A.A.o. USEJNOV, M.A.
Chairman of the Supreme Soviet - Vorsitzender des Obersten Sowjets - Predsedatel'Verchovnogo Soveta	- RUSTAM-ZADE, S.A.o.	
Deputies-Stellvertreter-Zamestiteli	- ADAMJAN, S.A. FATULLAEVA, F.A.k.	GORBAČEVA, A.A. SAFARALIEV, R.K.

Council of Ministers of the Azerbaijan SSR - Ministerrat der
Aserbaidschanischen SSR - Sovet Ministrov Azerbaidžanskoj SSR

Chairman-Vorsitzender-Predsedatel'	- IBRAGIMOV, A.I.	
First Deputy - Erster Stellvertreter - Pervyj Zamestitel'	- TATLIEV, S.B.o.	
Deputies-Stellvertreter-Zamestiteli	- KADIROV, A.M.o. GUSEJNOV, K.A.o. LEMBERANSKIJ, A.D.	RASIZADE, S.A.R.o. ŠČEGLOV, G.V.

Union Republican Ministries of - Unionsrepublikanische Ministerien für -
Sojuzno-respublikanskie Ministerstva:

Agriculture - Landwirtschaft - sel'skogo chozjajstva	- ASKEROV, M.G.o.
Communications - Post-u.Fernmeldewesen - svjazi	- RASULBEKOV, G.D.
Construction Materials Industry - Baustoffindustrie - promyšlennosti stroitel'nych materialov	- ISAEV, N.A.
Culture - Kultur - kul'tury	- BAGIROV, Z.N.o.
Education - Volksbildung - prosveščenija	- MECHTIZADE, M.M.
Finance - Finanzen - finansov	- BACHŠALIEV, B.G.o.
Food Industry - Nahrungsmittelindustrie - piščevoj promyšlennosti	- MAMEDOV, K.S.o.
Foreign Affairs - äußere Angelegenheiten - inostrannych del	- TAIROVA, T.A.
Health - Gesundheitswesen - zdravoochranenija	- ABDULLAEV, G.M.o.
Higher and Secondary Specialized Education - Hochschul-u.mittl. Fachschulbildung - vysšego i srednego special'nogo obrazovanija	-ALIEV, K.G.o.

State Structure 4.4.7
Staatsordnung

Industrial Construction - Industriebauwesen - promyšlennogo stroitel'stva	- PJATIBRAT, V.L.
Internal Affairs - innere Angelegenheiten - vnutrennich del	- --
Justice - Justiz - justicii	- MAMEDOV, A.A.o.
Land Reclamation and Water Resources - Melioration u.Wasserwirtschaft - melioracii i vodnogo chozjajstva	- RUSTAMOV, N.G.o.
Light Industry - Leichtindustrie - legkoj promyšlennosti	- MELIKOV, E.S.o.
Meat and Dairy Industry - Fleisch-und Milchindustrie - mjasnoj i močnoj promyšlennosti	- MAMEDOV, A.G.K.o.
Petroleum Refining and Petrochemical Industry - erdölverarbeitende Industrie und Petrochemie - neftepererabatyvajuščej i neftechimičeskoj promyšlennosti	- AKIMOV, K.A.o.
Procurement - Beschaffungen - zagotovok	- AZIZOV, S.G.o.
Rural Construction - Landbauwesen - sel'skogo stroitel'stva	- GUSEJN-ZADE, A.M.A.K.o.
Timber and Wood Processing Industry - Holz-u.holzbearbeitende Industrie - lesnoj i derevoobrabatyvajuščej promyšlennosti	- AJRIJAN, A.A.
Trade - Handel - torgovli	- ZEJNALOV, G.Ju.o.

Republican Ministries of - Republikanische Ministerien für - Respublikanskie Ministerstva:

Construction and Maintenance of Highways - Bau und Nutzung der Autobahnen - stroitel'stva i ekspluatacii avtomobil'nych dorog	- ASANOV, D.M.o.
Consumer Services - Dienstleistungen - bytovogo obsluživanija naselenija	- GASANOVA, Z.M.k.
Local Industry - lokale Industrie - mestnoj promyšlennosti	- ASADULLAEV, A.B.o.
Motor Transport - Kraftverkehr - avtomobil'nogo transporta	- BABAEV, M.A.o.
Municipal Services - Kommunalwirtschaft - kommunal'nogo chozjajstva	- TOPČIEV, A.R.
Social Security - Sozialfürsorge - social'nogo obespečenija	- KAZIEV, M.Ja.

Chairman/Chief
Vorsitzender/Leiter
Predsedatel'/Načalnik

State Planning Committee - Staatl. Plankomitee - Gosudarstvennyj Planovyj komitet - GOSPLAN	- KADIROV, A.M.o.[1]
State Committee for Construction Affairs - Staatskomitee für Bauwesen - Gosudarstvennyj komitet po delam stroitel'stva	- IZMAJLOV, Ja.A.A.
Committee for People's Control - Komitee für Volkskontrolle - Komitet narodnogo kontrolja	- EFENDIEV, G.Š.o.
State Committee for Vocational and Technical Education - Staatskomitee f.berufstechnische Ausbildung - Gosudarstvennyj komitet po professional'no-techničeskomu obrazovaniju	- ALLACHVERDIEV, T.A.-G.
State Committee for Labor - Staatskomitee für Arbeit - Gosudarstvennyj komitet po trudu	- KURMAKAEV, Z.A.
Committee for State Security - Komitee für Staatssicherheit - Komitet gosudarstvennoj bezopasnosti	- KRASILNIKOV, V.S.
State Committee for Forestry - Staatskomitee für Forstwirtschaft - Gosudarstvennyj komitet lesnogo chozjajstva	- MUSTAFAEV, M.G.
State Production Committee for Viticulture and Winemaking - Staatl.Produktionskomitee für Weinbau und Weinbereitung - Gosudarstvennyj proizvodstvennyj komitet po vinogradarstvu i vinodeliju	- RZAEV, Ju.K.
State Committee for the Protection of Nature - Staatskomitee für Naturschutz - Gosudarstvennyj komitet po ochrane prirody	- ADIGEZALOV, B.M.S.o.

[1] Also Deputy Chairman of the Council of Ministers
glz.stellv.Vorsitzender des Ministerrates

4.4.7 State Structure
4.4.8 Staatsordnung

State Committee for Television and Broadcasting - Staatskomitee
für Fernseh- und Rundfunkwesen - Gosudarstvennyj komitet po
televideniju i radioveščaniju — - JUSIFZADE, K.Ju.o.
State Committee for Cinematography - Staatskomitee für Film-
wesen - Gosudarstvennyj komitet po kinematografii — - KURBANOV, M.K.o.
State Committee for Publishing Houses, Printing Plants and the
Book Trade - Staatskomitee für Verlagswesen, Polygraphie und
Buchhandel - Gosudarstvennyj komitet po delam izdatelstv,
poligrafii i knižnoj torgovli — - ALLACHVERDIEV,M.A.o.
State Committee for Prices - Staatskomitee für Preispolitik -
Gosudarstvennyj komitet cen — - ZULFUGAROV, A.M.
Agrarian-Industrial Association for the Production, Procurement,
Industrial Processing and Sale of Vegetables and Fruits -
Agrar-industrielle Vereinigung für Produktion, Beschaffung,
Verarbeitung und Absatz von Gemüse und Obst - Agrarno-
promyšlennoe ob'edinenie po proizvodstvu, zagotovkam,
pererabotke i sbytu ovoščej i plodov "Azplodovoščprom" — - SAMIEV, I.S.
Main Administration for Material and Technical Supply -
Hauptverwaltung für materiell-technische Versorgung -
Glavnoe upravlenie po material'no-techničeskomu snabženiju — - GUSEJNOV, R.A.G.o.
Main Administration for Installation and Special Construction
Work - Hauptverwaltung für Montage-u.Spezialbauarbeiten -
Glavnoe upravlenie po montažnym i special'nym stroitel'nym
rabotam — - KJASIMOV, T.M.o.
Administration for Geology - Verwaltung für Geologie -
Upravlenie geologii — - ŠEKINSKIJ, E.M.M.
State Committee for Production-Technological Supply in
Agriculture - Staatskomitee für produktionstechnische Versor-
gung der Landwirtschaft - Gosudarstvennyj komitet po proiz-
vodstvenno-techničeskom obespečeniju sel'skogo chozjajstva — - MOLOTIEVSKIJ, L.A.
Association for Nonferrous Metallurgy - Verwaltung für
Buntmetallurgie - Ob'edinenie po cvetnoj metallurgii — - RIZAEV, K.N.o.
Central Statistical Administration - Statistische Zentral-
verwaltung - Central'noe statističeskoe upravlenie — - ABBASALIEV, S.k.o.

4.4.8 Litovskaja SSR

Supreme Soviet of the Lithuanian SSR - Oberster Sowjet der Litauischen SSR - Verchovnyj Sovet Litovskoj SSR

Presidium-Präsidium-Prezidija

Chairman-Vorsitzender-Predsedatel' — - BARKAUSKAS, A.S.

Deputy Chairmen-stellv.Vorsitzende-
Zamestiteli predsedatelja — - DIRŽINSKAITE-PILJUŠENKO, L.Ju.
                              MEŽELAITIS, E.B.

Secretary-Sekretär-Sekretar' — - NAUJALIS, S.S.

Presidium members-Mitglieder des
Präsidiums-Členy prezidiuma — - GRIŠKEVICIUS, P.P.   PETRONIS, P.P.
                                GURECKAS, J.J.   POVILAUSKAS, V.-P.
                                KULIKOV, Ju.I.   ŠPAKOVA, T.I.
                                MEŠKAUSKIENE, A.A.   VILEIKIS, A.A.P.
                                MIKUČIAUSKAS, V.K.   ZINKEVIČIENE, V.V.

Chairman of the Supreme Soviet -
Vorsitzender des Obersten Sowjets -
Predsedatel'Verchovnogo Soveta — - SONGAILA, R.-B.I.

Deputies-Stellvertreter-Zamestiteli — - GREIČUVIENE, Ja.P.   MARKEVICIENE, E.C.
                                        KORSAKAS, K.P.   SYČEV, G.A.

156

State Structure
Staatsordnung 4.4.8

Council of Ministers of the Lithuanian SSR - Ministerrat der Litauischen SSR - Sovet Ministrov Litovskoj SSR

Chairman-Vorsitzender-Predsedatel'	- MANIUŠIS, Jo.A.	
First Deputy - Erster Stellvertreter - Pervyj Zamestitel'	- KAIRIS, K.K.	
Deputies-Stellvertreter-Zamestiteli	- ČESNAVIČIUS, A.J.	RUSENKO, Ju.L.
	DROBNIS, A.A.	VAZALINSKAS, V.M.

Union Republican Ministries of - Unionsrepublikanische Ministerien für - Sojuzno-respublikanskie Ministerstva:

Agriculture - Landwirtschaft - sel'skogo chozjajstva — - GRIGALIUNAS, M.Ju.

Communications - Post-und Fernmeldewesen - svjazi — - ONAITIS, K.K.

Construction - Bauwesen - stroitel'stva — - SEŠPLAUKIS, B.A.

Construction Materials Industry - Baustoffindustrie - promyšlennosti stroitel'nych materialov — - JASIUNAS, S.P.
Culture - Kultur - kul'tury — - BELINIS, J.L.

Education - Volksbildung - prosveščenija — - RIMKUS, A.S.

Finance - Finanzen - finansov — - SIKORSKIS, R.A.

Food Industry - Nahrungsmittelindustrie - piščevoj promyšlennosti-DULSKAS, S.A.

Foreign Affairs - äußere Angelegenheiten - inostrannych del — - ZENKIAVIČIUS, V.

Forestry and Timber Industry - Forstwirtschaft u.Holzindustrie - lesnogo chozjajstva i lesnoj promyšlennosti — - LUKAŠEVIČIUS, V.-P.V.
Furniture and Woodworking Industry - Möbel-u.holzbearbeitende Industrie - mebel'noj i derevoobrabatyvajuščej promyšlennosti - KURIS, Povilas M.
Health - Gesundheitswesen - zdravoochranenija — - KLEIZA, V.-A.J.

Higher and Secondary Specialized Education - Hochschul-u.mittl. Fachschulbildung - vysšego i srednego special'nogo obrazovanija-ZABULIS, G.K.
Internal Affairs - innere Angelegenheiten - vnutrennich del — - MIKALAUSKAS, Ju.V.

Justice - Justiz - justicii — - KURIS, Pranas M.

Land Reclamation and Water Resources - Melioration und Wasserwirtschaft - melioracii i vodnogo chozjajstva — - VELIČKA, J.J.
Light Industry - Leichtindustrie - legkoj promyšlennosti — - RAMANAUSKAS, J.K.

Meat and Dairy Industry - Fleisch-u.Milchindustrie - mjasnoj i moločnoj promyšlennosti — - BUKLIS, M.V.
Procurement - Beschaffungen - zagotovok — - KARECKAS, L.J.

Rural Construction - Landbauwesen - sel'skogo stroitel'stva — - BAGDONAS, A.I.

Trade - Handel - torgovli — - MICKUNAS, P.P.

Republican Ministries of - Republikanische Ministerien für - Respublikanskie Ministerstva:

Consumer Services - Dienstleistungen - bytovogo obsluživanija naselenija — - PLECHAVIČIUS, K.P.
Local Industry - lokale Industrie - mestnoj promyšlennosti — - SIMENENKO, G.K.

Motor Transport and Roads - Kraftverkehr und Landstraßen - avtomobil'nogo transporta i šossejnych dorog — - ČERNIKOV, I.S.
Municipal Services - Kommunalwirtschaft - kommunal'nogo chozjajstva — - ŠERIS, Ju.M.
Social Security - Sozialfürsorge - social'nogo obespečenija — - PACEVIČIENE, Ja.B.

157

4.4.8 State Structure
4.4.9 Staatsordnung

Chairman/Chief
Vorsitzender/Leiter
Predsedatel'/Načalnik

State Planning Committee - Staatl. Plankomitee - Gosudarstvennyj Planovyj komitet - GOSPLAN — DROBNIS, A.A.[1]
State Committee for Construction Affairs - Staatskomitee für Bauwesen - Gosudarstvennyj komitet po delam stroitel'stva — AKSOMITAS, A.Ju.
Committee for People's Control - Komitee für Volkskontrolle - Komitet narodnogo kontrolja — BARAUSKAS, A.B.
State Committee for Labor - Staatskomitee für Arbeit - Gosudarstvennyj komitet po trudu — GAIGALAS, B.P.
State Committee for Cinematography - Staatskomitee für Filmwesen - Gosudarstvennyj komitet po kinematografii — JUŠKIS, E.Ju.
State Committee for Publishing Houses, Printing Plants and the Book Trade - Staatskomitee für Verlagswesen, Polygraphie und Buchhandel - Gosudarstvennyj komitet po delam izdatel'stv, poligrafii i knižnoj torgovli — NEKROŠIUS, Ju.P.
State Committee for Vocational and Technical Education - Staatskomitee f.berufstechnische Ausbildung - Gosudarstvennyj komitet po professional'no-techničeskomu obrazovaniju — MORKUNAS, V.A.
State Committee for Television and Broadcasting - Staatskomitee für Fernseh- und Rundfunkwesen - Gosudarstvennyj komitet po televideniju i radioveščaniju — JANUITIS, J.J.
State Committee for Prices - Staatskomitee für Preispolitik - Gosudarstvennyj komitet cen — GRUODIS, M.
Committee for State Security - Komitee für Staatssicherheit - Komitet gosudarstvennoj bezopasnosti — PETKEVIČIUS, Ju.Ju.
State Committee for Production-Technological Supply in Agriculture - Staatskomitee für produktionstechnische Versorgung der Landwirtschaft - Gosudarstvennyj komitet po proizvodstvenno-techničeskom obespečeniju sel'skogo chozjajstva — ZORSKAS, A.T.
Central Statistical Administration - Statistische Zentralverwaltung - Central'noe statističeskoe upravlenie — LENGVINAS, K.K.
Main Administration for Material and Technical Supply - Hauptverwaltung für materiell-technische Versorgung - Glavnoe upravlenie po material'no-techničeskomu snabženiju — KIRJUŠČENKO, Ja.V.

4.4.9 Moldavskaja SSR

Supreme Soviet of the Moldavian SSR - Oberster Sowjet der Moldauischen SSR - Verchovnyj Sovet Moldavskoj SSR

Presidium-Präsidium-Prezidija

Chairman-Vorsitzender-Predsedatel'	— ILJAŠENKO, K.F.	
Deputy Chairmen - stellv.Vorsitzende - Zamestiteli predsedatelja	— AFTENJUK, G.T.	BOTEZAT, I.F.
Secretary - Sekretär - Sekretar'	— MELNIK, A.V.	
Presidium members - Mitglieder des Präsidiums - Členy prezidiuma	— BODJUL, I.I. BOCU, P.P. ČUTAK, D.I. GOCHBERG, A.Ja. GUCU, I.T. KIŠLAR, A.S. KOCHANSKIJ, V.I.	MARJASOV, N.P. PETRAŠKU, V.G. PLAMADJALA, A.D. PLATONOVA, A.P. RJABČIČ, V.A. SOLOMKO, F.M.

---

[1] Also Deputy Chairman of the Council of Ministers glz.stellv.Vorsitzender des Ministerrates

State Structure 4.4.9
Staatsordnung

Chairman of the Supreme Soviet –
Vorsitzender des Obersten Sowjets –
Predsedatel' Verchovnogo Soveta   – LAZAREV, A.M.

Deputies-Stellvertreter-Zamestiteli   – PANČENKO, G.P.   PROCENKO, V.A.
                                           PEREGUDOVA, V.A.   STRUŽUK, E.F.

Council of Ministers of the Moldavian SSR – Ministerrat der Moldauischen SSR – Sovet Ministrov Moldavskoj SSR

Chairman-Vorsitzender-Predsedatel'   – GROSSU, S.K.

First Deputy – Erster Stellvertreter –
Pervyj Zamestitel'   – EREMEJ, G.I.

Deputies-Stellvertreter-Zamestiteli   – DOBYNDE, I.G.   STEPANOV, G.A.
                                           POLJAKOV, N.D.   USTJAN, I.G.

Union Republican Ministries of – Unionsrepublikanische Ministerien für –
Sojuzno-respublikanskie Ministerstva:

Agriculture – Landwirtschaft – sel'skogo chozjajstva   – BEREŽNOJ, I.N.

Communications – Post-und Fernmeldewesen – svjazi   – RUSSU, V.P.

Construction – Bauwesen – stroitel'stva   – ZBARAZSKIJ, V.V.

Construction Materials Industry – Baustoffindustrie –
promyšlennosti stroitel'nych materialov   – AKINFIEV, V.I.
Culture – Kultur – kul'tury   – KONSTANTINOV, A.S.

Education – Volksbildung – narodnogo obrazovanija   – KERDIVARENKO, V.A.

Finance – Finanzen – finansov   – ARPENTEV, V.A.

Food Industry – Nahrungsmittelindustrie – piščevoj promyšlennosti – ČEKOJ, A.I.

Foreign Affairs – äußere Angelegenheiten – inostrannych del   – GROSSU, S.K.[1]
Forestry – Forstwirtschaft – lesnogo chozjajstva   – VASALATIJ, G.I.
Health – Gesundheitswesen – zdravoochranenija   – DRAGANJUK, K.A.
Internal Affairs – innere Angelegenheiten – vnutrennich del   – BRADULOV, N.M.

Justice – Justiz – justicii   – VOLOSJUK, V.M.

Land Reclamation and Water Resources – Melioration u.Wasser-
wirtschaft – melioracii i vodnogo chozjajstva   – OLEKSIĆ, V.N.

Furniture and Wood Processing Industry – Möbel-u.holzbearbeitende
Industrie – mebel'noj i derevoobrabatyvajuščej promyšlennosti   – TERECHOV, B.P.
Light Industry – Leichtindustrie – legkoj promyšlennosti   – ŽITNJUK, G.M.

Meat and Dairy Industry – Fleisch-und Milchindustrie –
mjasnoj i moločnoj promyšlennosti   – TIUNOV, A.I.
Procurement – Beschaffungen – zagotovok   – TUSLOV, M.I.

Rural Construction – Landbauwesen – sel'skogo stroitel'stva   – JARUTIN, V.K.

Trade – Handel – torgovli   – ČOLAK, M.I.

Republican Ministries of – Republikanische Ministerien für – Respublikanskie
Ministerstva:

Construction and Utilization of Highways – Bau und Nutzung
der Autobahnen – stroitel'stva i ekspluatacii avtomobil'-
nych dorog   – BOLBAT, I.S.
Consumer Services – Dienstleistungen – bytovogo
obsluživanija naselenija   – KUSKEVIČ, I.V.
Local Industry – lokale Industrie – mestnoj promyšlennosti   – NEČAENKO, A.V.

---

[1] Also Deputy Chairman of the Council of Ministers
glz.stellv.Vorsitzender des Ministerrates

4.4.9 State Structure
Staatsordnung

Motor Transport - Kraftverkehr - avtomobil'nogo transporta	- FOMIN, V.M.
Municipal Services - Kommunalwirtschaft - kommunal'nogo chozjajstva	- POLOŽENKO, N.V.
Social Security - Sozialfürsorge - social'nogo obespečenija	- BYKOVA, O.V.

Chairman/Chief
Vorsitzender/Leiter
Predsedatel'/Načalnik

State Planning Committee - Staatl. Plankomitee - Gosudarstvennyj Planovyj komitet - GOSPLAN	- USTJAN, S.G.[1]
State Committee for Construction Affairs - Staatskomitee für Bauwesen - Gosudarstvennyj komitet po delam stroitel'stva	- GRAFOV, S.S.
Committee for People's Control - Komitee für Volkskontrolle - Komitet narodnogo kontrolja	- VORONIN, P.V.
State Committee for Prices - Staatskomitee für Preispolitik - Gosudarstvennyj komitet cen	- KUTYRKIN, V.G.
State Committee for Vocational and Technical Education - Staatskomitee f.berufstechnische Ausbildung - Gosudarstvennyj komitet po professional'no-techničeskomu obrazovaniju	- SIDORENKO, S.S.
State Committee for Labor - Staatskomitee für Arbeit - Gosudarstvennyj komitet po trudu	- JAKUBOVSKIJ, P.I.
State Committee for Television and Broadcasting - Staatskomitee für Fernseh- und Rundfunkwesen - Gosudarstvennyj komitet po televideniju i radioveščaniju	- LOZAN, S.I.
State Committee for the Protection of Nature - Staatskomitee für Naturschutz - Gosudarstvennyj komitet po ochrane prirody	- KOTJACY, I.A.
State Committee for Cinematography - Staatskomitee für Filmwesen - Gosudarstvennyj komitet po kinematografii	- IORDANOV, I.E.
State Committee for Publishing Houses, Printing Plants and the Book Trade - Staatskomitee für Verlagswesen, Polygraphie und Buchhandel - Gosudarstvennyj komitet po delam izdatel'stv, poligrafii i knižnoj torgovli	- CHROPOTINSKIJ, V.P.
Committee for State Security - Komitee für Staatssicherheit - Komitet gosudarstvennoj bezopasnosti	- RAGOZIN, A.P.
Agrarian-Industrial Association for Viticulture and Winemaking - Agrar-industrielle Vereinigung für Weinbau und Weinbereitung - Agrarno-promyšlennoe ob'edinenie po vinogradarstvu i vinodeliju	- LUKJANOV, N.N.
Agrarian-Industrial Association for the Production, Procurement, Industrial Processing and Sale of Vegetables and Fruits - Agrar-Industrielle Vereinigung für Produktion, Beschaffung, industrielle Verarbeitung und Verkauf von Gemüse und Obst - Agrarno-promyšlennoe ob'edinenie po proizvodstvu,zagotovkam,promyšlennoj pererabotke i sbytu ovoščej i fruktov	- IVAŠČUK, D.I.
State Committee for Production-Technological Supply in in Agriculture - Staatskomitee für produktionstechnische Versorgung der Landwirtschaft - Gosudarstvennyj komitet po proizvodstvenno-techničeskom obespečeniju sel'skogo chozjajstva	- BONDARENKO, M.V.
State Committee for Material and Technical Supply - Staatskomitee für materiell-technische Versorgung - Gosudarstvennyj komitet po material'no-techničeskomu snabženiju	- PARFENOV, V.G.
Agrarian-Industrial Association for the Cultivation, Processing and Sale of Tobacco - Agrar-industrielle Vereinigung für Zucht, Verarbeitung und Verkauf von Tabak - Agrarno-promyšlennoe ob'edinenie po tabaku	- VERBICKIJ, N.F.
Central Statistical Administration - Statistische Zentralverwaltung - Central'noe statističeskoe upravlenie	- KOZUB, K.I.

1 also Deputy Chairman of the Council of Ministers
glz.stellv.Vorsitzender des Ministerrates

State Structure
Staatsordnung 4.4.10

4.4.10 Latvijskaja SSR

Supreme Soviet of the Latvian SSR - Oberster Sowjet der Lettischen SSR - Verchovnyj Sovet Latvijskoj SSR

Presidium-Präsidium-Prezidija

Chairman-Vorsitzender-Predsedatel'	- STRAUTMANIS, P.Ja.	
Deputy Chairmen - stellv.Vorsitzende - Zamestiteli predsedatelja	- BLUM, V.A.	DRIZUL, A.A.
Secretary - Sekretär - Sekretar'	- ZORIN, K.E.	
Presidium Members - Mitglieder des Präsidiums - Členy prezidiuma	- GRAUDS, L.Ju. GRIGULIS, A.P. IKAUNIEKS, A.E. KALNBERZIN, Ja.E. KRONBERG, V.V.	LENEV, O.K. PLAUDE, A.K. VOSS, A.E. ZIEMELIS, G.K. DUBRA, M.Ja.
Chairman of the Supreme Soviet - Vorsitzender des Obersten Sowjets - Predsedatel' Verchovnogo Soveta	- KLIBIK, V.S.	
Deputies-Stellvertreter-Zamestiteli	- EGOROV, I.T.	ZVAIGZNE, D.Ja.

Council of Ministers of the Latvian SSR - Ministerrat der Lettischen SSR - Sovet Ministrov Latvijskoj SSR

Chairman-Vorsitzender-Predsedatel'	- RUBEN, Ju.Ja.	
First Deputy - Erster Stellvertreter - Pervyj Zamestitel'	- VERRO, R.O.	
Deputies-Stellvertreter-Zamestiteli	- BONDALETOV, I.V. KRUMIN, V.M.	PETERSON, E.K. RAMAN, M.L.

Union Republican Ministries of - Unionsrepublikanische Ministerien für - Sojuzno-respublikanskie Ministerstva:

Agriculture - Landwirtschaft - sel'skogo chozjajstva	- ANSPOK, K.S.
Communications - Post- und Fernmeldewesen - svjazi	- STUNGREVIC, O.K.
Construction - Bauwesen - stroitel'stva	- ULMANIS, I.N.
Construction Materials Industry - Baustoffindustrie - promyšlennosti stroitel'nych materialov	- DOROFEEV, N.I.
Culture - Kultur - kul'tury	- KAUPUŽ, V.I.
Education - Volksbildung - prosveščenija	- KARKLIN, M.Ja.
Finance - Finanzen - finansov	- PRAUDE, R.V.
Food Industry - Nahrungsmittelindustrie - piščevoj promyšlennosti	-KUZNECOVA, I.D.
Foreign Affairs - auswärtige Angelegenheiten - inostrannych del-	KRUMIN, V.M.[1]
Forestry and Timber Industry - Forstwirtschaft und Holzindustrie - lesnogo chozjajstva i lesnoj promyšlennosti	- VITOL, L.P.
Health - Gesundheitswesen - zdravoochranenija	- KANEP, V.V.
Internal Affairs - innere Angelegenheiten - vnutrennich del	- DROZD, M.F.
Justice - Justiz - justicii	- DZENITIS, Ja.E.

[1] Also Deputy Chairman of the Council of Ministers
glz.stellv.Vorsitzender des Ministerrates

161

4.4.10 State Structure / Staatsordnung

Land Reclamation and Water Resources - Melioration u.Wasser-
wirtschaft - melioracii i vodnogo chozjajstva — SAMOLEVSKIJ, V.N.
Light Industry - Leichtindustrie - legkoj promyšlennosti — JABLONSKIJ, E.Ja.

Higher and Secondary Specialized Education - Hochschul-u.mittl.
Fachschulbildung - vysšego i srednego special'nogo obrazovanija — LINDE, E.V.
Meat and Dairy Industry - Fleisch-und Milchindustrie -
mjasnoj i moločnoj promyšlennosti — VANNACH, S.E.
Procurement - Beschaffungen - zagotovok — GIRGENSON, Z.V.

Trade - Handel - torgovli — AZAN, V.D.

Wood-Working Industry - holzbearbeitende Industrie -
derevoobrabatyvajuščej promyšlennosti — BIRKENFELD, V.Ja.

Republican Ministries of - Republikanische Ministerien für - Respublikanskie Ministerstva:

Consumer Services - Dienstleistungen - bytovogo
obsluživanija naselenija — TUMOVS-BEKIS, Ja.D.
Local Industry - lokale Industrie - mestnoj promyšlennosti — ALTUCHOV, N.G.

Motor Transport and Highways - Kraftverkehr und Landstraßen - avtomobil'nogo transporta i šossejnych dorog — SLIEDE, E.E.
Municipal Services - Kommunalwirtschaft - kommunal'nogo
chozjajstva — BERZIN, I.P.
Social Security - Sozialfürsorge - social'nogo obespečenija — PICHELS, V.S.

Chairman/Chief
Vorsitzender/Leiter
Predsedatel'/Načalnik

State Planning Committee - Staatl. Plankomitee -
Gosudarstvennyj Planovyj komitet - GOSPLAN — RAMAN, M.L.[1]
State Committee for Construction Affairs - Staatskomitee für
Bauwesen - Gosudarstvennyj komitet po delam stroitel'stva — RUBINS, Ja.F.
Committee for People's Control - Komitee für Volkskontrolle -
Komitet narodnogo kontrolja — BEMAN, E.K.
State Committee for Labor - Staatskomitee für Arbeit -
Gosudarstvennyj komitet po trudu — LEONOVA, V.V.
State Committee for Vocational and Technical Education -
Staatskomitee f.berufstechnische Ausbildung - Gosudarstvennyj
komitet po professional'no-techničeskomu obrazovaniju — BRODELIS, Ja.Ja.
State Committee for Television and Broadcasting - Staats-
komitee für Fernseh- und Rundfunkwesen - Gosudarstvennyj
komitet po televideniju i radioveščaniju — BARTKEVIČ, L.L.
State Committee for Cinematography - Staatskomitee für Film-
wesen - Gosudarstvennyj komitet po kinematografii — RUDNEV, O.A.
State Committee for Publishing Houses, Printing Plants and
the Book Trade - Staatskomitee für Verlagswesen, Poly-
graphie und Buchhandel - Gosudarstvennyj komitet po delam
izdatel'stv, poligrafii i knižnoj torgovli — REIMANE, I.A.
State Committee for Prices - Staatskomitee für Preispolitik -
Gosudarstvennyj komitet cen — SEDOLS, V.I.
Committee for State Security - Komitee für Staatssicherheit -
Komitet qosudarstvennoj bezopasnosti — AVDJUKEVIČ, L.I.
State Committee for Production-Technological Supply in
Agriculture - Staatskomitee für produktionstechnische Versor-
gung der Landwirtschaft - Gosudarstvennyj komitet po proiz-
vodstvenno-techničeskom obespečeniju sel'skogo chozjajstva — BABKIN, N.A.
State Committee for Material and Technical Supply - Staats-
komitee für materiell-technische Versorgung - Gosudarstvennyj
komitet po material'no-techničeskogo snabženija — PROŠKOVIČ, Ju.L.
Central Statistical Administration - Statistische Zentralverwaltung - Central'noe statističeskoe upravlenie — BALTIN, G.A.

[1] Also Deputy Chairman of the Council of Ministers -
glz.stellv.Vorsitzender des Ministerrates

State Structure 4.4.11
Staatsordnung

4.4.11 Kirgizskaja SSR

Supreme Soviet of the Kirgiz SSR - Oberster Sowjet der Kirgisischen SSR - Verchovnyj Sovet Kirgizskoj SSR

Presidium-Präsidium-Prezidija

Chairman-Vorsitzender-Predsedatel'	- IBRAIMOV, S.I.	
Deputy Chairmen - stellv.Vorsitzende - Zamestiteli predsedatelja	- AJTIEV, G.	BUSS, A.A.
Secretary - Sekretärin - Sekretar'	- TUMENBAEVA, D.	
Presidium members - Mitglieder des Präsidiums - Členy prezidiuma	- ALYMBEKOV, N.	DMITRIEV, A.I.
	ČYNYBAEV, K.	MOLDOBAEV, K.M.
	DŽOLDOŠEVA, A.	SULAJMANOVA, K.
	GANIN, P.A.	TRUŠKINA, M.N.
	KOŠOEV, T.Ch.	USUBALIEV, T.U.
	LEBEDEVA, R.I.	
Chairman of the Supreme Soviet - Vorsitzender des Obersten Sowjets - Predsedatel' Verchovnogo Soveta	- TABYŠALIEV, S.	
Deputies-Stellvertreter-Zamestiteli	- KRAVČENKO, P.I.	MUKAŠEVA, K.

Council of Ministers of the Kirgiz SSR - Ministerrat der Kirgisischen SSR - Sovet Ministrov Kirgizskoj SSR

Chairman-Vorsitzender-Predsedatel'	- SUJUMBAEV, A.S.	
First Deputy - Erster Stellvertreter - Pervyj Zamestitel'	- CHODOS, P.M.	
Deputies-Stellvertreter-Zamestiteli	- BEGMATOVA, S.	MOISEEV, S.G.
	BEGALIEV, S.	PONOMAREV, O.B.

Union Republican Ministries of - Unionsrepublikanische Ministerien für - Sojuzno-respublikanskie Ministerstva:

Agriculture - Landwirtschaft - sel'skogo chozjajstva	- TURSUNOV, S.T.
Communications - Post-und Fernmeldewesen - svjazi	- TJUREBAEV, V.N.
Construction - Bauwesen - stroitel'stva	- KUZNECOV, A.N.
Construction Materials Industry - Baustoffindustrie - promyšlennosti stroitel'nych materialov	- BESSMERTNYJ, I.S.
Culture - Kultur - kul'tury	- KONDUČALOVA, K.
Education - Volksbildung - narodnogo obrazovanija	-
Finance - Finanzen - finansov	- TOKTONALIEV, A.
Food Industry - Nahrungsmittelindustrie - piščevoj promyšlennosti	- USMANOV, R.B.
Foreign Affairs - auswärtige Angelegenheiten - inostrannych del	- BEGMATOVA, S.[1]
Health - Gesundheitswesen - zdravoochranenija	- PETROSJANC, V.A.
Internal Affairs - innere Angelegenheiten - vnutrennich del	- GABIDULIN, A.K.
Justice - Justiz - justicii	- DŽUMABAEV, M.A.

1 Also Deputy Chairman of the Council of Ministers - glz.stellv.Vorsitzender des Ministerrates

163

4.4.11 State Structure / Staatsordnung

Land Reclamation and Water Resources - Melioration u.Wasserwirtschaft - melioracii i vodnogo chozjajstva	- KOŽOMKULOV, A.
Light Industry - Leichtindustrie - legkoj promyšlennosti	- SATAROV, K.
Meat and Dairy Industry - Fleisch-und Milchindustrie - mjasnoj i moločnoj promyšlennosti	- SUETOV, I.G.
Procurement - Beschaffungen - zagotovok	- OROZBEKOV, T.
Rural Construction - Landbauwesen - sel'skogo stroitel'stva	- KIM, N.K.
Trade - Handel - torgovli	- ATAŠEV, K.K.

Republican Ministries of - Republikanische Ministerien für - Respublikanskie Ministerstva:

Consumer Services - Dienstleistungen - bytovogo obsluživanija naselenija	- DADABAEV, Ch.
Local Industry - lokale Industrie - mestnoj promyšlennosti	- KONURBAEV, M.O.
Motor Transport and Highways - Kraftverkehr und Landstraßen - avtomobil'nogo transporta i šossejnych dorog	- CHILIMONČIK, V.P.
Municipal Services - Kommunalwirtschaft - kommunal'nogo chozjajstva	- DŽUMANALIEV, K.
Social Security - Sozialfürsorge - social'nogo obespečenija	- SALIEVA, B.
	Chairman/Chief Vorsitzender/Leiter Predsedatel'/Načalnik
State Planning Committee - Staatl. Plankomitee - Gosudarstvennyj Planovyj komitet - GOSPLAN	- BEGALIEV, S.[1]
State Committee for Construction Affairs - Staatskomitee für Bauwesen - Gosudarstvennyj komitet po delam stroitel'stva	- CHOCHLAČEV, M.E.
Comitee for People's Control - Komitee für Volkskontrolle - Komitet narodnogo kontrolja	- MINIČ, N.G.
State Committee for Labor - Staatskomitee für Arbeit - Gosudarstvennyj komitet po trudu	- ENDOVICKIJ, M.V.
State Committee for Forestry - Staatskomitee für Forstwirtschaft - Gosudarstvennyj komitet lesnogo chozjajstva	- BEKBAEV, D.B.
State Committee for Vocational and Technical Education - Staatskomitee f.berufstechnische Ausbildung - Gosudarstvennyj komitet po professional'no-techničeskomu obrazovaniju	- KASENDEEV, I.
State Committee for Television and Broadcasting - Staatskomitee für Fernseh-und Rundfunkwesen - Gosudarstvennyj komitet po televideniju i radioveščaniju	- TOKOMBAEV, A.
State Committee for Cinematography - Staatskomitee für Filmwesen - Gosudarstvennyj komitet po kinematografii	- BAJALINOV, M.K.
State Committee for Publishing Houses, Printing Plants and the Book Trade - Staatskomitee für Verlagswesen, Polygraphie und Buchhandel - Gosudarstvennyj komitet po delam izdatel'stv, poligrafii i knižnoj torgovli	- ABAKIROV, A.
State Committee for Prices - Staatskomitee für Preispolitik - Gosudarstvennyj komitet cen	- ČONOEV, A.
Committee for State Security - Komitee für Staatssicherheit - Komitet gosudarstvennoj bezopasnosti	- LOMOV, N.P.
State Committee for Production-Technological Supply in Agriculture - Staatskomitee für produktionstechnische Versorgung der Landwirtschaft - Gosudarstvennyj komitet po proizvodstvenno-techničeskom obespečeniju sel'skogo chozjajstva	- IVANČENKO, M.L.
State Committee for Material and Technical Supply - Staatskomitee für materiell-technische Versorgung - Gosudarstvennyj komitet po material'no-techničeskom snabženiju	- PITENKOV, N.A.
Central Statistical Administration - Statistische Zentralverwaltung - Central'noe statističeskoe upravlenie	- ALMAEV, T.M.

[1] Also Deputy Chairman of the Council of Ministers - glz.stellv.Vorsitzender des Ministerrates

State Structure
Staatsordnung 4.4.12

4.4.12 Tadžikskaja SSR

Supreme Soviet of the Tadzhik SSR - Oberster Sowjet der Tadschikischen SSR - Verchovnyj Sovet Tadžikskoj SSR

Presidium-Präsidium-Prezidija

Chairman-Vorsitzender-Predsedatel'	- CHOLOV, M.	
Deputy Chairmen - stellv.Vorsitzende - Zamestiteli predsedatelja	- OPLANČUK, V.Ja.	ZARIPOVA, N.
Secretary - Sekretär - Sekretar'	- GADOEV, D.	
Presidium members - Mitglieder des Präsidiums - Členy prezidiuma	- ASURALIEV, F. JUSUPOV, A. KASIMOV, U. KOZLOVA, V.I. KURBANOVA, R. MACHMADALIEV, M.	MAMADNAZAROV, Ch. MUCHAMEDOV, D. RADŽABOV, Ch. RASULOV, D. USMANOV, U.G.
Chairman of the Supreme Soviet - Vorsitzender des Obersten Sowjets - Predsedatel' Verchovnogo Soveta	- DŽURAEV, K.S.	
Deputies-Stellvertreter-Zamestiteli	- ALOVIDDINOV, U.A.	SODYEVA, Z.

Council of Ministers of the Tadzhik SSR - Ministerrat der Tadschikischen SSR - Sovet Ministrov Tadžikskoj SSR

Chairman-Vorsitzender-Predsedatel'	- NABIEV, R.	
First Deputy - Erster Stellvertreter - Pervyj Zamestitel'	- NOVIČKOV, V.E.	
Deputies-Stellvertreter-Zamestiteli	- JUSUFBEKOV, R. MACHKAMOV, K.	MAKSUMOV, A.N.

Union Republican Ministries of - Unionsrepublikanische Ministerien für - Sojuzno-respublikanskie Ministerstva:

Agriculture - Landwirtschaft - sel'skogo chozjajstva	- ZAIROV, M.
Communications - Post-und Fernmeldewesen - svjazi	- POPOV, D.I.
Construction - Bauwesen - stroitel'stva	- ŠARIPOV, M.
Construction Materials Industry - Baustoffindustrie - promyšlennosti stroitel'nych materialov	- ŠEVČENKO, I.V.
Culture - Kultur - kul'tury	- NAZAROV, M.N.
Education - Volksbildung - narodnogo obrazovanija	- DADABOEV, R.
Finance - Finanzen - finansov	- LAFIZOV, D.
Food Industry - Nahrungsmittelindustrie - piščevoj promyšlennosti	- KURBANOV, I.I.
Foreign Affairs - auswärtige Angelegenheiten - inostrannych del	- NABIEV, R.
Health - Gesundheitswesen - zdravoochranenija	- SAŽENIN, I.A.
Internal Affairs - innere Angelegenheiten - vnutrennich del	- ABDULCHAKOV, N.
Justice - Justiz - justicii	- RADŽABOV, S.

165

4.4.12 State Structure / Staatsordnung

Land Reclamation and Water Resources - Melioration u.Wasserwirtschaft - melioracii i vodnogo chozjajstva	- KASIMOV, A.
Light Industry - Leichtindustrie - legkoj promyšlennosti	- MIR CHALIKOV, T.
Meat and Dairy Industry - Fleisch-und Milchindustrie - mjasnoj i močnoj promyšlennosti	- CHAEEV, I.
Procurement - Beschaffungen - zagotovok	- JACHŠIBAEV, U.
Rural Construction - Landbauwesen - sel'skogo stroitel'stva	- GAFUROV, R.
Trade - Handel - torgovli	- GRIŠINA, R.M.

Republican Ministries of - Republikanische Ministerien für - Respublikanskie Ministerstva:

Consumer Services - Dienstleistungen - bytovogo obsluživanija naselenija	- KASYMOVA, A.T.
Local Industry - lokale Industrie - mestnoj promyšlennosti	- BAJMATOV, A.
Municipal Services - Kommunalwirtschaft - kommunal'nogo chozjajstva	- KURBANOV, R.M.
Social Security - Sozialfürsorge - social'nogo obespečenija	- RACHIMOVA, A.M.
Transportation and Roads - Transport und Straßenwesen - transporta i dorožnogo chozjajstva	- JAKUBOV, N.Ch.

	Chairman/Chief Vorsitzender/Leiter Predsedatel'/Načalnik
State Planning Committee - Staatl. Plankomitee - Gosudarstvennyj Planovyj komitet - GOSPLAN	- MACHKAMOV, K.[1]
State Committee for Construction Affairs - Staatskomitee für Bauwesen - Gosudarstvennyj komitet po delam stroitel'stva	- AVGITOV, L.G.
State Committee for Forestry - Staatskomitee für Forstwirtschaft - Gosudarstvennyj komitet lesnogo chozjajstva	- ZACHVATOV, V.E.
Committee for People's Control - Komitee für Volkskontrolle - Komitet narodnogo kontrolja	- KARMYŠEV, L.
State Committee for Publishing Houses, Printing Plants and the Book Trade - Staatskomitee für Verlagswesen, Polygraphie und Buchhandel - Gosudarstvennyj komitet po delam izdatel'stv, poligrafii i knižnoj torgovli	- PULATOV, S.
State Committee for Cinematography - Staatskomitee für Filmwesen - Gosudarstvennyj komitet po kinematografii	- SAIDOV, S.
State Committee for Labor - Staatskomitee für Arbeit - Gosudarstvennyj komitet po trudu	- NARZIBEKOV, M.
State Committee for Vocational and Technical Education - Staatskomitee f.berufstechnische Ausbildung - Gosudarstvennyj komitet po professional'no-techničeskomu obrazovaniju	- CHASANOV, K.G.
State Committee for Television and Broadcasting - Staatskomitee für Fernseh-und Rundfunkwesen - Gosudarstvennyj komitet po televideniju i radioveščaniju	- KALANDAROV, G.
State Committee for Prices - Staatskomitee für Preispolitik - Gosudarstvennyj komitet cen	- RAFIEV, M.M.
Committee for State Security - Komitee für Staatssicherheit - Komitet gosudarstvennoj bezopasnosti	- PERVENCEV, E.I.
State Committee for Material and Technical Supply - Staatskomitee für materiell-technische Versorgung - Gosudarstvennyj komitet po material'no-techničeskom snabženiju	- MERZAEV, B.A.
Main Administration for Production, Processing and Sale of Fruit, Vegetables, Melons and Potatoes - Hauptverwaltung für Produktion, Verarbeitung und Verkauf von Obst, Gemüse, Melonen und Kartoffeln - Glavnoe upravlenie po proizvodstvu, zagotovke, pererabotke i realizacii fruktov, ovoščej, bachčevych kul'tur i kartofelja	- CHAKNAZAROV, S.

[1] Also Deputy Chairman of the Council of Ministers - glz.stellv.Vorsitzender des Ministerrates

State Structure 4.4.12
Staatsordnung 4.4.13

State Committee for Production-Technological Supply in
Agriculture - Staatskomitee für produktionstechnische Versor-
gung der Landwirtschaft - Gosudarstvennyj komitet po proiz-
vodstvenno-techničeskom obespečeniju sel'skogo chozjajstva — BABAEV, A.M.
Administration of Geology - Verwaltung für Geologie -
Upravlenie geologii — KOSLAKOV, G.V.
Administration of the Cotton-Cleaning Industry -
Verwaltung für die Baumwollreinigungsindustrie -
Upravlenie chlopkoočistitel'noj promyšlennosti — KOBILOV, U.
Central Statistical Administration - Statistische Zentral-
verwaltung - Central'noe statističeskoe upravlenie — KAPUSTIN, E.D.
Agrarian-Industrial Association for Fruit-Culture, Viticulture
and Winemaking - Agrar-industrielle Vereinigung für Obstbau,
Weinbau und Weinbereitung - Agrarno-promyšlennoe ob'edinenie
po plodovodstvu, vinogradarstvu i vinodeliju — KASIMOV, M.

4.4.13 Armjanskaja SSR

Supreme Soviet of the Armenian SSR - Oberster Sowjet der Armenischen SSR - Verchovnyj Sovet Armjanskoj SSR

Presidium-Präsidium-Prezidija

Chairman-Vorsitzender-Predsedatel'   — SARKISOV, B.E.

Deputy Chairmen - stellv.Vorsitzende -
Zamestiteli predsedatelja   — BAGDASARJAN, O.M.   BAJRAMOV, M.B.o.

Secretary - Sekretär - Sekretar'   — BACHČINJAN, M.M.

Presidium members - Mitglieder des
Präsidiums - Členy prezidiuma   — AJRAPETJAN, A.A.   DAVTJAN, P.M.
                                            ANDREASJAN, A.M.   DEMIRČJAN, K.S.
                                            ARUTJUNJAN, D.A.   DOLABČJAN, Z.L.
                                            ARUTJUNJAN, V.F.   MANUKJAN, A.G.
                                            ASATRJAN, N.O.   MINASJAN, R.A.
                                            AVETISJAN, S.S.   PETROSJAN, S.D.
                                            CHANDŽJAN, G.S.   VARDIKJAN, B.D.
Chairman of the Supreme Soviet -   OGANJAN, G.A.
Vorsitzender des Obersten Sowjets -   SARKISJAN, A.G.
Predsedatel' Verchovnogo Soveta   — AMBARCUMJAN, S.A.

Deputies-Stellvertreter-Zamestiteli   — ARAKELJAN, A.G.   NUŽNYJ, V.I.
                                            MSTOJAN, M.A.

Council of Ministers of the Armenian SSR - Ministerrat der Armenischen SSR - Sovet Ministrov Armjanskoj SSR

Chairman-Vorsitzender-Predsedatel'   — SARKISJAN, F.T.

First Deputy - Erster Stellvertreter -
Pervyj Zamestitel'   — KIRAKOSJAN, A.M.

Deputies-Stellvertreter-Zamestiteli   — AJRAPETJAN, G.A.   SAGOJAN, G.S.
                                            GAMBARJAN, K.A.   SVETLOVA, R.Ch.
                                            MOVSESJAN, V.M.

Union Republican Ministries of - Unionsrepublikanische Ministerien für -
Sojuzno-respublikanskie Ministerstva:

Agriculture - Landwirtschaft - sel'skogo chozjajstva   — TARDŽUMANJAN, G.V.

Communications - Post-und Fernmeldewesen - svjazi   — MINASJANC, T.S.

Construction Materials Industry - Baustoffindustrie -
promyšlennosti stroitel'nych materialov   — VARTANJAN, G.O.
Culture - Kultur - kul'tury   — PARSAMJAN, R.O.

Education - Volksbildung - prosveščenija   — ACHUMJAN, S.T.

4.4.13 State Structure
Staatsordnung

Finance - Finanzen - finansov	- DŽANOJAN, D.A.
Food Industry - Nahrungsmittelindustrie - piščevoj promyšlennosti	- ARAKELJAN, S.V.
Foreign Affairs - auswärtige Angelegenheiten - inostrannych del-	KIRAKOSJAN, A.M.[1]
Health - Gesundheitswesen - zdravoochranenija	- GABRIELJAN, E.S.
Higher and Secondary Spezialized Education - Hochschul-u.mittl. Fachschulbildung - vysšego i srednego special'nogo obrazovanija-	GARIBDŽANJAN, L.P.
Industrial Construction - Industriebauwesen - promyšlennogo stroitel'stva	- AKOPJAN, K.A.
Internal Affairs - innere Angelegenheiten - vnutrennich del	- PATALOV, E.G.
Justice - Justiz - justicii	- GEVORKJAN, A.A.
Land Reclamation and Water Resources - Melioration u.Wasserwirtschaft - melioracii i vodnogo chozjajstva	- SAGOJAN, R.A.
Light Industry - Leichtindustrie - legkoj promyšlennosti	- GEVORKJAN, A.A.
Meat and Dairy Industry - Fleisch-und Milchindustrie - mjasnoj i moločnoj promyšlennosti	- VARTANJAN, S.A.
Procurement - Beschaffungen - zagotovok	- OVAKIMJAN, O.T.
Rural Construction - Landbauwesen - sel'skogo stroitel'stva	- TATEVOSJAN, G.A.
Timber and Wood Processing Industry - Holz-und holzbearbeitende Industrie - lesnoj i derevoobrabatyvajuščej promyšlennosti	- STEPANJAN, A.A.
Trade - Handel - torgovli	- SAFARJAN, S.R.

Republican Ministries of - Republikanische Ministerien für - Respublikanskie Ministerstva:

Construction and Utilization of Highways - Bau und Nutzung der Autobahnen - stroitel'stva i ekspluatacii avtomobil'nych dorog	- MELKUMJAN, G.A.
Consumer Services - Dienstleistungen - bytovogo obslužzivanija naselenija	- TUMANJAN, S.A.
Local Industry - lokale Industrie - mestnoj promyšlennosti	- ZURABJAN, M.A.
Motor Transport - Kraftverkehr - avtomobil'nogo transporta	- DRAMPJAN, Ch.A.
Municipal Services - Kommunalwirtschaft - kommunal'nogo chozjajstva	-
Social Security - Sozialfürsorge - social'nogo obespečenija	- GALSTJAN, R.S.

Chairman/Chief
Vorsitzender/Leiter
Predsedatel'/Načalnik

State Planning Committee - Staatl. Plankomitee - Gosudarstvennyj Planovyj komitet - GOSPLAN	- SAGOJAN, G.S.[1]
State Committee for Construction Affairs - Staatskomitee für Bauwesen - Gosudarstvennyj komitet po delam stroitel'stva	- MARUTJAN, K.A.
Committee for People's Control - Komitee für Volkskontrolle - Komitet narodnogo kontrolja	- MARTIROSJAN, G.A.
State Committee for Utilization and Conservation of Surface and Underground Water Resources - Staatskomitee für Nutzung und Schutz der Wasserreserven auf und im Erdboden - Gosudarstvennyj komitet po ispol'zovaniju i ochrane poverchostnych i podzemnych vodnych resursov	- MOVSESJAN, K.M.
State Committee for Labor - Staatskomitee für Arbeit - Gosudarstvennyj komitet po trudu	- OGANESJAN, O.G.
State Committee for Cinematography - Staatskomitee für Filmwesen - Gosudarstvennyj komitet po kinematografii	- AJRJAN, G.A.
State Committee for Forestry - Staatskomitee für Forstwirtschaft - Gosudarstvennyj komitet lesnogo chozjajstva	- AVAKJAN, G.A.

1 Also Deputy Chairman of the Council of Ministers - glz.stellv.Vorsitzender des Ministerrates

State Structure 4.4.13
Staatsordnung 4.4.14

State Committee for Publishing Houses, Printing Plants and
 the Book Trade - Staatskomitee für Verlagswesen, Polygraphie
 und Buchhandel - Gosudarstvennyj komitet po delam izdatel'stv,
 poligrafii i knižnoj torgovli   - BAGDASARJAN, S.B.
State Committee for Vocational and Technical Education -
 Staatskomitee f.berufstechnische Ausbildung - Gosudarstvennyj
 komitet po professional'no-techničeskomu obrazovaniju   - MIKAELJAN, S.A.
State Committee for Television and Broadcasting - Staats-
 komitee für Fernseh- und Rundfunkwesen - Gosudarstvennyj
 komitet po televideniju i radioveščaniju   - POGOSJAN, S.K.
State Committee for Prices - Staatskomitee für Preis-
 politik - Gosudarstvennyj komitet cen   - ARUTJUNJAN, G.T.
Committee for State Security - Komitee für Staatssicherheit -
 Komitet gosudarstvennoj bezopasnosti   - JUZBASJAN, M.A.
State Committee for the Supervision of Labor Safety in
 Industry and Mining - Staatskomitee f.d.Überwachung
 d.Arbeitssicherheit i.d.Industrie u.f.Bergwerksaufsicht -
 Gosudarstvennyj komitet po nadzoru za bezopasnym vedeniem
 rabot v promyšlennosti i gornomu nadzoru   - GASPARJAN, G.A.
State Committee for Production-Technological Supply in
 Agriculture - Staatskomitee für produktionstechnische Versor-
 gung der Landwirtschaft - Gosudarstvennyj komitet po proiz-
 vodstvenno-techničeskom obespečeniju sel'skogo chozjajstva   - NAVASARDJAN, G.G.
Main Administration of Material and Technical Supply -
 Hauptverwaltung für materiell-technische Versorgung -
 Glavnoe upravlenie po material'no-techničeskomu snabženiju   - ASCATRJAN, E.T.
Main Administration for Installation and Special Construction
 Projects - Hauptverwaltung für Montage- und Spezialbau-
 arbeiten - Glavnoe upravlenie po montažnym i special'nym
 stroitel'nym rabotam   - GAMBARJAN, G.O.
Administration of Geology - Verwaltung für Geologie -
 Upravlenie po geologii   - GULJAN, E.Ch.
Administration of Nonferrous Metallurgy - Verwaltung für
 Buntmetallurgie - Upravlenie cvetnoj metallurgii   - PETROSJAN, F.A.
Main Administration for Gasification - Hauptverwaltung für
 Gasifizierung - Glavnoe upravlenie gazifikacii   - MUTAFJAN, St.G.
Central Statistical Administration - Statistische Zentral-
 verwaltung - Central'noe statističeskoe upravlenie   - PACHLEVANJAN, G.A.

4.4.14 Turkmenskaja SSR

Supreme Soviet of the Turkmen SSR - Oberster Sowjet der Turkmenischen SSR - Verchovnyj Sovet Turkmenskoj SSR

Presidium-Präsidium-Prezidija

Chairman-Vorsitzender-Predsedatel'   - KLYČEV, A.

Deputy Chairmen - stellv.Vorsitzende -
 Zamestiteli predsedatelja   - KARRYEVA, R.M.   TELKOV, N.T.

Secretary - Sekretärin - Sekretar'   - NAZAROVA, O.

Presidium members - Mitglieder des
 Präsidiums - Členy prezidiuma   - AKGAEV, A.   IVANOV, V.S.
                                              AMANBERDYEV, K.   MICHAJLOV, V.V.
                                              ATDAEV, Ch.   PIRKULIEV, A.
                                              CHAKIMOV, D.   POLIKAROVA, M.S.
                                              IŠANKULIEVA, D.I.   URAEV, K.
                                              GAPUROV, M.G.

---

1 Also Deputy Chairman of the Council of Ministers -
 glz.stellv.Vorsitzender des Ministerrates

169

4.4.14 State Structure
Staatsordnung

Chairman of the Supreme Soviet -
Vorsitzender des Obersten Sowjets -
Predsedatel' Verchovnogo Soveta — - DURDYEV, A.A.

Deputies-Stellvertreter-Zamestiteli — - ANNAEVA, S.   MIŠČENKO, G.S.

Council of Ministers of the Turkmen SSR - Ministerrat der Turkmenischen SSR - Sovet Ministrov Turkmenskoj SSR

Chairman-Vorsitzender-Predsedatel'   - JAZKULIEV, B.

First Deputy - Erster Stellvertreter -
Pervyj Zamestitel'   - BURAŠNIKOV, B.F.

Deputies-Stellvertreter-Zamestiteli   - ABRAMOV, V.E.   SUJUNOV, N.T.
    BAZAROVA, R.A.   ŽULENEV, V.F.

Union Republican Ministries of - Unionsrepublikanische Ministerien für -
Sojuzno-respublikanskie Ministerstva:

Agriculture - Landwirtschaft - sel'skogo chozjajstva   - SACHATMURADOV, K.

Communications - Post- und Fernmeldewesen - svjazi   - ABDYKERIMOV, A.

Culture - Kultur - kul'tury   - ESENOV, R.M.

Education - Volksbildung - prosveščenija   - PALVANOVA, B.

Finance - Finanzen - finansov   - SUCHANOV, CH.

Food Industry - Nahrungsmittelindustrie - piščevoj promyšl.   - NURMUCHAMEDOV, R.

Foreign Affairs - auswärtige Angelegenheiten - inostrannych del-JAZKULIEV, B.[1]

Construction Affairs - Bauwesen - stroitel'stva   - ŠEREMETEV, N.V.

Construction Materials Industry - Baustoffindustrie -
promyšlennosti stroitel'nych materialov   - BRJUŠKOV, I.V.
Cotton-Cleaning Industry - Baumwollreinigungsindustrie -
chlopkoočistitel'noj promyšlennosti   - IZOTOV, V.D.
Health - Gesundheitswesen - zdravoochranenija   - CHODŽAKULIEV, G.

Higher and Secondary Specialized Education - Hochschul-u.mittl.
Fachschulbildung-vysšego i srednego special'nogo obrazovanija-   --
Internal Affairs - innere Angelegenheiten - vnutrennich del   - BERDYEV, R.N.

Justice - Justiz - justicii   - AJMAMEDOV, A.

Land Reclamation and Water Resources - Melioration u.Wasser-
wirtschaft - melioracii i vodnogo chozjajstva   - ATAEV, K.
Light Industry - Leichtindustrie - legkoj promyšlennosti   - CHANAEV, K.

Meat and Dairy Industry - Fleisch- und Milchindustrie -
mjasnoj i moločnoj promyšlennosti   - GUKASOV, S.B.
Procurement - Beschaffungen - zagotovok   - BABAEV, S.

Rural Construction - Landbauwesen - sel'skogo stroitel'stva   - GULMANOV, B.

Trade - Handel - torgovli   - RYBALOV, E.G.

Republican Ministries of - Republikanische Ministerien für - Respublikanskie
Ministerstva:

Consumer Services - Dienstleistungen - bytovogo
obsluživanija naselenija   - CHODŽAMAMEDOV, K.
Local industry - lokale Industrie - mestnoj promyšlennosti   - BAJMACHANOVA, A.
Motor Transport and Highways - Kraftverkehr und Landstraßen -
avtomdil'nogo transporta i šossejnych dorog   - GURBANGELDYEV, Ch
Municipal Services - Kommunalwirtschaft - kommunal'nogo
chozjajstva   - ORAZMAMEDOV, S.
Social Security - Sozialfürsorge - social'nogo obespečenija   - MAMEDOVA, D.

State Structure 4.4.14
Staatsordnung

Chairman/Chief
Vorsitzender/Leiter
Predsedatel'/Načalnik

State Planning Committee - Staatl. Plankomitee -
Gosudarstvennyj Planovyj komitet - GOSPLAN — ABRAMOV, V.E.[1]
State Committee for Construction Affairs - Staatskomitee
für Bauwesen - Gosudarstvennyj komitet po delam stroitel'stva — ORAZMUCHAMEDOV, N.
Committee for People's Control - Komitee für Volkskontrolle -
Komitet narodnogo kontrolja — MAKARKIN, N.V.
State Committee for Television and Broadcasting - Staatskomitee für Fernseh- und Rundfunkwesen - Gosudarstvennyj
komitet po televideniju i radioveščaniju — ANNAKURBANOV, Č.
State Committee for Cinematography - Staatskomitee für
Filmwesen - Gosudarstvennyj komitet po kinematografii — REDŽEPOV, P.
State Committee for Forestry - Staatskomitee für Forstwirtschaft - Gosudarstvennyj komitet lesnogo chozjajstva — FROLOV, M.I.
State Committee for Publishing Houses, Printing Plants and
the Book Trade - Staatskomitee für Verlagswesen, Polygraphie und Buchhandel - Gosudarstvennyj komitet po delam
izdatel'stv, poligrafii i knižnoj torgovli — BADAEV, M.B.
State Committee for Vocational and Technical Education -
Staatskomitee f.berufstechnische Ausbildung - Gosudarstvennyj
komitet po professional'no-techničeskomu obrazovaniju — CHODŽAEV, E.
State Committee for Labor - Staatskomitee für Arbeit -
Gosudarstvennyj komitet po trudu — ALOVOV, N.
State Committee for Prices - Staatskomitee für Preispolitik -
Gosudarstvennyj komitet cen — ORAZOV, N.
Committee for State Security - Komitee für Staatssicherheit -
Komitet gosudarstvennoj bezopasnosti — KISELEV, Ja.P.
State Committee for Production-Technological Supply in
Agriculture - Staatskomitee für produktionstechnische Versorgung der Landwirtschaft - Gosudarstvennyj komitet po proizvodstvenno-techničeskom obespečeniju sel'skogo chozjajstva — ASLANOV, A.I.
State Committee for the Supervision of Labor Safety in
Industry and Mining - Staatskomitee f.d.Überwachung der
Arbeitssicherheit i.d.Industrie und für Bergwerksaufsicht -
Gosudarstvennyj komitet po nadzoru za bezopasnym vedeniem
rabot v promyšlennosti i gornomu nadzoru — KLYČEV, N.-D.
State Committee for Material and Technical Supply - Staatskomitee für materiell-technische Versorgung - Gosudarstvennyj
komitet po material'no-techničeskom snabženiju — ZUBRILIN, A.F.
Administration for Geology - Verwaltung für Geologie -
Upravlenie po geologii — --
Main Administration for Gasification - Hauptverwaltung für
Gasifizierung - Glavnoe upravlenie gazifikacii — SABASANOV, M.K.
Agrarian-Industrial Association for Production, Procurement,
Processing and Sale of Vegetables, Potatoes, Melons and
Berries - Agrar-Industrielle Vereinigung für Produktion,
Beschaffung, Verarbeitung und Verkauf von Gemüse, Kartoffeln,
Melonen und Beeren - Agrarno-promyšlennoe ob'edinenie po
proizvodstvu, zagotovkam, pererabotke i realizacii ovoščej,
kartofelja, bachčevych i plodojagodnych kul'tur —
Central Statistical Administration - Statistische Zentralverwaltung - Central'noe statističeskoe upravlenie — SAFARMAMEDOV, A.S.

---

1 Also Deputy Chairman of the Council of Ministers -
glz.stellv.Vorsitzender des Ministerrates

171

4.4.15 State Structure / Staatsordnung

4.4.15 Estonskaja SSR

Supreme Soviet of the Estonian SSR - Oberster Sowjet der Estnischen SSR - Verchovnyj Sovet Estonskoj SSR

Presidium-Präsidium-Prezidija

Chairman-Vorsitzender-Predsedatel'	- KEBIN, I.G.	
Deputy Chairmen - stellv.Vorsitzende - Zamestiteli predsedatelja	- RJUJTEL, A.F.	VANNAS, M.V.
Secretary - Sekretär - Sekretar'	- VACHT, V.A.	
Presidium members - Mitglieder des Präsidiums - Členy prezidiuma	- BEEKMAN, V.E.	NYMMIK, E.A.
	ILVES, H.I.	TAAL, A.E.
	KANTE, E.K.	TOOME, I.H.
	VAJNO, K.G.	VOCHMJANINA, G.K.
	LEBEDEV, K.V.	
Chairman of the Supreme Soviet - Vorsitzender des Obersten Sowjets - Predsedatel' Verchovnogo Soveta	- LOTT, I.A.	
Deputies - Stellvertreter - Zamestiteli	- ECHALA, E.S.	TIKK, V.A.

Council of Ministers of the Estonian SSR - Ministerrat der Estnischen SSR - Sovet Ministrov Estonskoj SSR

Chairman-Vorsitzender-Predsedatel'	- KLAUSON, V.I.	
First Deputy - Erster Stellvertreter - Pervyj Zamestitel'	- TYNURIST, E.G.	
Deputies-Stellvertreter-Zamestiteli	- GREN, A.K.	SAUL, B.E.
	TREGUBOV, A.I.	TYNSPOEG, G.A.

Union Republican Ministries of - Unionsrepublikanische Ministerien für - Sojuzno-respublikanskie Ministerstva:

Agriculture - Landwirtschaft - sel'skogo chozjajstva	- MJANNIK, H.A.
Communications - Post-und Fernmeldewesen - svjazi	- KALDMA, A.U.
Construction - Bauwesen - stroitel'stva	- PALU, P.K.
Construction Materials Industry - Baustoffindustrie - promyšlennosti stroitel'nych materialov	- VICHVELIN, L.A.
Culture - Kultur - kul'tury	- JURNA, Ju.-K.M.
Education - Volksbildung - prosveščenija	- EISEN, F.M.
Finance - Finanzen - finansov	- NORAK, A.A.
Food Industry - Nahrungsmittelindustrie - piščevoj promyšlennosti	- TEPANDI, Ja.Ja.
Foreign Affairs - auswärtige Angelegenheiten - inostrannych del	- GREN, A.K.[1]
Forestry and Protection of Nature - Forstwirtschaft und Naturschutz - lesnogo chozjajstva i ochrany prirody	- TEDER, H.O.
Health - Gesundheitswesen - zdravoochranenija	- RJATSEP, V.Jo.
Higher and Secondary Specialized Education - Hochschul-u.mittl. Fachschulbildung - vysšego i srednego special'nogo obrazovanija	-NUUT, I.Ju.
Internal Affairs - innere Angelegenheiten - vnutrennich del	- ANI, V.F.

[1] Also Deputy Chairman of the Council of Ministers - glz.stellv.Vorsitzender des Ministerrates

State Structure 4.4.15
Staatsordnung

Justice - Justiz - Justicii — SILVET, E.P.
Light Industry - Leichtindustrie - legkoj promyšlennosti — KRAFT, Ju.A.
Meat and Dairy Industry - Fleisch-u.Milchindustrie -
mjasnoj i moločnoj promyšlennosti — ESSENSON, A.R.
Procurement - Beschaffungen - zagotovok — PEDAJAS, A.A.
Timber and Wood Processing Industry - Holz-und holzbearbeitende
Industrie - lesnoj i derevoobrabaty-vajuščej promyšlennosti — ČERNYŠEV, V.V.
Trade - Handel - torgovli — TODESON, K.E.

Republican Ministries of - Republikanische Ministerien für - Respublikanskie Ministerstva:

Consumer Services - Dienstleistungen - bytovogo
obsluživanija naselenija — CHALMJAGI, V.A.
Local Industry - lokale Industrie - mestnoj promyšlennosti — JURGENS, F.E.
Motor Transport and Highways - Kraftverkehr und Landstraßen -
avtomobil'nogo transporta i šossejnych dorog — SIBUL, R.Ja.
Municipal Services - Kommunalwirtschaft - kommunal'nogo
chozjajstva — BLUM, A.I.
Social Security - Sozialfürsorge - social'nogo obespečenija — SARRI, G.E.

Chairman/Chief
Vorsitzender/Leiter
Predsedatel'/Načalnik

State Planning Committee - Staatl. Plankomitee -
Gosudarstvennyj Planovyj komitet - GOSPLAN — TYNSPOEG, G.A.[1]
State Committee for Construction Affairs - Staatskomitee
für Bauwesen - Gosudarstvennyj komitet po delam stroitel'stva — PAALMAN, E.R.
Committee for People's Control - Komitee für Volkskontrolle -
Komitet narodnogo kontrolja — MERIMAA, O.O.
State Committee for Prices - Staatskomitee für Preispolitik -
Gosudarstvennyj komitet cen — VLADYČIN, Ju.N.
State Committee for Cinematography - Staatskomitee für Film-
wesen - Gosudarstvennyj komitet po kinematografii — LIJVIK, F.Jo.
State Committee for Publishing Houses, Printing Plants and
the Book Trade - Staatskomitee für Verlagswesen, Poly-
graphie und Buchhandel - Gosudarstvennyj komitet po delam
izdatel'stv, poligrafii i knižnoj torgovli — KAJK, L.Ju.
State Committee for Vocational and Technical Education -
Staatskomitee f.berufstechnische Ausbildung - Gosudarstvennyj
komitet po professional'no-techničeskomu obrazovaniju — ŠIŠKIN, A.A.
State Committee for Land Reclamation and Water Resources -
Staatskomitee für Melioration und Wasserwirtschaft - Gosu-
darstvennyj komitet melioracii i vodnogo chozjajstva — VALING, O.Ja.
State Committee for Television and Broadcasting - Staats-
komitee für Fernseh-und Rundfunkwesen - Gosudarstvennyj
komitet po televideniju i radioveščaniju — PENU, R.A.
State Committee for Labor - Staatskomitee für Arbeit -
Gosudarstvennyj komitet po trudu — KONSTANTINOV, V.N.
Committee for State Security - Komitee für Staatssicherheit -
Komitet gosudarstvennoj bezopasnosti — PORK, A.P.
State Committee for Production-Technological Supply in
Agriculture - Staatskomitee für produktionstechnische Versor-
gung der Landwirtschaft - Gosudarstvennyj komitet po proiz-
vodstvenno-techničeskom obespečeniju sel'skogo chozjajstva — METTE, A.A.
Main Administration of Material and Technical Supply -
Hauptverwaltung für materiell-technische Versorgung -
Glavnoe upravlenie material'no-techničeskogo snabženija — TOOTS, E.Ja.
Central Statistical Administration - Statistische Zentral-
verwaltung - Central'noe statističeskoe upravlenie — KIMASK, G.K.

---

[1] Also Deputy Chairman of the Council of Ministers -
glz.stellv.Vorsitzender des Ministerrates

173

5.1.1 Economy
Wirtschaft

5. ECONOMY — WIRTSCHAFT —

5.1 INDUSTRY   -   INDUSTRIE   -

5.1.1 OUTPUT OF THE MOST IMPORTANT
PRODUKTION DER WICHTIGSTEN
PROIZVODSTVO VAŽNEJŠICH VIDOV
(1922-1977)

		1922	1928	1937	1940	1945	1950
1.	Electric power, '000 mill. kWh Elektroenergie, Mrd. Kw Elektroenergija, mrd. kvt-č	0.8	5.0	36.2	48.3	43.3	91.2
2.	Crude oil, mill. tons Erdöl, Mill. t Neft', mln. t	4.7	11.6	28.5	31.1	19.4	37.9
3.	Crude oil (incl. gas condensate), mill. tons Erdöl (einschl. Gaskondensat), Mill. t Neft' (vključaja gazovyj kondensat), mln. t	4.7	11.6	28.5	31.1	19.4	37.9
4.	Natural gas, '000 mill. cu.m. Erdgas, Mrd. m^3 Gaz estestvennyj, mrd. m^3	0.03	0.3	2.2	3.2	3.3	5.8
5.	Coal, mill. tons Kohle, Mill. t Ugol', mln. t	11.3	35.5	128.0	165.9	149.3	261.1
6.	Peat for fuel, mill. tons (of standard moisture) Heiztorf, Mill. t (bedingter Feuchtigkeit) Torf toplivnyj, mln. t (uslovnoj vlažnosti)	2.2	5.3	24.0	33.2	22.4	36.0
7.	Pig-Iron, mill. tons Roheisen, Mill. t Čugun, mln. t	0.2	3.3	14.5	14.9	8.8	19.2
8.	Steel, mill. tons Stahl, Mill. t Stal', mln. t	0.3	4.3	17.7	18.3	12.3	27.3
9.	Rolled steel, total, mill. tons Walzstahl - insg., Mill. t Prokat černych metallov - vsego, mln. t	0.26	3.4	13.0	13.1	8.5	20.9
10.	of which finished rolled steel darunter fertige Walzerzeugnisse v tom čisle gotovyj prokat	0.24	3.2	11.1	11.4	7.4	18.0
11.	Iron ore, mill. tons Eisenerz, Mill. t Železnaja ruda, mln. t	0.2	6.1	27.8	29.9	15.9	39.7
12.	Sulphuric acid in monohydrate, mill. tons Schwefelsäure als Monohydrat, Mill. t Sernaja kislota v monogidrate, mln. t	0.03	0.2	1.4	1.6	0.8	2.1

NARODNOE CHOZJAJSTVO

Economy 5.1.1
Wirtschaft

PROMYŠLENNOST'

INDUSTRIAL BRANCHES
INDUSTRIEZWEIGE
PROMYŠLENNOJ PRODUKCII
(1922-1977)

1955	1960	1965	1970	1971	1972	1973	1974	1975	1976	1977	
170	292	507	741	800	857	915	976	1,038	1.111	1.150	1.
70.8	147	242	349	372	393.8	421	451	482	--	--	2.
70.8	148	243	353	377	400.4	429	459	491	520	546	3.
9.0	45.3	128	198	212	221	236	261	289	321	346	4.
390	510	578	624	641	655	668	685	701	712	722	5.
50.8	53.6	45.7	57.4	54.3	61.2	58.5	39.8	53.8	32.8	--	6.
33.3	46.8	66.2	85.9	89.3	92.3	95.9	99.9	103	105	107	7.
45.3	65.3	91.0	116	121	126	131	136	141	145	147	8.
35.3	51.0	70.9	92.5	95.9	99.5	104	109	115	118	118	9.
30.6	43.7	61.7	80.6	84.1	87.5	91.5	94.3	98.6	101	102	10.
71.9	106	153	195	203	208	216	225	233	239	240	11.
3.8	5.4	8.5	12.1	12.8	13.7	14.9	16.7	18.6	20.0	21.1	12.

5.1.1 Economy
Wirtschaft

	1922	1928	1937	1940	1945	1950
13. Soda ash (95 per cent), '000 tons Kalzinierte Soda (95%ige), Tsd. t Soda kal'cinirovannaja (95%-naja), tys. t	32	217	528	536	235	749
14. Caustic soda (92 per cent), '000 tons Kaustische Soda (92%ige), Tsd. t Soda kausticeskaja (92%-naja), tys. t	10	59	164	190	128	325
15. Mineral fertilizers, mill. tons: Mineralische Düngemittel, Mill. t: Mineral'nye udobrenija, mln. t:						
in terms of 100 per cent content of nutrients umgerechnet auf 100% Reinnährstoffgehalt v perescete na 100%-noe soderzanie pitatel'nych vescestv	0.0	0.03	0.7	0.7	0.3	1.2
in conventional units in Bezugseinheitsmaßen v uslovnych edinicach	0.0	0.1	3.2	3.2	1.1	5.5
16. Herbicides, '000 tons: Chemische Pflanzenschutzmittel, Tsd. t: Chimiceskie sredstva zascity rastenij, tys. t:						
in terms of 100 per cent active base berechnet auf 100% Wirkstoffgehalt v 100%-nom iscislenii po dejstvujuscemu nacalu	...	...	...	...	...	5.1
in conventional units in Bezugseinheitsmaßen v uslovnych edinicach	...	...	...	...	...	13.0
17. Synthetic resins and plastics, '000 tons Kunstharze und Plaste, Tsd. t Sinteticeskie smoly i plasticeskie massy - tys. t	--	0.3	8.0	10.9	21.3	67.1
18. Synthetic fibres, '000 tons Chemische Fasern, Tsd. t Chimiceskie volokna, tys. t	--	0.2	8.6	11.1	1.1	24.2
19. Tires, mill. units Reifendecken, Mill. Stck. Avtopokryski, mln. st.	0.1	0.1	2.7	3.0	1.4	7.4

5.1.1 Economy / Wirtschaft

	1922	1928	1937	1940	1945	1950
69. Television sets, '000 Fernsehgeräte, Tsd.Stck. Televizory širokoveščatel'nye, tys.št.	--	--	--	0.3	--	11.9
70. Refrigerators, '000 Kühlschränke, Tsd.Stck. Cholodil'niki bytovye, tys.št.	--	--	--	3.5	0.3	1.2
71. Washing machines, '000 Waschmaschinen, Tsd.Stck. Stiralnye mašiny bytovye, tys.št.	--	--	--	--	--	0.3
72. Vacuum cleaners, '000 Elektr. Staubsauger, Tsd.Stck. Elektropylesosy bytovye, tys.št.	--	--	--	--	1.1	6.1
73. Sewing machines, '000 Nähmaschinen, Tsd.Stck. Švejnye mašiny bytovye, tys.št.	--	286	510	175	--	502
74. Motorcycles and scooters, '000 Motorräder und -roller, Tsd.Stck. Motocikly i motorollery, tys.št.	--	--	13.1	6.7	4.7	123
75. Granulated sugar, '000 tons Streuzucker, Tsd. t Sachar-pesok, tys. t	210	1,283	2,421	2,165	465	2,523
of which made from sugar beats darunter aus Zuckerrüben v tom čisle iz sacharnoj svekly	210	1,283	2,421	2,165	465	2,523
76. Meat (incl. subproducts of 1st category), '000 tons Fleisch (einschl. Subprodukte der 1.Güterklasse), Tsd. t Mjaso (vključaja subprodukty I kategorii), tys. t	260	678	1,002	1,501	663	1,556
77. Fish catch, incl. sea animals, whales, and other sea products, '000 tons Fischfang, Fang von Seetieren, Walen und anderen Meeresprodukten, Tsd. t Ulov ryby, dobyča morskogo zverja, kitov i moreproduktov, tys.t	483	840	1,609	1,404	1,125	1,755
78. Butter, '000 tons Butter, Tsd. t Maslo životnoe, tys.t	25	82	185	226	117	336
79. Dairy products in terms of milk, mill. tons Vollmilcherzeugnisse, umgerechnet auf Milch, Mill. t Cel'nomoločnaja produkcija v perescete na moloko, mln.t	0.0	0.1	0.8	1.3	0.6	1.1

Economy
Wirtschaft 5.1.1

1955	1960	1965	1970	1971	1972	1973	1974	1975	1976	1977	
1,848	2,334	3,231	4,185	4,407	4,613	4,908	5,040	5,215	5,389	5,500	56.
22.5	45.5	72.4	95.2	100.3	104.3	190.5	115.1	122	124	127	57.
5.0	30.2	56.1	84.6	90.8	96.1	102.9	108.5	114	117	121	58.
20.8	35.5	36.6	43.2	44.6	45.7	46.8	46.7	47	47	--	59.
4,227	4,838	5,499	6,152	6,397	6,421	6,578	6,624	6,635	6,775	6,800	60.
316	439	466	643	675	681	703	724	740	764	800	61.
272	516	548	707	760	775	796	796	778	807	800	62.
415	675	801	1,146	1,190	1,270	1,345	1,413	1,508	1,598	1,600	63.
772	964	1,350	1,338	1,309	1,337	1,411	1,469	1,494	1,538	--	64.
432	583	903	1,229	1,274	1,294	1,360	1,389	1,420	1,458	1,511	65.
271	419	486	679	682	647	666	684	698	725	735	66.
19.7	26.0	30.6	40.2	42.1	44.1	47.5	50.6	55.0	57.9	60.7	67.
8.0	16.3	14.8	21.7	23.3	24.6	26.6	28.9	31.3	--	--	
3,549	4,165	5,160	7,815	8,794	8,842	8,615	8,753	8,376	8,443	8,700	68.

5.1.1 Economy / Wirtschaft

	1922	1928	1937	1940	1945	1950
56. Paper, '000 tons / Papier, Tsd. t / Bumaga, tys. t	40	285	832	812	321	1,180
57. Cement, mill. tons / Zement, Mill. t / Cement, mln. t	0.1	1.8	5.5	5.7	1.8	10.2
58. Precast reinforced concrete structures and articles, mill. cu.m. of articles / Montierbare Stahlbetonkonstruktionen und Einzelteile, Mill. m^3 der Erzeugnisse / Sbornye železobetonnye konstrukcii i detali - mln. m^3 izdelij	--	--	0.0	0.3	0.5	1.2
59. Construction bricks, '000 mill.pcs / Bauziegel, Mrd.Stck. / Kirpič stroitel'nyj, mrd. št.	0.1	2.8	8.7	7.5	2.0	10.2
60. Cotton fabrics, mill.m^2 / Baumwollstoffe, Mill.m^2 / Chlopčatobumažnye tkani, mln.m^2	--	1,821	2,431	2,715	1,149	2,745
61. Woollen fabrics, mill.m^2 / Wollstoffe, Mill.m^2 / Šerstjanye tkani, mln.m^2	--	112	139	155	65	193
62. Linen fabrics, mill.m^2 / Leinenstoffe, Mill.m^2 / L'janye tkani, mln.m^2	--	177	274	272	98	257
63. Silk fabrics, mill.m^2 / Seidenstoffe, Mill.m^2 / Šelkovye tkani, mln.m^2	--	8.0	49.0	67	29.2	106
64. Hosiery, mill. pairs / Strumpf-u.Sockenwaren, Mill.Paar / Čuločno-nosočnye izdelija, mln.par	2.2	67.7	409	485	91.0	473
65. Knitted wear, mill. pcs. / Wäsche und Obertrikotagen, Mill.Stck. / Bel'evoj i verchnij trikotaž, mln.št.	1.9	8.3	157	183	50.0	197
66. Leather footwear, mill.pairs / Lederschuhe, Mill. Paar / Obuv' kožanaja, mln.par	6.8	58.0	183	211	63.1	203
67. Clocks and watches, mill.pcs. / Uhren, Mill.Stck. / Časy bytovye, mln.št.	0.02	0.9	4.0	2.8	0.3	7.6
of which wrist watches / darunter Armbanduhren / v tom čisle naručnye	--	--	--	0.2	0.1	1.5
68. Radios and radiogramophones, '000 / Rundfunkgeräte und -empfänger mit eing.Plattenspieler, Tsd.Stck. / Radiopriemniki i radioly širokoveščatel'nye, tys.št.	--	3.0	200	160	14	1,072

Economy
Wirtschaft 5.1.1

1955	1960	1965	1970	1971	1972	1973	1974	1975	1976	1977	
103	149	166	212	221	227	232	218	205	202	--	42.
115	112	262	163	141	145	160	178	180	191	--	43.
113	84.8	206	219	184	178	195	178	188	190	--	44.
22.6	87.5	122	144	150	155	131	93.0	83.9	89.4	--	45.
48.0	59.0	85.8	99.2	102	95.7	84.8	88.4	97.5	102	106	46.
5,242	12,589	21,565	30,844	33,164	34,875	35,831	37,059	38,965	40,400	41,500	47.
2,316	3,264	6,764	5,740	5,772	5,750	5,928	6,359	6,523	6,865	--	48.
5,505	6,695	11,141	15,397	16,231	16,369	17,186	18,989	19,681	20,162	--	49.
112	835	1,236	1,963	2,180	2,235	2,272	2,459	2,442	2,504	--	50.
2,040	2,679	3,227	4,027	3,855	4,442	4,761	5,149	5,359	--	--	51.
16.0	16.5	24.3	19.8	18.6	19.5	25.0	28.8	31.3	30.9	--	52.
212	262	274	299	298	298	304	304	311	303	--	53.
75.6	106	111	116	119	119	116	115	115	114	--	54.
1,742	2,282	3,234	5,110	5,412	5,684	6,070	6,340	6,840	7,200	7,400	55.

Economy 5.1.1
Wirtschaft

1955	1960	1965	1970	1971	1972	1973	1974	1975	1976	1977	
495	1,726	3,655	6,682	5,817	5,980	6,271	6,569	6,961	7,060	7,100	69.
151	529	1,675	4,140	4,557	5,030	5,423	5,426	5,606	5,834	5,800	70.
87	895	3,430	5,243	4,052	3,001	2,987	3,075	3,284	3,509	3,600	71.
131	501	800	1,509	1,738	2,168	2,658	3,319	2,920	2,655	--	72.
1,611	3,096	800	1,400	1,408	1,439	1,400	1,366	1,360	1,358		73.
235	533	711	833	872	898	932	960	1,029	1,059		74.
3,419	6,363	11,037	10,221	9,025	8,903	10,714	9,446	10,382	9,200	12,000	75.
3,239	5,266	8,924	8,139	7,805	7,307	8,449	7,848	7,445	--	--	
2,524	4,406	5,245	7,144	8,182	8,723	8,346	9,367	9,883	8,265	--	76.
2,737	3,541	5,774	7,828	7,785	8,209	9,005	9,622	10,357	--	--	77.
463	737	1,072	963	1,022	1,080	1,239	1,260	1,231	1,263	1,400	78.
2.6	8.3	11.7	19.7	19.7	19.9	21.2	23.0	23.6	23.4	24,3	79.

5.1.1 Economy / Wirtschaft

	1922	1928	1937	1940	1945	1950
80. Vegetable oil, '000 tons Pflanzliche Fette, Tsd. t Maslo rastitel'noe, tys.t	86	448	539	798	292	819
81. Canned food, '000 mill. conventional cans Konserven, Mrd. Normdosen Konservy, mrd. uslovnych banok	0.0	0.1	1.0	1.1	0.6	1.5
82. Mixed feed, mill. tons Mischfutter, Mill. t Kombikorma, mln. t	--	0.0	0.9	1.2	0.2	1.1

Economy
Wirtschaft 5.1.1

1955	1960	1965	1970	1971	1972	1973	1974	1975	1976	1977	
1,168	1,586	2,770	2,784	2,923	2,827	2,676	3,411	3,354	2,787	2,900	80.
3.2	4.9	7.1	10.7	11.3	12.1	13.0	14.2	14.5	14.5	15.0	81.
2.5	9.3	15.5	23.7	26.7	28.3	31.7	37.7	41.8	46.0	51.0	82.

5.1.2.1 Economy / Wirtschaft

5.1.2 ELECTRIC POWER – ELEKTROENERGIE – ELEKTROENERGETIKA

5.1.2.1 Capacity of Electric Power Stations and Output of Electric Power
Kapazität der Elektrizitätswerke und Elektroenergieerzeugung
Moščnost'elektrostancij i proizvodstvo elektroenergii

Year Jahr Gody	All electric power stations Gesamte Elektrizitätswerke Vse elektrostancii		Hydroelectric stations Wasserkraftwerke Gidroelektrostancii	
	Capacity Kapazität Moščnost' '000 kW 1.000 Kw tys.kvt	Output of electric power Elektroenergie-erzeugung Proizvodstvo elektroenergii mill.kWh Mill.Kwh mln.kvt-č	Capacity Kapazität Moščnost' '000 kW 1.000 Kw tys.kvt	Output of electric power Elektroenergie-erzeugung Proizvodstvo elektroenergii mill.kWh Mill.Kwh mln.kvt-č
1913[1]	1,098	1,945	16	35
1913[2]	1,141	2,039	16	35
1916	1,192	2,575	16	37
1921	1,228	520	18	10
1922	1,247	775	19	12
1928	1,905	5,007	121	430
1932	4,677	13,540	504	812
1937	8,235	36,173	1,044	4,184
1940	11,193	48,309	1,587	5,113
1945	11,124	43,257	1,252	4,841
1946	12,338	48,571	1,427	6,046
1950	19,614	91,226	3,218	12,691
1955	37,246	170,225	5,996	23,165
1960	66,721	292,274	14,781	50,913
1961	74,098	327,611	16,366	59,122
1962	82,461	369,275	18,622	71,944
1963	93,050	412,418	20,830	75,859
1964	103,584	458,902	21,251	77,361
1965	115,033	506,672	22,244	81,434
1966	123,007	544,566	23,077	91,823
1967	131,727	587,699	24,813	88,571
1968	142,504	638,661	27,035	104,040
1969	153,790	689,050	29,645	115,181
1970	166,150	740,926	31,368	124,377
1971	175,365	800,360	33,448	126,099
1972	186,239	857,435	34,846	122,899
1973	195,560	914,606	35,320	122,345
1974	205,442	975,754	36,978	132,030
1975	217,484	1,038,607	40,515	125,987

[1] within the borders of the U.S.S.R. up to 17.9.1939 – in den Grenzen der UdSSR bis 17.9.1939 – v granicach SSSR do 17 sentjabrja 1939 g.
[2] within the present borders of the U.S.S.R. – in den heutigen Grenzen der UdSSR – v sovremennych granicach SSSR

Economy / Wirtschaft 5.1.2.2

5.1.2.2 CONSUMPTION OF ELECTRIC POWER – VERBRAUCH AN ELEKTROENERGIE – POTREBLENIE ELEKTROENERGII

Territory of the U.S.S.R. / Territorium der UdSSR / Territorija SSSR	Year / Jahr / Gody	Total / Insgesamt / Vsego '000 mill. Mrd. kWh mlrd.kvt-č	%	Industry & Construct / Industrie u.Bauwesen / Promyšlennost'ju i stroitel'stvom '000 mill. Mrd. kWh mlrd.kvt-č	%	Transport / Transport / Transportom '000 mill. Mrd. kWh mlrd.kvt-č	%	Agriculture / Landwirtschaft / Sel'skim chozjajstvom '000 mill. Mrd. kWh mlrd.kvt-č	%	Communal Economy and other Consumers / Kommunalwirtschaft u. andere Konsumenten / Kommunal'nym chozjajstvom i pročimi potrebiteljami '000 mill. Mrd. kWh mlrd.kvt-č	%	Losses in the Distribution Network / Verluste im Netz d. allgemeinen Nutzung / Poteri v setjach obščego pol'zovanja '000 mill. Mrd. kWh mlrd.kvt-č	%
SSSR	1965	505.2	100	361.3	71.5	37.1	7.3	21.1	4.2	50.6	10	35.1	6.9
	1970	735.7	100	503.4	68.4	54.4	7.4	38.6	5.2	81.0	11	58.3	7.9
	1975	1027.0	100	678.0	65.9	74.0	7.2	74.0	7.2	119.0	11.7	82.0	8.0
RSFSR	1965	339.3	100	245.1	72.2	28.9	8.5	10.5	3.1	33.5	9.9	21.4	6.3
	1970	478.7	100	330.8	69.1	41.2	8.6	18.9	3.9	52.8	11.0	35.0	7.3
	1975	658.8	100	441.3	66.9	55.6	8.4	36.4	5.7	77.2	11.8	48.3	7.2
Ukrainskaja SSR	1965	92.2	100	67.7	73.4	5.3	5.7	4.5	4.9	8.0	8.7	6.7	7.3
	1970	134.5	100	94.8	70.5	8.1	6.0	7.8	5.8	12.9	9.6	10.9	8.1
	1975	182	100	124.4	68.2	10.4	5.8	13.9	7.8	18.3	10	15	8.2
Belorusskaja SSR	1965	7.55	100	4.8	63.6	0.23	3.0	0.52	6.9	1.17	15.5	0.79	10.5
	1970	14.3	100	9.1	63.6	0.63	4.4	1.14	8.0	2.0	14.0	1.4	9.8
	1975	22.7	100	14.5	63.9	0.8	3.5	2.3	10.1	3.17	13.7	2	8.8
Kazachskaja SSR	1965	19.6	100	13.7	69.9	0.99	5.1	1.7	8.7	2.1	10.7	1.1	5.6
	1970	36.4	100	25.3	69.5	2.0	5.5	2.5	6.9	3.9	10.7	2.7	7.4
	1975	57.7	100	38.9	67.4	3.1	5.4	5.3	9.2	6	10.4	4.4	7.6
Transcaucasian Republics / Transkaukasische Republiken / Respubliki Zakavkaz'ja	1965	19.35	100	12.9	66.7	0.85	4.4	1.0	5.2	2.1	10.9	2.5	12.9
	1970	27.1	100	17.2	63.5	1.3	4.8	1.66	6.1	3.2	11.8	3.7	13.7
	1975	35	100	20.4	58.3	2.3	6.6	2.8	8.0	4.7	13.3	4.8	13.8
Baltic Republics / Baltische Republiken / Pribaltijskie respubliki	1965	9.1	100	5.4	59.3	0.31	3.4	0.8	8.8	1.48	16.3	1.1	12.1
	1970	16.0	100	9.3	58.1	0.44	2.8	1.7	10.6	2.65	16.6	1.9	11.9
	1975	21.44	100	12.0	56	0.54	2.5	3.0	14	3.4	16.0	2.5	11.5
Middle Asiatic Republics / Mittelasiatische Republ. / Srednjeaziatskie respubliki	1965	16.2	100	10.5	64.8	0.48	3.0	1.82	11.2	2.0	12.3	1.39	8.6
	1970	26.6	100	16.2	60.9	0.7	2.6	4.0	15.0	3.4	12.8	2.3	8.6
	1975	42.8	100	23.7	55.4	1.2	2.8	8.5	19.8	5.2	12.2	4.2	9.8
Moldavskaja SSR	1965	1.9	100	0.91	47.9	0.06	3.2	0.36	18.9	0.37	19.5	0.22	11.6
	1970	3.8	100	1.67	43.9	0.08	2.1	0.93	24.5	0.64	16.8	0.48	12.6
	1975	6.5	100	2.9	44.6	0.1	1.6	1.6	24.6	1.0	15.4	0.9	13.8

5.1.2.3 Economy / Wirtschaft

ENERGETIC CAPACITY AND CONSUMPTION OF ELECTRIC POWER BY THE MOST IMPORTANT INDUSTRIAL BRANCHES
ENERGETISCHE KAPAZITÄTEN UND VERBRAUCH AN ELEKTROENERGIE NACH DEN WICHTIGSTEN INDUSTRIEZWEIGEN
ENERGETIČESKIE MOŠČNOSTI I POTREBLENIE ELEKTROENERGII PO VAŽNEJŠIM OTRASLJAM PROMYŠLENNOSTI

Industrial branches Industriezweige Otrasli promyšlennosti	Year Jahr Gody	Capacity, mill kW / Kapazität, Mio Kw / Moščnost', mln.kvt				Consumption of electric power, '000 mill.kWh / Verbrauch an Elektroenergie, Mrd.Kwh / Potreblenie elektroenergii, mlrd.kvt-č				Anzahl d. Stunden d. Nutzungskapazität / Čislo časov ispol'zovanija ustanovlennoj moščnosti	
		Total Insg. Vsego	Electro-motors Elektro-motoren Elektro-dvigatelej	Electric apparatus Elektro-apparate Elektro-apparatov		Total Insg. Vsego	Technological demand Technologi-scher Bedarf Technologi-českie nužy	Electro-motors Elektro-motoren Elektro-dvigatelej	Lighting Beleuchtung Osveščenie	Electric motors Elektro-motoren Elektro-dvigatelej	Electric apparatus Elektro-apparate Elektro-apparatov
Industry, total / Industrie, insg. / Vsego po promyšlennosti	1970 1975	218.0 295.5	175.2 236.9	42.8 58.6		437.9 588.0	125.0 170.6	275.0 367.0	37.9 50.4	1,570 1,560	2,920 2,920
of which-darunter-v tom čisle: fuel industry Brennstoffindustrie Toplivnaja prom.	1970 1975	25.2 33.2	24.3 32.2	0.9 1.0		46.0 60.8	0.9 1.7	42.5 56.0	2.6 3.1	1,750 1,740	1,000 1,700
Iron & steel industry Eisen-u.Stahlindustrie Černaja metallurgija	1970 1975	37.8 52.0	32.7 45.5	5.1 6.5		70.7 94.5	18.7 25.4	45.9 61.6	6.1 7.5	1,405 1,350	3,670 3,930
Buntmetallurgie Cvetnaja metallurgija	1970 1975	18.9 25.9	11.5 15.2	7.4 10.7		67.3 92.4	43.4 61.5	19.3 26.0	4.6 4.9	1,680 1,730	5,870 5,750
Chemical & petrolchem. Chemische u.petrolchem. Chimičeskaja i neftech.	1970 1975	23.3 31.6	19.1 26.5	4.2 5.1		64.2 91.6	15.7 21.1	44.8 65.1	3.7 5.4	2,350 2,470	3,740 4,140
Mach.build.& metal work. Masch.bau u.Metallbear. Mašinostroenie i metalloobrabotka	1970 1975	61.5 83.6	42.3 56.4	19.2 27.2		65.6 90.3	25.1 34.8	33.3 45.6	7.2 9.9	787 810	1,306 1,280

Economy 5.1.2.4
Wirtschaft 5.1.2.5

5.1.2.4
POWER CAPACITY OF THE POWER STATIONS IN THE USSR
ENERGETISCHE KAPAZITÄTEN IN DEN KRAFTWERKEN DER UdSSR
VVOD V DEJSTVIE ENERGETIČESKICH MOŠČNOSTEJ NA ELEKTROSTANCIJACH SSSR

	1971 - 1975 mill.kWh Mio Kwh mln.vKt	%	1976 - 1980 mill.kWh Mio Kwh mln.vKt	%	Increase in the X.Five-Year's Plan compared with the IX. Wachstum im X.Fünfjahrplan verglichen mit dem IX. Rost v desjatom pjatiletii po sravneniju s devjatym %
Total-Insg.-Vsego	58	100	71	100	122
of which-darunter- v tom čisle:					
nuclear power stations Kernkraftwerke na atomnych elektro- stancijach	3.8	6.5	1		
Hydroelectric stations Wasserkraftwerke na gidravličeskich elektrostancijach	9.0	15.5	1		
Thermal electric stations Wärmekraftwerke na teplovych elektrostancijach	45.2	78.0	4:		

Page 195

English translation of Russian headline
VVOD V DEJSTVIE ENERGETIČES-
KICH MOŠČNOSTEJ NA ELEKTRO-
STANCIJACH SSSR
should read:
Introduction of power capacity of the
power stations in the USSR.

Units given table 5.1.2.4 below 1971–
1975 and 1976–1980 should read:
mill kW (instead of mill kWh).

5.1.2.5   ELECTRIC POWER OUTPUT PER CAPITA
ELEKTROENERGIEERZEUGUNG PRO KOPF DER BEVÖLKERUNG
PROIZVODSTVO ELEKTROENERGII NA DUŠU NASELENIJA

Union Republics Unionsrepubliken Sojuznye respubliki	1965	1970	1975	1975 to-zu-k 1965	1975 to-zu-k 1970
	kWh-Kwh-kVt-č			%	
SSSR	2,194	3,052	4,082	185	133.7
RSFSR	2,625	3,607	4,764	181	132
Ukrainskaja SSR	2,083	2,909	3,968	191	136
Belorusskaja SSR	977	1,669	2,846	291	170
Uzbekskaja SSR	1,106	1,511	2,388	216	158
Kazachskaja SSR	1,655	2,682	3,642	220	136
Gruzinskaja SSR	1,350	1,904	2,341	173	123
Azerbajdžanskaja SSR	2,279	2,328	2,577	113	111
Litovskaja SSR	1,296	2,340	2,713	209	116
Moldavskaja SSR	926	2,117	3,563	385	168
Latvijskaja SSR	656	1,135	1,159	177	102
Kirgizskaja SSR	898	1,193	1,298	145	109
Tadžikskaja SSR	624	1,101	1,333	214	121
Armjanskaja SSR	1,295	2,426	3,235	250	133
Turkmenskaja SSR	742	842	1,743	235	207
Estonskaja SSR	5,502	8,482	11,622	211	137

5.1.2.6 ELECTRIC POWER OUTPUT IN THE UNION REPUBLICS
ELEKTROENERGIEERZEUGUNG IN DEN UNIONSREPUBLIKEN
PROIZVODSTVO ELEKTROENERGII PO SOJUZNYM RESPUBLIKAM
('000 mill.kWh - Mrd.Kwh - mlrd.kVt-č)

	1940	1965	1970	1971	1972	1973	1974	1975	1976	1977
SSSR	48	507	741	800	857	915	976	1,038	1,111	1,150
RSFSR	30.8	333	470	503	537	568	606	640	686	709
Ukrainskaja SSR	12.4	94.6	138	150	158	172	181	194	209	215
Belorusskaja SSR	0.5	8.4	15.1	18.5	21.0	23.0	24.7	26.7	29.0	30.1
Uzbekskaja SSR	0.5	11.5	18.3	21.3	23.8	26.1	30.0	33.6	35.1	34.9
Kazachskaja SSR	0.6	19.2	34.7	37.8	41.5	44.2	48.7	52.5	55.6	58.2
Gruzinskaja SSR	0.7	6.0	9.0	9.5	10.0	10.7	11.1	11.6	12.1	12.0
Azerbajdžanskaja SSR	1.8	10.4	12.0	12.3	12.7	13.5	14.2	14.7	15.3	15.7
Litovskaja SSR	0.04	3.9	7.4	7.5	9.5	9.9	9.2	9.0	9.7	10.7
Moldavskaja SSR	0.02	3.1	7.6	8.5	9.6	10.6	12.2	13.7	13.7	13.6
Latvijskaja SSR	0.13	1.5	2.7	2.5	2.3	2.2	2.5	2.5	2.5	3.3
Kirgizskaja SSR	0.05	2.3	3.5	3.9	4.0	4.3	4.4	4.4	4.8	4.9
Tadžikskaja SSR	0.06	1.6	3.2	3.4	3.6	3.8	3.9	4.7	5.2	7.3
Armjanskaja SSR	0.4	2.9	6.1	7.3	7.5	7.9	8.5	9.2	9.7	10.9
Turkmenskaja SSR	0.08	1.4	1.8	1.9	2.1	2.5	3.9	4.5	5.2	5.6
Estonskaja SSR	0.1	7.1	11.6	13.0	14.5	16.2	16.0	16.7	18.6	18.9

5.1.3
IRON AND STEEL INDUSTRY - EISEN- UND STAHLINDUSTRIE - ČERNAJA METALLURGIJA

5.1.3.1
OUTPUT OF PIG IRON, STEEL, FINISHED ROLLED STEEL AND STEEL TUBES
PRODUKTION VON ROHEISEN, STAHL, EISEN-U.STAHLWALZGUT UND STAHLROHREN
PROIZVODSTVO ČUGUNA, STALI, PROKATA ČEPNYCH METALLOV I STAL'NYCH TRUB

Year Jahr Gody	Pig iron Roheisen Čugun	Steel Stahl Stal'	Finished rolled steel Fertiges Walzgut Gotovyj prokat	Steel tubes Stahlrohre stal'nye truby '000 tons Tsd. t tys.tonn	mill.meters Mio m mln.metrov
	('000 tons-Tsd. t-tys.t)				
1913[1]	4.216	4.231	3.287	77.7	
1913[2]	4,216	4,307	3,372	77.7	
1928	3,282	4,251	3,213	171	
1932	6,161	5,927	4,060	310	
1937	14,487	17,730	11,108	923	
1940	14,902	18,317	11,430	966	
1945	8,803	12,252	7,358	571	
1946	9,862	13,346	8,263	796	
1950	19,175	27,329	17,973	2,001	
1955	33,310	45,272	30,556	3,549	
1960	46,757	65,294	43,679	5,805	883
1965	66,184	91,021	61,650	9,014	1,381
1966	70,264	96,907	66,139	9,905	1,503
1967	74,812	102,224	70,621	10,582	1,641
1968	78,788	106,537	74,079	11,215	1,751
1969	81,634	110,330	76,272	11,551	1,819
1970	85,933	115,889	80,645	12,434	1,917
1971	89,256	120,660	84,124	13,356	2,000
1972	92,327	125,592	87,470	13,829	2,148
1973	95,933	131,481	91,462	14,369	2,237
1974	99,868	136,230	94,295	14,961	2,305
1975	102,968	141,344	98,686	15,967	2,396
1976	105,374	144,825	101,442	16,806	2,478
1977	107,000	147,000	102,000	17,000	--

[1] within the borders of the U.S.S.R. up to 17.9.1939 - in den Grenzen der UdSSR bis 17.9.1939 - v granicach SSSR do 17 sentjabrja 1939 g.
[2] within the present borders of the U.S.S.R. - in den heutigen Grenzen der UdSSR - v sovremennych granicach SSSR

5.1.3.2 Economy
5.1.3.3 Wirtschaft

5.1.3.2 OUTPUT OF IRON AND MANGANESE ORE (commercial type)
GEWINNUNG VON EISEN- UND MANGANERZ (Handelsware)
DOBYČA ŽELEZNOJ I MARGANCEVOJ RUDY (tovarnoj)
('000 tons - Tsd. t - tvs. t)

Year Jahr Gody	Iron ore Eisenerz Železnaja ruda	Manganese ore Manganerz Margancevaja ruda	Year Jahr Gody	Iron ore Eisenerz Železnaja ruda	Manganese ore Manganerz Margancevaja ruda
1913	9,214	1,245	1967	168,246	7,175
1922	195	84	1968	176,616	6,564
1928	6,133	702	1969	186,134	6,551
1932	12,086	832	1970	195,492	6,841
1937	27,770	2,752	1971	203,008	7,318
1940	29,866	2,557	1972	208,127	7,819
1945	15,864	1,470	1973	216,104	8,245
1946	19,327	1,730	1974	224,831	8,155
1950	39,651	3,377	1975	232,803	8,459
1955	71,862	4,743	1976	239,110	8,636
1960	105,857	5,872	1977	240,000	8,548 (Plan)
1961	117,633	5,972			
1962	128,111	6,402			
1963	137,502	6,663			
1964	145,856	7,096			
1965	153,432	7,576			
1966	160,271	7,706			

5.1.3.3 PIG IRON OUTPUT IN THE UNION REPUBLICS
ROHEISENGEWINNUNG IN DEN UNIONSREPUBLIKEN
VYPLAVKA ČUGUNA PO SOJUZNYM RESPUBLIKAM
('000 tons - Tsd.t - tys.t)

	1940	1965	1970	1971	1972	1973	1974	1975	1976	1977
SSSR	14,902	66,184	85,933	89,256	92,327	95,933	99,868	102,968	105,000	107,000
RSFSR	5,260	31,158	41,972	44,000	45,146	48,169	51,037	52,183	52,700	--
Ukrainskaja SSR	9,642	32,582	41,411	41,982	43,105	43,511	44,642	46,367	47,300	--
Kazachskaja SSR	--	1,625	1,767	2,528	3,366	3,512	3,408	3,634	4,600	--
Gruzinskaja SSR	--	819	783	746	710	741	781	784	796	--

Economy 5.1.3.4
Wirtschaft 5.1.3.5

5.1.3.4 STEEL OUTPUT IN THE UNION REPUBLICS
STAHLGEWINNUNG IN DEN UNIONSREPUBLIKEN
VYPLAVKA STALI PO SOJUZNYM RESPUBLIKAM
('000 tons - Tsd.t - tys.t)

	1940	1965	1970	1971	1972	1973	1974	1975	1976	1977
SSSR	18,317	91,021	115,889	120,660	125,592	131,481	136,230	141,344	145,000	147,000
RSFSR	9,311	50,058	63,877	66,846	69,248	72,438	75,646	79,881	82,600	83,700
Ukrainskaja SSR	8,938	36,980	46,599	47,363	49,181	50,961	52,370	53,061	53,100	53,700
Belorusskaja SSR	5.2	163.8	196.2	206.6	214.2	221.9	240.0	257.5	--	--
Uzbekskaja SSR	11.4	367.6	389.0	399.1	400.5	404.4	408.2	409.0	410.6	--
Kazachskaja SSR	--	1123.4	2225.3	3252.3	4024.7	4791.2	4829.6	4907.3	5000.6	--
Gruzinskaja SSR	0.2	1364.2	1410.9	1395.3	1303.3	1387.1	1430.7	1471.6	1475.0	--
Azerbajdžanskaja SSR	23.7	811.0	732.6	730.2	748.4	790.4	806.7	824.6	788.0	--
Litovskaja SSR	--	3.0	6.2	6.14	6.2	6.2	6.7	6.5	--	--
Moldavskaja SSR	--	--	0.1	1.1	1.6	2.1	2.8	3.0	--	--
Latvijskaja SSR	27.9	139.2	442.7	444.8	447.3	460.2	464.1	496.2	502.0	--
Kirgizskaja SSR	--	1.9	2.0	6.3	6.1	6.9	8.3	8.9	--	--
Tadžikskaja SSR	--	1.9	2.3	2.6	3.6	4.3	7.9	7.3	--	--
Armjanskaja SSR	--	0.5	0.6	0.52	0.7	0.6	0.7	1.1	--	--
Estonskaja SSR	--	7.0	5.3	5.74	5.8	6.3	7.8	8.6	--	--

5.1.3.5
PRODUCTION OF FINISHED ROLLED STEEL IN THE UNION REPUBLICS
PRODUKTION VON FERTIGEM EISEN- UND STAHLWALZGUT IN DEN UNIONSREPUBLIKEN
PROIZVODSTVO GOTOVOGO PROKATA ČERNYCH METALLOV PO SOJUZNYM RESPUBLIKAM
('000 tons - Tsd.t - tys.t)

	1940	1965	1970	1971	1972	1973	1974	1975	1976	1977
SSSR	11,430	61,650	80,645	84,124	87,470	91,462	94,295	98,686	101,000	102,000
RSFSR	5,747	33,117	43,164	45,593	47,739	49,819	50,976	54,208	56,700	57,300
Ukrainskaja SSR	5,647	26,004	32,669	33,429	34,145	35,354	36,710	37,682	37,700	37,800
Belorusskaja SSR	4.1	57.0	60.3	61.8	61.7	64.9	64.9	65.3	--	--
Uzbekskaja SSR	--	255.0	321.8	331.4	336.2	342.9	349.1	354.8	360.7	--
Kazachskaja SSR	--	390.0	2432.6	2610.9	3081.6	3527.3	3749.4	3846.4	4,000	--
Gruzinskaja SSR	--	960.4	1142.9	1129.1	1046.0	1162.5	1206.0	1234.3	1,274	--
Azerbajdžanskaja SSR	8.5	604.0	585.0	602.6	626.0	665.0	661.0	670.2	--	--
Latvijskaja SSR	23.9	262.3	269.6	366.4	435.0	526.0	578.3	623.7	--	--

5.1.4.1 Economy / Wirtschaft

5.1.4 FUEL INDUSTRY - BRENNSTOFFINDUSTRIE - TOPLIVNAJA PROMYŠLENNOST'

5.1.4.1
FUEL OUTPUT BY TYPES (CONVERTED TO CONVENTIONAL UNITS OF 7000 GREAT CALORIES)
BRENNSTOFFGEWINNUNG NACH ARTEN (UMGERECHNET AUF DIE MASSEINHEIT 7000 KCAL)
DOBYČA TOPLIVA PO VIDAM (V PEREŠČETE NA USLOVNOE TOPLIVO 7000 KILOKALORIJ)

Year Jahr Gody	Total Insg. Vsego	Mineral oil (incl. gas condensate) Erdöl (inkl. Gaskondensat) Neft' (vključaja gazovyj kondensat)	Gas Gas Gaz	Coal Kohle Ugol'	Peat Torf Torf	Shale Schiefer Slancy	Firewood Brennholz Drova
A	B	C	D	E	F	G	H

Mill. tons - Mio t - mln. tonn

1913	48.2	14.7	--	23.1	0.7	--	9.7
1922	29.7	6.7	0.03	9.0	0.9	0.0	13.1
1940	237.7	44.5	4.4	140.5	13.6	0.6	34.1
1945	185.0	27.8	4.2	115.0	9.2	0.4	28.4
1946	202.7	31.0	4.5	127.3	11.2	0.7	28.0
1950	311.2	54.2	7.3	205.7	14.8	1.3	27.9
1955	479.9	101.2	11.4	310.8	20.8	3.3	32.4
1960	692.8	211.4	54.4	373.1	20.4	4.8	28.7
1961	732.7	237.5	70.8	370.1	19.5	5.2	29.6
1962	778.6	266.5	84.6	379.7	12.9	5.8	29.1
1963	847.1	294.7	105.1	388.4	21.7	6.5	30.7
1964	912.2	319.8	127.0	403.3	22.2	7.1	32.8
1965	966.6	346.4	149.8	412.5	17.0	7.4	33.5
1966	1,033.1	379.1	170.1	420.1	24.4	7.5	31.9
1967	1,088.4	411.9	187.4	428.6	22.4	7.5	30.6
1968	1,126.6	442.1	201.2	428.7	18.3	7.6	28.7
1969	1,177.4	469.6	215.5	439.6	16.7	8.0	28.0
1970	1,221.8	502.5	233.5	432.7	17.7	8.8	26.6
1971	1,284.9	537.3	250.6	444.2	16.7	9.5	26.6
1972	1,353.8	572.6	264.6	459.8	21.2	9.9	25.7
1973	1,420.6	613.5	282.4	468.8	20.2	10.6	25.1
1974	1,497.1	656.3	311.4	480.2	13.9	11.3	24.0
1975	1,590.3	701.8	345.7	490.4	16.9	11.7	23.8

Percent of total - Prozentsatz der Gesamtgewinnung - v procentach k itogu

1913	100	30.5	--	48.0	1.4	--	20.1
1922	100	22.5	0.1	30.3	3.0	0.0	44.1
1940	100	18.7	1.9	59.1	5.7	0.3	14.3
1945	100	15.0	2.3	62.2	4.9	0.2	15.4
1946	100	15.3	2.2	62.8	5.5	0.4	13.8
1950	100	17.4	2.3	66.1	4.8	0.4	9.0
1955	100	21.1	2.4	64.8	4.3	0.7	6.7

Economy   5.1.4.1
Wirtschaft 5.1.4.2

A	B	C	D	E	F	G	H
1960	100	30.5	7.9	53.9	2.9	0.7	4.1
1961	100	32.4	9.7	50.5	2.7	0.7	4.0
1962	100	34.2	10.9	48.8	1.7	0.7	3.7
1963	100	34.8	12.4	45.9	2.5	0.8	3.6
1964	100	35.1	13.9	44.2	2.4	0.8	3.6
1965	100	35.8	15.5	42.7	1.7	0.8	3.5
1966	100	36.7	16.5	40.7	2.3	0.7	3.1
1967	100	37.8	17.2	39.4	2.1	0.7	2.8
1968	100	39.2	17.9	38.0	1.6	0.7	2.6
1969	100	39.9	18.3	37.3	1.4	0.7	2.4
1970	100	41.1	19.1	35.4	1.5	0.7	2.2
1971	100	41.8	19.5	34.6	1.3	0.7	2.1
1972	100	42.3	19.4	34.0	1.6	0.7	1.9
1973	100	43.1	20.0	33.0	1.4	0.7	1.8
1974	100	43.8	20.8	32.1	0.9	0.7	1.6
1975	100	44.1	22.6	30.8	1.1	0.7	1.5

5.1.4.2
COAL OUTPUT BY TYPES-KOHLEGEWINNUNG NACH ARTEN-DOBYČA UGLJA PO VIDAM
('000 tons - Tsd.t - tys.tonn)

Year Jahr Gody	Total Insg. Vsego	Hard coal Steinkohle Kamennyj ugol'	Anthracite Anthrazit Antracit	Brown coal Braunkohle Buryj ugol'	of total coal output, in open pit mining v.d.gesamten Kohlegewinnung,gewonnen im Tagebau iz obščej dobyči uglja dobyto otkrytym sposobom
1913[1]	29,117	27,987	4,778	1,130	185
1913[2]	29,153	27,987	4,778	1,166	185
1922	11,324	9,318	2,221	2,006	150
1928	35,510	32,453	8,003	3,057	300
1932	64,360	57,471	18,139	6,889	366
1937	127,968	109,878	28,010	18,090	2,504
1940	165,923	139,974	35,657	25,949	6,309
1945	149,333	99,428	16,896	49,905	17,781
1946	164,063	114,295	21,576	49,768	17,928
1950	261,089	185,225	40,158	75,864	27,141
1955	389,868	276,615	57,834	113,253	64,466
1960	509,623	374,925	74,128	134,698	101,977
1961	506,364	377,019	73,585	129,345	106,625
1962	517,408	386,432	72,536	130,976	114,280
1963	531,722	395,132	72,729	136,590	121,254
1964	553,997	408,870	74,898	145,127	130,854
1965	577,731	427,881	76,467	149,850	140,517
1966	585,629	439,195	76,775	146,434	146,035
1967	595,237	451,422	77,139	143,815	151,164
1968	594,180	455,881	76,896	138,299	150,770
1969	607,802	467,316	76,711	140,486	156,670
1970	624,114	476,406	75,803	147,708	166,627
1971	640,881	487,539	75,760	153,342	179,153
1972	655,188	499,469	75,417	155,719	190,200
1973	667,581	510,621	76,433	156,960	199,440
1974	684,508	523,867	75,828	160,641	212,713
1975	701,280	537,647	76,965	163,633	225,751

5.1.4.3 Economy
5.1.4.4 Wirtschaft

5.1.4.3 COAL OUTPUT IN THE UNION REPUBLICS
KOHLEGEWINNUNG IN DEN UNIONSREPUBLIKEN
DOBYČA UGLJA PO SOJUZNYM RESPUBLIKAM
('000 tons - Tsd.t - tys.tonn)

	1940	1965	1970	1971	1972	1973	1974	1975	1976	1977
SSSR	165,923	577,731	624,114	640,881	655,188	667,581	684,508	701,280	712,000	722,000
RSFSR	72,798	325,889	344,827	353,318	358,749	363,952	372,076	381,059	387,000	394,000
Ukrainskaja SSR	83,841	194,298	207,082	209,461	211,184	212,607	213,674	215,736	218,000	217,000
Uzbekskaja SSR	3.4	4,533	3,747	3,811	3,908	4,275	4,722	5,263	5,412	
Kazachskaja SSR	6,972	45,820	61,578	67,339	74,457	79,819	86,972	92,225	93,700	
Gruzinskaja SSR	625	2,621	2,298	2,322	2,160	2,119	2,152	2,050	1,930	
Kirgizskaja SSR	1,475	3,666	3,695	3,741	3,830	3,912	3,980	4,079	4,270	
Tadžikskaja SSR	204	904	887	889	900	897	932	868	800	

5.1.4.4 MINERAL OIL OUTPUT (INCL. GAS CONDENSATE) IN THE UNION REPUBLICS
ERDÖLGEWINNUNG (MIT GASKONDENSAT) IN DEN UNIONSREPUBLIKEN
DOBYČA NEFTI (VKLJUČAJA GAZOVYJ KONDENSAT) PO SOJUZNYM RESPUBLIKAM
('000 tons - Tsd.t - tys.tonn)

	1940	1965	1970	1971	1972	1973	1974	1975	1976	1977
SSSR	31,121	242,888	353,039	377,075	400,440	429,037	458,948	490,801	520,000	546,000
RSFSR	7,039	199,929	284,753	304,417	325,556	351,002	379,793	411,325	445,000	478,000
Ukrainskaja SSR	353	7,580	13,909	14,330	14,500	14,107	13,494	12,770	11,600	10,500
Belorusskaja SSR	--	39	4,234	5,303	5,846	7,030	7,864	7,954	6,200	
Uzbekskaja SSR	119	1,800	1,805	1,753	1,595	1,535	1,395	1,352	1,282	
Kazachskaja SSR	697	2,022	13,161	16,023	18,112	20,433	22,308	23,889	23,200	
Gruzinskaja SSR	41	30	24	27	24	22	44	261		
Azerbajdžanskaja SSR	22,231	21,500	20,187	19,203	18,365	18,239	17,716	17,169	16,476	
Kirgizskaja SSR	24	305	298	292	277	243	235	230	225.2	
Tadžikskaja SSR	30	47	181	192	203	231	242	274	312	344
Turkmenskaja SSR	587	9,636	14,487	15,535	15,962	16,195	15,857	15,577	14,774	

5.1.4.5 NATURAL GAS OUTPUT IN THE UNION REPUBLICS
GASGEWINNUNG IN DEN UNIONSREPUBLIKEN
DOBYČA GAZA PO SOJUZNYM RESPUBLIKAM
(mill.cu.m. - Mio m³ - mill.ku.m.)

	1940	1965	1970	1971	1972	1973	1974	1975	1976	1977
SSSR	3,219	127,666	197,945	212,398	221,386	236,326	260,553	289,268	321,000	346,000
RSFSR	210	64,257	83,321	87,483	87,400	87,841	100,046	115,217	136,000	158,000
Ukrainskaja SSR	495	39,362	60,877	64,669	67,236	68,161	68,318	68,703	68,700	
Belorusskaja SSR	--	--	178	295	401	413	511	568		
Uzbekskaja SSR	0.7	16,474	32,094	33,653	33,739	37,104	37,064	37,211	36,100	
Kazachskaja SSR	4	29	2,092	2,747	3,525	4,847	5,372	5,199	5,200	
Azerbajdžanskaja SSR	2,498	6,180	5,521	5,822	6,880	8,399	9,151	9,890	10,989	
Kirgizskaja SSR	--	155	367	383	395	396	323	285	260.5	
Tadžikskaja SSR	2	52	388	447	498	520	496	419	319	
Turkmenskaja SSR	9	1,157	13,107	16,899	21,312	28,645	39,272	51,776	62,581	

5.1.5.1 Economy
Wirtschaft

5.1.5 MACHINE BUILDING AND METAL WORKING INDUSTRY
MASCHINENBAU UND METALLBEARBEITENDE INDUSTRIE
MAŠINOSTROENIE I METALLOOBRABOTKA

5.1.5.1 OUTPUT OF EQUIPMENT FOR VARIOUS BRANCHES OF THE INDUSTRY
PRODUKTION VON AUSRÜSTUNGEN FÜR VERSCHIEDENE INDUSTRIEZWEIGE
PROIZVODSTVO OBORUDOVANIJA DLJA RAZLIČNYCH OTRASLEJ PROMYŠLENNOSTI

	1940	1965	1970	1971	1972	1973	1974	1975
Metallurgical installations, '000 tons: Metallurgische Ausrüstungen, Tsd.t: Metallurgičeskoe oborudovanie, tys.t:								
Blast furnace equipment - Hochofen- ausrüstung - domennoe oborudovanie	7.0	83.9	110.8	111.4	120.1	119.4	124	124
Steel smelting equipment - Stahlschmelz- ausrüstung - staleplavil'noe oborudovanie	6.5	37.2	50.7	54.5	45.8	57.3	63.3	63.4
Installations for uninterrupted steel teeming- Anlagen für ununterbrochenes Stahlgießen - ustanovki nepreryvnoj razlivki stali	--	10.0	12.4	16.4	15.1	20.3	24.3	22.1
Installations for steel rolling - Walzwerk- ausrüstung - prokatnoe oborudovanie	10.2	111.2	140.1	140.7	141.1	144.8	127	132
Heading combines, units - Vortriebkombiner, Stck. - Prochodčeskie kombajny, št.	--	131	327	363	424	451	487	510
Coal cutting machines, units - Schrämmaschinen, Stck. - Vrubovye mašiny, št.	1,256	202	115	110	110	85	90	90
Mine loading machines, units - Schachtlade- maschinen, Stck. - Mašiny šachtnye pogruzočnye, št.	194	2,802	2,459	2,553	2,433	2,674	2,811	2,807
Mine electric locomotives, units - Grubenloko- motiven,Stck. - Elektrovozy rudničnye, št.	511	2,411	2,548	2,492	2,585	2,621	2,554	2,605
Oil drilling equipment,'000 tons - Erdölappa- raturen,Tsd.t - Nefteapparatura,tys.t	15.5	139.7	126.6	139.1	156.9	158.7	172	171
Deep-well pumps,'000 units - Tiefbrunnen- pumpen,Tsd.Stck. - Nasosy glubinnye,tys.št.	31.9	92.8	77.0	81.0	81.0	82.0	85.0	85.1
Turbo-drills,sections - Turbobohrer, Sektionen - Turbobury,sekcij	90	8,439	6,562	7,384	7,694	8,103	9,328	9,780

204

Economy
Wirtschaft 5.1.5.1

	1940	1965	1970	1971	1972	1973	1974	1975
Electric drills, units - Elektrotiefbohrgeräte, Stck. - Elektrobury, St.	--	220	115	114	86	112	104	97
Drilling installations for exploitation and deep prospecting, sets - Bohranlagen für Ausbeutungs-u.tiefe Schürfungsbohrungen, Satz - Ustanovki burovye dlja ekspluatacionnogo i glubokogo razvedočnogo burenija, komplektov	129	520	480	497	512	516	483	544
Pumps (except deep-well), '000 units - Pumpen (ohne Tiefbrunnenpumpen), Tsd.Stck. - Nasosy (krome glubinnych), tys.št.	27.0	774.3	1,160	1,199	1,191	1,213	1,328	1,378
Air and gas compressors, '000 units - Luftverdichter u.Gasantriebskompressoren, Tsd. Kompressory vozdušnye i gazovye privodnye, tys.	4.8	66.0	89.5	93.8	95.6	99.9	107	112
Industrial refrigerators, '000 sets-Kühlanlagen für Industriezwecke, Tsd. - Cholodil'nye ustanovki promyšlennogo tipa, tys.komplektov	1.1	141.9	237.5	267.5	291.3	307.9	338	360
Oxygen and liquified gas installations, sets - Anlagen zur Gewinnung von Sauerstoff u.seltener Gase, Satz - Kislorodnye ustanovki i ustanovki redkich gazov, komplektov	...	459	259	246	275	300	327	344
Production equipment for cellulose and paper industries, mill.rubles: Technologische Ausrüstung für Zellulose-u.Papierindustrie, Mio Rubel: Technologičeskoe oborudovanie dlja celljuloznobumažnoj promyšlennosti, mln.rub.:								
at factory wholesale prices of July 1,1955 zu Großhandelspreisen d.Betriebe z.1.Juli 1955 v optovych cenach predprijatij na 1 ijulja 1955	...	40.1						
at factory wholesale prices of July 1,1967 zu Großhandelspreisen d.Betriebe z.1.Juli 1967 v optovych cenach predprijatij na 1 ijulja 1967			84.1	91.8	100.1	114.2	128	143
Industrial fixtures, mill.pcs. - Industrielle Armaturen, Mio Stck. armatura promyšlennaja, mln.št.	...	54.1	74.1	76.8	73.1	78.6	84	86

205

5.1.5.2 Economy / Wirtschaft

5.1.5.2 OUTPUT OF INSTRUMENTS, MEANS OF AUTOMATION, AND COMPUTERS (MILL. RUBLES)
PRODUKTION VON GERÄTEN, AUTOMATISATIONSMITTELN UND EDV (MIO RUBEL)
PROIZVODSTVO PRIBOROV, SREDSTV AVTOMATIZACII I SREDSTV VYČISLITEL'NOJ TECHNIKI (MLN.RUB.)

	At factory wholesale prices of July 1, 1955 / In Großhandelspreisen der Betriebe zum 1.Juli 1955 / V optovych cenach predprijatij na 1 ijulja 1955 g.			At factory wholesale prices of July 1, 1967 / In Großhandelspreisen der Betriebe zum 1.Juli 1967 / V optovych cenach predprijatij na 1 ijulja 1967 g.							
	1940	1965	1967	1967	1970	1971	1972	1973	1974	1975
Instruments, means of automation, and their spare parts, total – Geräte, Automationsmittel u.Ersatzteile dazu, insg. – Pribory, sredstva avtomatizacii i zapasnye časti k nim, vsego	30.6	1850.7	2369.9	1631.4	2364.1	2610.4	2955.9	3354.3	3.798	4,254
Optic-mechanical instruments & apparatuses – Optisch-mechanische Geräte u.Apparaturen – pribory i apparatura optiko-mechaničeskie	5.8	277.6	341.2	256.0	331.6	356.9	392.1	438.3	482	520
Electric measurement instruments – Elektrische Meßgeräte – pribory elektroizmeritel'nye	3.9	229.5	320.4	224.2	314.2	350.5	402.3	460.7	533	623
Technological control instruments – Geräte zur Kontrolle u.Steuerung technischer Prozesse – pribory kontrolja i regulirovanija technologičeskich processov	5.0	442.8	570.2	416.5	565.3	627.2	710.1	807.0	921	1,041
Instruments for physical research – Geräte für physikalische Forschungen – pribory dlja fizičeskich issledovanij	2.0	109.4	106.9	86.7	121.1	131.3	146.6	151.0	159	173
Mechanical measurement instruments – Mechanische Meßgeräte – pribory dlja izmerenija mechaničeskich veličin	4.1	143.7	184.8	148.2	196.6	218.5	241.1	272.8	316	352

Economy   5.1.5.2
Wirtschaft 5.1.5.3

	1940	1965	1967	1967	1970	1971	1972	1973	1974	1975
Instruments for medicine, physiology, and biology - Medizinische, physiologische u.biologische Geräte - pribory dlja mediciny, fiziologii i biologii	0.2	69.1	87.4	73.5	91.1	93.9	101.3	114.0	128	145
Time measuring instruments - Zeitmeßgeräte - pribory vremeni	3.4	341.4	435.0	208.5	281.5	312.4	347.3	394.2	441	503
Instruments for mechanization and automation of engineering & technical jobs - Geräte zur Mechanisierung u.Automatisierung ingenieur-technischer Arbeiten - pribory dlja mechanizacii i avtomatizacii inženerno-techničeskogo truda	4.1	86.8	131.5	85.8	238.1	269.4	322.6	375.5	408	422
Computers and spare parts - EDV und Ersatzteile dazu - Sredstva vyčislitel'noj techniki i zapasnye časti k nim	0.3	245.3	376.1	260.8	709.7	904.9	1.213	1.699	2.221	2.927

5.1.5.3
PRODUCTION OF CHEMICAL EQUIPMENT - PRODUKTION VON CHEMISCHEN AUSRÜSTUNGEN - PROIZVODSTVO CHIMIČESKOGO OBORUDOVANIJA

	1965	1967	1970	1971	1972	1973	1974	1975
Chemical equipment and spare parts,total,mill.rub. Chemische Ausrüstungen u.Ersatzteile dazu,insg.,Mio Rub. Chimičeskoe oborudovanie i zapasnye časti k nemu, vsego, mln.rub.:								
1	340	357	399	453	488	542	607	675
2		361						
Of the total of chemical equipment: Aus der Gesamtmenge der chemischen Ausrüstungen: Iz obščego količestva chimičeskogo oborudovanija: Equipment made of alloy steel, mill.rubles - Ausrüstungen aus Sonderstahl, Mio Rubel - oborudovanie iz special'nych stalej, mln.rub.:								
1	87.4	105.3	113.1	127.4	135.1	159.7	175	194
2		107.4						

1 at factory wholesale prices of July 1, 1955 - in Großhandelspreisen der Betriebe zum 1.Juli 1955 - v optovych cenach predprijatij na 1 ijulja 1955 g.
2 at factory wholesale prices of July 1, 1967 - in Großhandelspreisen der Betriebe zum 1. Juli 1967 - v optovych cenach predprijatij na 1 ijulja 1967 g.

5.1.5.3 Economy
5.1.5.4 Wirtschaft

	1965	1967	1970	1971	1972	1973	1974	1975
Equipment made of non-ferrous metals (except of titanium and alloys), mill.rubles – Ausrüstungen aus Buntmetallen (ohne Ausrüstungen aus Titan und seinen Legierungen), Mio Rubel – oborudovanie iz cvetnych metallov (bez oborudovanija iz titana i ego splavov), mln.rub.								
1	16.7	16.3	15.0	13.6	10.9	12.8	10.4	10.3
2		15.0						
Equipment with chemically stable enamel coating, mill.rubles – Ausrüstungen mit chemisch beständigem Emailleüberzug, Mio Rubel – oborudovanie s chimičeski stojkim emalepokrytiem, mln.rub.								
1	7.6	13.7	27.8	38.8	43.3	46.1		
2		12.9						
Equipment for reprocessing of polymer materials and spare parts, mill.rubles – Ausrüstungen f.d.Verarbeitung von Polymeren u.Ersatzteile, Mio Rubel – oborudovanie dlja pererabotki polimernych materialov i zapasnye časti k nemu, mln.rub.								
1	42.7	66.6	65.2	76.5	81.4	92.0	92.3	96.0
2		68.3						

5.1.5.4 PRODUCTION OF MATERIAL-HANDLING EQUIPMENT (UNITS)
PRODUKTION VON HEBE- UND TRANSPORTAUSRÜSTUNGEN (STCK.)
PROIZVODSTVO PODEMNO-TRANSPORTNOGO OBORUDOVANIJA (ST.)

	1940	1965	1970	1971	1972	1973	1974	1975
Electric bridge cranes (incl.special) – Elektrische Brückenkräne (einschl. Spezialkräne) – Krany mostovye električeskie (vključaja special'nye)	302	6,764	5,740	5,772	5,750	5,928	6,359	6,523
Railway cranes – Eisenbahnkräne – Krany na železnodorožnom chodu	258	463	493	496	509	482	474	499
Truck hoists – Kräne mit Automobilfahrwerk – Krany na avtomobil'nom chodu	139	11,141	15,397	16,231	16,369	17,186	18,989	19,681

1 at factory wholesale prices of July 1, 1955 – in Großhandelspreisen der Betriebe zum 1.Juli 1955 – v optovych cenach predprijatij na 1 ijulja 1955 g.
2 at factory wholesale prices of July 1, 1967 – in Großhandelspreisen der Betriebe zum 1.Juli 1967 – v optovych cenach predprijatij na 1 ijulja 1967 g.

	1940	1965	1970	1971	1972	1973	1974	1975
Tower cranes – Turmkräne – Krany bašennye	57	3,455	3,925	4,161	4,393	4,593	4,589	4,641
Cranes on pneumatic wheels – Kräne mit Luftreifenfahrwerk – Krany na pnevmokolesnom chodu	--	1,236	1,963	2,180	2,235	2,272	2,459	2,442
Elevators – Aufzüge – Lifty	513	8,639	18,107	20,746	22,804	24,259	25,323	25,218

5.1.5.5 OUTPUT OF PRODUCTION EQUIPMENT FOR THE LIGHT, FOOD, AND PRINTING INDUSTRIES, AND TRADE AND PUBLIC CATERING ENTERPRISES
PRODUKTION VON TECHNOLOGISCHEN AUSRÜSTUNGEN FÜR DIE LEICHT-, NAHRUNGSMITTEL- UND POLYGRAPHISCHE INDUSTRIE UND FÜR BETRIEBE DES HANDELS UND DER ÖFFENTLICHEN ERNÄHRUNG
PROIZVODSTVO TECHNOLOGIČESKOGO OBORUDOVANIJA DLJA LEGKOJ, PIŠČEVOJ, POLIGRAFIČESKOJ PROMYŠLENNOSTI I PREDPRIJATIJ TORGOVLI I OBŠČESTVENNOGO PITANIJA

	1940	1965	1967	1970	1971	1972	1973	1974	1975
Production equipment for light industry and spare parts, mill.rubles – Technologische Ausrüstungen f.d.Leichtindustrie und Ersatzteile dazu, Mio Rubel – Technologičeskoe oborudovanie i zapasnye časti k nemu dlja legkoj promyšlennosti, mln.rub. [1] [2]	...	311	406 376	430	458	498	560	629	691
Production equipment for textile industry and spare parts, mill.rubles – Technologische Ausrüstungen f.d.Textilindustrie und Ersatzteile dazu, Mio Rubel – Technologičeskoe oborudovanie i zapasnye časti k nemu dlja tekstil'noj promyšlennosti, mln.rub. [1] [2]	...	188	238 231	265	285	316	361	423	476
Combing machines for cotton industry, units – Krempel f.d.Baumwollindustrie, Stck. – Česal'nye mašiny dlja chlopčatobumažnoj promyšlennosti, St.	1,312	3,796	4,564	5,177	5,902	4,153	3,637	3,300	2,500

1 at factory wholesale prices of July 1, 1955 – in Großhandelspreisen der Betriebe zum 1.Juli 1955 – v optovych cenach predprijatij na 1 ijulja 1955 g.
2 at factory wholesale prices of July 1, 1967 – in Großhandelspreisen der Betriebe zum 1.Juli 1967 – v optovych cenach predprijatij na 1 ijulja 1967 g.

5.1.5.5 Economy / Wirtschaft

	1940	1965	1967	1970	1971	1972	1973	1974	1975
Spinning machines, units – Spinnmaschinen,Stck.– prjadil'nye mašiny, št.	1,109	3,227	3,923	4,027	3,855	4,442	4,761	5,100	5,400
Winding machines (except those for silk), units Haspelmaschinen (ohne Seidenhaspelmaschinen),Stck. motalnye mašiny (bez šelkomotal'nych), št.	27	566	541	352	354	560	570	518	540
Looms, '000 Units – Webstühle, Tsd.Stck. – tkackie stanki, tys.št.	1.8	24.3	21.3	19.8	18.6	19.5	25.0	28.8	31.3
Production equipment for the knitted goods industry and spare parts, mill.rubles – Technologische Ausrüstungen f.d.Trikotagenindustrie und Ersatzteile dazu, Mio Rubel – Technologičeskoe oborudovanie i zapasnye časti k nemu dlja trikotažnoj promyšlennosti, mln.rub.									
1	...	24.8	38.4	36.0	36.1	37.7	40.8	41.2	43.7
2			31.6						
Automatic hosiery machines, units – Strumpf- u.Sockenrundstrickautomaten, Stck. – krugločuločno-nosočnye avtomaty, št.	1,243	3,249	4,707	3,135	2,654	2,679	2,836	2,800	2,900
Production equipment for the clothing industry and spare parts, mill.rubles – Technologische Ausrüstungen f.d.Bekleidungsindustrie u.Ersatzteile dazu, Mio Rubel – Technologičeskoe oborudovanie i zapasnye časti k nemu dlja švejnoj promyšlennosti, mln.rub.									
1	...	37.7	48.2	47.9	55.9	61.7	67.3	67.4	70.8
2			37.0						
Industrial sewing machines, '000 units – Nähmaschinen für Industriezwecke, Tsd.Stck. – švejnye promyšlennye mašiny, tys.št.	20	105	126	129	157	165	180	170	148
Dye and decoration work machinery and spare parts, mill.rubles – Färbe-u.Dekorationsausrüstungen u.Ersatzteile dazu, Mio Rubel –									

1 at factory wholesale prices of July 1, 1955 – in Großhandelspreisen der Betriebe zum 1.Juli 1955 – v optovych cenach predprijatij na 1 ijulja 1955 g.
2 at factory wholesale prices of July 1, 1967 – in Großhandelspreisen der Betriebe zum 1.Juli 1967 – v optovych cenach predprijatij na 1 ijulja 1967 g.

Economy
Wirtschaft 5.1.5.5

	1940	1965	1967	1970	1971	1972	1973	1974	1975
Krasil'no-otdeločnoe oborudovanie i zapasnye časti k nemu, mln.rub.									
1	...	18.8	30.5						
2			30.3	29.2	26.9	25.5	28.4	36.5	36.1
Production equipment for leather shoes, furs, and haberdashery industries and spare parts, mill.rubles – Technologische Ausrüstungen f.d. Leder-, Schuh-, Pelz- u. Lederkurzwarenindustrie u. Ersatzteile dazu, Mio Rubel – Technologičeskoe oborudovanie i zapasnye časti k nemu dlja koževenno-obuvnoj, mechovoj i kožgalanterejnoj promyšlennosti, mln.rub.									
1	...	15.8	22.2						
2			19.8	24.5	25.3	28.1	29.4	27.5	29.0
Production equipment for the food industry, and spare parts, mill.rubles – Technologische Ausrüstungen f.d. Nahrungsmittelindustrie u. Ersatzteile dazu, Mio Rubel – Technologičeskoe oborudovanie i zapasnye časti k nemu dlja piščevoj promyšlennosti, mln.rub.									
1	...	249	317						
2			279	344	354	388	420	465	501
Automatic pasteurization and cooling plate installations, with capacity of 3,000-10,000 litres p.hr., sets – Automatisierte plattenförmige Pasteurisier- u. Kühleinrichtungen mit einer Leistung von 3.000-10.000 l/h – Avtomatizirovannye plastinčatye pasterizacionno-ochladitel'nye ustanovki proizvoditel'nosti 3000-10000 l/čas, komplektov	--	871	1,692	2,187	1,034	1,531	1,916	2,319	2,661
Equipment lines for washing and bottling milk and milk products, with capacity of 2.000-12.000 bottles p.hr., sets –									

1 at factory wholesale prices of July 1, 1955 – in Großhandelspreisen der Betriebe zum 1.Juli 1955 – v optovych cenach predprijatij na 1 ijulja 1955 g.
2 at factory wholesale prices of July 1, 1967 – in Großhandelspreisen der Betriebe zum 1.Juli 1967 – v optovych cenach predprijatij na 1 ijulja 1967 g.

5.1.5.5 Economy / Wirtschaft

	1940	1965	1967	1970	1971	1972	1973	1974	1975
Einrichtungen f.Flaschenreinigung,Einfüllen von Milch u.Dickmilch u.Verschließen der Flaschen m.e.Leistung von 2.000-12.000 Flaschen/h,Satz – Linii oborudovanija dlja mojki butylok,razliva v nich moloka,prostokvaši i ukuporki proizvoditel' nostiju 2000-12000 butylok v čas, komplektov	–	89	174	329	140	216	234	194	79
Printing equipment and spare parts, mill.rub.– Polygraphische Ausrüstungen u.Ersatzteile dazu, Mio Rubel – Poligrafičeskoe oborudovanie i zapasnye časti k nemu, mln.rub.									
1			43.3	50.4	51.5	54.0	55.2	60.9	60.7
2	1	36.2	42.2						
Composing machines, units – Setzmaschinen, Stck. – nabornye mašiny, št.	145	1,314	1,306	1,626	1,683	1,841	1,814	1,493	1,019
Printing presses, units – Druckmaschinen, Stck. – pečatnye mašiny, št.	411	1,512	2,748	2,293	2,319	2,363	2,107	2,394	2,017
Production equipment for the trade and catering industries and spare parts, mill.rubles – Technologische Ausrüstungen f.d.Betriebe d.Handels u.d.öffentlichen Ernährung u.Ersatzteile dazu, Mio Rubel – Technologičeskoe oborudovanie i zapasnye časti k nemu dlja predprijatij torgovli i obščestvennogo pitanija, mln.rub.									
1	...	145.6	220.6	277	301	343	385	412	443
2			177.6						

1 at factory wholesale prices of July 1, 1955 – in Großhandelspreisen der Betriebe zum 1.Juli 1955 – v optovych cenach predprijatij na 1 ijulja 1955 g.
2 at factory wholesale prices of July 1, 1967 – in Großhandelspreisen der Betriebe zum 1.Juli 1967 – v optovych cenach predprijatij na 1 ijulja 1967 g.

5.1.5.6 OUTPUT OF SANITARY ENGINEERING EQUIPMENT
PRODUKTION VON SANITÄR-TECHNISCHEN AUSRÜSTUNGEN
PROIZVODSTVO SANITARNO-TECHNIČESKOGO OBORUDOVANIJA

	1965	1970	1971	1972	1973	1974	1975
Heating boilers, mill. standard sq.m - Heizungskessel, Mio m² - Kotly otopitel'nye, mln.uslovnych m²	2.8	3.7	3.7	3.8	3.9	4.1	4.3
Heating radiators and convectors, mill.equivalent sq.m - Heizkörper u.Konvektoren, Mio äquivalente m² - Radiatory i konvektory otopitel'nye,mln.ekvivalentnych m²	25.5	29.7	32.2	34.2	36.6	40.0	42.1
Air heaters, mill.sq.m - Kaliroferen, Mio m² - Kalorifery, mln.m²	8.0	10.6	11.3	12.0	12.1	11.9	12.2
Iron sewer pipes and moulded parts, '000 tons - Gußeiserne Kanalisationsrohre u.Formteile dazu,Tsd.t - Truby kanalizacionnye čugunnye i fasonnye časti k nim, tys.t	320.6	367.1	383.0	385.8	408.9	425	437
Gilled tubes, mill.sq.m - Rippenrohre, Mio m² - Truby rebristye, mln.m²	3.1	3.1	3.0	2.9	2.9	2.7	2.8
Enameled bathtubs, '000 units - Emaillierte Badewannen, Tsd.Stck. - Vanny emalirovannye, tys.št.	1,613	1,886	1,892	1,944	2,025	2,226	2,235
Water heaters for baths, '000 units - Badeöfen, Tsd.Stck. - Kolonki vodogrejnye dlja vann, tys.št.	659	890	957	995	970	763	765

5.1.5.7 Economy / Wirtschaft

OUTPUT OF AGRICULTURAL MACHINES - PRODUKTION VON LANDWIRTSCHAFTSMASCHINEN - PROIZVODSTVO SEL'SKOCHOZJAJSTVENNYCH MAŠIN

	1940	1965	1970	1971	1972	1973	1974	1975
Agricultural machinery, mill.rubles - Landwirtschaftsmaschinen, Mio Rubel - Sel'skochozjajstvennye mašiny, mln.rub.: at factory wholesale prices - in Großhandelspreisen d. Betriebe - v optovych cenach predprijatij								
of July 1 - zum 1.Juli - na 1 ijulja 1955	50							
of July 1 - zum 1.Juli - na 1 ijulja 1967		1,461	2,121	2,346	2,623	2,989	3,470	3,772
Basic types of agricultural machines, '000 units - Grundarten der Landwirtschaftsmaschinen, Tsd.Stck. - Osnovnye vidy sel'skochozjajstvennych mašin, tys.št.								
Tractor ploughs - Schlepperpflüge - Plugi traktornye	38.4	166	212	221	227	232	218	205
of which, mounted - darunter Anbaupflüge - v tom čisle navesnye	--	54.1	124	131	140	138	140	144
Tractor stubble breakers - Schlepperschälpflüge - Luščil'niki traktornye	3.8	18.4	22.8	26.4	26.6	28.7	30.1	32.1
Tractor drills - Traktor-Drillmaschinen - Sejalki traktornye	21.4	262	163	141	145	160	178	180
of which, mounted - darunter Anbaudrillmaschinen - v tom čisle navesnye	--	28.3	39.6	49.3	58.8	54.5	57.4	56.8
Potato planters - Kartoffellegemaschinen - Kartofelesažalki traktornye	3.6	16.1	18.0	13.0	6.9	2.3	7.2	9.1
Tractor cultivators - Traktor-Hackmaschinen - Kul'tivatory traktornye	32.3	206	219	184	178	195	178	188
of which, mounted - darunter Anbauhackmaschinen - v tom čisle navesnye	1.3	83.6	114	121	114	124	122	122
Sprayers and dusters - Kombinierte Spritz-u.Stäubegeräte - Opryskivateli i opylivateli traktornye	2.9	26.9	31.2	32.7	34.0	37.8	39.9	33.1
Windrowers - Mäher mit seitlichem Mähwerk - Žatki rjadkovye	--	97.8	47.7	51.8	60.4	63.7	83.5	92.1
Grain combines - Mähdrescher - Kombajny zernouboročnye	12.8	85.8	99.2	102	95.7	84.8	88.4	97.5

Economy
Wirtschaft 5.1.5.7

	1940	1965	1970	1971	1972	1973	1974	1975
Potato harvesting machines – Kartoffelvollerntemaschinen – Kombajny kartofeleuboročnye	--	4.9	7.0	8.0	8.6	8.8	8.8	9.4
Beet harvesters – Rübenvollerntemaschinen – Kombajny sveklouboročnye	--	17.5	9.1	10.1	11.4	14.1	15.9	17.1
Corn harvesters – Maisvollerntemaschinen – Kombajnye kukuruzouboročnye	--	6[1]	5.1	7.0	8.2	9.1	10.1	10.3
Grain cleaning machines – Getreidereinigungsmaschinen – Zernoočistitel'nye mašiny	4.3	24.1	22.0	20.6	19.1	19.0		
Cotton-picking machines (in physical units) – Baumwollerntemaschinen (in physikalischen Einheiten) – Chlopkouboročnye mašiny (v fizičeskich edinicach)	5[1]	7.7	5.9	6.7	6.8	6.7	7.4	7.6
Sprinkling machines – Bewässerungsmaschinen – Doždeval'nye mašiny	...	14.3	12.3	13.8	13.2	22.4	25.0	27.1
Tractor mowers – Schleppermähmaschinen – Kosilki traktornye	3.3	122	144	150	155	131	93.0	83.9
of which, mounted – darunter Anbaumähmaschinen – v tom čisle navesnye	--	53.6	99.2	115	124	101	77.5	73.8
Tractor rakes – Schlepperrechen – Grabli traktornye	0.9	39.9	61.7	49.6	48.0	59.1	53.0	46.1
Pick-up balers – Sammelpressen – Press-podborščiki	...	7.0	15.8	18.1	20.8	23.0	25.5	28.1
Forage harvesters – Silokombiner – Kombajny silosouboročnye	--	20.0	34.3	40.2	53.9	60.1	68.4	70.9
Loaders – Lademaschinen f.d.Landwirtschaft – Pogruzčiki universal'nye sel'skochozjajstvennogo naznačenija	...	68.7	78.2	82.0	87.4	85.8	85.9	90.1
Feed crushers – Futterzerkleinerungsmaschinen – Drobilki kormov	--	17.6	14.2	16.2	20.2	28.0	32.0	33.2
Automated troughs – Selbsttränken für Rindvieh – Avtopoilki dlja krupnogo rogatogo skota	--	3,831	5,305	5,560	5,366	5,301	5,339	5,169
Milking machines – Melkanlagen – Doil'nye ustanovki	--	6.7	39.2	56.1	57.1	55.3	54.0	53.3

1 pieces – Stück – štuk

5.1.5.8 Economy / Wirtschaft

5.1.5.8 OUTPUT OF TRACTORS BY TYPES – PRODUKTION VON TRAKTOREN NACH ARTEN – PROIZVODSTVO TRAKTOROV PO VIDAM
('000 units – Tsd.Stck. – tys.št.)

	1940	1965	1970	1971	1972	1973	1974	1975
Total – Insgesamt – Vsego	31.6	354.5	458.5	472.0	477.8	499.6	531.1	550.4
Caterpillars – Raupenschlepper – guseničnye	26.5	157.0	217.7	225.5	229.5	230.1	239.5	252.6
Wheel-type – Radschlepper – kolesnye	5.1	197.5	240.8	246.5	248.3	269.5	291.6	297.8
Of the total of tractors – Aus der Gesamtzahl der Traktoren – Iz obščego količestva traktorov:								
Cultivating – Ackerschlepper – propašnye	5.1	206.6	247.7	251.3	245.9	255.2	266.0	271.1
Ploughing – Pflugschlepper – pachotnye	26.5	133.9	193.8	203.3	213.6	226.8	246.0	259.4
Skidding – Holzrückschlepper – trelevočnye	--	14.0	17.0	17.4	18.3	17.6	19.1	19.9

5.1.6 CHEMICAL INDUSTRY - CHEMISCHE INDUSTRIE - CHIMIČESKAJA PROMYŠLENNOST'

5.1.6.1 OUTPUT OF MINERAL FERTILIZERS BY TYPES ('000 tons)
PRODUKTION VON MINERALDÜNGER NACH ARTEN (Tsd.t)
PROIZVODSTVO MINERAL'NYCH UDOBRENIJ PO VIDAM (tys.t)

	1940	1950	1960	1965	1970	1971	1972	1973	1974	1975
Converted to 100% consumable contents - Umgerechnet auf 100%igen Nährstoffgehalt - V peresčete na 100%-noe soderžanie pitatel'nych veščestv										
Mineral fertilizers, total - Mineraldünger,insg. - Mineral'nye udobrenija,vs.	746	1,236	3,281	7,389	13,099	14,670	15,931	17,429	19,352	21,998
of which - darunter - v tom čisle:										
nitrogen - Stickstoff - azotnye	199	392	1,003	2,712	5,423	6,055	6,551	7,241	7,856	8,535
phosphate - Phosphate - fosfatnye	253	440	912	1,599	2,500	2,772	2,929	3,236	3,868	4,452
potassium - Kali - kalijnye	221	312	1,084	2,368	4,087	4,807	5,433	5,918	6,586	7,944
ground phosphorite - Phosphoritmehl - fosforitnaja muka	73	92	280	701	1,085	1,030	1,011	1,025	1,034	1,059
In standard units - in Normeinheiten - V uslovnych edinicach										
Mineral fertilizers, total - Mineraldünger,insg. - Mineral'nye udobrenija,vs.	3,238	5,497	13,867	31,253	55,400	61,398	66,066	72,332	80,357	90,202
of which - darunter - v tom čisle:										
nitrogen - Stickstoff - azotnye	972	1,913	4,892	13,217	26,442	29,530	31,945	35,310	38,308	41,628
phosphate - Phosphate - fosfatnye	1,352	2,351	4,878	8,550	13,370	14,826	15,663	17,305	20,683	23,816
potassium - Kali - kalijnye	532	750	2,606	5,691	9,824	11,556	13,061	14,224	15,832	19,097
ground phosphorite - Phosphoritmehl - fosforitnaja muka	382	483	1,473	3,690	5,709	5,420	5,319	5,395	5,442	5,573

5.1.6.2 Economy
5.1.6.3 Wirtschaft

5.1.6.2
OUTPUT OF MINERAL FERTILIZERS IN THE UNION REPUBLICS (IN STANDARD UNITS, '000 tons)
PRODUKTION VON MINERALDÜNGER IN DEN UNIONSREPUBLIKEN (IN NORMEINHEITEN, Tsd.t)
PROIZVODSTVO MINERAL'NYCH UDOBRENIJ PO SOJUZNYM RESPUBLIKAM (V USLOVNYCH EDINICACH,tys.t)

	1940	1965	1970	1971	1972	1973	1974	1975	1976	1977
SSSR	3,238	31,253	55,400	61,398	66,066	72,332	80,357	90,202	92,300	96,700
RSFSR	2,164	16,197	27,277	29,669	31,341	33,797	36,771	42,444	43,200	45,900
Ukrainskaja SSR	1,012	7,312	11,541	12,310	13,023	14,052	16,349	18,265	19,400	20,000
Belorusskaja SSR	13	1,850	6,120	7,250	8,105	9,001	9,873	11,033	11,400	11,700
Uzbekskaja SSR	2	2,146	4,091	4,570	4,920	5,351	5,801	6,132	5,839	5,878
Kazachskaja SSR	--	776	1,957	2,822	3,348	4,186	5,334	5,822	5,800	6,500
Gruzinskaja SSR	--	436	467	561	560	648	672	696	713	749
Azerbajdžanskaja SSR	--	448	580	489	624	754	853	896	940	979
Litovskaja SSR	--	593	1,168	1,411	1,640	1,862	1,977	2,111	2,207	2,470
Tadžikskaja SSR	--	--	252	261	324	373	387	406	402	405
Armjanskaja SSR	--	103	253	299	345	393	400	401	385	416
Turkmenskaja SSR	--	257	368	395	404	402	397	431	430	428
Estonskaja SSR	--	804	1,326	1,361	1,432	1,513	1,543	1,565	1,400	1,382

5.1.6.3 OUTPUT OF SYNTHETIC RESINS AND PLASTICS
PRODUKTION VON SYNTHETISCHEN HARZEN UND KUNSTSTOFFEN
PROIZVODSTVO SINTETIČESKICH SMOL I PLASTIČESKICH MASS

Year Jahr Gody	'000 tons Tsd. t tys.tonn	Year Jahr Gody	'000 tons Tsd. t tys.tonn
1928	0.3	1967	1,113
1932	2.4	1968	1,291
1937	8.0	1969	1,453
1940	10.9	1970	1,673
1945	21.3	1971	1,864
1946	26.3	1972	2,042
1950	67.1	1973	2,320
1955	160.3	1974	2,493
1960	311.6	1975	2,842
1965	802.9	1976	3,100
1966	971.1	1977	3,300

5.1.6.4 OUTPUT OF CHEMICAL FIBRES – PRODUKTION VON CHEMISCHEN FASERN – PROIZVODSTVO CHIMIČESKICH VOLOKON
('000 tons – Tsd.t – tys.tonn)

Year Jahr Gody	Chemical fibres–chemische Fasern–chimičeskie volokna					Synthetic fibres–synthetische Fasern–sintetičeskie volokna			
	Total Insg. Vsego	Artificial fibres Kunst- fasern Iskusstven- nye volokna	Silk(with- out cord) Seide(ohne Seide f.Kord) Šelk(bez šel- ka dlja korda)	Silk for cord Seide für Kord Šelk dlja korda	Staple fibre Stapel- faser Stapel'noe volokno	Total Insg. Vsego	Silk (without cord and tech- nical articles) Seide (ohne Seide f.Kord u.techni- sche Erzeugnisse) Šelk(bez šelka dlja korda i tech- ničeskich izdelij)	Silk for cord and technical articles Seide f.Kord u.technische Erzeugnisse Šelk dlja korda i techničeskich izdelij	Staple fibre Stapel- faser Štapel'noe volokno
1928	0.2	0.2	0.2	--	--	--	--	--	--
1932	2.8	2.8	2.8	--	--	--	--	--	--
1937	8.6	8.6	7.6	--	1.0	--	--	--	--
1940	11.1	11.1	8.6	--	2.5	--	--	--	--
1945	1.1	1.1	0.7	--	0.4	--	--	--	--
1946	3.2	3.2	2.0	--	1.2	--	--	--	--
1950	24.2	22.9	11.2	2.2	9.5	1.3	1.2	--	0.1
1955	110.5	101.6	30.4	14.2	57.0	8.9	5.5	1.4	2.0
1960	211.2	196.2	47.4	53.7	95.1	15.0	6.6	4.1	4.3
1965	407.3	329.8	78.6	86.0	165.2	77.5	20.3	33.9	23.3
1966	458.3	362.0	82.1	99.2	180.7	96.3	22.4	47.4	26.5
1967	510.7	394.8	87.4	104.2	203.2	115.8	27.6	57.5	30.7
1968	553.7	424.0	88.8	117.1	218.1	129.7	31.2	63.0	35.5
1969	583.5	441.0	90.7	127.1	223.2	142.5	36.4	67.0	39.1
1970	623.0	456.4	93.1	129.0	234.3	166.5	39.5	75.6	51.4
1971	676.4	473.3	98.2	132.3	242.8	203.1	42.0	90.3	70.8
1972	746.1	507.5	105.4	139.8	262.3	238.6	47.9	109.3	81.4
1973	830.0	543.1	110.1	149.2	283.8	286.9	51.6	124.6	110.7
1974	887	569	111	156	302	318	54	141	123
1975	955	590	122	159	309	365	60	171	134
1976									
1977									

5.1.6.5 Economy / Wirtschaft

5.1.6.5 OUTPUT OF TIRES BY TYPES (mill.pics.)
PRODUKTION VON KRAFTFAHRZEUG- UND FAHRRADDECKEN (Mio Stck.)
PROIZVODSTVO AVTOPOKRYŠEK PO VIDAM I VELOSIPEDNYCH POKRYŠEK (mill.št.)

	1940	1965	1970	1971	1972	1973	1974	1975
Automobile tires – Kraftfahrzeugdecken – Avtopokryški	3.0	26.4	34.6	36.2	38.8	42.3	47.1	51.5
of which – darunter – v tom čisle: for trucks – für LKW – dlja gruzovych avtomobilej	1.1	16.0	17.2	17.9	18.5	19.5	20.6	21.3
for passenger cars – für PKW – dlja legkovych avtomobilej	1.8	3.8	5.2	6.2	7.5	9.2	11.5	13.9
for wheel tractors and agricultural machines – für Radschlepper u.Landwirtschaftsmaschinen – dlja kolesnych traktorov i sel'skochozjajstvennych mašin	—	3.6	6.0	6.8	7.6	8.2	9.0	9.7
for motorcycles and -rollers – für Motorräder und -roller – dlja motociklov i motorollerov	0.05	3.0	6.2	5.3	5.2	5.4	6.0	6.6
Bicycle tires – Fahrraddecken – Pokryški velosipednye	0.8	12.9	13.5	13.9	14.2	14.9	15.0	15.2

Economy   5.1.7.1
Wirtschaft 5.1.7.2

5.1.7 FORESTRY, WOOD WORKING AND CELLULOSE-PAPER INDUSTRY
FORST-, HOLZBEARBEITENDE UND ZELLULOSE-PAPIER-INDUSTRIE
LESNAJA, DEREVOOBRABATYVAJUSČAJA I CELLJULOZNO-BUMAŽNAJA PROMYŠLENNOST'

5.1.7.1
TIMBER LOGGING (mill.compact cu.m) - NUTZHOLZEINSCHLAG (Mio fm³) - VYVOZKA DREVESINY (mill.plotnych kubičeskich metrov)

Year Jahr Gody	Timber, total Holz, insg. Vsja drevesina	Commercial timber Nutzholz Delovaja drevesina	Firewood Brennholz Drova	Year Jahr Gody	Timber, total Holz, insg. Vsja drevesina	Commercial timber Nutzholz Delovaja drevesina	Firewood Brennholz Drova
1913[1]	60.6	27.2	33.4	1966	373.5	271.7	101.8
1913[2]	67.0	30.5	36.5	1967	383.0	286.9	96.1
1928	61.7	36.0	25.7	1968	380.4	289.9	90.5
1932	164.7	99.4	65.3	1969	374.2	286.3	87.9
1937	209.0	114.2	94.8	1970	385.0	298.5	86.5
1940	246.1	117.9	128.2	1971	384.7	298.3	86.4
1945	168.4	61.6	106.8	1972	382.9	297.6	85.3
1946	185.5	80.3	105.2	1973	387.8	304.3	83.5
1950	266.0	161.0	105.0	1974	388.5	303.7	82.3
1955	333.9	212.1	121.8	1975	395.1	312.9	81.7
1960	369.5	261.5	108.0	1976			
1965	378.9	273.8	105.1	1977			

5.1.7.2
EXPLOITATION OF DENSELY WOODED REGIONS - ERSCHLIESSUNG DER WALDREICHEN REGIONEN - OSVOENIE MNOGOLESNYCH RAJONOV

	1940	1965	1970	1971	1972	1973	1974	1975
Timber logging, mill.compact cu.m. - Holzeinschlag, Mio fm³ - Vyvozka drevesiny, mln.plotnych m³	246.1	378.9	385.0	384.7	383.0	387.6	388	395
in densely wooded regions-in waldreichen Regionen - iz mnogolesnych rajonov	132.2	263.3	276.5	276.4	277.2	282.8	285	290
in poorly wooded regions - in waldarmen Regionen - iz malolesnych rajonov	113.9	115.6	108.5	108.3	105.8	104.8	103	105

1 within the borders of the U.S.S.R. up to 17.9.1939 - in den Grenzen der UdSSR bis 17.9.1939 - v granicach SSSR do 17 sentjabrja 1939 g.
2 in the present borders of the U.S.S.R. - in den heutigen Grenzen der UdSSR - v sovremennych granicach SSSR

5.1.7.2 Economy
Wirtschaft

	1940	1965	1970	1971	1972	1973	1974	1975
Of the total timber logged, commercial timber, mill. compact cu.m. – vom gesamten Holzeinschlag, Nutzholz, Mio fm³ – iz obščej vyvozki drevesiny, delovaja drevesina, mln.plotnych m³	117.9	273.8	298.5	298.3	297.6	304.2	304	313
in densely wooded regions – in waldreichen Regionen – iz mnogolesnych rajonov	69.8	201.0	225.9	225.6	226.1	231.2	231	238
in poorly wooded regions – in waldarmen Regionen – iz malolesnych rajonov	48.1	72.8	72.6	72.7	71.5	73.0	73	75
Portion of total timber logged (percent of total) – Anteil am gesamten Holzeinschlag (in %) – Udel'nyj ves vo vsej vyvozke drevesiny (v procentach):								
Timber from densely wooded regions – Holz aus waldreichen Rayons – drevesiny iz mnogolesnych rajonov	54	69	72	72	72	73	73	73
Timber from poorly wooded Rayons – Holz aus waldarmen Rayons – drevesiny iz malolesnych rajonov	46	31	28	28	28	27	27	27
Portion of total commercial timber logged (percent of total) – Anteil am gesamten Nutzholzeinschlag (in %) – Udel'nyj ves vo vsej vyvozke delovoj drevesiny (v procentach):								
Timber from densely wooded regions – Holz aus waldreichen Regionen – drevesiny iz mnogolesnych rajonov	59	73	76	76	76	76	76	76
Timber from poorly wooded regions – Holz aus waldarmen Regionen – drevesiny iz malolesnych rajonov	41	27	24	24	24	24	24	24

The densely wooded regions are – Zu den waldreichen Regionen gehören – K mnogolesnym rajonam otneseny: Archangel'skaja, Vologodskaja i Murmanskaja oblasti, Karel'skaja ASSR, Komi ASSR, Kirovskaja oblast', Baškirskaja ASSR, Permskaja i Sverdlovskaja oblasti, Altajskij kraj, Kemerovskaja, Tomskaja i Tjumenskaja oblasti, Krasnojarskij kraj, Irkutskaja i Citinskaja oblasti, Burjatskaja ASSR, Tuvinskaja ASSR, Primorskij i Chabarovskij kraja, Amurskaja, Kamčatskaja, Magadanskaja i Sachalinskaja oblasti, Jakutskaja ASSR, Vostočno-Kazachstanskaja oblast'.

Economy 5.1.7.3
Wirtschaft 5.1.7.4

5.1.7.3 OUTPUT OF SAWED TIMBER AND PLYWOOD - PRODUKTION VON SCHNITTHOLZ UND FURNIERPLATTEN - PROIZVODSTVO PILOMATERIALOV I FANERY KLEENOJ

Year Jahr Gody	Sawed timber, mill.cu.m. Schnittholz, Mio m³ Pilomaterialy, mln.m³	Plywood, '000 cu.m. Furnierplatten, Tsd. m³ Fanera kleenaja, tys. m³	Year Jahr Gody	Sawed timber, mill.cu.m. Schnittholz, Mio m³ Pilomaterialy, mln.m³	Plywood, '000 cu.m. Furnierplatten, Tsd. m³ Fanera kleenaja, tys. m³
1913[1]	11.9	130.0	1966	106.7	1,830
1913[2]	14.2	203.5	1967	109.0	1,878
1928	13.6	185.4	1968	110.0	1,899
1932	24.4	423.6	1969	112.3	1,946
1937	33.8	678.9	1970	116.4	2,045
1940	34.8	731.9	1971	118.8	2,083
1945	14.7	192.2	1972	118.7	2,110
1946	19.6	251.6	1973	116.2	2,142
1950	49.5	657.5	1974	115	2,160
1955	75.6	1,049	1975	116	2,196
1960	105.6	1,354			
1965	111.0	1,756			

5.1.7.4 OUTPUT OF SAWED TIMBER IN THE UNION REPUBLICS ('000 compact cu.m.)
PRODUKTION VON SCHNITTHOLZ IN DEN UNIONSREPUBLIKEN (Tsd. fm³)
PROIZVODSTVO PILOMATERIALOV PO SOJUZNYM RESPUBLIKAM (tys.kubičeskich metrov)

	1940	1965	1970	1971	1972	1973	1974	1975
SSSR	34,831	110,975	116,391	118,842	118,709	116,193	114,748	116,219
RSFSR	28,755	89,924	91,829	93,401	93,786	92,678	91,725	93,513
Ukrainskaja SSR	2,981	9,036	10,377	10,680	10,698	10,024	9,568	9,479
Belorusskaja SSR	1,635	2,762	3,070	3,286	3,250	3,127	3,176	3,171
Uzbekskaja SSR	30	630	709	803	720	589	602	579
Kazachskaja SSR	320	2,694	2,551	2,671	2,727	2,639	2,694	2,645
Gruzinskaja SSR	258	633	659	667	658	595	619	577
Azerbajdžanskaja SSR	77	403	386	375	349	332	330	331
Litovskaja SSR	223	1,044	1,313	1,285	1,204	1,111	1,034	1,098
Moldavskaja SSR	19	540	624	624	592	589	505	526
Latvijskaja SSR	244	1,205	1,352	1,552	1,362	1,224	1,041	999
Kirgizskaja SSR	54	441	335	355	324	322	327	288
Tadžikskaja SSR	13	229	262	276	221	204	230	210
Armjanskaja SSR	52	236	197	173	162	136	129	128
Turkmenskaja SSR	12	171	237	156	131	103	114	171
Estonskaja SSR	158	730	798	814	838	828	901	796

5.1.7.5
TIMBER LOGGING IN THE UNION REPUBLICS - HOLZEINSCHLAG IN DEN UNIONSREPUBLIKEN -
('000 compact cu.m. - Tsd. fm^3 - tys.plotnych kubičeskich metrov)

	1940 Timber, total Holz, insg. Vsja drevesina A	of which, commercial timber darunter Nutzholz v tom čisle delovaja B	1965 A	B	1970 A	B	1971 A	B
SSSR	246,062	117,906	378,906	273,834	385,019	298,548	384,689	298,320
RSFSR	215,746	101,750	346,074	252,123	353,991	276,767	352,679	275,610
Ukrainskaja SSR	7,768	5,210	12,529	9,704	9,271	7,030	9,261	7,176
Belorusskaja SSR	10,208	6,108	7,183	4,884	6,262	4,707	6,663	4,941
Uzbekskaja SSR	165	10	64	5	67	1	75	0.4
Kazachskaja SSR	2,104	713	2,039	1,232	1,901	1,245	1,955	1,336
Gruzinskaja SSR	939	323	1,009	557	651	408	608.4	399
Azerbajdžanskaja SSR	185	89	222	86	160	59	146	65
Litovskaja SSR	3,000	1,260	2,530	1,277	2,685	1,519	2,698	1,527
Moldavskaja SSR	57	8	184	79	237	110	215	95
Latvijskaja SSR	3,969	1,344	4,991	2,659	7,307	5,012	7,854	5,481
Kirgizskaja SSR	261	137	40	22	41	22	40	19
Tadžikskaja SSR	82	1	21	2	22	3	22	2.4
Armjanskaja SSR	110	39	106	65	74	46	65.2	40
Turkmenskaja SSR	120	--	62	--	9	--	12	--
Estonskaja SSR	1,348	914	1,852	1,139	2,341	1,619	2,395	1,628

Economy 5.1.7.5
Wirtschaft

VYVOZKA DREVESINY PO SOJUZNYM RESPUBLIKAM

1972		1973		1974		1975	
A	B	A	B	A	B	A	B
382,930	297,602	387,792	304,325	388,468	303,650	395,054	312,902
353,176	276,515	358,982	283,527	360,746	283,295	366,915	292,024
9,199	7,146	9,330	7,338	9,280	7,398	9,635	7,715
6,475	4,852	6,387	4,927	6,161	4,912	6,190	5,054
80	0.2	86	3.5	73	--	60	--
1,956	1,402	2,110	1,538	2,259	1,618	2,210	1,584
658	403	605	368	638	401	564	345
124.1	52	122	58	137	62	119	68
2,598	1,602	2,775	1,812	2,515	1,787	2,685	1,835
217	98	210	94	211	97	206	97
5,937	3,851	4,767	2,960	4,037	2,350	3,937	2,287
42	20	44	25	41	21	39	19
21	3	20	3.7	22	4	25	4
65	40	65	41	63	40	58	39
8.4	--	8	--	5	--	5	--
2,373	1,618	2,281	1,630	2,280	1,665	2,406	1,831

5.1.7.6 Economy
5.1.7.7 Wirtschaft

5.1.7.6 OUTPUT OF CELLULOSE, NEWSPRINT, AND CARDBOARD ('000 tons) – PRODUKTION VON ZELLULOSE, PAPIER UND KARTON (Tsd.t) – PROIZVODSTVO ZELLJULOZY, BUMAGI I KARTONA (tys.tonn)

Year Jahr Gody	Cellulose Zellulose zelljuloza	Newsprint & cardboard Papier und Karton bumaga i karton	Newsprint Papier bumaga	Cardboard Karton karton	Year Jahr Gody	Cellulose Zellulose zelljuloza	Newsprint & cardboard Papier und Karton bumaga i karton	Newsprint Papier bumaga	Cardboard Karton karton
1913[1]	41	226	197	29	1966	3,599	5,231	3,568	1,663
1913[2]	258	310	269	41	1967	4,031	5,677	3,9P1	1,876
1928	86	332	285	47	1968	4,341	5,970	3,955	2,015
1932	185	544	471	73	1969	4,615	6,284	4,046	2,238
1937	426	976	832	144	1970	5,110	6,701	4,185	2,516
1940	592	991	838	153	1971	5,412	7,086	4,407	2,679
1945	276	377	321	56	1972	5,684	7,424	4,613	2,811
1946	328	614	514	100	1973	6,070	7,890	4,908	2,982
1950	1,100	1,485	1,180	305	1974	6,340	8,198	5,040	3,158
1955	1,742	2,408	1,848	560	1975	6,840	8,583	5,215	3,368
1960	2,282	3,227	2,334	893	1976	7,200	8,916	5,389	3,527
1965	3,234	4,680	3,231	1,449	1977	7,400	9,100	5,500	3,600

5.1.7.7 OUTPUT OF NEWSPRINT IN THE UNION REPUBLICS ('000 tons) – PAPIERERZEUGUNG IN DEN UNIONSREPUBLIKEN (Tsd.t) – PROIZVODSTVO BUMAGI PO SOJUZNYM RESPUBLIKAM (tys.tonn)

	1940	1965	1970	1971	1972	1973	1974	1975	1976	1977
SSSR	838	3,231	4,185	4,407	4,613	4,908	5,040	5,215	5,389	5,500
RSFSR	691	2,659	3,476	3,662	3,833	4,085	4,192	4,317	4,500	4,500
Ukrainskaja SSR	28	166	187	193	201	213	222	235	245	250
Belorusskaja SSR	51	90	103	122	139	158	165	178	174.6	178.4
Uzbekskaja SSR	1.9	17	23	23	24	24.5	24.7	26.1	26.1	26.2
Kazachskaja SSR	--	--	--	--	1.6	1	10	18.3	--	10.7
Gruzinskaja SSR	9.7	32	36	35	36	40	36	33	33.1	35.5
Litovskaja SSR	11	72	102	106	110	113	116	119	122	124
Latvijskaja SSR	24	98	148	157	159	164	162	174	169	169
Armjanskaja SSR	--	2	5	8	8	6	8.6	11.1	--	--
Estonskaja SSR	21.6	95	105	101	101	103	104	103	104	106

1 within the borders of the U.S.S.R. up to 17.9.1939 – in den Grenzen der UdSSR bis 17.9.1939 – v granicach SSSR do 17 sentjabrja 1939 g.
2 in the present borders of the U.S.S.R. – in den heutigen Grenzen der UdSSR – v sovremennych granicach SSSR

5.1.8
CONSTRUCTION MATERIALS INDUSTRY - BAUSTOFFINDUSTRIE - PROMYŠLENNOST' STROITEL'NYCH MATERIALOV

5.1.8.1 OUTPUT OF CEMENT BY TYPES, IN 1975 ('000 tons) - ZEMENTERZEUGUNG NACH SORTEN IM JAHRE 1975 (Tsd. t) -
PROIZVODSTVO CEMENTA PO MARKAM V 1975 G. (tys.tonn)

	Cement type Zementsorte Marka cementa					Average type of cement (kg/cm^2) Durchschnittl. Zementsorte (kg/cm^2) srednjaja marka cementa (kg/sm^2)
	200	300	400	500	600	
Cement, total Zement, insg. Cement, vsego	761	22,249	73,480	21,902	379	399
of which, portland darunter Portlandzement v tom čisle portlandskij	--	1,419	55,546	21,883	379	427

5.1.8.2 OUTPUT OF CEMENT IN THE UNION REPUBLICS ('000 tons) - ZEMENTERZEUGUNG IN DEN UNIONSREPUBLIKEN (Tsd.t) -
PROIZVODSTVO CEMENTA PO SOJUZNYM RESPUBLIKAM (tys.tonn)

	1940	1965	1970	1971	1972	1973	1974	1975	1976
SSSR	5,773	72,388	95,248	100,331	104,299	109,521	115,145	122,057	124,000
RSFSR	3,567	43,931	57,680	60,309	62,712	65,427	68,890	73,119	74,500
Ukrainskaja SSR	1,218	12,341	17,271	17,836	18,740	20,198	21,489	22,462	22,500
Belorusskaja SSR	200	1,748	1,929	1,940	1,952	1,987	2,040	2,169	2,180
Uzbekskaja SSR	267	2,465	3,196	3,222	3,360	3,434	3,480	3,536	3,572
Kazachskaja SSR	--	4,037	5,653	5,991	6,144	6,297	6,491	6,782	7,300
Gruzinskaja SSR	118	1,375	1,451	1,496	1,481	1,534	1,601	1,671	1,675
Azerbajdžanskaja SSR	112	1,274	1,409	1,455	1,346	1,439	1,453	1,398	1,381
Litovskaja SSR	--	798	1,121	1,875	2,060	2,157	2,279	2,993	3,308
Moldavskaja SSR	--	574	760	899	940	1,025	1,175	1,231	1,236
Latvijskaja SSR	125	762	862	869	875	887	853	903	877
Kirgizskaja SSR	--	508	990	1,013	1,029	1,048	1,076	1,131	1,180
Tadžikskaja SSR	--	940	872	941	967	975	993	1,010	995
Armjanskaja SSR	95	620	730	1,078	1,243	1,563	1,768	1,828	1,816
Turkmenskaja SSR	--	340	360	436	464	534	510	564	615
Estonskaja SSR	71	675	964	971	986	1,016	1,047	1,260	1,196

5.1.8.3 Economy / Wirtschaft

5.1.8.3 OUTPUT OF VARIOUS TYPES OF PRECAST CONCRETE STRUCTURES AND COMPONENTS ('000 cu.m. of articles) –
PRODUKTION EINZELNER ARTEN VON MONTIERBAREN STAHLBETONKONSTRUKTIONEN UND DETAILS (Tsd. m³ der Erzeugnisse) –
PROIZVODSTVO OTDEL'NYCH VIDOV SBORNYCH ŽELEZOBETONNYCH KONSTRUKCIJ I DETALEJ (tys.kubičeskich metrov izdelij)

	1965	1970	1971	1972	1973	1974	1975	1976
Precast concrete structure and components, total – Montierbare Stahlbetonkonstruktionen u.Details,insg.– Sbornye železobetonnye konstrukcii i detali-vsego	56,106	84,561	90,763	96,067	102,949	108,540	114,161	118,702
of which – davon – iz nich:								
Wall slabs – Wandplatten – Stenovye paneli	6,357	11,580	12,866	14,129	15,784	17,340	18,649	19,359
Concrete poles for electric power and tele-communication lines;precast components for the system of electrified roads & lighting networks – Stahlbetonstützen für Kraftübertragungsstrecken u.Fernmeldelinien; Elemente des Montagenetzes d. elektrifizierten Bahnen u.Lichtleitungsnetze – Železobetonnye opory dlja linij elektroperedači i svjazi;elementy montažnoj seti elektrificirovannych dorog i osvetitel'nych setej	809	1,362	1,408	1,402	1,444	1,460	1,537	1,585
Concrete railroad sleepers – Stahlbetonschwellen für Eisenbahn – Železobetonnye železnodorožnye špaly	278	744	834	902	945	1,086	989	1,030
Concrete blocks and tubing for tunnels and mining piles – Stahlbetonblöcke und -tübbings für Tunnelbau und Schachtausbau – Železobetonnye bloki i tjubingi dlja tonnelej i šachtnaja krep'	307	485	524	597	587	626	631	625
Concrete pipes – Stahlbetonrohre – Truby železobetonnye	958	1,185	1,298	1,384	1,490	1,649	1,774	1,838
Of the total of precast concrete structures and components,those of prestressed reinforced concrete – Aus der Gesamtmenge der montierbaren Stahlbeton-konstruktionen und Details, Spannbeton – Iz obščego količestva sbornych železobetonnych konstrukcij i detalej-s predvaritel'no naprjažennym armirovaniem	10,045	19,330	20,551	21,853	23,437	25,545	27,167	28,269

5.1.8.4 OUTPUT OF WALL CONSTRUCTION MATERIALS (mill.standard type bricks)
PRODUKTION VON BAUSTOFFEN NACH ARTEN (Mio Stck. Einheitsziegel)
PROIZVODSTVO STENOVYCH MATERIALOV PO VIDAM (mln.št. uslovnogo kirpiča)

	1965	1970	1971	1972	1973	1974	1975	1976
Wall construction materials, total – Baustoffe, insg. – Stenovye materialy, vsego	46,553	56,860	58,717	60,122	61,565	61,832	62,997	62,779
of which–darunter–v tom čisle: Bricks for construction – Bauziegel – Kirpič stroitel'nyj	36,574	43,153	44,561	45,650	46,709	46,727	47,212	46,447
of which baked bricks – davon gebrannte Ziegel – v tom čisle obožžennyj	28,177	32,378	33,239	33,876	34,257	33,788	33,726	32,477
Large concrete and silicate blocks (incl. concrete blocks for basement walls) – Große Beton- und Silikatblöcke (einschl. Betonblöcke für Kellermauern) – Stenovye krupnye betonnye i silikatnye bloki (vključaja betonnye bloki sten podvalov)	3,409	5,289	5,674	6,056	6,383	6,635	6,891	7,283
Small blocks (for walls) – Kleine Blöcke – Stenovye melkie bloki	1,962	2,595	2,580	2,674	2,768	2,368	2,416	2,307
Blocks of natural stone (for walls) – Blöcke aus Naturstein – Stenovye bloki iz estestvennogo kamnja	4,495	5,376	5,283	5,086	4,974	4,820	5,028	5,116
Blocks of cellular concrete (for walls) – Blöcke aus Zellenbeton – Stenovye bloki iz jačeistych betonov	113	447	619	656	731	1,282	1,450	1,626

5.1.8.5 Economy
5.1.8.6 Wirtschaft

5.1.8.5 OUTPUT OF ROOFING MATERIALS - PRODUKTION VON BEDACHUNGSMATERIALIEN - PROIZVODSTVO KROVEL'NYCH MATERIALOV

Year Jahr Gody	Soft roofing and insulating materials (mill.squ.m) Weiche Bedachungs-u. Isolationsmaterialien (Mio m^2) Mjagkie krovel'nye materialy i izol (mln.m^2)	Asbestos slate (mill.unit plates) Asbestschiefer (Mio Einheitsplatten) Sifer asbesto-cement-nyj (mln.uslovnych plitok)	Tiles (mill.squ.m roofage) Dachziegel (Mio m^2 Dachfläche) Čerepica (mln.m^2 krojuščej poverchnosti)
1913[1]	8.8	9.0	1.9
1913[2]	10.2	9.0	2.1
1928	19.2	38.5	...
1932	66.0	112	3.7
1937	161	187	8.9
1940	130	212	10.5
1945	71.2	83.6	1.8
1946	126	170	3.8
1950	286	546	13.1
1955	504	1,488	28.3
1960	750	2,991	51.1
1965	1,083	4,162	20.3
1966	1,157	4,512	19.6
1967	1,207	4,864	18.2
1968	1,182	5,145	16.3
1969	1,261	5,222	12.0
1970	1,334	5,840	8.7
1971	1,369	6,200	5.6
1972	1,417	6,571	4.9
1973	1,557	6,978	4.0
1974	1,684	7,367	2.9
1975	1,760	7,840	1.9
1976	1,885	8,114	1.2
1977(Plan)	1,904	8,310	--

5.1.8.6 OUTPUT OF LINOLEUM - PRODUKTION VON LINOLEUM - PROIZVODSTVO LINOLEUMA

Year Jahr Gody	mill.squ.m. Mio m^2 mln.m^2	Year Jahr Gody	mill.squ.m. Mio m^2 mln.m^2
1955	5.0	1970	57.4
1960	13.3	1971	59.8
1965	31.2	1972	60.1
1966	33.4	1973	61.1
1967	38.8	1974	64.2
1968	45.4	1975	71.9
1969	51.3	1976	78.7

---
1 within the borders of the U.S.S.R. up to 17.9.1939 - in den Grenzen der UdSSR bis 17.9.1939 - v granicach SSSR do 17 sentjabrja 1939 g.
2 within the present borders of the U.S.S.R. - in den heutigen Grenzen der UdSSR - v sovremennych granicach SSSR

5.1.9 LIGHT INDUSTRY – LEICHTINDUSTRIE – LEGKAJA PROMYŠLENNOST'

5.1.9.1 OUTPUT OF THE MOST IMPORTANT PRODUCTS OF THE LIGHT INDUSTRY
PRODUKTION DER WICHTIGSTEN ERZEUGNISSE DER LEICHTINDUSTRIE
PROIZVODSTVO VAŽNEJŠICH IZDELIJ LEGKOJ PROMYŠLENNOSTI

	1940	1965	1970	1971	1972	1973	1974	1975	1976	1977(Plan)
Cotton fibre, '000 tons – Baumwollfaser, Tsd.t – Chlopok-volokno, tys.t	849	1,835	2,129	2,361	2,360	2,471	2,476	2,648	2,590	2,611
Raw silk, tons – Rohseide, t – Šelk-syrec, t	1,816	2,645	3,020	3,078	3,119	3,303	3,435	3,461	3,414	3,610
Cotton yarn, '000 tons – Baumwollgarn, Tsd.t – Chlopčatobumažnaja prjaža, tys.t	655	1,292	1,435	1,495	1,505	1,535	1,557	1,573	1,583	1,655
Cotton fabrics – Baumwollgewebe – Chlopčatobumažnye tkani:										
mill.running m – Mio lfd.m – mln.pog.m	3,970	7,077	7,482	7,716	7,680	7,839	7,857	7,810	7,899	8,196
mill.squ.m – Mio m² – mln.m²	2,715	5,499	6,152	6,397	6,421	6,578	6,624	6,634	6,779	7,004
Cotton twists, mill.reels (in reels of 200 m) – Baumwollfäden, Mio Rollen (in 200-Meter-Rollen) – Chlopčatobumažnye nitki,mln.katušek (v 200-m-namotke)	1,212	2,256	2,594	2,685	2,751	2,853	2,879	2,887	– –	– –
Wool yarn, '000 tons – Wollgarn, Tsd.t – Šerstjanaja prjaža, tys.t	84.7	236	350	371	377	393	408	417	429	461
Wool fabrics – Wollgewebe – Šerstjanye tkani:										
mill.running m – Mio lfd.m – mln.pog.m	122	365	496	515	518	530	541	552	567	603
mill.squ.m – Mio m² – mln.m²	155	466	643	675	681	703	724	740	764	816
Linen yarn, '000 tons – Leinengarn, Tsd.t – L'njanaja prjaža, tys.t	114	209	252	264	264	267	267	260	268	280
Linen fabrics – Leinengewebe – L'njanye tkani:										
mill.running m – Mio lfd.m – mln.pog.m	289	587	725	773	776	795	797	768	781	794
mill.squ.m. – Mio m² – mln.m²	272	548	707	760	775	796	796	779	807	822
Silk fabrics – Seidenstoffe – Šelkovye tkani:										
mill.running m – Mio lfd.m – mln.pog.m	80.4	937	1,241	1,273	1,348	1,401	1,447	1,517	1,588	1,618
mill.squ.m. – Mio m² – mln.m²	66.7	801	1,146	1,190	1,270	1,345	1,413	1,508	1,599	1,648

5.1.9.1 Economy
Wirtschaft

	1940	1965	1970	1971	1972	1973	1974	1975	1976	1977 (Plan)
Ready-to-wear products, '000 mill.rubles (at factory wholesale prices of July 1, 1967) - Konfektionserzeugnisse, Mrd.Rubel (in Großhandelspreisen der Betriebe zum 1.7.1967 - Švejnye izdelija, mlrd.rub. (v optovych cenach predprijatij na 1 ijulja 1967 g.)	...	9.0	16.0	17.0	17.2	17.5	18.0	19.0	19.8	19.7
Hosiery and socks, mill.pairs - Strumpf-Socken-Erzeugnisse, Mio Paar - Čuločno-nosočnye izdelija,mln.par	489	1,350	1,338	1,309	1,337	1,411	1,469	1,495	1,540	1,542
Linen hosiery, mill.pcs. - Wäschetrikotagen, Mio Stck. - Bel'evoj trikotaž, mln.št.	127	715	814	828	843	900	920	955	990	1,031
Outer hosiery, mill.pcs. - Obertrikotagen, Mio Stck.- Verchnij trikotaž, mln.št.	58.9	188	415	446	451	460	469	465	472	491
Leather shoes, mill.pairs - Lederschuhe, Mio Paar - Kožanaja obuv', mln.par	212	486	679	682	647	666	684	698	724	742
Rubber shoes, mill.pairs - Gummischuhe, Mio Paar - Rezinovaja obuv', mln.par	71.4	161	173	179	180	194	205	205	203	204
Felt shoes, mill.pairs - Filzschuhe, Mio Paar - Valjanaja obuv'(vključaja fetrovuju), mln.par	18.0	33.3	31.8	31.5	30.9	30.8	30.5	30.1	29.2	29.8
Carpets and carpet products, mill.squ.m.- Teppiche und Teppicherzeugnisse, Mio m^2 - Kovry i kovrovye izdelija, mln.m^2	...	19.6	30.3	33.1	35.9	39.0	44.7	47.5	52.2	61.7

Economy 5.1.9.2
Wirtschaft 5.1.9.3

5.1.9.2 OUTPUT OF COTTON FABRICS IN THE UNION REPUBLICS (Mill.running meters)
PRODUKTION VON BAUMWOLLGEWEBEN NACH UNIONSREPUBLIKEN (Mio laufende Meter)
PROIZVODSTVO CHLOPCATOBUMAŽNYCH TKANEJ PO SOJUZNYM RESPUBLIKAM (mln.pogonnych metrov)

	1940	1965	1970	1971	1972	1973	1974	1975	1976[1]
SSSR	3969.6	7076.9	7481.9	7716.3	7679.7	7838.6	7856.8	7809.9	6,779
RSFSR	3707.2	6002.0	6144.0	6297.9	6226.8	6319.7	6265.9	6104.6	5,153
Ukrainskaja SSR	13.8	184.9	247.7	255.4	260.6	293.7	364.3	429.4	437
Belorusskaja SSR	9.1	8.4	86.1	100.2	108.4	110.9	111.7	100.5	116.5
Uzbekskaja SSR	107.4	254.1	210.1	210.7	212.0	215.7	217.7	223.1	184.2
Kazachskaja SSR	0.1	22.5	64.1	65.8	79.8	80.3	94.0	96.7	103.3
Gruzinskaja SSR	0.4	59.2	63.9	52.8	56.4	64.7	65.7	66.2	56.7
Azerbajdžanskaja SSR	49.1	132.2	132.9	132.1	125.8	122.8	127.0	125.5	107.4
Litovskaja SSR	2.4	23.1	33.7	38.4	39.5	55.6	76.6	86.3	85.8
Moldavskaja SSR	---	2.1	3.5	3.9	4.3	4.1	3.9	18.5	36.3
Latvijskaja SSR	20.6	59.7	63.5	65.6	69.1	69.2	61.5	62.8	55.0
Kirgizskaja SSR	0.04	1.8	1.7	35.8	40.0	44.9	46.0	64.0	71.9
Tadžikskaja SSR	0.2	78.7	99.9	97.9	99.8	108.0	109.4	113.1	93.3
Armjanskaja SSR	26.8	88.3	94.5	95.7	86.9	89.4	94.3	100.1	81.7
Turkmenskaja SSR	9.7	19.8	19.0	19.8	20.1	22.3	23.1	23.1	20.8
Estonskaja SSR	22.8	140.1	217.3	244.3	250.2	237.3	195.7	196.0	172.0

5.1.9.3 OUTPUT OF WOOLEN FABRICS IN THE UNION REPUBLICS (mill.running meters)
PRODUKTION VON WOLLGEWEBEN NACH UNIONSREPUBLIKEN (Mio laufende Meter)
PROIZVODSTVO ŠERST'JANYCH TKANEJ PO SOJUZNYM RESPUBLIKAM (mln.pogonnych metrov)

	1940	1965	1970	1971	1972	1973	1974	1975	1976[1]
SSSR	121.8	365.0	495.7	515.5	518.0	529.9	540.9	551.6	764
RSFSR	101.5	279.1	358.1	374.0	375.8	384.5	386.5	390.8	535
Ukrainskaja SSR	12.0	23.6	48.8	51.2	51.9	53.3	53.7	54.4	73.7
Belorusskaja SSR	0.3	19.8	24.8	26.1	26.5	27.3	28.1	29.0	42.7
Kazachskaja SSR	0.4	3.9	5.0	5.4	5.5	5.5	10.8	14.1	23.9
Gruzinskaja SSR	1.9	3.4	6.5	6.9	6.3	6.0	5.8	5.3	7.8
Azerbajdžanskaja SSR	0.5	5.2	8.5	9.0	9.9	10.8	11.8	12.4	16.1
Litovskaja SSR	2.0	8.4	10.8	10.5	10.8	11.1	11.9	12.4	18.4
Moldavskaja SSR	---	0.02	0.9	0.9	0.9	0.9	0.9	0.9	0.8
Latvijskaja SSR	1.8	10.6	13.4	13.0	12.9	13.3	13.8	14.0	18.0
Kirgizskaja SSR	0.3	2.6	8.3	8.0	7.0	6.3	6.8	6.9	11.4
Armjanskaja SSR	0.02	3.8	5.2	4.9	4.2	4.4	4.1	4.6	7.7
Turkmenskaja SSR	---	0.7	1.0	1.1	1.2	0.9	0.9	0.7	0.9
Estonskaja SSR	1.1	3.7	4.4	4.6	4.7	5.1	5.3	5.3	7.4

[1] mill.squ.m. - Mio m^2

5.1.9.4 Economy
5.1.9.5 Wirtschaft
5.1.9.6

5.1.9.4 OUTPUT OF LINEN FABRICS IN THE UNION REPUBLICS (mill.running meters)
PRODUKTION VON LEINENGEWEBEN NACH UNIONSREPUBLIKEN (Mio laufende Meter)
PROIZVODSTVO L'NJANYCH TKANEJ PO SOJUZNYM RESPUBLIKAM (mln.pogonnych metrov)

	1940	1965	1970	1971	1972	1973	1974	1975	1976[1]
SSSR	289.0	587.3	725.3	772.5	776.0	794.6	796.6	768.4	807
RSFSR	263.4	458.1	564.8	604.4	606.0	612.6	614.2	583.8	584
Ukrainskaja SSR	2.1	30.6	53.9	59.2	60.1	67.1	68.6	69.8	86.7
Belorusskaja SSR	15.8	57.0	60.9	62.3	63.0	64.4	65.4	68.4	86.3
Litovskaja SSR	1.6	18.3	20.8	21.3	20.1	21.2	20.5	19.0	24.3
Latvijskaja SSR	3.8	13.8	16.6	16.8	18.7	20.9	21.1	21.3	19.0
Estonskaja SSR	2.3	9.5	8.3	8.5	8.1	8.4	6.8	6.1	6.6

5.1.9.5 OUTPUT OF SILK FABRICS IN THE UNION REPUBLICS (mill.running meters)
PRODUKTION VON SEIDENGEWEBEN NACH UNIONSREPUBLIKEN (Mio laufende Meter)
PROIZVODSTVO ŠELKOVYCH TKANEJ PO SOJUZNYM RESPUBLIKAM (mln.pogonnych metrov)

	1940	1965	1970	1971	1972	1973	1974	1975	1976[1]
SSSR	80.4	937.1	1241.2	1272.6	1347.5	1401.0	1447.1	1517.0	1,599
RSFSR	61.6	728.1	903.5	892.6	925.9	936.9	952.8	973.1	978
Ukrainskaja SSR	---	48.8	84.4	105.7	126.7	149.2	150.7	159.2	189
Belorusskaja SSR	0.005	2.6	19.9	19.9	20.7	20.8	26.3	42.0	71.8
Uzbekskaja SSR	4.5	37.8	50.4	59.7	69.5	75.2	86.2	94.2	93.6
Gruzinskaja SSR	5.3	20.7	38.2	40.3	40.6	39.5	41.1	42.8	43.8
Azerbajdžanskaja SSR	0.2	10.5	18.5	20.0	22.3	25.1	29.6	31.7	34.6
Litovskaja SSR	1.7	16.2	25.7	27.0	28.4	29.7	30.1	30.9	34.7
Moldavskaja SSR	---	8.1	16.8	18.8	21.1	24.9	27.0	28.9	30.3
Latvijskaja SSR	3.7	10.5	11.4	12.2	14.0	14.7	17.3	19.9	24.0
Kirgizskaja SSR	0.04	8.5	8.6	8.8	8.3	8.9	8.8	9.4	9.7
Tadžikskaja SSR	1.6	34.2	43.2	44.5	45.3	49.2	49.2	54.0	56.2
Armjanskaja SSR	0.2	7.9	12.1	13.0	13.8	14.7	16.1	18.2	18.7
Turkmenskaja SSR	0.1	0.06	4.9	5.3	5.7	6.5	5.9	6.4	6.6
Estonskaja SSR	1.5	3.1	3.6	4.8	5.0	5.5	5.8	5.9	6.0

5.1.9.6 OUTPUT OF COTTON FIBRES IN THE UNION REPUBLICS ('000 tons)
PRODUKTION VON BAUMWOLLFASERN NACH UNIONSREPUBLIKEN (Tsd.t)
PROIZVODSTVO CHLOPKA-VOLOKNA PO SOJUZNYM RESPUBLIKAM (tys.t)

	1940	1965	1970	1971	1972	1973	1974	1975	1976	1977(
SSSR	849	1,835	2,129	2,361	2,360	2,471	2,476	2,648	2,590	2,611
Uzbekskaja SSR	534	1,237	1,384	1,541	1,515	1,583	1,581	1,659	1,673	1,759
Kazachskaja SSR	32.9	70.4	96.6	105.7	100.4	100.8	103.4	113.5	--	--
Azerbajdžanskaja SSR	58.2	118.5	131.4	139.9	147.1	158.4	146.9	177.8	--	--
Kirgizskaja SSR	27.9	60.0	59.2	68.5	68.9	66.5	71.7	69.8	--	70.5
Tadžikskaja SSR	60.9	195.0	235.0	252.3	257.7	255.8	258.4	277.6	273	266
Turkmenskaja SSR	71.5	150.3	222.7	253.3	271.4	307.0	314.5	350.1	--	--

[1] mill.squ.m. - Mio m^2

Economy   5.1.9.7
Wirtschaft 5.1.9.8

5.1.9.7 OUTPUT OF RAW SILK IN THE UNION REPUBLICS (tons)
PRODUKTION VON ROHSEIDE NACH UNIONSREPUBLIKEN (t)
PROIZVODSTVO SELKA-SYRCA PO SOJUZNYM RESPUBLIKAM (tonn)

	1940	1965	1970	1971	1972	1973	1974	1975	1976	1977
SSSR	1,816	2,645	3,020	3,078	3,119	3,303	3,435	3,461	3,414	3,610(Pla
Ukrainskaja SSR	---	150	167	169	171	174	176	176	172	--
Uzbekskaja SSR	693	936	1,172	1,144	1,162	1,287	1,379	1,399	1,430	1,582
Gruzinskaja SSR	312	345	424	426	426	437	439	441	436	--
Azerbajdžanskaja SSR	292	358	409	439	446	476	501	512	484	--
Moldavskaja SSR	---	111	127	126	126	126	126	125	121	--
Kirgizskaja SSR	84	109	123	117	118	118	122	124	127	--
Tadžikskaja SSR	254	313	322	355	375	376	363	355	326	--
Armjanskaja SSR	21	51	47	52	51	52	53	54	51	--
Turkmenskaja SSR	149	272	229	250	244	257	276	275	267	279

5.1.9.8 OUTPUT OF HOSIERY AND SOCKS IN THE UNION REPUBLICS (mill.pairs)
PRODUKTION VON STRUMPF-SOCKEN-ERZEUGNISSEN NACH UNIONSREPUBLIKEN (Mio Paar)
PROIZVODSTVO ČULOČNO-NOSOČNYCH IZDELIJ PO SOJUZNYM RESPUBLIKAM (mln.par)

	1940	1965	1970	1971	1972	1973	1974	1975	1976	1977
SSSR	489	1,350	1,338	1,309	1,337	1,411	1,469	1,495	1,540	1,542(Pla
RSFSR	278.8	651.3	570.5	542.0	541.4	579.1	600.7	600.0	619.4	--
Ukrainskaja SSR	79.4	270.6	282.8	284.5	292.6	304.9	318.8	323.9	331	336
Belorusskaja SSR	81.0	102.1	109.8	110.2	117.0	121.4	125.4	129.3	132.7	134.7
Uzbekskaja SSR	8.6	29.4	30.1	31.2	32.8	33.8	35.7	36.6	38.1	39.3
Kazachskaja SSR	0.2	42.2	56.3	54.7	59.0	62.0	64.6	66.5	67.2	67.2
Gruzinskaja SSR	2.8	12.6	15.7	17.2	16.1	20.6	22.1	24.3	25.4	22.2
Azerbajdžanskaja SSR	20.9	34.5	24.9	24.9	24.1	26.1	27.0	28.1	31.1	33.6
Litovskaja SSR	2.0	58.2	73.3	75.0	75.5	78.4	80.8	84.2	86.5	86.1
Moldavskaja SSR	---	23.5	29.0	27.7	29.7	30.2	32.1	32.2	33.6	34.0
Latvijskaja SSR	3.3	37.3	58.3	59.4	60.3	61.4	62.6	64.7	65.8	66.0
Kirgizskaja SSR	0.3	8.6	7.5	7.3	7.3	7.9	9.5	11.8	12.2	12.6
Tadžikskaja SSR	0.2	16.2	25.5	26.1	26.3	27.5	27.8	28.3	28.2	28.7
Armjanskaja SSR	9.8	49.3	42.0	36.6	41.4	43.1	45.4	47.9	52.1	51.5
Turkmenskaja SSR	0.6	4.9	3.8	3.0	2.8	3.0	3.7	4.0	3.6	3.7
Estonskaja SSR	1.6	9.3	8.3	9.3	10.6	12.0	12.5	13.0	13.3	13.6

5.1.9.9 Economy
5.1.9.10 Wirtschaft

5.1.9.9 OUTPUT OF LINEN HOSIERY IN THE UNION REPUBLICS (mill.pcs.)
PRODUKTION VON WÄSCHETRIKOTAGE NACH UNIONSREPUBLIKEN (Mio Stck.)
PROIZVODSTVO BEL'EVOGO TRIKOTAŽA PO SOJUZNYM RESPUBLIKAM (mln.št.)

	1940	1965	1970	1971	1972	1973	1974	1975	1976	1977
SSSR	127	715	814	828	843	900	920	955	990	1,031(Pla
RSFSR	60.5	326.8	346.9	347.5	346.3	370.4	375.7	388.3	397.3	--
Ukrainskaja SSR	30.3	147.2	147.0	158.4	168.8	186.1	188.2	194.3	201.4	205
Belorusskaja SSR	17.5	42.2	51.8	54.8	58.4	61.4	63.4	64.0	72.6	83.3
Uzbekskaja SSR	2.5	16.6	21.4	21.6	23.5	26.9	27.0	29.8	29.8	30.0
Kazachskaja SSR	0.1	30.1	37.4	37.3	41.5	45.0	45.5	47.2	50.6	55.0
Gruzinskaja SSR	2.4	17.7	20.5	19.4	16.7	17.5	18.4	20.1	21.5	21.7
Azerbajdžanskaja SSR	5.3	12.7	15.9	15.6	15.8	17.0	17.7	18.6	18.4	18.6
Litovskaja SSR	0.8	25.4	43.3	44.6	43.9	43.7	42.6	43.2	43.5	43.8
Moldavskaja SSR	0.0	8.6	24.0	25.5	25.8	29.6	36.9	44.7	45.9	--
Latvijskaja SSR	3.2	25.3	27.7	28.1	28.0	27.0	26.0	25.1	24.1	--
Kirgizskaja SSR	0.1	8.3	10.3	10.3	10.5	10.8	11.0	11.8	12.0	--
Tadžikskaja SSR	0.5	4.7	5.7	5.8	5.6	6.0	6.0	5.8	5.9	--
Armjanskaja SSR	2.0	36.7	44.6	41.7	40.8	43.1	44.7	46.5	51.4	54.5
Turkmenskaja SSR	0.5	5.4	4.2	4.4	4.5	4.6	4.5	4.8	5.1	5.4
Estonskaja SSR	1.3	7.1	13.7	13.2	12.7	11.3	12.5	10.9	11.0	11.6

5.1.9.10 OUTPUT OF OUTER HOSIERY IN THE UNION REPUBLICS (mill.pcs.)
PRODUKTION VON OBERTRIKOTAGEN NACH UNIONSREPUBLIKEN (Mio Stck.)
PROIZVODSTVO VERCHNEGO TRIKOTAŽA PO SOJUZNYM RESPUBLIKAM (mln.št.)

	1940	1965	1970	1971	1972	1973	1974	1975	1976	1977
SSSR	58.9	188	415	446	451	460	469	465	472	491(Pl
RSFSR	40.2	101.4	201.9	212.3	210.9	213.6	217.8	215.0	216.0	--
Ukrainskaja SSR	12.0	32.6	71.0	73.8	72.7	73.9	73.7	73.4	76.3	77.8
Belorusskaja SSR	1.2	9.9	31.0	36.3	37.9	38.4	39.8	39.1	39.9	38.1
Uzbekskaja SSR	1.0	5.4	11.0	11.2	12.0	12.6	12.8	13.2	14.8	17.2
Kazachskaja SSR	0.2	7.0	23.9	27.4	28.1	28.5	29.0	27.7	27.3	28.1
Gruzinskaja SSR	1.5	4.9	9.6	10.7	11.9	12.5	13.1	14.1	13.6	15.0
Azerbajdžanskaja SSR	0.7	1.2	4.6	5.3	5.7	6.7	7.4	8.8	10.4	11.3
Litovskaja SSR	0.3	6.7	12.8	13.5	14.5	14.5	14.5	14.5	14.5	14.7
Moldavskaja SSR	0.1	2.6	5.7	5.7	6.0	6.8	7.4	7.7	7.8	--
Latvijskaja SSR	0.2	6.5	12.6	15.6	18.8	19.6	19.3	19.1	18.5	--
Kirgizskaja SSR	0.1	2.3	5.4	6.4	7.0	6.8	6.9	6.5	6.2	--
Tadžikskaja SSR	0.0	0.0	3.6	4.1	2.8	3.3	3.7	3.7	3.8	--
Armjanskaja SSR	1.0	4.1	15.4	15.8	15.3	14.0	15.6	15.4	16.0	16.4
Turkmenskaja SSR	0.2	0.8	2.0	2.1	1.8	2.3	2.0	1.8	1.8	1.9
Estonskaja SSR	0.2	2.5	4.7	5.4	6.0	6.3	5.6	5.5	5.3	9.8

PRODUCTION OF WOVEN FABRICS AND HOSIERY CONTAINING SYNTHETIC FIBRES
5.1.9.11 PRODUKTION VON GEWEBEN UND TRIKOTAGENERZEUGNISSEN UNTER VERWENDUNG VON CHEMISCHEN FASERN
PROIZVODSTVO TKANEJ I TRIKOTAŽNYCH IZDELIJ S PRIMENENIEM CHIMIČESKICH VOLOKON

Economy 5.1.9.11
Wirtschaft

	1965	1970	1971	1972	1973	1974	1975	1976	Portion (in per cent) of type of woven and knitted fabric of total production in % zum Gesamtumfang der Produktion jedes Gewebe- und Trikotagenerzeugnisses v procentach k obščemu ob'emu proizvodstva každogo vida tkanej i trikotažnych izdelij 1965	1970	1971	1972	1973	1974	1975	1976
Cotton fabrics,mill.runn.m— Baumwollgewebe,Mio lfd.m — Chlopčatobumažnye tkani, mln.pog.m	891	1,036	1,100	1,130	1,156	1,159	1,146	1,117	12.6	13.8	14.2	14.7	14.8	14.8	14.7	14.1
Wool fabrics,mill.runn.m — Wollgewebe, Mio lfd.m — Serstjanye tkani,mln.pog.m	311	425	437	433	435	448	450	461	85	86	85	84	82	83	82	81
worsted yarn — Kammgarn — kamvol'nye	140	201	206	208	215	219	232	239	85	83	82	83	82	83	82	81
Fine cloth — Feintuch — tonkosukonnye	157	204	211	206	203	211	201	203	90	89	88	85	83	84	82	82
Coarse cloth — Grobtuch — grubosukonnye	14	20	20	19	17	18	17	19	55	78	78	76	73	72	72	73
Silk fabrics,mill.runn.m — Seidengewebe, Mio lfd.m — Šelkovye tkani,mln.pog.m	900	1,198	1,228	1,301	1,355	1,400	1,470	1,541	96	97	96	97	97	97	97	97
Linen fabrics,mill.runn.m — Leinengewebe, Mio lfd.m — L'njanye tkani,mln.pog.m	255	339	346	352	378	388	377	391	43	47	45	45	48	49	49	50
Hosiery and socks (all-synthetic), mill.pairs — Strumpf-Socken-Erzeugnisse (reinsynthetisch),Mio Paar— Čuločno-nosočnye izdelija (čistosintetičeskie), mln.par	275	476	497	518	569	585	590	575	20	36	38	39	40	40	39	37
Linen hosiery,mill.pcs. — Wäschetrikotage, Mio Stck.— Bel'evoj trikotaž,mln.št.	281	358	374	394	418	403	424	444	39	44	45	47	46	44	44	45
Outer hosiery,mill.pcs. — Obertrikotage, Mio Stck.— Verchnij trikotaž,mln.št.	34	126	141	157	178	200	202	215	18	30	32	35	39	43	43	46

5.1.10.1 Economy / Wirtschaft

5.1.10 FOOD INDUSTRY – NAHRUNGSMITTELINDUSTRIE – PIŠČEVAJA PROMYŠLENNOSTI

5.1.10.1 OUTPUT OF THE MOST IMPORTANT PRODUCTS OF THE FOOD INDUSTRY (without those listed on pages 239-242)
PRODUKTION DER WICHTIGSTEN ERZEUGNISSE DER NAHRUNGSMITTELINDUSTRIE (ohne die auf S.239-242 aufgezählten)
PROIZVODSTVO VAŽNEJŠICH VIDOV PRODUKCII PIŠČEVOJ PROMYŠLENNOSTI

	1940	1965	1970	1971	1972	1973	1974	1975	1976	1977 (Plan)
Animal fats, '000 tons – Tierische Fette, Tsd.t – Maslo životnoe, tys.t	252	1,072	963	1,022	1,080	1,239	1,260	1,231	1,263	1,340
Fat and sheep cheese, '000 tons – Fett-u.Schafskäse, Tsd.t Syr i brynza žirnye, tys.t	53	310	478	463	483	536	565	562	613	620
Margarine, '000 tons – Margarine, Tsd.t – Margarinovaja produkcija, tys.t	121	670	762	850	850	883	997	999	1,040	1,150
Dried fruit, '000 tons – Trockenobst, Tsd.t – Suchie frukty, tys.t	23.4	57.3	34.7	36.2	40.1	43.9	37.8	45.2	33.2	--
Deep-frozen vegetables, '000 tons – Tiefkühlgemüse, Tsd.t – Svežezamorožennye ovošči, tys.t	...	1.1	4.0	3.9	3.4	2.8	3.6	2.6	3.1	--
Confectionery, '000 tons – Konditoreierzeugnisse, Tsd.t – Konditerskie tovary, tys.t	797	2,315	2,896	2,890	2,961	3,144	3,267	3,247	3,387	3,610
of which candies – davon Zuckerwaren – iz nich sacharistye	...	1,351	1,745	1,737	1,759	1,858	1,959	1,934	1,989	--
Farinaceous pastes, '000 tons – Teigwaren, Tsd.t – Makaronnye izdelija, tys.t	325	1,251	1,184	1,191	1,328	1,342	1,224	1,337	1,476	1,440
Beer, mill.gall. – Bier, Mio Gal. – Pivo,mln.gal.	124	317	419	441	469	508	540	571	592	675
Salt (extraction), mill.tons – Salz (Gewinnung), Mio t – Sol' (dobyča), mln.t	4.4	9.5	12.4	12.0	12.2	12.9	13.4	14.3	14.2	15.5
Flour, mill.tons – Mehl, Mio t – Muka, mln.t	29	37	42	43	44	43	42	42	42	42

5.1.10.2 PRODUCTION OF CASTOR AND REFINED SUGAR – PRODUKTION VON STREUZUCKER UND RAFFINADE – PROIZVODSTVO SACHARA-PESKA I SACHARA-RAFINADA
('000 tons – Tsd.t – tys.t)

Year Jahr Gody	Castor sugar Streuzucker Sachar-pesok	Refined sugar Raffinade Sachar-rafinad	Year Jahr Gody	Castor sugar Streuzucker Sachar-pesok	Refined sugar Raffinade Sachar-rafinad
1913[1]	1,352	828	1966	9,740	1,960
1913[2]	1,363	846	1967	9,939	1,976
1928	1,283	656	1968	10,766	1,781
1932	828	438	1969	10,347	1,766
1937	2,421	1,032	1970	10,221	2,005
1940	2,165	628	1971	9,025	2,027
1945	465	54	1972	8,903	1,934
1946	466	100	1973	10,714	2,265
1950	2,523	701	1974	9,446	2,330
1955	3,419	1,285	1975	10,382	2,478
1960	6,363	1,915	1976	9,249	2,525
1965	11,037	2,197	1977	12,000	--

5.1.10.3 PRODUCTION OF CASTOR SUGAR BY UNION REPUBLICS – PRODUKTION VON STREUZUCKER IN DEN UNIONSREPUBLIKEN – PROIZVODSTVO SACHARA-PESKA PO SOJUZNYM RESPUBLIKAM
('000 tons – Tsd.t – tys.t)

	1940	1965	1970	1971	1972	1973	1974	1975	1976	1977
USSR – UdSSR – SSSR of which-darunter-v tom čisle:	2,165	11,037	10,221	9,025	8,903	10,714	9,446	10,382	9,249	12,000
RSFSR	359	3,086	2,915	2,254	2,034	2,978	2,693	2,844	2,725	3,600
Ukrainskaja SSR	1,580	6,686	5,973	5,479	5,549	6,222	5,429	6,035	5,032	6,800
Belorusskaja SSR	--	127.5	180.5	201.0	191.5	229.9	221.3	248.9	244.2	298.0
Kazachskaja SSR	70.9	171.3	176.2	149.1	172.7	184.8	169.3	147.3	154.2	120.2
Gruzinskaja SSR	13.1	60.2	40.2	30.9	16.7	30.9	34.7	38.5	42.6	--
Litovskaja SSR	24.0	167.4	147.8	150.0	145.3	170.0	161.9	203.2	198.1	207.0
Moldavskaja SSR	11.8	344.9	356.5	341.2	322.8	409.8	282.0	395.1	339.4	424.7
Latvijskaja SSR	41.0	186.2	217.6	228.7	257.7	259.1	234.0	256.1	251.4	271.0
Kirgizskaja SSR	65.5	173.8	198.0	171.1	197.8	219.7	211.1	205.8	249.1	270.9
Armjanskaja SSR	--	32.9	16.1	19.5	14.4	9.5	9.8	8.7	11.9	--

[1] within the borders of the U.S.S.R. up to 17.9.1939 – in den Grenzen der UdSSR bis 17.9.1939 – v granicach SSSR do 17 sentjabrja 1939 g.
[2] in the present borders of the U.S.S.R. – in den heutigen Grenzen der UdSSR – v sovremennych granicach SSSR

5.1.10.4 Economy
5.1.10.5 Wirtschaft

5.1.10.4 MEAT PRODUCTION BY TYPES - FLEISCHPRODUKTION NACH ARTEN - PROIZVODSTVO MJASA PO VIDAM
('000 tons - Tsd.t - tys.t)

	1940	1965	1970	1971	1972	1973	1974	1975	1976
Meat (incl.subproducts of the 1st quality category)-Fleisch (einschl.Subprodukte I.Güteklasse)-Mjaso (vključaja subprodukty I kategorii) total - insg. - vsego	1,544	5,245	7,144	8,182	8,723	8,346	9,367	9,862	8,368
Beef and veal - Rind-u.Kalbfleisch - Govjadina i teljatina	850	2,412	3,463	3,667	3,889	3,911	4,365	4,511	4,434
Mutton - Hammelfleisch - Baranina	169	425	422	408	367	386	421	427	379
Pork - Schweinefleisch - Svinina	373	1,783	2,249	2,925	3,179	2,751	3,114	3,335	2,108
Poultry - Geflügelfleisch - Mjaso pticy	52	167	357	432	480	522	625	705	695
Other meat types and subproducts of the 1st quality category - Andere Fleischarten und Subprodukte der I.Güteklasse - Pročie vidy mjasa i subprodukty I kategorii	100	458	653	750	808	776	842	884	752

5.1.10.5 MEAT PRODUCTION BY UNION REPUBLICS (including subproducts of the 1st quality category)
FLEISCHPRODUKTION NACH UNIONSREPUBLIKEN (einschl.Subprodukte der I.Güterklasse)
PROIZVODSTVO MJASA PO SOJUZNYM RESPUBLIKAM (vključaja subprodukty I kategorii)
('000 tons - Tsd.t - tys.t)

	1940	1965	1970	1971	1972	1973	1974	1975	1976	1977
SSSR	1,544	5,245	7,144	8,182	8,723	8,346	9,367	9,862	8,368	14,800
RSFSR	859	2,830	3,693	4,315	4,584	4,173	4,792	5,032	4,131	7,400
Ukrainskaja SSR	299	1,107	1,565	1,791	1,955	1,929	2,104	2,215	1,858	3,500
Belorusskaja SSR	60.3	232.1	427.6	465.4	489.9	510.1	553.9	586.2	536.6	585
Uzbekskaja SSR	26.7	90.8	94.2	99.7	106.9	107.4	120.4	147.4	160.2	100.8
Kazachskaja SSR	97.0	411.4	525.0	568.4	578.5	609.0	694.2	694.2	537.6	596.5
Gruzinskaja SSR	11.5	30.5	48.4	54.3	59.3	58.4	67.5	75.5	78.1	71.3
Azerbajdžanskaja SSR	17.7	30.0	47.9	54.0	58.3	57.3	61.0	63.6	60.4	56.0
Litovskaja SSR	56.3	149.1	238.8	265.9	287.8	295.2	317.2	331.2	324.6	347.0
Moldavskaja SSR	5.6	79.6	106.2	124.7	127.1	136.2	154.3	161.5	140.1	144.6
Latvijskaja SSR	53.8	86.7	143.0	160.1	176.0	162.8	179.8	193.2	188.7	193.0
Kirgizskaja SSR	16.8	68.3	78.8	88.5	90.1	94.9	102.5	111.2	97.2	89.7
Tadžikskaja SSR	7.0	26.7	32.9	35.1	36.7	39.3	42.6	44.5	45.5	43.7
Armjanskaja SSR	8.6	22.2	27.3	28.9	37.0	43.0	46.6	47.9	45.6	46.7
Turkmenskaja SSR	8.5	16.1	16.8	21.1	21.0	22.4	25.1	28.8	27.4	26.0
Estonskaja SSR	16.7	65.1	98.6	110.6	115.4	108.2	122.2	130.1	137.3	136.0

Economy 5.1.10.6
Wirtschaft 5.1.10.7

5.1.10.6 PRODUCTION OF ANIMAL FATS BY UNION REPUBLICS – PRODUKTION VON TIERISCHEN FETTEN NACH UNIONSREPUBLIKEN – PROIZVODSTVO MASLA ŽIVOTNOGO PO SOJUZNYM RESPUBLIKAM

('000 tons – Tsd.t – tys.t)

	1940	1965	1970	1971	1972	1973	1974	1975	1976	1977
SSSR	252	1,072	963	1,022	1,080	1,239	1,260	1,231	1,263	1,400
RSFSR	141.1	559.0	486.3	515.9	546.3	631.4	644.6	628.1	614.6	683.0
Ukrainskaja SSR	33.3	281.0	245.2	265.9	280.7	329.0	327.7	313.7	340.5	386.0
Belorusskaja SSR	7.3	57.4	62.4	64.6	71.3	81.9	84.1	88.1	93.7	105
Uzbekskaja SSR	1.0	6.8	6.4	7.0	7.3	8.4	8.9	8.6	8.4	9.5
Kazachskaja SSR	12.1	45.1	42.2	43.7	45.3	50.1	48.0	44.9	47.0	55.6
Gruzinskaja SSR	0.5	1.0	0.9	0.9	0.9	1.0	1.1	1.2	1.3	1.4
Azerbajdžanskaja SSR	1.4	3.2	3.0	3.6	3.8	4.3	4.5	4.1	4.0	–
Litovskaja SSR	16.0	36.2	39.2	39.6	43.6	45.4	47.9	49.4	55.3	58.0
Moldavskaja SSR	0.1	11.9	10.4	10.6	11.1	13.5	13.6	14.3	14.1	16.7
Latvijskaja SSR	23.0	34.3	32.8	33.8	33.3	33.4	36.6	34.6	37.2	40.0
Kirgizskaja SSR	1.2	7.5	6.9	7.7	7.9	8.4	8.2	8.4	8.7	9.2
Tadžikskaja SSR	0.1	2.1	2.1	2.4	2.7	2.8	3.2	3.6	3.6	4.1
Armjanskaja SSR	1.6	3.0	1.7	2.0	1.7	1.8	1.7	1.7	1.5	–
Turkmenskaja SSR	0.3	1.9	1.9	2.0	2.1	2.4	2.6	2.6	2.7	2.9
Estonskaja SSR	13.2	21.6	21.6	22.0	22.6	24.9	27.1	28.0	30.8	30.4

5.1.10.7 PRODUCTION OF VEGETABLE FATS BY UNION REPUBLICS – PRODUKTION VON PFLANZLICHEN FETTEN NACH UNIONSREPUBLIKEN – PROIZVODSTVO MASLA RASTITEL'NOGO PO SOJUZNYM RESPUBLIKAM .

('000 tons – Tsd.t – tys.t)

	1940	1965	1970	1971	1972	1973	1974	1975	1976	1977
SSSR	804	2,770	2,784	2,923	2,827	2,676	3,411	3,344	2,775	2,900
RSFSR	421.6	1185.9	983.5	1134.6	986.7	915.6	1326.7	1265.9	945.4	1,200
Ukrainskaja SSR	158.7	872.2	1071.3	956.0	976.7	879.1	1149.8	1143.9	906.9	–
Belorusskaja SSR	10.3	25.8	22.1	17.9	21.2	15.7	20.0	21.4	21.0	–
Uzbekskaja SSR	141.7	308.6	293.6	367.0	380.2	391.6	403.7	430.9	439.2	450.0
Kazachskaja SSR	4.7	58.2	61.8	72.9	77.4	79.2	82.0	69.1	81.7	87.2
Gruzinskaja SSR	4.6	6.8	8.8	11.3	12.1	10.2	16.1	16.7	9.3	9.2
Azerbajdžanskaja SSR	10.8	24.1	28.1	33.3	33.8	28.0	32.2	36.0	40.2	40.9
Litovskaja SSR	9.0	7.2	5.4	5.3	4.5	3.9	5.3	5.5	3.9	–
Moldavskaja SSR	14.0	132.7	154.7	146.6	147.3	163.4	177.0	147.5	123.6	108.0
Latvijskaja SSR	2.5	20.3	21.7	22.9	22.4	23.1	25.2	25.0	20.4	–
Kirgizskaja SSR	0.4	17.2	16.9	19.4	20.5	20.1	20.8	20.6	20.8	20.1
Tadžikskaja SSR	3.5	62.7	68.8	76.5	84.4	84.7	90.9	94.5	93.5	88.0
Armjanskaja SSR	6.1	8.8	11.0	12.3	11.0	12.9	13.0	13.0	12.8	11.8
Turkmenskaja SSR	15.2	39.6	36.8	46.7	48.4	49.1	48.9	53.4	56.7	57.3

241

5.1.10.8 Economy / Wirtschaft

5.1.10.8 PRODUCTION OF CANNED GOODS BY TYPES - KONSERVENPRODUKTION NACH ARTEN - PROIZVODSTVO KONSERVOV PO VIDAM
(mill.standard cans - Mio Normdosen - mln.uslovnych banok)

	1940	1965	1970	1971	1972	1973	1974	1975	1976
Canned goods, total - Konserven, insg. - Konservy, vsego	1,118	7,078	10,678	11,304	12,057	13,037	14,155	14,565	14,520
of which-darunter-v tom čísle:									
Meat and meat dishes - Fleisch u.Fleischgerichte - mjasnye i mjaso-rastitel'nye	109	723	817	971	1,293	1,153	1,136	1,395	920
Fish - Fisch - rybnye	124	977	1,393	1,500	1,660	1,735	1,936	2,207	2,377
Vegetables - Gemüse - ovoščnye	110	1,484	2,611	2,723	2,894	3,285	3,372	3,016	2,960
Tomatoes - Tomaten - tomatnye	341	1,067	1,303	1,408	1,633	1,744	2,286	2,351	2,289
Fruit - Obst - fruktovye	264	1,380	1,526	1,540	1,285	1,509	1,474	1,434	1,637
of which marmalade, preserves, jam - davon Marmelade, Konfitüre, Jam - iz nich povidlo, varen'e, džem	...	796	629	638	.567	623	616	562	666
Milk - Milch - moločnye	71	707	1,104	1,151	1,169	1,278	1,384	1,465	1,459
Natural juices - Natursäfte - soki natural'nye	44	729	1,892	1,987	2,105	2,297	2,508	2,644	2,809

Economy 5.2.1
Wirtschaft

5.2 AGRICULTURE - LANDWIRTSCHAFT - SEL'SKOE CHOZJAJSTVO

5.2.1 GROSS AGRICULTURAL OUTPUT BY UNION REPUBLICS
(in all types of agricultural enterprises[1]; in prices compared to those of 1965)
BRUTTOPRODUKTION DER LANDWIRTSCHAFT NACH UNIONSREPUBLIKEN
(in allen landwirtschaftlichen Betrieben[1]; in Vergleichspreisen von 1965)
VALOVAJA PRODUKCIJA SEL'SKOGO CHOZJAJSTVA PO SOJUZNYM RESPUBLIKAM
(vo vsech kategorijach chozjajstv[1]; v sopostavimych cenach 1965 g.)
(in mill.rubles - in Mio Rubel - mln.rub.)

	1965	1970	1971	1972	1973	1974	1975
SSSR	70,867	86,992	87,928	84,314	97,919	95,242	89,215
RSFSR	34,926	43,502	42,941	39,202	47,967	45,776	42,755
Ukrainskaja SSR	17,355	19,615	20,805	20,032	23,150	22,750	20,359
Belorusskaja SSR	3,761	4,433	4,529	4,603	5,082	4,940	4,969
Uzbekskaja SSR	2,742	3,474	3,432	3,648	3,863	4,136	4,083
Kazachskaja SSR	3,680	5,673	5,664	6,358	6,462	5,844	5,066
Gruzinskaja SSR	913	1,173	1,075	1,066	1,181	1,294	1,372
Azerbajdžanskaja SSR	697	883	878	908	1,036	1,222	1,187
Litovskaja SSR	1,453	1,826	1,894	1,864	1,942	1,923	2,007
Moldavskaja SSR	1,498	1,720	1,861	1,882	2,130	2,064	2,051
Latvijskaja SSR	1,001	1,166	1,176	1,123	1,185	1,167	1,163
Kirgizskaja SSR	741	911	928	993	1,046	1,034	1,054
Tadžikskaja SSR	622	770	835	815	868	961	962
Armjanskaja SSR	353	445	448	432	481	489	524
Turkmenskaja SSR	500	692	716	699	794	863	863
Estonskaja SSR	625	709	746	689	732	779	800

[1] collective and state farms and individual subsidiary plots
Kolchosen, Sowchosen und private Nebenwirtschaften
Kolchozy, sovchozy i ličnye podsobnye chozjajstva

5.2.1.1 Economy / Wirtschaft

of which – davon – v tom čísle

5.2.1.1	\multicolumn{7}{c	}{Agricultural output / Produktion des Ackerbaus / Produkcija zemledelija}	\multicolumn{7}{c}{Output of livestock products / Produktion der Viehwirtschaft / Produkcija životnovodstva}
	1965	1970	1971	1972	1973	1974	1975	1965	1970	1971	1972	1973	1974	1975
SSSR	34,800	44,130	43,564	40,214	51,107	45,995	41,180	36,067	42,862	44,364	44,100	46,812	49,247	48,035
RSFSR	15,668	20,711	19,232	15,981	23,427	19,666	17,531	19,258	22,791	23,709	23,221	24,540	26,110	25,224
Ukrainskaja SSR	9,263	10,141	11,095	10,288	12,678	11,814	9,750	8,092	9,474	9,710	9,744	10,472	10,936	10,609
Belorusskaja SSR	1,953	2,182	2,241	2,213	2,488	2,259	2,335	1,808	2,251	2,288	2,390	2,594	2,681	2,634
Uzbekskaja SSR	2,091	2,640	2,565	2,743	2,889	3,126	3,073	651	834	867	905	974	1,010	1,010
Kazachskaja SSR	1,278	2,788	2,678	3,321	3,242	2,561	1,891	2,402	2,885	2,986	3,037	3,220	3,283	3,175
Gruzinskaja SSR	588	824	710	705	802	900	951	325	349	365	361	379	394	421
Azerbajdžanskaja SSR	423	545	543	567	652	815	776	274	338	335	341	384	407	411
Litovskaja SSR	563	664	692	667	724	666	724	890	1,162	1,202	1,197	1,218	1,257	1,283
Moldavskaja SSR	1,052	1,174	1,310	1,330	1,536	1,455	1,416	446	546	551	552	594	609	635
Latvijskaja SSR	368	460	430	377	443	385	370	633	706	746	746	742	782	793
Kirgizskaja SSR	335	435	434	497	514	500	512	406	476	494	496	532	534	542
Tadžikskaja SSR	461	569	616	591	631	706	698	161	201	219	224	237	255	264
Armjanskaja SSR	194	254	239	210	254	254	278	159	191	209	222	227	235	246
Turkmenskaja SSR	325	488	507	507	568	628	615	175	204	209	192	226	235	248
Estonskaja SSR	238	255	272	217	259	260	260	387	454	474	472	473	519	540

Economy 5.2.2
Wirtschaft

5.2.2 OUTPUT OF AGRICULTURAL PRODUCTS (in all types of agricultural enterprises[1])
ERZEUGUNG DER LANDWIRTSCHAFTLICHEN PRODUKTE (in allen landwirtschaftl.Betrieben[1])
PROIZVODSTVO SEL'SKOCHOZJAJSTVENNOJ PRODUKCII (vo vsech kategorijach chozjajstv[1])

Year Jahr Gody	A. Gross agricultural output (in prices compared to those of 1965), 000. mill.rubles Bruttoproduktion der Landwirtschaft (in Vergleichspreisen von 1965), Mrd.Rubel Valovaja produkcija sel'skogo chozjajstva (v sopostavimych cenach 1965 g.), Mlrd.rub.	B. Grain, mill.tons Getreide, Mio t Zerno, mln.t	C. Raw cotton, mill.tons Rohbaumwolle, Mio t Chlopok-syrec, mln.t	D. Sugar-beet (for factory processing), mill.tons Zuckerrüben (Fabrikrüben), Mio t Sacharnaja svekla (fabričnaja),mln.t	E. Sunflower seeds, mill.tons Sonnenblumenkerne, Mio t Podsolnečnik, mln.t	F. Flax fibre, '000 tons Flachsfaser, Tsd. t L'novolokno, tys.t	G. Potatoes, mill.tons Kartoffeln, Mio t Kartofel', mln.t	H. Vegetables, mill.tons Gemüse, Mio t Ovošči, mln.t	I. Meat (slaughter weight), mill.tons Fleisch (im Schlachtgewicht),Mio t Mjaso (v ubojnom vese), mln.t	J. Milk, mill.tons Milch, Mio t Moloko, mln.t	K. Eggs, '000 mill. Eier, Mrd.Stck. Jajca, mrd.št.	L. Wool, '000 tons Wolle, Tsd.t Šerst', tys.t
1913	28.1	86.0	0.74	11.3	0.75	401	31.9	5.5	5.0	29.4	11.9	192
1940	39.6	95.6	2.24	18.0	2.64	349	76.1	13.7	4.7	33.6	12.2	161
1945	24.1	47.3	1.16	5.5	0.84	150	58.3	10.3	2.6	26.4	4.9	111
1946	26.8	39.6	1.64	4.3	0.79	133	55.6	8.9	3.1	27.7	5.2	119
1947	34.5	65.9	1.70	14.0	1.39	170	74.5	14.9	2.5	30.2	4.9	125
1948	38.4	67.2	2.20	12.9	1.93	257	95.0	13.2	3.1	33.4	6.6	146
1949	39.3	70.2	2.53	15.7	1.85	310	89.6	10.8	3.8	34.9	9.1	163
1950	39.3	81.2	3.54	20.8	1.80	255	88.6	9.3	4.9	35.3	11.7	180
1951	36.6	78.7	3.73	23.6	1.74	193	58.8	8.8	4.7	36.2	13.3	192
1952	39.8	92.2	3.78	22.2	2.21	213	69.2	9.8	5.2	35.7	14.4	219
1953	41.0	82.5	3.85	23.2	2.63	162	72.6	11.4	5.8	36.5	16.1	235

[1] collective and state farms and individual subsidiary plots - Kolchosen, Sowchosen und private Nebenwirtschaften - Kolchozy, sovchozy i ličnye podsobnye chozjajstva

5.2.2 Economy / Wirtschaft

Year Jahr Gody	A.	B.	C.	D.	E.	F.	G.	H.	I.	J.	K.	L.
1954	43.1	85.6	4.20	19.8	1.91	218	75.0	11.9	6.3	38.2	17.2	230
1955	47.8	103.7	3.88	31.0	3.80	381	71.8	14.1	6.3	43.0	18.5	256
1956	54.3	125.0	4.33	32.5	3.95	521	96.0	14.3	6.6	49.1	19.5	261
1957	55.4	102.6	4.21	39.7	2.80	440	87.8	14.8	7.4	54.7	22.3	289
1958	61.4	134.7	4.34	54.4	4.63	438	86.5	14.9	7.7	58.7	23.0	322
1959	61.7	119.5	4.64	43.9	3.02	364	86.6	14.8	8.9	61.7	25.6	356
1960	63.0	125.5	4.29	57.7	3.97	425	84.4	16.6	8.7	61.7	27.4	357
1961	64.7	130.8	4.52	50.9	4.75	399	84.3	16.2	8.7	62.6	29.3	366
1962	65.7	140.2	4.30	47.4	4.80	432	69.7	16.0	9.5	63.9	30.1	371
1963	60.7	107.5	5.21	44.1	4.28	380	71.8	15.2	10.2	61.2	28.5	373
1964	69.5	152.1	5.28	81.2	6.06	346	93.6	19.5	8.3	63.3	26.7	341
1965	70.9	121.1	5.66	72.3	5.45	480	88.7	17.6	10.0	72.6	29.1	357
1966	77.0	171.2	5.98	74.0	6.15	461	87.9	17.9	10.7	76.0	31.7	371
1967	78.1	147.9	5.97	87.1	6.61	485	95.5	20.5	11.5	79.9	33.9	395
1968	81.6	169.5	5.95	94.3	6.68	402	102.2	19.0	11.6	82.3	35.7	415
1969	78.9	162.4	5.71	71.2	6.36	487	91.8	18.7	11.8	81.5	37.2	390
1970	87.0	186.8	6.89	78.9	6.14	456	96.8	21.2	12.3	83.0	40.7	419
1971	87.9	181.2	7.10	72.2	5.66	486	92.7	20.8	13.3	83.2	45.1	429
1972	84.3	168.2	7.30	76.4	5.05	456	78.3	19.9	13.6	83.2	47.9	420
1973	97.9	222.5	7.66	87.0	7.39	443	108.2	25.9	13.5	88.3	51.2	433
1974	95.2	195.7	8.41	77.9	6.78	402	81.0	24.8	14.6	91.8	55.5	461
1975	89.2	140.1	7.86	66.3	4.99	493	88.7	23.4	15.0	90.8	57.5	467
1976	--	223.8	8.28	99.9	5.28	507	85.1	25.0	13.4	89.1	55.6	433
1977	--	195.5	8.76	93.3	5.87	--	83.4	23.0	14.8	94.8	61.0	458

246

5.2.3 YIELD OF AGRICULTURAL CROPS (in all agricultural enterprises; mill.tons)
BRUTTOERNTEERTRAG DER LANDWIRTSCHAFTLICHEN KULTUREN (in allen landwirtschaftl.Betrieben; Mio t)
VALOVOJ SBOR SEL'SKOCHOZJAJSTVENNYCH KUL'TUR (vo vsech kategorijach chozjajstv; mln.t)

	1940	1965	1970	1971	1972	1973	1974	1975	1976	1977
Grain crops - Getreidekulturen - Zernovye kultury	95.6	121.1	186.8	181.2	168.2	222.5	195.7	140.1	223.8	195.5
of which-darunter-v tom čisle:										
wheat - Weizen - pšenica	31.8	59.7	99.7	98.8	86.0	109.8	83.9	66.2	96.9	92.0
rye - Roggen - rož'	21.1	16.2	13.0	12.8	9.6	10.8	15.2	9.1	14.0	8.5
maize (ripe) - Körnermais - kukuruza na zerno	5.2	8.0	9.4	8.6	9.8	13.2	12.1	7.3	10.1	11.0
barley - Gerste - jačmen'	12.0	20.3	38.2	34.6	36.8	55.0	54.2	35.8	69.5	52.7
oats - Hafer - oves	16.8	6.2	14.2	14.6	14.1	17.5	15.3	12.5	18.1	18.4
millet - Hirse - proso	4.39	2.20	2.10	2.04	2.12	4.42	2.91	1.13	3.2	2.0
buckwheat - Buchweizen - grečicha	1.31	0.95	1.08	1.17	0.81	1.30	0.97	0.49	0.90	1.0
rice - Reis - ris	0.30	0.58	1.28	1.43	1.65	1.77	1.91	2.01	2.0	2.2
legumes - Hülsenfrüchte - zernobobovye	2.18	6.69	7.62	6.95	7.10	8.45	8.71	5.32	8.65	7.5
Raw cotton - Rohbaumwolle - Chlopok-syrec	2.24	5.66	6.89	7.10	7.30	7.66	8.41	7.86	8.28	8.75
Sugar-beet(for factory processing) - Zuckerrüben (Fabrikrüben) - Sacharnaja svekla (fabričnaja)	18.0	72.3	78.9	72.2	76.4	87.0	77.9	66.3	99.9	93.1
Oil-seed - Ölsaatgut - Semena masličnych kul'tur	3.22	6.07	6.97	6.46	5.52	8.15	7.42	5.92	5.99	6.6
of which sunflower - darunter Sonnenblume - v tom čisle podsolnečnik	2.64	5.45	6.14	5.66	5.05	7.39	6.78	4.99	5.28	5.9
Flax fibre, '000 tons - Flachsfaser,Tsd.t - L'novolokno, tys.t	349	480	456	486	456	443	402	493	507	--
Potatoes - Kartoffeln - kartofel'	76.1	88.7	96.8	92.7	78.3	108.2	81.0	88.7	85.1	83.6

5.2.3 Economy
5.2.4 Wirtschaft

	1940	1965	1970	1971	1972	1973	1974	1975	1976	1977
Vegetables – Gemüse – ovošči	13.7	17.6	21.2	20.8	19.9	25.9	24.8	23.4	25.0	24.1
Maize for ensilage and feed Mais für Silos und Grünfutter – Kukuruza na silos i zelenyj korm	...	181	212	211	206	282	226	193	277	247
Hay and green fodder in terms of hay, total Heu u.Grünfutter umgerechnet auf Heu, insg. – Seno i zelenyj korm v peresčete na seno, vsego	75.0	82.5	110.3	112.7	114.5	126.1	130.7	115.8	131.2	-.-
Hay from perennial grass Heu von mehrjährigem Gras – seno mnogoletnich trav	10.2	18.3	34.3	35.8	40.5	45.8	50.9	45.4	50.3	-.-
Hay from annual grass Heu von einjährigem Gras – seno odnoletnich trav	4.1	20.1	26.5	27.9	27.0	32.3	31.5	25.3	35.0	-.-
Hay from natural meadows Heu von natürlichen Wiesen – seno estestvennych senokosov	60.7	44.1	49.5	49.0	47.0	48.0	48.3	45.1	45.9	-.-

SHARE OF TOTAL PRODUCTION OF AGRICULTURAL RAW PRODUCTS OF STATE FARMS, COLLECTIVE FARMS
AND OTHER STATE-OWNED ENTERPRISES –
5.2.4 ANTEIL DER PRODUKTION LANDWIRTSCHAFTLICHER GRUNDERZEUGNISSE DER KOLCHOSEN, SOWCHOSEN UND ANDEREN STAATLICHEN
LANDWIRTSCHAFTLICHEN BETRIEBEN AN DER GESAMTPRODUKTION (%)
UDEL'NYJ VES PROIZVODSTVA OSNOVNYCH SEL'SKOCHOZJAJSTVENNYCH PRODUKTOV KOLCHOZAMI, SOVCHOZAMI I DRUGIMI
GOSUDARSTVENNYMI CHOZJAJSTVAMI V OBŠČEM PROIZVODSTVE (%)

	1940	1965	1970	1971	1972	1973	1974	1975	1976
Among the collective and state farms and other state agricultural enterprises – Anteil der Kolchosen, Sowchosen und anderen staatlichen landwirtschaftl. Betrieben – Udel'nyj ves kolchozov, sovchozov i drugich gosudarstvennych chozjajstv									
Grain – Getreide – Zernovye kul'tury	88	98	99	99	99	99	99	99	99
Raw cotton – Rohbaumwolle – Chlopok-syrec	100	100	100	100	100	100	100	100	100
Sugar-beet (for factory processing) – Zuckerrüben (Fabrikrüben) – Sacharnaja svekla (fabričnaja)	94	100	100	100	100	100	100	100	100

Economy 5.2.4
Wirtschaft

	1940	1965	1970	1971	1972	1973	1974	1975	1976	1977
Sunflower seeds - Sonnenblumenkerne - Podsolnečnik	89	98	98	98	98	98	98	97	98	
Potatoes - Kartoffeln - Kartofel'	35	37	35	37	38	39	36	41	38	
Vegetables - Gemüse - ovošči	52	59	62	63	64	66	67	66	73	
Meat - Fleisch - mjaso	28	60	65	65	66	67	68	69	69	
Milk - Milch - moloko	23	61	64	65	66	67	68	69	70	
Eggs - Eier - jajca	6	33	47	50	53	57	59	61	63	
Wool - Wolle - šerst'	61	80	81	80	79	79	80	80	80	
of which state farms and other agricultural enterprises - darunter Anteil der Sowchosen und anderen staatlichen landwirtschaftl. Betrieben - v tom čisle udel'nyj ves sovchozov i drugich gosudarstvennych chozjajstv										
Grain - Getreide - Zernovye kul'tury	8	37	46	46	49	46	43	44	47	
Raw cotton - Rohbaumwolle - Chlopok-syrec	6	20	23	24	24	26	27	28	29	
Sugar-beet (for factory processing) - Zuckerrüben (Fabrikrüben) - Sacharnaja svekla (fabričnaja)	4	9	8	8	7	9	9	8	9	
Sunflower seeds - Sonnenblumenkerne - Podsolnečnik	2	14	20	20	20	21	19	20	23	
Potatoes - Kartoffeln - kartofel'	2	15	14	14	15	16	14	18	15	
Vegetables - Gemüse - ovošči	9	34	36	37	37	39	40	41	43	
Meat - Fleisch -mjaso	9	30	32	32	33	33	34	35	36	
Milk - Milch - moloko	6	26	28	29	29	29	30	30	31	
Eggs - Eier - jajca	2	20	33	36	39	43	46	49	54	
Wool - Wolle - šerst'	12	39	42	42	42	43	45	45	45	

5.2.5 Economy / Wirtschaft

PRODUCTION OF MARKETABLE AGRICULTURAL PRODUCTS
MARKTPRODUKTION DER LANDWIRTSCHAFT
TOVARNAJA PRODUKCIJA SEL'SKOGO CHOZJAJSTVA

	1940	1965	1970	1971	1972	1973	1974	1975	1976
Production of marketable agricultural products (harvest of year given above).mill.tons Marktproduktion des Ackerbaus (Ernte des entsprechenden Jahres), Mio t Tovarnaja produkcija zemledelija (iz urožaja sootvetstvujuščego goda), mln.t									
Grain crops - Getreidekulturen - zernovye kul'tury	38.3	41.1	80.8	70.5	67.2	100.0	80.8	55.3	101.5
of which wheat - darunter Weizen - v tom čisle pšenica	16.2	24.7	56.3	52.1	47.2	64.1	42.2	32.5	54.3
Raw cotton - Rohbaumwolle - Chlopok-syrec	2.24	5.66	6.89	7.10	7.30	7.66	8.41	7.86	8.28
Sugar-beet (for factory processing) - Zuckerrüben (Fabrikrüben) - Sacharnaja svekla	17.4	67.5	71.4	64.3	68.0	77.8	67.5	61.9	85.3
Sunflower seeds - Sonnenblumenkerne - Podsolnečnik	1.87	4.27	5.16	4.71	4.02	6.14	5.64	4.17	4.05
Potatoes - Kartoffeln - Kartofel'	12.9	15.8	18.1	18.0	16.4	23.1	17.3	20.7	20.6
Vegetables - Gemüse - Ovošči	6.1	9.9	13.8	14.0	13.7	17.3	17.0	16.4	18.4
Production of marketable livestock products (during calender year) Marktproduktion der Viehwirtschaft (im Kalenderjahr) - Tovarnaja produkcija životnovodstva (za kalndarnyj god)									
Meat (slaughter weight), mill.tons - Fleisch (im Schlachtgewicht), Mio t - mjaso (v ubojnom vese), mln.t	2.6	7.0	9.4	10.4	10.9	10.7	11.8	12.2	10.9
Milk and milk products (converted to milk), mill.tons - Milch u.Milchprodukte (umgerechnet auf Milch), Mio t - Moloko i moločnye produkty (v peresčete na moloko), mln.t	10.8	40.9	48.0	49.4	50.8	55.6	58.3	58.5	58.4
Eggs,'000 mill. - Eier, Mrd.Stck. - Jajca,mrd .št.	4.7	13.9	22.1	25.6	28.2	31.5	34.6	36.5	36.3
Wool, '000 tons - Wolle, Tsd.t - Šerst', tys.t	120	331	395	406	400	416	447	454	424

250

Economy 5.2.6
Wirtschaft

5.2.6 SHARE OF TOTAL MARKETABLE PRODUCTION OF THE CO-OPERATIVE AGRICULTURE OF STATE AND COLLECTIVE FARMS AND OTHER STATE-OWNED ENTERPRISES (in percent)
ANTEIL DER WARENPRODUKTION DER GESELLSCHAFTLICHEN LANDWIRTSCHAFT DER KOLCHOSEN, SOWCHOSEN UND ANDEREN STAATLICHEN WIRTSCHAFTEN AN DER GEMEINSAMEN WARENPRODUKTION (%)
UDEL'NYJ VES TOVARNOJ PRODUKCII OBŠČESTVENNOGO SEL'SKOGO CHOZJAJSTVA KOLCHOZOV, SOVCHOZOV I DRUGICH GOSUDARSTVENNYCH CHOZJAJSTV V OBŠČEJ TOVARNOJ PRODUKCII (%)

	1940	1965	1970	1971	1972	1973	1974	1975	1976
Share of state and collective farms and other state-owned enterprises Anteil der Kolchosen, Sowchosen und anderen staatlichen Wirtschaften – Udel'nyj ves kolchozov, sovchozov i drugich gosudarstvennych chozjajstv									
of the total marketable agricultural production – an der gesamten Warenproduktion der Landwirtschaft – vo vsej tovarnoj produkcii sel'skogo chozjajstva	73	87	88	88	87	89	88	88	--
of the total marketable field-crop production – an der gesamten Warenproduktion des Ackerbaus – vo vsej tovarnoj produkcii zemledelija	87	89	92	91	91	92	91	90	--
of the marketable production of – An der Warenproduktion von – v tovarnoj produkcii:									
Grain – Getreide – zerna	97	100	100	100	100	100	100	100	100
Raw cotton – Rohbaumwolle – chlopka-syrca	100	100	100	100	100	100	100	100	100
Sugar-beet – Zuckerrüben – sacharnoj svekly	94	100	100	100	100	100	100	100	100
Potatoes – Kartoffeln – kartofelja	46	55	60	62	61	60	58	63	58
Vegetables – Gemüse – ovoščej	82	88	87	86	86	87	86	87	90
of the total marketable livestock production – an der gesamten Warenproduktion der Viehwirtschaft – vo vsej tovarnoj produkcii životnovodstva	46	85	86	85	85	86	86	86	--
of the marketable production of – An der Warenproduktion von – v tovarnoj produkcii:									
Meat – Fleisch – mjasa	45	83	83	82	81	83	83	83	84
Milk – Milch – moloka	49	93	95	95	94	94	94	95	94

5.2.6 Economy / Wirtschaft

	1940	1965	1970	1971	1972	1973	1974	1975	1976
Eggs – Eier – jaic	7	64	81	84	86	88	89	91	93
Wool – Wolle – šersti	74	86	85	84	83	82	82	82	81
Share of state farms and other state-owned enterprises – Darunter Anteil der Sowchosen und anderen staatlichen Wirtschaften – V tom čisle udel'nyj ves sovchozov i drugich gosudarstvennych chozjajstv									
of the total marketable agricultural production – an der gesamten Warenproduktion der Landwirtschaft – Vo vsej tovarnoj produkcii sel'skogo chozjajstva	12	36	40	40	41	41	41	42	--
of the total marketable field-crop production – an der gesamten Warenproduktion des Ackerbaus – Vo vsej tovarnoj produkcii zemledelija	10	28	36	35	36	37	36	36	--
of the marketable production of – An der Warenproduktion von – V tovarnoj produkcii:									
Grain – Getreide – zerna	10	38	52	50	58	50	46	44	51
Raw cotton – Rohbaumwolle – chlopka-syrca	6	20	23	24	24	26	27	28	29
Sugar-beet – Zuckerrüben – sacharnoj svekly	4	9	9	8	8	9	8	10	9
Potatoes – Kartoffeln – kartofelja	5	27	29	30	28	30	26	30	28
Vegetables – Gemüse – ovoščej	16	53	53	53	52	53	53	56	56
of the total marketable livestock production – an der gesamten Warenproduktion der Viehwirtschaft – vo vsej tovarnoj produkcii životnovodstva	16	41	42	43	43	44	45	46	--
of the marketable production of – An der Warenproduktion von – V tovarnoj produkcii:									
Meat – Fleisch – mjasa	16	42	41	41	41	42	43	43	44
Milk – Milch – moloka	15	41	42	42	42	42	42	42	42
Eggs – Eier – jaic	3	39	58	61	64	67	70	74	80
Wool – Wolle – šersti	15	42	44	44	44	45	46	46	46

Economy   5.2.7
Wirtschaft 5.2.8

5.2.7   GROSS YIELD OF GRAIN CROPS BY UNION REPUBLICS[1]
         BRUTTOERNTEERTRAG AN GETREIDE NACH UNIONSREPUBLIKEN[1]
         VALOVOJ SBOR ZERNOVYCH KUL'TUR PO SOJUZNYM RESPUBLIKAM

	1940	1965	1970	1971	1972	1973	1974	1975	1976	1977
SSSR	95,638	121,141	186,795	181,175	168,238	222,530	195,708	140,118	223,755	195,500
RSFSR	55,637	69,665	113,457	104,810	91,568	128,990	111,815	77,521	127,059	108,600
Ukrainskaja SSR	26,420	31,651	36,392	39,398	32,566	48,422	45,873	33,803	44,567	48,600
Belorusskaja SSR	2,727	3,335	4,239	5,440	4,592	5,732	6,826	5,121	7,404	6,615
Uzbekskaja SSR	601	628	980	655	970	1,326	1,234	1,079	2,001	1,730
Kazachskaja SSR	2,516	7,604	22,240	21,085	29,039	27,687	18,490	12,007	29,826	17,700
Gruzinskaja SSR	538	658	621	580	666	796	813	715	766	704
Azerbajdžanskaja SSR	567	645	723	609	860	870	910	893	1,184	1,073
Litovskaja SSR	1,536	1,691	2,099	2,526	1,872	1,944	2,773	2,143	3,220	2,880
Moldavskaja SSR	1,810	2,494	2,438	2,170	2,777	2,890	2,485	2,677	2,258	3,071
Latvijskaja SSR	1,372	946	1,323	1,606	972	1,261	1,643	1,243	1,889	1,547
Kirgizskaja SSR	588	560	1,014	868	1,172	1,252	1,087	1,055	1,360	1,132
Tadžikskaja SSR	324	226	222	144	227	233	186	227	305	237
Armjanskaja SSR	223	244	252	250	261	286	224	296	314	317
Turkmenskaja SSR	124	83	69	100	120	127	182	224	258	199.8
Estonskaja SSR	655	711	726	934	576	714	1,167	1,114	1,344	1,243

5.2.8   GROSS YIELD OF WINTER AND SUMMER WHEAT BY UNION REPUBLICS[1]
         BRUTTOERNTEERTRAG AN WINTER- UND SOMMERWEIZEN NACH UNIONSREPUBLIKEN[1]
         VALOVOJ SBOR OZIMOJ I JAROVOJ PŠENICY PO SOJUZNYM RESPUBLIKAM[1]

	1940	1965	1970	1971	1972	1973	1974	1975
SSSR	31,781	59,686	99,734	98,760	85,993	109,784	83,913	66,224
RSFSR	19,306	34,282	62,870	57,070	46,865	58,558	48,725	35,515
Ukrainskaja SSR	8,407	16,148	15,606	21,977	13,249	26,681	18,949	18,247
Belorusskaja SSR	191	255	794	939	683	719	591	456
Uzbekskaja SSR	272	276	409	185	294	344	189	123
Kazachskaja SSR	1,644	5,842	17,173	15,802	21,716	19,891	12,487	8,421
Gruzinskaja SSR	117	177	190	206	212	295	259	263
Azerbajdžanskaja SSR	298	446	504	442	589	592	617	629
Litovskaja SSR	166	311	322	376	359	374	514	447

[1] in all types of agricultural enterprises; '000 tons - in allen landwirtschaftlichen Betrieben; Tsd.t - vo vsech kategorijach chozjajstv; tys.t

5.2.8
5.2.9 Economy
5.2.10 Wirtschaft
5.2.11

	1940	1965	1970	1971	1972	1973	1974	1975
Moldavskaja SSR	343	1,094	710	726	839	1,047	428	964
Latvijskaja SSR	197	193	189	222	204	229	283	226
Kirgizskaja SSR	332	279	595	479	603	638	524	477
Tadžikskaja SSR	221	145	127	68	109	115	76	96
Armjanskaja SSR	144	134	171	159	154	174	100	186
Turkmenskaja SSR	62	43	28	45	56	44	56	53
Estonskaja SSR	81	61	46	64	61	83	115	121

5.2.9 GROSS YIELD OF WINTER AND SUMMER RYE BY UNION   REPUBLICS[1]
BRUTTOERNTEERTRAG AN WINTER- UND SOMMERROGGEN NACH UNIONSREPUBLIKEN[1]
VALOVOJ SBOR OZIMOJ I JAROVOJ RŽI PO SOJUZNYM RESPUBLIKAM[1]

	1940	1965	1970	1971	1972	1973	1974	1975
SSSR	21,125	16,228	12,972	12,787	9,633	10,759	15,223	9,064
RSFSR	14,277	11,185	9,819	9,353	6,638	6,385	10,992	5,568
Ukrainskaja SSR	4,102	1,885	1,176	1,241	1,002	1,783	1,411	1,108
Belorusskaja SSR	1,369	1,937	1,189	1,354	1,257	1,724	1,789	1,709
Kazachskaja SSR	89	88	201	143	76	74	313	37
Litovskaja SSR	623	572	284	326	340	376	397	320
Moldavskaja SSR	69	31	12	10	13	14	7	13
Latvijskaja SSR	399	365	197	232	208	276	208	196
Estonskaja SSR	191	162	86	123	90	115	98	108

5.2.10 GROSS YIELD OF MAIZE (RIPE) BY UNION   REPUBLICS[1]
BRUTTOERNTEERTRAG AN KÖRNERMAIS NACH UNIONSREPUBLIKEN[1]
VALOVOJ SBOR KUKURUZY NA ZERNO PO SOJUZNYM RESPUBLIKAM[1]

	1940	1965	1970	1971	1972	1973	1974	1975
SSSR	5,170	8,030	9,428	8,597	9,830	13,216	12,104	7,328
RSFSR	1,056	1,498	1,018	854	1,350	2,743	2,056	1,318
Ukrainskaja SSR	2,550	4,724	6,337	5,921	5,947	7,815	6,982	3,080
Uzbekskaja SSR	34	54	67	79	143	327	516	504
Kazachskaja SSR	10	106	154	162	204	299	218	286
Gruzinskaja SSR	325	392	333	277	361	371	428	342
Azerbajdžanskaja SSR	10	34	22	18	27	24	42	28
Moldavskaja SSR	1,150	1,113	1,387	1,183	1,649	1,568	1,642	1,450
Kirgizskaja SSR	31	98	103	95	138	151	154	191
Tadžikskaja SSR	2	5	5	6	9	12	24	41
Armjanskaja SSR	1	4	1	1	1	1	1	1
Turkmenskaja SSR	--	2	1	1	1	5	41	87

5.2.11   GROSS YIELD OF MILLET BY UNION   REPUBLICS[1]
BRUTTOERNTEERTRAG AN HIRSE NACH UNIONSREPUBLIKEN[1]
VALOVOJ SBOR PROSA PO SOJUZNYM RESPUBLIKAM[1]

	1940	1965	1970	1971	1972	1973	1974	1975
SSSR	4,391	2,205	2,100	2,043	2,123	4,416	2,907	1,125
RSFSR	2,707	1,354	1,123	1,163	1,102	3,364	1,661	597
Ukrainskaja SSR	1,400	688	694	523	722	629	773	435
Kazachskaja SSR	206	149	277	353	293	421	470	91

[1] in all types of agricultural enterprises; '000 tons - in allen landwirtschaftlichen Betrieben; Tsd.t - vo vsech kategorijach chozjajstv; tys.t

Economy 5.2.12
Wirtschaft 5.2.13
5.2.14

5.2.12 GROSS YIELD OF BUCKWHEAT BY UNION REPUBLICS[1]
BRUTTOERNTEERTRAG AN BUCHWEIZEN NACH UNIONSREPUBLIKEN[1]
VALOVOJ SBOR GREČICHI PO SOJUZNYM RESPUBLIKAM[1]

	1940	1965	1970	1971	1972	1973	1974	1975
SSSR	1,314	950	1,081	1,170	811	1,304	974	485
RSFSR	569	552	679	677	380	897	620	308
Ukrainskaja SSR	581	338	285	322	253	300	304	133
Belorusskaja SSR	145	50	25	21	23	28	10	5
Kazachskaja SSR	0.1	8	92	150	155	79	40	39

5.2.13 GROSS YIELD OF RICE BY UNION REPUBLICS[1]
BRUTTOERNTEERTRAG AN REIS NACH UNIONSREPUBLIKEN[1]
VALOVOJ SBOR RISA PO SOJUZNYM RESPUBLIKAM[1]

	1940	1965	1970	1971	1972	1973	1974	1975
SSSR	303.1	583.4	1279.3	1429.5	1647.2	1765.0	1913.3	2009.3
RSFSR	43.2	256.9	603.2	696.9	788.4	850.7	972.6	1154.1
Ukrainskaja SSR	4.9	62.2	164.7	169.4	199.3	154.6	170.8	217.2
Uzbekskaja SSR	125.5	115.3	184.9	204.2	238.9	280.6	280.6	291.2
Kazachskaja SSR	55.5	93.3	276.7	307.6	371.3	428.4	436.6	283.4
Azerbajdžanskaja SSR	48.5	17.3	5.6	4.4	3.8	2.7	2.2	2.9
Kirgizskaja SSR	9.0	3.1	1.7	1.4	1.4	1.6	1.2	1.7
Tadžikskaja SSR	10.5	23.2	27.2	29.0	25.9	30.0	30.2	31.4
Turkmenskaja SSR	3.5	12.0	15.3	16.6	18.2	16.4	19.1	27.4

5.2.14 GROSS YIELD OF LEGUMES BY UNION REPUBLICS[1]
BRUTTOERNTEERTRAG AN HÜLSENFRÜCHTEN NACH UNIONSREPUBLIKEN[1]
VALOVOJ SBOR ZERNOBOBOVYCH KUL'TUR PO SOJUZNYM RESPUBLIKAM[1]

	1940	1965	1970	1971	1972	1973	1974	1975
SSSR	2,181	6,689	7,619	6,948	7,103	8,447	8,714	5,321
RSFSR	1,117	3,982	4,910	4,364	4,355	5,729	5,505	2,927
Ukrainskaja SSR	809	2,041	2,141	1,939	2,072	2,001	2,517	1,905
Belorusskaja SSR	70	281	192	214	229	252	191	145
Kazachskaja SSR	1	45	36	70	112	153	93	62
Gruzinskaja SSR	26	19	13	9	6	13	12	11
Azerbajdžanskaja SSR	10	9	7	6	8	9	9	9
Litovskaja SSR	73	149	149	216	168	160	224	163
Moldavskaja SSR	22	109	144	102	123	100	134	75
Latvijskaja SSR	33	27	15	16	12	13	13	10
Kirgizskaja SSR	1	4	2	2	3	2	1	1
Tadžikskaja SSR	6	8	5	4	7	5	6	6
Armjanskaja SSR	2	3	2	3	2	4	2	1
Estonskaja SSR	5	11	3	3	4	5	6	5

1 in all types of agricultural enterprises; '000 tons - in allen landwirtschaftlichen Betrieben; Tsd.t - vo vsech kategorijach chozjajstv; tys.t

5.2.15
5.2.16 Economy
5.2.17 Wirtschaft
5.2.18

5.2.15 GROSS YIELD OF SUGAR-BEET (FOR FACTORY PROCESSING) BY UNION REPUBLICS[1]
BRUTTOERNTEERTRAG AN ZUCKERRÜBEN (FABRIKRÜBEN) NACH UNIONSREPUBLIKEN[1]
VALOVOJ SBOR SACHARNOJ SVEKLY (FABRIČNOJ) PO SOJUZNYM RESPUBLIKAM[1]

	1940	1965	1970	1971	1972	1973	1974	1975	1976	1977
SSSR	18,018	72,276	78,942	72,185	76,424	87,047	77,948	66,314	99,872	93,300
RSFSR	3,239	20,655	23,903	17,957	16,057	30,443	20,378	19,226	27,832	28,500
Ukrainskaja SSR	13,052	43,793	46,309	46,101	49,563	47,520	48,258	38,342	61,840	55,500
Belorusskaja SSR	--	856	1,030	797	1,349	1,172	1,077	1,138	1,068	1,353
Kazachskaja SSR	385	1,930	2,223	2,129	2,478	2,363	2,044	1,959	2,140	--
Gruzinskaja SSR	72	124	124	142	131	119	127	141	132	135
Litovskaja SSR	255	569	526	553	1,007	760	897	801	641	756
Moldavskaja SSR	119	2,019	2,816	2,626	3,599	2,438	2,965	2,549	4,089	3,009
Latvijskaja SSR	251	330	236	229	302	262	268	205	194	336
Kirgizskaja SSR	628	1,875	1,685	1,562	1,829	1,854	1,799	1,799	1,768	1,802
Armjanskaja SSR	17	125	90	89	109	116	135	154	168	188

5.2.16 GROSS YIELD OF FLAX FIBRE BY UNION REPUBLICS[1]
BRUTTOERNTEERTRAG AN FLACHSFASER NACH UNIONSREPUBLIKEN[1]
VALOVOJ SBOR L'NOVOLOKNA PO SOJUZNYM RESPUBLIKAM[1]

	1940	1965	1970	1971	1972	1973	1974	1975	1976
SSSR	349	480	456	486	456	443	402	493	507
RSFSR	239	262	248	241	213	172	164	244	207
Ukrainskaja SSR	19	78	89	103	116	139	123	118	155
Belorusskaja SSR	36	114	102	121	107	116	99	113	131
Litovskaja SSR	30	17	12	15	13	10	12	13	20
Latvijskaja SSR	18	7	4	5	6	5	3	4	5
Estonskaja SSR	7	2	1	1	1	1	1	1	2

5.2.17 GROSS YIELD OF SUNFLOWER SEEDS BY UNION REPUBLICS[1]
BRUTTOERNTEERTRAG AN SONNENBLUMENSAMEN NACH UNIONSREPUBLIKEN[1]
VALOVOJ SBOR SEMJAN PODSOLNEČNIKA PO SOJUZNYM RESPUBLIKAM[1]

	1940	1965	1970	1971	1972	1973	1974	1975	1976	1977
SSSR	2,636	5,449	6,144	5,663	5,048	7,385	6,784	4,990	5,277	5,870
RSFSR	1,430	2,365	3,066	2,611	2,145	3,698	3,407	2,193	2,831	2,700
Ukrainskaja SSR	946	2,629	2,654	2,634	2,398	3,154	2,989	2,385	2,111	2,670
Kazachskaja SSR	23	54	78	90	91	92	11	75	87	--
Gruzinskaja SSR	11	19	11	6	23	22	25	14	17	12
Moldavskaja SSR	162	378	331	319	387	415	347	319	226	334

5.2.18 GROSS YIELD OF POTATOES BY UNION REPUBLICS[1]
BRUTTOERNTEERTRAG AN KARTOFFELN NACH UNIONSREPUBLIKEN[1]
VALOVOJ SBOR KARTOFELJA PO SOJUZNYM RESPUBLIKAM[1]

	1940	1965	1970	1971	1972	1973	1974	1975	1976	1977
SSSR	76,130	88,676	96,783	92,655	78,329	108,201	81,022	88,703	85,102	83,400
RSFSR	36,424	49,795	53,933	48,106	34,797	61,851	39,580	51,112	38,902	44,900
Ukrainskaja SSR	20,664	18,157	19,726	23,437	22,115	22,167	20,908	16,469	23,724	18,800
Belorusskaja SSR	11,879	12,116	13,234	12,316	13,020	14,472	12,437	12,736	14,126	11,256

[1] in all types of agricultural enterprises; '000 tons - in allen landwirtschaftlichen Betrieben; Tsd.t - vo vsech kategorijach chozjajstv; tys.t

Economy 5.2.18
Wirtschaft 5.2.19
5.2.20

	1940	1965	1970	1971	1972	1973	1974	1975	1976	1977
Uzbekskaja SSR	113	167	180	158	186	195	222	214	190	208
Kazachskaja SSR	394	1,131	1,896	1,710	2,049	1,917	1,689	1,728	1,747	--
Gruzinskaja SSR	139	228	299	177	209	233	298	267	276	320
Azerbajdžanskaja SSR	82	166	130	91	102	131	158	89	161	176
Litovskaja SSR	2,726	2,601	2,721	2,543	2,402	2,884	2,203	2,547	2,251	1.912
Moldavskaja SSR	147	321	297	287	312	300	358	238	393	--
Latvijskaja SSR	2,093	2,007	2,328	1,904	1,525	1,993	1,328	1,491	1,554	1.402
Kirgizskaja SSR	105	248	278	280	324	290	324	280	268	272
Tadžikskaja SSR	38	51	67	76	97	95	123	113	110	120
Armjanskaja SSR	97	198	267	139	143	246	277	190	207	280
Turkmenskaja SSR	6	9	13	12	12	12	12	13	12	--
Estonskaja SSR	1,223	1,481	1,414	1,419	1,036	1,415	1,105	1,216	1,181	1.156

5.2.19   GROSS YIELD OF VEGETABLES BY UNION REPUBLICS[1]
BRUTTOERNTEERTRAG AN GEMÜSE NACH UNIONSREPUBLIKEN[1]
VALOVOJ SBOR OVOŠČEJ PO SOJUZNYM RESPUBLIKAM[1]

	1940	1965	1970	1971	1972	1973	1974	1975	1976	1977
SSSR	13,732	17,627	21,212	20,840	19,941	25,927	24,811	23,351	25,008	23,000
RSFSR	6,391	8,289	10,066	9,381	8,020	11,894	10,777	10,600	9,346	9,100
Ukrainskaja SSR	5,486	5,350	5,807	6,231	5,944	7,557	7,117	6,038	8,213	6,600
Belorusskaja SSR	673	820	855	616	880	851	705	710	699	621
Uzbekskaja SSR	311	483	781	894	983	1,027	1,317	1,412	1,710	1,805
Kazachskaja SSR	172	590	798	792	847	957	956	918	885	--
Gruzinskaja SSR	104	261	327	317	325	369	446	406	491	499
Azerbajdžanskaja SSR	63	271	410	419	466	555	607	604	793	795
Litovskaja SSR	170	292	366	277	390	385	359	355	228	241
Moldavskaja SSR	98	479	553	629	724	897	1,028	930	1,136	984
Latvijskaja SSR	87	187	275	206	238	243	224	196	155	176
Kirgizskaja SSR	45	134	194	218	252	245	332	310	308	317
Tadžikskaja SSR	44	72	206	242	246	237	274	284	298	324
Armjanskaja SSR	33	187	280	317	306	381	339	299	432	384
Turkmenskaja SSR	32	121	156	168	178	197	199	182	233	228
Estonskaja SSR	23	91	138	133	142	132	131	107	81	--

5.2.20   GROSS YIELD OF GRAPES BY UNION REPUBLICS[1]
BRUTTOERNTEERTRAG AN WEINTRAUBEN NACH UNIONSREPUBLIKEN[1]
VALOVOJ SBOR VINOGRADA PO SOJUZNYM RESPUBLIKAM[1]

	1940	1965	1970	1971	1972	1973	1974	1975	1976
SSSR	1,131	3,723	4,011	4,467	2,786	4,583	4,608	5,400	5,435
RSFSR	73	712	724	690	364	671	681	748	834
Ukrainskaja SSR	161	958	904	1,034	706	1,254	940	1,187	810
Uzbekskaja SSR	130	215	290	259	305	320	367	373	390
Kazachskaja SSR	2	54	81	91	134	98	123	88	133
Gruzinskaja SSR	150	385	579	461	258	412	450	563	448
Azerbajdžanskaja SSR	81	158	352	322	233	440	631	706	765
Moldavskaja SSR	403	980	700	1,224	550	1,043	987	1,263	1,585

1 in all types of agricultural enterprises; '000 tons - in allen landwirtschaftlichen Betrieben; Tsd.t - vo vsech kategorijach chozjajstv; tys.t

257

5.2.20 Economy
5.2.21 Wirtschaft
5.2.22

	1940	1965	1970	1971	1972	1973	1974	1975	1976
Kirgizskaja SSR	0.4	22	21	25	41	39	46	56	62
Tadžikskaja SSR	49	71	95	114	64	109	137	147	167
Armjanskaja SSR	66	142	229	209	106	142	186	206	201
Turkmenskaja SSR	16	26	36	38	25	55	60	63	40

5.2.21 GROSS YIELD OF FRUIT AND BERRIES (INCL. GRAPES) BY UNION REPUBLICS[1]
BRUTTOERNTEERTRAG AN OBST UND BEERENOBST (EINSCHL.WEINTRAUBEN) NACH UNIONSREPUBLIKEN[1]
VALOVOJ SBOR FRUKTOV I JAGOD (VKLJUČAJA VINOGRAD) PO SOJUZNYM RESPUBLIKAM[1]

	1940	1965	1970	1971	1972	1973	1974	1975	1976
SSSR	3,873	8,100	11,690	12,307	9,570	13,351	12,441	14,235	15,252
RSFSR	1,093	1,857	3,045	3,169	1,988	2,977	3,048	3,293	3,618
Ukrainskaja SSR	951	2,818	3,254	3,578	2,888	4,520	3,583	3,697	3,927
Belorusskaja SSR	70	125	439	681	243	315	125	693	541
Uzbekskaja SSR	266	423	696	499	777	744	850	1,015	985
Kazachskaja SSR	37	107	284	185	380	253	294	284	427
Gruzinskaja SSR	293	593	1,088	796	656	846	950	1,085	970
Azerbajdžanskaja SSR	196	240	509	417	348	575	812	858	965
Litovskaja SSR	36	58	131	247	95	165	36	231	209
Moldavskaja SSR	580	1,304	1,321	1,891	1,431	2,036	1,770	1,870	2,314
Latvijskaja SSR	19	19	101	78	46	76	38	45	178
Kirgizskaja SSR	42	76	106	92	190	163	156	244	244
Tadžikskaja SSR	170	212	241	251	275	300	355	423	370
Armjanskaja SSR	95	221	375	301	178	260	288	367	346
Turkmenskaja SSR	21	40	57	61	50	89	86	101	60
Estonskaja SSR	4	7	43	61	25	32	50	29	98

5.2.22 SOWING AREA OF GRAIN BY UNION REPUBLICS[2]
GETREIDEANBAUFLÄCHE NACH UNIONSREPUBLIKEN[2]
POSEVNYE PLOSČADI ZERNOVYCH KUL'TUR PO SOJUZNYM RESPUBLIKAM[2]

	1940	1965	1970	1971	1972	1973	1974	1975	1976
SSSR	110,728	128,024	119,261	117,937	120,158	126,738	127,187	127,920	127,760
RSFSR	70,143	77,594	72,689	71,801	73,131	76,623	76,486	77,023	77,196
Ukrainskaja SSR	21,385	16,495	15,518	15,503	15,288	16,648	16,692	16,540	15,942
Belorusskaja SSR	3,475	2,890	2,505	2,537	2,659	2,621	2,603	2,603	2,766
Uzbekskaja SSR	1,480	1,252	1,160	1,057	1,114	1,129	1,117	1,124	1,182
Kazachskaja SSR	5,817	24,320	22,603	22,407	23,154	24,778	25,441	25,568	25,518
Gruzinskaja SSR	749	501	389	386	379	392	379	373	365
Azerbajdžanskaja SSR	797	658	621	493	648	615	623	611	626
Litovskaja SSR	1,638	1,043	856	948	924	942	1,029	1,070	1,096

1 in all types of agricultural enterprises; '000 tons - in allen landwirtschaftlichen Betrieben; Tsd.t - vo vsech kategorijach chozjajstv; tys.t
2 '000 hectares - Tsd. ha - tys.gektarov

Economy 5.2.22
Wirtschaft 5.2.23
5.2.24

	1940	1965	1970	1971	1972	1973	1974	1975	1976
Moldavskaja SSR	1,672	968	832	806	809	793	751	911	788
Latvijskaja SSR	1,132	623	573	610	579	615	627	645	703
Kirgizskaja SSR	778	607	583	562	576	628	573	546	596
Tadžikskaja SSR	567	397	321	223	285	300	211	200	262
Armjanskaja SSR	340	219	186	170	166	174	161	172	165
Turkmenskaja SSR	183	133	84	84	106	115	106	116	121
Estonskaja SSR	572	324	341	350	340	365	388	418	434

5.2.23   SOWING AREA OF WINTER WHEAT BY UNION   REPUBLICS[1]
         WINTERWEIZENANBAUFLÄCHE NACH UNIONSREPUBLIKEN[1]
         POSEVNYE PLOSCADI OZIMOJ PSENICY PO SOJUZNYM RESPUBLIKAM[1]

	1940	1965	1970	1971	1972	1973	1974	1975
SSSR	14,318	19,794	18,505	20,694	14,979	18,340	18,610	19,593
RSFSR	5,045	9,069	9,004	10,095	6,448	6,592	9,377	8,936
Ukrainskaja SSR	6,317	7,346	5,960	7,310	5,144	8,330	5,953	7,953
Belorusskaja SSR	76	171	437	423	341	302	217	190
Uzbekskaja SSR	616	523	540	415	417	368	411	367
Kazachskaja SSR	213	809	908	942	1,046	1,148	1,261	574
Gruzinskaja SSR	233	186	127	143	129	137	132	140
Azerbajdžanskaja SSR	449	429	418	344	415	398	407	409
Litovskaja SSR	142	166	129	143	139	126	154	156
Moldavskaja SSR	447	416	288	258	253	270	112	317
Latvijskaja SSR	70	80	75	82	76	79	88	84
Kirgizskaja SSR	243	206	274	272	271	285	260	224
Tadžikskaja SSR	230	206	181	104	141	147	97	85
Armjanskaja SSR	128	100	102	94	86	92	71	92
Turkmenskaja SSR	84	69	43	44	48	36	36	28
Estonskaja SSR	25	18	19	25	25	30	34	38

5.2.24   SOWING AREA OF SUMMER WHEAT BY UNION   REPUBLICS[1]
         SOMMERWEIZENANBAUFLÄCHE NACH UNIONSREPUBLIKEN[1]
         POSEVNYE PLOSCADI JAROVOJ PSENICY PO SOJUZNYM RESPUBLIKAM[1]

	1940	1965	1970	1971	1972	1973	1974	1975
SSSR	25,984	50,411	46,725	43,341	43,513	44,815	41,066	42,392
RSFSR	20,427	31,473	29,909	27,471	27,581	28,282	24,582	25,091
Ukrainskaja SSR	901	493	70	47	77	33	33	24
Belorusskaja SSR	186	16	5	7	8	6	5	6
Uzbekskaja SSR	396	212	124	74	78	129	70	147
Kazachskaja SSR	3,234	17,916	16,492	15,650	15,692	16,288	16,327	17,085
Gruzinskaja SSR	39	9	3	2	2	1	1	1
Azerbajdžanskaja SSR	22	10	2	1	3	3	3	3
Litovskaja SSR	61	2	1	1	0.3	0.2	0.3	0.3
Moldavskaja SSR	62	3	--	--	0.2	0.1	--	--
Latvijskaja SSR	88	26	2	1	1	1	0.3	0.3
Kirgizskaja SSR	207	105	52	38	30	29	16	11
Tadžikskaja SSR	180	82	39	32	24	29	16	11
Armjanskaja SSR	100	31	15	11	9	7	7	5
Turkmenskaja SSR	36	23	8	5	8	6	3	3
Estonskaja SSR	45	10	3	1	0.5	1	1	1

1 in all types of agricultural enterprises; '000 hectares - in allen landwirtschaftlichen Betrieben; Tsd. ha - vo vsech kategorijach chozjajstv; tys.gektarov

5.2.25
5.2.26 Economy
5.2.27 Wirtschaft
5.2.28

5.2.25 TOTAL SOWING AREA OF WINTER AND SUMMER RYE BY UNION REPUBLICS[1]
GESAMTANBAUFLÄCHE AN WINTER- UND SOMMERROGGEN NACH UNIONSREPUBLIKEN[1]
POSEVNYE PLOSCADI OZIMOJ I JAROVOJ RZI PO SOJUZNYM RESPUBLIKAM[1]

	1940	1965	1970	1971	1972	1973	1974	1975
SSSR	23,362	16,030	10,020	9,507	8,160	7,012	9,810	8,010
RSFSR	16,740	11,813	7,751	7,451	6,288	4,880	7,623	5,933
Ukrainskaja SSR	3,691	1,424	833	740	630	858	705	755
Belorusskaja SSR	1,583	1,715	858	731	693	749	728	808
Kazachskaja SSR	216	232	244	241	189	153	433	186
Litovskaja SSR	594	453	159	168	174	174	171	161
Moldavskaja SSR	84	16	7	6	6	6	3	7
Latvijskaja SSR	295	277	109	110	120	129	99	105
Estonskaja SSR	148	93	45	50	47	47	38	44

5.2.26 SOWING AREA OF MAIZE (RIPE) BY UNION REPUBLICS[1]
ANBAUFLÄCHE AN KÖRNERMAIS NACH UNIONSREPUBLIKEN[1]
POSEVNYE PLOSCADI KUKURUZY NA ZERNO PO SOJUZNYM RESPUBLIKAM[1]

	1940	1965	1970	1971	1972	1973	1974	1975
SSSR	3,690	3,177	3,353	3,332	4,012	4,031	3,955	2,652
RSFSR	865	630	421	454	666	1,058	714	532
Ukrainskaja SSR	1,560	1,814	2,262	2,192	2,597	2,220	2,391	1,247
Uzbekskaja SSR	17	25	25	30	45	66	97	94
Kazachskaja SSR	10	48	45	55	69	59	62	78
Gruzinskaja SSR	355	216	184	165	172	174	171	156
Azerbajdžanskaja SSR	10	19	12	10	13	13	17	12
Moldavskaja SSR	842	382	372	389	407	392	450	463
Kirgizskaja SSR	27	37	29	34	38	40	38	42
Tadžikskaja SSR	2	2	2	2	4	5	4	8
Armjanskaja SSR	2	1	0.3	0.3	0.5	0.3	0.3	0.2
Turkmenskaja SSR	--	3	1	1	1	4	11	20

5.2.27 SOWING AREA OF MILLET BY UNION REPUBLICS[1]
HIRSEANBAUFLÄCHE NACH UNIONSREPUBLIKEN[1]
POSEVNYE PLOSCADY PROSA PO SOJUZNYM RESPUBLIKAM[1]

	1940	1965	1970	1971	1972	1973	1974	1975
SSSR	5,970	3,253	2,691	2,397	2,724	2,850	2,970	2,774
RSFSR	3,995	2,055	1,449	1,376	1,601	1,852	1,778	1,615
Ukrainskaja SSR	955	438	521	306	395	326	427	327
Kazachskaja SSR	903	742	716	711	724	671	754	831

5.2.28 SOWING AREA OF BUCKWHEAT BY UNION REPUBLICS[1]
ANBAUFLÄCHE AN BUCHWEIZEN NACH UNIONSREPUBLIKEN[1]
POSEVNYE PLOSCADI GRECICHI PO SOJUZNYM RESPUBLIKAM[1]

	1940	1965	1970	1971	1972	1973	1974	1975
SSSR	2,063	1,794	1,879	1,768	1,720	1,648	1,589	1,459
RSFSR	1,066	1,184	1,296	1,151	1,097	1,076	1,085	1,012
Ukrainskaja SSR	723	395	364	292	304	277	276	239
Belorusskaja SSR	245	96	40	48	62	51	37	30
Kazachskaja SSR	1	115	178	277	257	244	191	178

[1] in all types of agricultural enterprises; '000 hectares - in allen landwirtschaftlichen Betrieben; Tsd.ha - vo vsech kategorijach chozjajstv; tys.gektarov

5.2.29   SOWING AREA OF RICE BY UNION   REPUBLICS[1]
         REISANBAUFLÄCHE NACH UNIONSREPUBLIKEN[1]
         POSEVNYE PLOSČADI RISA PO SOJUZNYM RESPUBLIKAM[1]

	1940	1965	1970	1971	1972	1973	1974	1975
SSSR	175	217	350	390	421	462	495	500
RSFSR	19	81	153	175	194	220	248	270
Ukrainskaja SSR	2	12	32	35	39	39	39	39
Uzbekskaja SSR	83	56	63	70	71	78	79	66
Kazachskaja SSR	28	42	82	90	99	107	112	105
Azerbajdžanskaja SSR	25	11	4	3	2	2	2	2
Kirgizskaja SSR	6	1	1	1	1	1	0.5	0.7
Tadžikskaja SSR	8	9	7	8	7	7	7	7
Turkmenskaja SSR	3	5	8	8	8	8	8	10

5.2.30   SOWING AREA OF LEGUMES BY UNION   REPUBLICS[1]
         ANBAUFLÄCHE AN HÜLSENFRÜCHTEN NACH UNIONSREPUBLIKEN[1]
         POSEVNYE PLOSČADI ZERNOBOBOVYCH KUL'TUR PO SOJUZNYM RESPUBLIKAM[1]

	1940	1965	1970	1971	1972	1973	1974	1975
SSSR	3,184	6,759	5,070	5,178	5,855	6,083	5,780	5,670
RSFSR	1,955	4,853	3,403	3,521	4,115	4,403	4,015	4,025
Ukrainskaja SSR	836	1,199	1,280	1,174	1,196	1,127	1,200	1,131
Belorusskaja SSR	166	290	168	178	200	183	156	146
Kazachskaja SSR	5	158	42	93	123	155	172	162
Gruzinskaja SSR	14	15	8	8	9	9	9	10
Azerbajdžanskaja SSR	27	11	9	9	8	8	8	6
Litovskaja SSR	86	95	59	94	99	101	115	113
Moldavskaja SSR	24	76	78	78	77	66	80	51
Latvijskaja SSR	36	20	6	6	9	8	6	6
Kirgizskaja SSR	2	6	1	2	2	2	1	1
Tadžikskaja SSR	13	16	9	8	10	10	9	9
Armjanskaja SSR	4	4	2	2	1	2	2	2
Estonskaja SSR	5	7	2	2	2	4	3	3

5.2.31   TOTAL SOWING AREA OF INDUSTRIAL CROPS BY UNION   REPUBLICS[1]
         GESAMTANBAUFLÄCHE AN TECHNISCHEN KULTUREN NACH UNIONSREPUBLIKEN[1]
         POSEVNYE PLOSČADI VSECH TECHNIČESKICH KUL'TUR PO SOJUZNYM RESPUBLIKAM[1]

	1940	1965	1970	1971	1972	1973	1974	1975
SSSR	11,789	15,333	14,486	14,233	14,361	14,665	14,710	14,122
RSFSR	6,201	7,211	6,528	6,253	6,245	6,614	6,511	5,947
Ukrainskaja SSR	2,700	4,248	3,939	3,897	4,049	4,042	4,075	4,027
Belorusskaja SSR	313	354	313	309	315	312	312	302
Uzbekskaja SSR	1,022	1,582	1,741	1,739	1,713	1,712	1,759	1,800
Kazachskaja SSR	341	448	406	458	426	386	364	348
Gruzinskaja SSR	52	44	40	43	45	46	45	44
Azerbajdžanskaja SSR	213	232	210	222	214	216	228	231
Litovskaja SSR	114	89	69	76	78	78	80	80
Moldavskaja SSR	261	399	381	369	409	387	391	392

[1] in all types of agricultural enterprises; '000 hectares - in allen landwirtschaftlichen Betrieben; Tsd.ha - vo vsech kategorijach chozjajstv; tys.gektarov

5.2.31
5.2.32 Economy
5.2.33 Wirtschaft
5.2.34

	1940	1965	1970	1971	1972	1973	1974	1975
Latvijskaja SSR	75	48	29	29	29	29	29	29
Kirgizskaja SSR	114	148	149	144	144	143	139	138
Tadžikskaja SSR	161	244	266	272	269	270	273	279
Armjanskaja SSR	36	20	12	13	13	13	14	14
Turkmenskaja SSR	160	261	400	405	408	413	485	487
Estonskaja SSR	26	5	3	4	4	4	5	4

5.2.32 SOWING AREA OF COTTON BY UNION REPUBLICS[1]
BAUMWOLLANBAUFLÄCHE NACH UNIONSREPUBLIKEN[1]
POSEVNYE PLOSČADI CHLOPČATNIKA PO SOJUZNYM RESPUBLIKAM[1]

	1940	1965	1970	1971	1972	1973	1974	1975	1976
SSSR	2,076	2,442	2,746	2,770	2,735	2,742	2,880	2,924	2,949
Uzbekskaja SSR	924	1,550	1,709	1,707	1,681	1,683	1,731	1,773	1,778
Kazachskaja SSR	102	112	118	118	116	115	115	110	110
Azerbajdžanskaja SSR	188	215	193	206	197	198	210	211	216
Kirgizskaja SSR	64	73	75	77	75	74	74	72	72
Tadžikskaja SSR	106	228	254	261	261	262	265	271	282
Turkmenskaja SSR	150	257	397	401	405	410	485	487	491

5.2.33 SOWING AREA OF SUGAR-BEET (FOR FACTORY PROCESSING) BY UNION REPUBLICS[1]
ANBAUFLÄCHE AN ZUCKERRÜBEN (FABRIKRÜBEN) NACH UNIONSREPUBLIKEN[1]
POSEVNYE PLOSČADI SACHARNOJ SVEKLY (FABRIČNOJ) PO SOJUZNYM RESPUBLIKAM[1]

	1940	1965	1970	1971	1972	1973	1974	1975	1976
SSSR	1,226	3,882	3,368	3,321	3,486	3,553	3,610	3,666	3,754
RSFSR	336	1,669	1,398	1,356	1,460	1,524	1,523	1,557	1,613
Ukrainskaja SSR	820	1,863	1,659	1,657	1,696	1,701	1,759	1,769	1,788
Belorusskaja SSR	--	59	49	49	54	50	47	51	50
Kazachskaja SSR	15	67	70	70	73	79	81	75	79
Gruzinskaja SSR	6	4	4	3	3	4	3	4	4
Litovskaja SSR	13	36	25	32	34	35	35	35	34
Moldavskaja SSR	4	103	98	94	104	98	100	112	123
Latvijskaja SSR	15	23	10	10	10	10	10	10	10
Kirgizskaja SSR	15	54	51	46	48	48	47	48	48
Armjanskaja SSR	2	4	4	4	4	4	5	4	5

5.2.34 SOWING AREA OF LONG-FIBRE FLAX BY UNION REPUBLICS[1]
ANBAUFLÄCHE AN FASERLEIN NACH UNIONSREPUBLIKEN[1]
POSEVNYE PLOSČADI L'NA-DOLGUNCA PO SOJUZNYM RESPUBLIKAM[1]

	1940	1965	1970	1971	1972	1973	1974	1975	1976
SSSR	2,099	1,476	1,284	1,244	1,251	1,248	1,210	1,215	1,214
RSFSR	1,525	888	727	691	692	688	641	664	656
Ukrainskaja SSR	118	224	230	230	235	237	241	237	238
Belorusskaja SSR	275	282	261	256	258	258	261	247	253
Litovskaja SSR	96	52	44	44	43	42	44	44	43
Latvijskaja SSR	59	25	19	19	19	19	19	19	18
Estonskaja SSR	26	5	3	4	4	4	4	4	6

1 in all types of agricultural enterprises; '000 hectares - in allen landwirtschaftlichen Betrieben; Tsd.ha - vo vsech kategorijach chozjajstv; tys.gektarov

5.2.35 SOWING AREA OF SUNFLOWER SEEDS BY UNION REPUBLICS[1]
ANBAUFLÄCHE AN SONNENBLUMENSAMEN NACH UNIONSREPUBLIKEN[1]
POSEVNYE PLOSČADI PODSOLNEČNIKA PO SOJUZNYM RESPUBLIKAM[1]

	1940	1965	1970	1971	1972	1973	1974	1975	1976
SSSR	3,543	4,870	4,777	4,498	4,394	4,745	4,686	4,045	4,534
RSFSR	2,452	2,734	2,744	2,520	2,303	2,693	2,656	2,060	2,528
Ukrainskaja SSR	720	1,777	1,710	1,662	1,748	1,728	1,718	1,672	1,703
Kazachskaja SSR	165	94	93	102	103	100	88	99	97
Gruzinskaja SSR	15	21	17	16	17	18	17	16	14
Moldavskaja SSR	178	239	208	193	218	202	202	194	188

5.2.36 SOWING AREA OF POTATOES BY UNION REPUBLICS[1]
KARTOFFELANBAUFLÄCHE NACH UNIONSREPUBLIKEN[1]
POSEVNYE PLOSČADI KARTOFELJA PO SOJUZNYM RESPUBLIKAM[1]

	1940	1965	1970	1971	1972	1973	1974	1975	1976
SSSR	7,738	8,612	8,064	7,894	7,960	8,017	7,983	7,912	7,087
RSFSR	4,078	4,723	4,391	4,335	4,404	4,467	4,457	4,449	3,890
Ukrainskaja SSR	2,060	2,108	1,988	1,899	1,900	1,901	1,890	1,857	1,702
Belorusskaja SSR	929	1,003	956	949	945	918	897	879	845
Uzbekskaja SSR	23	26	21	19	21	26	26	25	21
Kazachskaja SSR	100	180	193	190	193	200	205	203	170
Gruzinskaja SSR	25	24	25	25	25	26	28	28	26
Azerbajdžanskaja SSR	22	16	15	16	15	17	17	17	18
Litovskaja SSR	210	209	174	172	171	170	169	167	146
Moldavskaja SSR	29	46	37	37	38	39	41	40	41
Latvijskaja SSR	139	140	131	119	119	120	121	120	107
Kirgizskaja SSR	14	24	26	26	27	27	27	26	19
Tadžikskaja SSR	9	7	8	7	8	9	9	9	8
Armjanskaja SSR	13	17	18	18	17	19	19	19	18
Turkmenskaja SSR	4	2	2	2	2	2	2	2	2
Estonskaja SSR	83	87	79	80	75	76	75	71	74

5.2.37 SOWING AREA OF VEGETABLES BY UNION REPUBLICS[1]
GEMÜSEANBAUFLÄCHE NACH UNIONSREPUBLIKEN[1]
POSEVNYE PLOSČADI OVOSČEJ PO SOJUZNYM RESPUBLIKAM[1]

	1940	1965	1970	1971	1972	1973	1974	1975	1976
SSSR	1,507	1,404	1,499	1,519	1,578	1,621	1,642	1,652	1,562
RSFSR	827	632	676	676	706	731	732	735	645
Ukrainskaja SSR	486	464	466	476	486	496	496	499	493
Belorusskaja SSR	62	48	48	48	51	47	47	46	47
Uzbekskaja SSR	25	36	53	58	61	63	73	76	84
Kazachskaja SSR	23	48	51	53	56	59	60	61	55
Gruzinskaja SSR	14	24	30	29	29	31	32	33	35
Azerbajdžanskaja SSR	14	25	32	32	35	36	38	38	42
Litovskaja SSR	14	21	21	21	21	22	22	22	17
Moldavskaja SSR	11	48	52	56	61	62	68	67	69
Latvijskaja SSR	9	14	15	12	13	12	12	13	11
Kirgizskaja SSR	5	11	12	13	13	13	14	14	13

1 in all types of agricultural enterprises; '000 hectares - in allen landwirtschaftlichen Betrieben; Tsd.ha - vo vsech kategorijach chozjajstv; tys.gektarov

5.2.37 Economy
5.2.38 Wirtschaft
5.2.39

	1940	1965	1970	1971	1972	1973	1974	1975	1976
Tadžikskaja SSR	5	6	12	12	12	13	13	14	14
Armjanskaja SSR	5	11	14	15	15	16	16	16	17
Turkmenskaja SSR	5	10	11	12	13	14	13	13	15
Estonskaja SSR	2	6	6	6	6	6	6	5	5

5.2.38 SOWING AREA OF FODDER CROPS BY UNION REPUBLICS[1]
ANBAUFLÄCHE AN VIEHFUTTER NACH UNIONSREPUBLIKEN[1]
POSEVNYE PLOSČADI KORMOVYCH KUL'TUR PO SOJUZNYM RESPUBLIKAM[1]

	1940	1965	1970	1971	1972	1973	1974	1975	1976
SSSR	18,088	55,178	62,846	65,201	66,066	63,387	64,417	65,587	66,308
RSFSR	10,432	33,554	37,427	38,661	39,221	37,104	37,642	38,179	38,474
Ukrainskaja SSR	4,441	10,292	10,733	10,927	11,016	10,166	10,201	10,527	11,088
Belorusskaja SSR	433	1,738	2,224	2,213	2,173	2,270	2,324	2,342	2,238
Uzbekskaja SSR	447	395	452	516	544	580	573	636	595
Kazachskaja SSR	494	5,496	7,675	8,410	8,537	8,706	9,051	9,472	9,450
Gruzinskaja SSR	53	174	251	264	278	267	270	276	267
Azerbajdžanskaja SSR	66	207	308	356	352	362	360	402	379
Litovskaja SSR	520	1,078	1,165	1,110	1,161	1,140	1,069	1,035	1,035
Moldavskaja SSR	76	460	519	561	502	540	576	413	510
Latvijskaja SSR	609	730	793	770	834	806	805	795	760
Kirgizskaja SSR	141	376	490	504	511	494	529	517	511
Tadžikskaja SSR	55	105	151	186	171	173	207	192	191
Armjanskaja SSR	38	129	174	183	182	184	188	193	200
Turkmenskaja SSR	48	94	116	140	143	156	169	173	189
Estonskaja SSR	235	350	368	400	441	439	453	435	426

5.2.39 SOWING AREA OF SEASONAL AND PERENNIAL GRASS INCL. WINTER SOWING
FOR GREEN FODDER BY UNION REPUBLICS[1]
ANBAUFLÄCHE AN MEHR- UND EINJÄHRIGEN GRÄSERN EINSCHL. WINTERAUSSAAT
FÜR GRÜNFUTTER NACH UNIONSREPUBLIKEN[1]
POSEVNYE PLOSČADI MNOGOLETNICH I ODNOLETNICH TRAV, VKLJUČAJA POSEVY
OZIMYCH NA ZELENYJ KORM, PO SOJUZNYM RESPUBLIKAM[1]

	1940	1965	1970	1971	1972	1973	1974	1975
SSSR	16,314	30,009	39,684	41,770	42,264	40,517	41,571	42,068
RSFSR	9,496	18,041	23,645	24,355	24,716	23,142	23,823	23,741
Ukrainskaja SSR	3,831	5,084	5,368	5,797	5,725	5,256	5,193	5,367
Belorusskaja SSR	414	1,033	1,667	1,737	1,708	1,785	1,846	1,925
Uzbekskaja SSR	445	233	295	338	375	415	417	441
Kazachskaja SSR	459	3,154	5,519	6,213	6,344	6,484	6,810	7,134
Gruzinskaja SSR	46	84	151	153	180	175	184	185
Azerbajdžanskaja SSR	59	91	197	241	237	246	245	278
Litovskaja SSR	450	815	914	862	843	855	783	780
Moldavskaja SSR	54	171	249	305	306	310	328	298
Latvijskaja SSR	562	558	645	633	662	657	644	659
Kirgizskaja SSR	137	269	394	409	417	409	443	422
Tadžikskaja SSR	55	55	106	141	128	132	165	149
Armjanskaja SSR	35	98	143	149	148	152	156	162
Turkmenskaja SSR	47	51	77	89	90	104	125	129
Estonskaja SSR	224	272	314	348	385	395	409	398

[1] in all types of agricultural enterprises; '000 hectares - in allen landwirtschaftlichen Betrieben; Tsd.ha - vo vsech kategorijach chozjajstv; tys.gektarov

Economy   5.2.40
Wirtschaft 5.2.43

5.2.40 AREA OF IRRIGATED GROUND IN COLLECTIVE AND STATE FARMS AND OTHER
        STATE ENTERPRISES BY UNION   REPUBLICS ('000 hectares)
        BEWÄSSERTE BODENFLÄCHE IN KOLCHOSEN, SOWCHOSEN UND ANDEREN STAAT-
        LICHEN WIRTSCHAFTEN NACH UNIONSREPUBLIKEN (Tsd.ha)
        PLOŠČAD' OROŠAEMYCH ZEMEL' V KOLCHOZACH, SOVCHOZACH I DRUGICH
        GOSUDARSTVENNYCH CHOZJAJSTVACH PO SOJUZNYM RESPUBLIKAM (tys.gektarov)

	1940	1965	1970	1971	1972	1973	1974	1975	1976
SSSR	8,318	9,812	10,891	11,270	11,774	12,533	13,437	14,241	15,073
RSFSR	1,063	1,510	1,955	2,127	2,393	2,810	3,278	3,684	4,068
Ukrainskaja SSR	156	503	923	1,011	1,096	1,195	1,332	1,483	1,650
Belorusskaja SSR	--	--	--	--	10	61	108	139	170
Uzbekskaja SSR	2,276	2,639	2,696	2,721	2,774	2,832	2,915	3,006	3,132
Kazachskaja SSR	1,393	1,368	1,451	1,479	1,509	1,551	1,601	1,648	1,707
Gruzinskaja SSR	282	348	347	353	360	368	370	368	380
Azerbajdžanskaja SSR	1,160	1,278	1,108	1,111	1,117	1,122	1,128	1,141	1,148
Moldavskaja SSR	17	74	115	124	129	139	148	156	165
Kirgizskaja SSR	937	861	883	891	897	905	904	911	924
Tadžikskaja SSR	361	468	518	528	535	543	552	567	582
Armjanskaja SSR	219	249	252	253	256	265	275	283	258
Turkmenskaja SSR	454	514	643	672	698	727	796	819	846

5.2.41 see page 266 - siehe Seite 266
5.2.42 see page 267 - siehe Seite 267

5.2.43 AREA OF VITICULTURE OF ALL GROWING PHASES BY UNION   REPUBLICS[1]
        WEINBAUFLÄCHE ALLER WACHSTUMSPHASEN NACH UNIONSREPUBLIKEN[1]
        PLOŠČAD' VINOGRADNYCH NASAŽDENIJ VSECH VOZRASTOV PO SOJUZNYM RESPUBLIKAM[1]

	1940	1965	1970	1971	1972	1973	1974	1975	1976
SSSR	425	1,064	1,087	1,118	1,083	1,093	1,138	1,203	1,258
RSFSR	42	169	164	169	158	159	168	175	184
Ukrainskaja SSR	103	330	287	288	263	267	277	275	265
Uzbekskaja SSR	28	51	56	58	59	59	61	62	66
Kazachskaja SSR	2	17	20	21	22	22	22	23	22
Gruzinskaja SSR	70	106	118	119	116	117	121	126	134
Azerbajdžanskaja SSR	33	89	122	133	152	150	159	178	195
Moldavskaja SSR	118	235	251	260	242	247	257	289	315
Kirgizskaja SSR	1	6	6	6	6	6	7	7	7
Tadžikskaja SSR	8	16	18	19	20	21	21	22	23
Armjanskaja SSR	16	36	36	36	35	35	35	35	36
Turkmenskaja SSR	4	9	9	9	10	10	10	11	11

[1] in all types of agricultural enterprises; '000 hectares - in allen landwirtschaftlichen Betrieben; Tsd.ha - vo vsech kategorijach chozjajstv; tys.gektarov

5.2.41 Economy / Wirtschaft

5.2.41 SOWING AREA OF AGRICULTURAL CROPS ON IRRIGATED GROUND IN COLLECTIVE AND STATE FARMS AND OTHER STATE ENTERPRISES BY UNION REPUBLICS, 1975
ANBAUFLÄCHE AN LANDWIRTSCHAFTLICHEN KULTUREN AUF DEM BEWÄSSERTEN BODEN IN KOLCHOSEN, SOWCHOSEN UND ANDEREN STAATLICHEN WIRTSCHAFTEN NACH UNIONSREPUBLIKEN, 1975
POSEVNYE PLOŠČADI SEL'SKOCHOZJAJSTVENNYCH KUL'TUR NA OROŠAEMYCH ZEMLJACH V KOLCHOZACH, SOVCHOZACH I DRUGICH GOSUDARSTVENNYCH CHOZJAJSTVACH PO SOJUZNYM RESPUBLIKAM V 1975 G.

('000 hectares – Tsd.ha – tys.gektarov)

	Total sowing area, crop 1975 / Gesamte Anbaufläche für Ernte 1975 / Vsja posevnaja ploščad' pod urožaj 1975 g.	Agricultural crops / Getreidekulturen / Zernovye kul'tury	Winter & summer wheat / Winter-u. Sommerweizen / pšenica ozimaja i jarovaja	Maize (Ripe) / Körnermais / kukuruza na zerno	Rice / Reis / ris	Industrial crops / Technische Kulturen / techn. kul'tury	of which sugar-beet (for factory processing) / darunter Zuckerrüben (Fabrikrüben) / v tom čisle sacharnaja svekla (fabričnaja)	Potatoes, Vegetables and Melons / Kartoffeln, Gemüse u.Melonen / Kartofel'i ovošče-bachčevye kul'tury	Fodder crops / Futterkulturen / Kormovye kul'tury
	of which–darunter–v tom čisle								
SSSR	10746.4	2866.1	1206.0	371.8	497.0	3228.0	165.5	895.9	3756.4
RSFSR	2097.9	786.1	272.1	78.2	270.0	45.5	19.3	304.5	961.8
Ukrainskaja SSR	1207.2	375.3	195.7	53.6	38.7	28.5	11.1	197.4	606.0
Uzbekskaja SSR	2675.7	249.6	28.4	78.7	64.9	1798.6	--	99.4	528.1
Kazachskaja SSR	1408.4	507.4	197.2	71.0	105.1	196.4	74.7	89.7	614.9
Gruzinskaja SSR	170.9	69.5	37.2	15.0	--	10.4	3.1	26.7	64.3
Azerbajdžanskaja SSR	868.0	362.6	247.6	7.0	2.6	225.9	--	31.9	247.6
Moldavskaja SSR	121.1	31.7	16.0	11.6	--	10.6	4.6	40.0	38.8
Kirgizskaja SSR	782.8	272.4	135.4	30.2	0.4	136.3	47.9	21.6	352.5
Tadžikskaja SSR	448.8	40.2	12.0	6.4	5.1	275.8	--	17.9	114.9
Armjanskaja SSR	154.2	59.5	37.0	0.1	--	12.4	4.7	21.3	61.0
Turkmenskaja SSR	790.2	108.0	26.7	20.0	10.2	487.6	--	36.3	158.3

266

5.2.42 FRUIT-GROWING AND VITICULTURE (in all agricultural enterprises; '000 hectares)
OBST- UND WEINBAU (in allen landwirtschaftlichen Betrieben; Tsd.ha)
SADOVODSTVO I VINOGRADARSTVO (vo vsech kategorijach chozjajstv; tys.gektarov)

	1940	1965	1970	1971	1972	1973	1974	1975	1976
Sowing area of fruit and berries (incl. citrus fruits) Anbaufläche von Obst und Beeren (einschl. Zitrusfrüchte) Ploščad'plodovo-jagodnych nasaždenij (vključaja citrusovye)	1,790	3,626	3,848	3,815	3,773	3,734	3,690	3,628	3,571
of which at fruit-bearing state – darunter in fruchttragendem Alter – v tom čisle v plodonosjaščem vozraste	1,042	1,495	2,431	2,444	2,483	2,509	2,555	2,561	2,529
Area of viticulture – Weinbaufläche – Ploščad' vinogradnych nasaždenij	425	1,064	1,087	1,118	1,083	1,093	1,138	1,203	1,258
of which at fruit-bearing state – darunter in fruchttragendem Alter – v tom čisle v plodonosjaščem vozraste	330	765	813	828	781	759	784	818	827

5.2.44 Economy
5.2.45 Wirtschaft

5.2.44 AREA OF VITICULTURE AT FRUIT-BEARING STATE BY UNION REPUBLICS[1]
WEINBAUFLÄCHE IM FRUCHTTRAGENDEN STADIUM NACH UNIONSREPUBLIKEN[1]
PLOŠČAD' VINOGRADNYCH NASAŽDENIJ V PLODONOSJAŠČEM VOZRASTE PO SOJUZNYM RESPUBLIKAM[1]

	1940	1965	1970	1971	1972	1973	1974	1975	1976
SSSR	330	765	813	828	781	759	784	818	827
RSFSR	24	125	127	129	124	120	116	114	111
Ukrainskaja SSR	74	262	237	232	213	200	198	195	185
Uzbekskaja SSR	22	30	38	40	42	43	46	47	47
Kazachskaja SSR	1	11	14	15	15	15	16	17	17
Gruzinskaja SSR	53	74	93	96	92	87	94	98	100
Azerbajdžanskaja SSR	30	41	70	81	89	88	98	106	113
Moldavskaja SSR	105	179	178	178	148	148	157	181	194
Kirgizskaja SSR	0.2	3	5	5	4	5	5	6	5
Tadžikskaja SSR	7	9	14	15	16	16	16	16	17
Armjanskaja SSR	11	25	29	30	30	29	30	30	30
Turkmenskaja SSR	3	6	8	7	8	8	8	8	8

5.2.45 SOWING AREA OF TEA BY UNION REPUBLICS[1]
TEEANBAUFLÄCHE NACH UNIONSREPUBLIKEN[1]
PLOŠČAD' ČAJNYCH NASAŽDENIJ PO SOJUZNYM RESPUBLIKAM[1]

	1940	1965	1970	1971	1972	1973	1974	1975	1976
SSSR	55.3	71.0	74.4	75.5	74.7	73.9	75.5	76.0	76.8
RSFSR	0.6	2.0	1.7	1.7	1.6	1.7	1.7	1.7	1.7
Gruzinskaja SSR	49.6	62.6	64.8	65.6	65.0	64.8	65.6	65.8	66.1
Azerbajdžanskaja SSR	5.1	6.4	7.9	8.2	8.1	7.4	8.2	8.5	9.0

---

1 in all types of agricultural enterprises; '000 hectares - in allen landwirtschaftlichen Betrieben; Tsd.ha - vo vsech kategorijach chozjajstv; tys.gektarov

Economy
Wirtschaft 5.2.46.1

5.2.46 LIVESTOCK-BREEDING - VIEHWIRTSCHAFT - ŽIVOTNOVODSTVO

5.2.46.1 LIVESTOCK - VIEHBESTAND - POGOLOV'E SKOTA
(in all agricultural enterprises; January 1; million head)
(in allen landwirtschaftlichen Betrieben; Stand 1.Januar; Mio Stck.)
(vo vsech kategorijach chozjajstv; na 1 janvarja; mln.golov)

Year Jahr Gody	Cattle Rinder Krupnyj rogatyj skot	of which cows davon Kühe v tom čisle korovy	Pigs Schweine Svin'i	Sheep Schafe Ovcy	Goats Ziegen Kozy	Horses Pferde Lošadi
1916	58.4	28.8	23.0	89.7	6.6	38.2
1941	54.8	28.0	27.6	80.0	11.7	21.1
1951	57.1	24.3	24.4	82.6	16.4	13.8
1956	58.8	27.7	34.0	103.3	12.9	13.0
1961	75.8	34.5	58.7	133.0	7.3	9.9
1966	93.4	39.3	59.6	129.8	5.5	8.0
1967	97.1	40.3	58.0	135.5	5.5	8.0
1968	97.2	40.5	50.9	138.4	5.6	8.0
1969	95.7	40.1	49.0	140.6	5.5	8.0
1970	95.2	39.6	56.1	130.7	5.1	7.5
1971	99.2	39.8	67.5	138.0	5.4	7.4
1972	102.4	40.0	71.4	139.9	5.4	7.3
1973	104.0	40.6	66.6	139.1	5.6	7.1
1974	106.3	41.5	70.0	142.6	5.9	6.8
1975	109.1	41.9	72.3	145.3	5.9	6.8
1976	111.0	41.9	57.9	141.4	5.7	6.4
1977	110.3	42.0	63.1	139.8	5.5	--

5.2.46.2 Economy / Wirtschaft

5.2.46.2 DAIRY CATTLE AND LIVESTOCK IN INDIVIDUAL AGRICULTURAL ENTERPRISES (January 1; '000 head)
NUTZVIEHBESTAND IN DEN EINZELNEN LANDWIRTSCHAFTLICHEN BETRIEBEN (zum 1.Januar; Tsd.Stck.)
POGOLOV'E PRODUKTIVNOGO SKOTA PO KATEGORIJAM CHOZJAJSTV (na 1 janvarja; tys.golov)

	1941	1966	1971	1972	1973	1974	1975	1976	1977
Cattle – Rinder – Krupnyj rogatyj skot									
A. all agricultural enterprises – alle landwirtschaftlichen Betriebe – Vse kategorii chozjajstv of which-darunter-v tom čisle:	54,773	93,436	99,225	102,434	104,006	106,266	109,122	111,034	110,346
B. State farms and other state enterprises – Sowchosen u.andere staatl.Wirtschaften – Sovchozy i drugie gosudarstvennye chozjajstva	3,528	27,222	32,539	34,369	35,259	36,718	38,293	39,402	39,706
C. of which state farms – davon Sowchosen – iz nich sovchozy	2,462	24,501	29,073	30,658	31,435	33,288	34,605	35,588	37,049
D. collective farms-Kolchosen-kolchozy	20,096	38,341	41,733	43,142	44,071	44,933	46,320	48,167	47,827
E. Individual subsidiary plots of collective farmers,workers,employees and other population groups – Private Nebenwirtschaften der Kolchosbauern,Arbeiter,Angestellten u. anderen Bevölkerungsgruppen – Ličnye podsobnye chozjajstva kolchoznikov,rabočich,služaščich i drugich grupp naselenija	31,149	27,873	24,953	24,923	24,676	24,615	24,509	23,465	22,813
Cows – Kühe – Korovy									
A.	27,993	39,347	39,762	39,969	40,569	41,421	41,910	41,917	41,987
B.	1,308	9,520	10,696	11,153	11,634	12,212	12,611	12,854	13,062
C.	952	8,918	10,005	10,374	10,739	11,482	11,874	12,096	12,784
D.	5,678	13,182	13,546	13,746	14,243	14,723	15,067	15,323	15,537
E.	21,007	16,645	15,520	15,070	14,602	14,486	14,232	13,740	13,388

Economy / Wirtschaft 5.2.46.2

	1941	1966	1971	1972	1973	1974	1975	1976	1977
Pigs – Schweine – Svin'i									
A.	27,603	59,576	67,483	71,434	66,593	70,032	72,273	57,899	63,055
B.	3,260	16,745	21,366	23,725	22,607	24,385	25,498	19,943	22,812
C.	1,910	12,535	16,603	18,607	17,991	19,447	20,494	16,151	19,700
D.	8,235	24,629	29,555	31,855	30,677	32,089	33,124	25,729	28,475
Sheep – Schafe – Ovcy									
A.	80,030	129,764	138,059	139,916	139,086	142,634	145,305	141,436	139,834
B.	7,125	48,266	55,752	57,744	58,697	62,388	65,121	64,862	64,959
C.	5,841	46,207	53,106	55,219	55,989	59,666	62,478	62,398	63,684
D.	39,148	53,926	53,488	53,853	52,649	52,833	52,907	51,576	50,380
E.	33,757	27,572	28,819	28,319	27,740	27,413	27,277	24,998	24,495
Goats – Ziegen – Kozy									
A.	11,682	5,552	5,362	5,417	5,604	5,900	5,927	5,655	5,539
B.	124	232	386	421	495	565	618	665	776
C.	67	224	379	415	488	557	611	660	769
D.	2,800	663	615	599	582	612	588	575	477
E.	8,758	4,657	4,361	4,397	4,527	4,723	4,721	4,415	4,286

5.2.46.3 Economy
5.2.46.4 Wirtschaft

5.2.46.3 BEEF CATTLE BY UNION REPUBLICS[1]
RINDERBESTAND NACH UNIONSREPUBLIKEN[1]
POGOLOV'E KRUPNOGO ROGATOGO SKOTA PO SOJUZNYM RESPUBLIKAM[1]

	1941	1966	1971	1972	1973	1974	1975	1976	1977
SSSR	54,773	93,436	99,225	102,434	104,006	106,266	109,122	111,034	110,346
RSFSR	27,855	48,207	51,602	53,180	53,691	54,747	56,508	57,615	56,928
Ukrainskaja SSR	10,997	21,324	21,352	22,255	22,662	23,042	23,548	24,180	24,196
Belorusskaja SSR	2,844	4,704	5,383	5,581	5,769	5,987	6,261	6,406	6,494
Uzbekskaja SSR	1,672	2,494	2,907	2,951	2,996	3,095	3,182	3,218	3,217
Kazachskaja SSR	3,356	6,833	7,285	7,470	7,648	7,890	7,955	7,723	7,645
Gruzinskaja SSR	1,607	1,514	1,475	1,487	1,516	1,528	1,513	1,537	1,493
Azerbajdžanskaja SSR	1,357	1,460	1,577	1,576	1,565	1,637	1,653	1,667	1,646
Litovskaja SSR	1,054	1,526	1,814	1,857	1,897	1,961	2,023	2,121	2,136
Moldavskaja SSR	514	914	905	987	1,050	1,053	1,064	1,084	1,062
Latvijskaja SSR	986	1,108	1,203	1,266	1,289	1,326	1,359	1,389	1,385
Kirgizskaja SSR	556	857	912	925	939	949	973	942	940
Tadžikskaja SSR	580	818	1,008	1,036	1,063	1,075	1,090	1,095	1,101
Armjanskaja SSR	599	662	666	690	714	719	694	704	721
Turkmenskaja SSR	268	405	444	455	463	486	511	532	556
Estonskaja SSR	528	610	692	718	744	771	788	821	826

5.2.46.4 DAIRY CATTLE BY UNION REPUBLICS[1]
KÜHEBESTAND NACH UNIONSREPUBLIKEN[1]
POGOLOV'E KOROV PO SOJUZNYM RESPUBLIKAM[1]

	1941	1966	1971	1972	1973	1974	1975	1976	1977
SSSR	27,993	39,347	39,762	39,969	40,569	41,421	41,910	41,917	41,987
RSFSR	14,250	20,701	20,595	20,677	20,958	21,408	21,766	21,760	21,795
Ukrainskaja SSR	5,965	8,484	8,563	8,623	8,785	8,899	8,969	8,978	9,002
Belorusskaja SSR	1,956	2,331	2,490	2,510	2,550	2,611	2,608	2,680	2,688
Uzbekskaja SSR	622	1,012	1,140	1,133	1,148	1,190	1,216	1,214	1,230
Kazachskaja SSR	1,259	2,526	2,533	2,575	2,622	2,718	2,727	2,624	2,626
Gruzinskaja SSR	575	602	595	595	602	602	592	596	585
Azerbajdžanskaja SSR	489	576	605	595	592	620	623	622	614
Litovskaja SSR	782	807	839	834	835	858	873	890	887
Moldavskaja SSR	181	342	342	351	361	368	378	388	386
Latvijskaja SSR	797	580	571	571	580	587	589	586	584
Kirgizskaja SSR	219	343	360	361	363	370	375	366	366
Tadžikskaja SSR	188	315	372	375	389	394	397	403	403
Armjanskaja SSR	212	260	262	270	278	280	268	272	279
Turkmenskaja SSR	96	162	186	190	192	197	204	208	213
Estonskaja SSR	402	306	309	309	314	319	325	330	329

[1] in all agricultural enterprises; January 1; '000 head - in allen landwirtschaftlichen Betrieben; Stand 1.Januar; Tsd.Stck. - vo vsech kategorijach chozjajstv; na 1 janvarja; tys.golov

5.2.46.5 PIGS BY UNION REPUBLICS[1]
SCHWEINEBESTAND NACH UNIONSREPUBLIKEN[1]
POGOLOV'E SVINEJ PO SOJUZNYM RESPUBLIKAM[1]

	1941	1966	1971	1972	1973	1974	1975	1976	1977
SSSR	27,602	59,576	67,483	71,434	66,593	70,032	72,273	57,899	63,055
RSFSR	12,090	29,497	33,225	35,557	32,722	34,981	36,460	27,771	30,611
Ukrainskaja SSR	9,186	18,920	20,746	21,397	19,600	20,197	20,802	16,847	18,195
Belorusskaja SSR	2,520	3,688	4,004	4,072	4,115	4,291	4,328	3,999	4,158
Uzbekskaja SSR	103	230	296	338	363	377	393	305	217
Kazachskaja SSR	451	1,735	2,266	2,710	2,732	2,791	2,619	1,678	2,218
Gruzinskaja SSR	615	574	687	726	694	699	746	762	732
Azerbajdžanskaja SSR	120	85	113	122	129	143	151	135	141
Litovskaja SSR	1,068	1,731	2,297	2,334	2,223	2,365	2,346	2,141	2,326
Moldavskaja SSR	339	1,187	1,574	1,626	1,549	1,563	1,652	1,633	1,570
Latvijskaja SSR	588	913	1,075	1,196	1,136	1,230	1,273	1,195	1,275
Kirgizskaja SSR	87	224	244	291	284	290	290	216	220
Tadžikskaja SSR	21	61	78	93	97	99	106	86	99
Armjanskaja SSR	59	86	121	156	152	145	163	174	173
Turkmenskaja SSR	36	53	69	89	103	113	128	122	129
Estonskaja SSR	319	592	688	727	694	748	816	835	891

5.2.46.6 SHEEP AND GOATS BY UNION REPUBLICS[1]
SCHAF- UND ZIEGENBESTAND NACH UNIONSREPUBLIKEN[1]
POGOLOV'E OVEC I KOZ PO SOJUZNYM RESPUBLIKAM[1]

	1941	1966	1971	1972	1973	1974	1975	1976	1977
SSSR	91,712	135,316	143,421	145,333	144,690	148,534	151,232	147,091	145,373
RSFSR	51,235	61,416	66,964	67,659	66,256	67,304	68,673	66,109	65,361
Ukrainskaja SSR	7,325	9,342	8,971	9,069	9,082	9,301	9,547	9,115	8,911
Belorusskaja SSR	2,578	846	692	657	661	629	604	565	554
Uzbekskaja SSR	5,792	7,956	7,978	7,955	7,756	8,326	8,539	8,235	7,986
Kazachskaja SSR	8,132	30,120	31,776	32,596	33,555	34,609	35,386	34,579	34,438
Gruzinskaja SSR	2,194	2,174	1,955	1,997	2,052	2,094	1,984	2,080	1,984
Azerbajdžanskaja SSR	2,907	4,035	4,371	4,478	4,692	5,078	5,164	5,128	5,145
Litovskaja SSR	627	198	161	153	146	134	113	96	78
Moldavskaja SSR	1,464	1,676	1,419	1,400	1,333	1,266	1,253	1,230	1,158
Latvijskaja SSR	613	386	328	334	340	311	292	280	251
Kirgizskaja SSR	2,529	8,303	9,455	9,521	9,698	9,816	9,890	9,851	9,906
Tadžikskaja SSR	2,174	2,431	2,634	2,713	2,660	2,786	2,861	2,896	2,908
Armjanskaja SSR	1,221	2,222	2,063	2,192	2,321	2,363	2,285	2,331	2,290
Turkmenskaja SSR	2,596	4,036	4,489	4,439	3,956	4,337	4,465	4,423	4,251
Estonskaja SSR	325	175	165	170	182	180	176	173	152

1 in all agricultural enterprises; January 1; '000 head -
in allen landwirtschaftlichen Betrieben; Stand 1.Januar; Tsd.Stck. -
vo vsech kategorijach chozjajstv; na 1 janvarja; tys.golov

5.2.46.7 Economy
5.2.46.8 Wirtschaft

5.2.46.7 SHEEP BY UNION REPUBLICS ('000 head)[1]
SCHAFBESTAND NACH UNIONSREPUBLIKEN (Tsd.Stck.)[1]
POGOLOV'E OVEC PO SOJUZNYM RESPUBLIKAM (tys.golov)[1]

	1941	1966	1971	1972	1973	1974	1975	1976	1977
SSSR	80,030	129,764	138,059	139,916	139,086	142,634	145,305	141,436	139,834
RSFSR	46,716	58,695	64,245	64,862	63,355	64,233	65,586	63,218	62,554
Ukrainskaja SSR	6,700	8,646	8,614	8,748	8,779	9,022	9,281	8,863	8,669
Belorusskaja SSR	2,539	789	663	631	635	603	579	541	531
Uzbekskaja SSR	4,245	7,617	7,541	7,521	7,287	7,803	7,995	7,685	7,428
Kazachskaja SSR	6,988	29,632	31,254	32,032	32,947	33,950	34,725	33,955	33,827
Gruzinskaja SSR	1,692	2,011	1,814	1,867	1,924	1,968	1,867	1,973	1,886
Azerbajdžanskaja SSR	2,269	3,864	4,192	4,297	4,499	4,872	4,962	4,924	4,843
Litovskaja SSR	611	187	154	147	140	129	108	92	74
Moldavskaja SSR	1,450	1,613	1,389	1,373	1,309	1,244	1,233	1,211	1,142
Latvijskaja SSR	602	368	318	324	330	302	284	272	244
Kirgizskaja SSR	1,844	8,111	9,240	9,322	9,502	9,621	9,688	9,654	9,712
Tadžikskaja SSR	1,054	2,065	2,182	2,250	2,188	2,279	2,334	2,369	2,376
Armjanskaja SSR	999	2,151	1,999	2,128	2,255	2,303	2,233	2,281	2,245
Turkmenskaja SSR	1,999	3,844	4,291	4,246	3,756	4,127	4,256	4,226	4,052
Estonskaja SSR	322	171	163	168	180	178	174	172	151

5.2.46.8 POULTRY BY UNION REPUBLICS (mill.head)[1]
GEFLÜGELBESTAND NACH UNIONSREPUBLIKEN (Mio Stck.)[1]
POGOLOV'E PTICY PO SOJUZNYM RESPUBLIKAM (mln.golov)[1]

	1941	1966	1971	1972	1973	1974	1975	1976	1977
SSSR	255.7	490.7	652.7	686.5	700.0	747.7	792.4	734.9	778.9
RSFSR	135.2	269.7	358.2	380.5	382.9	408.0	434.3	394.6	422.2
Ukrainskaja SSR	69.6	120.5	155.2	160.8	163.7	177.3	185.3	168.3	177.1
Belorusskaja SSR	14.7	20.6	27.0	28.3	29.6	30.8	32.0	31.9	32.1
Uzbekskaja SSR	2.4	8.1	13.8	14.6	15.5	17.5	18.6	16.9	17.4
Kazachskaja SSR	6.7	19.9	29.5	31.8	33.2	35.1	37.4	36.7	38.0
Gruzinskaja SSR	7.1	8.3	11.7	12.3	13.9	13.3	14.2	14.9	15.5
Azerbajdžanskaja SSR	3.8	6.9	8.8	8.9	10.6	12.4	13.2	12.8	13.4
Litovskaja SSR	3.8	7.3	9.6	9.4	9.5	9.7	10.3	10.8	11.1
Moldavskaja SSR	4.4	11.0	12.1	11.5	11.3	12.1	12.7	13.3	13.9
Latvijskaja SSR	2.0	4.0	5.9	6.4	6.6	7.0	7.6	7.5	8.3
Kirgizskaja SSR	1.1	5.3	7.3	6.9	7.2	7.6	7.9	7.8	8.2
Tadžikskaja SSR	0.9	1.6	2.7	3.2	3.2	3.4	4.0	4.1	4.6
Armjanskaja SSR	1.7	3.1	4.5	5.0	5.8	6.1	6.6	7.0	7.8
Turkmenskaja SSR	0.7	1.9	2.7	3.0	3.1	3.3	3.9	3.6	4.1
Estonskaja SSR	1.6	2.5	3.7	3.9	3.9	4.1	4.4	4.7	5.2

[1] in all agricultural enterprises; January 1 - in allen landwirtschaftlichen Betrieben; Stand 1.Januar - vo vsech kategorijach chozjajstv; na 1 janvarja

5.2.46.9 BASIC LIVESTOCK PRODUCTS - GRUNDERZEUGNISSE DER VIEHWIRTSCHAFT - OSNOVNYE PRODUKTY ŽIVOTNOVODSTVA

Year Jahr Gody	Meat (slaughter weight), mill.tons Fleisch (Schlachtgewicht), Mio t Mjaso (v ubojnom vese), mln.t	Milk (mill.tons) Milch (Mio t) Moloko (mln.t)	Eggs ('000 mill.) Eier (Mrd.Stck.) Jajca (mrd.št.)	Wool ('000 tons) Wolle (Tsd.t) Šerst' (tys.t)
A.	B.	C.	D.	E.

All agricultural enterprises
Alle landwirtschaftlichen Betriebe
Vse kategorii chozjajstv

1940	4.7	33.6	12.2	161
1945	2.6	26.4	4.9	111
1950	4.9	35.3	11.7	180
1955	6.3	43.0	18.5	256
1960	8.7	61.7	27.4	357
1965	10.0	72.6	29.1	357
1966	10.7	76.0	31.7	371
1967	11.5	79.9	33.9	395
1968	11.6	82.3	35.7	415
1969	11.8	81.5	37.2	390
1970	12.3	83.0	40.7	419
1971	13.3	83.2	45.1	429
1972	13.6	83.2	47.9	420
1973	13.5	88.3	51.2	433
1974	14.6	91.8	55.5	461
1975	15.0	90.8	57.5	467
1976	13.4	89.1	55.6	433
1977	14.7	95.0	61.2	459

Collective and state farms and other state enterprises
Kolchosen, Sowchosen und andere staatliche Unternehmen
Kolchozy, sovchozy i drugie gosudarstvennye chozjajstva

1940	1.3	7.5	0.7	98
1945	1.0	4.7	0.5	75
1950	1.6	8.9	1.3	141
1955	3.0	17.0	2.3	207
1960	5.1	32.6	5.3	279
1965	6.0	43.9	9.5	284
1966	6.3	45.8	10.8	295
1967	7.0	48.8	12.6	315
1968	7.2	51.0	14.5	332
1969	7.6	51.2	16.3	307
1970	8.0	53.2	19.0	337
1971	8.7	53.9	22.4	343
1972	9.1	54.8	25.5	333
1973	9.1	59.4	29.1	343
1974	10.0	62.7	32.5	369
1975	10.3	62.9	34.8	373
1976	9.3	62.2	35.1	346

5.2.46.9 Economy
Wirtschaft

A.	B.	C.	D.	E.
Collective farms and inter-farm enterprises - Kolchosen und zwischen-wirtschaftliche Betriebe - Kolchozy i mežchozjajstvennye predprijatija					
1940	0.9	5.6	0.5	79
1945	0.8	3.6	0.4	62
1950	1.1	6.8	1.0	119
1955	2.2	13.6	1.7	170
1960	3.2	22.5	2.9	183
1965	3.0	25.3	3.8	147
1966	3.2	26.1	4.1	151
1967	3.6	27.6	4.5	158
1968	3.8	29.3	4.9	164
1969	4.0	29.3	5.0	152
1970	4.1	30.2	5.5	163
1971	4.4	30.1	6.2	163
1972	4.6	30.6	6.6	157
1973	4.6	33.4	7.0	155
1974	5.0	35.2	7.1	163
1975	5.0	35.3	6.4	161
1976	4.5	34.7	4.9	150
State farms and other state enterprises Sowchosen und andere staatliche Unternehmen Sovchozy i drugie gosudarstvennye chozjajstva					
1940	0.4	1.9	0.2	19
1945	0.2	1.1	0.1	13
1950	0.5	2.1	0.3	22
1955	0.8	3.4	0.6	37
1960	1.9	10.1	2.4	96
1965	3.0	18.6	5.7	137
1966	3.1	19.7	6.7	144
1967	3.4	21.2	8.1	157
1968	3.4	21.7	9.6	168
1969	3.6	21.9	11.3	155
1970	3.9	23.0	13.5	174
1971	4.3	23.8	16.2	180
1972	4.5	24.2	18.9	176
1973	4.5	26.0	22.1	188
1974	5.0	27.5	25.4	206
1975	5.3	27.6	28.4	212
1976	4.8	27.5	30.2	196

5.2.46.10 BASIC LIVESTOCK PRODUCTS BY UNION REPUBLICS (in all agricultural enterprises; annual average)
GRUNDERZEUGNISSE DER VIEHWIRTSCHAFT NACH UNIONSREPUBLIKEN (in allen landwirtschaftl.Betrieben; Jahresdurchschnitt)
OSNOVNYE PRODUKTY ŽIVOTNOVODSTVA PO SOJUZNYM RESPUBLIKAM (vo vsech kategorijach chozjajstv; v srednem za god)

	Meat (slaughter weight),'000 tons Fleisch (Schlachtgewicht), Tsd.t Mjaso (v ubojnom vese), tys.t			Milk, '000 tons Milch, Tsd.t Moloko, tys.t			Eggs, mill.pcs. Eier, Mio Stck. Jajca, mln.št.			Wool, '000 tons Wolle, Tsd.t Šerst', tys.t		
	1961–1965	1966–1970	1971–1975	1961–1965	1966–1970	1971–1975	1961–1965	1966–1970	1971–1975	1961–1965	1966–1970	1971–1975
SSSR	9,320	11,583	14,004	64,714	80,553	87,446	28,737	35,840	51,427	361.6	397.8	442.1
RSFSR	4,839	5,949	7,108	36,177	44,541	46,710	16,450	20,757	29,942	177.1	194.6	218.7
Ukrainskaja SSR	2,177	2,677	3,280	14,525	17,937	20,360	7,237	8,293	11,215	24.5	24.2	26.6
Belorusskaja SSR	454	642	789	3,538	4,907	5,720	997	1,437	2,289	1.8	1.3	1.2
Uzbekskaja SSR	155	188	240	843	1,169	1,610	530	704	1,128	22.0	21.9	23.3
Kazachskaja SSR	675	815	987	2,930	3,812	4,059	972	1,383	2,430	76.9	90.4	101.0
Gruzinskaja SSR	92	100	123	461	498	527	274	346	479	4.5	5.0	5.1
Azerbajdžanskaja SSR	80	86	104	397	465	575	306	362	496	8.3	7.9	8.7
Litovskaja SSR	232	357	429	1,821	2,385	2,586	478	641	795	0.9	0.4	0.3
Moldavskaja SSR	130	173	212	606	752	913	379	527	618	3.3	3.3	2.7
Latvijskaja SSR	151	192	237	1,449	1,745	1,737	360	433	619	1.0	0.8	0.7
Kirgizskaja SSR	99	123	145	436	522	591	186	230	326	18.8	25.1	30.2
Tadžikskaja SSR	48	57	75	213	270	346	88	110	192	4.5	4.9	5.0
Armjanskaja SSR	39	48	62	327	363	403	183	212	306	3.9	4.0	4.4
Turkmenskaja SSR	49	50	64	142	178	218	67	105	160	13.5	13.6	13.8
Estonskaja SSR	100	126	149	849	1,009	1,091	230	300	432	0.6	0.4	0.4

5.2.46.11 Economy
5.2.46.12 Wirtschaft

5.2.46.11 MEAT PRODUCTION BY UNION REPUBLICS (slaughter weight)[1]
FLEISCHERZEUGUNG NACH UNIONSREPUBLIKEN (Schlachtgewicht)[1]
PROIZVODSTVO MJASA PO SOJUZNYM RESPUBLIKAM (v ubojnom vese)[1]

	1940	1965	1970	1971	1972	1973	1974	1975	1976	1977
SSSR	4,695	9,956	12,278	13,272	13,633	13,527	14,620	14,968	13,395	14,800
RSFSR	2,373	5,203	6,213	6,836	6,970	6,763	7,421	7,548	6,700	7,400
Ukrainskaja SSR	1,127	2,221	2,850	3,035	3,199	3,213	3,438	3,516	3,100	3,500
Belorusskaja SSR	275	508	685	734	765	789	815	842	825	895
Uzbekskaja SSR	84	162	208	223	225	236	250	268	263	268
Kazachskaja SSR	224	768	916	927	923	976	1,032	1,075	893	975
Gruzinskaja SSR	75	93	104	112	117	122	127	136	141	136
Azerbajdžanskaja SSR	41	70	94	96	97	104	110	115	115	119
Litovskaja SSR	134	267	390	432	429	410	437	438	439	472
Moldavskaja SSR	51	140	176	190	200	214	229	230	228	245
Latvijskaja SSR	123	160	205	222	241	222	244	255	254	266
Kirgizskaja SSR	41	116	134	137	135	145	150	157	248	260
Tadžikskaja SSR	30	51	64	68	71	73	78	84	86	89
Armjanskaja SSR	23	40	52	54	59	63	68	67	69	73
Turkmenskaja SSR	22	50	51	62	55	60	65	75	63	79
Estonskaja SSR	72	107	136	144	147	137	156	162	173	182

5.2.46.12 MILK PRODUCTION BY UNION REPUBLICS[1]
MILCHERZEUGUNG NACH UNIONSREPUBLIKEN[1]
PROIZVODSTVO MOLOKA PO SOJUZNYM RESPUBLIKAM[1]

	1940	1965	1970	1971	1972	1973	1974	1975	1976	1977
SSSR	33,640	72,563	83,016	83,183	83,181	88,300	91,760	90,804	89,158	94,800
RSFSR	17,832	40,149	45,371	45,228	44,310	47,015	48,930	48,066	46,800	49,800
Ukrainskaja SSR	7,114	16,629	18,712	18,947	19,339	20,718	21,511	21,287	21,200	22,200
Belorusskaja SSR	2,005	4,124	5,264	5,168	5,467	5,813	6,044	6,109	6,087	6,534
Uzbekskaja SSR	461	923	1,333	1,453	1,543	1,638	1,709	1,708	1,857	1,842
Kazachskaja SSR	1,089	3,328	3,932	3,900	3,943	4,192	4,218	4,045	4,055	4,331
Gruzinskaja SSR	358	471	518	530	487	509	532	575	578	612
Azerbajdžanskaja SSR	275	408	478	486	502	604	625	658	666	701
Litovskaja SSR	1,383	2,042	2,490	2,459	2,527	2,578	2,661	2,703	2,750	2,817
Moldavskaja SSR	182	676	792	802	818	931	978	1,035	1,042	1,070
Latvijskaja SSR	1,537	1,654	1,713	1,718	1,703	1,686	1,792	1,787	1,806	1,880
Kirgizskaja SSR	210	481	548	562	573	599	608	611	616	632
Tadžikskaja SSR	135	230	285	305	322	347	372	383	408	418
Armjanskaja SSR	170	338	363	388	406	401	409	411	439	463
Turkmenskaja SSR	107	155	192	195	197	218	237	245	218	256
Estonskaja SSR	782	955	1,025	1,042	1,044	1,051	1,134	1,181	1,202	1,217

1 in all agricultural enterprises; '000 tons - in allen landwirtschaftlichen Betrieben; Tsd.t - vo vsech kategorijach chozjajstv; tys.t

5.2.46.13   EGG PRODUCTION BY UNION REPUBLICS (mill.pcs.)[1]
            EIERPRODUKTION NACH UNIONSREPUBLIKEN (Mio Stck.)[1]
            PROIZVODSTVO JAIC PO SOJUZNYM RESPUBLIKAM (mln.št.)[1]

	1940	1965	1970	1971	1972	1973	1974	1975	1976	1977
SSSR	12,214	29,068	40,740	45,100	47,910	51,154	55,509	57,463	55,626	61,000
RSFSR	6,577	16,794	23,594	26,350	27,993	29,654	32,343	33,371	32,500	35,400
Ukrainskaja SSR	3,272	6,941	9,202	9,858	10,464	11,266	12,059	12,429	12,000	13,100
Belorusskaja SSR	612	1,106	1,669	1,867	2,067	2,289	2,528	2,694	2,544	2,741
Uzbekskaja SSR	139	558	860	990	1,031	1,122	1,247	1,247	1,238	1,227
Kazachskaja SSR	307	1,052	1,708	2,013	2,200	2,413	2,691	2,835	2,913	3,144
Gruzinskaja SSR	251	305	397	422	429	494	516	537	558	577
Azerbajdžanskaja SSR	158	290	413	429	447	498	528	578	573	642
Litovskaja SSR	187	541	701	768	761	776	827	844	838	909
Moldavskaja SSR	235	369	578	601	594	608	613	672	682	777
Latvijskaja SSR	174	346	500	566	614	619	636	662	637	700
Kirgizskaja SSR	47	190	268	297	300	325	347	361	394	408
Tadžikskaja SSR	38	85	131	157	166	190	210	236	261	284
Armjanskaja SSR	46	193	238	251	273	312	340	353	371	391
Turkmenskaja SSR	37	80	122	145	136	151	174	194	160	224
Estonskaja SSR	134	218	359	386	435	437	450	450	444	461

5.2.46.14   WOOL PRODUCTION BY UNION REPUBLICS ('000 tons)[1]
            ERZEUGUNG VON WOLLE NACH UNIONSREPUBLIKEN (Tsd.t)[1]
            PROIZVODSTVO ŠERSTI PO SOJUZNYM RESPUBLIKAM (tys.t)[1]

	1940	1965	1970	1971	1972	1973	1974	1975	1976	1977
SSSR	161.1	356.9	418.9	428.8	420.1	433.3	461.6	466.6	432.8	458.0
RSFSR	98.0	172.0	209.1	218.5	213.0	208.4	226.9	226.6	208.0	226.0
Ukrainskaja SSR	13.4	22.1	24.9	25.1	25.6	25.9	27.6	28.8	24.9	29.6
Belorusskaja SSR	3.3	1.4	1.2	1.2	1.2	1.2	1.2	1.0	1.0	1.1
Uzbekskaja SSR	7.1	21.4	22.0	21.9	21.0	23.4	24.6	25.4	25.0	24.1
Kazachskaja SSR	13.4	80.0	95.0	94.1	93.0	101.5	107.1	109.6	102.1	102.8
Gruzinskaja SSR	3.5	4.5	4.7	5.1	4.7	5.2	5.2	5.5	5.3	5.1
Azerbajdžanskaja SSR	4.2	6.7	7.6	7.6	7.9	9.2	9.2	9.5	9.9	10.0
Litovskaja SSR	1.6	0.6	0.4	0.4	0.3	0.3	0.3	0.2	--	--
Moldavskaja SSR	2.2	3.2	3.1	2.8	2.7	2.6	2.6	2.6	2.4	2.4
Latvijskaja SSR	2.3	0.8	0.7	0.7	0.8	0.7	0.7	0.6	--	--
Kirgizskaja SSR	3.3	22.7	27.1	28.3	28.5	30.9	31.2	32.1	31.3	31.6
Tadžikskaja SSR	1.6	4.3	4.9	4.8	4.7	5.0	5.1	5.3	--	--
Armjanskaja SSR	1.5	3.9	3.9	4.2	4.1	4.6	4.5	4.9	4.6	4.5
Turkmenskaja SSR	4.9	12.8	14.0	13.7	12.1	14.0	15.0	14.1	13.8	15.0
Estonskaja SSR	0.8	0.5	0.3	0.4	0.5	0.4	0.4	0.4	--	--

1 in all agricultural enterprises - in allen landwirtschaftlichen Betrieben - vo vsech kategorijach chozjajstv

5.2.47.1 Economy
Wirtschaft

5.2.47 COLLECTIVE FARMS - KOLCHOSEN - KOLCHOZY

5.2.47.1 BASIC INDICATORS OF COLLECTIVE FARM DEVELOPMENT - HAUPTKENNZIFFERN DER ENTWICKLUNG DER KOLCHOSEN - OSNOVNYE POKAZATELI RAZVITIJA KOLCHOZOV

	1965	1970	1971	1972	1973	1974	1975	1976
Total number of collective farms (end-of-year figures), '000 - Gesamtzahl der Kolchosen (zum Jahresende), Tsd. - Čislo vsech kolchozov (na konec goda), tys.	36.9	33.6	32.8	32.1	31.4	30.0	29.0	27.7
of which (without fishing co-operatives) - darunter (ohne Fischfangkolchosen) - v tom čisle bez rybolovectkich	36.3	33.0	32.3	31.6	30.9	29.6	28.5	27.3
number of households at collective farms, mill. - darin vorhandene Kolchosbauernhöfe, Mio - v nich naličnych kolchoznych dvorov, mln.	15.4	14.4	14.1	14.0	13.9	13.7	13.5	13.3
Average annual number of persons engaged at the collective farms[1], mill. - Jahresdurchschnittszahl aller an der Arbeit in Kolchosen beteiligten Kolchosbauern[1], Mio - Srednegodovaja čislennost' vsech kolchoznikov, prinimavšich učastie v rabotach kolchozov[1], mln.	18.6	16.7	16.3	16.1	15.9	15.7	15.2	14.8
Gross agricultural production (compared to prices of 1965), '000 mill.rubles - Bruttoproduktion der Landwirtschaft (in Vergleichspreisen von 1965), Mrd.Rubel - Valovaja produkcija sel'skogo chozjajstva (v sopostavimych cenach 1965 g.), mlrd.rub.	29.0	34.6	34.5	32.9	39.0	37.9	33.6	--
Non-distributable assets of collective farms[1] in fixed and circulating means (end-of-year figures), '000 mill.rubles - Unteilbare Fonds der Kolchosen[1] in Grund-u.Umlaufmitteln (zum Jahresende), Mrd.Rubel - Nedelimye fondy kolchozov[1] v osnovnych i oborotnych sredstvach (na konec goda), mlrd.rub.	42.3	60.0	64.2	69.2	79.4	85.0	91.7	95.4

[1] without fishing co-operatives - ohne Fischfangkolchosen - bez rybolovectkich

Economy 5.2.47.1
Wirtschaft

	1965	1970	1971	1972	1973	1974	1975	1976
Gross income of collective farms[1] in prices of corresponding years, '000 mill.rubles - Bruttoeinkommen der Kolchosen[1] in Preisen des jeweiligen Jahres, Mrd.Rubel - Valovoj dochod kolchozov[1] v cenach sootvetstvujuščich let, mlrd.rub.	17.9	22.8	22.8	22.1	24.3	24.1	22.3	23.1
Payments in cash and kind for collective farmers' work, '000 mill.rubles - Arbeitsentgelt der Kolchosbauern in bar und Waren, Mrd.Rubel - Vydano v oplatu truda kolchoznikam deneg i produktov,mlrd.rub.	11.5	15.0	15.3	15.6	16.6	17.1	16.7	17.5
per one working day, rubles - umgerechnet auf 1 Arbeitstag, Rubel - v rasčete na 1 otrabotannyj čeloveko-den', rub.	2.68	3.90	4.03	4.11	4.38	4.50	4.54	4.77
Mutually-owned crops sown, mill.hectares - Gesamte genossenschaftl.Anbaufläche, Mio ha - Ploščad'vsech obščestvennych posevov, mln.ga	105.1	99.1	96.9	97.6	98.6	98.4	98.2	98.2
of which - darunter - v tom čisle:								
grain crops - Getreidekulturen - zernovych kul'tur	62.6	55.8	54.0	54.5	57.0	56.6	56.6	56.2
industrial crops-techn.Kulturen-techničeskich kul'tur	11.7	10.6	10.3	10.3	10.6	10.6	10.1	10.5
potatoes, vegetables and melons - Kartoffel-,Gemüseund Melonenkulturen - kartofelja i ovošče-bachčevych kul'tur	3.2	2.8	2.7	2.8	2.8	2.8	2.7	2.6
fodder crops - Futterpflanzen - kormovych kul'tur	27.6	29.9	29.9	30.0	28.2	28.4	28.8	28.9
Productive mutually-owned livestock (end-of-year figures), mill.head - Genossenschaftlicher Nutzviehbestand (zum Jahresende), Mio Stck. - Pogolov'e obščestvennogo produktivnogo skota (na konec goda), mln.golov:								
cattle - Rinder - krupnyj rogatyj skot	38.3	41.7	43.2	44.1	44.9	46.3	48.2	47.0
of which cows-darunter Kühe-v tom čisle korovy	13.2	13.5	13.7	14.2	14.7	15.1	15.3	15.5
Pigs - Schweine - svin'i	24.6	29.6	31.9	30.7	32.1	33.1	25.7	26.2
Sheep - Schafe - ovcy	53.9	53.5	53.9	52.6	52.8	52.9	51.5	49.9
Goats - Ziegen - kozy	0.7	0.6	0.6	0.6	0.6	0.6	0.6	0.4

[1] without fishing co-operatives - ohne Fischfangkolchosen - bez ryboloveckich

5.2.47.1 Economy / Wirtschaft

	1965	1970	1971	1972	1973	1974	1975	1976
Tractors (end-of-year figures) – Traktoren (zum Jahresende) – Číslo traktorov (na konec goda): '000 – Tsd.Stck. – tys.št.	756	942	965	1,001	1,029	1,049	1,064	1,071
aggregate capacity of tractor engines, mill.hp – summarische Motorleistung, Mill. PS – summarnaja moščnost' dvigatelej, mln.L.S.	34.8	50.3	52.6	55.8	59.5	63.6	66.1	69.3
Number of grain harvesters (end-of-year figures), '000 – Anzahl der Mähdrescher (zum Jahresende), Tsd.Stck. – Číslo zernouboročnych kombajnov(na konec goda), tys.št.	224	292	295	297	294	299	298	296
Lorries (end-of-year figures) – Lastkraftwagen (zum Jahresende) – Číslo gruzovych avtomobilej(na konec goda): '000 – Tsd.Stck. – tys.št.	426	479	478	494	505	513	520	516
Load capacity, '000 tons – Summarische Ladefähigkeit, Tsd. t – summarnaja gruzopod'emnost', tys.t	1,127	1,279	1,299	1,348	1,379	1,398	1,446	1,465
Average per collective farm – Durchschnittliche Größe der Kolchose – Prichoditsja v srednem na odin kolchoz								
Collective-farm households (end-of-year figures) – Kolchosbauernhöfe (zum Jahresende) – Kolchoznych dvorov (na konec goda)	426	435	439	443	449	463	473	
Agricultural area, '000 hectares – landwirtschaftliche Nutzfläche, Tsd.ha – sel'skochozjajstvennych ugodij,tys.ga	6.1	6.1	6.2	6.2	6.2	6.3	6.4	
Arable land, '000 hectares – Ackerland, Tsd.ha – Pašin, tys.ga	3.1	3.2	3.2	3.2	3.3	3.4	3.6	
Tractors, pc. – Traktoren, Stck. – Traktorov, štuk	21	29	30	32	33	35	37	
Mutually-owned crops sown, '000 hectares – Genossenschaftliche Anbaufläche, Tsd.ha – Obščestvennych posevov, tys.ga	2.9	3.0	3.0	3.1	3.2	3.3	3.4	
Mutually-owned livestock (end-of-year figures), head – Genossenschaftlicher Nutzviehbestand (zum Jahresende),Stck.– Obščestvennogo skota (na konec goda), golov:								
cattle – Rinder – krupnogo rogatogo skota	1,056	1,258	1,332	1,388	1,447	1,556	1,664	
of which cows–darunter Kühe–v tom čisle korov	363	409	426	450	475	508	535	

	1965	1970	1971	1972	1973	1974	1975
Pigs - Schweine - sviny	667	891	983	964	1,022	1,089	844
Sheep and goats - Schafe und Ziegen - ovec i koz	1,506	1,633	1,684	1,680	1,724	1,801	1,813
Non-distributable fixed and circulating assets, '000 rubles - Unteilbare Fonds in Grund-u.Umlaufmitteln, Tsd.Rub. - Nedelimych fondov v osnovnych i oborotnych sredstvach, tys.rub.	1,166	1,815	1,991	2,190	2,569	2,875	3,216
Gross income, '000 rubles - Bruttoeinkommen, Tsd.Rub. - Valovogo dochoda, tys.rub.	494	689	705	700	788	816	781

5.2.47.2 BREAKDOWN OF COLLECTIVE FARMS BY AMOUNT OF GROSS INCOME PER 100 HECTARES' ARABLE LAND (in percent)
GLIEDERUNG DER KOLCHOSEN NACH HÖHE DES BRUTTOEINKOMMENS PRO 100 HA ACKERLAND (in Prozent)
GRUPPIROVKA KOLCHOZOV PO RAZMERU VALOVOGO DOCHODA NA 100 GA PAŠIN (v procentach)

	1965	1970	1971	1972	1973	1975	1976
Total collective farms - alle Kolchosen - vsego kolchozov	100	100	100	100	100	100	100
of which collective farms with gross income per 100 ha arable land - davon Kolchosen mit Bruttoeinkommen umgerechnet auf 100 ha Ackerland - iz nich kolchozov, imejuščich valovoj dochod v rasčete na 100 ga pašin:							
- 1,000 Rub.	1.1	0.7	0.7	0.7	0.3	1.0	1.0
1,000 - 5,000 Rub.	8.3	2.8	3.0	3.2	1.9	5.2	4.2
5,000 - 10,000 Rub.	19.4	10.6	12.6	11.4	9.8	12.3	12.9
10,000 - 15,000 Rub.	17.7	15.0	14.4	13.2	13.5	12.4	13.5
15,000 - 20,000 Rub.	16.6	15.4	13.6	12.8	12.9	11.9	12.0
20,000 - 30,000 Rub.	} 36.9	23.8	21.9	19.6	23.2	19.4	19.3
30,000 - 40,000 Rub.		12.4	12.8	12.4	14.1	12.2	12.7
40,000 Rub.and more-und mehr-svyše		19.3	21.0	26.7	24.3	25.6	24.4

5.2.47.3 Economy / Wirtschaft

5.2.47.3 BREAKDOWN OF COLLECTIVE FARMS BY NUMBER OF HOUSEHOLDS (in percent)
GLIEDERUNG DER KOLCHOSEN NACH ANZAHL DER HÖFE (in Prozent)
GRUPPIROVKA KOLCHOZOV PO ČISLU DVOROV (v procentach)

	1940	1965	1970	1971	1972	1973	1975	1976
Total collective farms – alle Kolchosen – vsego kolchozov	100	100	100	100	100	100	100	100
of which collective farms with households – davon Kolchosen mit Kolchoshöfen – iz nich kolchozov, imejuščich kolchoznych dvorov:								
– 100	73.7	4.3	3.0	2.7	2.8	2.7	2.3	2.3
101 – 200	19.1	18.4	17.8	17.0	16.4	15.9	13.7	12.6
201 – 300	4.9	19.5	19.8	20.0	20.0	20.3	19.7	19.2
301 – 500	2.0	28.1	29.0	29.4	29.4	29.7	30.3	30.4
501 and more – und mehr – svyše	0.3	29.7	30.4	30.9	31.4	31.4	34.0	35.5

5.2.47.4   BREAKDOWN OF COLLECTIVE FARMS BY LIVESTOCK (in percent)
           GLIEDERUNG DER KOLCHOSEN NACH VIEHBESTAND (in Prozent)
           GRUPPIROVKA KOLCHOZOV PO POGOLOVJU SKOTA (v procentach)
           (end-of-year figures - zum Jahresende - na konec goda)

	1965	1976
Beef cattle - Rindvieh - Krupnyj rogatyj skot		
Collective farms with beef cattle - Kolchosen mit Rindviehbestand - Kolchozy imejuščie krupnyj rogatyj skot	99.8	99.6
Head - Stück - golov:		
- 600	34.2	9.8
600 - 999	27.3	16.1
1,000 - 3,000	35.1	62.9
over-über-svyše 3,000	3.2	10.8
Cows - Kühe - Korovy		
Collective farms with cows - Kolchosen mit Kühebestand - Kolchozy imejuščie korov	99.8	98.5
Head - Stück - golov:		
- 300	47.9	20.6
300 - 499	28.4	26.4
500 - 1,000	19.9	40.9
over-über-svyše 1,000	3.6	10.6
Pigs - Schweine - Svini		
Collective farms with pigs - Kolchosen mit Schweinebestand - Kolchozy imejuščie svinej	83.9	65.4
Head - Stück - golov:		
- 500	39.2	19.9
500 - 999	23.1	13.6
1,000 - 3,000	19.8	25.5
over-über-svyše 3,000	1.8	6.4
Sheep and goats - Schafe und Ziegen - Ovcy i kozy		
Collective farms with sheep and goats - Kolchosen mit Schaf- und Ziegenbestand - Kolchozy imejuščie ovec i koz	73.8	53.3
Head - Stück - golov:		
- 500	30.8	11.4
500 - 999	17.8	12.2
1,000 - 2,999	15.9	16.6
3,000 - 9,999	6.2	8.5
10,000 - 20,000	1.6	2.6
over-über-svyše 20,000	1.5	2.0

5.2.47.5 BASIC INDICATORS OF COLLECTIVE FARM DEVELOP
HAUPTKENNZIFFERN DER ENTWICKLUNG DER KOLCHO
OSNOVNYE POKAZATELI RAZVITIJA KOLCHOZOV PO

	All collective farms (end-of-year figures) Alle Kolchosen (zum Jahresende) Čislo vsech kolchozov (na konec goda)	of which (without fishing cooperatives) darunter (ohne Fischfangkolchosen) v tom čisle bez rybolovečkich	Collective farm households[1], '000 Kolchosbauernhöfe in den Kolchosen[1], Tsd. Čislo naličnych kolchoznych dvorov v kolchozach[1], tys.	Non-distributable assets of collective farms[1] in fixed and circulating means (end-of-year) '000 rubles Unteilbare Fonds d. Kolchosen[1] in Grundu. Umlaufmitteln (zum Jahresende, Tsd. Rub. Nedelimye fondy kolchozov[1] v osnovnych i oborotnych sredstva (na konec goda), mln. rub.
SSSR	28,953	28,515	13,496	91,704
RSFSR	12,871	12,579	4,766	37,647
Ukrainskaja SSR	7,688	7,603	4,791	28,297
Belorusskaja SSR	2,070	2,070	804	5,152
Uzbekskaja SSR	953	948	802	3,663
Kazachskaja SSR	422	404	201	2,044
Gruzinskaja SSR	877	872	327	1,142
Azerbajdžanskaja SSR	873	867	252	776
Litovskaja SSR	967	966	247	3,268
Moldavskaja SSR	467	467	471	2,644
Latvijskaja SSR	403	392	128	1,822
Kirgizskaja SSR	216	216	169	1,322
Tadžikskaja SSR	242	242	216	1,213
Armjanskaja SSR	371	371	88	380
Turkmenskaja SSR	334	330	175	1,353
Estonskaja SSR	199	188	59	981

1 without fishing cooperatives - ohne Fischfangkolchosen - bez rybolovečkich

Economy 5.2.47.5
Wirtschaft

MENT BY UNION REPUBLICS, 1975
SEN NACH UNIONSREPUBLIKEN, 1975
SOJUZNYM RESPUBLIKAM V 1975 G.

Gross income of collective farms[1] (mill.Rubles) Bruttoeinkommen der Kolchosen[1] (Mio Rubel) Valovoj dochod kolchozov[1] (mln.rub.)	Mutually-owned sowing area of all crops, '000 ha Genossenschaftliche Anbaufläche aller Kulturen,Tsd.ha Ploščad'obščestvennych posevov vsech kul'tur, tys.ga	of which- darunter- grain crops Getreidekulturen zernovych kul'tur	Mutually-owned productive livestock (end-of-year figures), '000 head Genossenschaftlicher Nutzviehbestand (zum Jahresende), Tsd.Stck. Pogolov'e obščestvennogo produktivnogo skota (na konec goda),tys.golov			
			Cattle Rinder krupnyj rogatyj skot	cows Kühe korovy	Pigs Schweine svin'i	Sheep and goats Schafe und Ziegen ovcy i kozy
22,280	98,231	56,552	48,167	15,323	25,729	52,151
7,622	57,374	36,152	22,988	7,546	10,510	25,091
6,735	24,016	12,366	15,431	4,741	9,742	6,580
1,281	3,529	1,635	3,317	1,084	1,622	319
1,791	1,694	278	835	208	57	1,435
380	4,296	3,010	936	250	183	5,553
380	355	187	389	103	165	870
430	848	395	499	129	49	1,895
648	1,445	671	1,001	356	1,160	9
815	1,353	680	670	221	1,100	472
302	871	373	588	228	526	38
389	693	306	396	119	74	5,621
465	436	120	330	81	33	1,142
143	180	84	210	70	45	603
688	719	101	247	62	104	2,520
211	422	194	330	125	359	3

5.2.48.1 Economy / Wirtschaft

5.2.48 STATE FARMS — SOWCHOSEN — SOVCHOZY

5.2.48.1
NUMBER OF STATE FARMS (END-OF-YEAR FIGURES) — ANZAHL DER SOWCHOSEN (ZUM JAHRESENDE) — ČISLO SOVCHOZOV (NA KONEC GODA)

	1965	1970	1971	1972	1973	1974	1975	1976
Number of state farms — Anzahl der Sowchosen — Čislo sovchozov	11,681	14,994	15,502	15,747	17,300	17,717	18,064	19,617
of which — darunter — v tom čisle:								
grain crops (incl. seed-growing) — Getreidesowchosen (einschl.Saatzuchtsowchosen) — zernovye (vključaja semenovodčeskie)	1,261	1,467	1,502	1,519	1,526	1,579	1,510	1,494
beet state farms — Rübensowchosen — sveklovičnye	320	283	292	294	291	282	314	313
cotton state farms — Baumwollsowchosen — chlopkovye	156	212	223	235	244	300	309	322
other state farms for special crops (essential oils, tobacco, tea) — andere Sowchosen für spezielle Kulturen (ätherische Öle, Tabak, Tee) — cial'nych kul'tur (efirnomasličnye, tabačnye, čajnye)	119	128	150	152	160	158	152	147
state farms for fruit and grapes, fruit and vegetables, and potatoes-vegetables — Obst-u.Weintrauben-, Obst-Gemüse- und Kartoffel-Gemüsesowchosen — plodovo-vinogradnye, plodovo-ovoščnye i kartofele-ovoščnye	1,668	2,368	2,519	2,577	2,602	2,643	2,878	3,094
Dairy and meat-dairy state farms — Milch-u.Fleisch-Milch-Sowchosen — moločnye i mjasomoločnye	4,633	6,210	6,528	6,571	6,672	6,814	6,815	6,892
Pig-breeding state farms — Schweinezucht-Sowchosen — svinovodčeskie	636	853	842	873	875	952	972	992
Sheep-breeding state farms (incl. Karakul sheep-breeding) — Schafzucht-Sowchosen(einschl.Karakulschafzucht) — ovcevodčeskie (vključaja karakulevodčeskie)	1,008	1,189	1,226	1,250	1,298	1,385	1,506	1,542
Horse-breeding state farms — Pferdezucht-Sowchosen — konevodčeskie	74	94	95	97	97	94	93	99

	1965	1970	1971	1972	1973	1974	1975	1976
Deer-breeding state farms – Hirschzucht-Sowchosen – olenevodčeskie	61	95	99	92	92	108	123	129
Fur state farms – Pelztierzucht-Sowchosen – zverovodčeskie	102	139	141	147	148	135	125	128
Poultry state farms – Geflügelzucht-Sowchosen – pticevodčeskie	716	1,006	1,054	1,083	1,113	1,128	1,104	1,145

5.2.48.2 BASIC INDICATORS ON STATE FARM DEVELOPMENT – GRUNDKENNZIFFERN DER ENTWICKLUNG DER SOWCHOSEN – OSNOVNYE POKAZATELI RAZVITIJA SOVCHOZOV

	1965	1970	1971	1972	1973	1974	1975	1976
Number of state farms (end-of-year figures) – Anzahl der Sowchosen (zum Jahresende) – Čislo sovchozov (na konec. goda)	11,681	14,994	15,502	15,747	17,300	17,717	18,064	19,617
Average annual number of persons engaged in all branches of production, thousands – Jahresdurchschnittszahl der in allen Bereichen Beschäftigten, Tsd. – Srednegodovaja čislennost'rabotnikov,zanjatych vo vsech otrasljach chozjajstva sovchozov, tys.čelovek	8,230	8,888	9,212	9,328	9,830	10,107	10,260	10,960
of whom in agriculture – darunter in der Landwirtschaft – v tom čisle v sel'skom chozjajstve	7,350	7,688	7,951	8,040	8,544	8,728	8,825	9,392
workers – Arbeiter – iz nich rabočich	6,882	7,040	7,287	7,354	7,783	7,931	7,991	8,485
Gross agricultural output (in prices compared to 1965), '000 mill.rubles – Bruttoproduktion der Landwirtschaft (in Vergleichspreisen zu 1965),Mrd.Rub. – Valovaja produkcija sel'skogo chozjajstva (v sopostavimych cenach 1965 g.), mlrd.rub.	16.9	24.3	25.0	24.8	29.8	30.1	28.6	--
Wages of state farm workers, rubles – Arbeitslohn der Sowchosarbeiter, Rubel – Zarabotnaja plata rabotnikov sovchozov, rub.: average monthly wages – durchschnittl.Monatslohn – srednemesjačnaja	74.6	101.1	106.6	112.1	117.9	124.7	127.3	135.0
converted to one worker's day – umgerechnet auf 1 Arbeitskräftetag – v rasčete na 1 otrabotannyj čelověko-děn'	3.21	4.43	4.65	4.89	5.13	5.42	5.51	5.83

5.2.48.2 Economy / Wirtschaft

	1965	1970	1971	1972	1973	1974	1975	1976
Total sowing area, '000 hectares – Gesamte Anbaufläche, Tsd.ha – Vsja posevnaja ploščad', tys.ga	89,062	91,749	94,417	96,561	103,973	105,844	107,240	111,431
of which – darunter – v tom čisle: grain crops – Getreidekulturen – zernovye kul'tury	59,643	57,383	57,886	59,345	65,636	66,597	67,367	69,486
industrial crops – techn.Kulturen-techničeskie kul't.	3,391	3,535	3,644	3,684	3,777	3,807	3,697	3,944
Potatoes and vegetable-melon crops – Kartoffeln und Gemüse-Melonenkulturen – kartofel' i ovošče-bachčevye kul'tury	1,925	1,838	1,879	1,977	2,121	2,154	2,169	2,309
Fodder crops – Futterkulturen – kormovye kul'tury	24,103	28,993	31,008	31,555	32,439	33,286	34,007	35,692
Livestock (end-of-year figures), '000 head – Viehbestand (zum Jahresende), Tsd.Stck. – Pogolov'e skota (na konec goda), tys.golov:								
Cattle – Rinder – krupnyj rogatyj skot	24,501	29,073	30,658	31,435	33,288	34,605	35,588	37,049
of which cows – darunter Kühe – v tom čisle korovy	8,918	10,005	10,374	10,739	11,482	11,874	12,096	12,784
Pigs – Schweine – sviny	12,535	16,603	18,607	17,991	19,447	20,494	16,151	19,700
Sheep and goats – Schafe u.Ziegen – ovcy i kozy	46,431	53,485	55,634	56,477	60,223	63,089	63,058	64,453
of which sheep – darunter Schafe – v tom čisle ovcy	46,207	53,106	55,219	55,989	59,666	62,478	62,398	63,684
Number of tractors (end-of-year figures) – Anzahl der Traktoren (zum Jahresende) – Čislo traktorov (na konec goda): '000 – Tsd.Stck. – tys.št.	681	803	837	865	942	994	1,038	1,125
aggregate capacity of tractor engines, mill.hp – summarische Motorleistung, Mio PS – summarnaja moščnost'dvigatelej, mln.l.s.	33.7	47.4	50.6	53.8	60.7	66.5	70.9	79.2
Number of grain harvesters (end-of-year figures), '000 – Anzahl der Mähdrescher (zum Jahresende), Tsd.Stck. – Čislo zernouboročnych kombajnov (na konec goda),tys.št.	265	294	306	320	338	346	351	369
Number of lorries (end-of-year figures) – Anzahl der Lastkraftwagen (zum Jahresende) – Čislo gruzovych avtomobilej (na konec goda): '000 – Tsd.Stck. – tys.št.	335	381	387	407	430	453	468	509
load capacity, '000 tons – summarische Ladefähigkeit, Tsd.t-summarnaja gruzopod'emnost', tys.t	914	1,069	1,113	1,154	1,258	1,354	1,406	1,562

5.2.48.3 NUMBER OF STATE FARMS BY UNION REPUBLICS (END-OF-YEAR FIGURES)[1]
ANZAHL DER SOWCHOSEN NACH UNIONSREPUBLIKEN (ZUM JAHRESENDE)[1]
ČISLO SOVCHOZOV PO SOJUZNYM RESPUBLIKAM (NA KONEC GODA)[1]

	1965	1970	1971	1972	1973	1974	1975
SSSR	11,681	14,994	15,502	15,747	17,300	17,717	18,064
RSFSR	6,321	8,594	8,897	9,015	10,308	10,502	10,624
Ukrainskaja SSR	1,343	1,605	1,615	1,621	1,635	1,674	1,763
Belorusskaja SSR	630	820	834	835	839	840	830
Uzbekskaja SSR	283	361	392	412	445	537	572
Kazachskaja SSR	1,521	1,625	1,631	1,653	1,783	1,826	1,864
Gruzinskaja SSR	168	231	265	265	269	282	310
Azerbajdžanskaja SSR	285	406	428	428	465	467	496
Litovskaja SSR	316	300	299	293	286	282	270
Moldavskaja SSR	81	145	213	213	239	242	224
Latvijskaja SSR	187	230	230	236	235	233	230
Kirgizskaja SSR	84	103	109	111	121	146	154
Tadžikskaja SSR	55	89	107	115	123	124	147
Armjanskaja SSR	203	261	265	338	340	354	358
Turkmenskaja SSR	47	53	53	53	55	55	56
Estonskaja SSR	157	171	164	159	157	153	166

1 All state farms of the USSR Ministry of Agriculture were completely transferred on full profit and loss account in 1975 -
Seit 1975 arbeiten alle Sowchosen des Ministeriums für Landwirtschaft der UdSSR nach wirtschaftlicher Rechnungsführung -
S.1975 g. vse sovchozy Ministerstva sel'skogo chozjajstva SSSR rabotajut na polnyj chozjajstvennyj rasčet.

5.2.49 STATE PURCHASES OF AGRICULTURAL PRODUCTS
STAATLICHE AUFKÄUFE VON LANDWIRTSCHAFTLICHEN ERZEUGNISSEN
GOSUDARSTVENNYE ZAKUPKI PRODUKTOV SEL'SKOGO CHOZJAJSTVA

5.2.49.1 STATE PURCHASES OF BASIC AGRICULTURAL PRODUCTS FROM THE COLLECTIVE AND STATE FARMS AND OTHER STATE AGRICULTURAL ENTERPRISES (percentage of total)
ANTEIL DER AUFKÄUFE DER LANDWIRTSCHAFTLICHEN GRUNDERZEUGNISSE IN DEN KOLCHOSEN, SOWCHOSEN UND ANDEREN STAATLICHEN BETRIEBEN AN DEN GESAMTEN STAATLICHEN AUFKÄUFEN (in Prozent)
UDEL'NYJ VES ZAKUPOK OSNOVNYCH SEL'SKOCHOZJAJSTVENNYCH PRODUKTOV U KOLCHOZOV, SOVCHOZOV I DRUGICH GOSUDARSTVENNYCH CHOZJAJSTV V OBŠCICH ZAKUPKACH (v procentach)

	1940	1965	1970	1971	1972	1973	1974	1975	1976
Collective and state farms and other state agricultural enterprises – Anteil der Kolchosen, Sowchosen und anderen staatlichen Betriebe – Udel'nyj ves kolchozov, sovchozov i drugich gosudarstvennych chozjajstv
Grain – Getreide – Zernovye kul'tury	97	100	100	100	100	100	100	100	100
Raw cotton – Rohbaumwolle – Chlopok-syrec	100	100	100	100	100	100	100	100	100
Sugar-beet – Zuckerrüben – Sacharnaja svekla	94	100	100	100	100	100	100	100	100
Sunflower seeds – Sonnenblumensamen – Podsolnečnik	95	100	100	100	100	100	100	100	100
Potatoes – Kartoffeln – Kartofel'	61	73	84	87	80	80	82	83	77
Vegetables – Gemüse – Ovošči	98	93	94	94	94	94	94	95	95
Cattle and poultry – Schlachtvieh und Geflügel – Skot i ptica	63	90	89	87	86	87	87	87	89
Milk – Milch – Moloko	66	96	97	96	95	95	95	95	95
Eggs – Eier – Jajca	7	74	89	90	92	93	93	94	96
Wool – Wolle – Šerst'	76	86	86	85	84	84	84	84	83
of which state farms and other agricultural enterprises – darunter Anteil der Sowchosen und anderen staatlichen Betriebe – v tom čisle udel'nyj ves sovchozov i drugich gosudarstvennych chozjajstv
Grain – Getreide – Zernovye kul'tury	10	37	50	49	57	49	44	43	50
Raw cotton – Rohbaumwolle – Chlopok-syrec	6	20	23	24	24	26	27	28	29
Sugar-beet – Zuckerrüben – Sacharnaja svekla	4	9	9	8	8	9	8	10	9
Sunflower seeds – Sonnenblumensamen – Podsolnečnik	2	14	19	20	19	21	19	20	23
Potatoes – Kartoffeln – Kartofel'	2	33	39	39	35	36	36	39	35
Vegetables – Gemüse – Ovošči	6	57	57	56	56	56	57	60	37

	1940	1965	1970	1971	1972	1973	1974	1975	1976
Cattle and poultry - Schlachtvieh und Geflügel - Skot i ptica	22	45	43	43	43	44	44	45	46
Milk - Milch - Moloko	16	41	42	43	42	42	42	42	42
Eggs - Eier - Jajca	3	45	65	66	69	71	73	77	84
Wool - Wolle - Šerst'	18	42	44	45	44	46	47	47	47

5.2.49.2 STATE PURCHASES OF AGRICULTURAL PRODUCTS (IN ALL AGRICULTURAL ENTERPRISES)
STAATLICHE AUFKÄUFE VON LANDWIRTSCHAFTLICHEN ERZEUGNISSEN (IN ALLEN LANDWIRTSCHAFTL.BETRIEBEN)
GOSUDARSTVENNYE ZAKUPKI PRODUKTOV SEL'SKOGO CHOZJAJSTVA (VO VSECH KATEGORIJACH CHOZJAJSTV)

	1940	1965	1970	1971	1972	1973	1974	1975	1976
Agricultural products (crops of the corresponding year) Erzeugnisse des Ackerbaus (Ernte des jeweiligen Jahres) Produkty zemledelija (iz urožaja sootvetstvujuščego goda)									
Grain, mill.tons - Getreide, Mio t - Zernovye kul'tury, mln.t	36.4	36.3	73.3	64.1	60.0	90.5	73.3	50.2	92.1
Raw cotton, mill.tons - Rohbaumwolle, Mio t - Chlopok-syrec, mln.t	2.24	5.66	6.89	7.10	7.30	7.66	8.41	7.86	8.28
Sugar-beet, mill.tons - Zuckerrüben, Mio t - Sacharnaja svekla, mln.t	17.4	67.5	71.4	64.3	68.0	77.8	67.5	61.9	85.3
Oil seeds, '000 tons - Ölsaat, Tsd.t - Semena masličnych kul'tur, tys.t	1,867	4,271	5,220	4,861	3,933	5,994	5,568	4,456	4,197
of which sunflower seeds - davon Sonnenblumensamen - v tom čisle podsolnečnik	1,500	3,888	4,613	4,359	3,753	5,553	5,228	3,841	3,763
Flax fibre, '000 tons - Flachsfaser, Tsd.t - L'novolokno, tys.t	245	433	431	461	439	421	364	478	473
Hemp, '000 tons - Hanf, Tsd.t - Pen'ka, tys.t	44	74	67	69	67	50	55	47	26
Tobacco, '000 tons - Tabak, Tsd.t - Tabak, tys.t	73	169	228	230	275	273	292	287	299
Machorka-tobacco, '000 tons - Machorka-Tabak, Tsd.t - Machorka, tys.t	168	43	30	24	17	26	18	9	12
Potatoes, mill.tons - Kartoffeln, Mio t - Kartofel', mln.t	8.6	9.9	11.2	11.5	11.1	15.4	11.1	14.5	13.6
Vegetables, mill.tons - Gemüse, Mio t - Ovošči, mln.t	3.0	7.7	10.9	11.5	11.2	14.1	14.7	13.9	16.2
Fruit (incl.berries), '000 tons - Obst (einschl. Beeren), Tsd.t - Frukty i jagody, tys.t	596	4,477	6,180	6,351	5,325	7,793	7,933	8,541	9,628

5.2.49.2 Economy / Wirtschaft

	1940	1965	1970	1971	1972	1973	1974	1975	1976
of which - darunter - v tom čisle:									
stone fruit - Kern-und Steinobst - plody semečkovye i kostočkovye	262	1,533	2,900	2,719	3,204	4,149	4,040	4,008	5,112
grapes - Weintrauben - vinograd	306	2,875	3,145	3,544	2,026	3,544	3,722	4,329	4,404
citruses - Zitrusfrüchte - plody citrusovye	23.4	28.6	86.2	33.2	46.1	45.1	114.3	143.0	112.4
Tea, '000 tons - Tee, Tsd.t - čajnyj list, tys.t	52	197	273	280	291	305	330	352	375
Livestock products (per calendar year) Erzeugnisse der Viehwirtschaft (pro Kalenderjahr) Produkty životnovodstva (za kalendarnyj god)									
Cattle and poultry (live weight), mill.tons - Schlachtvieh und Geflügel (Lebendgewicht),Mio t - Skot i ptica (v vese živogo skota i pticy),mln.t	2.2	9.3	12.6	14.2	15.0	14.7	16.2	16.8	14.7
in terms of slaughter weight, mill.tons - umgerechnet auf Schlachtgewicht, Mio t - v peresčete na ubojnyj ves, mln.t	1.3	5.8	8.1	9.2	9.7	9.5	10.5	10.9	9.4
Milk and dairy products (in terms of milk), mill.t - Milch und Milchprodukte (umgerechnet auf Milch), Mio t - Moloko i moločnye produkty (v peresčete na moloko), mln.t	6.5	38.7	45.7	47.1	48.4	53.0	55.8	56.3	56.2
Eggs, '000 mill. - Eier, Mrd.Stck. - Jajca, mlrd.št.	2.7	10.5	18.1	21.6	24.3	27.6	30.9	33.1	32.9
Wool (in weight charged), '000 tons - Wolle (in Anrechnungsgewicht), Tsd.t - Šerst' (v začetnom vese), tys.t	120	368	441	457	452	470	507	511	480
Silk cocoons, '000 tons - Seidenkokons, Tsd.t - Kokony, tys.t	20.5	34.8	33.7	36.7	41.4	39.9	38.7	39.1	45.0

5.2.49.3 STATE PURCHASES OF STAPLE AGRICULTURAL PRODUCTS (IN ALL AGRICULTURAL ENTERPRISES), mill.t
STAATLICHE AUFKÄUFE VON GRUNDERZEUGNISSEN DER LANDWIRTSCHAFT (IN ALLEN LANDWIRTSCHAFTL.BETRIEBEN), Mio t
GOSUDARSTVENNYE ZAKUPKI OSNOVNYCH PRODUKTOV SEL'SKOGO CHOZJAJSTVA (VO VSECH KATEGORIJACH CHOZJAJSTV), mln.t

Year Jahr Gody	Grain Getreide Zerno	Raw cotton Rohbaumwolle Chlopok-syrec	Sugar-beet Zuckerrüben Sacharnaja svekla	Sunflower seeds Sonnenblumensamen Podsolnečnik	Flax fibre, '000 tons Flachsfaser, Tsd.t L'novolokno, tys.t	Potatoes Kartoffeln Kartofel'	Vegetables Gemüse Ovošči	Cattle & poultry (live weight) Schlachtvieh u. Geflügel (Lebendgewicht) Skot i ptica (v vese živogo skota i pticy)	Milk & dairy products (in terms of milk) Milch u.Milchprodukte (umger.auf Milch) Moloko i moločnye produkty (v peresčete na moloko)	Eggs, '000 mill. Eier, Mrd.Stck. Jajca, mrd.št.
	A.	B.	C.	D.	E.	F.	G.	H.	I.	J.
1940	36.4	2.24	17.4	1.5	245.2	8.6	3.0	2.2	6.5	2.7
1945	20.0	1.16	4.7	0.5	64.5	4.5	1.8	1.3	2.9	1.1
1946	17.5	1.64	3.8	0.5	74.6	4.6	1.5	1.4	4.9	1.2
1947	27.5	1.70	12.2	0.8	92.8	5.2	2.1	1.4	5.3	0.7
1948	30.2	2.20	11.8	1.1	162.4	7.2	2.0	1.7	6.7	1.1
1949	32.1	2.53	15.3	1.2	208.5	7.0	1.9	1.8	7.5	1.4
1950	32.3	3.54	19.7	1.1	174.4	6.9	2.0	2.3	8.5	1.9
1951	33.6	3.73	23.4	1.2	159.0	5.2	1.8	2.6	9.4	2.3
1952	34.7	3.78	22.0	1.3	188.7	5.6	1.8	3.2	10.1	2.4
1953	31.1	3.85	22.9	1.8	145.5	5.4	2.5	3.6	10.6	2.6
1954	34.6	4.20	19.5	1.2	192.2	6.6	3.0	4.0	11.3	2.7
1955	36.9	3.88	30.7	2.3	347.1	5.9	3.9	4.2	13.5	2.9
1956	54.1	4.33	31.5	2.4	426.5	9.2	3.8	4.4	17.3	3.3
1957	35.4	4.21	38.5	1.8	386.7	7.9	4.2	5.1	20.5	4.3
1958	56.6	4.34	51.0	2.6	392.1	7.0	4.2	5.7	22.1	4.5
1959	46.6	4.64	41.4	1.9	332.8	6.8	4.5	7.5	25.0	5.7
1960	46.7	4.29	52.2	2.3	369.0	7.1	5.1	7.9	26.3	6.5
1961	52.1	4.52	47.7	2.9	368.6	7.0	5.5	7.3	28.3	7.4
1962	56.6	4.30	43.9	3.1	394.8	5.7	6.2	8.6	29.2	8.5
1963	44.8	5.21	41.5	3.0	368.5	8.0	6.3	9.3	28.5	8.7
1964	68.3	5.28	76.1	3.9	316.8	11.1	7.9	8.3	31.4	8.3
1965	36.3	5.66	67.5	3.9	432.6	9.9	7.7	9.3	38.7	10.5
1966	75.0	5.98	69.7	4.7	426.3	9.3	8.0	10.3	40.1	11.6

5.2.49.3 Economy
5.2.49.4 Wirtschaft

	A.	B.	C.	D.	E.	F.	G.	H.	I.	J.
1967	57.2	5.97	81.6	4.9	446.9	11.7	9.5	11.5	42.5	12.9
1968	69.0	5.95	84.2	4.9	355.5	11.7	9.1	11.9	44.0	14.1
1969	55.5	5.71	65.3	4.3	447.2	10.6	9.6	11.7	43.8	15.4
1970	73.3	6.89	71.4	4.6	431.4	11.2	10.9	12.6	45.7	18.1
1971	64.1	7.10	64.3	4.4	461.3	11.5	11.5	14.2	47.1	21.6
1972	60.0	7.30	68.0	3.8	439.1	11.1	11.2	15.0	48.4	24.3
1973	90.5	7.66	77.8	5.6	420.7	15.4	14.1	14.7	53.0	27.6
1974	73.3	8.41	67.5	5.2	364.1	11.1	14.7	12.2	55.8	30.9
1975	50.2	7.86	61.9	3.8	477.7	14.5	13.9	16.8	56.3	33.1
1976	92.1	--	85.3	3.8	472.9	13.6	16.2	14.7	56.2	32.9

5.2.49.4 STATE PURCHASES OF GRAIN CROPS BY UNION REPUBLICS (IN ALL AGRICULTURAL ENTERPRISES), '000 tons
STAATLICHE AUFKÄUFE AN GETREIDEKULTUREN NACH UNIONSREPUBLIKEN (IN ALLEN LANDWIRTSCHAFTL. BETRIEBEN), Tsd.t
GOSUDARSTVENNYE ZAKUPKI ZERNOVYCH KUL'TUR PO SOJUZNYM RESPUBLIKAM (VO VSECH KATEGORIJACH CHOZJAJSTV), tys.t

	1940	1965	1970	1971	1972	1973	1974	1975	1976
SSSR	36,446	36,331	73,284	64,119	59,971	90,529	73,285	50,213	92,107
RSFSR	24,238	21,848	45,672	36,521	29,503	52,186	42,965	26,231	52,580
Ukrainskaja SSR	9,368	10,343	11,659	12,573	9,237	17,521	16,507	14,013	14,922
Belorusskaja SSR	436	346	521	675	1,003	1,106	1,154	1,501	1,301
Uzbekskaja SSR	238	211	387	255	448	624	545	536	1,024
Kazachskaja SSR	1,282	2,373	13,377	12,306	17,413	16,658	9,868	5,080	19,608
Gruzinskaja SSR	35	72	100	105	140	170	172	204	201
Azerbajdžanskaja SSR	130	131	170	168	231	243	268	271	349
Litovskaja SSR	--	126	186	246	280	249	365	371	345
Moldavskaja SSR	356	546	555	609	915	1,003	651	1,063	824
Latvijskaja SSR	--	125	207	242	255	235	253	331	286
Kirgizskaja SSR	208	63	236	196	293	266	260	300	315
Tadžikskaja SSR	75	40	56	35	67	58	49	59	74
Armjanskaja SSR	40	22	35	43	54	56	46	63	70
Turkmenskaja SSR	40	26	26	34	38	42	46	48	55
Estonskaja SSR	--	59	97	111	94	112	136	142	153

Economy 5.2.49.5
Wirtschaft 5.2.49.6
5.2.49.7

5.2.49.5 STATE PURCHASES OF WHEAT BY UNION REPUBLICS[1]
STAATLICHE AUFKÄUFE AN WEIZEN NACH UNIONSREPUBLIKEN[1]
GOSUDARSTVENNYE ZAKUPKI PŠENICY PO SOJUZNYM RESPUBLIKAM[1]

	1940	1965	1970	1971	1972	1973	1974	1975
SSSR	15,645	21,840	51,046	47,338	42,106	57,995	38,268	29,522
RSFSR	10,268	12,351	31,878	26,360	20,434	29,323	21,232	14,499
Ukrainskaja SSR	3,831	6,843	6,498	9,420	5,236	13,377	8,785	9,562
Belorusskaja SSR	19	13	80	138	155	167	121	155
Uzbekskaja SSR	140	111	199	82	175	214	92	50
Kazachskaja SSR	953	1,962	11,573	10,520	14,963	13,721	7,108	3,911
Gruzinskaja SSR	20	36	67	77	91	123	113	134
Azerbajdžanskaja SSR	85	103	139	136	186	189	215	228
Litovskaja SSR	--	28	72	94	120	90	158	178
Moldavskaja SSR	82	258	205	231	348	419	123	410
Latvijskaja SSR	--	27	57	66	86	69	78	96
Kirgizskaja SSR	136	48	179	124	186	177	134	149
Tadžikskaja SSR	54	29	42	22	46	40	32	38
Armjanskaja SSR	28	10	29	31	38	43	22	51
Turkmenskaja SSR	29	15	10	17	19	20	22	23
Estonskaja SSR	--	6	18	20	23	23	33	38

5.2.49.6 STATE PURCHASES OF RYE BY UNION REPUBLICS[1]
STAATLICHE AUFKÄUFE AN ROGGEN NACH UNIONSREPUBLIKEN[1]
GOSUDARSTVENNYE ZAKUPKI RŽI PO SOJUZNYM RESPUBLIKAM[1]

	1940	1965	1970	1971	1972	1973	1974	1975
SSSR	7,992	5,451	5,399	4,809	2,978	3,188	6,618	2,865
RSFSR	6,231	4,457	4,502	3,847	2,045	1,789	5,347	1,595
Ukrainskaja SSR	1,386	429	275	288	205	536	339	277
Belorusskaja SSR	282	296	294	333	418	548	454	704
Kazachskaja SSR	53	35	122	84	23	24	196	7
Litovskaja SSR	--	93	81	108	136	124	159	132
Moldavskaja SSR	38	3	0.4	0.7	0.7	0.7	0.3	0.7
Latvijskaja SSR	--	86	77	87	97	99	70	88
Estonskaja SSR	--	50	46	61	53	66	49	60

5.2.49.7 STATE PURCHASES OF SUGAR-BEET BY UNION REPUBLICS[1]
STAATLICHE AUFKÄUFE AN ZUCKERRÜBEN NACH UNIONSREPUBLIKEN[1]
GOSUDARSTVENNYE ZAKUPKI SACHARNOJ SVEKLY PO SOJUZNYM RESPUBLIKAM[1]

	1940	1965	1970	1971	1972	1973	1974	1975	1976
SSSR	17,357	67,500	71,385	64,329	68,043	77,799	67,484	61,880	85,294
RSFSR	3,044	18,955	21,362	16,127	14,421	26,095	18,680	17,838	24,659
Ukrainskaja SSR	12,669	41,153	41,847	40,632	43,700	43,303	40,364	35,925	51,203
Belorusskaja SSR	--	768	932	726	1,206	1,054	960	1,057	961
Kazachskaja SSR	384	1,840	2,127	2,030	2,350	2,236	1,948	1,864	2,014
Gruzinskaja SSR	71	123	122	139	130	118	121	134	130
Litovskaja SSR	220	545	483	499	876	650	740	700	553
Moldavskaja SSR	119	1,935	2,612	2,398	3,284	2,260	2,649	2,360	3,812
Latvijskaja SSR	216	305	208	205	253	218	195	182	167
Kirgizskaja SSR	618	1,755	1,604	1,487	1,717	1,750	1,695	1,672	1,634
Armjanskaja SSR	16	121	88	86	106	115	132	148	161

1 in all agricultural enterprises; '000 tons - in allen landwirtschaftlichen Betrieben; Tsd.t - vo vsech kategorijach chozjajstv; tys.t

5.2.49.8 Economy
5.2.49.9 Wirtschaft
5.2.49.10

5.2.49.8 STATE PURCHASES OF FLAX FIBRES BY UNION REPUBLICS[1]
STAATLICHE AUFKÄUFE AN FLACHSFASER NACH UNIONSREPUBLIKEN[1]
GOSUDARSTVENNYE ZAKUPKI L'NOVOLOKNA PO SOJUZNYM RESPUBLIKAM[1]

	1940	1965	1970	1971	1972	1973	1974	1975	1976
SSSR	245.2	432.6	431.4	461.3	439.1	420.7	364.1	477.7	472.9
RSFSR	178.9	228.6	233.9	223.3	205.6	157.2	149.6	231.4	166.4
Ukrainskaja SSR	10.4	70.6	84.1	98.9	112.7	135.5	118.3	116.2	154.0
Belorusskaja SSR	21.6	110.4	98.7	118.5	104.3	113.4	82.5	112.8	126.1
Litovskaja SSR	16.4	15.0	10.6	14.0	10.1	9.6	10.0	13.2	19.2
Latvijskaja SSR	12.9	6.2	3.0	5.1	5.1	4.2	3.0	3.3	5.1
Estonskaja SSR	5.0	1.8	1.1	1.5	1.3	0.8	0.7	0.8	2.1

5.2.49.9 STATE PURCHASES OF SUNFLOWER SEEDS BY UNION REPUBLICS[1]
STAATLICHE AUFKÄUFE AN SONNENBLUMENSAMEN NACH UNIONSREPUBLIKEN[1]
GOSUDARSTVENNYE ZAKUPKI SEMJAN PODSOLNECNIKA PO SOJUZNYM RESPUBLIKAM[1]

	1940	1965	1970	1971	1972	1973	1974	1975	1976
SSSR	1,500	3,888	4,613	4,359	3,753	5,553	5,228	3,841	3,763
RSFSR	911	1,799	2,303	2,010	1,594	2,831	2,634	1,675	2,095
Ukrainskaja SSR	486	1,767	1,982	2,017	1,795	2,359	2,340	1,875	1,435
Kazachskaja SSR	12	38	58	67	68	72	4	54	62
Gruzinskaja SSR	3	11	8	4	16	16	16	10	12
Moldavskaja SSR	86	273	262	261	280	275	234	227	159

5.2.49.10 STATE PURCHASES OF POTATOES BY UNION REPUBLICS[1]
STAATLICHE AUFKÄUFE AN KARTOFFELN NACH UNIONSREPUBLIKEN[1]
GOSUDARSTVENNYE ZAKUPKI KARTOFELJA PO SOJUZNYM RESPUBLIKAM[1]

	1940	1965	1970	1971	1972	1973	1974	1975	1976
SSSR	8,642	9,946	11,233	11,482	11,087	15,410	11,156	14,527	13,636
RSFSR	5,192	6,429	7,221	6,676	4,424	9,963	5,424	9,061	6,977
Ukrainskaja SSR	1,823	1,620	1,706	2,387	2,731	2,500	2,483	2,023	3,064
Belorusskaja SSR	1,296	1,157	1,259	1,360	2,412	1,655	1,920	2,069	2,073
Uzbekskaja SSR	21	58	63	61	76	81	98	96	108
Kazachskaja SSR	37	60	206	219	329	296	246	196	310
Gruzinskaja SSR	19	59	68	37	68	60	96	102	101
Azerbajdžanskaja SSR	26	19	18	16	18	21	31	29	33
Litovskaja SSR	10	139	177	198	291	222	218	278	261
Moldavskaja SSR	10	9	13	22	29	22	23	10	24
Latvijskaja SSR	146	168	206	212	342	238	178	238	248
Kirgizskaja SSR	12	56	63	63	72	64	73	69	74
Tadžikskaja SSR	8	9	21	21	32	34	56	49	53
Armjanskaja SSR	11	14	44	24	36	53	76	61	70
Estonskaja SSR	30	149	165	182	224	197	231	242	235

[1] in all agricultural enterprises; '000 tons - in allen landwirtschaftlichen Betrieben; Tsd.t - vo vsech kategorijach chozjajstv; tys.t

5.2.49.11 STATE PURCHASES OF VEGETABLES BY UNION REPUBLICS[1]
STAATLICHE AUFKÄUFE AN GEMÜSE NACH UNIONSREPUBLIKEN[1]
GOSUDARSTVENNYE ZAKUPKI OVOŠČEJ PO SOJUZNYM RESPUBLIKAM[1]

	1940	1965	1970	1971	1972	1973	1974	1975	1976
SSSR	2,970	7,724	10,918	11,467	11,234	14,125	14,657	13,883	16,180
RSFSR	1,335	3,273	4,720	4,693	4,177	5,718	5,960	5,829	6,064
Ukrainskaja SSR	1,329	2,679	3,364	3,630	3,515	4,343	4,354	3,836	5,203
Belorusskaja SSR	68	118	233	178	251	333	276	255	279
Uzbekskaja SSR	70	352	614	738	811	865	993	1,027	1,169
Kazachskaja SSR	25	299	452	456	503	573	580	547	597
Gruzinskaja SSR	23	101	157	159	155	184	229	215	272
Azerbajdžanskaja SSR	25	185	268	296	338	413	447	455	586
Litovskaja SSR	--	30	60	53	91	80	75	86	77
Moldavskaja SSR	47	315	414	523	611	757	808	750	911
Latvijskaja SSR	--	41	84	87	92	102	102	89	84
Kirgizskaja SSR	8	84	118	141	158	158	195	178	206
Tadžikskaja SSR	5	33	88	101	117	111	148	159	168
Armjanskaja SSR	9	108	188	230	221	281	266	250	321
Turkmenskaja SSR	12	76	109	131	139	153	162	154	191
Estonskaja SSR	--	30	49	51	55	55	62	53	52

5.2.49.12 STATE PURCHASES OF FRUITS AND BERRIES (INCL. GRAPES) BY UNION REPUBLICS[1]
STAATLICHE AUFKÄUFE AN OBST UND BEEREN (EINSCHL. WEINTRAUBEN) NACH UNIONSREPUBLIKEN[1]
GOSUDARSTVENNYE ZAKUPKI FRUKTOV I JAGOD (VKLJUČAJA VINOGRAD) PO SOJUZNYM RESPUBLIKAM[1]

	1940	1965	1970	1971	1972	1973	1974	1975	1976
SSSR	596	4,477	6,180	6,351	5,325	7,793	7,933	8,541	9,628
RSFSR	116	1,108	1,593	1,469	1,129	1,812	1,966	1,990	2,435
Ukrainskaja SSR	140	1,235	1,446	1,649	1,396	2,287	1,962	2,101	2,135
Belorusskaja SSR	2	33	124	46	19	17	11	49	174
Uzbekskaja SSR	59	186	266	199	351	357	401	479	531
Kazachskaja SSR	7	71	148	117	232	165	194	184	257
Gruzinskaja SSR	71	354	658	478	397	474	669	778	716
Azerbajdžanskaja SSR	59	166	370	316	276	466	694	757	818
Litovskaja SSR	--	29	59	75	37	93	17	98	108
Moldavskaja SSR	84	998	1,004	1,524	1,091	1,637	1,432	1,403	1,754
Latvijskaja SSR	--	7	16	17	13	21	12	18	41
Kirgizskaja SSR	2	38	55	55	112	94	95	124	126
Tadžikskaja SSR	12	82	130	116	93	115	159	189	179
Armjanskaja SSR	36	142	272	249	147	198	249	295	289
Turkmenskaja SSR	8	25	30	33	24	50	56	66	41
Estonskaja SSR	--	3	9	8	8	7	16	10	24

5.2.49.13 STATE PURCHASES OF GRAPES BY UNION REPUBLICS[1]
STAATLICHE AUFKÄUFE VON WEINTRAUBEN NACH UNIONSREPUBLIKEN[1]
GOSUDARSTVENNYE ZAKUPKI VINOGRADA PO SOJUZNYM RESPUBLIKAM[1]

	1940	1965	1970	1971	1972	1973	1974	1975	1976
SSSR	306	2,875	3,145	3,544	2,026	3,544	3,722	4,329	4,404
RSFSR	47	635	662	632	322	633	628	698	785
Ukrainskaja SSR	52	711	685	778	474	913	701	936	625

1 in all agricultural enterprises; '000 tons - in allen landwirtschaftlichen Betrieben; Tsd.t - vo vsech kategorijach chozjajstv; tys.t

5.2.49.13 Economy
5.2.49.14 Wirtschaft
5.2.49.15

	1940	1965	1970	1971	1972	1973	1974	1975	1976
Uzbekskaja SSR	42	137	173	150	201	220	241	246	293
Kazachskaja SSR	1	48	73	87	126	90	115	80	124
Gruzinskaja SSR	36	245	392	307	160	226	322	409	291
Azerbajdžanskaja SSR	40	133	307	284	212	397	599	668	709
Moldavskaja SSR	42	765	513	967	339	798	755	910	1,187
Kirgizskaja SSR	--	18	21	24	39	31	38	32	39
Tadžikskaja SSR	7	54	83	84	31	61	91	98	119
Armjanskaja SSR	31	111	213	203	103	135	182	200	195
Turkmenskaja SSR	8	18	23	28	19	40	50	52	37

5.2.49.14 GROSS YIELD (PURCHASES) OF RAW TEA (HIGH GRADE) BY UNION REPUBLICS[1]
BRUTTOERNTEERTRAG (AUFKÄUFE) AN SORTENTEEBLÄTTERN NACH UNIONSREPUBLIKEN[1]
VALOVOJ SBOR (ZAKUPKI) OSNOVNOGO (SORTOVOGO) ČAJNOGO LISTA PO SOJUZNYM RESPUBLIKAM[1]

	1940	1965	1970	1971	1972	1973	1974	1975	1976	1977
SSSR	51.6	197.0	272.7	280.2	291.1	305.4	329.9	352.3		
RSFSR	0.01	2.7	4.0	4.3	4.0	4.4	4.6	4.6		
Gruzinskaja SSR	51.3	186.1	258.8	265.8	276.4	289.4	312.2	334.6		
Azerbajdžanskaja SSR	0.24	8.2	9.9	10.1	10.7	11.6	13.1	13.1		

5.2.49.15 STATE PURCHASES OF BASIC LIVESTOCK PRODUCTS IN INDIVIDUAL
AGRICULTURAL ENTERPRISES
STAATLICHE AUFKÄUFE VON GRUNDERZEUGNISSEN DER VIEHWIRTSCHAFT
IN DEN EINZELNEN LANDWIRTSCHAFTLICHEN BETRIEBEN
GOSUDARSTVENNYE ZAKUPKI OSNOVNYCH PRODUKTOV ŽIVOTNOVODSTVA PO
KATEGORIJAM CHOZJAJSTV

Year Jahr Gody	Cattle & poultry (live weight), mill.tons Vieh u.Geflügel (Lebendgewicht), Mio t Skot i ptica (v vese živogo skota i pticy),mln.t A.	Milk & dairy products (in terms of milk),mill.tons Milch u.Milchprodukte(umgerechnet auf Milch),Mio t Moloko i močnye produkty(v peresčete na moloko), mln.t B.	Eggs '000 mill. Eier Mrd.Stck. Jajca mlrd.št. C.	Wool (charging weight),'000 tons Wolle (Anrechnungsgewicht), Tsd.t Šerst' (v začetnom vese), tys.t D.
	All agricultural enterprises - alle landwirtschaftlichen Betriebe - vse kategorii chozjajstv			
1940	2.2	6.5	2.7	120
1945	1.3	2.9	1.1	67
1950	2.3	8.5	1.9	136
1955	4.2	13.5	2.9	230
1960	7.9	26.3	6.5	358
1965	9.3	38.7	10.5	368
1966	10.3	40.1	11.6	380
1967	11.5	42.5	12.9	410
1968	11.9	44.0	14.1	429
1969	11.7	43.8	15.4	402
1970	12.6	45.7	18.1	441

1 in all agricultural enterprises; '000 tons - in allen landwirtschaftlichen Betrieben; Tsd.t - vo vsech kategorijach chozjajstv; tys.t

	A.	B.	C.	D.		A.	B.	C.	D.
1971	14.2	47.1	21.6	457	1975	16.8	56.3	33.1	511
1972	15.0	48.4	24.3	452	1976	14.7	56.2	32.9	480
1973	14.7	53.0	27.6	470					
1974	16.2	55.8	30.9	507					

Collective and state farms and other state enterprises -
Kolchosen, Sowchosen und andere staatliche Betriebe -
Kolchozy, sovchozy i drugie gosudarstvennye chozjajstva

	A.	B.	C.	D.		A.	B.	C.	D.
1940	1.4	4.3	0.2	91	1969	10.8	42.7	13.5	345
1945	0.9	1.9	0.2	54	1970	11.3	44.2	16.1	380
1950	1.6	4.8	0.8	116	1971	12.3	45.2	19.5	391
1955	3.5	11.2	1.4	212	1972	12.9	46.2	22.3	380
1960	6.8	24.4	4.1	307	1973	12.8	50.6	25.6	395
1965	8.4	37.0	7.8	320	1974	14.2	53.2	28.8	427
1966	8.9	38.6	8.9	329	1975	14.6	53.7	31.1	427
1967	10.0	41.0	10.4	357	1976	13.1	53.4	31.7	400
1968	10.3	42.8	11.9	373					

Collective farms - Kolchosen - Kolchozy

	A.	B.	C.	D.		A.	B.	C.	D.
1940	0.9	3.3	0.1	69	1969	5.6	24.3	3.8	171
1945	0.8	1.6	0.2	45	1970	5.8	24.9	4.4	184
1950	1.0	3.5	0.6	95	1971	6.1	25.1	5.2	186
1955	2.5	8.7	0.9	171	1972	6.5	25.7	5.5	179
1960	4.3	16.0	2.2	198	1973	6.4	28.4	6.0	180
1965	4.2	21.1	3.0	164	1974	7.0	29.7	6.1	190
1966	4.6	21.9	3.2	168	1975	7.1	29.9	5.6	186
1967	5.1	23.1	3.5	179	1976	6.4	29.6	4.1	175
1968	5.3	24.5	3.7	184					

State farms and other state enterprises -
Sowchosen und andere staatliche Betriebe -
Sovchozy i drugie gosudarstvennye chozjajstva

	A.	B.	C.	D.		A.	B.	C.	D.
1940	0.5	1.0	0.1	22	1969	5.2	18.4	9.7	174
1945	0.1	0.3	--	9	1970	5.5	19.3	11.7	196
1950	0.6	1.3	0.2	21	1971	6.2	20.1	14.3	205
1955	1.0	2.5	0.5	41	1972	6.4	20.5	16.8	201
1960	2.5	8.4	1.9	109	1973	6.4	22.2	19.6	215
1965	4.2	15.9	4.8	156	1974	7.2	23.5	22.7	237
1966	4.3	16.7	5.7	161	1975	7.5	23.8	25.5	241
1967	4.9	17.9	6.9	178	1976	6.7	23.8	27.6	225
1968	5.0	18.3	8.2	189					

5.2.49.16 STATE PURCHASES OF CATTLE AND POULTRY BY UNION REPUBLICS (LIVE WEIGHT)[1]
STAATLICHE AUFKÄUFE VON VIEH UND GEFLÜGEL NACH UNIONSREPUBLIKEN (LEBENDGEWICHT)[1]
GOSUDARSTVENNYE ZAKUPKI SKOTA I PTICY PO SOJUZNYM RESPUBLIKAM
(V VESE ŽIVOGO SKOTA I PTICY)[1]

	1940	1965	1970	1971	1972	1973	1974	1975	1976
SSSR	2,217	9,280	12,595	14,163	15,023	14,695	16,187	16,756	14,706
RSFSR	1,194	4,909	6,404	7,358	7,832	7,350	8,237	8,482	7,360
Ukrainskaja SSR	516	1,841	2,626	2,938	3,235	3,229	3,503	3,632	3,134
Belorusskaja SSR	141	410	750	812	855	891	954	1,010	937
Uzbekskaja SSR	38	149	147	153	164	168	180	197	200
Kazachskaja SSR	162	979	1,201	1,245	1,218	1,321	1,423	1,490	1,113

[1] in all agricultural enterprises; '000 tons - in allen landwirtschaftlichen Betrieben; Tsd.t - vo vsech kategorijach chozjajstv; tys.t

5.2.49.16 Economy
5.2.49.17 Wirtschaft
5.2.49.18

	1940	1965	1970	1971	1972	1973	1974	1975	1976
Gruzinskaja SSR	21	53	74	86	95	97	111	120	130
Azerbajdžanskaja SSR	23	58	84	92	91	97	103	106	106
Litovskaja SSR	18	250	442	510	511	501	536	532	543
Moldavskaja SSR	12	125	173	197	205	222	241	243	244
Latvijskaja SSR	15	144	234	258	288	272	300	313	317
Kirgizskaja SSR	23	134	158	174	170	188	201	213	185
Tadžikskaja SSR	12	47	57	62	64	66	70	75	77
Armjanskaja SSR	13	38	50	57	66	72	81	82	84
Turkmenskaja SSR	10	34	36	44	45	47	50	53	54
Estonskaja SSR	19	109	159	177	184	174	197	208	222

5.2.49.17 STATE PURCHASES OF CATTLE AND POULTRY BY UNION REPUBLICS (SLAUGHTER WEIGHT) - STAATLICHE AUFKÄUFE VON VIEH UND GEFLÜGEL NACH UNIONS-REPUBLIKEN (UMGERECHNET AUF SCHLACHTGEWICHT) - GOSUDARSTVENNYE ZAKUPKI SKOTA I PTICY PO SOJUZNYM RESPUBLIKAM (V PERESČETE NA UBOJNYJ VES)[1]

	1965	1970	1971	1972	1973	1974	1975	1976
SSSR	5,813	8,110	9,184	9,712	9,471	10,474	10,861	9,361
RSFSR	3,085	4,111	4,763	5,036	4,731	5,325	5,478	4,598
Ukrainskaja SSR	1,191	1,728	1,957	2,134	2,123	2,313	2,432	2,074
Belorusskaja SSR	260	502	540	559	581	629	678	621
Uzbekskaja SSR	88	88	94	102	104	112	123	123
Kazachskaja SSR	551	699	728	728	779	836	858	643
Gruzinskaja SSR	31	52	54	60	61	72	78	84
Azerbajdžanskaja SSR	32	48	53	53	56	60	61	62
Litovskaja SSR	174	312	357	358	350	374	369	380
Moldavskaja SSR	86	123	141	144	154	170	171	167
Latvijskaja SSR	96	161	181	201	191	208	218	221
Kirgizskaja SSR	76	90	100	99	107	115	122	105
Tadžikskaja SSR	26	34	35	40	40	43	46	45
Armjanskaja SSR	21	29	33	41	44	49	49	51
Turkmenskaja SSR	19	20	24	27	28	30	31	31
Estonskaja SSR	77	113	124	130	122	138	147	156

5.2.49.18 STATE PURCHASES OF MILK AND DAIRY PRODUCTS BY UNION REPUBLICS (IN TERMS OF MILK) - STAATLICHE AUFKÄUFE VON MILCH UND MILCHPRODUKTEN NACH UNIONS-REPUBLIKEN (UMGERECHNET AUF MILCH) - GOSUDARSTVENNYE ZAKUPKI MOLOKA I MOLOČNYCH PRODUKTOV PO SOJUZNYM RESPUBLIKAM (V PERESČETE NA MOLOKO)[1]

	1940	1965	1970	1971	1972	1973	1974	1975	1976
SSSR	6,453	38,700	45,681	47,078	48,444	52,978	55,768	56,296	56,220
RSFSR	4,239	21,399	25,339	26,018	26,359	28,749	30,351	30,692	30,154
Ukrainskaja SSR	1,006	9,171	10,545	11,002	11,467	12,829	13,325	13,179	13,184
Belorusskaja SSR	231	1,939	2,549	2,609	2,850	3,208	3,381	3,530	3,592
Uzbekskaja SSR	31	291	354	380	403	445	479	506	534
Kazachskaja SSR	271	1,560	1,783	1,784	1,835	1,986	2,001	1,923	1,988
Gruzinskaja SSR	24	141	175	183	179	193	211	224	234
Azerbajdžanskaja SSR	39	156	182	197	204	231	243	248	259
Litovskaja SSR	126	1,121	1,440	1,455	1,612	1,664	1,797	1,895	2,003

1 in all agricultural enterprises; '000 tons - in allen landwirtschaftlichen Betrieben; Tsd.t - vo vsech kategorijach chozjajstv; tys.t

Economy 5.2.49.18
Wirtschaft 5.2.49.19
5.2.49.20

	1940	1965	1970	1971	1972	1973	1974	1975	1976
Moldavskaja SSR	3	411	492	512	523	600	624	664	675
Latvijskaja SSR	263	1,203	1,286	1,325	1,332	1,345	1,471	1,463	1,531
Kirgizskaja SSR	27	265	315	331	343	359	368	373	384
Tadžikskaja SSR	6	85	114	125	131	142	156	165	177
Armjanskaja SSR	20	155	186	202	214	220	227	239	254
Turkmenskaja SSR	8	66	81	85	90	99	107	114	118
Estonskaja SSR	159	737	840	870	902	909	1,027	1,081	1,133

5.2.49.19 STATE PURCHASES OF EGGS BY UNION REPUBLICS (mill.)[1]
STAATLICHE AUFKÄUFE VON EIERN NACH UNIONSREPUBLIKEN (Mio Stck.)[1]
GOSUDARSTVENNYE ZAKUPKI JAIC PO SOJUZNYM RESPUBLIKAM (mln.št.)[1]

	1940	1965	1970	1971	1972	1973	1974	1975	1976
SSSR	2,679	10,478	18,054	21,570	24,299	27,544	30,892	33,065	32,897
RSFSR	1,454	6,380	11,202	13,495	15,185	17,019	19,131	20,410	20,142
Ukrainskaja SSR	1,039	2,566	3,786	4,425	5,000	5,771	6,400	6,800	6,554
Belorusskaja SSR	112	262	483	586	699	885	994	1,106	1,167
Uzbekskaja SSR	--	154	304	353	392	456	518	558	620
Kazachskaja SSR	38	325	717	877	1,047	1,203	1,427	1,539	1,606
Gruzinskaja SSR	14	97	161	180	191	260	275	292	327
Azerbajdžanskaja SSR	10	81	133	152	162	180	201	223	220
Litovskaja SSR	--	94	212	251	283	310	345	386	406
Moldavskaja SSR	6	97	205	242	261	288	311	353	376
Latvijskaja SSR	--	143	268	327	356	370	397	426	433
Kirgizskaja SSR	--	71	138	163	162	178	199	207	232
Tadžikskaja SSR	--	44	85	105	113	131	148	169	195
Armjanskaja SSR	6	55	102	108	114	146	171	200	217
Turkmenskaja SSR	--	28	61	81	81	88	101	117	113
Estonskaja SSR	--	81	197	225	253	259	274	279	289

5.2.49.20 STATE PURCHASES OF WOOL BY UNION REPUBLICS (WEIGHT CHARGED), '000 tons[1]
STAATLICHE AUFKÄUFE VON WOLLE NACH UNIONSREPUBLIKEN (ANRECHNUNGSGEW.),Tsd.t[1]
GOSUDARSTVENNYE ZAKUPKI ŠERSTI PO SOJUZNYM RESPUBLIKAM (V ZAČETNOM VESE), tys.t[1]

	1940	1965	1970	1971	1972	1973	1974	1975	1976
SSSR	119.8	368.5	440.9	457.4	451.6	470.1	506.8	510.9	480.5
RSFSR	67.9	173.2	216.6	230.1	226.2	225.9	251.5	250.8	234.2
Ukrainskaja SSR	12.2	23.2	26.0	26.7	27.1	27.8	30.0	31.1	27.5
Belorusskaja SSR	1.2	1.1	1.1	1.1	1.2	1.2	1.2	1.2	1.1
Uzbekskaja SSR	7.9	20.4	21.5	21.2	20.5	23.1	24.3	25.0	24.5
Kazachskaja SSR	13.8	88.6	105.2	104.7	104.5	113.6	119.2	120.6	112.2
Gruzinskaja SSR	2.6	5.0	5.2	5.7	5.2	5.5	5.6	5.9	5.7
Azerbajdžanskaja SSR	3.1	7.2	8.0	8.6	8.8	9.6	9.6	9.8	10.6
Moldavskaja SSR	0.6	1.8	1.8	1.9	1.9	1.9	1.9	2.1	1.9
Kirgizskaja SSR	3.7	27.9	32.6	34.2	34.7	37.8	38.8	39.6	38.3
Tadžikskaja SSR	1.1	4.5	5.0	5.0	5.0	5.3	5.4	5.6	5.7
Armjanskaja SSR	1.0	3.6	4.0	4.5	4.5	4.5	4.5	4.9	4.7
Turkmenskaja SSR	4.7	12.0	13.9	13.7	12.0	13.9	14.8	14.3	14.1

1 in all agricultural enterprises - in allen landwirtschaftlichen Betrieben - vo vsech kategorijach chozjajstv

5.2.50 Economy / Wirtschaft

SUPPLY OF TRACTORS, LORRIES AND AGRICULTURAL MACHINES TO AGRICULTURE (thousands)
BELIEFERUNG DER LANDWIRTSCHAFT MIT TRAKTOREN, LASTKRAFTWAGEN UND LANDMASCHINEN (Tsd.Stck.)
POSTAVKA SEL'SKOMU CHOZJAJSTVU TRAKTOROV, GRUZOVYCH AVTOMOBILEJ I SEL'SKOCHOZJAJSTVENNYCH MAŠIN (tys.št.)

	1940	1965	1970	1971	1972	1973	1974	1975	1976	1977
Tractors, total – Traktoren, insg. – Traktory, vsego	20.3	239.5	309.3	313.2	312.8	323.0	348.0	370.4	368.6	364.6
aggregate capacity of tractor engines, mill.hp – summarische Motorleistung, Mio PS – summarnaja moščnost' dvigatelej vsech traktorov,mln.l.s.	0.9	12.8	19.0	20.0	21.2	22.6	25.3	27.3	28.5	28.3
Lorries – Lastkraftwagen – gruzovye avtomobili	17.5	70.2	125.8	137.3	152.7	188.4	212.4	228.5	226.1	224.2
Specialized automobiles – Spezialkraftfahrzeuge – Specializirovanye avtomobili	...	24.1	30.8	32.1	34.8	36.4	38.3	40.9	43.0	43.9
Tractor ploughs – Traktorenpflüge – Plugi traktornye	38.4	158.5	207.2	217.0	219.0	215.1	203.4	191.1	184.6	176.2
Tractor stubbler ploughs – Traktorenschälpflüge – Luščil'niki traktornye	12.8	44.2	38.2	28.0	27.6	26.5	30.5	31.3	28.7	31.7
Tractor drills – Traktorendrillmaschinen – sejalki traktornye	21.4	259.5	187.0	170.1	175.7	194.4	211.0	213.7	222.6	-.-
Tractor cultivators – Traktorengrubber – Kul'tivatory traktornye	32.3	208.3	204.6	183.0	176.3	190.0	176.2	181.7	186.6	181.6
Grain harvesters – Mähdrescher – Zernouboročnye kombajny	12.8	79.4	97.1	99.0	92.8	81.5	83.4	92.0	97.5	100.8
Windrowers – Schwadenmähmaschinen – Žatki rjadovye	-.-	97.7	47.7	51.4	59.2	63.3	82.9	91.5	92.1	-.-
Maize harvesters – Maisvollerntemaschinen – Kukuruzouboročnye kombajny	-.-	0.1	5.0	7.0	8.2	8.9	10.0	10.1	10.9	10.8
Potato harvesters – Kartoffelvollerntemaschinen – Kartofeleuboročnye kombajny	-.-	6.1	8.0	9.7	11.3	11.9	12.1	12.0	12.2	12.1
Beet harvesters – Rübenvollerntemaschinen – Svekjouboročnye kombajny	-.-	17.3	9.6	10.4	11.9	14.7	16.0	17.3	14.3	14.4
Silage harvesters – Silofeldheckler – Silosouboročnye kombajny	-.-	22.9	32.9	39.7	55.7	66.3	67.7	70.1	53.6	57.3
Cotton-pickers – Baumwollerntemaschinen – Chlopkouboročnye kombajny	-.-	8.0	5.9	6.8	6.7	6.5	7.3	7.5	7.9	-.-
Tractor mowers – Traktormähmaschinen – Kosilki traktornye	3.3	120.9	142.6	148.7	150.7	128.8	92.0	82.7	87.2	96.3

Economy 5.2.50
Wirtschaft 5.2.51

	1940	1965	1970	1971	1972	1973	1974	1975	1976	1977
Tractor rakers - Traktorrechen - Grabli traktornye	0.9	39.8	61.0	52.1	51.3	60.7	53.9	46.6	41.1	47.4
Press pickers - Räum-und Sammelpressen - Press-podborščiki	--	6.0	13.9	17.4	23.9	26.8	29.9	33.4	33.1	31.5
Loaders (universal) - Universalladevorrichtungen - Pogruzčiki universal'nye	--	68.9	75.3	78.8	86.0	84.2	83.8	87.3	93.0	--
Milking machines - Melkanlagen - Doilnye ustanovki	--	6.1	50.0	58.5	65.6	64.8	57.6	54.5	54.5	56.0
Sprinklers and sprinkling plants - Beregungsmaschinen und -anlagen - Doždeval'nye mašiny i ustanovki	--	13.5	12.7	13.5	13.3	22.5	25.0	27.9	28.3	--

5.2.51   NUMBER OF TRACTORS IN AGRICULTURE BY UNION REPUBLICS (END-OF-YEAR FIGURES)
TRAKTORENPARK IN DER LANDWIRTSCHAFT NACH UNIONSREPUBLIKEN (ZUM JAHRESENDE)
PARK TRAKTOROV V SEL'SKOM CHOZJAJSTVE PO SOJUZNYM RESPUBLIKAM (NA KONEC GODA)

In physical units, '000 - in physischen Einheiten, Tsd.Stck. - v fizičeskich edinicach, tys.št.

	1940	1965	1970	1971	1972	1973	1974	1975	1976
SSSR	530.8	1613.8	1977.5	2045.7	2111.9	2188.5	2266.5	2336.0	2402.0
RSFSR	342.2	840.4	1012.6	1045.4	1079.4	1119.7	1157.7	1191.3	1227.8
Ukrainskaja SSR	94.6	257.0	317.1	329.1	340.8	349.2	359.7	371.7	382.9
Belorusskaja SSR	10.4	55.4	81.6	85.4	90.8	95.9	99.4	102.5	105.9
Uzbekskaja SSR	23.0	89.9	121.3	127.2	130.6	138.8	144.0	147.6	149.5
Kazachskaja SSR	30.8	194.8	198.6	200.4	201.5	206.9	216.5	226.1	233.0
Gruzinskaja SSR	3.0	12.9	18.4	18.8	19.4	19.7	20.6	20.8	22.9
Azerbajdžanskaja SSR	6.1	21.1	25.3	26.7	27.9	28.8	29.8	30.8	31.6
Litovskaja SSR	1.2	28.3	40.3	42.5	44.4	45.7	47.8	48.7	48.8
Moldavskaja SSR	1.4	23.1	35.4	37.9	40.0	42.4	44.4	45.9	47.3
Latvijskaja SSR	1.3	19.6	29.1	29.8	30.5	31.2	31.9	32.2	31.9
Kirgizskaja SSR	5.2	19.3	23.2	24.3	24.6	25.0	25.5	25.4	25.6
Tadžikskaja SSR	3.9	15.8	22.0	22.6	24.3	25.4	26.7	28.4	29.2
Armjanskaja SSR	1.5	7.2	9.4	9.7	10.4	10.8	11.2	11.7	12.0
Turkmenskaja SSR	4.4	15.5	25.7	27.7	28.6	30.1	32.1	33.5	34.1
Estonskaja SSR	1.8	12.9	17.5	18.2	18.7	18.9	19.2	19.4	19.5

5.2.51 Economy
5.2.52 Wirtschaft

Total capacity of tractor engines, mill.hp – Summarische Motorleistung, Mio PS –
Summarnaja moščnost' dvigatelej vsech traktorov, mln.l.s.

	1940	1965	1970	1971	1972	1973	1974	1975	1976
SSSR	17.6	77.6	111.6	117.6	124.3	133.8	144.5	152.5	163.0
RSFSR	11.7	41.6	59.8	63.2	67.0	72.0	77.6	81.4	86.7
Ukrainskaja SSR	3.0	11.8	16.9	17.7	18.7	20.0	21.5	23.0	24.8
Belorusskaja SSR	0.3	2.5	4.0	4.2	4.4	4.8	5.2	5.5	5.9
Uzbekskaja SSR	0.6	3.3	5.7	6.1	6.4	7.1	7.9	8.2	8.7
Kazachskaja SSR	1.1	11.2	13.6	13.8	14.4	15.7	16.8	18.1	19.4
Gruzinskaja SSR	0.09	0.5	0.9	0.9	1.0	1.1	1.1	1.1	1.2
Azerbajdžanskaja SSR	0.2	0.9	1.3	1.4	1.5	1.6	1.7	1.8	1.9
Litovskaja SSR	0.03	1.2	1.9	2.1	2.2	2.3	2.5	2.6	2.8
Moldavskaja SSR	0.04	1.0	1.8	1.9	2.0	2.2	2.3	2.4	2.6
Latvijskaja SSR	0.03	0.8	1.2	1.3	1.4	1.5	1.7	1.8	1.9
Kirgizskaja SSR	0.2	0.8	1.1	1.2	1.2	1.3	1.4	1.4	1.4
Tadžikskaja SSR	0.1	0.6	1.0	1.1	1.2	1.2	1.4	1.5	1.6
Armjanskaja SSR	0.1	0.3	0.5	0.5	0.6	0.6	0.6	0.7	0.7
Turkmenskaja SSR	0.1	0.6	1.2	1.4	1.5	1.6	1.9	2.0	2.3
Estonskaja SSR	0.04	0.5	0.7	0.8	0.8	0.8	0.9	1.0	1.1

5.2.52
NUMBER OF GRAIN HARVESTERS IN AGRICULTURE BY UNION REPUBLICS (IN PHYSICAL UNITS; END-OF-YEAR FIGURES), thousands
MÄHDRESCHERPARK IN DER LANDWIRTSCHAFT NACH UNIONSREPUBLIKEN (IN PHYSISCHEN EINHEITEN; ZUM JAHRESENDE), Tsd.
PARK ZERNOUBOROČNYCH KOMBAJNOV V SEL'SKOM CHOZJAJSTVE PO SOJUZNYM RESPUBLIKAM (V FIZIČ.EDINICACH; NA KONEC GODA), tys.

	1940	1965	1970	1971	1972	1973	1974	1975	1976
SSSR	181.7	519.7	622.6	639.1	655.8	658.5	673.0	679.8	684.8
RSFSR	130.1	320.3	381.0	389.6	398.6	399.1	408.8	411.1	414.8
Ukrainskaja SSR	33.4	56.9	81.2	83.6	81.8	79.7	81.9	82.5	81.7
Belorusskaja SSR	1.7	13.5	24.5	26.8	29.0	29.6	29.8	29.9	30.0
Uzbekskaja SSR	1.6	4.7	6.8	6.6	6.4	6.6	6.7	6.9	7.0
Kazachskaja SSR	11.8	98.8	94.6	97.7	104.9	107.9	108.8	111.6	113.6
Gruzinskaja SSR	0.5	1.7	1.6	1.6	1.4	1.4	1.4	1.4	1.6
Azerbajdžanskaja SSR	0.7	4.0	4.1	4.0	4.1	4.2	4.3	4.4	4.4
Litovskaja SSR	--	4.0	9.0	9.4	9.8	10.0	10.4	10.6	10.5
Moldavskaja SSR	0.2	3.1	3.4	3.5	3.2	3.3	3.3	3.2	3.1

	1940	1965	1970	1971	1972	1973	1974	1975	1976
Latvijskaja SSR	--	3.7	6.1	6.0	6.1	6.2	6.7	7.0	6.9
Kirgizskaja SSR	1.1	3.0	3.4	3.5	3.8	3.8	3.9	4.0	4.0
Tadžikskaja SSR	0.1	1.3	1.2	1.2	1.2	1.2	1.2	1.2	1.3
Armjanskaja SSR	0.3	1.6	1.6	1.5	1.5	1.5	1.5	1.5	1.5
Turkmenskaja SSR	0.2	0.8	1.0	1.0	1.0	0.9	1.0	1.0	1.0
Estonskaja SSR	--	2.3	3.1	3.1	3.0	3.1	3.3	3.5	3.4

5.2.53 SUPPLY OF MINERAL FERTILIZERS TO AGRICULTURE ('000 tons) – BELIEFERUNG DER LANDWIRTSCHAFT MIT MINERALISCHEN DÜNGEMITTELN (Tsd.t) – POSTAVKA MINERAL'NYCH UDOBRENIJ SEL'SKOMU CHOZJAJSTVU (tys.t)

	1940	1965	1970	1971	1972	1973	1974	1975	1976
In conventional units – umgerechnet auf Bezugseinheiten – v peresčete na uslovnye edinicy	3,159	27,066	45,649	50,547	54,795	59,988	65,884	75,265	77,169
of which – darunter – v tom čisle:									
nitrogenous – Stickstoffdünger – azotnye	789	11,132	22,463	25,279	27,436	30,519	32,908	36,132	35,750
phosphate – Phosphatdünger – fosfatnye	1,371	8,044	11,821	13,584	14,741	15,964	19,320	22,325	24,068
phosphorite meal – Phosphoritmehl – fosforitnaja muka	473	3,246	5,122	4,916	4,756	4,740	4,650	4,731	4,395
potash – Kalidünger – kalijnye	526	4,547	6,187	6,703	7,784	8,667	8,914	11,991	12,875
In terms of 100 per cent content of nutrients – umgerechnet auf 100% Reinnährstoffgehalt – v peresčete na 100% pitatel'nych veščestv	727	6,303	10,368	11,451	12,530	13,756	14,572	17,477	18,028
of which – darunter – v tom čisle:									
nitrogenous – Stickstoffdünger – azotnye	162	2,282	4,605	5,182	5,606	6,224	6,696	6,746	7,427
phosphate – Phosphatdünger – fosfatnye	256	1,474	2,160	2,442	2,612	2,731	3,276	4,175	4,501
phosphorite meal – Phosphoritmehl – fosforitnaja muka	90	617	973	934	904	901	884	899	835
potash – Kalidünger – kalijnye	219	1,891	2,574	2,788	3,238	3,605	3,708	4,988	5,356

5.2.54.1 Economy
Wirtschaft

5.2.54 CADRES IN AGRICULTURE – KADER IN DER LANDWIRTSCHAFT – KADRY V SEL'SKOM CHOZJAJSTVE

5.2.54.1 AVERAGE ANNUAL NUMBER OF PERSONS ENGAGED AT COLLECTIVE AND STATE FARMS, SUBSIDIARY AND OTHER AGRICULTURAL PRODUCTION ENTERPRISES (mill.head) – JAHRESDURCHSCHNITTSZAHL DER BESCHÄFTIGTEN IN KOLCHOSEN, SOWCHOSEN, NEBEN- UND ANDEREN LANDWIRTSCHAFTLICHEN PRODUKTIONSBETRIEBEN (Mio Personen) – SREDNEGODOVAJA ČISLENNOST' RABOTNIKOV, ZANJATYCH V KOLCHOZACH, SOVCHOZACH, PODSOBNYCH I PROČICH PROIZVODSTVENNYCH SEL'SKOCHOZJAJSTVENNYCH PREDPRIJATIJACH (mln.čelovek)

	1940	1965	1970	1971	1972	1973	1974	1975	1976
Persons engaged in all branches of production of the collective and state farms, subsidiary and other agricultural production enterprises, total – Beschäftigte in allen Wirtschaftszweigen der Kolchosen,Sowchosen,Neben-u. anderen landwirtschaftl.Produktionsbetriebe,insg. – Zanjato rabotnikov vo vsech otrasljach chozjajstva kolchozov,sovchozov,podsobnych i pročich proizvodstvennych sel' skochozjajstvennych predprijatij, vsego	31.3	28.0	26.8	26.6	26.5	26.6	26.7	26.4	26.6
of which – darunter – v tom čisle: in collective farms (social production) – in Kolchosen (gesellschaftliche Wirtschaft) – v kolchozach (obščestvennoe chozjajstvo)	29.0	18.9	17.0	16.5	16.2	16.1	15.9	15.4	15.0
in state farms,subsidiary and other agricultural production enterprises – in Sowchosen,Neben-u.anderen landwirtschaftl.Produktionsbetrieben – v sovchozach, podsobnych i pročich proizvodstvennych sel'skochozjajstvennych predprijatijach	1.8	9.1	9.8	10.1	10.3	10.5	10.8	11.0	11.4
in engine-tractors and repair-technical stations – in Maschinen-Traktoren-u.reparaturtechnischen Stationen – v mašinno-traktornych i remontno-techničeskich stancijach	0.5	--	--	--	--	--	--	--	--
Moreover Persons engaged in other enterprises and organizations drafted to work on collective and state farms – Außerdem zur Arbeit in Kolchosen u.Sowchosen herangezogene Beschäftigte aus anderen Betrieben u.Organisationen – Krome togo,privlečeno rabotnikov iz drugich predprijatij i organizacij dlja raboty v kolchozach i sovchozach	0.1	0.5	0.6	0.7	0.8	0.9	0.9	1.0	1.0
From the total of persons (incl.persons drafted to) working in agriculture, total – Aus der Gesamtzahl der Beschäftigten(einschl.der herangezogenen Personen) arbeiten i.d.									

	1940	1965	1970	1971	1972	1973	1974	1975	1976
Landwirtschaft, insg. - Iz obščego čisla rabotnikov (vključaja privlečennych lic) zanjato v sel'skom chozjajstve, vsego	28.1	25.6	23.8	23.3	23.5	23.6	23.6	23.5	23.3

5.2.54.2 AVERAGE ANNUAL NUMBER OF ALL COLLECTIVE FARMERS PARTICIPATING IN WORK ON COLLECTIVE FARMS[1], BY UNION REPUBLICS (thousands) - JAHRESDURCHSCHNITTSZAHL ALLER KOLCHOSBAUERN, DIE SICH AN DER ARBEIT DER KOLCHOSEN[1] BETEILIGTEN, NACH UNIONSREPUBLIKEN (Tsd.) - SREDNEGODOVAJA ČISLENNOST' VSECH KOLCHOZNIKOV, PRINIMAVŠICH, UČASTIE V RABOTACH KOLCHOZOV[1], PO SOJUZNYM RESPUBLIKAM (tys.)

	1965	1970	1971	1972	1973	1974	1975
SSSR	18,644	16,715	16,313	16,108	15,919	15,697	15,173
RSFSR	7,343	6,303	6,035	5,903	5,833	5,665	5,492
Ukrainskaja SSR	6,042	5,427	5,357	5,321	5,216	5,190	4,948
Belorusskaja SSR	1,144	1,028	1,010	997	975	958	928
Uzbekskaja SSR	972	1,029	1,059	1,060	1,067	1,047	1,047
Kazachskaja SSR	301	288	286	284	285	281	280
Gruzinskaja SSR	429	384	373	364	379	380	345
Azerbajdžanskaja SSR	320	274	276	283	282	296	292
Litovskaja SSR	327	307	301	295	286	279	268
Moldavskaja SSR	671	633	570	577	567	558	530
Latvijskaja SSR	182	155	154	149	149	143	137
Kirgizskaja SSR	216	215	213	212	207	213	204
Tadžikskaja SSR	285	263	264	262	258	262	265
Armjanskaja SSR	121	104	105	87	89	89	90
Turkmenskaja SSR	217	244	254	259	272	283	295
Estonskaja SSR	74	61	56	55	54	53	52

[1] without fishing cooperatives - ohne Fischfangkolchosen - bez ryboloveckich

5.2.54.3 Economy
Wirtschaft

5.2.54.3

NUMBER OF SPECIALISTS WITH HIGHER AND SPECIALIZED SECONDARY EDUCATION ENGAGED AT COLLECTIVE AND STATE FARMS, SUBSIDIARY AND OTHER AGRICULTURAL PRODUCTION ENTERPRISES (thousands) -
ANZAHL DER SPEZIALISTEN MIT HOCHSCHUL- UND MITTLERER FACHSCHULBILDUNG, DIE IN KOLCHOSEN, SOWCHOSEN, NEBEN- UND ANDEREN LANDWIRTSCHAFTLICHEN PRODUKTIONSBETRIEBEN BESCHÄFTIGT SIND (Tsd.) -
ČISLENNOST' SPECIALISTOV S VYSŠIM I SREDNIM SPECIAL'NYM OBRAZOVANIEM, ZANJATYCH V KOLCHOZACH, SOVCHOZACH, PODSOBNYCH I PROČICH PROIZVODSTVENNYCH SEL'SKOCHOZJAJSTVENNYCH PREDPRIJATIJACH (tys.čelovek)

	1970	1973	1975
At collective farms - in Kolchosen - v kolchozach			
A. Specialists with higher and specialized secondary education of all branches - Spezialisten mit Hoch-u.mittlerer Fachschulbildung aller Fachrichtungen - Specialistov s vysšim i srednim special'nym obrazovaniem vsech special'nostej	390	482	548
B. of which agricultural specialists - darunter landwirtschaftl.Spezialisten - v tom čisle sel'skochozjajstvennych special'nostej	352	431	479
C. of which agriculturists, zoo engineers, veterinary staff - davon Agronomen, Zootechniker, veterinärmedizinisches Personal - iz nich agronomov, zootechnikov i veterinarnych rabotnikov	234	274	297
At state farms, subsidiary and other agricultural production enterprises - In Sowchosen, Neben-u.anderen landwirtschaftl.Produktionsbetrieben - V sovchozach,podsobnych i pročich proizvodstvennych sel'skochozjajstvennych predprijatijach			
A.	431	555	659
B.	364	456	525
C.	255	307	344
Total at collective and state farms,subsidiary and other agricultural production enterprises - Insgesamt in Kolchosen,Sowchosen,Neben-u.anderen landwirtschaftl.Produktionsbetrieben - Vsego v kolchozach,sovchozach,podsobnych i pročich proizvodstvennych sel'skochozjajstvennych predprijatijach			
A.	821	1,037	1,207
B.	716	887	1,004
C.	489	581	641

5.2.54.4

NUMBER OF SPECIALISTS WITH HIGHER AND SPECIALIZED SECONDARY EDUCATION ENGAGED AT COLLECTIVE AND STATE FARMS, SUBSIDIARY AND OTHER AGRICULTURAL PRODUCTION ENTERPRISES, BY UNION REPUBLICS (November 15, 1973 and November 14, 1975)
ANZAHL DER SPEZIALISTEN MIT HOCH-UND MITTLERER FACHSCHULBILDUNG, DIE IN KOLCHOSEN, SOWCHOSEN, NEBEN- UND ANDEREN LANDWIRTSCHAFTLICHEN PRODUKTIONSBETRIEBEN BESCHÄFTIGT SIND, NACH UNIONSREPUBLIKEN (15.11.1973 und 14.11.1975)
ČISLENNOST' SPECIALISTOV S VYSŠIM I SREDNIM SPECIAL'NYM OBRAZOVANIEM, ZANJATYCH V KOLCHOZACH, SOVCHOZACH, PODSOBNYCH I PROČICH PROIZVODSTVENNYCH SEL'SKOCHOZJAJSTVENNYCH PREDPRIJATIJACH, PO SOJUZNYM RESPUBLIKAM (na 15.11.1973 i 14.11.1975 g.)

	Specialists with high and specialized secondary education, total Spezialisten mit Hoch-u. mittl.Fachschulbildung, insg. Vsego specialistov s vysšim i srednim special'nym obrazovaniem		of which - darunter - v tom čisle			
			Specialists with higher education Spezialisten mit Hochschulbildung specialistov s vysšim obrazovaniem		Specialists with specialized secondary education Spezialisten mit mittl.Fachschulbildung specialistov so sred. special'nym obrazov.	
	1973	1975	1973	1975	1973	1975
SSSR	1,037,334	1,207,450	294,847	341,246	742,487	866,204
RSFSR	496,130	578,115	142,789	163,896	353,341	414,219
Ukrainskaja SSR	233,940	267,027	57,729	66,506	176,211	200,521
Belorusskaja SSR	51,030	60,156	13,483	15,855	37,547	44,301
Uzbekskaja SSR	42,647	51,966	14,739	17,405	27,908	34,561
Kazachskaja SSR	65,358	76,781	19,990	23,618	45,368	53,163
Gruzinskaja SSR	20,689	21,945	9,525	10,221	11,164	11,724
Azerbajdžanskaja SSR	20,765	24,559	5,905	6,951	14,860	17,608
Litovskaja SSR	25,015	28,022	4,373	5,069	20,642	22,953
Moldavskaja SSR	19,547	26,395	6,111	8,146	13,436	18,249
Latvijskaja SSR	17,817	20,176	3,852	4,503	13,965	15,673
Kirgizskaja SSR	11,366	13,157	4,393	4,987	6,973	8,170
Tadžikskaja SSR	7,454	9,028	3,222	3,817	4,232	5,211
Armjanskaja SSR	7,220	8,045	3,172	3,584	4,048	4,461
Turkmenskaja SSR	6,139	6,856	2,470	2,732	3,669	4,124
Estonskaja SSR	12,217	15,222	3,094	3,956	9,123	11,266

5.2.54.5 Economy / Wirtschaft

NUMBER OF LEADING CADRES ON COLLECTIVE FARMS[1] BY JOBS AND UNION REPUBLICS (April 1, 1976; persons)
ANZAHL DER LEITENDEN KADER DER KOLCHOSEN[1] NACH IHREN POSTEN, NACH UNIONSREPUBLIKEN (zum 1.April 1976; Personen)
ČISLENNOST' RUKOVODJAŠČICH RABOTNIKOV KOLCHOZOV PO ZANIMAEMYM DOLŽNOSTJAM PO SOJUZNYM RESPUBLIKAM
(na 1 aprelja 1976 g.; čelovek)

	Collective farm's chairmen – Predsedateli kolchozov – Kolchosovorsitzende	Chief deputies of collective farm's chairmen – Hauptamtliche Stellvertreter der Kolchosvorsitzenden – Osvoboždennye zamestiteli predsedatelej kolchozov	Chief specialists (chief agriculturists, chief zoo engineers, chief veterinarians, chief engineers) – Hauptspezialisten (Chefagronomen, Chefzootechniker, Chefttierärzte, Chefingenieure) – Glavnye specialisty (gl.agronomy, gl.zootechniki, gl.vetvrači, gl.inženery)	Agriculturists – Agronomen – Agronomy	Zoo engineers Zootechniker Zootechniki	Veterinarians, asst. veterinarians, veterinary engineers – Tierärzte, Tierunterärzte, Veterinärtechniker – Vetvrači, vetfel'dšery, vettechniki	Engineers and technicians – Ingenieure und Techniker – Inženery i techniki	Brigadiers in production brigades in agriculture – Brigadiere der Produktionsbrigaden im Ackerbau – Brigadiry proizvodstvennych brigad v zemledelii	Chiefs and brigadiers of cattle-breeding farms – Leiter und Brigadiere der Viehzuchtfarmen – Zavedujuščie i brigadiry životnovodčeskich farm
SSSR	27,737	17,888	88,726	44,854	35,433	51,675	89,007	136,582	83,685
davon Frauen – v tom čisle ženščiny									
RSFSR	12,473	6,222	39,773	18,407	16,954	23,692	40,850	47,315	39,630
Ukrainskaja SSR	7,307	6,502	25,011	14,019	10,632	17,638	23,914	32,996	23,104
Belorusskaja SSR	2,014	1,429	6,843	1,212	1,229	1,835	3,697	8,037	5,114
Uzbekskaja SSR	943	948	2,906	2,751	474	928	4,739	17,091	1,988
Kazachskaja SSR	403	255	1,592	712	940	1,663	2,255	1,787	1,352
Gruzinskaja SSR	744	61	1,175	1,186	329	608	605	5,082	2,361
Azerbajdžanskaja SSR	860	22	1,815	1,113	561	817	1,566	5,696	2,361
Litovskaja SSR	870	975	3,191	1,341	1,407	985	2,664	2,230	2,973
Moldavskaja SSR	462	432	1,416	1,179	490	909	1,753	3,451	1,147
Latvijskaja SSR	378	247	1,382	744	790	684	2,009	1,087	914
Kirgizskaja SSR	214	163	833	475	557	1,046	1,283	1,496	910
Tadžikskaja SSR	212	137	690	572	238	291	1,309	3,736	606
Armjanskaja SSR	372	6	556	142	94	236	254	1,188	770
Turkmenskaja SSR	333	356	967	480	166	69	1,100	4,951	792
Estonskaja SSR	152	133	576	521	572	274	1,009	439	662

1 without fishing cooperatives – ohne Fischfangkolchosen – bez rybolovetskich

Economy 5.2.54.6
Wirtschaft

5.2.54.6 NUMBER OF LEADING CADRES ON STATE FARMS BY JOBS AND UNION REPUBLICS (April 1, 1976; persons)
ANZAHL DER LEITENDEN KADER DER SOWCHOSEN NACH IHREN POSTEN, NACH UNIONSREPUBLIKEN (1.April 1976;Personen)
ČISLENNOST' RUKOVODJAŠČICH RABOTNIKOV SOVCHOZOV PO ZANIMAEMYM DOLŽNOSTJAM PO SOJUZNYM RESPUBLIKAM
(na 1 aprelja 1976 g.; čelovek)

	Directors of the state farms – Direktoren der Sowchosen – Direktora sovchozov	Heads of departments (farms) – Leiter der Abteilungen (Farmen) – Upravljajuščie otdelenijami (fermami)	Chief specialists (chief agriculturists,chief zoo engineers, chief veterinarians, chief engineers – Hauptspezialisten (Chefagronomen, Chefzootechniker, Chefleiterärzte, Chefingenieure) – Glavnye specialisty (gl.agronomy, gl.zootechniki, gl.vetvrači, gl.inženery)	Agriculturists – Agronomen – Agronomy	Zoo engineers – Zootechniker – Zootechniki	Veterinarians, sub-veterinarians, veterinary engineers – Tierärzte, Tierunterärzte, Veterinärtechniker – Vetvrači, vetfel'dšery, vettechniki	Engineers and technicians – Ingenieure und Techniker – Inženery i techniki	Brigadiers of the production brigades in agriculture – Brigadiere der Produktionsbrigaden im Ackerbau – Brigadiry proizvodstvennych brigad v zemledelii	Chiefs and brigadiers of cattle-breeding farms – Leiter und Brigadiere der Viehzuchtfarmen – Zavedujuščie i brigadiry životnovodčeskich ferm
SSSR	18,876	40,769	70,732	43,375	42,416	57,755	110,315	99,187	69,753
of which females – davon Frauen – v tom čisle ženščiny	295	2,072	8,247	12,428	19,358	21,687	8,203	17,652	28,247
RSFSR	11,176	24,798	41,931	24,096	25,821	34,788	63,238	45,659	44,561
Ukrainskaja SSR	1,711	4,006	6,774	4,554	3,376	5,325	13,356	9,735	7,887
Belorusskaja SSR	901	405	3,450	1,118	1,295	2,520	4,103	4,275	3,044
Uzbekskaja SSR	583	2,337	2,035	2,900	1,042	1,585	6,055	13,714	1,370
Kazachskaja SSR	1,873	4,900	7,340	5,436	7,280	8,479	12,849	7,930	4,475
Gruzinskaja SSR	379	1,093	1,128	1,113	271	673	971	3,949	1,254
Azerbajdžanskaja SSR	507	247	1,765	1,113	348	726	1,368	4,159	1,237
Litovskaja SSR	345	1,163	1,381	545	602	599	1,320	903	1,507
Moldavskaja SSR	257	191	891	622	206	281	1,790	2,058	435
Latvijskaja SSR	246	423	942	566	586	618	1,790	873	983
Kirgizskaja SSR	158	324	559	276	493	865	919	1,117	412
Tadžikskaja SSR	161	254	537	280	199	402	845	1,984	429
Armjanskaja SSR	358	11	1,164	185	202	397	376	1,472	1,041
Turkmenskaja SSR	56	122	170	73	126	111	195	546	23
Estonskaja SSR	165	495	665	498	569	386	1,140	813	1,095

313

5.2.54.7 Economy / Wirtschaft

5.2.54.7 NUMBER OF MECHANIST-CADRES AT COLLECTIVE AND STATE FARMS (April 1; thousands)
ANZAHL DER MECHANISATOREN-KADER IN DEN KOLCHOSEN UND SOWCHOSEN (zum 1.April; Tsd.Personen)
ČISLENNOST' MECHANIZATORSKICH KADROV V KOLCHOZACH I SOVCHOZACH (na 1 aprelja; tys.čelovek)

	1940	1965	1971	1972	1973	1974	1975	1976	1977
Number of tractorists-machinists, tractorists, harvester drivers and motorcar drivers, total – Zahl der Traktoristen-Maschinisten, Traktoristen, Kombineführer und Kraftfahrer, insg. – Čislennost' traktoristov-mašinistov, traktoristov, kombajnerov i šoferov, vsego	1,401	3,094	3,503	3,532	3,595	3,798	3,941	4,074	4,161.8
of which – darunter – v tom čisle:									
at collective farms – in Kolchosen – v kolchozach	1,298	1,876	2,068	2,053	2,087	2,148	2,181	2,181	2,203.1
at state farms – in Sowchosen – v sovchozach	103	1,218	1,435	1,479	1,508	1,650	1,732	1,850	1,958.7
From the total number of mechanist-cadres – Aus der Gesamtzahl der Mechanisatoren-Kader – Iz obščej čislennosti mechanizatorskich kadrov:									
Tractorists-machinists, tractorists, harvester drivers, total – Traktoristen-Maschinisten, Traktoristen, Kombineführer, insg. – traktoristov-mašinistov, traktoristov, kombajnerov, vsego	1,237	2,245	2,449	2,459	2,494	2,636	2,736	2,810	2,853.7
of which – darunter – v tom čisle:									
at collective farms – in Kolchosen – v kolchozach	1,153	1,383	1,476	1,457	1,473	1,518	1,542	1,541	1,549.0
at state farms – in Sowchosen – v sovchozach	84	862	973	1,002	1,021	1,118	1,176	1,242	1,304.7
Motorcar drivers, total – Kraftfahrer, insg. – šoferov, vsego	164	849	1,054	1,073	1,101	1,162	1,205	1,264	1,308.1
of which – darunter – v tom čisle:									
at collective farms – in Kolchosen – v kolchozach	145	493	592	596	614	630	639	646	654.1
at state farms – in Sowchosen – v sovchozach	19	356	462	477	487	532	556	608	654.0

Economy 5.2.54.8
Wirtschaft

5.2.54.8 NUMBER OF MECHANIST-CADRES AT COLLECTIVE AND STATE FARMS
BY UNION REPUBLICS (April 1, 1976; thousands
ANZAHL DER MECHANISATOREN-KADER IN DEN KOLCHOSEN UND SOWCHOSEN
NACH UNIONSREPUBLIKEN (zum 1.April 1976; Tsd.Personen)
ČISLENNOST' MECHANIZATORSKICH KADROV V KOLCHOZACH I SOVCHOZACH
PO SOJUZNYM RESPUBLIKAM (na 1 aprelja 1976 g.; tys.čelovek)

	at collective farms-in Kolchosen- v kolchozach		at state farms - in Sowchosen - v sovchozach		
	Tractorists-machinists, tractorists, harvester drivers Traktoristen-Maschinisten, Traktoristen, Kombineführer traktoristov-mašinistov, traktoristov, kombajnerov	Motorcar drivers Kraftfahrer Šoferov			Total (A,B) Insg. (A,B) Vsego (A,B)
	A.	B.	A.	B.	
SSSR	1540.8	640.4	1242.1	608.2	4074.0
RSFSR	674.0	268.7	734.3	341.7	2029.4
Ukrainskaja SSR	466.2	203.8	125.4	74.7	874.4
Belorusskaja SSR	85.1	34.6	49.5	24.2	194.0
Uzbekskaja SSR	94.6	23.6	60.7	20.5	201.2
Kazachskaja SSR	37.8	18.5	177.9	87.2	321.8
Gruzinskaja SSR	6.9	7.4	8.4	7.3	30.9
Azerbajdžanskaja SSR	14.8	10.3	10.2	8.9	44.6
Litovskaja SSR	29.3	14.3	14.0	7.3	64.9
Moldavskaja SSR	36.9	15.5	17.1	8.0	99.7
Latvijskaja SSR	15.9	8.9	12.0	6.4	43.2
Kirgizskaja SSR	16.5	9.1	10.0	6.6	42.6
Tadžikskaja SSR	19.0	8.3	8.2	5.1	40.9
Armjanskaja SSR	4.1	3.8	3.9	4.7	16.6
Turkmenskaja SSR	31.9	9.3	2.1	1.4	45.1
Estonskaja SSR	7.8	4.3	8.4	4.2	24.7

5.3 TRANSPORT AND COMMUNICATIONS — TRANSPORT-, POST- UND FERNMELDEWESEN — TRANSPORT I SVJAZ'

5.3.1 Economy / Wirtschaft

FREIGHT TRANSPORT BY ALL TYPES OF PUBLIC TRANSPORT ('000 million ton-kilometres)
GÜTERTRANSPORTLEISTUNG ALLER TRANSPORTZWEIGE DES ÖFFENTLICHEN VERKEHRS (Mrd.Tonnen-Kilometer)
GRUZOOBOROT VSECH VIDOV TRANSPORTA OBSČEGO POL'ZOVANIJA (mlrd. tonno-kilometrov)

Year Jahr Gody	All types of transport Alle Transportzweige Vse vidy transporta A.	Railway Eisenbahn Železnodorožnyj B.	Marine Seeschiffahrt morskoj C.	Inland navigation Binnenschiffahrt rečnoj D.	Pipelines (oil and oil products) Rohrfernleitungen (Erdöl und Erdölprodukte) truboprovodnyj (nefte-i nefteproduktoprovody) E.	Motor transport Kraftverkehr avtomobil'nyj F.	Air transport Luftverkehr vozdušnyj G.
1913[1]	114.5	65.7	19.9	28.5	0.3	0.1	--
1913[2]	126.0	76.4	20.3	28.9	0.3	0.1	--
1928	119.5	93.4	9.3	15.9	0.7	0.2	--
1932	218.4	169.3	20.1	25.0	2.9	1.1	0.0
1937	434.4	354.8	36.8	33.3	3.6	5.9	0.02
1940	487.6	415.0	23.8	36.1	3.8	8.9	0.02
1945	374.8	314.0	34.2	18.8	2.7	5.0	0.06
1946	395.5	335.0	29.4	20.6	2.9	7.5	0.08
1950	713.3	602.3	39.7	46.2	4.9	20.1	0.14
1955	1,165.0	970.9	68.9	67.7	14.7	42.5	0.25
1960	1,885.7	1,504.3	131.5	99.6	51.2	98.5	0.56
1965	2,764.0	1,950.2	388.8	133.9	146.7	143.1	1.34
1966	2,918.3	2,016.0	442.8	137.7	165.0	155.3	1.45
1967	3,186.8	2,160.5	527.1	143.9	183.4	170.2	1.66
1968	3,421.8	2,274.8	586.8	155.4	215.9	187.1	1.80
1969	3,575.1	2,367.1	601.3	160.1	244.6	200.1	1.95
1970	3,829.2	2,494.7	656.1	174.0	281.7	220.8	1.88
1971	4,088.0	2,637.3	696.0	183.8	328.5	240.4	1.98

1 within the borders of the U.S.S.R. up to 17.9.1939 – in den Grenzen der UdSSR bis 17.9.1939 – v granicach SSSR do 17 sentjabrja 1939 g.
2 in the present borders of the U.S.S.R. – in den heutigen Grenzen der UdSSR – v sovremennych granicach SSSR

Economy 5.3.1
Wirtschaft 5.3.2

	A.	B.	C.	D.	E.	F.	G.
1972	4,275.7	2,760.8	698.4	180.3	375.9	258.1	2.19
1973	4,623.8	2,958.0	750.7	189.5	439.4	283.8	2.37
1974	4,936.5	3,097.7	778.1	212.3	533.4	312.5	2.49
1975	5,200.8	3,236.5	736.2	221.7	665.8	338.0	2.59
1976	5,432.3	3,295.4	762.1	222.7	794.6	354.8	2.71
1977 (Plan)	5,787.8	3,440.0	824.1	239.9	896.0	385.0	2.82

5.3.2 PASSENGER TRANSPORT BY ALL TYPES OF PUBLIC TRANSPORT ('000 million ton-kilometres)
PERSONENBEFÖRDERUNGSLEISTUNG ALLER TRANSPORTZWEIGE DES ÖFFENTLICHEN VERKEHRS (Mrd.Passagier-Kilometer)
PASSAŽIROOBOROT VSECH VIDOV TRANSPORTA OBŠČEGO POL'ZOVANIJA (milliardov passažiro-kilometrov)

Year Jahr Gody	All types of transport Alle Transportzweige Vse vidy transporta A.	Railway Eisenbahn Železnodorožnyj B.	Marine Seeschiffahrt morskoj C.	Inland navigation Binnenschiffahrt rečnoj D.	Motor transport (buses) Autoverkehr (Öffentliche Busse) avtomobil'nyj (avtobusy obščego pol'zovanija) E.	Air transport Luftverkehr vozdušnyj F.
1913[1]	27.6	25.2	1.0	1.4	--	--
1913[2]	32.7	30.3	1.0	1.4	--	--
1928	27.1	24.5	0.3	2.1	--	--
1932	89.9	83.7	1.0	4.5	0.2	0.0
1937	97.3	90.9	0.9	3.2	0.7	0.01
1940	106.3	98.0	0.9	3.8	2.2	0.1
1945	69.8	65.9	0.6	2.3	3.4	0.2
1946	105.3	97.9	1.4	3.2	0.5	0.5
1950	98.3	88.0	1.2	2.7	1.8	1.0
1955	170.2	141.4	1.5	3.6	5.2	1.2
1960	249.5	170.8	1.3	4.3	20.9	2.8
1965	366.6	201.6	1.5	4.9	61.0	12.1
1966	408.3	219.4	1.6	5.2	120.5	38.1
1967	447.9	234.4	1.7	5.3	137.0	45.1
1968	492.0	254.1	1.8	5.5	153.0	53.5
					168.5	62.1

1 within the borders of the U.S.S.R. up to 17.9.1939 - in den Grenzen der UdSSR bis 17.9.1939 - v granicach SSSR do 17 sentjabrja 1939 g.
2 in the present borders of the U.S.S.R. - in den heutigen Grenzen der UdSSR - v sovremennych granicach SSSR

317

5.3.2 Economy
5.3.3.1 Wirtschaft

	A.	B.	C.	D.	E.	F.
1969	523.0	261.3	1.7	5.5	183.0	71.5
1970	553.1	265.4	1.6	5.4	202.5	78.2
1971	586.6	274.6	1.7	5.7	215.8	88.8
1972	624.9	285.8	1.9	5.7	235.6	95.9
1973	657.1	296.6	1.9	5.9	253.9	98.8
1974	702.4	306.3	2.1	6.1	279.1	108.8
1975	747.1	312.5	2.1	6.3	303.6	122.6
1976	779.6	315.1	2.4	6.0	325.3	130.8
1977 (Plan)	811.6	323.0	2.4	6.4	342.3	137.5

5.3.3 RAILWAY TRANSPORT — EISENBAHNTRANSPORT — ŽELEZNODOROŽNYJ TRANSPORT

5.3.3.1 LENGTH OF RAILWAY NETWORK FROM THE MINISTRY OF RAILWAYS (END-OF-YEAR FIGURES); '000 kilometres
LÄNGE DES BENUTZTEN EISENBAHNNETZES DES MINISTERIUMS FÜR VERKEHRSWESEN (ZUM JAHRESENDE); Tsd. km
EKSPLUATACIONNAJA DLINA ŽELEZNYCH DOROG MINISTERSTVA PUTEJ SOOBŠČENIJA (NA KONEC GODA); tys.km

	Total length of railway network Gesamtlänge des benutzten Eisenbahnnetzes Vsja ekspluatacionnaja dlina železnych dorog	of which electrified davon elektrifiziert iz nich elektrificirovannych	Year Jahr Gody		
Year Jahr Gody	A.	B.		A.	B.
1913[1]	58.5	--	1966	132.5	27.0
1913[2]	71.7	--	1967	133.3	29.1
1928	76.9	--	1968	133.6	30.8
1932	81.8	0.06	1969	134.6	32.4
1937	84.9	1.6	1970	135.2	33.9
1940	106.1	1.9	1971	135.4	35.0
1945	112.9	2.0	1972	136.3	36.2
1946	114.1	2.1	1973	136.8	37.2
1950	116.9	3.0	1974	137.5	38.1
1955	120.7	5.4	1975	138.3	38.9
1960	125.8	13.8	1976	138.5	39.7
1965	131.4	24.9			

1 within the borders of the U.S.S.R. up to 17.9.1939 — in den Grenzen der UdSSR bis 17.9.1939 — v granicach SSSR

5.3.3.2 LENGTH OF RAILWAY NETWORK FROM THE MINISTRY OF RAILWAYS BY UNION REPUBLICS (END-OF-YEAR FIGURES); '000 kilometres

LÄNGE DES BENUTZTEN EISENBAHNNETZES DES MINISTERIUMS FÜR VERKEHRSWESEN NACH UNIONSREPUBLIKEN (ZUM JAHRESENDE); Tsd. km

EKSPLUATACIONNAJA DLINA ŽELEZNYCH DOROG MINISTERSTVA PUTEJ SOOBŠCENIJA PO SOJUZNYM RESPUBLIKAM (NA KONEC GODA); tys. km

	1940	1965	1970	1971	1972	1973	1974	1975	1976
SSSR	106.1	131.4	135.2	135.4	136.3	136.8	137.5	138.3	138.5
RSFSR	58.68	75.44	77.55	77.59	78.21	78.64	78.93	79.75	79.87
Ukrainskaja SSR	20.10	21.73	22.06	22.09	22.12	22.15	22.23	22.27	22.24
Belorusskaja SSR	6.44	5.35	5.43	5.45	5.44	5.46	5.46	5.46	5.47
Uzbekskaja SSR	1.91	2.71	2.95	2.95	3.28	3.29	3.34	3.38	3.38
Kazachskaja SSR	6.58	12.47	13.77	13.89	14.09	14.08	14.12	14.12	14.14
Gruzinskaja SSR	1.13	1.41	1.41	1.42	1.42	1.42	1.42	1.42	1.42
Azerbajdžanskaja SSR	1.21	1.73	1.81	1.81	1.84	1.85	1.85	1.85	1.85
Litovskaja SSR	2.01	2.02	2.02	2.02	1.95	1.96	2.00	2.00	2.00
Moldavskaja SSR	0.82	1.03	1.07	1.11	1.11	1.11	1.11	1.11	1.11
Latvijskaja SSR	3.21	2.82	2.61	2.60	2.48	2.48	2.45	2.43	2.46
Kirgizskaja SSR	0.22	0.37	0.37	0.37	0.37	0.37	0.37	0.37	0.37
Tadžikskaja SSR	0.25	0.26	0.26	0.26	0.26	0.26	0.43	0.43	0.45
Armjanskaja SSR	0.40	0.55	0.56	0.56	0.58	0.58	0.59	0.59	0.71
Turkmenskaja SSR	1.75	2.10	2.11	2.11	2.12	2.12	2.12	2.12	2.12
Estonskaja SSR	1.39	1.40	1.20	1.18	1.02	1.00	1.03	1.00	0.95

5.3.3.3 PASSENGER TRAFFIC BY RAILWAY – PERSONENBEFÖRDERUNG PER BAHN – PASSAŽIROOBOROT ŽELEZNODOROŽNYM TRANSPORTOM

	1940	1965	1970	1971	1972	1973	1974	1975	1976
Passenger traffic, '000 mill.passenger-kilom. – Personenbeförderung, Mrd.Passagier-km – Passažirooborot, mlrd.passažiro-kilometr.	100.4	201.6	265.4	274.6	285.8	296.6	306.3	312.5	315.1
A.of which in suburban traffic-darunter im Vorortverkehr-v tom čisle v prigorodnom soob.	26.5	51.6	71.8	75.7	79.8	83.7	85.9	88.7	91.0
Passengers carried, mill.persons – Beförderte Passagiere, Mio Personen – Perevezeno passažirov, mln.čelovek	1,377	2,301	2,930	3,053	3,167	3,306	3,389	3,470	3,545
A.	1,025	2,049	2,616	2,729	2,837	2,970	3,048	3,130	3,201
Average travel distance of passengers, km – Durchschnittl.Reiseentfernung d.Passagiere,km – Srednjaja dal'nost'poezdki passažirov, km	73	88	91	90	90	90	90	90	89
A.	26	25	27	28	28	28	28	28	28

5.3.4.1 Economy / Wirtschaft

5.3.4 MARINE TRANSPORT - SEETRANSPORT - MORSKOJ TRANSPORT

5.3.4.1 BASIC INDICATORS OF MARINE TRANSPORT FROM THE MINISTRY OF THE HIGH-SEA FLEET[1]
GRUNDKENNZIFFERN DES SEETRANSPORTS DES MINISTERIUMS FÜR HOCHSEESCHIFFAHRT[1]
OSNOVNYE POKAZATELI MORSKOGO TRANSPORTA MINISTERSTVA MORSKOGO FLOTA[1]

	1940	1965	1970	1971	1972	1973	1974	1975	1976
Freight turnover, '000 mill.tons nautical miles - Frachtumsatz, Mrd.t Seemeilen - Gruzooborot, mlrd. tonnomil'	13.4	209.9	354.3	375.8	377.1	405.4	420.2	397.5	411.5
Goods carried, mill.tons - Beförderte Güter, Mio t - Perevezeno gruzov, mln.t	32.9	119.3	161.9	170.9	178.0	186.7	192.2	200.0	214.5
Average transport distance, 1 ton goods-nautical mile - durchschnittl.Transportentfernung, 1 t Güter-Seemeile - srednjaja dal'nost' perevozki 1 t gruza-mil'	409	1,759	2,188	2,199	2,118	2,171	2,186	1,988	1,919
Passenger turnover, mill.passenger-nautical miles - Passagierumsatz, Mio Passagier-Seemeilen - Passažirooborot,mln.passažiro-mil'	480	796	859	928	1,012	1,048	1,127	1,153	1,306
Passengers carried, mill.persons - Beförderte Passagiere, Mio Personen - Perevezeno passažirov, mln.čelovek	9.7	37.2	38.5	38.4	43.3	45.3	48.9	51.6	49.9
Average travel distance per passenger, nautical mile - durchschnittl.Reiseentfernung pro Passagier, Seemeile - srednjaja dal'nost' poezdki odonogo passažira, mil'	50	21	22	24	23	23	23	22	26

1 without Central Asian steam navigation - ohne Mittelasiatische Dampfschiffahrt - bez Sredneaziatskogo parochodstva

5.3.6.1 Economy
5.3.6.2 Wirtschaft

5.3.6 PIPELINE – ROHRFERNLEITUNGEN – MAGISTRAL'NYJ TRUBOPROVODNYJ TRANSPORT

5.3.6.1 PIPELINE FOR PETROLEUM AND PETROLEUM PRODUCTS – ROHRFERNLEITUNGEN FÜR ERDÖL UND ERDÖLPRODUKTE – NEFTE- I NEFTEPRODUKTOPROVODY

Year Jahr Gody	Length (end-of-year figures), '000 km Länge (zum Jahresende), Tsd.km Protjažennost' (na konec goda), tys.km A.	Transfer of petroleum and petroleum products, mill.tons Umpumpen von Erdölprodukten, Mio t Perekačka nefti i nefteproduktov, mln.t B.	Freight turnover, '000 mill.t/km Frachtumsatz, Mrd.t/km Gruzooborot, mlrd. tkm C.
1913	1.1	0.4	0.3
1928	1.6	1.1	0.7
1932	2.9	4.8	2.9
1937	3.9	7.5	3.6
1940	4.1	7.9	3.8
1945	4.4	5.6	2.7
1946	4.4	6.0	2.9
1950	5.4	15.3	4.9
1955	10.4	51.7	14.7
1960	17.3	129.9	51.2
1965	28.2	225.7	146.7
1966	29.5	247.7	165.0

Year Jahr Gody	A.	B.	C.
1967	32.4	273.3	183.4
1968	34.1	301.3	215.9
1969	36.9	324.0	244.6
1970	37.4	339.9	281.7
1971	41.0	352.5	328.5
1972	42.9	388.5	375.9
1973	47.2	421.4	439.4
1974	53.0	457.2	533.4
1975	56.9	497.6	665.8
1976	58.6	531.7	794.6

5.3.6.2 GAS LINES – GASLEITUNGEN – GAZOPROVODY

	1950	1965	1970	1971	1972	1973	1974	1975	1976
Length (end-of-year figures), '000 km – Länge (zum Jahresende), Tsd.km – Protjažennost' (na konec goda), tys.km	2.3	41.8	67.5	71.5	77.7	83.5	92.1	99.2	103.5
Gas transport, '000 mill.cu.m, – Gasförderung, Mrd.m^3 – Podača gaza, mlrd.m^3	1.5	112.1	181.5	209.8	219.9	231.1	245.7	279.4	309.5

Economy
Wirtschaft 5.3.5.2

5.3.5.2 FREIGHT CARRIED AND PASSENGER TRAFFIC IN PUBLIC INLAND WATER TRANSPORT, BY UNION REPUBLICS
GÜTERTRANSPORT UND PERSONENBEFÖRDERUNG IM ÖFFENTLICHEN BINNENWASSERTRANSPORT, NACH UNIONSREPUBLIKEN
PEREVOZKI GRUZOV I PASSAŽIROV REČNYM TRANSPORTOM OBŠČEGO POL'ZOVANIJA PO SOJUZNYM RESPUBLIKAM

	1940	1965	1970	1971	1972	1973	1974	1975
Freight carried, '000 tons – Beförderte Güter, Tsd.t – Perevezeno gruzov, tys.t								
SSSR	73,934	269,443	357,760	381,231	395,728	419,162	452,378	475,457
RSFSR	65,006	238,169	311,039	330,043	340,219	359,011	386,823	405,905
Ukrainskaja SSR	4,637	17,351	27,283	29,781	32,163	35,424	38,590	42,303
Belorusskaja SSR	1,681	3,480	5,295	5,991	6,751	7,466	8,646	8,770
Kazachskaja SSR	628	3,936	5,647	6,451	7,221	7,605	7,758	7,559
Litovskaja SSR	146	1,035	1,578	1,652	1,854	2,022	2,157	2,249
Moldavskaja SSR	9	728	1,378	1,479	1,901	1,909	2,217	2,343
Latvijskaja SSR	637	1,613	2,233	2,422	2,434	2,475	2,657	2,648
Central Asian Shipping Company of the Ministry of High-Sea Fleet – Mittelasiatische Reederei des Ministeriums für Hochseeschiffahrt – Sredneaziatskoe parochodstvo Ministerstva morskogo flota	873	2,749	2,752	2,810	2,590	2,638	2,885	3,054
Passengers carried, thousands – Beförderte Passagiere, Tsd.Personen – Perevezeno passažirov, tys.čelovek								
SSSR	73,401	133,901	145,202	146,466	150,403	146,666	152,289	161,425
RSFSR	63,909	109,073	116,738	116,372	118,298	114,501	118,822	124,084
Ukrainskaja SSR	6,810	18,692	21,379	22,587	23,715	23,514	24,681	27,914
Belorusskaja SSR	1,964	1,759	1,324	1,296	1,363	1,315	1,358	1,293
Kazachskaja SSR	177	438	1,135	1,268	1,501	1,545	1,638	1,662
Litovskaja SSR	150	1,230	1,989	2,265	2,409	2,699	2,509	2,872
Moldavskaja SSR	39	1,708	1,604	1,595	2,091	2,170	2,362	2,442
Latvijskaja SSR	190	702	784	835	837	773	782	1,010
Central Asian Shipping Company of the Ministry of High-Sea Fleet – Mittelasiatische Reederei des Ministeriums für Hochseeschiffahrt – Sredneaziatskoe parochodstvo Ministerstva morskogo flota	78	–	–	–	–	–	–	–

323

5.3.5.1 Economy / Wirtschaft

	1940	1965	1970	1971	1972	1973	1974	1975	1976
dry cargoes – trockene Güter – suchogruzy	31.0	167.3	252.5	274.7	294.6	319.0	346.4	371.2	378.8
of which – davon – iz nich:									
Wood and timber in boats – Holz und Brennholz in Schiffen – les i drova v sudach	7.6	20.0	19.4	19.7	19.3	19.1	20.1	20.2	19.4
Bituminous coal and coke – Steinkohle und Koks – kamennyj ugol' i koks	2.2	14.4	17.6	18.6	18.8	20.4	22.1	23.4	24.0
Ore – Erz – ruda	0.1	3.4	5.2	5.2	5.9	6.5	7.8	8.9	–
Mineral construction materials – Mineralbaustoffe – mineral'nye stroitel'nye materialy	7.6	107.8	180.9	200.1	219.8	239.3	259.6	281.0	288.5
of which cement–darunter Zement– v tom čisle cement	0.4	1.1	1.7	1.7	1.8	2.2	2.2	2.4	–
Chemical cargoes and mineral fertilizers – chemische Güter und Mineraldünger – chimičeskie gruzy i mineral'nye udobrenija	0.4	1.2	1.7	1.8	2.1	2.1	2.6	2.9	–
Metals and scrap iron – Metalle und Schrott – metally i metallolom	0.5	1.1	2.0	2.3	2.6	2.7	3.2	3.6	3.6
Grain – Getreide – chlebnye gruzy	5.2	5.6	6.8	7.1	5.5	7.3	7.0	6.0	6.6
Fruits and vegetables – Früchte und Gemüse – plody i ovošči	0.8	0.6	0.6	0.6	0.6	0.7	0.8	0.7	–
Average transport distance of 1 t cargo, km – durchschnittl.Transportentfernung von 1 t Güter,km – srednjaja dal'nost'perevozki 1 t gruza, km	489	497	486	482	456	452	469	466	459
Passenger turnover, '000 mill.passenger-km – Passagierumsatz, Mrd.Passagier-km – Passažirooborot, mlrd.passažiro-kilometrov	3.8	4.9	5.4	5.7	5.7	5.9	6.1	6.3	6.0
Passengers carried, mill.persons – Beförderte Passagiere, Mio Personen – Perevezeno passažirov, mln.čelovek	73.0	133.9	145.2	146.5	150.4	146.7	152.3	161.4	145.3
Average travel distance per passenger, km – durchschnittl.Reiseentfernung pro Passagier, km – srednjaja dal'nost'poezdki odnogo passažira, km	52	37	37	39	38	40	40	39	42

5.3.5 INLAND WATER TRANSPORT – BINNENWASSERTRANSPORT – REČNOJ TRANSPORT

5.3.5.1 BASIC INDICATORS ON PUBLIC INLAND WATERWAY TRANSPORT
GRUNDKENNZIFFERN DES ÖFFENTLICHEN BINNENWASSERTRANSPORTS
OSNOVNYE POKAZATELI REČNOGO TRANSPORTA OBŠČEGO POL'ZOVANIJA

(Ministry of Inland Navigation of the RSFSR, Administrations and shipping companies of the union republics, district administrations of inland navigation,and the Central Asian Shipping Company of the Ministry of the High-Sea Fleet)
(Ministerium für Binnenschiffahrt der RSFSR, Verwaltungen und Reedereien der Binnenschiffahrt der Unionsrepubliken, Gebietsverwaltungen der Binnenschiffahrt und die Mittelasiatische Reederei des Ministeriums für Hochseeschiffahrt)
(Ministerstvo rečnogo flota RSFSR, upravlenija i parochodstva rečnogo transporta sojuznych respublik, oblrečtransy i Sredneaziatskoe parochodstvo Ministerstva morskogo flota)

	1940	1965	1970	1971	1972	1973	1974	1975	1976
Length of the navigable inland waterways used by all organizations, '000 kilometres – Länge der schiffbaren Binnenwasserstraßen, die von allen Organisationen benutzt werden, Tsd.km – Protjažennost'vnutrennich vodnych sudochodnych putej soobščenija, ekspluatirovavšichsja vsemi organizacijami, tys.km	108.9	142.7	144.5	144.6	146.1	145.6	146.3	145.4	146.4
Length of the artificial navigable waterways, '000 kilometres – Länge der künstlichen schiffbaren Wasserstraßen, Tsd.km – Protjažennost' iskusstvennych vodnych sudochodnych putej soobščenija, tys.km	4.2	16.6	18.6	18.8	18.8	19.0	19.1	19.6	20.4
Freight turnover, '000 mill.tons/kilometres – Frachtumsatz, Mrd. t/km – Gruzooborot, mlrd.tkm	36.1	133.9	174.0	183.8	180.3	189.5	212.3	221.7	222.7
Goods carried, mill.tons – beförderte Güter, Mio t – perevezeno gruzov, mln.t	73.9	269.4	357.8	381.2	395.7	419.2	452.4	475.5	484.9
of which – darunter – v tom čisle: Petroleum and petrpleum products – Erdöl und Erdölprodukte – neft' i nefteprodukty	9,6	25,0	33.5	35.2	33.7	33.9	37.8	39.0	38.1
Wood and timber in rafts – Holz und Brennholz in Flößen – les i drova v plotach	33.3	77.1	71.8	71.3	67.5	66.3	68.2	65.3	68.0

Economy 5.3.7.1
Wirtschaft 5.3.7.2

5.3.7 MOTOR TRANSPORT - KRAFTVERKEHR - AVTOMOBIL'NYJ TRANSPORT

5.3.7.1 BASIC INDICATORS FOR FREIGHT TRANSPORT
GRUNDKENNZIFFERN DES VOLKSWIRTSCHAFTLICHEN KRAFTVERKEHRS
OSNOVNYE POKAZATELI AVTOMOBIL'NOGO TRANSPORTA NARODNOGO CHOZJAJSTVA

Year Jahr Gody	Freight turnover, '000 mill.t/km Frachtumsatz, Mrd. t/km Gruzooborot, mlrd. tkm	Goods carried, mill.tons Beförderte Güter, Mio t Perevezeno gruzov, mln.t	Average transport distance of 1 t goods, km Durchschnittl.Beförderungs- entfernung pro t Güter,km Srednjaja dal'nost' pere- vozki 1 t gruza, km
1940	8.9	858.6	10.4
1945	5.0	420.0	12.0
1946	7.5	610.0	12.3
1950	20.1	1,859.2	10.8
1955	42.5	3,730.0	11.4
1960	98.5	8,492.7	11.6
1965	143.1	10,746.0	13.3
1966	155.3	11,457.3	13.6
1967	170.2	11,947.0	14.2
1968	187.1	12,800.4	14.6
1969	200.1	13,392.1	14.9
1970	220.8	14,622.8	15.1
1971	240.4	15,688.2	15.3
1972	258.1	16,703.8	15.5
1973	283.8	18,243.5	15.6
1974	312	19,600	15.9
1975	338	21,000	16.1
1976	355	21,500	16.5

5.3.7.2 LENGTH OF MOTOR ROADS WITH HARD PAVEMENT (END-OF-YEAR FIGURES); '000 km
LÄNGE DER AUTOSTRASSEN MIT HARTER DECKE (ZUM JAHRESENDE); Tsd.km
PROTJAŽENNOST' AVTOMOBIL'NYCH DOROG S TVERDYM POKRYTIEM (NA KONEC GODA); tys.km

Year Jahr Gody	Total roads with hard pavement Alle Straßen mit harter Decke Vse dorogi s tverdym pokrytiem	of which improved (with cement-asphalt concrete and bituminous pavement) davon verbesserte (mit Zement-Asphalt- beton- und Schwarzdecke) iz nich usoveršenstvovannye (s cementno- asfal'tobetonnym pokrytiem i černoe šosse)
1940	143.4	7.1
1945	155.3	10.2
1946	164.6	13.4
1950	177.3	19.2
1955	206.8	41.1
1960	270.8	77.1
1965	378.3	131.7
1966	405.6	146.0
1967	433.0	161.1
1968	456.4	176.7
1969	483.2	191.0
1970	511.6	207.0
1971	540.4	224.3
1972	567.3	241.5
1973	598.4	260.1
1974	628.3	277.8
1975	660.5	296.7
1976	689.7	315.1

5.3.7.3 Economy / Wirtschaft

5.3.7.3 LENGTH OF MOTOR ROADS BY UNION REPUBLICS
LÄNGE DER AUTOSTRASSEN NACH UNIONSREPUBLIKEN
PROTJAŻENNOST' AVTOMOBIL'NYCH DOROG PO SOJUZNYM

	1940 A. All roads / Alle Straßen / Vse dorogi	1940 B. of which with hard pavement / darunter mit harter Decke / v tom čisle s tverdym pokrytiem	1965 A.	1965 B.	1970 A.	1970 B.	1971 A.	1971 B.
SSSR	1531.2	143.4	1362.7	378.3	1363.9	511.6	1369.6	540.4
RSFSR	872.9	67.8	747.4	168.1	751.7	221.5	757.5	233.2
Ukrainskaja SSR	270.7	29.3	236.1	67.2	223.5	90.8	221.3	96.7
Belorusskaja SSR	69.7	11.2	65.2	18.6	65.8	25.8	66.0	27.1
Uzbekskaja SSR	31.6	4.3	27.5	13.7	28.3	20.7	29.1	23.0
Kazachskaja SSR	106.6	1.5	109.3	24.4	110.3	41.1	110.0	44.
Gruzinskaja SSR	13.6	8.1	19.5	14.7	20.9	16.4	21.1	16.
Azerbajdżanskaja SSR	11.0	3.0	19.3	10.3	21.1	13.4	21.2	13.
Litovskaja SSR	37.8	2.2	33.2	11.9	33.5	14.5	33.4	14.
Moldavskaja SSR	15.0	1.1	12.9	5.4	10.2	7.1	10.2	7.
Latvijskaja SSR	36.0	2.6	24.0	8.1	24.2	11.1	24.2	11.
Kirgizskaja SSR	11.5	1.2	17.8	8.4	19.6	11.4	19.6	11.
Tadżikskaja SSR	13.5	0.9	12.3	4.8	13.4	8.0	13.4	8.
Armjanskaja SSR	7.2	2.6	8.1	4.9	8.3	5.4	8.4	5.
Turkmenskaja SSR	11.9	0.5	7.7	2.4	8.7	4.7	8.7	5.
Estonskaja SSR	22.2	7.1	22.4	15.4	24.4	19.7	25.4	21.

(END-OF-YEAR FIGURES); '000 kilometres
(ZUM JAHRESENDE); Tsd. km
RESPUBLIKAM (NA KONEC GODA); tys.km

1972		1973		1974		1975		1976	
A.	B.	A.	B.	A.	B.	A.	B.	A.	B.
1359.8	567.3	1398.0	598.4	1421.6	628.3	1403.0	660.5	1405.6	689.7
758.5	245.3	796.5	258.6	829.5	273.5	840.3	291.4	847.2	306.5
209.7	102.0	206.8	108.4	193.2	112.8	173.8	116.7	167.4	120.8
65.9	28.9	66.2	30.8	68.1	32.6	71.0	33.9	71.1	35.6
29.3	24.5	29.4	25.7	30.1	26.8	30.5	27.6	30.7	28.3
109.9	47.7	111.4	51.7	111.5	55.0	96.7	58.4	96.9	61.6
21.1	16.9	21.1	17.1	21.3	17.4	21.5	17.7	21.6	18.0
21.4	13.7	21.6	14.0	22.1	14.4	22.1	14.7	22.9	15.9
33.3	15.6	33.3	16.3	33.3	17.2	33.2	18.0	33.1	18.9
10.2	7.6	10.2	7.9	10.2	8.0	10.3	8.3	10.3	8.4
24.2	11.9	24.2	12.4	24.2	13.0	24.2	13.5	24.2	14.0
20.2	12.3	20.6	13.0	21.1	13.7	21.3	14.2	21.7	14.6
13.3	8.3	13.5	8.9	13.5	9.3	13.4	9.7	13.3	9.9
8.4	5.6	8.4	5.8	8.5	5.9	8.5	6.0	8.6	6.1
8.7	5.3	8.8	5.4	8.8	5.8	9.5	6.7	9.9	7.0
25.7	21.7	26.0	22.4	26.2	22.9	26.7	23.7	27.0	24.1

5.3.7.4 Economy
5.3.7.5 Wirtschaft

5.3.7.4 PASSENGER BUS TRANSPORT IN THE PUBLIC TRANSPORTATION SYSTEM, BY UNION REPUBLICS (millions)
PERSONENBEFÖRDERUNG MIT AUTOBUSSEN DER ÖFFENTLICHEN VERKEHRSMITTEL, NACH UNIONSREPUBLIKEN (Mio Personen)
PEREVOZKA PASSAŽIROV AVTOBUSAMI TRANSPORTA OBŠČEGO POL'ZOVANIJA PO SOJUZNYM RESPUBLIKAM (mln.čelovek)

	1940	1965	1970	1971	1972	1973	1974	1975	1976
SSSR	590.0	18656.6	27343.8	28752.1	30347.9	32133.1	34251.5	36468.8	37866.6
RSFSR	429.1	10967.5	15053.5	15647.3	16556.6	17588.1	18828.7	20039.3	20918.4
Ukrainskaja SSR	29.4	2885.3	5060.9	5514.5	5933.7	6285.2	6688.0	7089.3	7223.2
Belorusskaja SSR	10.5	629.5	1117.0	1146.8	1171.3	1218.3	1307.6	1397.2	1434.7
Uzbekskaja SSR	8.8	629.7	1042.9	1100.2	1155.2	1237.3	1349.8	1462.0	1552.5
Kazachskaja SSR	10.3	1278.9	1926.7	2063.7	2151.7	2316.9	2435.2	2634.9	2735.4
Gruzinskaja SSR	17.0	373.2	475.9	495.0	508.3	498.3	511.3	541.9	553.5
Azerbajdžanskaja SSR	3.8	245.3	351.4	382.4	395.3	413.8	439.3	462.4	480.7
Litovskaja SSR	30.7	389.5	569.5	590.8	611.9	644.7	658.6	675.0	689.4
Moldavskaja SSR	0.5	142.3	204.2	222.2	237.3	244.0	255.6	268.6	276.8
Latvijskaja SSR	4.4	224.6	302.2	304.0	317.5	328.4	348.6	362.6	373.9
Kirgizskaja SSR	2.9	257.6	353.9	365.4	386.5	390.0	406.1	433.8	449.1
Tadžikskaja SSR	6.2	139.4	194.7	214.4	216.5	230.0	246.8	269.0	293.1
Armjanskaja SSR	3.3	164.3	249.3	250.6	233.2	261.4	286.0	306.6	330.0
Turkmenskaja SSR	17.5	137.7	170.0	175.0	180.8	186.5	193.3	213.7	237.1
Estonskaja SSR	15.6	191.8	271.7	279.8	282.1	290.2	296.6	312.0	318.8

5.3.7.5 MUNICIPAL PASSENGER TRANSPORT WITH BUSES OF THE PUBLIC TRANSPORT SYSTEM
STÄDTISCHE PERSONENBEFÖRDERUNG MIT AUTOBUSSEN DER ÖFFENTLICHEN VERKEHRSMITTEL
VNUTRIGORODSKIE PASSAŽIRSKIE PEREVOZKI AVTOBUSAMI TRANSPORTA OBŠČEGO POL'ZOVANIJA

	1965	1970	1971	1972	1973	1974	1975	1976
Number of cities and city settlements with intercity bus lines – Zahl der Städte u.Stadtsiedlungen mit innerstädtischen Buslinien – Čislo gorodov i poselkov gorodskogo tipa, imejuščich vnutrigorodskoe avtobusnoe soobščenie	1,618	2,002	2,056	2,075	2,100	2,136	2,209	2,233
Passengers carried, '000 millions – Beförderte Passagiere, Mrd.Personen – Perevezeno passažirov, mlrd.čelovek	14.4	20.5	21.3	22.2	23.6	25.1	26.9	27.8

Economy 5.3.7.5
Wirtschaft 5.3.7.6
5.3.7.7

	1965	1970	1971	1972	1973	1974	1975	1976
Passenger turnover, '000 million passenger-km – Passagierumsatz, Mrd.Passagier-km – Passažirooborot, mlrd.passažiro-kilometrov	57.1	97.5	102.2	110.3	120.8	135.3	149.7	159.2
Average travel distance per passenger, km – Durchschnittl.Reiseentfernung pro Passagier, km – Srednjaja dal'nost' poezdki odnogo passažira, km	4.0	4.8	4.8	5.0	5.1	5.4	5.6	5.7

5.3.7.6 SUBURBAN PASSENGER TRANSPORT WITH BUSES OF THE PUBLIC TRANSPORT SYSTEM
VORORT-PERSONENBEFÖRDERUNG MIT AUTOBUSSEN DER ÖFFENTLICHEN VERKEHRSMITTEL
PRIGORODNYE PEREVOZKI PASSAŽIROV AVTOBUSAMI TRANSPORTA OBŠČEGO POL'ZOVANIJA

	1965	1970	1971	1972	1973	1974	1975	1976
Passengers carried, millions – Beförderte Passagiere, Mio Personen – Perevezeno passažirov, mln.čelovek	3,385	5,401	5,950	6,546	6,858	7,324	7,716	8,094
Passenger turnover, '000 million passenger-km – Passagierumsatz, Mrd. Passagier-km – Passažirooborot, mlrd.passažiro-kilometrov	34.0	56.0	61.7	69.3	73.3	78.8	83.6	91.9
Average travel distance per passenger, km – Durchschnittl.Reiseentfernung pro Passagier, km – Srednjaja dal'nost' poezdki odnogo passažira, km	10.1	10.4	10.4	10.6	10.7	10.8	10.8	11.4

5.3.7.7 UTILIZATION OF PASSENGER TAXIS IN THE PUBLIC TRANSPORT SYSTEM
NUTZUNG DER PERSONENTAXI DER ÖFFENTLICHEN VERKEHRSMITTEL
ISPOL'ZOVANIE LEGKOVYCH TAKSOMOTOROV TRANSPORTA OBŠČEGO POL'ZOVANIJA

	1940	1965	1970	1971	1972	1973	1974	1975	1976
Total distance covered, mill. kilometres – Gesamte durchlaufene Strecke, Mio km – Obščij probeg, mln.km	107	4,644	7,222	7,924	8,622	9,206	10,055	10,995	11,865
of which paid distance covered – davon bezahlte durchlaufene Strecke – v tom čisle platnyj probeg	89	3,515	5,951	6,570	7,179	7,695	8,444	9,291	10,097

329

5.3.8.1 Economy / Wirtschaft

5.3.8 MUNICIPAL ELECTRIFIED PASSENGER TRANSPORTATION
STÄDTISCHE ELEKTRIFIZIERTE PERSONENVERKEHRSMITTEL
GORODSKOJ PASSAŽIRSKIJ ELEKTRIČESKIJ TRANSPORT

5.3.8.1 DEVELOPMENT OF MUNICIPAL ELECTRIFIED PASSENGER TRANSPORTATION
ENTWICKLUNG DER STÄDTISCHEN ELEKTRIFIZIERTEN PERSONENVERKEHRSMITTEL
RAZVITIE GORODSKOGO PASSAŽIRSKOGO ELEKTRIČESKOGO TRANSPORTA

	1940	1965	1970	1971	1972	1973	1974	1975	1976
Length of lines (end-of-year figures), in kilometres – Länge der Linien (zum Jahresende), km – Protjažennost' putej (na konec goda), km:									
Length of single tramlines in operation – Länge der benutzten Straßenbahneinzellinie – Protjažennost' ekspluatacionnogo odinočnogo tramvajnogo puti	4,475	7,312	8,261	8,358	8,456	8,572	8,666	8,769	8,810
Length of single trolley lines in operation – Länge der benutzten Trolleybuseinzellinie – Protjažennost' ekspluatacionnoj odinočnoj trollejbusnoj linii	329	5,016	8,142	8,707	9,317	9,908	10,548	11,253	11,912
Length of subway lines in operation (double lines) – Länge der benutzten U-Bahn-Linie in zweigleisiger Berechnung – Protjažennost' ekspluatacionnogo puti metropolitenov v dvuchputnom isčislenii	23	147	214	224	240	240	243	274	278
Movable stock (end-of-year figures) – Beweglicher Bestand (zum Jahresende) – Podvižnoj sostav (na konec goda):									
Number of tramway passenger cars – Zahl der Straßenbahnpersonenwagen – Čislo tramvajnych passažirskich vagonov	11,391	20,921	22,051	21,793	21,614	21,080	21,000	20,800	20,700
Number of trolley passenger buses – Zahl der Personentrolleybusse – Čislo passažirskich trollejbussov	795	10,172	15,767	16,941	17,946	18,778	19,600	20,300	21,300
Number of subway passenger cars – Zahl der U-Bahn-Personenwagen – Čislo passažirskich vagonov metropolitenov	278	1,691	2,544	2,808	3,035	3,278	3,500	3,500	3,700

Economy 5.3.8.1
Wirtschaft 5.3.8.2

	1940	1965	1970	1971	1972	1973	1974	1975	1976
Passengers carried, in millions - Beförderte Passagiere, Mio Personen - Perevezeno passažirov, mln.čelovek:									
Tramway - Straßenbahn - Tramvajami	7,283	8,242	7,962	7,975	7,952	7,998	8,074	8,235	8,343
Trolley bus - Trolleybus(O-Bus) - Trollejbusami	294	4,298	6,122	6,588	6,974	7,298	7,639	7,963	8,345
Subway - U-Bahn - Metropolitenami	377	1,652	2,294	2,443	2,592	2,727	2,836	2,972	3,229

At the end of 1976 109 cities had tramway and 146 cities trolley bus connections. Moscow, Leningrad, Kiev, Charkov, Tbilisi and Baku have subways.
Ende 1976 hatten 109 Städte Straßenbahn- und 146 Trolleybusverbindungen. In Moskau, Leningrad, Kiew, Charkov, Tbilisi und Baku gibt es U-Bahnen.
K koncu 1976 g. tramvajnoe soobščenie imeli 109 gorodov, trollejbusnoe - 146. B. Moskve, Leningrade, Kieve, Charkove, Tbilisi i Baku imejutsja metropoliteny.

5.3.8.2 PASSENGER TRANSPORT ON SUBWAYS BY UNION REPUBLICS (millions)
PASSAGIERBEFÖRDERUNG IN U-BAHNEN NACH UNIONSREPUBLIKEN (Mio Personen)
PEREVOZKI PASSAŽIROV METROPOLITENAMI PO SOJUZNYM RESPUBLIKAM (mln. čelovek)

	1965	1970	1971	1972	1973	1974	1975	1976
SSSR	1652.4	2294.4	2443.3	2591.7	2727.0	2836.3	2972.0	3228.6
RSFSR	1592.0	2046.5	2156.2	2253.7	2344.1	2431.0	2520.4	2696.2
of which - darunter - v tom čisle:								
City of Moscow - Stadt Moskau - g.Moskva	1328.7	1628.1	1696.4	1770.4	1841.0	1906.8	1966.4	2083.4
City of Leningrad - Stadt Leningrad - g. Leningrad	263.3	418.4	459.8	483.3	503.1	524.2	554.0	612.8
Ukrainskaja SSR	60.4	126.8	144.2	177.7	189.0	197.4	236.3	307.8
City of Kiev - Stadt Kiev - g.Kiev	60.4	126.8	144.2	177.7	189.0	197.4	204.4	210.7
City of Charkov - Stadt Charkov - g.Charkov	--	--	--	--	--	--	31.9	97.1
Gruzinskaja SSR (Tbilisi)	--	74.4	87.5	97.4	102.3	106.9	110.5	114.9
Azerbajdžanskaja SSR (Baku)	--	46.7	55.4	62.9	91.6	101.0	104.8	109.7

331

5.3.8.3 Economy / Wirtschaft

5.3.8.3

LENGTH OF PUBLIC TRANSPORTATION ROUTES BY UNION REPUBLICS (END-OF-YEAR FIGURES; km)
LÄNGE DER BENUTZTEN VERKEHRSWEGE NACH UNIONSREPUBLIKEN (ZUM JAHRESENDE; km)
PROTJAŽENNOST' EKSPLUATACIONNYCH PUTEJ PO SOJUZNYM RESPUBLIKAM (NA KONEC GODA; km)

	1965	1970	1971	1972	1973	1974	1975	1976
Single tramlines - Straßenbahneinzellinien - Odinočnye tramvajnye puti:								
SSSR	7,312	8,261	8,358	8,456	8,572	8,666	8,769	8,810
RSFSR	4,649	5,312	5,383	5,448	5,540	5,627	5,702	5,758
Ukrainskaja SSR	1,685	1,869	1,893	1,925	1,951	1,964	1,986	1,996
Belorusskaja SSR	111	109	109	107	110	117	117	117
Uzbekskaja SSR	136	226	226	233	231	242	244	244
Kazachskaja SSR	216	234	236	235	235	238	242	224
Gruzinskaja SSR	106	90	90	96	96	86	86	86
Azerbajdžanskaja SSR	148	141	141	128	127	110	109	101
Litovskaja SSR	--	--	--	--	--	--	--	--
Moldavskaja SSR	--	--	--	--	--	--	--	---
Latvijskaja SSR	138	143	143	147	145	145	146	147
Kirgizskaja SSR	--	---	--	--	--	--	--	--
Tadžikskaja SSR	--	--	--	--	--	--	--	--
Armjanskaja SSR	86	99	99	99	99	99	99	99
Turkmenskaja SSR	--	--	--	--	--	--	--	--
Estonskaja SSR	37	38	38	38	38	38	38	38
Single trolley lines - Trolleybuseinzellinien - Odinočnye trollejbusnye linii:								
SSSR	5,016	8,142	8,707	9,317	9,908	10,548	11,253	11,912
RSFSR	2,708	4,309	4,541	4,854	5,218	5,543	5,925	6,317
Ukrainskaja SSR	1,241	2,032	2,148	2,277	2,364	2,508	2,660	2,783
Belorusskaja SSR	120	226	250	281	293	348	364	402
Uzbekskaja SSR	126	206	268	291	329	367	454	491
Kazachskaja SSR	94	211	248	282	318	337	346	361
Gruzinskaja SSR	111	185	211	213	231	234	241	251
Azerbajdžanskaja SSR	109	145	163	166	174	184	186	190
Litovskaja SSR	66	144	147	155	158	158	158	181
Moldavskaja SSR	63	114	110	141	149	175	182	188
Latvijskaja SSR	127	159	166	166	170	171	171	171
Kirgizskaja SSR	88	109	109	111	112	119	129	133
Tadžikskaja SSR	41	87	101	103	109	115	129	129
Armjanskaja SSR	79	129	132	164	169	170	180	186
Turkmenskaja SSR	35	55	74	74	74	79	88	88
Estonskaja SSR	8	31	39	39	40	40	40	41
Subways in double lines - U-Bahn-Linie in zweigleisiger Berechnung - Puti metropolitenov v dvuchputnom isčislenii:								
SSSR	147	214	224	240	240	243	274	278
RSFSR	134	179	182	193	193	196	217	217
Ukrainskaja SSR	13	14	18	18	18	18	28	30
Gruzinskaja SSR	--	10	13	13	13	13	13	13
Azerbajdžanskaja SSR	--	11	11	16	16	16	16	18

Economy
Wirtschaft 5.3.8.4

5.3.8.4 MOVABLE STOCK OF THE MUNICIPAL ELECTRIFIED PASSENGER TRANSPORTATION
SYSTEM BY UNION REPUBLICS (END-OF-YEAR FIGURES)
BEWEGLICHER BESTAND DER STÄDTISCHEN ELEKTRIFIZIERTEN VERKEHRSMITTEL
NACH UNIONSREPUBLIKEN (ZUM JAHRESENDE)
PODVIŽNOJ SOSTAV GORODSKOGO PASSAŽIRSKOGO ELEKTRIČESKOGO TRANSPORTA
PO SOJUZNYM RESPUBLIKAM (NA KONEC GODA)

	1965	1970	1971	1972	1973	1974	1975	1976
Number of tramway passenger cars - Zahl der Straßenbahnpersonenwagen - Čislo tramvajnych passažirskich vagonov:								
SSSR	20,921	22,051	21,793	21,614	21,080	20,987	20,766	20,664
RSFSR	13,394	14,260	14,078	13,976	13,613	13,616	13,508	13,491
Ukrainskaja SSR	4,944	5,285	5,225	5,174	5,099	5,142	5,171	5,159
Belorusskaja SSR	350	385	375	354	348	344	323	298
Uzbekskaja SSR	496	481	482	473	457	436	419	443
Kazachskaja SSR	387	404	414	440	428	371	335	295
Gruzinskaja SSR	285	233	214	214	177	142	124	134
Azerbajdžanskaja SSR	296	181	179	168	164	166	153	135
Litovskaja SSR	--	--	--	--	--	--	--	--
Moldavskaja SSR	--	--	--	--	--	--	--	--
Latvijskaja SSR	384	436	440	432	425	410	407	409
Kirgizskaja SSR	--	--	--	--	--	--	--	--
Tadžikskaja SSR	--	--	--	--	--	--	--	--
Armjanskaja SSR	221	236	236	233	217	208	176	156
Turkmenskaja SSR	--	--	--	--	--	--	--	--
Estonskaja SSR	164	150	150	150	152	152	150	144
Number of trolley passenger buses - Zahl der Personentrolleybusse - Čislo passažirskich trollejbusov:								
SSSR	10,172	15,767	16,941	17,946	18,778	19,618	20,289	21,344
RSFSR	5,616	8,274	8,871	9,391	9,764	10,135	10,446	10,989
Ukrainskaja SSR	2,509	4,016	4,341	4,627	4,827	5,040	5,159	5,503
Belorusskaja SSR	238	548	607	664	692	732	802	857
Uzbekskaja SSR	249	418	449	476	522	565	603	636
Kazachskaja SSR	160	279	334	370	410	477	505	515
Gruzinskaja SSR	215	295	317	330	357	341	370	374
Azerbajdžanskaja SSR	194	221	220	239	241	244	247	245
Litovskaja SSR	124	297	326	340	347	380	392	414
Moldavskaja SSR	140	288	301	343	372	397	430	458
Latvijskaja SSR	257	354	364	368	387	398	403	408
Kirgizskaja SSR	156	190	177	170	176	188	202	197
Tadžikskaja SSR	79	195	196	188	205	209	217	225
Armjanskaja SSR	191	257	277	279	323	333	344	346
Turkmenskaja SSR	35	66	76	76	65	75	65	59
Estonskaja SSR	9	69	85	85	90	104	104	118
Number of subway passenger cars - Zahl der U-Bahn-Personenwagen - Čislo passažirskich vagonov metropolitenov:								
SSSR	1,691	2,544	2,808	3,035	3,278	3,507	3,539	3,740
RSFSR	1,624	2,292	2,512	2,691	2,919	3,088	3,024	3,192
Ukrainskaja SSR	67	142	179	215	225	242	334	345
Gruzinskaja SSR	--	62	69	69	69	87	87	95
Azerbajdžanskaja SSR	--	48	48	60	65	90	94	108

5.3.9.1 Economy / Wirtschaft

5.3.9 AIR TRAFFIC - LUFTVERKEHR - VOZDUŠNYJ TRANSPORT

5.3.9.1 BASIC INDICATORS ON AIR TRAFFIC FROM THE MINISTRY OF CIVIL AVIATION
GRUNDKENNZIFFERN DES LUFTVERKEHRS DES MINISTERIUMS FÜR ZIVILE LUFTFAHRT
OSNOVNYE POKAZATELI VOZDUŠNOGO TRANSPORTA MINISTERSTVA GRAŽDANSKOJ AVIACII

	1940	1965	1970	1971	1972	1973	1974	1975	1976
Total length of airways (without intersecting lines), '000 kilometres - Gesamtlänge der Luftlinien (ohne die sich überschneidenden Strecken), Tsd.km - Obščaja protjažennost' vozdušnych linij (bez perekryvajuščichsja učastkov), tys.km	146.3	481.1	773.4	778.0	780.0	798.0	824	827	860
of which length of airways within the USSR territory - darunter Länge der Linien innerhalb des Territoriums der UdSSR - v tom čisle protjažennost'linij v predelach territorii SSSR	143.9	435.0	596.0	596.5	615.7	623.8	630	645	652
of which airways of union importance - davon Luftlinien von Unionsbedeutung - iz nich vozdušnye linii sojuznogo značenija	51.3	157.9	254.0	254.2	264.8	269.4	273	285	287
Freight turnover (incl. mail), mill.tons/km - Frachtumsatz (einschl.Post), Mio t/km - Gruzooborot (vključaja počtu),mln.tkm	23.2	1,338	1,877	1,982	2,188	2,372	2,485	2,590	2,710
Goods carried and mail, '000 tons - Beförderte Güter und Post, Tsd.t - Perevezeno gruzov i počty, tys.t	58.4	1,228	1,844	1,960	2,087	2,206	2,331	2,472	2,603
Passenger turnover, '000 millions passenger-km - Passagierumsatz, Mrd.Passagier-km - Passažirooborot, mlrd.passažirov-kilometrov	0.2	38.1	78.2	88.8	95.9	98.8	108.8	122.6	130.8
Passengers carried, millions - Beförderte Passagiere, Mio Personen - Perevezeno passažirov, mln.čelovek	0.4	42.1	71.4	78.1	82.5	84.3	90.5	98.1	100.9

Economy 5.3.9.1
Wirtschaft 5.3.9.2

	1940	1965	1970	1971	1972	1973	1974	1975	1976
Size of air-chemical works in agriculture and forestry, mill.hectares – Umfang der flugchemischen Arbeiten in Land-u.Forstwirtschaft, Mio ha – Ob-em aviachimičeskich rabot v sel'skom i lesnom chozjajstve, mln.ga	0.9	55.0	83.3	85.8	83.4	86.6	90.4	84.9	84.8

5.3.9.2   BASIC INDICATORS ON AIR TRAFFIC ON AN INTERNATIONAL BASIS
GRUNDKENNZIFFERN DES LUFTVERKEHRS AUF INTERNATIONALER EBENE
OSNOVNYE POKAZATELI VOZDUŠNOGO TRANSPORTA V MEŽDUNARODNOM SOOBŠČENII

	1965	1970	1971	1972	1973	1974	1975	1976
Freight turnover (incl.mail), mill.tons/km – Frachtumsatz (einschl.Post), Mio t/km – Gruzooborot (vključaja počtu),mln.tkm	50.1	97.3	145.2	171.0	172.1	190.7	231.3	253.6
Goods carried and mail, '000 tons – Beförderte Güter und Post, Tsd.t – Perevezeno gruzov i počty, tys.t	13.2	28.3	46.0	52.9	47.8	46.6	56.6	65.0
Passenger turnover, '000 mill. passenger-km – Passagierumsatz, Mrd.Passagier-km – Passažirooborot, mlrd.passažiro-kilometrov	1.1	2.7	3.7	4.6	4.8	5.6	6.9	7.1
Passengers carried, millions – Beförderte Passagiere, Mio Personen – Perevezeno passažirov, mln.čelovek	0.3	0.9	1.4	1.6	1.5	1.7	2.1	2.1

5.3.10.1 Economy / Wirtschaft

5.3.10 COMMUNICATIONS - POST- UND FERNMELDEWESEN - SVJAZ'

5.3.10.1 BASIC INDICATORS ON COMMUNICATION DEVELOPMENT - GRUNDKENNZIFFERN DER ENTWICKLUNG DES POST- UND FERNMELDEWESENS - OSNOVNYE POKAZATELI RAZVITIJA SVJAZI

	1940	1965	1970	1971	1972	1973	1974	1975	1976
Number of Post, telegraph and telephone offices (end-of-year figures), '000 - Anzahl der Post-, Telegraphen- und Telephonämter (zum Jahresende), Tsd. Číslo predprijatij pošty, telegrafa i telefona (na konec goda), tys.	51	72	81	83	84	85	86	88	88
of which in rural areas - darunter in ländlichen Gebieten - v tom čisle v sel'skich mestnostjach	44	54	60	60	61	62	62	63	63
Air mail, '000 tons - Postbeförderung auf dem Luftwege, Tsd.t - Perevezeno pošty aviacionnym transportom, tys.t	12.1	263.1	323.8	305.3	326.4	340.7	356	375	386
Services rendered by communications enterprises, '000 mill.rubles - Leistungen des Post- u. Fernmeldewesens, Mrd.Rubel - Produkcija svjazi, mlrd.rub.	0.6	2.0	3.3	3.5	3.8	4.1	4.5	4.8	5.1
Number of items posted, mill. - abgeliefert wurden, Mio - Otpravleno, mln.:									
letters - Briefsendungen - pisem	2,580	5,241	8,020	8,341	8,532	8,714	8,868	8,969	9,000
newspapers and magazines - Zeitungen u. Zeitschriften - gazet i žurnalov	6,698	22,599	33,242	35,092	36,892	38,264	39,500	41,100	41,700
parcels - Pakete - posylok	45	128	176	180	187	197	203	215	229
money orders and pension payments - Geldüberweisungen u.Rentenauszahlungen - denežnych perevodov i pensionnych vyplat	99	494	655	675	687	697	709	724	732
telegrams - Telegramme - telegramm	141	273	365	372	385	404	421	443	458

Economy 5.3.10.1
Wirtschaft

	1940	1965	1970	1971	1972	1973	1974	1975	1976
Number of long-distance calls, mill. – Zahl der Ferngespräche, Mio – Količestvo meždugorodnych telefonnych razgovorov, mln.	92	257	431	479	535	604	684	768	868
Number of telephones within public service network (end-of-year figures), '000 – Anzahl der Fernsprechapprate im öffentlichen Fernsprechnetz (zum Jahresende), Tsd.– Čislo telefonnych apparatov na obščej telefonnoj seti (na konec goda), tys.	1,729	6,399	10,987	12,078	13,199	14,463	15,825	17,167	18,422
of which – darunter – v tom čisle:									
within municipal service network – im städtischen Fernsprechnetz – na gorodskoj telefonnoj seti	1,548	5,490	9,504	10,436	11,380	12,450	13,589	14,694	15,712
within rural service network – im ländlichen Fernsprechnetz – na sel'skoj telefonnoj seti	181	909	1,483	1,642	1,819	2,013	2,236	2,473	2,710
automatic telephones, '000 – Wählapparate, Tsd. – avtomatičeskie apparaty, tys.	414	4,450	9,471	10,657	11,821	13,116	14,631	16,050	17,385
of which – darunter – v tom čisle:									
within municipal service network – im städtischen Fernsprechnetz – na gorodskoj telefonnoj seti	414	4,110	8,473	9,472	10,442	11,511	12,767	13,912	14,983
within rural service network – im ländlichen Fernsprechnetz – na sel'skoj telefonnoj seti	– –	340	998	1,185	1,379	1,605	1,864	2,138	2,402
Number of TV stations (end-of-year figures) – Anzahl der Fernsehsender (zum Jahresende) – Čislo programmnych televizijonnych stancij	2	653	1,233	1,344	1,466	1,620	1,749	1,957	2,116
Number of radio receivers (end-of-year figures), mill. – Anzahl der Funkempfangsanschlüsse (zum Jahresende), Mio – Čislo radiopriemnych toček (na konec goda), mln.	7.0	89.5	129.6	139.2	150.7	159.5	168.6	177.7	185.5

5.3.10.1 Economy
5.3.10.2 Wirtschaft

	1940	1965	1970	1971	1972	1973	1974	1975	1976
radio sets – Rundfunkgeräte – radiopriemnikov	1.1	38.2	48.6	50.8	53.2	54.8	57.1	59.8	61.5
TV sets – Fernsehgeräte – televizorov	400 sets-St.	15.7	34.8	39.3	45.4	49.2	52.5	55.2	57.6
rediffusion loudspeakers – Drahtfunkleitstellen – transljacionnych radiotoček	5.9	35.6	46.2	49.1	52.1	55.5	59.0	62.7	66.4

5.3.10.2 NUMBER OF POST, TELEGRAPH AND TELEPHONE OFFICES BY UNION REPUBLICS
ANZAHL DER POST-, TELEGRAPH- UND TELEPHONÄMTER NACH UNIONSREPUBLIKEN
ČISLO PREDPRIJATIJ POČTY, TELEGRAFA I TELEFONA PO SOJUZNYM RESPUBLIKAM

	1940	1965	1970	1971	1972	1973	1974	1975	1976
SSSR	51,353	72,179	81,435	82,595	83,857	85,092	86,332	87,579	88,418
RSFSR	32,278	42,483	46,057	46,447	46,927	47,399	47,910	48,413	48,711
Ukrainskaja SSR	8,370	11,667	14,114	14,471	14,824	15,163	15,496	15,790	16,001
Belorusskaja SSR	2,163	3,259	3,735	3,815	3,921	4,031	4,150	4,279	4,346
Uzbekskaja SSR	752	2,297	2,974	3,033	3,090	3,142	3,196	3,264	3,334
Kazachskaja SSR	2,252	4,137	4,667	4,740	4,823	4,907	4,987	5,078	5,156
Gruzinskaja SSR	663	1,226	1,430	1,471	1,511	1,552	1,587	1,624	1,660
Azerbajdžanskaja SSR	524	1,098	1,555	1,598	1,640	1,675	1,712	1,751	1,786
Litovskaja SSR	716	1,150	1,161	1,167	1,172	1,174	1,179	1,190	1,184
Moldavskaja SSR	293	1,008	1,252	1,277	1,301	1,322	1,336	1,353	1,362
Latvijskaja SSR	1,566	1,128	1,167	1,173	1,175	1,173	1,175	1,177	1,178
Kirgizskaja SSR	352	682	887	907	924	944	964	986	991
Tadžikskaja SSR	263	482	650	676	698	718	737	750	760
Armjanskaja SSR	242	469	621	644	667	693	719	742	764
Turkmenskaja SSR	247	412	476	487	493	505	516	524	531
Estonskaja SSR	672	681	689	689	691	694	668	658	654

5.3.10.3

NUMBER OF RADIO RECEIVERS (RADIO SETS, TV SETS AND REDIFFUSION LOUDSPEAKERS) BY UNION REPUBLICS (thousands)
ANZAHL DER FUNKEMPFANGSANSCHLÜSSE (RUNDFUNKGERÄTE, FERNSEHGERÄTE UND DRAHTFUNKLEITSTELLEN) NACH UNIONSREPUBLIKEN (Tsd.)
ČISLO RADIOPRIEMNYCH TOČEK (RADIOPRIEMNIKOV, TELEVIZOROV I TRANSLJACIONNYCH RADIOTOČEK) PO SOJUZNYM RESPUBLIKAM (tys.)

Economy
Wirtschaft 5.3.10.3

	1940	1965	1970	1971	1972	1973	1974	1975	1976
SSSR	6,976	89,559	129,604	139,164	150,701	159,468	168,615	177,658	185,549
RSFSR	4,641	54,294	77,590	83,329	90,255	95,419	100,819	106,162	110,992
Ukrainskaja SSR	1,303	17,724	25,591	27,260	29,359	31,099	32,808	34,574	36,065
Belorusskaja SSR	191	2,688	4,507	4,958	5,399	5,748	6,120	6,483	6,769
Uzbekskaja SSR	72	2,822	4,066	4,347	4,703	5,006	5,273	5,495	5,676
Kazachskaja SSR	151	3,765	5,609	6,074	6,611	7,080	7,645	8,189	8,657
Gruzinskaja SSR	67	1,295	1,748	1,829	1,989	2,069	2,162	2,257	2,349
Azerbajdžanskaja SSR	64	1,241	1,701	1,791	1,926	2,010	2,123	2,224	2,296
Litovskaja SSR	96	841	1,341	1,474	1,625	1,733	1,816	1,883	1,947
Moldavskaja SSR	18	1,014	1,611	1,756	1,918	2,037	2,164	2,315	2,433
Latvijskaja SSR	167	1,030	1,491	1,615	1,708	1,727	1,788	1,858	1,885
Kirgizskaja SSR	24	606	952	1,042	1,144	1,229	1,310	1,390	1,453
Tadžikskaja SSR	17	560	873	957	1,052	1,128	1,199	1,255	1,299
Armjanskaja SSR	38	586	866	939	1,056	1,109	1,182	1,247	1,307
Turkmenskaja SSR	28	481	780	866	948	1,020	1,095	1,179	1,240
Estonskaja SSR	99	612	878	927	1,008	1,054	1,111	1,147	1,181

5.4.1 Economy
Wirtschaft

5.4 CAPITAL CONSTRUCTION - INVESTITIONSBAU - KAPITAL'NOE STROITEL'STVO

5.4.1 COMMISSIONED FIXED ASSETS (in comparable prices; '000 million rubles)[1]
INANSPRUCHNAHME DER GRUNDFONDS (in Vergleichspreisen; Mrd.Rubel)[1]
VVOD V DEJSTVIE OSNOVNYCH FONDOV (v sopostavimych cenach; mlrd.rub.)[1]

	Total fixed assets commissioned by state and co-operative enterprises and organizations, collective farms and population Gesamtinanspruchnahme der Grundfonds durch staatl.u.genossenschaftliche Betriebe u.Organisationen, Kolchosen u.Bevölkerung Vsego vvedeno osnovnych fondov gosudarstvennymi i kooperativnymi predprijatijami i organizacijami, kolchozami i naseleniem A.	of which state and co-operative enterprises and organizations darunter durch staatl. u.genossenschaftliche Betriebe u.Organisationen v tom čisle gosudarstvennymi i kooperativnymi predprijatijami i organizacijami B.
1918-1977 insgesamt-total-vsego	1575.8	1372.0
1918-1928 (excl.fourth quarter-ohne 4.Quartal - bez IV kvartala 1928)	3.9	1.5
First Five-Year Plan(1929-1932, incl.fourth quarter of 1928) - 1. Fünfjahrplan (1929-1932, einschl.4.Quartal 1928) - Pervaja pjatiletka (1929-1932, vključaja IV kvartal 1928)	9.3	8.5
Second Five-Year Plan(1933-1937)- 2.Fünfjahrplan (1933-1937) - Vtoraja pjatiletka (1933-1937)	17.2	15.5
Three and a half years of the Third Five-Year Plan (1938-first half of 1941) - Dreieinhalb Jahre des 3.Fünfjahrplanes (1938-1.Halbjahr 1941) Tri s polovinoj goda tret'ej pjatiletki (1938 g.-I polugodie 1941 g.)	18.3	15.7

[1] On capital construction the comparable prices represent current estimated prices as of January 1, 1969 in this and in all other tables - Hier und in allen folgenden Tabellen über Investitionsbauwesen sind als Vergleichspreise die veranschlagten Preise vom 1.1.1969 zugrundegelegt - Zdes' i vo vsech tablicach po kapital'nomu stroitel'stvu v kačestve sopostavimych cen prinjaty smetnye ceny na 1 janvarja 1969 g.

Economy 5.4.1
Wirtschaft 5.4.2

	A.	B.
Four and a half years (July 1,1941-Jan.1,1946) - Viereinhalb Jahre (1.Juli 1941-1.Jan.1946) - Cetyre s polovinoj goda (s 1 ijulja 1941 g. do 1 janvarja 1946 g.)	18.9	15.6
Fourth Five-Year Plan - 4. Fünfjahrplan - Cetvertaja pjatiletka (1946-1950)	42.2	34.7
Fifth Five-Year Plan - 5. Fünfjahrplan - Pjataja pjatiletka (1951-1955)	79.9	67.2
Sixth Five-Year Plan - 6. Fünfjahrplan - Šestaja pjatiletka (1956-1960)	155.8	128.5
Seventh Five-Year Plan - 7. Fünfjahrplan - Sed'maja pjatiletka (1961-1965)	228.4	199.6
of which-darunter-v tom čisle: 1965	51.4	45.3
Eighth Five-Year Plan - 8. Fünfjahrplan - Vos'maja pjatiletka (1966-1970)	319.0	280.1
of which-darunter-v tom čisle: 1970	76.4	67.7
Ninth Five-Year Plan - 9. Fünfjahrplan - Devjataja pjatiletka (1971-1975)	460.8	407.8
1971	81.3	72.0
1972	83.9	74.1
1973	92.8	82.1
1974	97.2	85.9
1975	105.6	93.7
1976	107.2	95.2
1977 (planned - geplant)	114.9	102.1

5.4.2 PRODUCTIVE CAPACITIES COMMISSIONED BY EXPANDING AND RECONSTRUCTING
EXISTING AND BUILDING NEW ENTERPRISES
ANTEIL DER PRODUKTIONSKAPAZITÄTEN DURCH ERWEITERUNG UND REKONSTRUKTION
VON BESTEHENDEN UND BAU VON NEUEN BETRIEBEN
VVOD V DEJSTVIE PROIZVODSTVENNYCH MOŠČNOSTEJ ZA SČET RASŠIRENIJA I
REKONSTRUKCII DEJSTVUJUŠČICH I STROITEL'STVA NOVYCH PREDPRIJATIJ

	1961- 1965	1966- 1970	1971- 1975	1975	1976	1977
Electric power stations, mill.kW - Kraftwerke, Mio kW - Elektrostancii, mln.kVt	48.2	54.6	58.1	12.9	11.9	
Capacities for the production of - Kapazitäten für die Förderung von - Moščnosti po dobyče: coal,mill.tons p.year - Kohle, Mio t pro Jahr - uglja, mln.t v god	80	95.1	114.2	24.4	12.6	
iron ore,mill.tons per year - Eisenerz, Mio t pro Jahr - Železnoj rudy, mln.t v god	129.9	120.5	131.5	19.8	46.4	

341

5.4.2 Economy / Wirtschaft

	1961-1965	1966-1970	1971-1975	1975	1976
Capacities for the production of - Kapazitäten für die Erzeugung von - Možnosti po proizvodstvu:					
pig-iron, mill.tons per year - Roheisen, Mio t pro Jahr - čuguna, mln.t v god	12.6	9.7	12.9	1.8	2.25
steel, mill.tons per year - Rohstahl, Mio t pro Jahr - stali, mln.t v god	15.6	18.1	10.9	4.0	1.2
rolled ferrous metals(finished), mill.tons per year - Walzstahl (Fertigerzeugnisse),Mio t pro Jahr - prokata černych metallov (gotovogo), mln.t v god	9.1	14.3	12.2	3.5	4.0
steel pipes, '000 tons per year - Stahlrohre, Tsd.t pro Jahr - stal'nych trub, tys.t v god	2,432	2,469	2,383	425	340
mineral fertilizers (conventional units),mill.tons per year - mineralische Düngemittel (in Bezugseinheiten), Mio t pro Jahr - mineral'nych udobrenij (v uslovnych edinicach), mln.t v god	23.3	33.2	38	11.6	7.3
sulphuric acid,mill.tons per year - Schwefelsäure, Mio t pro Jahr - sernoj kisloty, mln.t v god	4.1	4.2	8.6	1.8	2.6
soda ash, '000 tons per year - kalzinierte Soda, Tsd.t pro Jahr - sody kal'cinirovannoj, tys.t v g.	720	1,221	1,038	347	244
plastic and synthetic resins, '000 tons per year - synthetische Harze u.Plaste, Tsd.t pro Jahr - sintetičeskich smol i plastičeskich mass, tys.t v god	548	706	981	142	310
chemical fibre and threads, '000 tons per year - chemische Fasern u.Fäden, Tsd.t pro Jahr - chimičeskich volokon i nitej,tys.t v g.	221	151	349	63	32
automobile tires, mill.per year - Kraftfahrzeugdecken, Mio Stck.p.J.- avtomobil'nych šin,mln.št.v.god	10	8.3	12.9	0.5	3.9
turbines, '000 kW per year - Turbinen, Tsd.kW pro Jahr - turbin, tys.kVt v god	3,092	4,257	5,600	1,130	399
power transformers, mill.kVA p.y.- Leistungstransformatoren,Mio kVA pro Jahr - transformatorov silovych, mln.kV A v god	55.1	28.2	20.6	6.0	0.8
excavators, '000 per year - Bagger, Tsd.Stck. pro Jahr - ekskavatorov, tys.št.v god	4.6	5.2	6.7	0.6	3.0

Economy 5.4.2
Wirtschaft

	1961-1965	1966-1970	1971-1975	1975	1976
metal-cutting lathes, '000 per year- spanabhebende Werkzeugmaschinen, Tsd.pro Jahr - metallorežuščich stankov, tys.št. v god	35.1	21.5	25.4	6.9	4.0
automobiles (incl.buses), '000 p.y.- Kraftfahrzeuge (einschl.Busse), Tsd. Stck.p.J. - avtomobilej (vključaja avtobusy), tys.št. v god	158.7	423.9	973.9	71.4	92.4
tractors, '000 per year - Traktoren, Tsd.Stck. pro Jahr - traktorov, tys.št. v god	135.1	121.0	79.6	16.0	26.7
cement, mill.tons per year - Zement, Mio t pro Jahr - cementa, mln.t v god	28.2	17.4	20.7	4.4	1.2
cellulose, mill.tons per year - Zellulose, Mio t pro Jahr - celljulozy, mln. t v god	1.3	2.2	2.1	0.5	0.2
paper, '000 tons per year - Papier, Tsd.t pro Jahr - bumagi, tys.t v god	1,291	502	509	65	2
Installed-installiert-Ustanovleno:					
Spinning spindles, mill. - Spindeln von Spinnmaschinen,Mio - prjadil'nych vereten, mln.št.	3.2	3.1	2.2	0.2	0.3
Looms, '000 - Webstühle, Tsd.Stck. - tkackich stankov, tys.št.	52.3	47.6	41.6	6.8	0.7
Capacities for the production of - Kapazitäten für die Erzeugung von - Moščnosti po proizvodstvu:					
leather footwear,mill.pairs per year- Lederschuhe, Mio Paar pro Jahr - kožanoj obuvi, mln.par v god	55.1	149.0	67.4	9.2	2.2
knitted outerwear and underwear, mill.per year - Ober-u.Untertrikota- gen,Mio Stck.pro Jahr - verchnego i bel'evogo trikotaža,mln.št.v god	108.9	410.3	162.5	93.3	2.3
porcelain and china ware,mill.p.year- Erzeugnisse aus Porzellan u.Stein- gut,Mio Stck.pro Jahr - farforo- fajansovych izdelij, mln.št.v god	36.5	176.5	487.2	178.9	35.0
granulated sugar,'000 centners of beet processed daily-Streuzucker, Tsd.dz verarbeitete Zuckerrüben pro Tag-sachara-peska, tys.c pererabotki svekly v sutki	1,180	682	861	253	92
vegetable oil,'000 t of oil seeds ex- tracting processed daily - Pflanzen- öle,Tsd.t pro Tag im Extraktions- verfahren verarbeitete Ölsamen - rastitel'nogo masla, tys.t pererabotki maslosemjan v sutki metodom ekstrakcii	3.7	4.4	2.8	0.1	0.3

5.4.2 Economy / Wirtschaft

	1961–1965	1966–1970	1971–1975	1975	1976
meat, '000 tons per shift - Fleisch, Tsd.t pro Schicht - mjasa, tys.t v smenu	4.9	2.2	4.1	1.1	1.0
whole milk products, '000 tons of milk per shift - Vollmilcherzeugnisse,Tsd.t Milch pro Schicht - cel'nomoločnoj produkcii,tys.t moloka v smenu	12.3	12.4	12.3	1.7	1.1
cheese, tons per shift - Käse, t pro Schicht - syra, tonn v smenu	133.5	312.6	260.9	20.2	12.5
Constructed-gebaut-postroeno:					
gas pipelines,mains and branches, '000 km - Erdgashaupt-u.Nebenfernleitungen,Tsd.km - gazoprovodov magistral'nych i otvodov ot nich, tys.km	21.9	25.5	33.7	7.3	4.7
oil and oil product pipelines,mains, '000 km - Erdölhaupt-u.Erdölproduktfernleitungen, Tsd.km - nefteprovodov i nefteproduktoprovodov magistral'nych, tys.km	11.8	10.1	22.6	5.0	3.0
new railways, '000 km - neue Eisenbahnstrecken, Tsd.km - novych železnodorožnych linij, tys.km	5.1	3.8	3.6	0.8	0.3
Electrified railways, '000 km - Elektrifizierte Eisenbahnstrecken, Tsd.km - Elektrificirovano železnych dorog, tys.km	10.8	8.7	4.8	0.8	0.7
Grain elevators, mill.tons - Elevatoren, Mio t - Elevatory, mln.t	3.5	8.7	16.6	4.2	4.3
Grain and grain-seed shops, mill.tons - Getreide-u.Getreidesamenspeicher,Mio t- Zernosklady i zernosemenochranilišča, mln.t	42.3	48.2	30.4	6.6	5.7
Irrigated land, mill.hectares - Bewässerter Boden, Mio ha - Orošaemye zemli, mln.ha	1.5	1.8	4.6	1.2	0.8
Reclaimed land, mill.hectares - Entwässerter Boden, Mio ha - Osušennye zemli, mln.ha	3.0	3.9	4.4	1.0	0.7

5.4.3 INVESTMENTS BY THE STATE AND COLLECTIVE FARMS IN AGRICULTURE (in comparable prices; mill.rubles)
INVESTITIONEN DES STAATES UND DER KOLCHOSEN IN DER LANDWIRTSCHAFT (in Vergleichspreisen; Mio Rubel)
KAPITAL'NYE VLOŽENIJA GOSUDARSTVA I KOLCHOZOV V SEL'SKOE CHOZJAJSTVO (v sopostavimych cenach; mln.rub.)

	Total investments Gesamt-investitionen Vse kapital'nye vloženija	of which for productive purposes davon für Produktions-zwecke iz nich po ob'ektam proizvodstvennogo naznačenija	of the total investments – von den Gesamtinvestitionen – iz obščego ob'ema kapital'nych vloženij			
			State investments Staatl. Investitionen gosudarstvennye kapital'nye vloženija	of which for productive purposes davon für Produktions-zwecke iz nich po ob'ektam proizvodstvennogo naznačenija	collective farm investments Investitionen der Kolchose kapital'nye vloženija kolchozov	of which for productive purposes davon für Produktions-zwecke iz nich po ob'ektam proizvodstvennogo naznačenija
	A.	B.	C.	D.	E.	F.
1918-1976 total-insg.-vsego	324,536	271,133	195,207	160,946	129,329	110,187
1918-1928 (without fourth quarter-ohne 4.Quartal-bez IV kvartala 1928)	145	137	115	109	30	28
First Five-Year Plan – 1.Fünfjahrplan – Pervaja pjatiletka	1,522	1,357	1,157	1,001	365	356
Second Five-Year Plan – 2. Fünfjahrplan – Vtoraja pjatiletka	2,605	2,331	1,443	1,243	1,162	1,088
Three and a half years of Third Five-Year Plan – Dreieinhalb Jahre des 3. Fünfjahrplanes – Tri s polovinoj goda tret'ej pjatiletki July 1,1941-Jan.1,1946 – 1.Juli 1941-1.Jan.1946 – S 1 ijulja 1941 g. do	2,413	2,195	880	770	1,533	1,425
1 janvarja 1946 g.	2,015	1,923	287	266	1,728	1,657

345

5.4.3 Economy / Wirtschaft

	A.	B.	C.	D.	E.	F.
Fourth Five-Year Plan – 4. Fünfjahrplan – Četvertaja pjatiletka	6,099	5,617	2,554	2,370	3,545	3,247
Fifth Five-Year Plan – 5. Fünfjahrplan – Pjataja pjatiletka	14,621	12,754	7,184	6,256	7,437	6,498
Sixth Five-Year Plan – 6. Fünfjahrplan – Šestaja pjatiletka	28,319	23,984	13,304	10,985	15,015	12,999
Seventh Five-Year Plan – 7. Fünfjahrplan – Sed'maja pjatiletka	45,311	37,759	26,679	21,253	18,632	16,506
of which–darunter–v tom čisle: 1965	11,465	9,471	7,085	5,699	4,380	3,772
Eighth Five-Year Plan – 8. Fünfjahrplan – Vos'maja pjatiletka	74,108	59,667	44,930	36,205	29,178	23,462
of which–darunter–v tom čisle: 1970	17,458	14,281	10,913	8,895	6,545	5,386
Ninth Five-Year Plan – 9. Fünfjahrplan – Devjataja pjatiletka	118,278	99,059	77,174	64,188	41,104	34,871
1971	19,692	16,414	12,587	10,357	7,105	6,057
1972	21,453	17,969	13,788	11,435	7,665	6,534
1973	23,528	19,840	15,229	12,752	8,299	7,088
1974	25,703	21,561	16,933	14,122	8,770	7,439
1975	27,902	23,275	18,637	15,522	9,265	7,753
1976	29,100	24,350	19,500	16,300	9,600	8,050

5.4.4 STRUCTURE OF INVESTMENTS IN FIXED ASSETS (percentage) — STRUKTUR DER INVESTITIONEN (in Prozent) — STRUKTURA KAPITAL'NYCH VLOŽENIJ (v procentach)

	1940	1965	1970	1971	1972	1973	1974	1975	1976
Total — Insgesamt — Vsego	100	100	100	100	100	100	100	100	100
of which — davon — v tom čisle:									
building and installation work — Bau- und Montagearbeiten — stroitel'no-montažnye raboty	82	63	61	62	62	60	60	59	57
equipment, tools and implements — Ausrüstungen, Instrumente und Inventar — oborudovanie, instrument i inventar'	13	31	31	30	30	32	32	33	34
project prospecting — Forschungs-, Projektierungs-u.Schürfarbeiten— proektno-izyskatel'skie raboty	2	1	2	2	2	2	2	2	2
other capital works and expenditures — übrige Investitionsarbeiten und Aufwendungen— pročie kapital'nye raboty i zatraty	3	5	6	6	6	6	6	6	7

5.4.5 Economy / Wirtschaft

5.4.5
NUMBER OF PLANTS, BUILDING AND OTHER PROJECTS WHICH WERE CONSTRUCTED, ARE BEING CONSTRUCTED OR ARE PLANNED WITH THE TECHNICAL AID OF THE USSR SINCE 1945 (up to January 1, 1977)
ANZAHL DER BETRIEBE, BAUTEN UND ANDEREN OBJEKTE, DIE SEIT 1945 MIT TECHNISCHER HILFE DER UdSSR IM AUSLAND GEBAUT WURDEN, SICH IM BAU BEFINDEN ODER GEBAUT WERDEN SOLLEN (zum 1. Januar 1977)
ČISLO PREDPRIJATIJ, SOORUŽENIJ I DRUGICH OB'EKTOV, POSTROENNYCH POSLE 1945 G., STROJAŠČICHSJA I PODLEŽAŠČICH STROITEL'STVU ZA GRANICEJ PRI TECHNIČESKOM SODEJSTVII SSSR (na 1 janvarja 1977)

	Total Insg. Vsego A.	of which in operation davon in Betrieb genommen v tom čisle vvedeno v ekspluataciju B.
Total - Insgesamt - Vsego	3,103	2,001
in the socialist countries - in den sozialistischen Ländern	2,137	1,487
Albania - Albanien	45	45
Bulgaria - Bulgarien	302	152
China	256	256
Cuba - Kuba	239	143
Czechoslovakia - Tschechoslowakei	35	21
Democratic Republic of Vietnam - Demokratische Republik Vietnam	245	175
German Democratic Republic - DDR	35	20
Hungary - Ungarn	93	67
Korean People's Democratic Republic - Volksdemokratische Republik Korea	73	53
Mongolian People's Republic - Mongolei	389	294
Poland - Polen	187	116
Romania - Rumänien	132	110
Yugoslavia - Jugoslawien	106	35
in the developing countries - in den Entwicklungsländern	954	507
Afghanistan	114	67
Algeria - Algerien	91	49
Bangladesh - Bangladesch	17	3
Burma - Birma	7	5
Egypt - Ägypten	103	86
Ethiopia - Äthiopien	9	3
Guinea	28	16
India - Indien	68	40
Iran	108	58
Iraq - Irak	104	45
Mali	14	12
Morocco - Marokko	3	1
Nepal	7	6
Pakistan	12	6
Somalia	35	14
Sri Lanka	8	6

Economy   5.4.5
Wirtschaft 5.4.6

	A.	B.
Sudan	15	8
Syria - Syrien	38	19
Turkey - Türkei	10	6
Yemen - Jemen	13	10
Yemen (People's Democratic Republic of) - Jemen (Volksdemokratische Republik)	21	10

5.4.6
NUMBER OF ENTERPRISES, BUILDINGS AND OTHER PROJECTS WHICH WERE CONSTRUCTED, ARE BEING CONSTRUCTED OR ARE PLANNED IN FOREIGN COUNTRIES WITH THE TECHNICAL AID OF THE USSR SINCE 1945 (up to Jan. 1977)
ANZAHL DER BETRIEBE, BAUTEN UND ANDEREN OBJEKTE, DIE SEIT 1945 MIT TECHNISCHER HILFE DER UdSSR IM AUSLAND GEBAUT WURDEN, SICH IM BAU BEFINDEN ODER GEBAUT WERDEN SOLLEN, NACH WIRTSCHAFTSZWEIGEN (zum 1. Januar 1977)
ČISLO PREDPRIJATIJ, SOORUŽENIJ I DRUGICH OB'EKTOV, POSTROENNYCH POSLE 1945 G., STROJAŠČICHSJA I PODLEŽAŠČICH STROITEL'STVU ZA GRANICEJ PRI TECHNIČESKOM SODEJSTVII SSSR, PO OTRASLJAM CHOZJAJSTVA (na 1 janvarja 1977)

	Total Insg. Vsego A.	of which in operation davon in Betrieb genommen v tom čisle vvedeno v ekspluatac. B.	of which-darunter-v tom čisle			
			in socialist countries in sozialist. Ländern		in developing countries in Entwicklungsländern	
			total insg. C.	of which in operation davon in Betrieb genommen D.	total insg. E.	of which in operation davon in Betrieb genommen F.
Total - Insg. - Vsego	3,103	2,001	2,137	1,487	954	507
by economic branches - nach Wirtschaftszweigen - po otrasljam chozjajstva:						
Industry - Industrie - promyšlennost'	1,957	1,314	1,523	1,103	426	208
electric power - Elektroenergie - elektroenergetika	332	228	251	193	74	33
ferrous metallurgy - Eisenhüttenindustrie - černaja metallurgija	100	64	78	51	21	12
nonferrous metallurgy - Buntmetallurgie - cvetnaja metallurgija	125	75	108	72	17	3
coal industry - Kohlenindustrie - ugol'naja promyšlennost'	82	54	68	48	14	6
petroleum refining and petrochemical industry-erdölverarbeitende Industrie u.Petrochemie-neftepererabatyvajuščaja i neftechimičeskaja promyšlennost'	95	51	83	42	12	9

5.4.6 Economy / Wirtschaft

	A.	B.	C.	D.	E.	F.
chemical industry - chemische Industrie - chimičeskaja promyšlennost'	121	66	107	60	14	6
machine building and metal industry- Maschinenbau und Metallindustrie - mašinostroenie i metalloobrabotka	270	199	217	159	53	40
construction materials industry - Baustoffindustrie - promyšlennost' stroitel'nych materialov	170	78	139	70	31	8
light industry - Leichtindustrie - legkaja promyšlennost'	71	41	46	34	25	7
food industry - Nahrungsmittelindustrie - piščevaja promyšlennost'	259	201	203	179	56	22
mill and mixed provender industry - Mühlen- und Mischfutterindustrie - mukomol'no-krupjanaja i kombikormovaja promyšlennost'	108	75	40	37	68	38
Agriculture - Landwirtschaft - Sel'skoe chozjajstvo	342	192	204	126	138	66
Transport and communications - Transport, Post-u.Fernmeldewesen - Transport i svjaz'	310	228	218	166	88	58
Education, culture, health, sporting grounds - Volksbildung, Kultur, Gesundheitswesen, Sportanlagen - Prosveščenie, kul'tura, zdravoochranenie, sportivnye sooruženija	329	169	114	40	215	129
Housing and municipal services - Wohnungs- und Kommunalwirtschaft - ziliščnoe i kommunal'noe chozjajstvo	53	38	44	32	9	6

Economy
Wirtschaft 5.5.1

5.5 FOREIGN TRADE - AUSSENWIRTSCHAFTLICHE BEZIEHUNGEN - VNEŠNJAJA TORGOVLJA

5.5.1 FOREIGN TRADE TURNOVER - AUSSENHANDELSUMSATZ - OB'EM VNEŠNEJ TORGOVLI

(in prices of the corresponding years; '000 million rubles -
in Preisen der entsprechenden Jahre; Mrd.Rubel -
v cenach sootvetstvujuščich let; mlrd.rub.)

Year Jahr Gody	Turnover Umsatz Oborot	Export Eksport	Import
1938	0.5	0.2	0.3
1946	1.3	0.6	0.7
1950	2.9	1.6	1.3
1955	5.8	3.1	2.7
1956	6.5	3.3	3.2
1957	7.5	3.9	3.6
1958	7.8	3.9	3.9
1959	9.5	4.9	4.6
1960	10.1	5.0	5.1
1961	10.6	5.4	5.2
1962	12.1	6.3	5.8
1963	12.9	6.5	6.4
1964	13.9	6.9	7.0
1965	14.6	7.4	7.2
1966	15.1	8.0	7.1
1967	16.4	8.7	7.7
1968	18.0	9.6	8.4
1969	19.8	10.5	9.3
1970	22.1	11.5	10.6
1971	23.6	12.4	11.2
1972	26.0	12.7	13.3
1973	31.3	15.8	15.5
1974	39.6	20.8	18.8
1975	50.7	24.0	26.7
1976	56.8	28.0	28.8

5.5.2 Economy / Wirtschaft

FOREIGN TRADE BY COUNTRY GROUPS – AUSSENHANDEL NACH LÄNDERGRUPPEN – VNESNJAJA TORGOVLJA PO GRUPPAN STRAN
('000 mill.rubles – Mrd.Rubel – mlrd.rub.)

	1946	1965	1970	1971	1972	1973	1974	1975	1976
Total foreign trade – Gesamter Außenhandel	1.3	14.6	22.1	23.6	26.0	31.3	39.6	50.7	56.8
of which with – darunter mit the socialist countries – den sozialistischen Ländern	0.7	10.1	14.4	15.4	16.8	18.3	21.4	28.6	31.5
of which with the CMEA countries – davon mit den RGW-Mitgliedsländern	0.5	8.5	12.3	13.3	15.5	16.9	19.4	26.3	28.8
the developed capitalist countries – den industriell entwickelten kapitalistischen Ländern	0.5	2.8	4.7	5.1	5.9	8.3	12.4	15.8	18.7
the developing countries – den Entwicklungsländern	0.1	1.7	3.0	3.1	3.3	4.7	5.8	6.3	6.6
Exports – Ausfuhr	0.6	7.4	11.5	12.4	12.7	15.8	20.8	24.0	28.0
of which to – darunter in the socialist countries – die sozialistischen Länder	0.4	5.0	7.5	8.1	8.3	9.1	11.1	14.6	16.4
of which to the CMEA countries – davon in die RGW-Mitgliedsländer	0.3	4.2	6.3	6.7	7.5	8.3	9.9	13.4	14.9
the developed capitalist countries – die industriell entwickelten kapitalistischen Länder	0.2	1.4	2.2	2.5	2.4	3.7	6.3	6.1	7.9
the developing countries – die Entwicklungsländer	0.0	1.0	1.8	1.8	2.0	3.0	3.4	3.3	3.7
Imports – Einfuhr	0.7	7.2	10.6	11.2	13.3	15.5	18.8	26.7	28.8
of which from – darunter aus the socialist countries – den sozialistischen Ländern	0.3	5.1	6.9	7.3	8.5	9.2	10.3	14.0	15.1
of which from the CMEA countries – davon aus den RGW-Mitgliedsländern	0.2	4.3	6.0	6.6	8.0	8.6	9.5	12.9	13.9
the developed capitalist countries – den industriell entwickelten kapitalistischen Ländern	0.3	1.4	2.5	2.6	3.5	4.6	6.1	9.7	10.8
the developing countries – den Entwicklungsländern	0.1	0.7	1.2	1.3	1.3	1.7	2.4	3.0	2.9

5.5.3 FOREIGN TRADE BY COUNTRIES — AUSSENHANDELSUMSATZ NACH LÄNDERN — OB'EM VNEŠNEJ TORGOVLI PO STRANAM
(mill.rubles — Mio Rubel — mln.rub.)

Country Land		1970	1971	1972	1973	1974	1975	1976
Total – Insg.	A. Turnover-Umsatz	22,078.6	23,656.5	26,043.6	31,342.6	39,567.0	50,704.3	56,752.9
	B. Export	11,520.1	12,425.6	12,734.4	15,801.8	20,737.8	24,033.7	28,022.2
	C. Import	10,558.5	11,230.9	13,309.2	15,540.8	18,829.2	26,670.6	28,730.7
Europe – Europa:								
Austria – Österreich	A.	154.9	172.3	163.5	189.3	339.6	444.8	466.5
	B.	66.7	90.9	82.7	99.6	166.0	218.2	274.1
	C.	88.2	81.4	80.8	89.7	173.6	226.6	192.4
Belgium – Belgien	A.	149.0	157.7	174.5	354.3	603.4	529.8	541.3
	B.	74.0	97.9	108.1	194.3	297.9	243.6	323.1
	C.	75.0	59.8	66.4	160.0	305.5	286.2	218.2
Bulgaria – Bulgarien	A.	1,816.5	2,068.7	2,345.2	2,554.8	2,904.1	3,990.8	4,465.5
	B.	844.0	984.0	1,121.4	1,230.8	1,478.5	2,059.6	2,276.7
	C.	972.5	1,084.7	1,223.8	1,324.0	1,425.6	1,931.2	2,188.8
Czechoslovakia – Tschechoslowakei	A.	2,193.2	2,421.8	2,625.9	2,759.6	3,029.5	3,911.2	4,543.3
	B.	1,082.7	1,217.6	1,253.7	1,354.0	1,511.1	2,019.5	2,320.5
	C.	1,110.5	1,204.2	1,372.2	1,405.6	1,518.4	1,891.7	2,222.8
Denmark – Dänemark	A.	43.8	47.9	48.9	79.9	119.9	146.1	208.4
	B.	20.8	26.0	24.9	53.8	78.1	105.7	154.9
	C.	23.0	21.9	24.0	26.1	41.8	40.4	53.5
Finland – Finnland	A.	530.7	569.1	601.7	777.4	1,539.7	1,755.5	1,979.1
	B.	258.3	322.8	297.6	415.1	937.6	918.2	990.3
	C.	272.4	246.3	304.1	362.3	602.1	837.3	988.8
France – Frankreich	A.	412.8	476.2	544.3	721.6	941.0	1,296.5	1,697.0
	B.	126.0	194.3	194.0	272.2	397.9	495.7	773.8
	C.	286.8	281.9	350.3	449.4	543.1	800.8	923.2
German Democratic Republic – DDR	A.	3,295.0	3,443.4	3,705.5	3,965.3	4,315.3	5,623.4	5,997.2
	B.	1,738.1	1,715.9	1,670.8	1,856.4	2,164.6	2,980.3	3,217.9
	C.	1,556.9	1,727.5	2,034.7	2,108.9	2,150.7	2,643.1	2,779.3

5.5.3 Economy / Wirtschaft

Country / Land		1970	1971	1972	1973	1974	1975	1976
Germany, Federal Republic of – BRD	A. B. C.	544.0 223.4 320.6	666.6 254.7 411.9	827.3 255.9 571.4	1,210.2 453.8 756.4	2,208.7 834.5 1,374.2	2,777.3 857.9 1,919.4	3,008.8 1,069.2 1,939.6
Greece – Griechenland	A. B. C.	63.1 31.7 31.4	46.7 29.7 17.0	62.2 32.4 29.8	79.2 42.6 36.6	154.9 89.0 65.9	194.3 138.0 56.3	224.2 162.4 61.8
Hungary – Ungarn	A. B. C.	1,479.9 758.3 721.6	1,659.6 880.8 778.8	1,881.7 903.6 978.1	2,063.5 975.6 1,087.9	2,282.3 1,134.5 1,147.8	3,273.7 1,657.7 1,616.0	3,492.1 1,771.3 1,720.8
Iceland – Island	A. B. C.	17.4 8.3 9.1	21.3 10.2 11.1	22.1 10.7 11.4	23.2 15.7 7.5	56.2 38.1 18.1	60.9 36.8 24.1	54.2 36.9 17.3
Ireland – Irland	A. B. C.	2.1 2.0 0.1	4.6 4.3 0.3	3.4 2.9 0.5	6.2 5.6 0.6	28.5 12.6 15.9	31.1 10.7 20.4	20.0 12.2 7.8
Italy – Italien	A. B. C.	471.9 190.5 281.4	494.6 233.1 261.5	463.5 228.0 235.5	613.6 309.5 304.1	1,136.8 597.6 539.2	1,426.8 638.0 788.8	1,778.5 1,069.3 709.2
Luxembourg – Luxemburg	A. B. C.	0.3 0 0.3	11.7 0.5 11.2	15.3 0.6 14.7	17.0 3.9 13.1	22.6 7.3 15.3	21.8 6.0 15.8	29.2 5.7 23.5
Malta	A. B. C.	0.7 0.7 0	2.4 2.2 0.2	1.3 1.3 0	1.1 1.1 0	2.1 1.2 0.9	3.1 3.1 0	0.4 0.4 0
Netherlands – Niederlande	A. B. C.	222.9 151.2 71.7	224.1 153.6 70.5	222.3 154.6 67.7	356.3 260.6 95.7	570.7 394.3 176.4	451.0 303.8 147.2	541.7 366.8 174.9
Norway – Norwegen	A. B. C.	46.8 24.3 22.5	58.1 42.1 16.0	37.9 21.8 16.1	51.2 34.7 16.5	91.9 46.8 45.1	137.8 64.6 73.2	101.2 43.9 57.3
Poland – Polen	A. B. C.	2,349.8 1,214.9 1,134.9	2,519.9 1,292.4 1,227.5	2,802.7 1,306.9 1,495.8	3,000.3 1,445.0 1,555.3	3,583.6 1,838.2 1,745.4	4,853.3 2,447.2 2,406.1	5,235.0 2,750.1 2,484.9

Economy 5.5.3
Wirtschaft

Country Land		1970	1971	1972	1973	1974	1975	1976
Portugal	A.	--	--	--	--	6.9	77.9	115.5
	B.	--	--	--	--	6.3	64.9	75.1
	C.	--	--	--	--	0.6	13.0	40.4
Romania – Rumänien	A.	918.6	935.5	1,052.7	1,130.3	1,190.8	1,525.8	1,599.9
	B.	444.6	426.5	470.3	519.1	578.5	702.1	770.2
	C.	474.0	509.0	582.4	611.2	612.3	823.7	829.7
Spain – Spanien	A.	13.4	19.0	43.8	40.6	149.4	189.0	226.0
	B.	7.7	10.0	20.9	30.0	122.0	143.6	164.7
	C.	5.7	9.0	22.9	10.6	27.4	45.4	61.3
Sweden – Schweden	A.	234.9	196.5	188.6	232.3	435.5	545.4	539.4
	B.	105.4	111.0	108.9	130.7	285.8	289.5	280.5
	C.	129.5	85.5	79.7	101.6	149.7	255.9	258.9
Switzerland – Schweiz	A.	95.1	110.6	121.2	167.7	244.6	323.2	371.4
	B.	24.6	35.9	30.7	67.9	79.5	89.7	108.1
	C.	70.5	74.7	90.5	99.8	165.1	233.5	263.3
United Kingdom – Großbritannien	A.	641.4	606.8	557.8	715.2	889.8	959.3	1,231.8
	B.	418.2	406.8	371.1	540.6	690.2	591.1	824.9
	C.	223.2	200.0	186.7	174.6	199.6	368.2	406.9
West Berlin	A.	24.8	31.9	25.7	35.3	63.0	96.9	135.4
	B.	7.8	8.0	10.3	28.2	46.1	68.3	98.4
	C.	17.0	23.9	15.4	7.1	16.9	28.6	37.0
Yugoslavia – Jugoslawien	A.	519.8	548.4	569.3	670.9	1,239.6	1,558.4	1,821.1
	B.	293.5	293.5	281.7	336.8	680.1	782.4	920.9
	C.	226.3	254.9	287.6	334.1	559.5	776.0	900.2
Asia – Asien:								
Afghanistan	A.	66.9	79.9	68.9	68.1	122.4	132.2	154.3
	B.	36.0	45.3	38.1	33.7	61.8	67.9	87.5
	C.	30.9	34.6	30.8	34.4	60.6	64.3	66.8
Bangladesh – Bangladesch	A.	--	--	16.6	53.3	58.1	52.2	36.6
	B.	--	--	8.8	43.5	40.0	37.2	23.5
	C.	--	--	7.8	9.8	18.1	15.0	13.1

5.5.3 Economy / Wirtschaft

Country Land		1970	1971	1972	1973	1974	1975	1976
Burma – Birma	A.	4.4	5.0	6.6	2.4	3.4	4.9	2.0
	B.	3.0	3.2	3.9	1.9	3.1	4.5	1.3
	C.	1.4	1.8	2.7	0.5	0.3	0.4	0.7
China	A.	41.9	138.7	210.6	201.3	213.9	200.9	314.4
	B.	22.4	70.1	100.2	100.5	108.4	93.1	179.8
	C.	19.5	68.6	110.4	100.8	105.5	107.8	134.6
Cyprus – Zypern	A.	9.3	12.2	13.8	12.7	19.8	16.8	27.1
	B.	4.1	7.3	7.1	7.6	10.8	12.7	16.7
	C.	5.2	4.9	6.7	5.1	9.0	4.1	10.4
India – Indien	A.	364.9	372.1	457.2	588.8	615.5	685.6	647.5
	B.	122.3	116.3	138.5	222.8	269.4	292.1	271.0
	C.	242.6	255.8	318.7	366.0	346.1	393.5	376.5
Indonesia – Indonesien	A.	29.5	20.2	9.4	6.9	27.9	28.6	32.3
	B.	4.5	10.1	2.6	2.7	8.0	7.7	4.4
	C.	25.0	10.1	6.8	4.2	19.9	20.9	27.9
Iran	A.	231.2	239.4	229.5	275.0	495.7	509.7	444.6
	B.	169.0	139.3	95.5	137.3	265.8	281.5	217.9
	C.	62.2	100.1	134.0	137.7	229.9	228.2	226.7
Iraq – Irak	A.	63.5	104.6	151.7	332.1	453.1	599.5	714.5
	B.	59.4	99.1	90.1	141.5	182.3	274.1	341.6
	C.	4.1	5.5	61.6	190.6	270.8	325.4	372.9
Japan	A.	652.3	733.6	815.6	994.4	1,679.8	1,922.4	2,120.5
	B.	341.4	377.4	381.7	622.0	905.7	668.9	748.4
	C.	310.9	356.2	433.9	372.4	774.1	1,253.5	1,372.1
Jordan – Jordanien	A.	6.4	5.9	0.6	2.5	2.4	4.0	4.0
	B.	6.4	5.9	0.6	2.5	2.4	4.0	4.0
	C.	--	--	--	--	--	--	--
Kambodsha – Kambodscha	A.	1.7	0.1	--	--	--	--	--
	B.	0.3	0.1	--	--	--	--	--
	C.	1.4	--	--	--	--	--	--
Korea, People's Democratic Republic Koreanische Volksdemokratische Rep.	A.	329.3	452.3	380.0	357.3	343.2	338.2	300.5
	B.	207.0	330.1	251.6	224.0	194.3	186.8	181.8
	C.	122.3	122.2	128.4	133.3	148.9	151.4	118.7

Economy 5.5.3
Wirtschaft

Country Land		1970	1971	1972	1973	1974	1975	1976
Kuwait – Kuweit	A.	10.0	18.1	14.5	7.9	4.7	3.5	10.1
	B.	9.7	17.4	14.5	7.9	4.7	3.5	10.1
	C.	0.3	0.7	–	–	–	–	–
Laos	A.	–	–	–	–	–	–	10.6
	B.	–	–	–	–	–	–	10.6
	C.	–	–	–	–	–	–	–
Lebanon – Libanon	A.	17.5	22.0	18.2	19.1	32.9	21.4	10.8
	B.	13.7	18.4	13.8	11.5	25.5	15.2	6.8
	C.	3.8	3.6	4.4	7.6	7.4	6.2	4.0
Malaysia	A.	112.6	79.1	59.4	97.6	188.7	102.1	107.7
	B.	1.6	1.5	1.0	0.9	0.7	0.8	4.2
	C.	111.0	77.6	58.4	96.7	188.0	101.3	103.5
Mongolia – Mongolei	A.	230.9	235.3	287.2	338.5	404.3	480.4	614.5
	B.	178.3	163.8	210.2	250.6	285.2	355.1	474.7
	C.	52.6	71.5	77.0	87.9	119.1	125.3	139.8
Nepal	A.	1.3	1.6	1.2	1.0	2.1	5.5	6.4
	B.	0.7	0.6	0.6	0.7	2.1	5.0	6.4
	C.	0.6	1.0	0.6	0.3	–	0.5	–
Pakistan	A.	60.4	60.8	36.2	36.4	54.8	60.7	58.6
	B.	32.1	25.8	17.5	12.6	30.2	37.1	43.0
	C.	28.3	35.0	18.7	23.8	24.6	23.6	15.6
Philippines – Philippinen	A.	–	–	–	–	–	12.8	68.3
	B.	–	–	–	–	–	0.4	1.4
	C.	–	–	–	–	–	12.4	66.9
Saudi-Arabia – Saudi-Arabien	A.	5.4	5.4	4.5	2.9	2.8	5.6	13.2
	B.	5.4	5.4	4.5	2.9	2.8	5.6	13.2
	C.	–	–	–	–	–	–	–
Singapore – Singapur	A.	8.4	8.1	9.0	9.6	18.0	14.5	21.0
	B.	5.5	4.4	4.4	6.4	4.5	3.8	11.9
	C.	2.9	3.7	4.6	3.2	13.5	10.7	9.1
Sri Lanka	A.	17.0	23.0	13.0	13.1	34.2	22.4	28.6
	B.	5.0	8.5	3.1	6.3	22.2	12.0	14.6
	C.	12.0	14.5	9.9	6.8	12.0	10.4	14.0

357

5.5.3 Economy / Wirtschaft

Country / Land		1970	1971	1972	1973	1974	1975	1976
Syria – Syrien	A.	59.1	78.3	112.3	118.8	172.4	167.8	235.4
	B.	41.8	51.9	58.6	72.1	70.1	99.0	138.5
	C.	17.3	26.4	53.7	46.7	102.3	68.8	96.9
Thailand	A.	3.4	6.6	6.0	4.5	11.1	17.3	10.2
	B.	2.6	2.5	2.8	2.1	1.3	4.0	7.8
	C.	0.8	4.1	3.2	2.4	9.8	13.3	2.4
Turkey – Türkei	A.	83.3	102.0	144.7	132.8	129.1	95.3	114.5
	B.	56.2	68.4	110.8	93.9	72.3	38.2	54.5
	C.	27.1	33.6	33.9	38.9	56.8	57.1	60.0
Vereinigte Arabische Emirate	A.	--	--	--	--	--	1.9	4.6
	B.	--	--	--	--	--	1.9	4.6
	C.	--	--	--	--	--	--	--
Vietnam, Democratic Republic – Demokratische Republik Vietnam	A.	183.2	160.8	116.8	179.8	235.7	206.5	296.1
	B.	166.5	139.3	94.2	142.9	192.3	158.7	232.5
	C.	16.7	21.5	22.6	36.9	43.4	47.8	63.6
Yemen, Arab Republic – Arabische Republik Jemen	A.	11.0	7.5	2.7	3.6	8.6	5.6	9.2
	B.	10.0	7.2	2.3	3.4	8.5	5.0	8.8
	C.	1.0	0.3	0.4	0.2	0.1	0.6	0.4
Yemen (People's Democratic Republic) – Volksdemokratische Republik Jemen	A.	4.5	2.2	6.5	11.6	15.2	13.9	20.0
	B.	4.3	2.2	6.5	11.5	15.1	13.8	20.0
	C.	0.2	--	--	0.1	0.1	0.1	--
Africa – Afrika:								
Algeria – Algerien	A.	118.3	121.9	114.5	116.8	171.7	247.0	190.3
	B.	62.5	52.6	55.9	64.7	110.3	112.3	131.4
	C.	55.8	69.3	58.6	52.1	61.4	134.7	58.9
Angola	A.	--	--	--	--	--	--	19.7
	B.	--	--	--	--	--	--	5.3
	C.	--	--	--	--	--	--	14.4
Benin (formerly-früher: Tahomé)	A.	0.7	1.9	1.4	3.4	1.6	3.0	2.7
	B.	0.7	1.0	1.4	1.3	1.6	2.5	2.7
	C.	--	0.9	--	2.1	--	0.5	--

Economy 5.5.3
Wirtschaft

Country Land		1970	1971	1972	1973	1974	1975	1976
Cameroon – Kamerun	A. B. C.	7.5 0.6 6.9	5.1 1.4 3.7	4.1 0.9 3.2	4.2 0.7 3.5	12.3 1.0 11.3	36.6 1.9 34.7	36.7 3.3 33.4
Central African Empire – Zentralafrikanisches Reich (formerly-früher: Republic-Republik)	A. B. C.	-- -- --	1.4 1.4 --	0.1 0.1 --	0.4 0.4 --	0.5 0.5 --	0.1 0.1 --	0.1 0.1 --
Congo, People's Republic – Volksrepublik Kongo	A. B. C.	1.5 0.8 0.7	4.8 4.2 0.6	1.3 0.3 1.0	3.8 1.2 2.6	4.0 2.0 2.0	4.2 1.8 2.4	4.5 2.5 2.0
Egypt – Ägypten	A. B. C.	606.4 326.9 279.5	643.9 343.2 300.7	513.7 266.1 247.6	541.1 277.2 263.9	728.1 301.3 426.8	710.3 262.0 448.3	530.6 199.8 330.8
Equatorial Guinea – Äquatorial-Guinea	A. B. C.	-- -- --	0.9 0.9 --	0.1 0.1 --	3.1 -- 3.1	-- -- --	2.0 0.5 1.5	2.6 1.3 1.3
Ethiopia – Äthiopien	A. B. C.	2.1 1.3 0.8	4.2 1.3 2.9	3.7 1.6 2.1	3.8 1.6 2.2	6.2 2.6 3.6	5.3 3.2 2.1	4.3 3.6 0.7
Ghana	A. B. C.	49.7 9.9 39.8	19.6 12.7 6.9	39.9 9.2 30.7	37.7 9.7 28.0	49.9 25.3 24.6	57.0 10.7 46.3	81.2 16.9 64.3
Guinea	A. B. C.	14.2 11.2 3.0	36.2 31.2 5.0	50.5 44.9 5.6	43.7 41.8 1.9	27.3 22.4 4.9	34.1 19.7 14.4	50.1 23.3 26.8
Guinea-Bissau	A. B. C.	-- -- --	-- -- --	-- -- --	-- -- --	-- -- --	0.3 0.3 --	1.4 1.4 --
Ivory Coast – Elfenbeinküste	A. B. C.	1.9 0.4 1.5	12.4 1.2 11.2	5.3 1.7 3.6	10.1 3.9 6.2	28.2 8.6 19.6	32.7 13.2 19.5	24.3 9.6 14.7
Kenia	A. B. C.	1.8 1.4 0.4	3.4 1.2 2.2	1.4 0.7 0.7	0.2 0.2 --	1.0 0.4 0.6	3.3 0.3 3.0	1.1 0.1 1.0

359

5.5.3 Economy / Wirtschaft

Country / Land		1970	1971	1972	1973	1974	1975	1976
Liberia	A.	--	--	--	--	3.0	3.1	3.7
	B.	--	--	--	--	2.6	2.6	3.4
	C.	--	--	--	--	0.4	0.5	0.3
Libya – Libyen	A.	12.9	8.9	38.6	44.5	28.5	18.8	16.2
	B.	12.9	8.9	8.6	14.1	28.5	18.8	16.2
	C.	--	--	30.0	30.4	--	--	--
Madagascar – Madagaskar	A.	0.6	0.9	1.2	0.3	0.7	1.1	3.4
	B.	--	--	--	--	--	--	0.1
	C.	0.6	0.9	1.2	0.3	0.7	1.1	3.3
Mali	A.	6.4	4.1	2.3	3.2	4.9	6.6	5.5
	B.	4.7	2.3	1.1	2.7	4.2	5.8	4.9
	C.	1.7	1.8	1.2	0.5	0.7	0.8	0.6
Mauritania – Mauretanien	A.	0.4	0.1	--	--	--	--	--
	B.	0.4	0.1	--	--	--	--	--
	C.	--	--	--	--	--	--	--
Morocco – Marokko	A.	50.1	47.1	55.2	54.4	87.1	86.9	105.6
	B.	32.5	28.2	31.5	28.3	54.1	45.7	55.3
	C.	17.6	18.9	23.7	26.1	33.0	41.2	50.3
Nigeria – Nigerien	A.	31.2	56.7	28.8	39.9	91.9	108.3	50.5
	B.	10.9	15.7	9.0	11.0	21.5	24.3	23.9
	C.	20.3	41.0	19.8	28.9	70.4	84.0	26.6
Rwanda – Ruanda	A.	--	--	--	--	0.8	1.8	0.9
	B.	--	--	--	--	0.8	0.9	0.9
	C.	--	--	--	--	--	0.9	--
Senegal	A.	1.2	0.9	1.7	4.9	16.3	3.2	1.6
	B.	1.2	0.9	1.4	4.9	16.3	3.2	0.4
	C.	--	--	0.3	--	--	--	1.2
Sierra Leone	A.	1.6	2.3	2.4	2.7	1.1	2.2	2.1
	B.	1.6	2.3	0.8	1.2	1.1	1.7	2.1
	C.	--	--	1.6	1.5	--	0.5	--
Somalia	A.	3.2	7.3	14.6	12.6	18.8	26.5	23.4
	B.	2.8	5.5	11.7	11.5	16.8	22.2	18.7
	C.	0.4	1.8	2.9	1.1	2.0	4.3	4.7

Economy 5.5.3
Wirtschaft

Country Land		1970	1971	1972	1973	1974	1975	1976
Sudan	A.	77.4	67.1	18.2	2.5	6.2	12.6	19.0
	B.	32.5	20.1	17.1	2.5	3.8	4.7	4.5
	C.	44.9	47.0	1.1	--	2.4	7.9	14.5
Tanzania - Tansania	A.	1.8	2.2	1.4	3.1	5.1	8.5	4.0
	B.	1.1	0.6	0.6	0.6	2.3	2.6	1.2
	C.	0.7	1.6	0.8	2.5	2.8	5.9	2.8
Togo	A.	4.0	6.2	5.3	1.4	1.7	2.8	4.5
	B.	1.2	1.8	1.4	1.4	1.7	2.8	2.9
	C.	2.8	4.4	3.9	--	--	--	1.6
Tunisia - Tunesien	A.	5.7	9.9	9.6	11.2	17.1	10.5	14.8
	B.	3.1	3.6	2.7	5.8	8.1	3.5	9.9
	C.	2.6	6.3	6.9	5.4	9.0	7.0	4.9
Uganda	A.	3.9	3.9	4.1	3.3	5.7	6.1	1.5
	B.	1.1	3.9	3.4	0.9	0.9	1.4	1.5
	C.	2.8	--	0.7	2.4	4.8	4.7	--
Zambia - Sambia	A.	--	--	--	--	3.2	7.5	2.3
	B.	--	--	--	--	3.2	7.5	2.3
	C.	--	--	--	--	--	--	--
America - Amerika:								
Argentina - Argentinien	A.	29.9	32.3	24.7	76.7	137.5	304.4	233.9
	B.	1.7	1.9	1.8	4.5	6.0	10.7	8.5
	C.	28.2	30.4	22.9	72.2	131.5	293.7	225.4
Bolivia - Bolivien	A.	3.1	9.0	3.3	16.2	15.5	12.6	16.5
	B.	--	--	0.8	4.0	4.1	3.0	4.2
	C.	3.1	9.0	2.5	12.2	11.4	9.6	12.3
Brazil - Brasilien	A.	23.2	43.7	72.9	125.8	202.0	396.1	445.5
	B.	2.4	2.0	7.1	9.3	90.0	93.3	76.1
	C.	20.8	41.7	65.8	116.5	112.0	302.8	369.4
Canada - Kanada	A.	125.3	148.6	299.8	265.0	111.0	471.2	541.2
	B.	7.5	12.4	18.7	20.9	28.9	31.9	41.9
	C.	117.8	136.2	281.1	244.1	82.1	439.3	499.3
Chile	A.	0.8	7.8	18.9	28.6	--	--	--
	B.	0.5	7.0	11.6	16.0	--	--	--
	C.	0.3	0.8	7.3	12.6	--	--	--

5.5.3 Economy / Wirtschaft

Country / Land		1970	1971	1972	1973	1974	1975	1976
Colombia – Kolumbien	A.	10.9	5.4	3.9	10.1	5.3	9.0	5.0
	B.	1.5	1.1	2.7	0.8	1.0	1.9	1.7
	C.	9.4	4.3	1.2	9.3	4.3	7.1	3.3
Costa-Rica	A.	6.2	2.2	2.8	5.3	2.2	0.5	2.8
	B.	--	--	--	0.2	0.6	0.5	0.6
	C.	6.2	2.2	2.8	5.1	1.6	--	2.2
Cuba – Kuba	A.	1,045.0	890.9	821.7	1,109.7	1,642.3	2,589.0	2,872.1
	B.	580.0	602.0	616.2	679.2	926.1	1,141.3	1,351.3
	C.	465.0	288.9	205.5	430.5	716.2	1,447.7	1,520.8
Dominican Republic – Dominikanische Republik	A.	--	--	2.8	15.6	--	--	--
	B.	--	--	--	--	--	--	--
	C.	--	--	2.8	15.6	--	--	--
Ecuador	A.	0.8	3.3	2.4	0.9	4.9	13.5	7.8
	B.	0.1	--	0.1	0.2	0.5	0.6	0.4
	C.	0.7	3.3	2.3	0.7	4.4	12.9	7.4
Guatemala	A.	--	--	--	4.3	--	--	--
	B.	--	--	--	--	--	--	--
	C.	--	--	--	4.3	--	--	--
Guyana – Guayana	A.	--	--	0.3	6.9	4.7	24.5	--
	B.	--	--	0.3	--	0.2	--	--
	C.	--	--	--	6.9	4.5	24.5	--
Jamaica – Jamaika	A.	0.7	2.3	1.0	3.9	9.5	11.2	--
	B.	--	--	--	--	--	--	--
	C.	0.7	2.3	1.0	3.9	9.5	11.2	--
Mexico – Mexiko	A.	1.0	9.5	8.4	0.6	2.4	6.1	18.0
	B.	0.7	0.3	0.6	0.5	1.1	4.4	6.9
	C.	0.3	9.2	7.8	0.1	1.3	1.7	11.1
Panama	A.	--	--	--	--	--	2.6	3.8
	B.	--	--	--	--	--	2.6	3.8
	C.	--	--	--	--	--	--	--
Peru	A.	0.3	0.2	2.0	19.7	9.3	118.5	32.0
	B.	0.1	--	0.2	4.3	4.6	28.3	13.9
	C.	0.2	0.2	1.8	15.4	4.7	90.2	18.1

Economy
Wirtschaft 5.5.3

Country Land		1970	1971	1972	1973	1974	1975	1976
Salvador	A.	--	--	2.8	3.7	--	0.1	--
	B.	--	--	--	--	--	0.1	--
	C.	--	--	2.8	3.7	--	--	--
USA	A.	160.9	183.6	537.8	1,161.0	742.2	1,599.5	2,205.5
	B.	57.8	54.4	76.4	137.8	177.3	137.4	198.7
	C.	103.1	129.2	461.4	1,023.2	564.9	1,462.1	2,006.8
Uruguay	A.	1.8	2.2	3.4	6.1	25.5	15.0	5.4
	B.	0.8	0.9	1.2	0.8	0.8	1.0	1.3
	C.	1.0	1.3	2.2	5.3	24.7	14.0	4.1
Venezuela	A.	--	--	4.2	1.2	0.2	0.2	0.3
	B.	--	--	0.1	0.6	0.2	0.2	0.3
	C.	--	--	4.1	0.6	--	--	--
Australia and Oceania – Australien und Ozeanien:								
Australia – Australien	A.	61.8	69.4	73.0	198.0	183.9	329.4	409.7
	B.	1.5	1.3	1.8	3.2	5.4	2.1	3.1
	C.	60.3	68.1	71.2	194.8	178.5	327.3	406.6
New Zealand – Neuseeland	A.	19.6	27.4	22.6	38.7	60.4	32.5	81.1
	B.	0.7	1.3	1.0	1.4	2.4	2.0	2.4
	C.	18.9	26.1	21.6	37.3	58.0	30.5	78.7

5.5.4 Economy / Wirtschaft

5.5.4 EXPORT STRUCTURE – STRUKTUR DES EXPORTS – STRUKTURA EKSPORTA
(in percent – in Prozent – v procentach)

	1970	1971	1972	1973	1974	1975	1976
Total – Insgesamt – Vsego	100.0	100.0	100.0	100.0	100.0	100.0	100.0
of which – darunter – v tom čisle:							
machines, equipment and means of transportation – Maschinen, Ausrüstungen und Transportmittel – mašiny, oborudovanie i transportnye sredstva	21.5	21.8	23.6	21.8	19.2	18.7	19.4
combustibles and electric power – Brennstoffe und Elektroenergie – toplivo i elektroenergija	15.6	18.0	17.7	19.2	25.4	31.4	34.3
ores and concentrates, metals and metal products – Erze und Konzentrate, Metalle u.Metallerzeugnisse – rudy i koncentraty, metally i izdelija iz nich	19.6	18.7	19.0	17.1	14.7	14.3	13.2
chemical products, fertilizers, caoutchouc – chemische Produkte, Düngemittel, Kautschuk – chimičeskie produkty, udobrenija, kaučuk	3.5	3.4	3.3	3.0	3.6	3.5	3.0
timber, cellulose and paper products – Nutzholz, Zellulose- und Papiererzeugnisse – lesomaterialy i celljulozno-bumažnye izdelija	6.5	6.3	6.1	6.4	6.9	5.7	5.3
textile raw materials and semifinished goods – Textilrohstoffe und Halbfabrikate – tekstil'noe syr'e i polufabrikaty	3.4	3.3	3.8	3.3	3.3	2.9	2.9
furs and raw furs – Rauchwaren und Rohfelle – pušnina i mechovoe syr'e	0.4	0.4	0.4	0.3	0.3	0.2	0.3
food and luxuries and raw materials for their production – Nahrungs-u.Genußmittel u.Rohstoffe für deren Produkt.– piščevkusovye tovary i syr'e dlja ich proizvodstva	8.4	9.2	5.9	5.6	7.1	4.8	3.0
industrial consumer products – Industriegüter des Volksbedarfs – promyšlennye tovary narodnogo potreblenija	2.7	2.9	3.1	3.0	2.9	3.1	3.0

Economy 5.5.5
Wirtschaft

5.5.5 IMPORT STRUCTURE – STRUKTUR DES IMPORTS – STRUKTURA IMPORTA
(in percent – in Prozent – v procentach)

	1970	1971	1972	1973	1974	1975	1976	1977
Total – Insgesamt – Vsego of which – darunter – v tom čisle:	100.0	100.0	100.0	100.0	100.0	100.0	100.0	100.0
machines, equipment and means of transportation – Maschinen, Ausrüstungen und Transportmittel – mašiny, oborudovanie i transportnye sredstva	35.5	34.0	34.6	34.3	32.4	33.9	36.3	
combustibles and electric power – Brennstoffe und Elektroenergie – toplivo i elektroenergija	2.0	2.7	3.0	3.4	3.5	3.9	3.6	
ores and concentrates, metals and metal products – Erze und Konzentrate, Metalle u.Metallerzeugnisse – rudy i koncentraty, metally i izdelija iz nich	9.6	9.8	8.9	9.9	13.6	11.6	10.8	
chemical products, fertilizers, caoutchouc – chemische Produkte, Düngemittel, Kautschuk – chimičeskie produkty, udobrenija, kaučuk	5.7	5.4	4.9	4.3	6.3	4.7	4.3	
timber, cellulose and paper products – Nutzholz, Zellulose- und Papiererzeugnisse – lesomaterialy i celljulozno-bumažnye izdelija	2.1	2.1	1.8	1.6	1.9	2.2	1.8	
textile raw materials and semifinished goods – Textilrohstoffe und Halbfabrikate – tekstil'noe syr'e i polufabrikaty	4.8	4.5	3.3	3.7	4.1	2.4	2.3	
food and luxuries and raw materials for their production – Nahrungs-u.Genußmittel und Rohstoffe für deren Produktion – piščevkusovye tovary i syr'e dlja ich proizvodstva	15.8	15.2	18.0	20.2	17.1	23.0	22.8	
industrial consumer products – Industriegüter des Volksbedarfs – promyšlennye tovary narodnogo potreblenija	18.3	20.1	18.6	15.9	14.6	12.9	12.6	

5.5.6 Economy / Wirtschaft

SHARE OF THE MOST IMPORTANT PRODUCTS IN EXPORT — ANTEIL DER WICHTIGSTEN GÜTER AM EXPORT — UDEL'NYJ VES VAŽNEJŠICH TOVAROV V EKSPORTE
(in percent — in Prozent — v procentach)

Products-Güter-Tovary	1970	1971	1972	1973	1974	1975	1976	1977
Total – Insgesamt – Vsego	100.0	100.0	100.0	100.0	100.0	100.0	100.0	100.0
machines, equipment and means of transportation – Maschinen, Ausrüstungen und Transportmittel – mašiny, oborudovanie i transportnye sredstva	21.5	21.8	23.6	21.8	19.2	18.7	19.4	
of which – davon – iz nich:								
machine tools – Werkzeugmaschinen – stanki metallorežuščie	0.7	0.6	0.7	0.6	0.6	0.6	0.7	
energetic equipment – energetische Ausrüstungen – energetičeskoe oborudovanie	1.9	1.6	1.9	1.8	1.5	1.3	1.6	
electrotechnical equipment – elektrotechnische Ausrüstungen – elektrotechničeskoe oborudovanie	0.2	0.3	0.3	0.3	0.3	0.3	0.3	
equipment for underground and open-pit mining of mineral resources – Ausrüstungen für Untertage- u.Tagebau von Bodenschätzen – oborudovanie dlja podzemnoj i otkrytoj razrabotki poleznych iskopaemych	0.4	0.6	0.7	0.6	0.6	0.7	0.8	
hoisting devices – Hebetransportausrüstungen – pod'emno-transportnoe oborudovanie	0.4	0.4	0.4	0.4	0.4	0.4	0.3	
road and road construction equipment & machines – Straßen-u.Straßenbauausrüstungen und -maschinen – oborudovanie i mašiny dorožnye i dorožno-stroitel'nye	0.8	0.8	0.8	0.7	0.6	0.6	0.7	
tractors – Traktoren – traktory	0.7	0.6	0.7	0.7	0.6	0.6	0.7	
grain harvesters – Mähdrescher – kombajny	0.2	0.2	0.2	0.2	0.3	0.3	0.2	
Diesel locomotives – Diesellokomotiven – teplovozy	0.3	0.4	0.4	0.4	0.4	0.4	0.4	
trucks and garage equipments – Lastwagen und Garageausrüstungen – avtomobili gruzovye i garažnoe oborudovanie	2.3	2.4	2.5	2.1	1.7	1.9	2.0	
ships and ship equipment – Schiffe und Schiffsausrüstungen – suda i sudovoe oborudovanie	0.6	0.6	0.6	0.6	0.4	0.4	0.3	
air transport vehicles – Luftverkehrsmittel – sredstva vozdušnogo soobščenija	1.3	1.8	2.1	2.5	1.6	1.3	1.3	

Economy 5.5.6
Wirtschaft

	1970	1971	1972	1973	1974	1975	1976	1977
Passenger cars, motorcycles, motor scooters – Personenwagen, Motorräder, Motorroller – avtomobili legkovye, motocikly, motorollery	1.2	1.8	2.3	2.2	2.1	2.0	2.2	
Pit and anthracite coal – Stein-und Anthrazitkohle – Ugol'kamennyj i antracit	2.4	2.7	2.5	2.0	2.1	3.3	2.9	
Hard-coal coke – Steinkohlenkoks-Koks kamennougol'nyj	0.8	0.9	0.9	0.7	0.6	0.9	0.7	
Crude oil – Rohöl – Neft' syraja	7.2	8.5	8.6	8.5	11.2	15.6	18.3	
Mineral oil products, liquid synthetic combustibles – Erdölprodukte, synthetische flüssige Brennstoffe – Nefteprodukty, sintetičeskoe židkoe toplivo	4.3	4.8	4.4	6.7	9.8	9.0	9.1	
Fuel gas – Brenngas – Gaz gorjučij	0.4	0.5	0.4	0.6	1.0	1.9	2.6	
Electric power – Elektroenergie – Elektroenergija	0.4	0.6	0.6	0.6	0.5	0.7	0.6	
Iron ore – Eisenerz – Ruda železnaja	2.5	2.4	2.5	2.2	1.8	2.1	1.7	
Manganese ore – Manganerz – Ruda margancevaja	0.2	0.2	0.1	0.1	0.1	0.1	0.1	
Chromic ore – Chromerz – Ruda chromovaja								
Asbestos – Asbest – Asbest	0.4	0.4	0.4	0.3	0.3	0.4	– –	
Pig iron – Roheisen – Cugun	1.9	1.7	1.6	1.4	1.1	1.4	1.1	
Ferro alloys – Ferrolegierungen – Ferrosplavy	0.5	0.5	0.4	0.4	0.4	0.4	0.3	
Rolling stock of ferrous metals and steel – Walzgut aus Fe-Metallen – Prokat černych metallov	6.6	5.9	5.6	4.5	3.7	4.8	4.3	
Tubes – Rohre – Truby	0.5	0.7	0.5	0.4	0.3	0.4	0.6	
Copper – Kupfer – Med'	0.8	1.3	1.7	1.8	1.6	0.9	– –	
Aluminum – Aluminium – Aljuminij	1.4	1.4	1.6	1.5	1.3	1.1	– –	
Rolling stock of non-ferrous metals – Walzgut aus NE-Metallen – Prokat cvetnych metallov	0.9	0.7	0.8	0.6	0.5	0.4	0.4	
Chemical products – chemische Produkte – Chimičeskie produkty	1.5	1.4	1.3	1.2	1.4	1.1	1.1	
Fertilizers – Düngemittel – Udobrenija	0.9	0.9	0.9	0.8	1.4	1.5	1.1	
Synthetic caoutchouc – Synthesekautschuk – Kautschuk sintetičeskij	0.2	0.2	0.2	0.2	0.2	0.2	– –	
Tires – Reifen – Šiny	0.3	0.4	0.3	0.3	0.3	0.3	– –	
Cement – Zement – Cement	0.3	0.3	0.2	0.3	0.3	0.3	0.2	
Round wood – Rundholz – Kruglyj les	2.2	2.1	2.0	2.6	2.7	1.9	1.7	
Sawn timber – Schnittholz – Pilomaterialy	2.6	2.5	2.4	2.3	2.7	2.3	2.2	
Paper – Papier – Bumaga	0.6	0.5	0.6	0.5	0.5	0.5	0.4	
Cotton fibers – Baumwollfasern – Chlopok-volokno	2.9	2.9	3.4	3.0	3.1	2.7	2.7	
Wool – Wolle – Šerst'	0.2	0.2	0.1	0.1	0.1	0.1	– –	

5.5.6 Economy / Wirtschaft

	1970	1971	1972	1973	1974	1975	1976	1977
Furs and raw furs (without finished fur products) - Rauchwaren und Rohpelze (ohne fertige Pelzerzeugnisse - Pušnina i mechovoe syr'e (krome gotovych mechovych izdelij)	0.4	0.4	0.4	0.3	0.3	0.2	0.3	
Corn (without barley) - Korn (ohne Graupen) - Zerno (krome krupjanogo)	3.1	4.4	—	—	—	—	—	—
Sunflower seeds - Sonnenblumenkerne - Semja podsolnečnika	0.2	0.1	0.1	0.1	—	—	—	—
Meat and meat products - Fleisch u. Fleischprodukte - Mjaso i mjasoprodukty	0.3	0.2	0.3	0.3	0.2	0.2	0.1	
Butter - Maslo korov'e	0.5	0.2	0.1	0.1	0.1	0.1	0.1	
Fish and fish products - Fisch u. Fischprodukte - Ryba i ryboprodukty	0.6	0.7	0.6	0.6	0.6	0.6	0.5	
Flour - Mehl - Muka	0.5	0.4	0.2	0.3	0.4	0.3	0.3	
Refined sugar - Raffinadezucker - Sachar rafinirovannyj	0.8	0.8	—	—	—	—	—	—
Salad-oils - Speiseöle - Masla rastitel'nye prodovol'stvennye	0.8	1.0	0.9	0.6	1.3	0.9	0.5	
Cotton and cotton-like fabrics - Baumwoll- und baumwollähnliche Stoffe - Tkani chlopčatobumažnye i tipa chlopčatobumažnych	0.4	0.4	0.4	0.3	0.2	0.2	0.2	
Medicines - Medikamente - Medikamenty	0.3	0.4	0.4	0.3	0.3	0.3	0.3	
Household machines and appliances - Haushaltmaschinen und -geräte - Mašiny i pribory bytovye	0.9	0.9	0.9	0.8	0.9	1.1	1.1	

Economy 5.5.7
Wirtschaft

5.5.7　FOREIGN TRADE ORGANIZATIONS　-　AUSSENHANDELSORGANISATIONEN　-
VNEŠNETORGOVYE ORGANIZACII (V/O)

> The USSR Chamber of Commerce and Industry -
> Handels- und Industriekammer der UdSSR -
> Torgovo-promyšlennaja palata SSSR
> Moskva 103097, ul. Kuibyševa 6
> Tel.: 2210811, 223423
> Telex: 7126
>
>
> Bank for Foreign Trade of the USSR -
> Außenhandelsbank der UdSSR -
> Vneštorgbank SSSR
> Moskva K-16, Neglinnaja ul. 12
> Tel.: 296- 34- 77, 296- 31- 38
> and-und:
> Moskva K-16, Kopjevskij Per. 3/5
> Tel.: 296- 30- 12, 228- 48- 60
> Telex: 7174,7175,7176,7177,7178

ALMAZJUVELIREXPORT
Moskva 121019, Prospekt Kalinina 29
Tel.: 202-81-90, Telex: 7125
　　Exports and imports diamonds, jewellery articles with precious and semi-
　　precious gems, articles of silver, amber articles, precious gems, jewel gems
　　and natural semi-precious gems in jewellery made of gold, silver and platinum,
　　synthetic quartz, precious metals in nuggets and powder form, silver solder
　　for silver articles, industrial articles of precious metals and their
　　alloys -
　　Aus- und Einfuhr: Brillanten, Juwelierwaren mit Edelsteinen und Halbedel-
　　steinen, silberne Gegenstände, Bernsteinschmuck, Edelsteine, Schmucksteine
　　und natürliche Halbedelsteine in Schmuck aus Gold, Silber und Platin, synthe-
　　tischer Quarz, Edelmetalle in Barren und Pulverform, Silberlot für Silber-
　　waren, diverse Industrieerzeugnisse aus Edelmetallen und ihre Legierungen.

AVIAEXPORT
Moskva 121200, Smolenskaja-Sennaja pl. 32/34
Tel.: 244-26-86, Telex: 7257
　　Exports and imports aircrafts, helicopters, aircraft engines, aircraft units,
　　cockpit equipment , electrical and radio-navigation equipment, control and
　　testing apparatus and aircraft spare parts; ground equipment for the operation
　　and technical maintenance of aircraft and helicopters, propellers and para-
　　chutes; provides technical servicing of aircraft equipment and training
　　of aircraft specialists -
　　Aus- und Einfuhr: Flugzeuge, Hubschrauber, Flugmotoren, Aggregate, Flugzeug-
　　bordgeräte, elektrische und Funknavigationsgeräte, Kontroll- und Prüfgeräte
　　sowie Flugzeugersatzteile; ferner Bodenausrüstungen für den Betrieb und die
　　technische Wartung von Flugzeugen und Hubschraubern, Propeller und Fallschirme;
　　vermittelt die Durchführung der Reparatur, sichert die Wartung der verkauften
　　Maschinen und Ausrüstungen, veranstaltet die Schulung der Flugzeugfachleute.

5.5.7 Economy / Wirtschaft

AVTOEXPORT
Moskva 121019, ul. Volchonka 14
Tel.: 202-85-35, Telex: 7135, 7253
Exports and imports passenger cars and lorries, motor coaches, truck-tractors, tip-up lorries, motorcars for special purposes, motorcycles, motor scooters, bicycles and mopeds; exports garage and repair equipment. Buyers are guaranteed technical servicing of supplied vehicles and training of foreign specialists -
Aus- und Einfuhr: Personen- und Lastkraftwagen, Omnibusse, Zugmaschinen und Kipper, Kraftwagen für Sonderzwecke, Motorräder, Motorroller, Fahrräder und Mopeds; exportiert Garagen- und Reparaturwerkstättenausrüstungen. Erteilt den Kunden jegliche Unterstützung bei der technischen Bedienung der aus der UdSSR gelieferten Maschinen und führt Schulungen für ausländische Fachleute durch.

AVTOPROMIMPORT
Moskva 109017, Pjatnickaja ul. 50/2
Tel.: 231-81-26, Telex: 7264
Imports complete plants for the automobile industry including equipment for foundry, thermal treatment, stamping and pressing, mechanical, painting, plating, body building and assembly shops; complete production lines, welding and laboratory equipment, test sets and stands, factory transport facilities, universal equipment for plants and single departments, warehouse and other equipment for new buildings or modernization of motorcar plants or similar plants as well as test and repair equipment for motorcars -
Einfuhr: Komplette Ausrüstungen für Kraftwagenherstellerwerke einschl. zur Komplettierung von Härtereien, Schmieden und Pressereien, mechanischen Abteilungen, Anstreichereien, galvanischen Abteilungen, Karosseriefertigungsabteilungen und Montageschlossereien, komplette Taktstraßen, Schweißanlagen und Laboreinrichtungen, Prüfgeräte und Prüfeinrichtungen, innerbetriebliche Transportmittel, Universalausrüstungen für Werke und einzelne Abteilungen, Lager-und andere Einrichtungen für Neubauten oder zur Modernisierung von Kraftwagenherstellerwerken oder verwandter Werke sowie auch Anlagen zur Untersuchung und Wartung von Kraftwagen.

ELEKTRONORGTECHNIKA
Moskva 103006, Kaljaevskaja ul. 5
Tel.: 251-39-46, Telex: 7586
Exports and imports general-purpose digital and analogue electronic computers, peripheral devices for computers, management control equipment devices for acquisition and primary processing of data, including desk key-operated computers and calculating punches. Exports valves, semi-conductor devices, integrated circuits, S.H.F. instruments, gas-discharge devices, camera and oscillographic tubes, electronic multipliers, photocells, ferrite elements, resistors and condensators. Renders assistance to buyers in erecting, mounting and starting the equipment, in maintaining the equipment delivered from the USSR and in training personnel from different countries. -
Aus- und Einfuhr: Elektrische Digital- und Analogrechenmaschinen von allgemeiner Bestimmung, Außenanlagen zu diesen Rechenmaschinen, Vorrichtungen zum Sammeln bzw. zur primären Bearbeitung von Informationen einschl. Tischtastenund Perforationsrechenmaschinen. Ausfuhr von: Elektronenröhren, Halbleitergeräten, integrierten Schaltungen, Hochfrequenzgeräten, Gasentladungsgeräten, Fernsehröhren und Oszillographenröhren, Fotomultiplier, Fotozellen, Erzeugnisse aus Ferromaterialien, Kurzschluß-Strom-Begrenzungswiderstände und Kondensatoren. Erteilt den Kunden Unterstützung beim Erstellen, Bau und der Inbetriebnahme von Ausrüstungen, bei der Wartung der aus der UdSSR gelieferten Ausrüstungen und bei der Schulung von Personal aus verschiedenen Ländern.

ENERGOMASEXPORT
Moskva 117330, Mosfilmovskaja ul. 35
Tel.: 147-21-77, Telex: 7565

Economy
Wirtschaft 5.5.7

Exports equipment and component parts for thermal and hydro-electric stations, Diesel engines and Diesel generators, Diesel plants, gas-electric units, electric engines, rectifiers and equipment for low voltage, equipment for electric welding, induction-heating plants, gas welding equipment; equipment and installations for railways, rolling stock for railways and electric road traffic, spare parts, also exports electric power. Provides assistance in mounting, starting and maintenance of the equipment delivered from the USSR and in training foreign specialists. -
Ausfuhr: Komplette Ausrüstungen und Einzelteile für Wärmekraft- und Wasserkraftwerke; Dieselmotoren und Dieselgeneratoren, Dieselkraftwerke, benzinelektrische Aggregate, Elektromotoren, Gleichrichter und Ausrüstungen für Niederspannung, ferner Ausrüstungen für das Elektroschweißen, die Elektrothermie, Gasschweißen, Ausrüstungen und Einrichtungen für die Eisenbahn, rollendes Material für Eisenbahnen und den elektrischen Straßenverkehr, Ersatzteile, exportiert auch elektrischen Strom. Hilfe bei der Montage, Inbetriebnahme und Wartung der aus der UdSSR gelieferten Ausrüstungen und Ausbildung ausländischer Fachkräfte.

EXPORTCHLEB
Moskva 121200, Smolenskaja-Sennaja pl. 32/34
Tel.: 244-47-01, Telex: 7145, 7146, 7147
Exports and imports wheat, rye, barley, oats, maize, rice, pulse , flour, groats, oil seeds, oil cakes, oil-seed meal, and other grain and fodder products, as well as seeds and seedlings -
Aus- und Einfuhr: Weizen, Roggen, Gerste, Hafer, Mais, Reis, Hülsenfrüchte, Mehl, Grütze, Ölsamen, Ölkuchen, Schrot und sonstiges Tierfutter sowie Samen, Saat- und Pflanzengut.

EXPORTLES
Moskva 121200, Smolenskaja-Sennaja pl. 32/34
Tel.: 241-60-44, Telex: 7229
Exports and imports sawn timber of Sibirian larch, pine and fir timber, timber sleepers, pitprops, pulpwood, round wood, lumber, plywood, fibreboards and chipboards, cellulose, paper, carton, cardboard, furniture, prefabricated wooden houses and other goods -
Aus- und Einfuhr: Schnittholz von sibirischen Lärchen, Kiefern- und Tannenschnittholz, Holzschwellen, Grubenholz, Rundholz, Papierholz, Sägematerial, Sperrholz, Holzfaser- und Holzspanpreßplatten, Zellulose, Papier, Karton, Pappe, Möbel, zusammensetzbare Holzhäuser und verschiedene andere Artikel.

EXPORTLJON
Moskva 117393, ul. Architektora Vlasova 33
Tel.: 128-07-86, Telex: 205
Exports and imports cotton, linter, flax, flax tow, long hemp fibers, flax for spinning, sheep, goat and camel wool, goat fluff, cotton, wool, silk, spun rayon fabrics and products, linen, cotton yarn, nets for fishing and net materials, also waste from natural silk, cotton, linen, hemp and from the production of chemical fibers. Imports cotton, sheep wool, woollen yarn, jute and jute goods, sisal, raw silk, artificial and synthetic fibers, fabrics, rayon and acetate yarn, cord -
Aus- und Einfuhr: Baumwolle, Linters, Flachs, Flachshede, lange Hanffasern, spinnfertiger Flachs und Hanfwerg, Schaf-, Ziegen- und Kamelwolle, Ziegenflaum, Baumwoll-, Woll-, Seiden-, Zellwollstoffe und Erzeugnisse aus ihnen; Leinen, Baumwollgarn, Netze für den Fischfang und Netzmaterialien, Abfälle von Naturseide, Baumwolle, Leinen, Hanf und Abfälle der Chemiefaserproduktion. Importiert Baumwolle, Schafwolle, Wollgarn, Jute und Erzeugnisse aus Jute, Sisal, Rohseide, Kunstfasern und synthetische Fasern, Stoffe, Viskose- und Azetatgarn, Kord.

5.5.7 Economy
Wirtschaft

LICENSINTORG
   Moskva 113461, ul. Kachovka 31
   Tel.: 122-02-54, Telex: 7246
      Handles operations involving the sale of licenses for Soviet inventions in
      all fields of industry and undertakes obligations for rendering license pur-
      chasers skilled technical assistance, transfer of know-how and technical
      documents; purchases licenses for foreign inventions and scientific and tech-
      nical improvements; sells and buys machines, equipment, materials and manu-
      factured goods whose delivery as prototypes and samples is stipulated in the
      terms of license agreements; renders on a commercial basis engineering
      services in the fields of metallurgical, foundry, and chemical technology and
      some other fields of industry by carrying out research and planning work,
      giving recommendations on industrial construction and technical consultations,
      etc. -
      Verkauf von Lizenzen auf sowjetische Erfindungen in sämtlichen Bereichen der
      Industrieproduktion, Erwerb von Lizenzen auf ausländische Erfindungen und
      wissenschaftliche und technische Verbesserungen; Ausfuhr und Einfuhr von Ma-
      schinen, Ausrüstungen, Werkstoffen und Erzeugnissen, deren Lieferung als Proto-
      typen oder Musterstücke durch die Lizenzabkommen vorgesehen ist; technische
      Unterstützung auf dem Gebiet der Metallurgie, Gießerei, chemischen Technologie
      und anderen Gebieten der Industrieproduktion durch Forschungs- und Planungs-
      arbeit, Empfehlungen beim Bau von Industrieobjekten, technische Konsultationen
      usw. -

MAŠINOEXPORT
   Moskva 117330, Mosfilmovskaja ul. 35
   Tel.: 147-15-42, Telex: 7207
      Exports equipment and tools for oil and gas drilling, geological prospecting
      and geophysical operations, as well as for oil-fields; tanks for storage
      of oil and oil products, liquefied gases and equipment for them, conveyors,
      elevators, escalators, jacks, pulleys, tackles, winches, lifts, hoisting
      machines; various cranes and excavators, blast furnace, steel-smelting, foundry,
      rolling, drawing, finishing equipment, equipment for continuous steel pouring;
      sintering and coking equipment, equipment for non-ferrous metallurgy, equipment
      for the building material and building industries; crushing and grinding, ore-
      dressing equipment; material handling equipment, drilling and building machines;
      equipment for pipeline construction, for sinking mines and extraction of
      minerals, for loading minerals and mechanization of transportation work in
      mines, for building underground railway tunnels, as well as for underground
      and open-pit mining; peat extracting equipment; garage and repair equipment
      for technical servicing of excavators, cranes, loaders, pipe-layers and
      other machinery. Supplies spare parts for all machinery delivered. Renders
      technical assistance in the assembly, maintenance and servicing. Trains
      technical personnel of customers. -
      Ausfuhr: Ausrüstungen und Instrumente für Erdöl- und Naturgasbohrungen, für
      geologische Erkundungsarbeiten und geophysikalische Arbeiten, für den Erdölberg-
      bau und die erdölerzeugende Industrie; Behälter für Erdöl, Erdölprodukte und
      verflüssigte Gase sowie entsprechende Ausrüstungen; Fördermaschinen, Elevato-
      ren, Rolltreppen, Hebeböcke, Blöcke, Flaschenzüge, Fahrstühle, Aufzüge, ver-
      schiedene Kräne und Bagger, Hochofen-, Stahlschmelzerei-, Gießerei-, Walzwerk-
      ausrüstungen, Ziehbänke mit Zubehör, Adjustageausrüstungen; Ausrüstungen zum
      kontinuierlichen Vergießen von Stahl, Ausrüstungen zum Sintern und Verkoken,
      Ausrüstungen für die Buntmetallurgie, Ausrüstungen für die Baumaterialien- und
      Bauindustrie; Zerkleinerungs- und Mahlmaschinen, Aufbereitungsanlagen, Bela-
      dungs- und Entladungseinrichtungen, Bohr- und Baumaschinen für den Bergbau;
      Ausrüstungen für die Rohrverlegung; Ausrüstungen für den Streckenvortrieb und
      zur Förderung von Bodenschätzen; Ausrüstungen zum Verladen der Bodenschätze
      und zur Mechanisierung der Förderanlagen in den Bergwerken, Ausrüstungen für
      den Bau von U-Bahn-Tunnels, ferner für die Arbeiten unter Tage und des Tage-
      baus; Montangrubenausrüstungen und Ausrüstungen zur Torfgewinnung; Garagen-

und Reparaturwerkstättenausrüstungen zur technischen Wartung von Baggern, Kränen, Lademaschinen, Rohrbiegemaschinen und anderen Maschinen; Lieferung von Ersatzteilen; erteilt technische Unterstützung beim Zusammenbau, bei der Wartung und bei Vorsorgereparaturen; führt Schulungen für Kundenpersonal durch.

MASINOIMPORT
Moskva 121200, Smolenskaja-Sennaja pl. 32/34
Tel.: 244-33-09, Telex: 7231, 7232

Imports power engineering and electrotechnical equipment, hoisting and haulage, pumping and compressing equipment, excavators, railway rolling stock, oil extracting and oil refining equipment and industrial fittings -

Einfuhr: Kraftwerksausrüstungen, elektrotechnische Ausrüstungen, Hebe- und Förderausrüstungen, Pumpen- und Kompressorausrüstungen, Selbstfahrkräne, Bagger, rollendes Eisenbahnmaterial, Ausrüstungen für die Rohölförderung und Erdölraffinerie sowie Industriearmaturen.

MASPRIBORINTORG
Moskva 121200, Smolenskaja-Sennaja pl. 32/34
Tel.: 244-27-75, Telex: 7235, 7236

Exports and imports wire and radio communication equipment, electric and measuring instruments, checking and measuring instruments and automatic devices, material testing machines and instruments, meteorological, aerological, oceanographic and hydrological instruments and equipment, photographic and motion picture equipment, radio and TV sets, watches, optical instruments for industrial and scientific purposes -

Aus- und Einfuhr: Ausrüstungen zur Nachrichtenübermittlung über Leitungen und Funkverbindungen, Elektro- und Hochfrequenzmeßgeräte, Kontroll- und Meßgeräte, Ausrüstungen zur Automatisierung technologischer Prozesse, Maschinen und Geräte zur Werkstoffprüfung, meteorologische, aerologische, ozeanographische und hydrologische Geräte und Ausrüstungen, Fotokameras und Kinoapparate, Rundfunk- und Fernsehempfänger, Uhren, optische Geräte für industrielle und wissenschaftliche Zwecke.

MEDEXPORT
Moskva 113461, ul. Kachovka 31
Tel.: 121-01-54, Telex: 7247

Exports various medical preparations: antibiotics, vitamins, sulphanylamides, etc., pharmaceutical raw materials for manufacture of medicines; up-to-date medical equipment and surgical appliances, a wide assortment of medical instruments; Tibetan medicines; vaccines and serums. Imports medicines, medical equipment, instruments and other goods -

Ausfuhr: Verschiedene gebrauchsfertige medizinische Präparate: Antibiotika, Vitamine, Sulfanilamide usw., Ausgangsstoffe für die pharmazeutische Industrie, Vakzine und Seren, medizinische Einrichtungen, Geräte und Apparate, eine große Auswahl medizinischer und tierärztlicher Instrumente; Artikel der tibetanischen Medizin sowie Verbandszeug. Einfuhr: Arzneimittel, medizinische Ausrüstungen, Instrumente und andere Waren.

MEŽDUNARODNAJA KNIGA
Moskva 121200, Smolenskaja-Sennaja pl. 32/34
Tel.: 244-10-22, Telex: 7160

Exports books, newspapers, magazines, sheet music, postcards, colour reproductions, albums, gramophone records, postage stamps for collections, film strips and slides. Handles operations involving the publication of Soviet books and musical works abroad. Imports books, newspapers, magazines, gramophone records -

5.5.7 Economy
Wirtschaft

Ausfuhr: Bücher, Zeitungen, Zeitschriften, Musikalien (Notenwerke), künstlerische Druckwerke (Kunstblätter und Alben), Schallplatten, Briefmarken für philatelistische Sammlungen, Filmstreifen und Diapositive. Erledigt die mit der Veröffentlichung von sowjetischen Büchern und musikalischen Werken im Ausland zusammenhängenden Arbeiten. Import: Bücher, Zeitungen, Zeitschriften, Schallplatten.

METALLURGIMPORT
Moskvà 117393, ul. Architektora Vlasova 33
Tel.: 128-37-20, 128-07-75, Telex: 7588

Imports mining, ore-dressing and drilling equipment: tunnelling and extracting machines, timbering, drilling equipment for mines, handling and transporting machines, conveyors, rotor and multi-bucket excavators, crushing and milling equipment, ore-dressing equipment, coal and peat briquetting plants;
metallurgical and foundry equipment: sintering and ore pelletizing equipment, equipment for coke-oven, blast-furnace, steel-making and foundry plants, equipment for non-ferrous metallurgy;
rolling equipment: blooming and slabbing mill trains, steel-sheet and section mills, flattening mills, railway-wheel mills and other rolling equipment; drawing and finishing equipment for rolling and sizing shops at rolling plants: draw and push benches, pointing machines, automatic lines and equipment for sizing, straightening, cutting, trimming, grinding and polishing of rods, sheets and strips, packing lines and lines for other finishing operations;
handling and transporting equipment for metallurgical industry: cranes for metallurgical operations, ore and coal reloaders and other handling machinery for metallurgical plants;
equipment for integrated plants: equipment for mining, handling and dressing of iron and non-ferrous metal ores, equipment for mining and stripping operations, ferrous and non-ferrous plants, coke-oven plants, peat-briquetting plants. -

Einfuhr: Einrichtungen für Schacht- und Grubenausbau sowie Aufbereitung: Streckenvortriebs-, Gewinnungs-, Lade- und Fördermaschinen, Ausrüstungen für den Grubenausbau, Bohranlagen für den Bergbau, Bandförderer u.a. Steigförderer, Schaufelrad- und andere Mehrgefäßbagger, Zerkleinerungs- und Vermahlungsausrüstungen, Ausrüstungen zur Aufbereitung von Bodenschätzen, Anlagen zur Brikettierung von Kohle und Torf;
Hütten- und Gießereiausrüstungen: Ausrüstungen zur Agglomerierung von Erzen und Sinteranlage, Ausrüstungen für Kokereien und chemische Nebenbetriebe, Hochöfen, SM-Stahlwerke, Gießereien, ferner Ausrüstungen für verschiedene Metallhütten;
Walzwerkausrüstungen: Block- und Brammenstraßen, Blech- und Formstahlwalzwerke, Plattfederstahl-Radscheiben-, Rohrwalz- und Rohrschweißwalzwerke sowie andere Walzwerkausrüstungen;
Ziehbank- und Nachbearbeitungsausrüstungen für Walz- und Kalibrierungszwecke der Hüttenwerke: Ziehbänke, Zieh- und Wetzmaschinen, Kalibrierungs-, Richt-, Schneide-, Schleif- und Polierungsstraßen für Stangen, Blech und Stahlband, ferner Verpackungs- und andere Nachbearbeitungsausrüstungen;
Hebe- und Förderanlagen für Hüttenwerke: Krananlagen, Umladevorrichtungen für Erze und Kohle sowie andere Hebe- und Förderanlagen für Hüttenwerke; komplette Werke: Montan- und Aufbereitungswerke für Eisen- und Nichteisenerze, komplette Werkanlagen für den Aufschluß von Lagerstätten, Eisenhüttenwerke und verschiedene Metallhüttenwerke sowie Koks- und Torfbrikettierungswerke.

Economy
Wirtschaft 5.5.7

NEFTECHIMPROMEXPORT
Moskva 113324, Ovčinnikovskaja Nab. 18/1
Tel.: 220-11-09
Renders technical assistance in the projecting and building of complete plants for the oil refining, petrochemical, chemical and paper-and-pulp industries abroad. Handles surveying, research and designing work, exports equipment, materials and spare parts, undertakes author's supervision, assembly and adjustment work, commissioning of enterprises and training of customers' personnel in Soviet enterprises or in the customers' countries directly, delegates specialists -

Technische Unterstützung bei der Projektierung und beim Bau kompletter Werke der erdölverarbeitenden, petrolchemischen, chemischen, Zellstoff- und Papierindustrie im Ausland. Führt wissenschaftliche Forschungs- und Projektierungsarbeiten durch, exportiert Ausrüstungen, Materialien und Ersatzteile, übernimmt die technische Aufsicht, erledigt Montage- und Einrichtungsarbeiten, führt die Inbetriebnahme von Werkanlagen durch und bildet technisches Personal des Auftraggebers in den Betrieben der Sowjetunion oder direkt in den Ländern ihrer Kunden aus, entsendet Fachkräfte.

NOVOEXPORT
Moskva 103287, ul. Bašilovskaja 19
Tel.: 285-66-90, Telex: 7254
Exports and imports art handicraft articles of wood, metal, bone; handwoven carpets, uncut semiprecious and precious stones; works by Soviet painters, graphic artists and sculptors; ceramic articles; fishing tackle and hunting gear; model products; pearl paste; equipment for city transport and railway passengers; peat, household wooden articles and other goods. Assists foreign firms and merchant companies in setting up business contacts with Soviet foreign trade organizations in signing deals for commercial exchange -

Aus- und Einfuhr: Kunstgewerbeerzeugnisse aus Holz, Metall, Elfenbein, Stein; handgewebte Teppiche, rohe Schmucksteine; Werke sowjetischer Maler, Graphiker und Bildhauer; Kunstkeramik; Angel- und Jagdsportzubehör; Modellbauteile; Perlenpaste; Einrichtungen in den Fahrzeugen des Straßen- und Eisenbahnverkehrs; Torf, Holzerzeugnisse für den Wirtschaftsbedarf und andere Waren. Unterstützt ausländische Firmen und Handelsgesellschaften bei der Erstellung von Geschäftsbeziehungen mit sowjetischen Außenhandelsorganisationen durch die Unterzeichnung von Abkommen über Handelsaustausch.

PRODINTORG
Moskva 121200, Smolenskaja-Sennaja pl. 32/34
Tel.: 244-26-29, Telex: 7201, 7206
Exports and imports sugar, soft and pressed caviar, tinned fish and crabmeat, fresh and quick-frozen fish, seafood; trepang, squid, shrimp, frozen shark; meat, meat products, meat subproducts, tinned meat; endocrine and enzyme products; poultry, eggs and egg products, wild fowl; milk and tinned milk, dairy products and cheese; fats, butter and vegetable oils, sunflower seeds; pedigree, horses (for breeding, work and slaughter); pedigree cattle and animals for zoos -

Aus- und Einfuhr: Zucker, großkörnigen und Preßkaviar, Fisch- und Krabbenkonserven, frische und tiefgekühlte Fische, Produkte des Seefischfangs; Trepange, Kalmare, Garnelen, gefrorenes Haifischfleisch; Fleisch, Fleischprodukte, Fleischkonserven; Ausgangsstoffe zur Hormon- und Enzymegewinnung; Geflügel, Eier und Produkte aus Eiern, Wildfleisch; Milch und Kondensmilch, Milchprodukte und Käse; Fette, Butter und pflanzliche Öle, Sonnenblumenkerne; Zucht-, Arbeits- und Fleischpferde; Zuchtvieh und Tiere für zoologische Gärten.

5.5.7 Economy / Wirtschaft

PROMMAŠEXPORT
Moskva 113324, Ovčinnikovskaja Nab. 18/1
Tel.: 295-51-14, Telex: 7532
Renders technical assistance in the construction of industrial enterprises and projects for heavy and farm machine-building; ship, automobile, tractor building, machine-tool-making, electrical engineering and radio-engineering communications; fish processing factories; in organizing commercial fisheries and fishing, as well as in the construction of refrigerating plants; supplies complete equipment for motion picture studios. Undertakes designing and surveying, technical supervision of building and assembly work in conformity with design and technical documents. It renders technical assistance in setting up and organizing enterprises and other projects. Undertakes industrial training of personnel both in the USSR and in the client's country. -

Technische Unterstützung beim Bau von Werken und Betrieben für Schwer- und Landwirtschaftsmaschinenbau; Schiffs-, Automobil- und Traktorenbau, Werkzeugproduktion, Elektroindustrie und Rundfunktechnik; Einrichtungen für die Fischverarbeitung; bei der Einrichtung von Fischerei- und Fischzuchtbetrieben sowie beim Bau von Eisfabriken; liefert komplette Einrichtungen für Filmstudios. Übernimmt Entwurf und Überwachung, technische Aufsicht von Bau- und Montagearbeiten in Übereinstimmung mit Entwürfen und technischen Unterlagen, erteilt technische Unterstützung bei der Einrichtung und Inbetriebnahme von Werken und anderen Projekten. Führt industrielle Schulung von Personal sowohl in der UdSSR als auch im Kundenland durch.

PROMMAŠIMPORT
Moskva 121200, Smolenskaja-Sennaja pl. 32/34
Tel.: 244-43-57, Telex: 7260, 7261
Imports equipment for cellulose, paper and cardboards-making factories, equipment for the manufacture of corrugated cardboard and packaging materials, equipment for making semi-finished and finished paper goods, equipment for sawmills and furniture factories, chipboards and fibreboards, plywood and parquetry factories, woodworking tools and other equipment for the woodworking industry, installations for coating paper and other materials -

Einfuhr: komplette Ausrüstungen für Zellstoff-, Papier- und Kartonagenfabriken, für die Herstellung von Wellpappe und deren Weiterverarbeitung zu Verpackungsmaterial, für die Verarbeitung von Papier in Halbfabrikate und Fertigerzeugnisse, für Sägewerke und Möbelfabriken, für Betriebe zur Herstellung von Preßplatten aus Sägespänen und Holzfaserplatten, von Sperrholz, Parkett, Werkzeugmaschinen und andere Ausrüstungen für die holzverarbeitende Industrie, Ausrüstungen kompletter Anlagen zum Auftragen von Schutzschichten auf Papier und andere Materialien.

PROMSYRJOIMPORT
Moskva 121314, ul. Čajkovskogo 13
Tel.: 203-05-95, 203-05-77, Telex: 7151, 7152
Exports and imports pig-iron, ferro-alloys, steel billets, structural steel, quality and high-quality steels, sheets and plates, cast iron tubes and steel pipes, steel cylinders for gases, hot-rolled and cold-rolled strips, steel wire of various qualities and for various purposes, steel wire ropes, railway transport materials, chains, electrodes, bolts, nails, nuts, rivets and other small iron and steel products -

Aus- und Einfuhr: Roheisen, Ferrolegierungen, Stahlrohlinge, Form- und Profilstahl, Stahl-Grob- und Feinbleche, Qualitäts- und Edelstahl, Rohre aus Gußeisen und Stahl, Gasflaschen aus Stahl, warm- und kaltgewalzte Streifen, Stahldraht verschiedener Qualität und für zahlreiche Zwecke, Stahldrahtseile, Materialien für den Eisenbahntransport, Ketten, Elektroden, Bolzen, Nägel, Schrauben, Muttern, Nieten und diverse Eisen- und Stahlwaren.

Economy
Wirtschaft 5.5.7

RAZNOEXPORT
Moskva 107140, Verchne-Krasnosel'skaja ul. 15
Tel.: 264-56-56, Telex: 7163, 7161, 7162

Exports and imports portland cement, window, mirror, wire and ornamental glass, marble and granite, plaster, mica, perlite, products of cement asbestos, roofing felt, radiators, wall and floor tiles, products for sanitary-technical plants; refrigerators, washing machines, vacuum cleaners, floor polishers, flat irons, fans, and other electrical household appliances; electric and mechanic razors, razor blades and other accessories for hairdresser's shops; pen and sporting knives; electric lamps; insulators for high and low frequency, electric insulating materials ; household sewing machines, kerosene gas stoves, wind lanterns, tea-urns, kitchen equipment, hunting and sporting guns and ammunition, sporting and household accessories; porcelain, aluminum, enameled and zinced objects, glass ware, crystal products, tableware of stainless steel, musical instruments, office supplies and stationery, slide rules, drawing instruments, illustrative material for instruction purposes, pencils and fountain-pens; toys; sewn and knitted goods, embroideries and decorative woven goods; store and laundry equipment; fire-extinguishers and fire brigade equipment; gas cookers and gas-kitcheners; drafting machines; fiberglass laminated articles, various plastic foils and plastic articles; leather haberdashery and other ready-made leather goods, leather and rubber footwear; oriental types of leaf tobacco; matches and match sticks, cigarettes. -

Aus- und Einfuhr: Portlandzement, Fenster-, Spiegel-, Draht- und Ornamentglas, Marmor und Granit, Gips, Glimmer, Perlit, Zementasbesterzeugnisse, Dachpappe, Heizkörper, Wand- und Bodenfliesen, Erzeugnisse für sanitärtechnische Anlagen; Kühlschränke, Waschmaschinen, Staubsauger, Bohnermaschinen, Bügeleisen, Ventilatoren und andere elektrische Haushaltsgeräte; elektrische und mechanische Rasierapparate, Rasierklingen und anderes Zubehör für Frisiersalons; Feder- und Jagdmesser; elektrische Lampen; Isolatoren für Hoch- und Niederspannung, elektrische Installationsmaterialien und Isolierstoffe; Haushaltsnähmaschinen, Petroleumgaskocher, Windlaternen, Teemaschinen, Kücheneinrichtungen, Jagd-und Sportwaffen nebst Munition, Sport-und Haushaltswaren; Porzellan-, Aluminium-, emailliertes und verzinktes Geschirr, Glasgeschirr, Kristallerzeugnisse, Eßbestecke aus nichtrostendem Stahl, Musikinstrumente, Büro- und Schreibwaren, Rechenschieber, Reißzeuge, Anschauungsmaterial für Unterrichtszwecke, Bleistifte und Füllfederhalter; Spielzeug; Nähwaren und Trikotagen, Stickereien und Erzeugnisse der dekorativen Weberei; Geschäftseinrichtungen und Wäschereiausrüstungen; Feuerlöscher und Feuerwehrausrüstungen; Gaskocher und Gasherde; Zeichenmaschinen; Erzeugnisse aus Glasfaserstoffen, verschiedene Plastfolien und Erzeugnisse aus Plasten; Galanteriewaren aus Leder und andere Lederwaren, Leder- und Gummischuhwerk; orientalische Sorten von Blättertabak, Streichhölzer, Zündholzschachteln, Zigaretten.

RAZNOIMPORT
Moskva 121200, Smolenskaja-Sennaja pl. 32/34
Tel.: 244-34-72, 244-37-61, Telex: 7153, 7154

Imports and exports non-ferrous metals and alloys, foils and powders, cable articles, cable fittings and wires, non-ferrous rolled stock, natural and synthetic rubber, tires for lorries and passenger cars, buses, motorcycles, bicycles, tractors and farm machines, technical rubber goods, floor coatings -

Ein- und Ausfuhr: Buntmetalle und deren Legierungen, Metallfolien und -pulver, Kabel, Kabelarmaturen , Buntmetallwalzgut, Natur- und Synthesekautschuk, Reifen für Personen- und Lastkraftwagen, Omnibusse, Kraft- und Fahrräder, Traktoren und Landmaschinen, technische Gummierzeugnisse und Bodenbeläge.

5.5.7 Economy / Wirtschaft

SELCHOZPROMEXPORT
Moskva 113324, Ovčinnikovskaja Nab. 18/1
Tel.: 220-16-92, Telex: 7533
Renders technical assistance in the construction of hydro-engineering and irrigation projects, grain elevators, grain storages, flour mills, fodder factories, machine rental and pump stations, livestock farms, repair shops, research centers for dry and irrigated farming, as well as mechanized farms for growing cotton, grain and oil-bearing crops. Carries out various prospecting and research jobs, ground levelling and preliminary work for the building of agricultural enterprises and other projects. Supervises building and assembly work, renders technical assistance in assembly and starting up of equipment delivered. Trains national personnel in the client's country and in the USSR for the above mentioned enterprises -

Erteilt technische Hilfe beim Bau von Bewässerungsanlagen, Getreideelevatoren, Getreidespeichern, Mühlen, Futtermittelfabriken, Maschinenverleih- und Pumpstationen, Viehzuchtfarmen, Reparaturwerkstätten, Versuchsbetrieben für trockene und bewässerte Landwirtschaft sowie von maschinellen Baumwoll-, Getreide- und technischen Kulturen (Ölpflanzen). Führt verschiedene Untersuchungs- und Forschungsarbeiten, Bodennivellierungen und Vorkehrungen für den Bau von landwirtschaftlichen Betrieben und anderen Projekten durch. Überwacht den Bau und die Inbetriebnahme, erteilt technische Hilfe bei der Errichtung und Inbetriebnahme der gelieferten Ausrüstungen. Schult inländisches Personal im Kundenland und in der UdSSR für die oben erwähnten Unternehmungen.

SKOTOIMPORT
Moskva 103062, ul. Makarenko 6
Tel.: 297-22-32
Imports slaughter meat cattle, sheep, goats, pigs, horses for slaughter as well as meat of poultry and game -
Einfuhr von Schlachtvieh wie Rinder, Schafe, Ziegen, Schweine, Fleischpferde sowie Fleisch von Geflügel und Wildbret.

SOJUZATTRAKCION
Moskva 119034, ul. Ryleeva 25
Tel.: 241-59-98
Advises amusement park enterprises (equipment and facilities) -
Berät Schaustellergeschäfte, zuständig für Vergnügungseinrichtungen in Vergnügungsparks.

SOJUZCHIMEXPORT
Moskva 121200, Smolenskaja-Sennaja pl. 32/34
Tel.: 244-22-84, Telex: 7295, 7296
Exports and imports products of basic chemistry, gases and elements, soda products, inorganic acids and salts, products of organic synthesis, alcohols and solvents, organic acids, products for the chemical processing of coke and wood, synthetic resins and plastics, crop dusting, synthetic dyes and other auxiliary products for the textile industry, synthetic industrial detergents, chemicals for the rubber industry, lacquers and paints, inorganic pigments, chemical reagents and pure preparation, film and photographic materials, photographic chemicals, chemicals for color film production, volatile oil, synthetic aromatic substances, perfumes, soap, household chemical goods, glycol, silicon fluids and dopes for oil products -

Aus- und Einfuhr: Erzeugnisse der chemischen Grundstoffindustrie, Gase und Grundstoffe, Sodaprodukte, anorganische Säuren und deren Salze, Erzeugnisse der organischen Synthese, Alkohole und Lösungsmittel, organische Säuren, Produkte der chemischen Bearbeitung von Koks und Holz, synthetische Harze und Plaste, Schädlingsbekämpfungsmittel, synthetische Farbstoffe und andere Hilfsstoffe für die Textilindustrie, synthetische Waschmittel für den Industriebedarf, Chemikalien für die Gummiindustrie, Lackfarbstoffe, anorganische Pigmente, chemische Reagenzen und Reinpräparate, Film- und Fotoartikel, Fotochemikalien, Chemikalien für die Farbfilmproduktion, ätherische Öle und synthetische Duftstoffe, Parfüms, Seife, Gegenstände der Haushaltschemie, Glykole, Silikonöle und Zusätze für Erdölprodukte.

SOJUZGAZEXPORT
  Moskva 117071, Seninskij Prospekt 20
  Tel.: 234-39-50, 234-39-51, Telex: 7146, 7149
    Exports and imports specifically pipe line and liquefied natural gases -
    Aus- und Einfuhr von Leitungs- und flüssigem Erdgas.

SOJUZMEDTECHNIKA
  Moskva 129090, Vtoroj Troickij Pereulok 6 a
  Tel.: 281-98-41
    In charge of export and import, assembly and repair of medical equipment -
    Zuständig für die Aus- und Einfuhr, Montage und Reparatur medizinischer Einrichtungen.

SOJUZNEFTEEXPORT
  Moskva 121200, Smolenskaja-Sennaja pl. 32/34
  Tel.: 244-40-49, 244-40-48, Telex: 7148, 7149
    Exports crude oil, liquefied and natural gases, straight-run, automobile and
    aircraft fuel, kerosene, Diesel oils, masouts, lubricating oils,
    paraffin wax, benzene, toluene, ozokerite, petroleum coke, as well as imports
    various petroleum products -
    Ausfuhr: Roherdöl, Flüssig- und Naturgase, Destillatbenzin, Auto- und Flugzeugbenzin, Leuchtpetroleum, Dieselbrennstoffe, Masut, Schmieröle, Paraffinwachs, Benzol, Toluol, Erdwachs, Erdölkoks. Einfuhr: verschiedene Erdölprodukte.

SOJUZPLODOIMPORT
  Moskva 121200, Smolenskaja-Sennaja pl. 32/34
  Tel.: 244-36-36, Telex: 7262
    Imports and exports fresh, dried and quick-frozen fruits, berries and vegetables, canned fruits and vegetables, nuts, fruit and berry pulp and juices, wine additives, wines and liquors, brandies, mineral waters, various flavourings and spices, starches, confectionery goods, concentrated foods, baby foods and other foodstuffs. -

    Aus- und Einfuhr: Frisch-, Dörr- und Gefrierobst, Beeren und Gemüse, Obst- und Gemüsekonserven, Nüsse, Pulpe und Säfte von Früchten und Beeren, Zutaten zur Herstellung von Wein, Weine und Liköre, Weinbrand, Mineralwasser, verschiedene Gewürze und Würmittel, Stärke, Konditoreierzeugnisse, Speisekonzentrate, Kindernährmittel und andere Nahrungsmittel.

SOJUZPROMEXPORT
  Moskva 121200, Smolenskaja-Sennaja pl. 32/34
  Tel.: 244-19-79, Telex: 7268
    Exports and imports coal, coke, anthracite, coal pitch; manganese, chrome and iron ores, peroxide; asbestos and products thereof; mineral fertilizers; graphite, magnesite and magnesite clinker, refractories, crucibles and graphite retorts for metal smelting; electric carbons, sodium sulphate, sulphur pyrite; welding flux; sulphur; pyrite cinders, talcum, barite; precious metals and raw materials -

    Aus- und Einfuhr: Kohle, Koks, Anthrazit, Steinkohlenteerpech; Mangan-, Chrom- und Eisenerz, Braunstein; Asbest und Erzeugnisse davon; Mineraldünger; Graphit; Magnesit und Magnesitklinker, Schamotte und andere feuerfeste Materalien,

5.5.7 Economy / Wirtschaft

Elektrokohle, Natriumsulfat, Schwefelkies, Schweißpulver und -paste, Schwefel, Pyritabbrand, Talkum, Baryt, Edelmetalle und Rohstoffe.

SOJUZPUŠINA
Moskva 103012, ul. Kuibyševa 6
Tel.: 294-08-45, 223-09-23, Telex: 7150

Exports and imports mink, Persian lamb (karakul), sable and other furs, altogether more than 100 various kinds, raw skins, natural and artificial leather, bristles, animal hair, brushes and other products, wigs, slaughter cattle intestines and artificial skins for the sausage production, down and feathers, casein, glue and other goods of animal origin. Holds three fur actions a year in Leningrad, takes part in the Leipzig and London auctions, sells goods from warehouses in Moscow, Leningrad, London, Paris, and Stockholm, concludes long-term contracts for delivery of furs to foreign firms -

Aus- und Einfuhr: Nerz, Persianer (Karakul), Zobel und andere Rauchwaren, insgesamt über 100 verschiedene Sorten, Rohhäute, Natur- und künstliches Leder, Borsten, Tierhaare, Bürsten und andere Erzeugnisse, Perücken, Schlachttierdärme und künstliche Häute zur Verwendung in der Wurstfabrikation, Flaum und Federn, Kasein, Leim und andere Waren animalischen Ursprungs. Veranstaltet alljährlich drei Rauchwarenauktionen in Leningrad, beteiligt sich an den Auktionen in Leipzig und London, verkauft Waren aus ihren Lagern in Moskau, Leningrad, London, Paris und Stockholm und schließt mit ausländischen Firmen langfristige Abschlüsse über die Lieferung von Rauchwaren ab.

SOJUZVNEŠSTROJIMPORT
Moskva 121200, Smolenskaja-Sennaja pl. 2
Tel.: 241-49-27, Telex: 7261

Responsible for turn-key projects for which foreign companies will provide labor and equipment, such as hotel and gas pipeline construction -
Zuständig für Schlüsselprojekte, an denen sich ausländische Gesellschaften mit Arbeit und Ausrüstungen beteiligen, beispielsweise Hotels und Gasfernleitungsbau.

SOJUZVNEŠTRANS
Moskva 121200, Smolenskaja-Sennaja pl. 32/34
Tel.: 244-39-51, Telex: 7266, 7291

Renders transportation and expedition services for the foreign trade organizations of the USSR, fulfils orders for the transportation of export and import goods by sea, river, railway, highway and air; executes commissions in transportation and expedition of domestic, diplomatic and other goods for foreign companies, effects payments of expenditures for transportation, storage, transfer and expedition of these goods on the territory of the USSR at the expense of these companies. Undertakes shipment of transit goods through USSR territory from and to European and eastern (Asian) countries by all means of transportation; transit goods can be transported through Soviet territory to the frontiers, major inland cities as well as ports of destination at shippers' request -

Leistet Transport- und Speditionsdienste für die Außenhandelsorganisationen der UdSSR, erfüllt Aufträge zum Transport von Export- und Importgütern auf dem Seeweg, auf Binnenwasserstraßen, mit Eisenbahn, Kraftwagen und Flugzeugen; führt Transport- und Speditionsaufträge ausländischer Firmen von Nichtaußenhandelsgütern, diplomatischen und anderen Gütern durch, leistet für Rechnung dieser Gesellschaften Zahlungen für Kosten beim Transport, bei der Lagerung, beim Umladen und bei der Spedition dieser Güter auf dem Territorium der UdSSR. Übernimmt die Verschiffung von Transitgütern durch das Territorium der UdSSR aus europäischen in Ostländer und zurück mit allen Arten von Transportmitteln. Auf Wunsch des Verladers werden Transitgüter durch sowjetisches Territorium zu den Grenzen, inländischen Zentren und Bestimmungshäfen befördert.

Economy
Wirtschaft 5.5.7

SOVFRACHT
Moskva 121200, Smolenskaja-Sennaja pl. 32/34
Tel.: 244-24-11, Telex: 7168,7169,7170,7171,7172,7217,7541,7542
Carries out broker services involving chartering Soviet ships for the conveyance of goods of foreign charterers and charters foreign tonnage for the conveyance of cargoes of Soviet foreign trade organizations. Provides broker services in chartering foreign tonnage for the conveyance of cargoes of foreign charterers. Uses chartered foreign tonnage on time-charter terms. Books liner tonnage belonging to Soviet and foreign liner services in all directions. Delivers cargoes on direct Bills of Lading to any port of the world -

Frachtmakler, stellt unter anderem sowjetischen Schiffsraum zur Beförderung von Gütern ausländischer Befrachter bereit, frachtet ebenfalls ausländischen Schiffsraum zur Beförderung von Gütern sowjetischer Außenhandelsorganisationen. Frachtmakler für ausländischen Schiffsraum zur Beförderung von Gütern ausländischer Befrachter. Chartert ausländischen Schiffsraum zu den Bedingungen der Zeitcharter. Bucht Tonnage auf Linienschiffen in alle Richtungen, die sowjetischen und ausländischen Liniendiensten gehören. Spediert Güter auf direkten Seefrachtbriefen in jeden Hafen der Welt.

SOVEXPORTFILM
Moskva 103009, Kalašnyj Per. 14
Tel.: 290-50-09, Telex: 7143
Exports color and black-and-white full-length and short-reel films produced by all the studios of the Soviet Union on standard 35-mm film (ordinary and wide-screen versions), 70-mm (wide gauge) and 16-mm films. Documentaries and popular science films as well as newsreels can be supplied in their original language to be dubbed abroad or with a running commentary dubbed into any foreign language in the USSR. Imports full-length feature films and short-reels to be shown in the Soviet Union -

Ausfuhr: Farb- und Schwarzweißfilme, abendfüllende und Kurzfilme sämtlicher Filmstudios der Sowjetunion auf 35-mm-Normalfilm (mit Ausführungen für Normal- und Breitwand), 70-mm (Breitwand) und 16-mm-Filme. Dokumentar- und populärwissenschaftliche Filme sowie Wochenschauen können in ihrer Originalsprache zum Synchronisieren im Ausland oder mit einem in der UdSSR in eine ausländische Sprache synchronisierten Kommentar geliefert werden. Einfuhr: abendfüllende Spielfilme und Kurzfilme für den Filmverleih in der Sowjetunion.

SOVINFILM
Moskva 121069, ul. Vorovskogo 33
Tel.: 290-45-35, Telex: 7114
Coordinates commercial contacts of Soviet film studios with film organizations and motion picture firms in foreign countries in rendering and employing production and art services and in making joint film productions -

Koordinierung von kommerziellen Verbindungen sowjetischer Filmstudios mit ausländischen Filmgesellschaften und -organisationen, Erweisung filmtechnischer und schöpferischer Dienste sowie der Koproduktion von Filmen.

SOVINFLOT
Moskva 103012, ul. Ždanova 1/4
Tel.: 296-50-32, 296-53-76, Telex: 7217 (answer back-Rückantwort: "Sovfracht 2")
The main purpose of "Sovinflot" is to improve the services extended to Soviet ships that call at foreign ports, and also to raise the quality of services provided to foreign vessels in the ports of the Soviet Union. "Sovinflot", as the general agent of Soviet steamship companies, ensures proper negotiating, stevedoring and other services to Soviet ships in foreign ports, including their provision with bunkers and lubricants. It also sees to the legal interests of steamship companies abroad and handles individual

5.5.7 Economy / Wirtschaft

cases in courts of arbitration and law on their behalf. In Soviet ports it controls the activities of "Inflot" maritime agencies, which render assistance to captains and owners of foreign ships in going through port formalities, repairing ships, providing them with bunkers, supplies and food products -

Hauptaufgabe von "Sovinflot" ist die Verbesserung der Versorgung sowjetischer Schiffe, die in ausländischen Häfen anlegen, sowie eine qualitativ verbesserte Versorgung ausländischer Schiffe in sowjetischen Häfen. "Sovinflot" - als solche Generalagent der sowjetischen Schiffahrtsgesellschaften - garantiert die ordnungsmäßige Vermittlung, Stauerei und andere Leistungen für sowjetische Schiffe in ausländischen Häfen, einschließlich deren Versorgung mit Bunker und Schmierstoffen. Vertritt die Rechtsansprüche von Reedereien im Ausland und deren Interessen in Arbitrage- und Gerichtsstreitigkeiten. Kontrolliert in sowjetischen Häfen die Tätigkeit der "Inflot"-Schiffahrtsagenturen, die Schiffskapitänen und Eigentümern ausländischer Schiffe bei der Abwicklung von Hafenformalitäten, Schiffsreparaturen, Versorgung mit Bunker, Vorräten und Nahrungsmitteln behilflich sind.

SOVTRANSAVTO
Moskva 103012, Staropanskij Per. 1/5
Tel.: 221-36-53, Telex: 7251

International transport of goods and persons by motor vehicle, undertakes shipment for Soviet and foreign customers of foreign trade goods, diplomatic and personal baggage by truck to and from the Soviet Union and to European countries by transit through the Soviet Union -

Transport von Gütern und Personen im internationalen Kraftwagenverkehr, befördert für sowjetische und ausländische Auftraggeber Außenhandelsgüter, diplomatisches und persönliches Gepäck mit Lkw von und nach der Sowjetunion und nach europäischen Ländern im Transit durch die Sowjetunion.

STANKOIMPORT
Moskva 121200, Smolenskaja-Sennaja pl. 32/34
Tel.: 244-21-32, Telex: 7227, 7228

Exports and imports a wide range of metal-cutting machine-tools, wood-working machine-tools (export), forging and pressing equipment, measuring units and instruments, hand-operated electric and pneumatic tools, metal- and woodcutting tools, mechanical tools, chucks, machine-tool accessories, hard-alloy products, abrasive products, ball and roller bearings -

Aus- und Einfuhr: ein weiter Bereich von spanabhebenden Werkzeugmaschinen, Werkzeugmaschinen für die Holzverarbeitung (Export), Ausrüstungen für Schmieden und Pressereien, Meßgeräte und Instrumente, elektrische und pneumatische Handwerkzeuge, Schneidewerkzeuge für die Metall- und Holzbearbeitung, mechanische Werkzeuge, Spannfutter, Zubehör für Werkzeugmaschinen, Erzeugnisse aus Hartlegierungen, Schleifmittel, Kugel- und Rollenlager.

SUDOIMPORT
Moskva 103006, Kaljaevskaja ul. 5
Tel.: 251-05-05, Telex: 7587, 7272

Exports hydrofoil ships, tugs, buckets, suction dredgers, motor boats; ship equipment - pumps, compressors, deck machinery, electrical and navigational equipment. Imports sea-going, river vessels, fishing and auxiliary craft, undertakes repairs of ships abroad -

Ausfuhr: Wasserfaltboote, Schlepper, Becher, Saugbagger, Motorboote; Schiffsausrüstungen: Pumpen, Kompressoren, Deckmaschinen, elektrische und Navigationsausrüstungen. Einfuhr: Hochsee- und Flußschiffe, Fischerei- und Hilfsschiffe; übernimmt Schiffsreparaturen im Ausland.

Economy 5.5.7
Wirtschaft

TECHMASEXPORT
Moskva 117330, Mosfilmovskaja ul. 35
Tel.: 147-15-62, Telex: 7568
Exports modern textile, polygraphic, glass, paper-and-pulp, chemical, pump and compressor, oxygen and refrigeration equipment, industrial fittings and also technological equipment for the electronic and light engineering industries -

Ausfuhr: Ausrüstungen für die Textil-, polygraphische, Glas-, Papier- und Zellulose-, chemische, Pumpen- und Kompressoren-, Sauerstoff- und Kühlindustrie, Industriearmaturen sowie technologische Ausrüstungen für die elektronische und beleuchtungstechnische Industrie.

TECHMASIMPORT
Moskva 121200, Smolenskaja-Sennaja pl. 32/34
Tel.: 244-15-09, 244-11-41, Telex: 7194
Imports equipment and machines for the chemical and oil-refining industry, for the production of basic chemical products, for organic synthesis, for the manufacture of chemical fibres and plastics, synthetic rubbers, rubber and rubber goods, dyestuffs, lacquers and paints, plant protective agents as well as equipment for the manufacture of plastic goods, refrigerating equipment and laundries and cleaners -

Einfuhr: Ausrüstungen und Maschinen für die chemische Industrie und Petrolchemie, zur Herstellung von Erzeugnissen der Grundstoffchemie und organischen Synthese, Chemiefasern und Plaste, Synthesekautschuk, Gummi und Gummierzeugnissen, Farbstoffpigmenten, Lacken und Farben, Pflanzenschutzmitteln sowie Ausrüstungen für die Herstellung von Kunststofferzeugnissen, Ausrüstungen von Kühlanlagen sowie für chemische Reinigungsanstalten und industrielle Wäschereien.

TECHNOEXPORT
Moskva 113324, Ovčinnikovskaja Nab. 18/1
Tel.: 220-14-48, 220-16-70
Renders technical assistance in geological studies of regions and also integrated prospecting for all types of raw materials, the development of explored oil deposits, in the construction of subways, highways, and railways, bridges, tunnels, trestles, sea and river ports, apartment and administrative buildings, hotels, house building enterprises, building material factories, higher and secondary educational establishments, hospitals, polyclinics, stadiums and sports installations, textile and garment factories. Sends physicians and teachers to work at the Client's medical and educational establishments, sports instructors to work as coaches and recommends culture and art experts -

Technische Hilfe bei geologischen Studien von Regionen sowie bei der integrierten Schürfung nach allen Arten von Rohstoffen, beim Ausbau bereits erschlossener Ölvorkommen, beim Bau von U-Bahnen, Autobahnen und Eisenbahnen, Brücken, Tunnels, See- und Binnenhäfen, Wohn- und Geschäftshäusern, Hotels, Hausbauunternehmen, Baustoffbetrieben, Hoch- und Mittelschulen, Krankenhäusern, Polikliniken, Stadien und Sporteinrichtungen, Textil- und Konfektionsfabriken. Entsendung von Ärzten und Lehrern zu Arbeiten in medizinischen und Bildungsstätten, Sportlehrern zur Arbeit als Trainer sowie Kultur- und Kunstexperten.

TECHNOPROMEXPORT
Moskva 113324, Ovčinnikovskaja Nab. 18/1
Tel.: 220-15-23, 220-14-26, Telex: 7158
Renders technical assistance in the construction of thermal, atomic and hydro-power stations, transformer substations, electric power transmission lines, atomic power and other units for research and training purposes. Undertakes designing and surveying jobs, assembling, adjusting and building jobs -

383

5.5.7 Economy / Wirtschaft

Technische Unterstützung beim Bau von Wärme-, Atom- und Wasserkraftwerken, Umspannwerken, elektrischen Hochspannungsfernleitungen, Atomkraft- und sonstigen Einheiten für Forschungs- und Schulungszwecke. Projektierungs- und Erkundungsarbeiten, Montage- und Bauarbeiten sowie Inbetriebnahme von Anlagen.

TECHNOPROMIMPORT
Moskva 121200, Smolenskaja Sennaja pl. 32/34
Tel.: 244-27-87, 244-33-52, Telex: 7233

Imports equipment for the light, polygraphic, cable-making, glass, meat and dairy, confectionery, tobacco and winemaking industries, equipment for mills and elevators, packaging machines for the indicated industries as well as for medicines and vitamins, equipment for the electronic and light engineering and building materials industries, and for the production of ferments -

Einfuhr: Ausrüstungen für die polygraphische, Leicht-, Kabel-, Glas-, Fleisch- und Milchverarbeitungs-, Süßwaren-, Tabak- und Weinindustrie, Ausrüstungen für Mühlen und Getreideelevatoren, Verpackungsmaschinen für die erwähnten Industriezweige sowie für medizinische Präparate und Vitamine, Ausrüstungen für Elektronik und Lichttechnik, für die Baumaterialienindustrie sowie für die Produktion von Fermentpräparaten.

TECHSNABEXPORT
Moskva 121200, Smolenskaja-Sennaja pl. 32/34
Tel.: 244-32-85, Telex: 7628

Exports and imports rare and rare-earth metals and their alloys, isotopes, ionizing-radiation sources, deuterium and tritium targets, medical and flaw-detecting betatrons, elementary-particle accelerators, radio-isotope and dosimetric instruments, mass-spectrometers, medical radiological equipment, scientific and industrial X-ray equipment, biological shields and personal protective facilities for work with radioactive materials -

Aus- und Einfuhr: Seltene Metalle und Erdmetalle sowie deren Verbindungen, Isotopen, Strahlungsquellen, Deuterium- und Tritium-Antikathoden, Betatrone für medizinische Zwecke und Defektoskopie, Teilchenbeschleunigeranlagen, Radioisotopen- und dosimetrische Geräte, Massenspektrometer, radiologische medizinische Ausrüstungen, Röntgenausrüstungen für wissenschaftliche und industrielle Zwecke, Strahlenschutz- und Abschirmungsmittel für Einzelpersonen bei der Arbeit mit radioaktiven Stoffen.

TJAŽPROMEXPORT
Moskva 113324, Ovčinnikovskaja Nab. 18/1
Tel.: 220-16-10, 220-15-89, Telex: 7531

Renders technical assistance in the construction of complete industrial enterprises and buildings for the ferrous metallurgy and mining industries. Conducts surveying and research work, designs enterprises and buildings, exports and imports complete equipment, supervises building and erection work and mounting of equipment, renders technical assistance in starting up enterprises and in bringing them up to the projected capacity, carries out technical training of national personnel in the Client's country and in the enterprises of the USSR -

Technische Unterstützung beim Bau kompletter Industriebetriebe und Anlagen der Eisenhüttenmetallurgie und des Bergbaus. Überwachungs- und Forschungsarbeiten, Entwurf von Betrieben und Gebäuden, Aus- und Einfuhr kompletter Ausrüstungen, Überwachung von Bau- und Montagearbeiten, technische Unterstützung bei der Inbetriebnahme von Betrieben und beim Erreichen der veranschlagten Leistung, Ausbildung von einheimischem Personal im Kundenland und in den Betrieben der UdSSR.

Economy
Wirtschaft 5.5.7

TRAKTOREXPORT
Moskva 103031, Kuzneckij most 21/5
Tel.: 244-32-37, Telex: 7273
    Exports and imports tractors, farm and roadbuilding machines, special equipment, appliances and instruments for repairs and technical servicing of the indicated machines; renders technical assistance to its clients in the technical servicing of machines imported from the USSR and in training personnel -

    Aus- und Einfuhr: Traktoren, Land- und Straßenbaumaschinen, Spezialausrüstungen, Vorrichtungen und Geräte zur Reparatur und Wartung der angegebenen Maschinen; technische Unterstützung der Kunden bei der Wartung der aus der UdSSR importierten Maschinen und bei der Ausbildung des Personals.

CVETMETPROMEXPORT
Moskva 113324, Ovčinnikovskaja Nab. 18/1
Tel.: 220-18-61, Telex: 7158
    Renders technical assistance in surveying, designing, construction and erection projects, supplies equipment, sets up and puts enterprises into operation, and also trains clients' personnel both in their countries and in the USSR in the following industries: non-ferrous metallurgy - construction of pits, quarries, refining plants, metallurgical plants (for production of lead, copper, zink, aluminum and other non-ferrous metals), ferrous metals (aluminum, lead, etc.), treating plants, semiconductor materials (silicon, germanium, (etc.)production plants;coal industry - construction of coal pits, mines, refining plants; gas industry - laying of trunk gas pipelines, construction of gas-transfer stations, gas turbine installations, natural gasoline plants, laying of trunk oil pipelines, construction of oil transfer stations, and oil reservoirs -

    Technische Unterstützung bei Überwachungs-, Entwurfs-, Bau- und Montagearbeiten, Lieferung von Ausrüstungen, Erstellung und Inbetriebnahme von Betrieben, Schulung von Kundenpersonal sowohl in den entsprechenden Ländern als auch in der Sowjetunion in folgenden Industriezweigen: NE-Metallurgie - Bau von Schächten, Steinbrüchen, Raffinerieanlagen, Eisenhüttenanlagen (zur Herstellung von Blei, Kupfer, Zink, Aluminium und anderer Buntmetalle), Eisenerze (Aluminium, Blei usw.)-Bearbeitungsbetriebe, Halbleitermaterialien (Silikon, Germanium usw.)-Herstellungsbetriebe; Kohleindustrie: Bau von Kohleschächten, Minen und Raffinerieanlagen; Gasindustrie: Verlegung von Gasfernleitungen, Bau von Gasübertragungsstationen, Gasturbinenanlagen, Erdgasanlagen, Verlegung von Ölfernleitungen, Bau von Ölübertragungsstationen und Ölreservoirs.

VNEŠPOSYLTORG
Moskva 121200, Smolenskaja-Sennaja pl. 32/34
Tel.: 241-89-39, 243-47-92, Telex: 7250
    Exports and sells for freely convertible currency manufactured goods and foodstuffs in small wholesale lots offering: passenger cars, motorcycles, electric utensils for household and daily use, TV sets, radio sets, motion-picture cameras for amateurs, binoculars, watches, cottage pianos, fur clothing, handicraft products of the USSR peoples as well as various goods (fabrics, perfumery etc.) and foodstuffs. Exports of manufactured goods and foodstuffs to Soviet citizines working abroad and to foreigners, to Soviet citizens having received foreign currency by bank transfer as inheritance, royalties or for other reasons, as well as to various foreign and national institutions (embassies, legations, foreign firms, shops, restaurants etc.). "Vnešposyltorg" offers the indicated goods to the diplomatic staff of embassies, legations and agencies of international organizations as well as the resident agents of foreign firms in special commercial houses of the USSR trade network for payment by cheques of the Bank for Foreign Trade of the USSR ("D" series) -

5.5.7 Economy / Wirtschaft

Ausfuhr und Verkauf von Industrieerzeugnissen und Lebensmitteln in kleineren Großhandelsposten gegen Devisen. Die Vereinigung offeriert: Personenkraftwagen, Motorräder, Elektrogeräte für den Haushalt und den täglichen Gebrauch, Fernsehgeräte, Rundfunkempfänger, Kinokameras für Amateure, Ferngläser, Uhren, Pianinos, Pelzkonfektion, Erzeugnisse des Kunsthandwerks der Völker der UdSSR sowie die verschiedensten Gebrauchsartikel (Stoffe, Parfümerie usw.) und Lebensmittel. Export von Industrieerzeugnissen und Lebensmitteln an Sowjetbürger, die im Ausland tätig sind und an Ausländer, an Sowjetbürger, die ausländische Devisen durch eine Banküberweisung als Erbschaft, Honorar oder aus anderen Ursachen erhalten haben sowie auch verschiedenen Institutionen im Ausland und in der UdSSR (Botschaften, Gesandtschaften, ausländische Firmen, Geschäfte, Restaurants usw.). "Vnešposyltorg offeriert die genannten Waren dem Diplomatischen Personal der Botschaften, Gesandtschaften und Vertretungen internationaler Organisationen sowie den ständigen Vertretungen ausländischer Firmen in den speziellen Handelshäusern des Handelsnetzes der UdSSR gegen Bezahlung mit Schecks der Serie "D" der Außenhandelsbank der UdSSR.

VNEŠTECHNIKA
Moskva 119034, Starokonjušennyj Per.6 and/und ul. Gorkogo 11
Tel.: 229-16-20

"Vneštechnika for scientific and technical exchange with foreign countries, renders assistance to Soviet and foreign research, designing and technological organizations, industrial plants and firms in handling commercial, transportation and legal problems involving in implementing scientific and technical collaboration in joint and contractual research, designing and technological work, in filling orders from Soviet and foreign organizations and firms for drawing up and delivery of blueprints and scientific equipment, as well as experimental samples of products and materials, in carrying out scientific and technical research, consultations, testing of equipment and materials, in implementing other types of scientific and technical exchange in individual fields -

Zuständig für den wissenschaftlich-technischen Austausch mit ausländischen Staaten, Unterstützung sowjetischer und ausländischer Forschungs-, Projektierungs- und Entwicklungsorganisationen, Industriebetriebe und Firmen bei der Lösung von Handels-, Transport- und Rechtsfragen, die mit der Abwicklung gemeinsamer und vertraglicher Forschungs-, Planungs- und Entwicklungsvorhaben verbunden sind, bei der Erfüllung von Aufträgen sowjetischer und ausländischer Organisationen und Firmen für die Ausarbeitung und Lieferung von Entwürfen und wissenschaftlichen Ausrüstungen sowie von Versuchsproben für Erzeugnisse und Materialien, bei der Durchführung wissenschaftlich-technischer Untersuchungen und andere Arten von wissenschaftlich-technischem Austausch in verschiedenen Bereichen.

VNEŠTORGIZDAT
Moskva 125807, Oružejnyj Per. 25 a
Tel.: 250-51-62, Telex: 7238

Publishes in Russian and foreign languages foreign trade advertising matter, catalogues, prospectuses, posters, booklets, leaflets, etc. as well as technical documents on Soviet exports. Accepts from foreign organizations and companies orders for publishing in Russian (including translations from foreign languages) technical documents, advertising matter and other material on goods intended for export and for display at international exhibitions organized in the USSR. Places orders for Soviet organizations with foreign firms for printing books and advertising matter in Russian and foreign languages -

Verlagsunternehmen, das Außenhandelswerbeliteratur, Kataloge, Prospekte, Plakate, Broschüren, Flugblätter usw. sowie technische Schriftstücke über

Economy 5.5.7
Wirtschaft

sowjetische Exportgüter in russischer Sprache und in Fremdsprachen verlegt. Übernimmt von ausländischen Organisationen und Gesellschaften Aufträge zur Herausgabe von technischen Schriftstücken, Werbeliteratur und anderen Papieren in russischer Sprache (einschl. Übersetzung aus Fremdsprachen) für Waren, die zum Export und für in der UdSSR durchgeführte internationale Ausstellungen bestimmt sind. Läßt Bücher und Werbeschriften in russischer Sprache und in Fremdsprachen, die von sowjetischen Organisationen bestellt werden, im Ausland drucken.

VNESTORGREKLAMA
Moskva 113461, ul. Kachovka 31, Korp. 2
Tel.: 121-04-34, Telex: 7265
Carries out all kinds of commercial advertising for Soviet export goods abroad, including advertising in press, cinema, radio and TV, also handles matters connected with public relations; fills orders by foreign firms for all accepted types of commercial advertising within the USSR -

Vergabe von Werbeaufträgen ins Ausland für sowjetische Exportwaren einschl. Werbung in der Presse, im Kino, im Radio und Fernsehen, sowie Durchführung von Öffentlichkeitsarbeit; Übernahme von Werbeaufträgen ausländischer Firmen für alle zugelassenen Arten von Werbung innerhalb der UdSSR.

VOSTOKINTORG
Moskva 121200, Smolenskaja-Sennaja pl. 32/34
Tel.: 244-20-34, Telex: 7123
Handles operations involving export and import trade with the Mongolian People's Republic, Afghanistan, Iran, Turkey, the Arab Republic of Yemen and the People's Democratic Republic of Yemen. Exports rolled stock of ferrous and non-ferrous metals, building materials, cement, window glass, textile goods, clothing, leather and rubber footwear, sugar, tea, flour, fats and oils, tinned products and other foodstuffs, cigarettes, matches, porcelain, faience, glass and enamelled crockery, sewing machines, electric household appliances, sports and hunting gear, perfumery and haberdashery, musical instruments, sanitary-technical and other goods. Imports wool, cotton, skins and hides, fur pelts, coffee, fresh and dried fruit, citrus fruit, almonds, nuts, oilseeds, fats and oils, quick-frozen fish, caviar, gum tragacanth, henna, black dye, knitted wear, footwear and other traditional exports of the above-mentioned Eastern countries -

Unterstützung bei der Aus- und Einfuhr von und nach folgenden Ländern: Mongolische Volksrepublik, Afghanistan, Iran, Türkei, Arabische Republik Jemen und Volksdemokratische Republik Jemen. Ausfuhr: Walzgut aus Eisen- und Buntmetallen, Baustoffe, Zement, Fensterglas, Textilwaren, Kleidung, Leder- und Gummischuhwerk, Zucker, Tee, Mehl, Fette und Öle, Konserven und andere Nahrungsmittel, Zigaretten, Zündhölzer, Porzellan, Geschirr aus Glas und Email, Nähmaschinen, elektrische Haushaltgeräte, Sport- und Jagdzubehör, Parfümerie und Kurzwaren, Musikinstrumente, sanitär-technische und andere Waren. Einfuhr: Wolle, Baumwolle, Pelze und Felle, Kaffee, frisches und Dörrobst, Zitrusfrüchte, Mandeln, Nüsse, Ölsamen, Fette und Öle, tiefgefrorenen Fisch, Kaviar, Tragantgummi, Henna, schwarzer Farbstoff, Strickwaren, Schuhwerk und andere traditionelle Exportgüter aus den angegebenen Ostländern.

ZAPCASTEXPORT
Moskva 109029, ul. Vtoraja Skotoprogonnaja 35
Tel.: 278-63-05, Telex: 7243
Exports spare parts for cars, tractors, motorcycles, bicycles, road-building, farm and other special-purpose machines -
Ausfuhr: Ersatzteile für Kraftwagen, Traktoren, Motorräder, Fahrräder, Straßenbau-, Land- und andere Spezialmaschinen.

5.5.7.1 Economy
Wirtschaft

5.5.7.1 OTHER ORGANIZATIONS - ANDERE ORGANISATIONEN - DRUGIE ORGANIZACII

V/O ATOMENERGOEXPORT
Moskva 113324, Ovčinnikovskaja Nab. 18/1
Tel.: 220-14-36, Telex: 7158
  Exports atomic power plants, nuclear demineralization plants, research reactors, radio-chemical laboratories for the production of isotopes, acceleration of various systems, industrial cobalt plants, and nuclear physical laboratories; designing, prospecting and scientific research work, erection and construction work as well as training and delegation of specialists. Imports equipment and materials for atomic power plants; joint construction of atomic power plants with foreign firms -

  Ausfuhr: Atomkraftwerke, nukleare Entsalzungsanlagen, Untersuchungs- und Forschungsreaktoren, radiochemische Labors zur Isotopenerzeugung, Beschleunigung verschiedener Systeme, industrielle Kobaltanlagen und kernphysikalische Labors; Projektierungs-, Erkundungs- und wissenschaftliche Forschungsarbeiten, Montage- und Bauarbeiten sowie Ausbildung und Entsendung von Fachleuten. Einfuhr: Ausrüstungen und Materialien für Atomkraftwerke; Bau von Atomkraftwerken in Gemeinschaftsarbeit mit ausländischen Firmen.

V/K DALINTORG
Nachodka, Primorskij kraj 4
Tel.: 67-17
  Handles export and import transactions in the Eastern Siberian and coastal region involving trade with the Far East and Japan and the Korean People's Democratic Republic; exports coal, mine-chemical products, round timber, timber goods and wooden by-products, marble, granite, fish and fish products, sea food, tinned food, medicinal raw materials, skins and hides, deer horns and other goods; imports fishing equipment and outfits, equipment for the fish processing industry, medical equipment and instruments, stationery, photographic goods, ropes, wire ropes, wires, cable, building materials, sewn and knitted goods, fabrics, footwear, crockery, vegetables, fruit and other goods -

  Abwicklung des Küsten- und Grenzhandels bei Aus- und Einfuhr zwischen den östlichen Regionen Sibiriens und dem Fernen Osten mit Japan und der Volksdemokratischen Republik Korea; **Ausfuhr**: Kohle, grubenchemische Produkte, Rundholz, Holzwaren und Abfallprodukte aus Holz, Marmor, Granit, Fisch und Fischprodukte, Meerestiere, Nahrungsmittel in Konserven, medizinische Rohstoffe, Pelze und Felle, Hirschgeweihe und andere Waren; Einfuhr: Fischereiausrüstungen, Ausrüstungen für die fischverarbeitende Industrie, medizinische Ausrüstungen und Instrumente, Schreib- und Papierwaren, Fotoartikel, Seile, Drahtseile, Drähte, Kabel, Baustoffe, Strick- und Wirkwaren, Stoffe, Schuhwerk, Geshirr, Gemüse, Obst und andere Waren.

INGOSSTRACH
Moskva 103012, ul. Kuibyševa 11/10
Tel.: 223-49-27, Telex: 7144
  Undertakes all kinds of insurance and reinsurance, including transport insurance of cargo and ships, insurance of property against fire and natural calamities, insurance of motor vehicles as well as civil liability deriving from their use, insurance of airplanes and helicopters, and their owner's civil liability, accident insurance. Has a wide network of representatives and agents in the USSR and abroad -

"Ingosstrach" übernimmt alle Formen der Versicherung und Rückversicherung, darunter Transportversicherung von Frachten und Schiffen, Versicherung von Immobilien und Mobilien gegen Feuer und Naturkatastrophen, Kraftfahrzeug-Haftpflichtversicherung sowie Haftpflichtversicherung der Fahrzeuginsassen, Flugversicherung von Flugzeugen und Hubschraubern sowie die Inhaber-Haftpflichtversicherung, Unfallversicherung. Ingosstrach verfügt über ein weitverzweigtes Netz von Vertretungen und Agenturen in der UdSSR und im Ausland.

VA/O INTOURIST
Moskva 103009, Prospekt Marksa 16
Tel.: 292-29-89, 203-69-62, 292-27-67, Telex: 7211,7212,7213

Offers varied and fascinating itineraries by train, plane, motorship, by car and by boat, wonderful rest and medical treatment at the finest resorts on the Black Sea coast, at the Caucasian Spas, at Tskhaltubo in the Caucasus, camping trips in the country's most picturesque spots, car rental with or without the services of a chauffeur, hunting trips in the Northern Caucasus, Azerbaijan and Siberia, trips to the traditional art festival "Moscow Stars", "White Nights", "Russian Winter", boat cruises on the most beautiful rivers of Europe - the Volga and the Dnieper. Full information can be obtained at travel bureaus acting as agents of Intourist and also at information bureaus of Intourist in many countries of the world -

Organisation und Durchführung von Bahn-, Flug-, Motorschiff-, Auto- und Schiffsreisen, wunderbare Erholung und ärztliche Behandlung in den besten Kurorten an der Schwarzmeerküste, in den kaukasischen Heilbädern und in Tschaltubo (Kaukasus), Campingfahrten in die malerischsten Gegenden des Landes, Autoverleih mit und ohne Chauffeur, Jagdausflüge in den Nordkaukasus, nach Azerbaidschan und Sibirien, Reisen zu den traditionellen Kunstfestivals "Stars von Moskau", "Weiße Nächte" und "Russischer Winter", Kreuzfahrten auf den schönsten Flüssen Europas - Wolga und Dnjepr. Auskünfte erteilen die Reiseagenturen von Intourist sowie Auskunftbüros von Intourist in vielen Ländern der Welt.

V/K LENFINTORG
196084 Leningrad and/und Moskva, Moskovskij Prosp. 98
Tel.: 92-56-25, Telex: 518 (Leningrad)

Carries on barter trade in consumer goods with Finland and Norway. Exports bicycles, photographic goods, watches, electric bulbs, toys, refrigerators, art handicraft articles, aluminum and enamelled utensils, porcelain, cut glass, fabrics, soap, matches, hunting and sports gear, zoological goods, carpets, perfumery, musical instruments, tinned fish and crabmeat, salmon and sturgeon caviar, fruit and vegetables, juices, syrups, mineral water, wines and liquors, and other goods. Imports furniture, garments and knitted goods, footwear, plastic articles, household chemicals, cosmetics and perfumery, paper and cardboard goods, and other consumer goods -

Tauschhandel von Verbrauchsgütern mit Finnland und Norwegen. Ausfuhr: Fahrräder, Fotoartikel, Uhren, elektrische Glühbirnen, Spielzeug, Kühlschränke, Kunstgewerbeartikel, Aluminium- und Emailgeschirr, Porzellan, geschliffenes Glas, Stoffe, Seife, Zündhölzer, Jagd- und Sportzubehör, zoologische Artikel, Teppiche, Parfümerie, Musikinstrumente, Fisch- und Krabbenkonserven, Lachs und Störkaviar, Obst und Gemüse, Säfte, Sirup, Mineralwasser, Weine und Liköre, sowie andere Waren. Einfuhr: Möbel, Kleider und Strickwaren, Schuhbekleidung, Plastikartikel, Haushaltschemikalien, Kosmetik und Parfümerie, Papier- und Kartonagenartikel sowie andere Konsumgüter.

5.5.7.1 Economy / Wirtschaft

MORPASFLOT
Moskva, ul. Ždanova 1/4
Tel.: 291-93-31, 296-55-95, Telex: 7134
Central passenger agent, handles the chartering of passenger ships for Soviet organizations and foreign firms, concludes contracts with foreign firms on taking over the general agency for passenger traffic. The agency carries on negotiations and concludes contracts with foreign firms on the servicing of Soviet passenger ships in foreign ports. The agency reserves and sells tickets for passenger ships of the international lines in Moscow. "Morpasflot" together with the All-Union Corporation "Intourist" handles the transportation of foreign transit passengers through the USSR, reserves seats on ships and takes care of them in the ports. The Soviet ships travel on the various routes throughout the whole year -

Zentrale Fahrgastagentur, übernimmt das Verchartern von Fahrgastschiffen an sowjetische Organisationen und ausländische Firmen, schließt Verträge mit ausländischen Firmen zur Übernahme der Generalagentur im Fahrgastverkehr. Die Agentur führt Unterhandlungen und schließt Verträge mit ausländischen Firmen über die Bedienung sowjetischer Fahrgastschiffe in ausländischen Häfen. Sie reserviert und verkauft in Moskau Fahrkarten der Fahrgast-Seeschiffe des internationalen Linienverkehrs. "Morpasflot" übernimmt gemeinsam mit der Allunions-Aktiengesellschaft "Intourist" die Beförderung ausländischer Transit-Fahrgäste durch die UdSSR, ihre Versorgung mit Plätzen auf Seeschiffen sowie ihre Betreuung in den Häfen. Die sowjetischen Schiffe befahren das ganze Jahr hindurch die verschiedenen Reiserouten.

VKO SOJUZKOOPVNEŠTORG
Moskva 103003, Bolšoj Čerkasskij Per. 15/17
Tel.: 223-79-30, 225-09-14, Telex: 7127, 7128
"Sojuzkoopvneštorg" is a cooperative foreign trade organization in charge of foreign trade transactions with foreign cooperative organizations and firms. Exports honey, poppy seeds for cooking, cedar and hazel nuts, walnuts, dried vegetables and fruit, fruit compotes and jams, tomato-paste, dried mushrooms, salted and pickled mushrooms, salted and pickled cucumbers, onions, garlic, dried bilberries, cowberries in their own juice, cranberries, cloudberries, dried ashberries, pumpkin seeds, apple and bilberry pulp, potatoes and starc , live crawfish, and snails, salted and quick-frozen herring , canned fish, champagne, cognac, vodka, liquors, tea, medicinal and technical raw materials, non-standard skins and hides, horns and hooves, mackle-paper, rags, kitchen ware and household goods, petrol, kerosene, still cameras, radio sets, radiogramophones, record-players, TV sets, electric household appliances, bicycles, motorcycles, and other consumer goods. Imports clothing, knitted wear and underwear, footwear, hosiery, haberdashery, furniture, paints, carpets, sporting gear, tinned vegetables and fruit, fresh apples -

"Sojuzkoopvneštorg" ist eine konsumgenossenschaftliche Außenhandelsorganisation, die Außenhandelsgeschäfte mit ausländischen konsumgenossenschaftlichen Organisationen und Firmen tätigt. Ausfuhr: Honig, küchenfertiger Mohn, Zedar- und Haselnüsse, Walnüsse, Dörrgemüse und -obst, Fruchtkompotte und Marmelade, Tomatenmark, getrocknete, eingelegte und marinierte Pilze, gesalzene und eingelegte Gurken, Zwiebeln, Knoblauch, getrocknete Heidelbeeren, Sumpfbrombeeren im eigenen Saft, Preiselbeeren, Moosbeeren, getrocknete Ebereschenbeeren, Kürbiskerne, Apfel- und Heidelbeermark, Kartoffeln und Stärke, lebende Krebse und Frösche, gesalzene und tiefgefrorene Heringe, Fischkonserven, Champagner, Cognac, Wodka, Liköre, Tee, medizinische und technische Rohstoffe, Rohlederabfall, Hörner und Hufe, Altpapier, Lappen, Küchen- und Haushaltsartikel, Benzin, Kerosin, Fotokameras, Uhren, Radioapparate, Radiogeräte mit Plattenspieler, Plattenspieler, Fernsehgeräte, elektrische Haushaltsgeräte, Fahrräder, Motorräder und andere Konsumgüter. Einfuhr: Bekleidung, Ober- und Untertrikotagen, Schuhwerk, Strumpfwaren, Kurzwaren, Möbel, Farben, Teppiche, Sportartikel, Gemüse- und Obstkonserven, frische Äpfel.

V/K TECHVNESTRANS
Moskva 113324, Ovčinnikovskaja Nab. 18/1
Tel.: 220-19-53

Handles transports in connection with the organization, construction and operation of industrial enterprises and other projects abroad. Organizes the transportation of the export and import goods of the aforementioned organizations "Technoexport", "Technopromexport", "Tjašpromexport", "Prommašexport", "Neftechimpromexport", "Selchospromexport" and "Tsvetmetpromexport" by all means of transportation -

Übernimmt die Transporte, die bei der Organisierung, beim Bau und Betrieb von Industriebetrieben und anderen Objekten im Ausland verbunden sind. Organisiert die Beförderung der Export- und Importgüter der vorgenannten Organisationen "Technoexport", "Technopromexport", "Tjašpromexport", "Prommašexport", "Neftechimpromexport", "Selchospromexport" und "Tsvetmetpromexport" mit allen Transportmitteln.

6. LABOUR – ARBEITSRESERVEN – TRUDOVYE REZERVY

6.1 SHARE OF THE WORKING-AGE POPULATION ON TOTAL POPULATION
ANTEIL DER BEVÖLKERUNG IM ARBEITSFÄHIGEN ALTER AN DER GESAMTBEVÖLKERUNG
NASELENIE V TRUDOSPOSOBNOM VOZRASTE K OBŠČEJ ČISLENNOSTI NASELENIJA
(Census – Volkszählungen – Perepisi naselenija 1959, 1970)

	1959 Total Insg. Vsego A.	1959 males Männer mužčiny B.	1959 females Frauen ženščiny C.	1970 Total Insg. Vsego D.	1970 males Männer mužčiny E.	1970 females Frauen ženščiny F.	1970 % in relation to / % im Verhältnis zu / v & k 1959 Total Insg. Vsego G.	1959 m. M. m. H.	1959 f. F. ž. I.	per 1,000 inhabitants / je 1.000 Einwohner / na 1.000 žitelej 1959 m. M. m. J.	1959 f. F. ž. K.	1970 m. M. m. L.	1970 f. F. ž. M.
SSSR													
1.	208826650	94050303	114776347	241720134	111399377	130320757	116	118	114	450	550	461	539
2.	119821618	55076204	64745414	130486541	64003489	66483052	109	116	103	460	540	490	510
3.	99977695	45208278	54769417	135991514	63026095	72965419	136	139	133	452	548	463	537
4.	62187956	28744501	33443455	81363923	40034653	41329270	131	139	124	462	538	492	508
5.	108848955	48842025	60006930	105728620	48373282	57355338	97	99	96	449	551	458	542
6.	57633662	26331703	31301959	49122618	23968836	25153782	85	91	80	457	543	488	512
RSFSR													
1.	117534306	52424832	65109474	130079210	59324787	70754423	111	113	109	446	554	456	544
2.	68609392	31341607	37267785	72991608	35883808	37107800	106	114	100	457	543	492	508
3.	61611074	27652664	33958410	80981143	37137193	43843950	131	134	129	449	551	459	541
4.	38629448	17778237	20851211	49310122	24195823	25114299	128	136	120	460	540	491	509
5.	55923232	24772168	31151064	49098067	22187594	26910473	88	90	86	443	557	452	548
6.	29979944	13563370	16416574	23681486	11687985	11993501	79	86	73	452	548	494	506

1. Urban and rural population – Stadt- und Landbevölkerung – Gorodskoe i sel'skoe naselenie
2. of which at working age (males 16–59, females 15–54 years) – davon im arbeitsfähigen Alter (Männer 16–59, Frauen 15–54 Jahre) – iz nich v trudosposobnom vozraste (mužčiny 16–59, ženščiny 16–54 let)
3. Urban population – Stadtbevölkerung – Gorodskoe naselenie
4. of which at working age (males 16–59, females 15–54 years) – davon im arbeitsfähigen Alter (Männer 16–59, Frauen 15–54 Jahre) – iz nich v trudosposobnom vozraste (mužčiny 16–59, ženščiny 16–54 let)
5. Rural population – Landbevölkerung – Sel'skoe naselenie
6. of which at working age – davon im arbeitsfähigen Alter – iz nich v trudosposobnom vozraste

Labour
Arbeitsreserven 6.1

	A.	B.	C.	D.	E.	F.	G.	H.	I.	J.	K.	L.	M.
Ukrainskaja SSR													
1.	41869046	18575382	23293664	47126517	21305320	25821197	113	115	111	444	556	452	548
2.	24882425	11272424	13610001	26191662	12654644	13537018	105	112	99	453	547	483	517
3.	19147419	8664550	10482869	25688560	11881383	13807177	134	137	132	453	547	463	537
4.	12188934	5645185	6543749	15544366	7624337	7920029	128	135	121	463	537	490	510
5.	22721627	9910832	12810795	21437957	9423937	12014020	94	95	94	436	564	440	560
6.	12693491	5627239	7066252	10647296	5030307	5616989	84	89	79	443	557	472	528
Belorusskaja SSR													
1.	8055714	3581485	4474229	9002338	4137816	4864522	112	116	109	445	555	460	540
2.	4447035	1994653	2452382	4765681	2303780	2461901	107	115	100	449	551	483	517
3.	2480505	1105079	1375426	3907783	1835603	2072180	158	166	151	446	554	470	530
4.	1532642	679553	853089	2410140	1169441	1240699	157	172	145	443	557	485	515
5.	5575209	2476406	3098803	5094555	2302213	2792342	91	93	90	444	556	452	548
6.	2911393	1315100	1599293	2355541	1134339	1221202	81	86	76	451	549	482	518
Uzbekskaja SSR													
1.	8119103	3897342	4221761	11799429	5743956	6055473	145	147	143	480	520	487	513
2.	3989406	1943388	2046018	4979189	2474731	2504458	125	127	122	487	513	497	503
3.	2728580	1284590	1443990	4321603	2089086	2232517	158	163	155	471	529	483	517
4.	1532505	725516	806989	2218425	1114401	1104024	145	154	137	473	527	502	498
5.	5390523	2612752	2777771	7477826	3654870	3822956	139	140	138	485	515	489	511
6.	2456901	1217872	1239029	2760764	1360330	1400434	112	112	113	496	504	493	507
Kazachskaja SSR													
1.	9294741	4414699	4880042	13008726	6262721	6746005	140	142	138	475	525	481	519
2.	4972625	2403588	2569037	6484030	3254007	3230023	130	135	126	483	517	502	498
3.	4067224	1922760	2144464	6538652	3151725	3386927	161	164	158	473	527	482	518
4.	2380101	1143233	1236868	3723723	1884869	1838854	156	165	149	480	520	506	494
5.	5227517	2491939	2735578	6470074	3110996	3359078	124	125	123	477	523	481	519
6.	2592524	1260355	1332169	2760307	1369138	1391169	106	109	104	486	514	496	504
Gruzinskaja SSR													
1.	4044045	1865345	2178700	4686358	2200580	2483778	116	118	114	461	539	470	530
2.	2268737	1054736	1214001	2466222	1204923	1261299	109	114	104	465	535	489	511
3.	1712897	779420	933477	2239738	1046903	1192835	131	134	128	455	545	467	533
4.	1071833	491196	580637	1299146	630483	668663	121	128	115	458	542	485	515
5.	2331148	1085925	1245223	2446620	1155677	1290943	105	106	104	466	534	472	528
6.	1196904	563540	633364	1167076	574440	592636	98	102	94	471	529	492	508

393

6.1 Labour / Arbeitsreserven

	A.	B.	C.	D.	E.	F.	G.	H.	I.	J.	K.	L.	M.
Azerbajdžanskaja SSR													
1.	3697717	1756561	1941156	5117081	2433035	2634046	138	141	136	475	525	485	515
2.	1902263	912051	990212	2242755	1118616	1124139	118	123	114	479	521	499	501
3.	1767270	836017	931253	2564551	1254991	1309560	145	150	141	473	527	489	511
4.	1004277	479636	524641	1313886	669631	644255	131	140	123	478	522	510	490
5.	1930447	920544	1009903	2552530	1228044	1324486	132	133	131	477	523	481	519
6.	897986	432415	465571	928869	448985	479884	103	104	103	482	518	483	517
Litovskaja SSR													
1.	2711445	1244678	1466767	3128236	1467950	1660286	115	118	113	459	541	469	531
2.	1536538	730425	806113	1677938	820706	857232	109	112	106	475	525	489	511
3.	1045965	472738	573227	1571737	741258	830479	150	157	145	452	548	472	528
4.	654192	304512	349680	954373	468393	485980	146	154	139	465	535	491	509
5.	1665480	771940	893540	1556499	726692	829807	93	94	93	463	537	467	533
6.	882346	425913	456433	723565	352313	371252	82	83	81	483	517	487	513
Moldavskaja SSR													
1.	2884477	1333794	1550683	3568873	1662275	1906598	124	125	123	462	538	466	534
2.	1593878	744861	849017	1899135	904158	994977	119	121	117	467	533	476	524
3.	642244	293768	348476	1130048	529339	600709	176	180	172	457	543	468	532
4.	392791	181586	211205	692681	333615	359066	176	184	170	462	538	482	518
5.	2242233	1040026	1202207	2438825	1132936	1305889	109	109	109	464	536	465	535
6.	1201087	563275	637812	1206454	570543	635911	100	101	100	469	531	473	527
Latvijskaja SSR													
1.	2093458	919008	1174450	2364127	1080616	1283511	113	118	109	439	561	457	543
2.	1218258	564458	653800	1329172	658358	670814	109	117	103	463	537	495	505
3.	1173976	508815	665161	1476602	675437	801165	126	133	120	433	567	457	543
4.	722994	330036	392958	901353	444280	457073	125	135	116	456	544	493	507
5.	919482	410193	509289	887525	405179	482346	97	99	95	446	554	457	543
6.	495264	234422	260842	427819	214078	213741	86	91	82	473	527	500	500
Kirgizskaja SSR													
1.	2065837	974620	1091217	2932805	1401557	1531248	142	144	140	472	528	478	522
2.	1030041	492012	538029	1325192	651340	673852	129	132	125	478	522	492	508
3.	696207	326442	369765	1097498	515622	581876	158	158	157	469	531	470	530
4.	400324	188409	211915	603981	292012	311969	151	155	147	471	529	483	517
5.	1369630	648178	721452	1835307	885935	949372	134	137	132	473	527	483	517
6.	629717	303603	326114	721211	359328	361883	115	118	111	482	518	498	502

Labour 6.1
Arbeitsreserven

	A.	B.	C.	D.	E.	F.	G.	H.	I.	J.	K.	L.	M.
Tadžikskaja SSR													
1.	1980547	964728	1015819	2899602	1426255	1473347	146	148	145	487	513	492	508
2.	993121	486843	506278	1222906	610843	612063	123	125	121	490	510	500	500
3.	646178	308021	338157	1076700	527776	548924	167	171	162	477	523	490	510
4.	367751	175831	191920	545612	276418	269194	148	157	140	478	522	507	493
5.	1334369	656707	677662	1822902	898479	924423	137	137	136	492	508	493	507
6.	625370	311012	314358	677294	334425	342869	108	108	109	497	503	494	506
Armjanskaja SSR													
1.	1763048	842406	920642	2491873	1217163	1274710	141	144	138	478	522	488	512
2.	921052	440802	480250	1202280	598575	603705	131	136	126	479	521	498	502
3.	881844	422307	459537	1481532	725022	756510	168	172	165	479	521	489	511
4.	495124	238026	257098	791020	396496	394524	160	167	153	481	519	501	499
5.	881204	420099	461105	1010341	492141	518000	115	117	112	477	523	487	513
6.	425928	202776	223152	411260	202079	209181	97	100	94	476	524	491	509
Turkmenskaja SSR													
1.	1516375	730333	786042	2158880	1063151	1095729	142	146	139	482	518	492	508
2.	768582	373230	395352	946739	483173	463566	123	129	117	486	514	510	490
3.	700797	335199	365598	1034199	512621	521578	148	153	143	478	522	496	504
4.	394808	189353	205455	521583	271148	250435	132	143	122	480	520	520	480
5.	815578	395134	420444	1124681	550530	574151	138	139	137	484	516	489	511
6.	373774	183877	189897	425156	212025	213131	114	115	112	492	508	499	501
Estonskaja SSR													
1.	1196791	525090	671701	1356079	620195	735884	113	118	110	439	561	457	543
2.	688265	321126	367139	762032	381827	380205	111	119	104	467	533	501	499
3.	675515	295908	379607	881168	402136	479032	130	136	126	438	562	456	544
4.	420232	194192	226040	533512	263306	270206	127	136	120	462	538	494	506
5.	521276	229182	292094	474911	218059	256852	91	95	88	440	560	459	541
6.	268033	126934	141099	228520	118521	109999	85	93	78	474	526	519	481

6.2 Labour
Arbeitsreserven

6.2 EDUCATIONAL LEVEL OF THE WORKING-AGE POPULATION
BILDUNGSSTAND DER BEVÖLKERUNG IM ARBEITSFÄHIGEN ALTER
UROVEN' OBRAZOVANIJA ZANJATOGO NASELENIJA
(Census - Volkszählungen - Perepisi naselenija 1959, 1970)

	per 1,000 people engaged - auf 1.000 Beschäftigte - na 1.000 zanjatych							
	1959				1970			
	A.	B.	C.	D.	A.	B.	C.	D.

A. Higher education (complete and incomplete) and secondary specialized education / Hochschulbildung (abgeschlossene u.nicht abgeschlossene) u.mittl.Fachschulbildung / Vysšee, nezakončennoe vysšee i srednee special'noe obrazovanie
B. Secondary education[1] / Mittelschulbildung[1] / Srednee obrazovanie
C. Incomplete secondary education / Nicht abgeschlossene Mittelschulbildung / Nepolnoe srednee obrazovanie
D. Primary education / Grundschulbildung / Načal'noe obrazovanie

USSR

1. Urban and rural population -
Stadt-und Landbevölkerung -
Gorodskoe i sel'skoe naselenie

1.1 All social groups -
Alle gesellschaftl.Gruppen -
Vse obščestvennye gruppy

Total-Insg.-Vsego	109	64	260	331	183	159	311	248
Males-Männer-mužčiny	103	60	271	386	171	156	327	268
Females-Frauen-ženščiny	116	68	247	272	194	162	295	228

1.2 Workers-Arbeiter-rabočie

Total-Insg.-Vsego	22	62	312	412	37	162	387	308
Males-Männer-mužčiny	23	57	314	458	39	169	399	315
Females-Frauen-ženščiny	20	68	309	346	33	155	372	299

1.3 Employees-Angestellte-služaščie

Total-Insg.-Vsego	520	144	243	81	594	196	164	39
Males-Männer-mužčiny	521	124	222	115	647	159	137	49
Females-Frauen-ženščiny	519	162	260	51	557	221	184	32

1.4 Collective farmers-Kolchosbauern-kolchozniki

Total-Insg.-Vsego	9	23	194	355	28	75	290	393
Males-Männer-mužčiny	14	29	218	413	37	91	307	398
Females-Frauen-ženščiny	6	18	174	308	19	61	275	389

[1] in the German Democratic Republic: high school - in der DDR: Oberschule

Labour 6.2
Arbeitsreserven

	1959				1970			
	A.	B.	C.	D.	A.	B.	C.	D.
2. Urban population-Stadtbevölkerung-Gorodskoe naselenie								
2.1 All social groups - Alle gesellschaftl.Gruppen - Vse obščestvennye gruppy								
Total-Insg.-Vsego	167	94	303	307	237	192	319	192
Males-Männer-mužčiny	153	82	302	362	225	181	334	214
Females-Frauen-ženščiny	184	109	304	243	250	201	304	170
2.2 Workers-Arbeiter-rabočie								
Total-Insg.-Vsego	26	73	333	403	44	189	409	275
Males-Männer-mužčiny	28	68	336	447	48	193	420	282
Females-Frauen-ženščiny	23	81	328	343	40	184	395	266
2.3 Employees-Angestellte-služaščie								
Total-Insg.-Vsego	522	151	240	76	609	196	156	33
Males-Männer-mužčiny	545	128	207	105	681	153	120	39
Females-Frauen-ženščiny	502	171	267	52	560	225	180	30
3. Rural population - Landbevölkerung - Sel'skoe naselenie								
3.1 All social groups - Alle gesellschaftl.Gruppen - Vse obščestvennye gruppy								
Total-Insg.-Vsego	59	36	221	352	95	106	298	338
Males-Männer-mužčiny	56	40	241	408	86	115	316	354
Females-Frauen-ženščiny	60	34	200	295	103	97	281	322
3.2 Workers-Arbeiter-rabočie								
Total-Insg.-Vsego	13	38	269	430	20	103	337	382
Males-Männer-mužčiny	15	37	271	478	21	116	350	389
Females-Frauen-ženščiny	12	40	265	354	18	87	320	374
3.3 Employees-Angestellte-služaščie								
Total-Insg.-Vsego	516	125	250	94	535	195	198	62
Males-Männer-mužčiny	464	114	260	139	519	181	197	89
Females-Frauen-ženščiny	569	136	239	49	548	206	199	41
3.4 Collective farmers - Kolchosbauern - kolchozniki								
Total-Insg.-Vsego	9	23	194	355	27	74	289	396
Males-Männer-mužčiny	13	29	218	412	36	89	305	402
Females-Frauen-ženščiny	6	18	174	309	19	61	275	391
RSFSR								
1.1 Total - Insg.	117	60	263	353	189	141	326	257
Males - Männer	108	52	268	424	173	132	341	289
Females - Frauen	127	68	257	277	207	149	311	224
1.2 Total - Insg.	20	54	304	435	33	137	397	329
Males - Männer	22	48	303	494	36	141	409	343
Females - Frauen	19	61	305	358	31	133	383	311
1.3 Total - Insg.	511	129	257	91	585	178	187	44
Males - Männer	517	105	230	131	644	139	152	57
Females - Frauen	506	148	280	58	548	202	209	36
1.4 Total - Insg.	8	16	177	392	27	44	289	435
Males - Männer	11	19	199	485	33	53	310	455
Females - Frauen	6	14	159	316	21	34	267	415

6.2 Labour / Arbeitsreserven

	1959 A.	1959 B.	1959 C.	1959 D.	1970 A.	1970 B.	1970 C.	1970 D.
2.1 Total - Insg.	163	84	304	326	231	170	336	206
Males - Männer	150	70	299	390	216	158	350	235
Females - Frauen	177	99	310	255	245	182	323	177
2.2 Total - Insg.	24	64	326	423	40	163	422	294
Males - Männer	25	58	327	479	43	165	433	307
Females - Frauen	22	72	325	354	36	161	409	277
2.3 Total - Insg.	516	136	253	84	602	181	175	37
Males - Männer	545	110	213	117	630	138	133	43
Females - Frauen	493	156	285	58	551	208	203	33
3.1 Total - Insg.	65	32	216	383	101	80	305	363
Males - Männer	59	31	231	464	81	81	324	399
Females - Frauen	72	33	201	300	123	79	285	327
3.2 Total - Insg.	13	32	256	460	17	72	334	418
Males - Männer	14	29	255	524	18	80	349	435
Females - Frauen	12	36	258	367	16	62	316	397
3.3 Total - Insg.	497	108	270	110	515	165	237	74
Males - Männer	443	92	275	167	490	143	239	114
Females - Frauen	546	123	266	58	531	179	235	49
3.4 Total-Insg.	8	16	176	392	26	43	288	438
Males - Männer	11	18	198	484	32	51	308	459
Females - Frauen	5	14	159	317	20	34	267	416
Ukrainskaja SSR								
1.1 Total - Insg.	99	67	272	315	175	191	302	233
Males - Männer	97	65	297	357	170	192	323	238
Females - Frauen	101	71	244	270	181	189	282	228
1.2 Total - Insg.	25	84	357	370	45	231	389	251
Males - Männer	27	74	359	408	47	233	399	254
Females - Frauen	23	101	353	308	42	228	377	247
1.3 Total - Insg.	551	158	222	60	627	224	119	25
Males - Männer	540	133	222	91	671	179	109	34
Females - Frauen	562	181	221	31	594	257	126	19
1.4 Total - Insg.	9	22	213	356	28	72	297	399
Males - Männer	13	27	249	401	37	96	322	386
Females - Frauen	6	18	186	322	21	52	277	410
2.1 Total - Insg.	169	113	318	275	246	244	299	157
Males - Männer	153	96	328	323	240	233	317	168
Females - Frauen	188	135	306	213	254	255	280	145
2.2 Total - Insg.	30	98	370	358	53	260	397	221
Males - Männer	32	86	375	396	57	262	408	222
Females - Frauen	27	115	362	299	49	258	384	220
2.3 Total - Insg.	547	170	218	56	639	223	112	21
Males - Männer	563	141	202	82	707	170	93	25
Females - Frauen	533	196	233	33	589	261	127	19
3.1 Total - Insg.	48	34	237	344	78	118	307	337
Males - Männer	48	37	271	386	70	133	331	339
Females - Frauen	47	32	207	305	86	103	284	336
3.2 Total - Insg.	14	51	325	398	22	155	368	328
Males - Männer	14	44	322	437	21	160	376	336
Females - Frauen	14	62	330	332	24	150	357	317

Labour
Arbeitsreserven 6.2

	1 9 5 9				1 9 7 0			
	A.	B.	C.	D.	A.	B.	C.	D.
3.3 Total - Insg.	564	124	230	70	569	229	149	44
Males - Männer	481	110	275	115	504	223	183	75
Females - Frauen	651	138	184	23	616	234	124	22
3.4 Total - Insg.	9	21	215	356	27	71	298	402
Males - Männer	13	26	251	400	36	95	322	389
Females - Frauen	6	18	188	323	21	52	278	411
Belorusskaja SSR								
1.1 Total - Insg.	80	52	199	364	167	154	273	298
Males - Männer	77	49	226	431	157	150	307	307
Females - Frauen	82	54	175	304	176	158	241	289
1.2 Total - Insg.	16	65	292	435	31	176	361	334
Males - Männer	17	55	298	488	31	176	386	336
Females - Frauen	15	79	284	367	32	176	331	332
1.3 Total - Insg.	542	147	236	69	615	207	142	31
Males - Männer	505	131	244	110	633	171	143	46
Females - Frauen	574	163	229	31	601	235	141	20
1.4 Total - Insg.	6	19	133	395	25	38	200	505
Males - Männer	8	23	163	474	30	50	245	506
Females - Frauen	4	17	111	336	20	29	163	504
2.1 Total - Insg.	176	108	304	297	253	226	307	169
Males - Männer	161	93	308	351	246	212	331	180
Females - Frauen	192	124	298	241	260	240	283	159
2.2 Total - Insg.	24	90	349	403	44	237	408	249
Males - Männer	25	76	354	448	44	234	432	249
Females - Frauen	22	107	342	349	44	242	381	248
2.3 Total - Insg.	529	160	244	61	632	208	134	23
Males - Männer	519	147	232	94	676	169	122	29
Females - Frauen	538	172	255	32	599	238	142	17
3.1 Total - Insg.	43	30	159	390	83	84	240	423
Males - Männer	41	31	190	465	71	89	283	431
Females - Frauen	44	29	132	326	94	79	200	415
3.2 Total - Insg.	8	38	232	470	13	91	295	453
Males - Männer	9	33	243	528	13	99	326	451
Females - Frauen	7	45	216	388	14	81	259	454
3.3 Total - Insg.	564	125	222	82	563	206	167	56
Males - Männer	484	102	264	137	507	178	204	96
Females - Frauen	643	146	181	28	605	227	138	27
3.4 Total - Insg.	5	19	133	395	24	38	199	507
Males - Männer	7	23	163	475	29	49	243	509
Females - Frauen	4	17	110	337	20	29	163	505
Uzbekskaja SSR								
1.1 Total - Insg.	87	80	280	203	155	213	295	191
Males - Männer	93	99	275	206	174	245	278	179
Females - Frauen	79	56	287	199	134	178	313	204
1.2 Total - Insg.	21	69	295	282	43	218	345	243
Males - Männer	25	82	300	287	50	255	339	227
Females - Frauen	15	45	286	273	31	160	355	268

399

6.2 Labour / Arbeitsreserven

	1959				1970			
	A.	B.	C.	D.	A.	B.	C.	D.
1.3 Total - Insg.	507	188	214	66	575	233	136	39
Males - Männer	515	194	189	72	619	217	107	39
Females - Frauen	497	180	246	59	529	250	166	40
1.4 Total - Insg.	9	54	289	180	19	196	347	232
Males - Männer	16	83	279	166	39	254	310	213
Females - Frauen	2	26	299	193	5	154	374	246
2.1 Total - Insg.	178	107	277	248	249	212	273	169
Males - Männer	157	106	277	272	236	222	280	176
Females - Frauen	210	108	276	213	264	201	264	160
2.2 Total - Insg.	30	79	308	339	57	212	354	248
Males - Männer	32	86	315	347	62	237	356	239
Females - Frauen	26	66	294	324	49	173	351	262
2.3 Total - Insg.	516	170	219	72	587	212	146	40
Males - Männer	533	167	185	83	645	184	112	42
Females - Frauen	501	173	251	60	543	233	172	38
3.1 Total - Insg.	45	68	282	182	89	213	311	207
Males - Männer	61	95	273	173	128	263	276	182
Females - Frauen	27	35	291	193	48	162	346	233
3.2 Total - Insg.	12	58	282	224	25	224	335	238
Males - Männer	16	77	285	223	36	277	318	213
Females - Frauen	6	25	278	227	11	145	360	274
3.3 Total - Insg.	491	220	205	57	551	275	116	39
Males - Männer	492	228	194	58	586	259	100	36
Females - Frauen	488	201	230	56	483	306	148	43
3.4 Total - Insg.	9	54	291	178	19	198	349	231
Males - Männer	15	83	281	164	39	256	311	212
Females - Frauen	2	26	300	192	5	155	377	245
Kazachskaja SSR								
1.1 Total - Insg.	106	67	274	310	175	155	324	239
Males - Männer	95	66	284	344	163	155	342	253
Females - Frauen	124	70	258	259	188	155	303	223
1.2 Total - Insg.	19	51	302	384	30	137	388	315
Males - Männer	21	52	312	408	33	153	405	310
Females - Frauen	17	49	284	335	26	115	363	322
1.3 Total - Insg.	466	154	270	89	543	209	192	46
Males - Männer	455	143	251	120	596	176	160	56
Females - Frauen	477	165	291	57	505	233	215	39
1.4 Total - Insg.	14	31	198	315	35	107	285	332
Males - Männer	22	41	222	332	51	128	301	322
Females - Frauen	6	19	170	297	16	83	266	343
2.1 Total - Insg.	147	86	307	307	221	173	336	200
Males - Männer	125	77	302	354	203	168	354	220
Females - Frauen	179	99	315	236	239	178	317	177
2.2 Total - Insg.	25	60	323	390	40	159	420	284
Males - Männer	26	59	324	420	43	172	433	283
Females - Frauen	22	63	320	335	36	140	400	285
2.3 Total - Insg.	470	153	269	88	569	196	186	41
Males - Männer	475	143	234	119	644	157	143	46
Females - Frauen	465	163	303	59	519	222	214	37

Labour
Arbeitsreserven 6.2

	1 9 5 9				1 9 7 0			
	A.	B.	C.	D.	A.	B.	C.	D.
3.1 Total - Insg.	75	53	246	312	113	131	307	292
Males - Männer	71	57	269	336	108	138	327	298
Females - Frauen	81	47	212	277	119	123	284	286
3.2 Total - Insg.	13	41	279	375	17	107	345	357
Males - Männer	15	45	298	395	19	126	366	350
Females - Frauen	11	33	240	336	15	84	319	366
3.3 Total - Insg.	459	155	272	91	485	238	205	60
Males - Männer	428	144	273	122	505	212	193	75
Females - Frauen	501	169	269	51	468	260	216	46
3.4 Total - Insg.	14	31	197	313	35	107	284	333
Males - Männer	21	41	222	327	51	128	298	324
Females - Frauen	6	19	170	297	16	83	268	343
Gruzinskaja SSR								
1.1 Total - Insg.	152	140	200	209	237	270	204	181
Males - Männer	150	139	225	232	238	265	223	182
Females - Frauen	154	140	170	182	236	276	184	179
1.2 Total - Insg.	41	162	295	280	66	312	277	224
Males - Männer	44	167	314	294	71	317	298	217
Females - Frauen	33	154	258	250	59	304	246	234
1.3 Total - Insg.	620	246	87	33	678	253	48	16
Males - Männer	620	220	95	46	704	214	54	21
Females - Frauen	621	273	78	20	655	286	43	11
1.4 Total - Insg.	28	82	184	234	56	200	261	295
Males - Männer	38	81	200	252	78	189	264	295
Females - Frauen	20	82	169	218	38	209	259	295
2.1 Total - Insg.	251	207	211	185	334	322	172	115
Males - Männer	230	197	233	210	322	313	195	121
Females - Frauen	279	221	180	149	348	332	146	107
2.2 Total - Insg.	43	186	297	275	76	372	272	192
Males - Männer	47	193	312	287	80	379	287	185
Females - Frauen	35	173	269	254	70	363	249	202
2.3 Total - Insg.	607	261	86	33	678	258	44	15
Males - Männer	625	229	85	43	719	214	44	17
Females - Frauen	589	293	86	23	643	296	44	12
3.1 Total - Insg.	89	97	193	224	141	218	237	246
Males - Männer	91	97	219	247	148	214	254	246
Females - Frauen	87	97	164	200	132	223	220	246
3.2 Total - Insg.	36	110	291	289	52	228	284	269
Males - Männer	38	113	317	309	59	231	313	262
Females - Frauen	29	102	228	240	43	222	242	279
3.3 Total - Insg.	653	210	90	32	679	236	60	19
Males - Männer	607	197	120	52	663	216	82	31
Females - Frauen	698	223	59	13	695	255	39	8
3.4 Total - Insg.	28	80	184	234	56	198	260	297
Males - Männer	37	79	200	252	78	186	261	299
Females - Frauen	19	82	170	218	38	208	260	295

6.2 Labour
Arbeitsreserven

	1959				1970			
	A.	B.	C.	D.	A.	B.	C.	D.
Azerbajdžanskaja SSR								
1.1 Total - Insg.	119	89	265	209	204	208	262	182
Males - Männer	130	104	290	220	225	239	265	163
Females - Frauen	105	70	233	195	176	170	259	206
1.2 Total - Insg.	32	91	321	293	51	224	333	230
Males - Männer	36	101	352	305	63	268	343	207
Females - Frauen	22	69	254	265	32	153	316	267
1.3 Total - Insg.	560	191	175	51	629	234	99	28
Males - Männer	582	185	151	55	676	207	79	27
Females - Frauen	533	197	205	47	575	264	121	29
1.4 Total - Insg.	15	49	259	207	36	132	309	277
Males - Männer	29	73	287	201	73	187	300	235
Females - Frauen	3	29	233	213	6	87	317	311
2.1 Total - Insg.	192	125	274	222	274	242	243	144
Males - Männer	175	124	294	248	272	252	257	145
Females - Frauen	221	126	243	180	277	228	224	144
2.2 Total - Insg.	33	95	322	304	65	247	333	217
Males - Männer	38	104	350	317	76	278	345	202
Females - Frauen	24	76	265	275	47	191	312	243
2.3 Total - Insg.	536	195	190	57	623	233	104	29
Males - Männer	565	188	157	63	686	197	79	27
Females - Frauen	505	202	224	51	563	267	128	30
3.1 Total - Insg.	62	61	258	199	112	164	287	232
Males - Männer	87	85	287	195	159	219	275	190
Females - Frauen	34	36	227	204	59	103	300	278
3.2 Total - Insg.	23	76	317	248	25	181	332	255
Males - Männer	28	90	358	260	38	247	338	218
Females - Frauen	9	37	191	211	8	91	323	305
3.3 Total - Insg.	644	174	125	33	650	236	80	24
Males - Männer	625	178	135	37	651	232	81	25
Females - Frauen	687	166	101	25	649	244	77	21
3.4 Total - Insg.	15	49	261	206	35	132	310	279
Males - Männer	28	73	291	198	72	187	298	237
Females - Frauen	3	29	236	212	6	88	321	312
Litovskaja SSR								
1.1 Total - Insg.	75	41	134	409	160	98	238	371
Males - Männer	65	36	139	446	139	84	264	387
Females - Frauen	87	46	128	366	183	113	211	353
1.2 Total - Insg.	13	31	185	510	26	81	314	442
Males - Männer	12	28	183	540	23	78	337	440
Females - Frauen	14	36	189	461	30	85	285	444
1.3 Total - Insg.	460	179	242	109	585	209	156	45
Males - Männer	426	160	240	157	615	174	145	61
Females - Frauen	492	198	243	63	563	234	165	34
1.4 Total - Insg.	4	5	60	424	41	11	132	565
Males - Männer	6	5	64	444	36	11	160	551
Females - Frauen	3	5	56	406	45	11	104	580

Labour
Arbeitsreserven 6.2

| | 1 9 5 9 |||| 1 9 7 0 ||||
	A.	B.	C.	D.	A.	B.	C.	D.
2.1 Total - Insg.	156	87	229	370	227	146	283	271
Males - Männer	135	75	226	417	206	129	311	289
Females - Frauen	182	102	232	312	248	164	253	253
2.2 Total - Insg.	17	44	227	496	34	107	357	397
Males - Männer	17	41	227	526	31	103	387	392
Females - Frauen	18	48	226	454	37	110	322	404
2.3 Total - Insg.	465	187	247	92	595	215	148	38
Males - Männer	447	170	238	132	632	182	134	48
Females - Frauen	481	204	255	55	567	239	158	32
3.1 Total - Insg.	30	15	82	431	76	36	182	497
Males - Männer	25	13	88	463	56	28	207	507
Females - Frauen	36	17	75	394	96	46	154	486
3.2 Total - Insg.	5	11	119	533	12	32	231	527
Males - Männer	5	11	120	561	9	32	248	527
Females - Frauen	5	11	117	476	16	34	207	527
3.3 Total - Insg.	445	158	227	155	539	183	195	76
Males - Männer	362	130	249	233	528	134	200	127
Females - Frauen	523	183	207	83	546	213	191	46
3.4 Total - Insg.	4	4	60	424	40	11	130	567
Males - Männer	6	4	63	444	35	10	157	554
Females - Frauen	3	5	56	406	45	11	104	581
Moldavskaja SSR								
1.1 Total - Insg.	60	29	191	331	123	104	281	280
Males - Männer	59	30	224	389	116	107	309	300
Females - Frauen	62	28	158	276	128	102	255	261
1.2 Total - Insg.	22	48	274	398	29	134	368	294
Males - Männer	21	44	284	437	30	138	388	302
Females - Frauen	23	55	258	333	28	130	344	284
1.3 Total - Insg.	562	155	217	60	625	206	130	32
Males - Männer	517	144	237	92	638	170	134	48
Females - Frauen	605	165	198	29	615	232	128	20
1.4 Total - Insg.	6	8	165	348	17	36	267	365
Males - Männer	10	10	201	412	25	47	294	391
Females - Frauen	4	6	135	295	9	26	243	343
2.1 Total - Insg.	176	89	259	289	244	191	290	180
Males - Männer	150	80	271	339	230	181	315	196
Females - Frauen	209	101	243	225	257	202	265	163
2.2 Total - Insg.	27	65	300	390	43	186	390	257
Males - Männer	27	58	307	428	45	187	411	260
Females - Frauen	28	74	290	331	40	184	365	253
2.3 Total - Insg.	545	170	220	58	632	212	125	25
Males - Männer	524	162	220	84	676	171	112	33
Females - Frauen	564	177	221	34	601	242	134	19
3.1 Total - Insg.	34	15	175	341	60	59	277	331
Males - Männer	34	16	212	402	55	67	306	356
Females - Frauen	34	14	142	285	63	52	251	309
3.2 Total - Insg.	14	25	238	408	13	75	343	336
Males - Männer	14	24	254	448	12	82	362	350
Females- Frauen	15	26	209	336	14	66	319	320

403

6.2 Labour / Arbeitsreserven

	1959				1970			
	A.	B.	C.	D.	A.	B.	C.	D.
3.3 Total - Insg.	587	134	211	62	608	192	143	47
Males - Männer	507	120	260	103	548	167	185	84
Females - Frauen	665	147	164	21	650	211	113	21
3.4 Total - Insg.	6	8	166	348	16	36	268	366
Males - Männer	9	9	203	413	24	47	295	392
Females - Frauen	3	6	136	295	9	26	245	343
Latvijskaja SSR								
1.1 Total - Insg.	127	78	297	332	210	147	304	251
Males - Männer	120	63	308	367	198	123	328	271
Females - Frauen	135	94	284	295	222	171	280	231
1.2 Total - Insg.	39	64	370	387	62	135	381	321
Males - Männer	45	56	378	407	68	127	400	322
Females - Frauen	32	74	360	357	55	145	358	320
1.3 Total - Insg.	512	203	232	49	581	217	156	42
Males - Männer	540	163	218	73	658	154	134	48
Females - Frauen	492	232	242	32	531	256	170	38
1.4 Total - Insg.	18	17	209	430	67	35	305	404
Males - Männer	23	16	203	464	64	33	326	409
Females - Frauen	15	18	214	401	70	38	283	399
2.1 Total - Insg.	182	116	335	277	256	184	297	205
Males - Männer	172	93	350	311	252	156	323	220
Females - Frauen	191	141	319	241	260	210	272	191
2.2 Total - Insg.	46	78	395	367	70	161	388	297
Males - Männer	55	70	406	383	79	153	411	293
Females - Frauen	35	89	379	347	59	170	362	301
2.3 Total - Insg.	511	216	221	48	591	224	142	39
Males - Männer	549	173	205	68	674	159	119	42
Females - Frauen	485	248	233	33	536	266	157	37
3.1 Total - Insg.	61	32	250	399	114	69	319	347
Males - Männer	57	29	257	434	94	56	337	371
Females - Frauen	67	36	242	360	138	83	299	320
3.2 Total - Insg.	24	31	316	430	39	64	360	388
Males - Männer	26	29	321	455	38	58	371	397
Females - Frauen	21	34	305	385	41	72	347	376
3.3 Total - Insg.	516	147	276	57	529	179	228	59
Males - Männer	507	121	271	93	565	125	220	82
Females - Frauen	523	167	279	30	509	210	232	46
3.4 Total - Insg.	18	16	207	430	63	33	303	409
Males - Männer	21	15	201	464	58	31	321	416
Females - Frauen	15	17	213	401	68	37	284	401
Kirgizskaja SSR								
1.1 Total - Insg.	103	69	257	246	169	175	299	210
Males - Männer	102	79	268	266	166	188	311	212
Females - Frauen	105	57	242	221	171	162	287	208
1.2 Total - Insg.	21	65	303	341	36	174	367	268
Males - Männer	22	68	308	363	40	189	379	265
Females - Frauen	20	59	295	303	32	155	351	272

Labour
Arbeitsreserven 6.2

	1 9 5 9				1 9 7 0			
	A.	B.	C.	D.	A.	B.	C.	D.
1.3 Total - Insg.	537	158	225	64	607	204	150	31
Males - Männer	529	161	204	83	646	185	122	37
Females - Frauen	546	154	247	44	576	218	172	27
1.4 Total - Insg.	11	39	228	230	30	136	301	277
Males - Männer	19	59	251	230	51	165	312	262
Females - Frauen	4	19	205	230	9	108	290	292
2.1 Total - Insg.	180	97	290	265	246	192	302	172
Males - Männer	154	92	289	305	227	190	316	190
Females - Frauen	216	105	293	208	266	194	287	153
2.2 Total - Insg.	27	76	324	356	46	190	387	253
Males - Männer	27	75	324	384	48	197	399	257
Females - Frauen	28	79	322	309	44	180	371	247
2.3 Total - Insg.	584	151	232	68	617	190	154	31
Males - Männer	537	148	202	91	673	163	119	35
Females - Frauen	531	154	259	47	579	208	178	28
3.1 Total - Insg.	67	55	240	237	108	163	298	239
Males - Männer	74	72	.258	245	120	186	308	229
Females - Frauen	58	35	220	227	96	137	287	250
3.2 Total - Insg.	15	51	279	323	25	158	345	285
Males - Männer	17	59	288	339	30	181	357	274
Females - Frauen	12	37	265	295	19	128	330	299
3.3 Total - Insg.	543	166	215	58	588	229	142	33
Males - Männer	521	176	206	73	607	217	126	40
Females - Frauen	574	153	227	37	569	240	159	26
3.4 Total - Insg.	11	39	229	229	30	136	301	277
Males - Männer	19	59	252	228	51	166	312	262
Females - Frauen	4	19	206	230	9	109	291	292
Tadžikskaja SSR								
1.1 Total - Insg.	83	53	271	216	140	164	298	214
Males - Männer	90	63	271	224	154	183	296	209
Females - Frauen	75	40	270	205	124	141	301	221
1.2 Total - Insg.	22	53	285	314	35	170	352	256
Males - Männer	23	56	294	326	39	195	359	244
Females - Frauen	20	45	266	291	27	125	339	278
1.3 Total - Insg.	533	162	215	68	564	216	158	43
Males - Männer	551	168	183	72	599	212	124	44
Females - Frauen	511	155	255	63	523	221	197	42
1.4 Total - Insg.	8	27	277	200	13	126	325	274
Males - Männer	14	40	280	194	25	140	319	275
Females - Frauen	2	13	274	206	3	114	330	273
2.1 Total - Insg.	168	86	262	263	226	177	286	185
Males - Männer	145	83	259	294	210	188	294	195
Females - Frauen	203	91	266	217	247	163	277	172
2.2 Total - Insg.	24	57	281	349	42	163	356	265
Males - Männer	24	58	286	368	47	187	365	257
Females - Frauen	24	54	271	314	34	124	341	277
2.3 Total - Insg.	514	155	231	78	572	199	170	42
Males - Männer	531	157	192	91	626	185	124	44
Females - Frauen	498	153	267	67	531	210	206	40

405

6.2 Labour / Arbeitsreserven

	1959 A.	B.	C.	D.	1970 A.	B.	C.	D.
3.1 Total - Insg.	46	39	274	195	75	154	307	237
Males - Männer	64	54	277	190	112	179	298	218
Females - Frauen	24	19	271	200	29	125	319	259
3.2 Total - Insg.	17	44	295	240	22	184	345	241
Males - Männer	20	53	310	245	27	208	350	224
Females - Frauen	9	20	252	225	10	125	332	282
3.3 Total - Insg.	573	176	182	48	544	254	128	46
Males - Männer	576	181	173	47	564	246	123	43
Females - Frauen	562	161	209	49	473	284	147	55
3.4 Total - Insg.	8	26	279	199	12	125	326	275
Males - Männer	13	40	282	193	24	138	318	278
Females - Frauen	2	13	276	204	2	114	332	273
Armjanskaja SSR								
1.1 Total - Insg.	129	124	274	247	203	253	241	184
Males - Männer	127	123	294	260	206	243	259	188
Females - Frauen	134	125	245	229	198	264	221	181
1.2 Total - Insg.	25	118	344	307	47	251	319	245
Males - Männer	26	121	364	316	51	255	334	241
Females - Frauen	23	112	299	286	40	246	298	251
1.3 Total - Insg.	577	259	117	36	598	300	69	24
Males - Männer	574	232	131	48	638	243	77	30
Females - Frauen	581	289	100	23	560	353	61	19
1.4 Total - Insg.	17	67	282	288	33	131	317	293
Males - Männer	27	71	290	294	57	139	312	292
Females - Frauen	8	62	274	282	11	124	322	294
2.1 Total - Insg.	202	172	267	220	262	301	217	144
Males - Männer	176	159	293	243	254	283	241	154
Females - Frauen	248	195	222	180	273	322	188	133
2.2 Total - Insg.	28	135	346	307	57	298	318	222
Males - Männer	29	136	363	315	60	297	333	220
Females - Frauen	27	133	308	288	53	300	296	225
2.3 Total - Insg.	573	262	115	38	608	298	64	22
Males - Männer	575	234	125	50	653	242	69	27
Females - Frauen	572	293	103	24	568	348	59	18
3.1 Total - Insg.	66	82	280	270	97	168	285	255
Males - Männer	76	86	296	277	117	168	294	251
Females - Frauen	55	78	261	263	77	167	275	259
3.2 Total - Insg.	17	71	336	307	25	153	321	292
Males - Männer	20	76	368	319	32	160	335	286
Females - Frauen	12	62	276	283	17	143	303	299
3.3 Total - Insg.	589	247	123	32	551	305	95	33
Males - Männer	570	228	148	42	583	244	110	42
Females - Frauen	616	275	88	16	511	383	75	22
3.4 Total - Insg.	17	66	284	288	32	128	318	297
Males - Männer	26	70	292	294	57	133	310	299
Females - Frauen	8	62	275	282	11	124	324	294

Labour
Arbeitsreserven 6.2

	1959				1970			
	A.	B.	C.	D.	A.	B.	C.	D.
Turkmenskaja SSR								
1.1 Total - Insg.	103	65	329	191	158	176	348	179
Males - Männer	105	74	320	209	176	190	342	174
Females - Frauen	100	53	340	167	137	159	355	184
1.2 Total - Insg.	23	55	309	303	45	176	395	241
Males - Männer	25	63	331	310	48	205	407	224
Females - Frauen	17	39	259	286	40	124	372	271
1.3 Total - Insg.	499	144	257	77	575	200	169	43
Males - Männer	509	152	229	81	623	186	135	41
Females - Frauen	486	135	290	73	523	214	205	46
1.4 Total - Insg.	10	43	377	144	24	159	426	205
Males - Männer	18	54	352	147	43	174	403	196
Females - Frauen	2	32	401	141	8	146	445	213
2.1 Total - Insg.	168	82	291	249	228	173	312	178
Males - Männer	142	83	301	277	219	184	325	182
Females - Frauen	207	80	275	206	242	159	295	171
2.2 Total - Insg.	24	54	302	330	48	167	391	254
Males - Männer	27	61	325	340	53	193	405	242
Females - Frauen	19	41	254	306	41	121	366	274
2.3 Total - Insg.	478	143	269	87	564	194	182	48
Males - Männer	483	150	236	99	622	175	142	47
Females - Frauen	472	136	300	76	516	210	215	48
3.1 Total - Insg.	49	52	360	143	80	178	388	180
Males - Männer	71	66	338	146	124	196	363	164
Females - Frauen	22	34	387	139	32	159	414	197
3.2 Total - Insg.	17	58	336	200	34	209	407	197
Males - Männer	20	68	352	207	32	242	413	168
Females - Frauen	7	25	283	177	37	137	394	260
3.3 Total - Insg.	581	149	211	38	616	222	119	26
Males - Männer	572	156	213	38	626	212	118	26
Females - Frauen	615	122	202	40	585	250	123	26
3.4 Total - Insg.	10	43	378	142	23	157	428	207
Males - Männer	17	54	354	144	43	171	404	198
Females - Frauen	2	32	403	140	8	146	447	213
Estonskaja SSR								
1.1 Total - Insg.	125	86	237	470	203	153	304	310
Males - Männer	116	68	246	499	191	128	325	331
Females - Frauen	135	103	228	440	215	178	284	289
1.2 Total - Insg.	37	62	295	531	56	129	383	395
Males - Männer	38	54	299	549	57	122	400	394
Females - Frauen	36	74	288	506	55	138	362	396
1.3 Total - Insg.	469	216	214	99	545	228	160	63
Males - Männer	499	174	191	132	628	170	130	67
Females - Frauen	448	245	230	75	492	265	180	60
1.4 Total - Insg.	15	17	113	678	82	35	265	573
Males - Männer	21	16	117	675	76	33	291	557
Females - Frauen	11	17	110	681	89	37	234	591

6.2 Labour
6.3 Arbeitsreserven

	1 9 5 9				1 9 7 0			
	A.	B.	C.	D.	A.	B.	C.	D.
2.1 Total - Insg.	169	124	290	370	234	187	312	243
Males - Männer	158	97	300	409	231	159	336	257
Females - Frauen	181	152	279	329	239	212	289	230
2.2 Total - Insg.	42	78	327	489	62	154	404	346
Males - Männer	44	69	339	503	66	149	427	339
Females - Frauen	39	89	313	472	57	161	378	355
2.3 Total - Insg.	468	233	209	87	552	237	152	54
Males - Männer	509	187	186	114	645	176	121	54
Females - Frauen	439	267	225	67	492	277	172	54
3.1 Total - Insg.	68	36	170	598	129	75	287	465
Males - Männer	60	30	177	616	107	61	301	488
Females - Frauen	76	42	163	580	156	90	272	439
3.2 Total - Insg.	25	29	225	621	42	61	324	527
Males - Männer	25	25	224	638	35	57	331	533
Females - Frauen	26	35	227	592	51	68	313	519
3.3 Total - Insg.	473	150	233	142	510	180	199	106
Males - Männer	462	127	211	196	545	144	170	135
Females - Frauen	481	166	248	105	488	203	216	89
3.4 Total - Insg.	15	16	112	682	80	32	259	583
Males - Männer	21	15	115	677	72	28	281	573
Females - Frauen	11	17	109	685	88	35	233	594

6.3 EDUCATIONAL LEVEL OF THE POPULATION OF THE USSR BY PROFESSIONS
BILDUNGSSTAND DER BEVÖLKERUNG DER UdSSR NACH BERUFEN
UROVEN' OBRAZOVANIJA NASELENIJA SSSR PO ZANJATIJAM
(Census - Volkszählung - Perepis' naselenija 1970)

	per 1,000 people - je 1.000 Personen - na 1.000 čelovek				
	A. Higher education / Hochschulbildung / Vysšee obrazovanie	B. Incomplete higher & secondary specialized education / Nicht abgeschl.Hochschul-u. mittlere Fachschulbildung / Nezakončennoe vysšee i srednee special'noe obrazovanie	C. Secondary education / Mittelschulbildung / Srednee obrazovanie	D. Incompl.secondary education / Nicht abgeschl.Mittelschulb. / Nepolnoe srednee obrazovanie	E. Primary education(complete and incomplete) / Grundschulbildung (mit und ohne Abschluß) / Načal'noe i nezakončennoe načal'noe obrazovanie
Total population employed - Beschäftigte insgesamt - Vse zanjatoe naselenie	65	118	159	311	347
Mainly with physical work - vorwiegend mit körperlicher Arbeit - zanjatye preimuščestvenno fizičeskim trudom	1	30	143	366	460

Labour
Arbeitsreserven 6.3

	A.	B.	C.	D.	E.
In power plants - in Kraftwerken - Zanjatye na silovych ustanovkach	2	36	107	335	520
Miners - Bergarbeiter - Gornjaki	3	40	145	404	408
Foundrymen and smelters - Hüttenarbeiter und Metallgießer - Metallurgi i litejščiki	4	51	184	402	359
In machine-building and metal industry - Im Maschinenbau und in der Metallindustrie - Zanjatye v mašinostroenni i metalloobrabotke	2	55	254	431	258
Chemical workers - Chemiearbeiter - Chimiki	4	79	270	388	259
In the production of construction materials, concrete and reinforced concrete, glass, porcelain and crockery products - In der Produktion von Baustoffen, Beton-, Eisenbeton-, Glas-, Porzellan-u.Steinguterzeugnissen- Zanjatye v proizvodstve stroitel'nych materialov, betonnych i železnobetonnych, stekol'nych i farforo-fajansovych izdelij	1	25	154	402	418
In production of wood and timber - In Holzbeschaffung und Abharzung - Zanjatye na lesozagotovkach i podsočke lesa	1	13	56	312	618
In wood working - in der Holzbearbeitung - Derevoobrabotčiki	1	21	130	386	462
Paper and cardboard workers - Papier-u.Kartonagearbeiter - Bumažniki i kartonažniki	2	40	173	389	396
In the printing industry - Polygraphiearbeiter - Poligrafisty	4	59	298	448	191
Textile workers - Textilarbeiter - Tekstil'ščiki	1	30	209	440	320
Clothing industry workers - Konfektionsarbeiter - Šveiniki	1	36	236	460	267
Leather workers and furriers - Lederarbeiter u.Kürschner - Koževniki i mechovščiki	2	25	157	391	425
Shoe workers - Schuharbeiter - Obuvščiki	1	22	181	412	384
Food industry workers - Arbeiter der Lebensmittelindustrie - piščeviki	2	30	149	386	433
Construction workers-Bauarbeiter-Stroiteli	1	19	116	405	459
Agricultural professions - landwirtschaftliche Berufe - Sel'skochozjajstvennye zanjatija	1	9	61	277	652
In fishing, fish-hatching and hunting - In Fischfang, Fischzucht und Jagd - Zanjatye v rybolovstve, rybovodstve i ochote	2	20	59	238	681
Railwaymen - Eisenbahner - Železnodorožniki	2	52	144	397	405
In navigation - in der Schiffahrt - Vodniki	4	65	203	456	272
In motor transport and municipal electrified transport - im Kraftverkehr und städtischen elektrifizierten Kraftverkehr - Zanjatye na avtotransporte i gorodskom elektrotransporte	1	18	153	511	317

409

6.3 Labour
Arbeitsreserven

	A.	B.	C.	D.	E.
Other transport workers - andere Transportarbeiter - pročie rabočie na transporte	1	13	75	279	632
Postmen - Briefträger - Počtal'ony	1	17	143	471	368
On elevating and conveying machines - Auf Hebe- und Transportmechanismen - Zanjatye na pod'emno-transportnych mechanizm.	1	26	181	446	346
In Trade and communal canteens - in Handel und Gemeinschaftsverpflegung - Rabočie v torgovle i obščestvennom pitanii	3	81	227	451	238
In municipal economy and public services - in der Kommunalwirtschaft und Dienstleistungsbetrieben - Rabočie kommunal' nogo i bytovogo obsluživanija	1	12	51	218	718
Nurses - Krankenpflegerinnen - Sanitarki, sidelki, njani	0.5	13	88	335	564
Machinists and enginemen - Maschinisten und Motorwärter - Mašinisty i motoristy	2	40	153	405	400
Laboratory assistants (workers) - Laboranten (Arbeiter) - Laboranty (rabočie)	5	127	479	306	83
Controllers, goods' examiners, assorters - Kontrolleure, Warenprüfer, Sortierer - Kontrolery, brakovščiki, sortirovščiki	3	87	324	400	186
Stockmen, weighing foremen, surveyors, distributors - Lageristen, Wiegemeister, Abnehmer, Ausgeber - Kladovščiki, vesovščiki, priemščiki, razdatčiki	3	53	201	482	261
Unskilled and warehouse hands - Hilfs-u.Lagerarbeiter - Raznorabočie, skladskie rabočie	1	15	109	324	551
Mainly with mental work - vorwiegend mit geistiger Arbeit - zanjatye preimuščestvenno umstvennym trudom		235	354	195	168	48
Heads of the municipal executives and their structural subdivisions - Leiter der Organe der Stadtverwaltung und ihrer strukturellen Unterabteilungen - Rukovoditeli organov gosudarstvennogo upravlenija i ich strukturnych podrazdelenij		354	244	207	164	31
Leaders of party, Komsomol, labor union and other social organizations - Leiter der Partei-,Komsomol-,Gewerkschafts-u.anderen gesellschaftl.Organisationen - Rukovoditeli partijnych,komsomol'skich,profsojuznych i drugich obščestvennych organizacij		370	317	214	84	15
Works managers(industry,architecture,agriculture,forestry,transport,communications) and their structural subdivisions - Betriebsleiter(Industrie,Bauwesen,Land-u.Forstwirtschaft,Transport-,Post-u.Fernmeldewesen) und ihrer strukturellen Unterabteilungen -					

Labour
Arbeitsreserven 6.3

	A.	B.	C.	D.	E.
Rukovoditeli predprijatij(promyšlennosti, stroitel'stva,sel'skogo i lesnogo chozjajstva, transporta,svjazi)i ich strukturnych podraz.	341	370	103	122	64
Technical engineering cadres - Ingenieur-technische Kader - Inženerno-techničeskie rabotn.	247	437	168	116	32
Agriculturists, zoo engineers, veterinarians and foresters(incl.chief specialists) - Agronomen,Zootechniker,Veterinäre und Förster (einschl.Hauptspezialisten) - Agronomy,zootechniki,veterinarnye rabotniki i lesničie (vključaja glavnych specialistov)	306	503	54	88	49
Physicians and medical staff - Ärzte und medizinisches Personal - Medicinskie rabotniki	222	585	98	73	22
Scientists, teachers, tutors - Wissenschaftler, Lehrer, Erzieher - Naučnye rabotniki, pedagogi, vospitateli	494	351	116	31	8
Men of letters and journalists - Literaten und Presseleute - Rabotniki literatury i pečati	549	191	216	37	7
In cultural and information work - Kultur- und Aufklärungsschaffende - Kul'turno-prosvetitel'nye rabotniki	128	275	326	225	46
Artists - Kunstschaffende - Rabotniki iskusstva	202	312	287	162	37
Juristic staff - juristisches Personal - Juridičeskij personal	703	158	93	39	7
In communications - im Post-u.Fernmeldewesen - Rabotniki svjazi	9	100	343	442	106
In trade, public catering, procurement , supply, and sale - in Handel, Gemeinschaftsverpflegung, Beschaffungen,Versorgung und Absatz - Rabotniki torgovli,obščestvennogo pitanija, zagotovok, snabženija i sbyta	78	276	215	313	118
In planning and statistics - in Planung und Statistik - Rabotniki planirovanija i učeta	80	273	298	302	47
In municipal economy and public services - in Kommunalwirtschaft und Dienstleistungsbetrieben - Rabotniki kommunal'nych predprijatij i bytovogo obsluživanija	58	183	221	361	177
Shorthand typists and stenographers - Stenotypisten u.Stenographen - Mašinistki i stenografistki	8	76	513	355	48
Secretaries and other secretarial staff - Sekretäre,Schriftführer u.anderes Schriftführerpersonal - Sekretari, deloproizvoditeli i pročij deloproizvodstvennyj personal	22	123	484	335	36
Agents and forwarding agents - Agenten und Expediteure - Agenty i ekspeditory	21	141	267	410	161

6.4 Labour
Arbeitsreserven

6.4 AVERAGE ANNUAL NUMBER OF WORKERS AND EMPLOYEES BY BRANCHES OF THE NATIONAL ECONOMY
JAHRESDURCHSCHNITTSZAHL DER ARBEITER UND ANGESTELLTEN NACH VOLKSWIRTSCHAFTSBEREICHEN
SREDNEGODOVAJA ČISLENNOST' RABOČICH I SLUŽAŠČICH PO OTRASLJAM NARODNOGO CHOZJAJSTVA
(thousands – Tsd. – tys.)

	1940	1965	1970	1975	1976
Total number of workers and employees in the national economy – Arbeiter und Angestellte in der Volkswirtschaft, insgesamt – Vsego rabočich i služaščich v narodnom chozjajstve	33,926	76,915	90,186	102,160	104,235
Industry (industrial production staff) – Industrie (Industrieproduktionspersonal) – Promyšlennost' (promyšlenno-proizvodstvennyj personal)	13,079	27,447	31,593	34,054	34,815
Agriculture – Landwirtschaft – Sel'skoe chozjajstvo	2,703	8,926	9,418	10,519	10,767
of which state farms, subsidiary and other agricultural enterprises – darunter Sowchosen, Neben- und sonstige landwirtschaftliche Betriebe – v tom čisle sovchozy, podsobnye i pročie proizvodstvennye sel'skochozjajstvennye predprijatija	1,760	8,471	8,832	9,785	9,970
Forestry – Forstwirtschaft – Lesnoe chozjajstvo	280	402	433	453	449
Transport – Verkehr – Transport	3,525	7,252	7,985	9,215	9,378
Railway – Eisenbahn – Železnodorožnyj	1,767	2,319	2,331	2,459	2,460
Waterways – See- und Binnenschiffahrt – vodnyj	206	348	370	404	411
Motor transport, municipal electrified and other transport, loading and unloading enterprises – Kraftverkehr, städtischer elektrifizierter und sonstiger Verkehr, Be-u.Entladeorganisationen – Avtomobil'nyj, gorodskoj električeskij i pročij transport, pogruzočno-razgruzočnye organizacii	1,552	4,585	5,284	6,352	6,507
Communications – Post-und Fernmeldewesen – Svjaz'	484	1,007	1,330	1,528	1,555
Construction – Bauwesen – Stroitel'stvo	1,993	7,301	9,052	10,574	10,716
of which building and installation work – darunter Bau- und Montagearbeiten – v tom čisle stroitel'no-montažnye raboty	1,620	5,685	6,994	7,930	7,999

412

Labour
Arbeitsreserven 6.4

	1940	1965	1970	1975	1976
Trade, public catering, material and technical supply, distribution and procurements - Handel, Gemeinschaftsverpflegung, materiell-technische Versorgung, Absatz und Erfassung - Torgovlja, obščestvennoe pitanie, material'no-techničeskoe snabženie i sbyt, zagotovki	3,351	6,009	7,537	8,857	9,010
Other activity in material production - Sonstige Tätigkeit in der materiellen Produktion - Pročie vidy dejatel'nosti sfery materiel'nogo proizvodstva	166	775	998	1,250	1,290
Housing and communal services - Wohnungs- und Kommunalwirtschaft, Dienstleistungen für die Bevölkerung - Žiliščno-kommunal'noe chozjajstvo i bytovoe obslužuvanie naselenija	1,516	2,386	3,052	3,805	3,896
Public health, physical culture and social security - Gesundheitswesen, Körperkultur und Sozialfürsorge - Zdravoochranenie, fizkul'tura i social'noe obespečenie	1,512	4,277	5,080	5,769	5,878
Public education - Volksbildung - Prosveščenie	2,482	6,044	7,201	8,080	8,239
Culture - Kultur - Kul'tura	196	556	824	1,056	1,097
Art - Kunst - Iskusstvo	173	370	412	446	448
Science and scientific services - Wissenschaft und wissenschaftliche Dienstleistungen - Nauka i naučnoe obslužuvanie	362	2,403	3,000	3,792	3,860
Credit and state insurance institutions - Kreditwesen und staatliche Versicherung - Kreditovanie i gosudarstvennoe strachovanie	267	300	388	519	546
State administration and economic management, administration of cooperative and mass organizations - Staats- und Wirtschaftsverwaltung, Verwaltung der genossenschaftlichen und gesellschaftlichen Organisationen - Apparat organov gosudarstvennogo i chozjajstvennogo upravlenija, organov upravlenija kooperativnych i obščestvennych organizacij	1,837	1,460	1,883	2,243	2,291

6.5 Labour
Arbeitsreserven

6.5 AVERAGE ANNUAL NUMBER OF WORKERS AND EMPLOYEES IN THE NATIONAL ECONOMY
JAHRESDURCHSCHNITTSZAHL DER ARBEITER UND ANGESTELLTEN IN DER VOLKSWIRTSCHAFT
SREDNEGODOVAJA ČISLENNOST' RABOČICH I SLUŽAŠČICH V NARODNOM CHOZJAJSTVE
(millions - Millionen - mln.)

Year Jahr Gody	Total number of workers & employees - Arbeiter und Angestellte insgesamt - Vsego rabočich i služaščich	of whom workers (incl. junior service staff and guards) - darunter Arbeiter (einschl. Hilfspersonal der unteren Stufe u. Personal für den Betriebsschutz) - v tom čisle rabočich (vkl. mladšij obsluživajuščij personal i rabotnikov ochrany)
1913 within the borders of the U.S.S.R. up to 17.9.1939 - in den Grenzen der UdSSR bis 17.9.1939 - v granicach SSSR do 17 sentjabrja 1939 g.	11.4	9.8
in the present borders of the U.S.S.R. - in den heutigen Grenzen der UdSSR - v sovremennych granicach SSSR	12.9	11.0
1928	11.4	8.7
1940	33.9	23.7
1950	40.4	28.7
1955	50.3	36.8
1960	62.0	45.9
1965	76.9	55.9
1970	90.2	64.3
1971	92.8	66.2
1972	95.2	67.5
1973	97.5	68.8
1974	99.8	70.2
1975	102.2	71.7
1976	104.3	73
1977 (planned-geplant)	106.2	74

Labour
Arbeitsreserven 6.6

6.6 PERCENTAGE OF FEMALES IN RELATION TO TOTAL NUMBER OF WORKERS AND EMPLOYEES BY BRANCHES OF THE NATIONAL ECONOMY
PROZENTUALER ANTEIL DER FRAUEN AN DER GESAMTZAHL DER ARBEITER UND ANGESTELLTEN NACH VOLKSWIRTSCHAFTSZWEIGEN
PROCENT ŽENŠČIN V OBŠČEJ ČISLENNOSTI RABOČICH I SLUŽAŠČICH PO OTRASLJAM NARODNOGO CHOZJAJSTVA

Branch of the national economy – Volkswirtschaftszweig – Otrasl' narodnogo chozjajstva	1940	1950	1960	1965	1970	1971	1972	1975
Total national economy – Gesamte Volkswirtschaft – Vse narodnoe chozjajstvo	39	47	47	49	51	51	51	51
Industry (industrial production staff) – Industrie (Industrie-Produktionspersonal) – Promyšlennost' (promyšlenno-proizvodstvennyj personal)	38	46	45	46	48	48	49	49
Agriculture – Landwirtschaft – Sel'skoe chozjajstvo	30	42	41	44	44	45	45	44
State farms, subsidiary and other agricultural production enterprises – Sowchosen, Neben- u.andere landwirtschaftliche Produktionsbetriebe – Sovchozy, podsobnye i pročie proizvodstvennye sel'skochozjajstvennye predprijatija	34	49	43	44	45	45	45	45
Transport – Verkehr – Transport	21	28	24	24	24	24	24	24
Communications – Post-und Fernmeldewesen – Svjaz'	48	59	64	65	68	68	68	68
Construction – Bauwesen – Stroitel'stvo	24	32	30	30	29	29	29	28
Building and installation work – Bau-und Montagearbeiten – Stroitel'no-montažnye raboty	23	33	29	29	26	26	26	25
Trade, public catering, material and technical supply and distribution, procurement – Handel, Gemeinschaftsverpflegung, materiell-technische Versorgung und Absatz, Beschaffung – Torgovlja, obščestvennoe pitanie, material'no-techničeskoe snabženie i sbyt, zagotovki	44	57	66	72	75	76	76	76
Housing and communal services, consumer services – Wohnungs-u.Kommunalwirtschaft, Dienstleistungen f.d.Bevölkerung – Žiliščno-kommunal'noe chozjajstvo i bytovoe obsluživanie naselenija	43	53	53	53	51	53	53	53

415

6.6 Labour
Arbeitsreserven

Branch of the national economy – Volkswirtschaftszweig – Otrasl' narodnogo chozjajstva	1940	1950	1960	1965	1970	1971	1972	1975
Public health, physical culture and social security – Gesundheitswesen, Körperkultur und Sozialfürsorge – Zdravoochranenie, fizkul'tura i social'noe obespečenie	76	84	85	86	85	85	85	84
Public education and culture – Volksbildung und Kultur – Prosveščenie i kul'tura	59	69	70	72	72	73	72	73
Kunst – Art – Iskusstvo	39	37	36	40	44	45	45	47
Science and science services – Wissenschaft und wissenschaftliche Betreuung – Nauka i naučnoe obsluživanie	42	43	42	44	47	48	48	50
Credit and state insurance institutions – Kreditwesen und staatliche Versicherung – Kreditovanie i gosudarstvennoe strachovanie	41	58	68	72	78	78	79	82
State administration and economic management, administration of cooperative and mass organizations – Staats- und Wirtschaftsverwaltung, Verwaltung der genossenschaftlichen u.gesellschaftlichen Organisationen – Apparat organov gosudarstvennogo i chozjajstvennogo upravlenija organov upravlenija kooperativnych i obščestvennych organizacij	34	43	51	55	61	62	62	65

Labour 6.7
Arbeitsreserven 6.8

6.7 PERCENTAGE OF FEMALES IN RELATION TO TOTAL NUMBER OF WORKERS AND EMPLOYEES
BY UNION REPUBLICS - PROZENTUALER ANTEIL DER FRAUEN AN DER GESAMTZAHL DER
ARBEITER UND ANGESTELLTEN NACH UNIONSREPUBLIKEN - PROCENT ŽENŠČIN V OBŠČEJ
ČISLENNOST' RABOČICH I SLUŽAŠČICH PO SOJUZNYM RESPUBLIKAM

	1928	1940	1950	1960	1970	1975	1976	1977
SSSR	24	39	47	47	51	51	51	51.5
RSFSR	27	41	50	50	53	53	53	53
Ukrainskaja SSR	21	37	43	45	50	52	52	52
Belorusskaja SSR	22	40	45	49	52	53	53	53
Uzbekskaja SSR	18	31	40	39	41	42	43	43
Kazachskaja SSR	15	30	40	38	47	48	48	49
Gruzinskaja SSR	19	35	40	40	43	45	46	46
Azerbajdžanskaja SSR	14	34	40	38	41	43	42	42
Litovskaja SSR		30	38	43	49	51	51	51
Moldavskaja SSR	21	35	38	43	51	51	51	51
Latvijskaja SSR		36	45	49	53	54	55	55
Kirgizskaja SSR	11	29	41	41	47	48	48	48
Tadžikskaja SSR	7	29	39	37	38	38	38	38
Armjanskaja SSR	15	34	40	38	41	45	46	46
Turkmenskaja SSR	25	36	41	36	39	40	40	40
Estonskaja SSR		35	48	50	53	54	54	54

6.8 PERCENTAGE OF FEMALES IN RELATION TO AVERAGE ANNUAL NUMBER OF ALL COLLECTIVE
FARMERS HAVING PARTICIPATED IN THE WORK AT COLLECTIVE FARMS, BY UNION REPUBLICS-
PROZENTUALER ANTEIL DER FRAUEN AN DER JAHRESDURCHSCHNITTSZAHL ALLER KOLCHOS-
BAUERN, DIE SICH AN ARBEITEN IN DEN KOLCHOSEN BETEILIGT HABEN, NACH UNIONSREPUBLIKEN
PROCENT ŽENŠČIN V SREDNEGODOVOJ ČISLENNOSTI VSECH KOLCHOZNIKOV, PRINIMAVŠICH
UČASTIE V RABOTACH KOLCHOZOV, PO SOJUZNYM RESPUBLIKAM

	1960	1965	1970	1975	1976	1977
SSSR	52	50	50	48	48	
RSFSR	53	50	49	46	46	
Ukrainskaja SSR	54	53	52	50	51	
Belorusskaja SSR	55	53	52	50	50	
Uzbekskaja SSR	45	46	48	49	49	
Kazachskaja SSR	43	41	40	40	40	
Gruzinskaja SSR	47	46	48	50	51	
Azerbajdžanskaja SSR	47	47	46	48	50	
Litovskaja SSR	47	46	46	45	45	
Moldavskaja SSR	50	49	51	50	52	
Latvijskaja SSR	52	51	47	45	46	
Kirgizskaja SSR	44	43	43	43	42	
Tadžikskaja SSR	42	41	43	44	45	
Armjanskaja SSR	43	43	44	46	46	
Turkmenskaja SSR	50	50	48	48	48	
Estonskaja SSR	56	51	47	44	44	

6.9 Labour
6.10 Arbeitsreserven

6.9 NUMBER OF FEMALE SPECIALISTS WITH HIGHER AND SPECIALIZED SECONDARY EDUCATION, ENGAGED IN THE NATIONAL ECONOMY - ZAHL DER IN DER VOLKSWIRTSCHAFT BESCHÄFTIGTEN FRAUEN-SPEZIALISTEN MIT HOCHSCHUL- UND MITTLERER FACHSCHULBILDUNG - ČISLENNOST' ŽENŠČIN-SPECIALISTOV S VYSŠIM I SREDNIM SPECIAL'NYM OBRAZOVANIEM, ZANJATYCH V NARODNOM CHOZJAJSTVE

Year Jahr Gody	Total Insg. Vsego	with higher education mit Hochschulbildung s vysšim obrazovaniem	with specialized second.education mit mittl.Fachschulbildung so srednim special'nym obrazovaniem	% of females in relation to total of specialists with higher and special. secondary education Proz.Anteil d.Frauen a.d. Gesamtzahl d.Spezialisten mit Hochschul-u.mittl. Fachschulbildung Procent ženščin v obščej čislennosti specialistov s vysšim i srednim special'nym obrazovaniem
		(in thousands - Tsd. - tys.)		
1928	151	65	86	29
1941	864	312	552	36
1955	3,115	1,155	1,960	61
1960	5,189	1,865	3,324	59
1965	6,941	2,518	4,423	58
1970	9,900	3,568	6,332	59
1973	11,998	4,397	7,601	59
1975	13,411	4,962	8,449	59
1976	14,100	5,230	8,870	59
1977				

6.10 NUMBER OF WOMAN DOCTORS IN ALL SPECIAL BRANCHES (END-OF-YEAR FIGURES)
ZAHL DER ÄRZTINNEN ALLER FACHRICHTUNGEN (ZUM JAHRESENDE)
ČISLENNOST' ŽENŠČIN-VRAČEJ VSECH SPECIAL'NOSTEJ (NA KONEC GODA)

Year Jahr Gody	Thousands Tausend Tysjač	% in relation to total number of doctors % im Verhältnis zur Gesamtzahl der Ärzte V % k obščej čislennosti vračej
1913	2.8	10
1940	96.3	62
1950	204.9	77
1955	254.8	76
1960	327.1	76
1965	408.9	74
1970	479.6	72
1975	583.5	70
1976	600.6	69
1977		

6.11 PERCENTAGE OF WORKERS AND EMPLOYEES OF 55 YEARS OF AGE AND OLDER BY BRANCHES OF THE NATIONAL ECONOMY
PROZENTUALER ANTEIL VON ARBEITERN UND ANGESTELLTEN, DIE 55 JAHRE ALT UND ÄLTER SIND, NACH VOLKSWIRTSCHAFTSZWEIGEN
RASPREDELENIE RABOČICH I SLUŽAŠČICH V VOZRASTE 55 LET I STARŠE PO OTRASLJAM NARODNOGO CHOZJAJSTVA (v procentach)

Labour
Arbeitsreserven 6.11

	55-59 years-Jahre-let			60 and older-u.älter-i starše		
	1967	1973	1973 in relation to im Verhältnis zu po sravneniju s 1967	1967	1973	1973 in relation to im Verhältnis zu po sravneniju s 1967
Industry – Industrie – Promyšlennost'	3.0	2.9	– 0.1	1.1	2.0	+ 0.9
Agriculture – Landwirtschaft – Sel'skoe chozjajstvo	5.1	4.4	– 0.7	2.5	3.1	+ 0.6
Transport	4.5	4.2	– 0.3	1.2	2.5	+ 1.3
Railway – Eisenbahn – Železnodorožnyj	5.4	4.8	– 0.6	1.0	2.4	+ 1.4
Waterways – Schiffahrt – vodnyj	4.2	3.6	– 0.6	1.4	2.7	+ 1.3
Motor transport – Kraftverkehr – avtomobil'nyj	3.9	3.8	– 0.1	1.2	2.2	+ 1.0
Communications – Post-u.Fernmeldewesen – Svjaz'	2.8	3.3	+ 0.5	1.4	2.6	+ 1.2
Construction – Bauwesen – Stroitel'stvo	2.8	2.6	– 0.2	1.1	1.7	+ 0.6
Trade,public catering,material & technical supply & distribution,procurement – Handel,gesell.Verpflegung,materiell-techn.Versorgung u.Absatz,Beschaffungsw.– Torgovija, obščestvennoe pitanie,material'no-techn.snabženie i sbyt,zagotovki	4.1	4.3	+ 0.2	2.2	3.7	+ 1.5
Public health,physical culture & social security – Gesundheitswesen, Körperkultur u.Sozialfürsorge – Zdravoochranenie,fizkul'tura i social'noe obespečenie[1]	3.8	4.6	+ 0.8	2.4	4.0	+ 1.6
Education and culture-Bildungswesen u.Kultur – Prosveščenie i kul'tura[2]	3.7	4.1	+ 0.4	2.1	3.2	+ 1.1
Science & scientific services – Wissenschaft u.wissenschaftliche Dienstleistungen – Nauka i naučnoe obsluživanie	3.7	3.3	– 0.4	1.9	3.2	+ 1.3
Credit & state insurance – Kreditwesen u.staatliche Versicherung – Kreditovanie i gosudarstvennoe strachovanie	4.5	5.0	+ 0.5	2.1	3.9	+ 1.8
Apparatus of the organs for state & economic management of cooperative & mass organizations – Apparat der Organe der staatl.u.wirtschaftl.Leitung der genossenschaftl.u.gesellschaftl.Organisationen – Apparat organov gosudarstvennogo i chozjajstvennogo upravlenija kooperativnych i obščestv.organ.	5.0	4.6	– 0.4	2.8	3.2	+ 0.4

[1] 1967: only includes public health – nur Gesundheitswesen – tol'ko zdravoochranenie
[2] 1967: only includes education – nur Bildungswesen – tol'ko prosveščenie

7. SOCIAL STRUCTURE – SOZIALE STRUKTUR – SOCIAL'NAJA STRUKTURA

7.1 Social Structure / Soziale Struktur

7.1 BREAKDOWN OF THE POPULATION OF THE USSR AND THE UNION REPUBLICS BY SOCIAL GROUPS[1]
AUFTEILUNG DER BEVÖLKERUNG DER UdSSR UND DER UNIONSREPUBLIKEN NACH GESELLSCHAFTLICHEN GRUPPEN[1]
RASPREDELENIE NASELENIJA SSSR I SOJUZNYCH RESPUBLIK PO OBŠČESTVENNYM GRUPPAM[1]

(Census – Volkszählungen – Perepisi naselenija 1959, 1970)

	A. Total population / Gesamtbevölkerung / Vse naselenie	1970 of which – darunter – v tom čisle			% in relation to total population / im Verhältnis zur Gesamtbevölkerung / v procentach ko vsemu naseleniju						
		B. Workers / Arbeiter / Rabočie	C. Employees / Angestellte / Služaščie	D. Collective Farmers / Kolchosbauern / Kolchozniki	1959 E. Workers	F. Employees	G. Collective Farmers	1970 H. Workers	I. Employees	J. Collective Farmers
SSSR										
Urban & rural population Stadt-u.Landbevölkerung Gorodskoe i sel'skoe nas.	241436013	136930781	54551734	49461551	49.5	18.8	31.4	56.7	22.6	20.5
Males–Männer–mužčiny	111182265	66969787	23277923	20810291	51.8	18.0	29.9	60.2	21.0	18.7
Females–Frauen–ženščiny	130253748	69960994	31273811	28651260	47.6	19.5	32.6	53.7	24.0	22.0
Urban population – Stadtbevölkerung – Gorodskoe naselenie	135330189	89247466	42676887	3228191	68.0	28.5	3.3	66.0	31.5	2.4
Males–Männer–mužčiny	62677636	43626203	17888621	1123559	69.9	26.5	3.4	69.6	28.5	1.8
Females–Frauen–ženščiny	72652553	45621263	24788266	2104632	66.5	30.1	3.2	62.8	34.1	2.9

[1] persons engaged and non-working dependants – Beschäftigte und abhängige Familienmitglieder – rabotajuščie i iždivency

Social Structure
Soziale Struktur 7.1

	A.	B.	C.	D.	E.	F.	G.	H.	I.	J.
3. Rural population – Landbevölkerung – Sel'skoe naselenie	106105824	47683315	11874847	46233360	32.5	9.9	57.3	44.9	11.2	43.6
Males–Männer–mužčiny	48504629	23343584	5389302	19686732	35.1	10.0	54.5	48.1	11.1	40.6
Females–Frauen–ženščiny	57601195	24339731	6485545	26546628	30.5	9.7	59.5	42.2	11.3	46.1
RSFSR										
1.	129941212	79617464	31528248	18634111	55.4	20.2	24.2	61.3	24.3	14.3
Males–Männer–mužčiny	59160721	38460469	13021671	7636144	57.6	19.3	22.8	65.0	22.0	12.9
Females–Frauen–ženščiny	70780491	41156995	18506577	10997967	53.6	20.9	25.3	58.2	26.1	15.5
2.	80631371	53725406	25506889	1339420	69.8	28.2	1.8	66.6	31.6	1.7
Males–Männer–mužčiny	36930897	26078725	10465382	373332	71.5	26.4	1.9	70.6	28.4	1.0
Females–Frauen–ženščiny	43700474	27646681	15041507	966088	68.4	29.8	1.7	63.3	34.4	2.2
3.	49309841	25892058	6021359	17294691	39.5	11.3	48.9	52.5	12.2	35.1
Males–Männer–mužčiny	22229824	12381744	2556289	7262812	42.1	11.4	46.1	55.7	11.5	32.7
Females–Frauen–ženščiny	27080017	13510314	3465070	10031879	37.5	11.2	51.0	49.9	12.8	37.0
Ukrainskaja SSR										
1.	47055852	23429542	9281475	14230270	42.1	16.1	41.4	49.8	19.7	30.3
Males–Männer–mužčiny	21284158	11519051	4006364	5727633	45.4	15.7	38.5	54.1	18.8	26.9
Females–Frauen–ženščiny	25771694	11910491	5275111	8502637	39.5	16.4	43.8	46.2	20.5	33.0
2.	25545650	16697867	7711579	1093887	66.4	27.1	6.2	65.4	30.2	4.3
Males–Männer–mužčiny	11823177	8107735	3308203	398657	68.5	25.3	5.9	68.6	28.0	3.3
Females–Frauen–ženščiny	13722473	8590132	4403376	695230	64.6	28.7	6.4	62.6	32.1	5.1
3.	21510202	6731675	1569896	13136383	21.7	6.7	71.1	31.3	7.3	61.1
Males–Männer–mužčiny	9460981	3411316	698161	5328976	25.2	7.3	67.0	36.1	7.4	56.3
Females–Frauen–ženščiny	12049221	3320359	871735	7807407	19.0	6.3	74.3	27.6	7.2	64.8
Belorusskaja SSR										
1.	8992190	4700161	17338519	2536091	35.7	15.1	48.5	52.3	19.3	28.2
Males–Männer–mužčiny	4129064	2281744	776521	1065771	37.8	14.9	46.5	55.3	18.8	25.8
Females–Frauen–ženščiny	4863126	2418417	961998	1470320	34.0	15.2	50.1	49.7	19.8	30.2
2.	3890580	2457684	1301929	126103	60.1	32.6	6.9	63.2	33.5	3.2
Males–Männer–mužčiny	1826626	1199560	578399	47588	61.2	31.3	7.0	65.7	31.6	2.6
Females–Frauen–ženščiny	2063954	1258124	723530	78515	59.2	33.6	6.8	61.0	35.0	3.8

421

7.1 Social Structure
Soziale Struktur

	A.	B.	C.	D.	E.	F.	G.	H.	I.	J.
3.										
Males-Männer-mužčiny	5101610	2242477	436590	2409988	24.9	7.3	67.0	44.0	8.6	47.2
Females-Frauen-ženščiny	2302438	1082184	198122	1018183	27.4	7.6	64.2	47.0	8.6	44.2
	2799172	1160293	238468	1391805	22.9	7.0	69.3	41.5	8.5	49.7
Uzbekskaja SSR										
1.										
Males-Männer-mužčiny	11773869	5358748	2345927	3997722	40.7	16.4	42.6	45.5	19.9	34.0
Females-Frauen-ženščiny	5732096	2750015	1134011	1833047	42.2	15.6	41.9	47.9	19.8	32.0
	6041773	2608733	1211916	2164675	39.3	17.2	43.2	43.2	20.1	35.8
2.										
Males-Männer-mužčiny	4297953	2725168	1375430	175260	62.9	30.6	5.9	63.4	32.0	4.1
Females-Frauen-ženščiny	2076961	1383067	603419	85221	65.1	27.6	6.7	66.6	29.0	4.1
	2220992	1342101	772011	90039	60.9	33.2	5.2	60.4	34.8	4.0
3.										
Males-Männer-mužčiny	7475916	2633580	970497	3822462	29.4	9.3	61.2	35.2	13.0	51.1
Females-Frauen-ženščiny	3655135	1366948	530592	1747826	30.9	9.7	59.3	37.4	14.5	47.8
	3820781	1266632	439905	2074636	28.0	8.8	63.1	33.2	11.5	54.3
Kazachskaja SSR										
1.										
Males-Männer-mužčiny	13009272	8854938	3056672	1074330	59.5	19.7	20.7	68.1	23.5	8.2
Females-Frauen-ženščiny	6265985	4433409	1337959	490515	61.1	18.4	20.4	70.7	21.4	7.8
	6743287	4421529	1718713	583815	58.0	20.9	21.0	65.6	25.5	8.6
2.										
Males-Männer-mužčiny	6512238	4496772	1930885	74443	72.0	26.2	1.7	69.1	29.6	1.1
Females-Frauen-ženščiny	3139425	2300698	813037	24097	74.0	23.9	2.0	73.3	25.9	0.7
	3372813	2196074	1117848	50346	70.3	28.2	1.4	65.1	33.1	1.5
3.										
Males-Männer-mužčiny	6497034	4358166	1125787	999887	49.8	14.6	35.5	67.1	17.3	15.4
Females-Frauen-ženščiny	3126560	2132711	524922	466418	51.2	14.1	34.6	68.2	16.8	14.9
	3370474	2225455	600865	533469	48.5	15.2	36.3	66.1	17.8	15.8
Gruzinskaja SSR										
1.										
Males-Männer-mužčiny	4674591	2185731	1163779	1307630	33.2	22.5	44.0	46.7	24.9	28.0
Females-Frauen-ženščiny	2195490	1102759	518595	569674	36.5	20.3	42.9	50.2	23.6	26.0
	2479101	1082972	645184	737956	30.3	24.4	45.0	43.7	26.0	29.8
2.										
Males-Männer-mužčiny	2210973	1272206	875742	56508	54.6	38.5	6.4	57.5	39.6	2.6
Females-Frauen-ženščiny	1032535	626021	378734	25953	58.7	34.2	6.6	60.6	36.7	2.5
	1178438	646185	497008	30555	51.1	42.1	6.4	54.8	42.2	2.6
3.										
Males-Männer-mužčiny	2463618	913525	288037	1251122	17.5	10.7	71.6	37.1	11.7	50.8
Females-Frauen-ženščiny	1162955	476738	139861	543721	20.5	10.3	69.0	41.0	12.0	46.8
	1300663	436787	148176	707401	14.8	11.1	74.0	33.6	11.4	54.4

Social Structure 7.1
Soziale Struktur

	A.	B.	C.	D.	E.	F.	G.	H.	I.	J.
Azerbajdžanskaja SSR										
1.										
Males-Männer-mužčiny	5116525	2662635	1188076	1255528	36.4	21.1	42.4	52.1	23.2	24.5
Females-Frauen-ženščiny	2483631	1346408	571693	562276	38.8	19.6	41.4	54.2	23.0	22.7
	2632894	1316227	616883	691252	34.2	22.5	43.2	50.0	23.4	26.3
2.										
Males-Männer-mužčiny	2549597	1643091	340564	60093	61.5	32.9	5.4	64.4	33.0	2.4
Females-Frauen-ženščiny	1247303	834458	382265	29012	64.6	29.1	6.1	66.9	30.7	2.3
	1302294	808633	458299	31081	58.7	36.2	4.9	62.1	35.2	2.4
3.										
Males-Männer-mužčiny	2566928	1019544	347512	1193435	13.4	10.3	76.2	39.7	13.5	46.5
Females-Frauen-ženščiny	1236328	511950	189428	533264	15.5	10.9	73.5	41.4	15.3	43.2
	1330600	507594	158084	660171	11.5	9.8	78.6	38.1	11.9	49.6
Litovskaja SSR										
1.										
Males-Männer-mužčiny	3118941	1684664	605643	816822	40.9	14.9	43.3	54.0	19.4	26.2
Females-Frauen-ženščiny	1462850	827832	261702	366905	42.4	14.2	42.4	56.6	17.9	25.2
	1656091	856832	343941	447917	39.7	15.5	44.0	51.7	20.8	27.1
2.										
Males-Männer-mužčiny	1557731	1021170	496228	36466	65.3	29.7	4.2	65.6	31.9	2.3
Females-Frauen-ženščiny	733683	501549	215839	15119	66.5	28.6	4.0	68.3	29.4	2.1
	824048	519621	280389	21347	64.4	30.5	4.4	63.1	34.0	2.6
3.										
Males-Männer-mužčiny	1561210	663494	109415	780356	25.6	5.7	67.8	42.5	7.0	50.0
Females-Frauen-ženščiny	729167	326283	45863	353786	27.6	5.5	65.9	44.8	6.3	48.5
	832043	337211	63552	426570	23.8	5.9	69.4	40.5	7.6	51.3
Moldavskaja SSR										
1.										
Males-Männer-mužčiny	3569846	1295839	497073	1768791	21.9	10.1	67.5	36.1	13.9	49.6
Females-Frauen-ženščiny	1669166	652202	214328	799505	23.7	9.4	66.4	39.1	12.8	47.9
	1900680	643637	282745	969286	20.4	10.8	68.4	33.8	14.9	51.0
2.										
Males-Männer-mužčiny	1123512	672353	356795	91679	59.5	29.2	10.7	56.8	31.8	8.2
Females-Frauen-ženščiny	525339	331764	151957	40795	62.0	26.4	11.0	63.1	28.9	7.8
	598173	340589	204838	50884	57.3	31.6	10.6	56.9	34.3	8.5
3.										
Males-Männer-mužčiny	2446334	623486	140278	1677112	11.2	4.7	83.7	25.5	5.7	68.6
Females-Frauen-ženščiny	1143827	320438	62371	758710	12.9	4.6	82.1	28.0	5.5	66.3
	1302507	303048	77907	918402	9.7	4.7	85.2	23.3	6.0	70.5
Latvijskaja SSR										
1.										
Males-Männer-mužčiny	2351903	1331971	600027	413523	53.1	20.3	26.1	56.6	25.5	17.6
Females-Frauen-ženščiny	1073060	648165	244270	179002	56.1	18.6	24.8	60.4	22.7	16.7
	1278842	683806	355757	234521	50.7	21.7	27.1	53.5	27.8	18.3

423

7.1 Social Structure / Soziale Struktur

	A.	B.	C.	D.	E.	F.	G.	H.	I.	J.
2.										
Males-Männer-mužčiny	1463872	930863	502447	27542	64.7	29.7	5.1	63.6	34.3	1.9
Females-Frauen-ženščiny	669067	451718	206093	10532	67.3	27.4	4.8	67.5	30.8	1.6
	794805	479145	296354	17010	62.7	31.4	5.4	60.3	37.3	2.1
3.										
Males-Männer-mužčiny	888031	401108	97580	385981	38.2	8.4	52.9	45.2	11.0	43.4
Females-Frauen-ženščiny	403993	196447	38177	168470	42.2	7.8	49.5	48.6	9.5	41.7
	484038	204661	59403	217511	35.0	8.9	55.6	42.3	12.3	44.9
Kirgizskaja SSR										
1.										
Males-Männer-mužčiny	2933732	1517173	573585	833711	40.9	17.1	41.7	51.7	19.6	28.4
Females-Frauen-ženščiny	1402186	753375	259581	386785	41.9	16.4	41.4	53.7	18.5	27.6
	1531546	763798	314004	446926	40.0	17.8	42.0	49.9	20.5	29.2
2.										
Males-Männer-mužčiny	1095444	724127	333586	35190	65.5	28.6	5.5	66.1	30.5	3.2
Females-Frauen-ženščiny	514626	356965	141597	15351	66.8	26.6	6.2	69.4	27.5	3.0
	580818	367162	191989	19839	64.3	30.4	4.9	63.2	33.1	3.4
3.										
Males-Männer-mužčiny	1838288	793046	239999	798521	28.5	11.2	60.1	43.1	13.1	43.4
Females-Frauen-ženščiny	887560	396410	117984	371434	29.5	11.2	59.1	44.7	13.3	41.8
	950728	396636	122015	427087	27.6	11.2	61.0	41.7	12.9	44.9
Tadžikskaja SSR										
1.										
Males-Männer-mužčiny	2898317	1171877	528298	1189529	31.1	15.2	53.5	40.4	18.2	41.1
Females-Frauen-ženščiny	1426928	614770	265227	545135	32.3	14.5	53.0	43.1	18.6	38.2
	1471389	557107	263071	644394	30.1	15.8	53.9	37.8	17.9	43.8
2.										
Males-Männer-mužčiny	1073506	708799	317083	44671	64.5	28.9	6.1	66.0	29.5	4.2
Females-Frauen-ženščiny	526361	359120	142290	24412	66.2	26.1	7.2	68.2	27.0	4.7
	547145	349679	174793	20259	63.0	31.4	5.1	63.9	32.0	3.7
3.										
Males-Männer-mužčiny	1824811	463078	211215	1144858	15.0	8.5	76.4	25.4	11.6	62.7
Females-Frauen-ženščiny	900567	255650	122937	520723	16.4	9.0	74.5	28.4	13.7	57.8
	924244	207428	88278	624135	13.6	8.1	78.2	22.4	9.6	67.5
Armjanskaja SSR										
1.										
Males-Männer-mužčiny	2492616	1446098	604553	427133	41.1	21.2	37.5	58.0	24.3	17.1
Females-Frauen-ženščiny	1217463	734756	283583	196755	43.5	19.8	36.4	60.3	23.3	16.2
	1275153	711342	320970	230378	38.9	22.5	38.4	55.8	25.2	18.0
2.										
Males-Männer-mužčiny	1472723	953006	484216	29628	62.1	32.0	5.5	64.7	32.9	2.0
Females-Frauen-ženščiny	721546	484929	221185	14493	65.0	29.0	5.6	67.2	30.7	2.0
	751177	468077	263031	15135	59.4	34.8	5.5	62.3	35.0	2.0

Social Structure 7.1
Soziale Struktur

	A.	B.	C.	D.	E.	F.	G.	H.	I.	J.
3.										
Males-Männer-mužčiny	1019893	493092	120337	397505	20.1	10.4	69.4	48.3	11.8	39.0
Females-Frauen-ženščiny	495917	249827	62398	182262	21.9	10.6	67.4	50.4	12.6	36.7
	523976	243265	57939	215243	18.5	10.2	71.2	46.4	11.1	41.1
Turkmenskaja SSR										
1.										
Males-Männer-mužčiny	2152534	860366	479778	800549	37.6	19.8	42.1	40.0	22.3	37.2
Females-Frauen-ženščiny	1059540	448703	234955	373765	39.6	18.5	41.5	42.3	22.2	35.3
	1092994	411663	244823	426784	35.8	20.9	42.8	37.7	22.4	39.0
2.										
Males-Männer-mužčiny	1028429	654572	345910	24047	63.7	32.3	3.5	63.7	33.6	2.3
Females-Frauen-ženščiny	509400	336545	158288	13977	66.3	28.9	4.4	66.1	31.1	2.7
	519029	318027	187622	10070	61.3	35.5	2.7	61.3	36.2	1.9
3.										
Males-Männer-mužčiny	1124105	205794	133868	776502	15.2	9.0	75.3	18.3	11.9	69.1
Females-Frauen-ženščiny	550140	112158	76667	359788	16.8	9.8	72.9	20.4	13.9	65.4
	573965	93636	57201	416714	13.7	8.3	77.5	16.3	10.0	72.6
Estonskaja SSR										
1.										
Males-Männer-mužčiny	1354613	813574	360081	177811	56.9	21.9	20.6	60.1	26.6	13.1
Females-Frauen-ženščiny	619927	396129	147463	75379	60.5	20.0	19.0	63.9	23.8	12.2
	734686	417445	212618	102432	54.0	23.4	22.0	55.8	29.0	13.9
2.										
Males-Männer-mužčiny	876610	564382	297604	13254	67.2	30.3	2.1	64.4	33.9	1.5
Females-Frauen-ženščiny	400690	273349	121933	5020	69.8	27.8	2.1	68.2	30.4	1.3
	475920	291033	175671	8234	65.3	32.2	2.1	61.2	36.9	1.7
3.										
Males-Männer-mužčiny	478003	249192	62477	164557	43.5	11.0	44.7	52.1	13.1	34.4
Females-Frauen-ženščiny	219237	122780	25530	70359	48.5	9.9	40.8	56.0	11.6	32.1
	258766	126412	36947	94198	39.5	11.9	47.8	48.8	14.3	36.4

7.2 Social Structure / Soziale Struktur

BREAKDOWN OF GAINFULLY EMPLOYED POPULATION OF THE USSR AND THE UNION REPUBLICS BY SOCIAL GROUPS
AUFTEILUNG DER BESCHÄFTIGTEN BEVÖLKERUNG DER UdSSR UND DER UNIONSREPUBLIKEN NACH GESELLSCHAFTLICHEN GRUPPEN
RASPREDELENIE ZANJATOGO NASELENIJA SSSR I SOJUZNYCH RESPUBLIK PO OBŠČESTVENNYM GRUPPAM
(Census – Volkszählungen – Perepisi naselenija 1959, 1970)

	A. Total gainfully employed population – Gesamte beschäftigte Bevölkerung – Vse zanjatoe naselenie	1970 of which – darunter – v tom čisle			% in relation to total gainfully employed population – % im Verhältnis zur gesamten beschäftigten Bevölkerung – V procentach k vsemu zanjatomu naseleniju					
		B. Workers Arbeiter Raboč́ie	C. Employees Angestellte Služašč́ie	D. Collective farmers Kolchosbauern Kolchozniki	1959			1970		
					E. Workers	F. Employees	G. Collective farmers	H. Workers	I. Employees	J. Collective farmers
SSSR										
1. Urban & rural population – Stadt-u.Landbevölkerung – Gorodskoe i sel'skoe nas.	115204076	66321222	30617865	17899838	47.9	18.5	33.3	57.6	26.6	15.5
Males–Männer–mužč́iny	57828454	36708783	12554160	8494957	53.9	16.8	29.0	63.5	21.7	14.7
Females–Frauen–ženšč́iny	57375622	29612439	18063705	9404881	41.4	20.4	38.0	51.6	31.5	16.4
2. Urban population – Stadtbevölkerung – Gorodskoe naselenie	70900220	45911714	24367480	502440	68.6	28.6	2.7	64.7	34.4	0.7
Males–Männer–mužč́iny	35490325	25338321	9858017	277418	73.0	24.3	2.5	71.4	27.8	0.8
Females–Frauen–ženšč́iny	35409895	20573393	14509463	225022	63.5	33.6	2.8	58.1	41.0	0.6
3. Rural population – Landbevölkerung – Sel'skoe naselenie	44303856	20409508	6250385	17397398	29.4	9.4	60.8	46.1	14.1	39.3

Social Structure 7.2
Soziale Struktur

	A.	B.	C.	D.	E.	F.	G.	H.	I.	J.
RSFSR										
1.										
Males-Männer-mužčiny	22336129	11370462	2696143	8217539	35.6	9.6	54.4	50.9	12.1	36.8
Females-Frauen-ženščiny	21965727	9039046	3554242	9179859	23.1	9.4	67.2	41.1	16.2	41.8
Males-Männer-mužčiny	64818232	39902049	18425442	6379093	54.3	20.5	25.0	61.6	28.4	9.8
Females-Frauen-ženščiny	32240036	21781667	7190367	3245181	59.8	18.0	21.9	67.5	22.3	10.1
	32578196	18120382	11235075	3133912	48.5	23.0	28.3	55.6	34.5	9.6
2.										
Males-Männer-mužčiny	43732720	28603799	14964863	127487	70.1	28.4	1.4	65.4	34.2	0.3
Females-Frauen-ženščiny	21525027	15580840	5850444	88683	74.3	24.2	1.4	72.4	27.2	0.4
	22207693	13022959	9114419	38800	65.6	33.1	1.2	58.7	41.0	0.2
3.										
Males-Männer-mužčiny	21085512	11298250	3460579	6251606	36.3	11.4	52.0	53.6	16.4	29.6
Females-Frauen-ženščiny	10715009	6200827	1339923	3156498	42.7	10.8	46.1	57.9	12.5	29.4
	10370503	5097423	2120656	3095108	29.8	12.0	58.0	49.2	20.4	29.8
Ukrainskaja SSR										
1.										
Males-Männer-mužčiny	23270653	12059267	5400180	5725250	39.5	15.5	44.7	51.8	23.2	24.6
Females-Frauen-ženščiny	11528128	6644352	2280308	2585834	47.1	14.8	37.8	57.6	19.8	22.4
	11742525	5414915	3119872	3139416	31.5	16.2	52.0	46.1	26.6	26.7
2.										
Males-Männer-mužčiny	13388366	8683567	4432525	241523	66.7	27.2	5.9	64.9	33.1	1.8
Females-Frauen-ženščiny	6751648	4753761	1877171	116721	71.7	23.3	4.8	70.4	27.8	1.7
	6636718	3929806	2555354	124802	60.4	32.2	7.3	59.2	38.5	1.9
3.										
Males-Männer-mužčiny	9882287	3375700	967655	5483727	19.5	6.9	73.2	34.1	9.8	55.5
Females-Frauen-ženščiny	4776480	1890591	403137	2469113	25.8	7.5	66.3	39.6	8.4	51.7
	5105807	1485109	564518	3014614	13.9	6.3	79.4	29.1	11.1	59.0
Belorusskaja SSR										
1.										
Males-Männer-mužčiny	4299658	2319374	994231	972805	33.2	13.1	53.1	54.0	23.1	22.6
Females-Frauen-ženščiny	2106810	1230314	428776	444575	38.8	13.2	47.3	58.4	20.4	21.1
	2192848	1089060	565455	528230	28.1	13.1	58.3	49.6	25.8	24.1
2.										
Males-Männer-mužčiny	2101672	1349107	739840	9460	62.9	30.6	6.2	64.2	35.2	0.4
Females-Frauen-ženščiny	1030834	704220	320385	5729	66.1	28.0	5.4	68.3	31.1	0.6
	1070838	644887	419455	3731	59.5	33.2	7.1	60.2	39.2	0.3
3.										
Males-Männer-mužčiny	2197986	970267	254391	963345	21.8	6.5	71.0	44.1	11.6	43.8
Females-Frauen-ženščiny	1075976	526094	108391	438846	27.3	7.0	64.9	48.9	10.1	40.8
	1122010	444173	146000	524499	17.0	6.0	76.3	39.6	13.0	46.7

7.2 Social Structure
Soziale Struktur

	A.	B.	C.	D.	E.	F.	G.	H.	I.	J.
Uzbekskaja SSR										
1.										
Males-Männer-mužčiny	4238002	1938959	973330	1267614	39.2	14.9	45.7	45.7	23.0	29.9
Females-Frauen-ženščiny	2211336	1172399	495466	534545	44.4	14.9	40.4	53.0	22.4	24.2
	2026666	766560	477864	733069	32.6	14.8	52.4	37.8	23.6	36.2
2.										
Males-Männer-mužčiny	1756197	1059661	643991	37520	63.9	30.9	4.6	60.3	36.7	2.1
Females-Frauen-ženščiny	947589	650840	277476	17130	69.2	25.5	4.7	68.7	29.3	1.8
	808608	408821	366515	20390	55.8	39.2	4.5	50.6	45.3	2.5
3.										
Males-Männer-mužčiny	2481805	879298	329339	1230094	27.9	7.5	64.5	35.4	13.3	49.6
Females-Frauen-ženščiny	1263747	521559	217990	517415	31.7	9.6	58.5	41.3	17.3	40.9
	1218058	357739	111349	712679	23.3	4.9	71.7	29.4	9.1	58.5
Kazachskaja SSR										
1.										
Males-Männer-mužčiny	5492078	3639432	1519851	313919	58.4	19.9	21.6	66.3	27.7	5.7
Females-Frauen-ženščiny	2927805	2116953	638199	170123	63.6	17.2	19.1	72.3	21.8	5.8
	2564273	1522479	881652	143796	50.6	23.9	25.4	59.4	34.4	5.6
2.										
Males-Männer-mužčiny	3128810	2073404	1041289	6539	71.2	27.5	1.2	66.3	33.3	0.2
Females-Frauen-ženščiny	1663861	1242764	415896	4416	76.3	22.1	1.5	74.7	25.0	0.3
	1464949	830640	625393	2123	63.3	35.8	0.8	56.7	42.7	0.1
3.										
Males-Männer-mužčiny	2363268	1566028	478562	307380	48.2	13.8	37.9	66.3	20.2	13.0
Females-Frauen-ženščiny	1263944	874189	222303	165707	53.4	13.2	33.3	69.2	17.6	13.1
	1099324	691839	256259	141673	40.5	14.6	44.8	62.9	23.3	12.9
Gruzinskaja SSR										
1.										
Males-Männer-mužčiny	2101734	956780	608736	521575	31.7	20.2	47.8	45.5	29.0	24.8
Females-Frauen-ženščiny	1090852	569129	283443	235007	38.8	19.0	41.8	52.2	26.0	21.5
	1010882	387651	325293	286568	23.1	21.8	54.9	38.4	32.2	28.3
2.										
Males-Männer-mužčiny	1035524	558775	457263	15001	56.4	37.0	6.2	54.0	44.2	1.4
Females-Frauen-ženščiny	551529	332853	209475	8217	61.9	32.0	5.6	60.3	38.0	1.5
	483995	225922	247788	6784	48.5	44.2	7.1	46.7	51.2	1.4
3.										
Males-Männer-mužčiny	1066210	398005	151473	506574	15.9	9.6	74.3	37.3	14.2	47.5
Females-Frauen-ženščiny	539323	236276	73968	226790	22.0	9.5	68.2	43.8	13.7	42.1
	526887	161729	77505	279784	9.4	9.7	80.7	30.7	14.7	53.1

Social Structure 7.2
Soziale Struktur

	A.	B.	C.	D.	E.	F.	G.	H.	I.	J.
Azerbajdžanskaja SSR										
1.	1774737	914485	486630	364556	34.4	18.1	47.4	51.5	27.4	20.6
Males-Männer-mužčiny	986293	563884	258534	162050	42.1	17.9	39.8	57.2	26.2	16.4
Females-Frauen-ženščiny	788444	350601	228096	202506	24.4	18.4	57.1	44.5	28.9	25.7
2.	994337	597655	380592	12252	63.2	32.0	4.7	60.1	38.3	1.2
Males-Männer-mužčiny	571827	381783	183627	5721	68.8	26.4	4.6	66.8	32.1	1.0
Females-Frauen-ženščiny	422510	215872	196965	6531	54.0	41.1	4.8	51.1	46.6	1.6
3.	780400	316830	106038	352304	11.8	7.3	80.8	40.6	13.6	45.1
Males-Männer-mužčiny	414466	182101	74907	156329	17.0	9.9	72.9	43.9	18.1	37.7
Females-Frauen-ženščiny	365934	134729	31131	195975	6.3	4.5	89.2	36.8	8.5	53.6
Litovskaja SSR										
1.	1531249	833930	365002	324137	37.8	14.7	46.5	54.5	23.8	21.2
Males-Männer-mužčiny	787024	469079	151992	163592	43.4	13.3	42.3	59.6	19.3	20.8
Females-Frauen-ženščiny	744225	364851	213010	160545	31.3	16.3	51.5	49.0	28.6	21.6
2.	850719	547562	298357	2392	66.1	31.0	2.2	64.3	35.1	0.3
Males-Männer-mužčiny	429616	300666	126753	1728	69.9	27.3	2.0	70.0	29.5	0.4
Females-Frauen-ženščiny	421103	246898	171604	664	61.5	35.5	2.5	58.6	40.7	0.2
3.	680530	286368	66645	321745	22.2	5.7	71.0	42.1	9.8	47.3
Males-Männer-mužčiny	357408	168413	25239	161864	28.1	5.2	65.6	47.1	7.1	45.3
Females-Frauen-ženščiny	323122	117955	41406	159881	15.6	6.3	77.0	36.5	12.8	49.5
Moldavskaja SSR										
1.	1788606	682266	300705	800926	19.4	9.1	71.2	38.1	16.8	44.8
Males-Männer-mužčiny	868443	371578	126099	369298	24.6	9.0	66.0	42.8	14.5	42.5
Females-Frauen-ženščiny	920163	310688	174606	431628	14.3	9.2	76.2	33.7	19.0	46.9
2.	597768	365737	210603	19990	60.7	28.9	10.0	61.2	35.2	3.4
Males-Männer-mužčiny	295505	197619	88458	9156	65.8	24.8	8.8	66.9	29.9	3.1
Females-Frauen-ženščiny	302263	168118	122145	10834	54.1	34.0	11.7	55.6	40.4	3.6
3.	1190838	316529	90102	780936	9.9	4.6	85.2	26.6	7.5	65.6
Males-Männer-mužčiny	572938	173959	37641	360142	13.4	4.7	81.5	30.4	6.6	62.8
Females-Frauen-ženščiny	617900	142570	52461	420794	6.7	4.4	88.6	23.1	8.5	68.1

7.2 Social Structure / Soziale Struktur

	A.	B.	C.	D.	E.	F.	G.	H.	I.	J.
Latvijskaja SSR										
1.	1258382	729741	363868	160189	52.0	19.8	27.6	58.0	28.9	12.7
Males-Männer-mužčiny	626543	400199	141572	83802	58.8	16.4	24.3	63.8	22.6	13.4
Females-Frauen-ženščiny	631839	329542	222296	76387	44.7	23.5	31.2	52.1	35.2	12.1
2.	850351	538134	305719	4597	66.0	29.3	4.2	63.3	36.0	0.5
Males-Männer-mužčiny	415432	290582	120946	3549	71.5	24.3	3.8	69.9	29.1	0.9
Females-Frauen-ženščiny	434919	247552	184773	1048	60.1	34.8	4.6	56.9	42.5	0.2
3.	408031	191607	58149	155592	35.0	8.3	56.0	47.0	14.2	38.1
Males-Männer-mužčiny	211111	109617	20626	80253	43.4	6.9	49.1	51.9	9.8	38.0
Females-Frauen-ženščiny	196920	81990	37523	75339	25.9	9.8	63.6	41.6	19.0	38.3
Kirgizskaja SSR										
1.	1123774	602328	261791	252430	39.7	16.7	43.4	53.6	23.3	22.5
Males-Männer-mužčiny	579566	338837	115515	123715	44.8	15.9	39.0	58.5	19.9	21.3
Females-Frauen-ženščiny	544208	263491	146276	128715	33.4	17.6	48.9	48.4	26.9	23.6
2.	489867	314225	169829	4125	65.8	30.2	3.7	64.2	34.7	0.8
Males-Männer-mužčiny	250494	178565	69066	2500	70.7	25.1	3.8	71.3	27.6	1.0
Females-Frauen-ženščiny	239373	135660	100763	1625	58.8	37.5	3.5	56.7	42.1	0.7
3.	633907	288103	91962	248305	27.1	10.1	62.6	45.4	14.5	39.2
Males-Männer-mužčiny	329072	160272	46449	121215	31.2	11.0	57.5	48.7	14.1	36.8
Females-Frauen-ženščiny	304835	127831	45513	127090	22.3	9.0	68.6	41.9	14.9	41.7
Tadžikskaja SSR										
1.	1003906	421370	219341	356679	29.1	13.6	57.1	42.0	21.9	35.5
Males-Männer-mužčiny	551634	271435	118337	160929	34.4	13.7	51.7	49.2	21.4	29.2
Females-Frauen-ženščiny	452272	149935	101004	195759	22.0	13.6	64.3	33.2	22.3	43.3
2.	431530	269931	152467	7226	65.1	29.8	4.7	62.6	35.3	1.7
Males-Männer-mužčiny	234610	164454	65979	4019	70.6	24.2	4.8	70.1	28.1	1.7
Females-Frauen-ženščiny	196920	105477	86488	3207	57.0	38.2	4.5	53.6	43.9	1.6
3.	572376	151439	66874	349453	13.2	6.5	80.2	26.5	11.7	61.0
Males-Männer-mužčiny	317024	106981	52358	156910	17.4	8.7	73.8	33.8	16.5	49.5
Females-Frauen-ženščiny	255352	44458	14516	192543	7.9	3.8	88.3	17.4	5.7	75.4

430

Social Structure 7.2
Soziale Struktur

	A.	B.	C.	D.	E.	F.	G.	H.	I.	J.
Armjanskaja SSR										
1.	980140	551735	285383	132644	39.3	19.5	41.0	56.3	29.1	13.5
Males-Männer-mužčiny	526844	324583	138285	62852	45.7	18.3	35.7	61.6	26.3	11.9
Females-Frauen-ženščiny	453296	227152	147098	69792	30.4	21.1	48.4	50.1	32.5	15.4
2.	618152	372549	235261	6339	62.2	32.1	5.4	60.3	38.1	1.0
Males-Männer-mužčiny	338790	223927	110344	4178	67.7	27.1	4.8	66.1	32.6	1.2
Females-Frauen-ženščiny	279362	148622	124917	2161	52.6	40.9	6.4	53.2	44.7	0.8
3.	361988	179186	50122	126305	19.5	8.5	71.9	49.5	13.8	34.9
Males-Männer-mužčiny	188054	100656	27941	58674	23.2	9.4	67.2	53.5	14.9	31.2
Females-Frauen-ženščiny	173934	78530	22181	67631	15.1	7.5	77.3	45.1	12.8	38.9
Turkmenskaja SSR										
1.	800529	330107	194930	264541	37.3	18.1	44.2	41.2	24.4	33.0
Males-Männer-mužčiny	435803	213418	101697	115002	44.4	17.1	38.1	49.0	23.3	27.3
Females-Frauen-ženščiny	364726	116689	93233	145539	27.7	19.4	52.5	32.0	25.6	39.9
2.	419143	256347	153773	5622	65.3	31.7	2.6	61.2	36.7	1.3
Males-Männer-mužčiny	237564	162859	70662	3689	71.6	25.3	2.8	68.6	29.7	1.6
Females-Frauen-ženščiny	181579	93488	83111	1933	55.3	41.9	2.2	51.5	45.8	1.0
3.	381386	73760	41157	258919	14.1	6.8	78.7	19.3	10.8	67.9
Males-Männer-mužčiny	198239	50559	31035	115313	19.3	9.6	70.6	25.5	15.6	58.2
Females-Frauen-ženščiny	183147	23201	10122	143606	7.8	3.3	88.6	12.7	5.5	78.4
Estonskaja SSR										
1.	722396	439399	218445	63480	56.9	21.5	21.1	60.8	30.2	8.8
Males-Männer-mužčiny	361337	240956	85570	34452	64.1	17.6	17.9	66.7	23.7	9.5
Females-Frauen-ženščiny	361059	198443	132875	29028	49.4	25.5	24.6	55.0	36.8	8.0
2.	505064	321261	181108	2367	69.0	29.9	0.9	63.6	35.8	0.5
Males-Männer-mužčiny	245999	172588	71335	1982	74.3	24.5	1.0	70.2	29.0	0.8
Females-Frauen-ženščiny	259065	148673	109773	385	63.4	35.5	0.9	57.4	42.4	0.1
3.	217332	118138	37337	61113	41.4	10.6	47.2	54.4	17.2	28.1
Males-Männer-mužčiny	115338	68368	14235	32470	50.9	8.4	39.9	59.3	12.3	28.2
Females-Frauen-ženščiny	101994	49770	23102	28643	31.7	12.8	54.6	48.8	22.6	28.1

7.3 Social Structure / Soziale Struktur

BREAKDOWN OF THE POPULATION OF THE USSR AND THE UNION REPUBLICS BY MEANS OF INCOME
AUFTEILUNG DER BEVÖLKERUNG DER UdSSR UND DER UNIONSREPUBLIKEN NACH EINKOMMENS-QUELLEN
RASPREDELENIE NASELENIJA SSSR I SOJUZNYCH RESPUBLIK PO ISTOČNIKAM SREDSTV SUSČESTVOVANIJA
(Census – Volkszählungen – Perepisi naselenija 1959, 1970)

(% IN RELATION TO TOTAL POPULATION – % IM VERHÄLTNIS ZUR GESAMTBEVÖLKERUNG – V PROCENTACH KO VSEMU NASELENIJU)

A. Gainfully employed population – Beschäftigte Bevölkerung – Zanjatoe naselenie
B. Persons engaged in private agricultural subsid. enterprises – Beschäftigte i.d. privaten land-wirtschaftl. Nebenwirtschaften – Zanjatye v ličnom podsobnom sel'skom chozjajstve
C. Persons living on state welfare (pensioners and others) – Von der Staatsfürsorge lebende Personen (Rentner u.a.) – Lica, nachodjaščiesja na obespečenii gosudarstva (pensionery i drugie)
D. Scholars – Stipendiaten – Stipendiaty
E. Dependants of single persons – Abhängige Familienmitglieder einzelner Personen – Iždivency otdel'nych lic
F. Persons with other means of income, not indicated by them – Personen mit anderen, von ihnen nicht angegebenen Einkommens-quellen – Lica imejuščie drugie istočniki sredstv suščestvovanija i ne ukazavšie istočnik

	1959						1970					
	A.	B.	C.	D.	E.	F.	A.	B.	C.	D.	E.	F.
SSSR												
1.	47.5	4.7	6.0	0.8	40.9	0.1	47.7	0.8	13.5	1.5	36.4	0.1
Males-Männer	54.8	1.0	5.9	1.0	37.2	0.1	52.0	0.2	9.8	1.5	36.4	0.1
Females-Frauen	41.5	7.8	6.0	0.7	43.9	0.1	44.0	1.3	16.7	1.4	36.5	0.1
2.	46.8	1.1	8.2	1.6	42.1	0.2	52.4	0.2	11.8	2.3	33.2	0.1
Males-Männer	55.8	0.1	8.1	1.9	34.0	0.1	56.6	0.0	9.3	2.4	31.6	0.1
Females-Frauen	39.4	1.9	8.3	1.3	48.9	0.2	48.7	0.5	13.9	2.3	34.6	0.2
3.	48.0	8.1	3.9	0.1	39.8	0.1	41.8	1.5	15.8	0.3	40.5	0.1
Males-Männer	53.8	1.8	3.9	0.2	40.2	0.1	46.1	0.3	10.6	0.4	42.5	0.1
Females-Frauen	43.4	13.2	3.8	0.1	39.4	0.1	38.1	2.5	20.2	0.3	38.8	0.1

1. Urban and rural population – Stadt-u.Landbevölkerung – Gorodskoe i sel'skoe naselenie
2. Urban population – Stadtbevölkerung – Gorodskoe naselenie
3. Rural population – Landbevölkerung – Sel'skoe naselenie

Social Structure 7.3
Soziale Struktur

	1959							1970						
	A.	B.	C.	D.	E.	F.		A.	B.	C.	D.	E.	F.
RSFSR													
1.													
Males-Männer	47.8	4.2	7.0	0.9	40.0	0.1		49.9	0.5	14.3	1.5	33.7	0.1
Females-Frauen	55.0	0.6	6.8	1.0	36.5	0.1		54.5	0.1	9.9	1.5	33.9	0.1
2.													
Males-Männer	41.9	7.1	7.2	0.8	42.8	0.2		46.0	0.9	18.0	1.5	33.5	0.1
Females-Frauen	48.6	0.8	8.8	1.5	40.1	0.2		54.2	0.1	12.6	2.2	30.8	0.1
Males-Männer	56.5	0.1	8.3	1.7	33.3	0.1		58.3	0.0	9.4	2.1	30.1	0.1
Females-Frauen	42.1	1.4	9.2	1.4	45.7	0.2		50.8	0.2	15.3	2.3	31.3	0.1
3.													
Males-Männer	46.9	7.9	5.1	0.2	39.8	0.1		42.8	1.2	17.1	0.4	38.4	0.1
Males-Männer	53.4	1.2	5.2	0.2	40.0	0.0		48.2	0.2	10.8	0.4	40.3	0.1
Females-Frauen	41.8	13.3	5.1	0.1	39.6	0.1		38.3	2.1	22.3	0.3	36.9	0.1
Ukrainskaja SSR													
1.													
Males-Männer	49.8	6.2	5.5	0.8	37.6	0.1		49.5	1.1	15.7	1.4	32.2	0.1
Females-Frauen	57.5	1.5	6.0	1.1	33.8	0.1		54.2	0.3	11.9	1.5	32.0	0.1
2.													
Males-Männer	43.6	9.8	5.2	0.8	40.6	0.1		45.6	1.8	18.8	1.3	32.4	0.1
Females-Frauen	46.1	1.8	8.3	1.6	42.0	0.2		52.4	0.3	12.5	2.3	32.3	0.2
Males-Männer	57.2	0.2	9.1	2.1	31.3	0.1		57.1	0.1	10.9	2.5	29.3	0.1
Females-Frauen	36.8	3.1	7.7	1.3	50.8	0.3		48.4	0.6	13.8	2.2	34.8	0.2
3.													
Males-Männer	53.0	9.8	3.2	0.1	33.8	0.1		45.9	2.1	19.6	0.3	32.0	0.1
Males-Männer	57.8	2.7	3.4	0.2	35.9	0.1		50.5	0.5	13.3	0.4	35.2	0.1
Females-Frauen	49.3	15.3	3.1	0.1	32.2	0.0		42.4	3.3	24.5	0.2	29.5	0.1
Belorusskaja SSR													
1.													
Males-Männer	51.6	5.7	3.6	0.8	38.2	0.1		47.8	0.9	14.7	1.5	35.0	0.1
Females-Frauen	55.4	1.4	4.2	0.9	38.0	0.1		51.0	0.2	10.8	1.5	36.4	0.1
2.													
Males-Männer	48.6	9.2	3.2	0.7	38.2	0.1		45.1	1.5	18.1	1.5	33.7	0.1
Females-Frauen	46.5	1.8	6.9	2.6	42.4	0.2		54.0	0.2	9.4	3.0	33.3	0.2
Males-Männer	53.3	0.2	7.8	2.6	36.0	0.1		56.4	0.2	7.0	2.9	32.6	0.1
Females-Frauen	41.0	3.0	6.2	2.0	47.5	0.3		51.9	0.3	10.7	3.1	33.9	0.1
3.													
Males-Männer	53.9	7.5	2.2	0.1	36.3	0.0		43.1	1.5	18.8	0.3	36.2	0.1
Males-Männer	56.3	1.9	2.6	0.2	39.0	0.0		46.7	0.3	13.0	0.4	39.5	0.1
Females-Frauen	51.9	11.9	1.9	0.1	34.1	0.1		40.1	2.5	23.5	0.3	33.5	0.1
Uzbekskaja SSR													
1.													
Males-Männer	40.3	3.9	2.9	0.6	52.2	0.1		36.0	0.5	8.6	1.4	53.3	0.2
Females-Frauen	47.1	1.8	3.1	0.9	47.0	0.1		38.6	0.1	7.2	1.7	52.2	0.2
2.													
Males-Männer	33.9	5.9	2.7	0.4	57.0	0.1		33.5	0.8	9.9	1.1	54.5	0.2
Females-Frauen	37.6	0.6	5.5	1.7	54.3	0.3		40.9	0.2	7.7	3.2	47.7	0.3
Males-Männer	48.1	0.2	5.8	2.5	43.1	0.3		45.6	0.1	6.8	3.9	43.3	0.3
Females-Frauen	28.3	1.0	5.1	1.1	64.2	0.3		36.4	0.3	8.5	2.6	51.9	0.3

7.3 Social Structure
    Soziale Struktur

	1959							1970						
	A.	B.	C.	D.	E.	F.	A.	B.	C.	D.	E.	F.
3.												
Males-Männer	41.5	5.6	1.6	0.1	51.1	0.1	33.2	0.7	9.0	0.3	56.6	0.2
Females-Frauen	46.7	2.6	1.8	0.1	48.8	0.0	34.6	0.2	7.4	0.4	57.2	0.2
	36.7	8.4	1.5	0.0	53.3	0.1	31.9	1.1	10.6	0.2	56.0	0.2
Kazachskaja SSR												
1.												
Males-Männer	40.0	5.2	4.2	1.0	49.5	0.1	42.2	0.8	8.9	1.4	46.6	0.1
Females-Frauen	50.7	0.7	4.7	1.3	42.5	0.1	46.7	0.1	7.8	1.4	43.9	0.1
	30.4	9.1	3.9	0.7	55.8	0.1	38.0	1.5	9.9	1.5	49.0	0.1
2.												
Males-Männer	40.7	1.5	5.7	1.7	50.2	0.2	48.1	0.2	8.6	2.4	40.6	0.1
Females-Frauen	52.0	0.2	6.4	2.0	39.3	0.1	53.0	0.1	7.7	2.2	36.9	0.1
	30.6	2.6	5.2	1.4	60.0	0.2	43.4	0.4	9.3	2.6	44.2	0.1
3.												
Males-Männer	39.4	8.1	3.1	0.4	48.9	0.1	36.4	1.4	9.2	0.4	52.5	0.1
Females-Frauen	49.6	1.1	3.4	0.7	45.1	0.1	40.4	0.2	7.8	0.5	51.0	0.1
	30.2	14.3	2.8	0.2	52.4	0.1	32.6	2.7	10.4	0.3	53.9	0.1
Gruzinskaja SSR												
1.												
Males-Männer	46.0	6.1	4.1	0.4	43.3	0.1	44.9	1.3	11.6	1.0	41.0	0.2
Females-Frauen	54.3	2.0	4.3	0.5	38.8	0.1	49.7	0.4	9.0	1.1	39.6	0.2
	38.8	9.7	4.0	0.2	47.2	0.1	40.8	2.2	14.0	0.8	42.0	0.2
2.												
Males-Männer	42.2	1.6	7.5	0.7	47.8	0.2	46.8	0.3	10.0	1.7	40.9	0.3
Females-Frauen	54.8	0.4	7.4	1.0	36.2	0.2	53.4	0.1	8.2	1.9	36.1	0.3
	31.7	2.6	7.5	0.5	57.5	0.2	41.1	0.4	11.6	1.5	45.1	0.3
3.												
Males-Männer	48.7	9.5	1.7	0.1	40.0	0.0	43.3	2.3	13.1	0.3	40.9	0.1
Females-Frauen	54.0	3.2	2.0	0.1	40.7	0.0	46.4	0.7	9.6	0.5	42.7	0.1
	44.2	15.0	1.4	0.0	39.4	0.0	40.5	3.7	16.2	0.3	39.2	0.1
Azerbajdžanskaja SSR												
1.												
Males-Männer	41.3	3.1	3.4	0.5	51.6	0.1	34.7	1.2	8.6	1.2	54.2	0.1
Females-Frauen	48.9	0.8	3.4	0.8	46.1	0.0	39.7	0.2	6.3	1.6	52.1	0.1
	34.5	5.2	3.4	0.3	56.5	0.1	30.0	2.1	10.7	0.9	56.2	0.1
2.												
Males-Männer	38.0	1.0	6.2	1.0	53.7	0.1	39.0	0.3	8.7	2.3	49.5	0.2
Females-Frauen	49.8	0.2	6.1	1.6	42.2	0.1	45.8	0.1	7.1	2.9	43.9	0.2
	27.4	1.7	6.2	0.6	64.0	0.1	32.4	0.5	10.1	1.8	55.0	0.2
3.												
Males-Männer	44.4	5.0	0.9	0.0	49.7	0.0	30.4	2.1	8.4	0.2	58.8	0.1
Females-Frauen	48.1	1.3	0.9	0.0	49.7	0.0	30.4	0.4	5.4	0.3	60.3	0.1
	41.0	8.4	0.9	0.0	49.7	0.0	27.5	3.7	11.3	0.1	57.3	0.1
Litovskaja SSR												
1.												
	49.9	5.9	2.9	0.8	40.2	0.3	49.1	2.0	12.3	1.9	34.4	0.3

Social Structure 7.3
Soziale Struktur

	1959						1970					
	A.	B.	C.	D.	E.	F.	A.	B.	C.	D.	E.	F.
Moldavskaja SSR												
Males-Männer	58.5	1.7	3.1	1.0	35.5	0.2	53.8	0.6	10.0	1.9	33.4	0.3
Females-Frauen	42.6	9.4	2.8	0.7	44.1	0.4	44.9	3.3	14.3	1.9	35.3	0.3
2.												
Males-Männer	45.9	1.1	5.4	2.0	45.0	0.6	54.6	0.2	8.0	3.1	33.8	0.3
Females-Frauen	56.5	0.3	5.7	2.4	34.8	0.3	58.6	0.1	6.6	3.0	31.5	0.2
3.												
Males-Männer	37.2	1.8	5.2	1.7	53.4	0.7	51.1	0.4	9.2	3.3	35.7	0.3
Females-Frauen	52.4	8.8	1.4	0.1	37.1	0.2	43.6	3.8	16.5	0.7	35.1	0.3
Males-Männer	59.7	2.5	1.4	0.2	36.0	0.2	49.0	1.0	13.4	0.9	35.4	0.3
Females-Frauen	46.0	14.3	1.3	0.1	38.1	0.2	38.8	6.2	19.3	0.6	34.8	0.3
Moldavskaja SSR												
1.												
Males-Männer	54.0	3.1	2.2	0.5	40.1	0.1	50.1	1.0	9.7	1.6	37.5	0.1
Females-Frauen	57.3	0.6	2.4	0.6	39.0	0.1	52.0	0.2	7.5	1.7	38.5	0.1
2.												
Males-Männer	51.1	5.1	2.1	0.4	41.1	0.2	48.4	1.6	11.6	1.6	36.7	0.1
Females-Frauen	45.2	1.1	5.4	2.0	46.0	0.3	53.2	0.3	8.9	4.3	33.1	0.2
3.												
Males-Männer	55.4	0.1	6.3	2.3	35.7	0.2	56.2	0.1	8.2	4.0	31.3	0.2
Females-Frauen	36.7	1.9	4.6	1.7	54.7	0.4	50.5	0.6	9.5	4.5	34.7	0.2
Males-Männer	56.5	3.6	1.3	0.1	38.4	0.1	48.7	1.3	10.0	0.4	39.5	0.1
Females-Frauen	57.9	0.7	1.2	0.1	40.0	0.1	50.1	0.3	7.2	0.6	41.7	0.1
	55.3	6.1	1.4	0.0	37.1	0.1	47.4	2.1	12.6	0.3	37.5	0.1
Latvijskaja SSR												
1.												
Males-Männer	51.6	4.7	7.2	1.0	35.3	0.2	53.5	1.1	15.4	1.5	28.3	0.2
Females-Frauen	61.0	1.3	6.5	1.0	30.1	0.1	58.4	0.3	12.0	1.7	27.4	0.2
2.												
Males-Männer	44.3	7.3	7.8	0.9	39.4	0.3	49.4	1.8	18.2	1.3	29.1	0.2
Females-Frauen	50.4	1.0	9.8	1.3	37.2	0.3	58.1	0.0	12.2	2.0	27.5	0.2
3.												
Males-Männer	60.1	0.3	8.6	1.3	29.5	0.2	62.1	0.0	9.2	2.2	26.3	0.2
Females-Frauen	43.0	1.7	10.6	1.3	43.1	0.3	54.7	0.1	14.7	1.8	28.5	0.2
Males-Männer	53.1	9.4	4.0	0.5	32.9	0.1	45.9	2.8	20.1	0.7	29.7	0.2
Females-Frauen	62.1	2.6	3.8	0.6	30.8	0.1	52.3	0.8	16.6	0.8	29.3	0.2
	45.9	14.8	4.1	0.5	34.5	0.2	40.7	4.5	24.0	0.5	30.1	0.2
Kirgizskaja SSR												
1.												
Males-Männer	40.5	5.3	3.3	0.7	50.1	0.1	38.3	0.7	9.6	1.3	50.0	0.1
Females-Frauen	47.7	1.9	3.8	1.0	45.5	0.1	41.3	0.2	8.1	1.3	49.0	0.1
2.												
Males-Männer	34.0	8.3	2.9	0.5	54.2	0.1	35.5	1.2	11.0	1.4	50.8	0.1
Females-Frauen	39.1	1.5	5.6	2.0	51.5	0.3	44.7	0.2	8.9	3.2	42.8	0.2
3.												
Males-Männer	49.2	0.3	6.3	2.6	41.4	0.2	48.7	0.1	8.2	3.1	39.7	0.1
Females-Frauen	30.4	2.6	4.9	1.4	60.4	0.3	41.2	0.3	9.6	3.2	45.5	0.2
Males-Männer	41.1	7.1	2.2	0.1	49.4	0.1	34.5	1.0	10.0	0.2	54.2	0.1
Females-Frauen	47.0	2.6	2.6	0.1	47.6	0.1	37.1	0.2	7.9	0.3	54.4	0.1
	35.8	11.2	1.9	0.0	51.0	0.1	32.1	1.8	11.8	0.2	54.0	0.1

435

7.3 Social Structure / Soziale Struktur

	1959 A.	B.	C.	D.	E.	F.	1970 A.	B.	C.	D.	E.	F.
Tadžikskaja SSR												
1.												
Males-Männer	41.8	5.0	2.1	0.8	50.2	0.1	34.7	2.3	7.7	1.3	53.8	0.2
Females-Frauen	48.9	1.4	2.4	1.2	46.0	0.1	38.7	0.2	6.6	1.8	52.5	0.2
2.												
Males-Männer	35.0	8.5	1.8	0.4	54.2	0.1	30.8	4.4	8.7	0.8	55.1	0.2
Females-Frauen	39.1	1.9	4.1	2.2	52.5	0.2	40.2	0.9	6.7	3.1	48.9	0.2
3.												
Males-Männer	49.0	0.3	4.6	3.3	42.6	0.2	44.6	0.1	6.2	4.4	44.6	0.1
Females-Frauen	30.1	3.4	3.6	1.1	61.6	0.2	36.0	1.6	7.2	2.0	53.0	0.2
Males-Männer	43.1	6.6	1.1	0.1	49.1	0.0	31.4	3.2	8.2	0.2	56.7	0.3
Females-Frauen	48.8	1.9	1.4	0.2	47.7	0.0	35.2	0.3	6.8	0.3	57.1	0.3
Males-Männer	37.5	11.1	0.9	0.0	50.5	0.0	27.6	6.0	9.6	0.1	56.4	0.3
Armjanskaja SSR												
1.												
Males-Männer	39.8	4.3	3.8	0.3	51.6	0.2	39.3	0.9	8.3	1.5	49.7	0.3
Females-Frauen	48.5	1.0	3.9	0.5	46.0	0.1	43.3	0.1	6.3	1.8	48.2	0.3
2.												
Males-Männer	32.0	7.2	3.7	0.2	56.7	0.2	35.5	1.5	10.2	1.3	51.2	0.3
Females-Frauen	36.9	0.7	6.0	0.7	55.4	0.3	42.0	0.2	7.7	2.3	47.5	0.3
3.												
Males-Männer	48.8	0.2	6.2	1.0	43.6	0.2	47.0	0.0	6.3	2.6	43.8	0.3
Females-Frauen	26.1	1.2	5.8	0.4	66.2	0.3	37.2	0.3	9.0	2.1	51.1	0.3
Males-Männer	42.7	7.9	1.6	0.0	47.8	0.0	35.5	1.8	9.1	0.4	52.9	0.3
Females-Frauen	48.1	1.9	1.6	0.1	48.3	0.0	37.9	0.4	6.2	0.5	54.7	0.3
Males-Männer	37.8	13.3	1.6	0.0	47.3	0.0	33.2	3.2	11.8	0.3	51.2	0.3
Turkmenskaja SSR												
1.												
Males-Männer	39.7	4.9	2.9	0.8	51.6	0.1	37.2	0.7	7.4	1.3	53.3	0.1
Females-Frauen	47.7	2.2	3.0	1.2	45.8	0.1	41.1	0.2	6.0	1.7	50.9	0.1
2.												
Males-Männer	32.2	7.5	2.8	0.5	56.9	0.1	33.4	1.2	8.7	0.9	55.7	0.1
Females-Frauen	39.0	1.4	4.9	1.6	52.9	0.2	40.8	0.3	6.6	2.4	49.8	0.1
3.												
Males-Männer	49.8	0.3	5.1	2.3	42.3	0.2	46.6	0.1	5.7	3.1	44.4	0.1
Females-Frauen	29.0	2.5	4.8	1.0	62.5	0.2	35.0	0.5	7.4	1.8	55.1	0.2
Males-Männer	40.4	8.0	1.1	0.1	50.4	0.0	33.9	1.1	8.2	0.2	56.5	0.1
Females-Frauen	46.0	3.9	1.2	0.3	48.6	0.0	36.0	0.3	6.3	0.4	56.9	0.1
Males-Männer	35.1	11.8	1.0	0.0	52.1	0.0	31.9	1.8	9.9	0.1	56.2	0.1
Estonskaja SSR												
1.												
Males-Männer	51.4	2.8	7.4	0.9	37.4	0.1	53.3	0.7	15.8	1.4	28.6	0.2
Females-Frauen	59.6	1.1	6.5	1.0	31.7	0.1	58.3	0.2	11.7	1.4	28.2	0.2
2.												
Males-Männer	44.9	4.2	8.1	0.8	41.8	0.2	49.2	1.1	19.1	1.4	29.0	0.2
Females-Frauen	51.3	0.3	8.9	1.2	38.1	0.2	57.6	0.1	12.1	1.7	28.3	0.2
3.												
Males-Männer	59.9	0.1	7.7	1.4	30.8	0.1	61.6	0.0	8.9	1.6	27.9	0.2
Females-Frauen	44.6	0.3	10.0	1.1	43.8	0.2	54.4	0.1	14.8	1.8	28.7	0.2
Males-Männer	51.5	6.1	5.5	0.4	36.4	0.1	45.5	1.9	22.4	0.7	29.2	0.3
Females-Frauen	59.2	2.3	5.1	0.4	32.9	0.1	52.6	0.7	16.9	0.9	28.7	0.2
Males-Männer					29.8		39.4	3.0	27.1	0.6	29.6	0.3

7.4 BREAKDOWN OF THE POPULATION OF THE USSR AND THE UNION REPUBLICS BY MEANS OF INCOME AND SOCIAL GROUPS
AUFTEILUNG DER BEVÖLKERUNG DER USSR UND DER UNIONSREPUBLIKEN NACH EINKOMMENS-QUELLEN UND GESELLSCHAFTL.GRUPPEN
RASPREDELENIE NASELENIJA SSSR I SOJUZNYH RESPUBLIK PO ISTOČNIKAM SREDSTV SUŠČESTVOVANIJA I OBŠČESTVENNYM GRUPPAM

Social Structure 7.4
Soziale Struktur

	Both sexes – beide Geschlechter – Oba pola				Males – Männer – Mužčiny				Females – Frauen – Ženščiny			
	A. All social groups / Alle gesellschaftl. Gruppen / Vse obščestvennye gruppy	B. Workers Arbeiter rabočie	C. Employees Angestellte služaščie	D. Collective farmers Kolchosbauern kolchozniki	A.	B.	C.	D.	A.	B.	C.	D.
SSSR												
1.	241436013	136930781	54551734	49461551	111182265	66969787	23277923	20810291	130253748	69960994	31273811	28651260
1.1.	115204076	6631222	30617865	17899838	57828454	36708783	12554160	8494957	57375622	29612439	18063705	9404881
1.2.	1823499	917599	66606	828896	161874	64000	2925	92673	1661625	853599	63681	736223
1.3.	32641210	16607907	3962743	12050188	10923885	6147511	1736816	3032539	21717325	10460396	2225927	9017649
1.4.	3522580	1606681	1380593	533877	1682575	765795	632958	282995	1840005	840886	747635	250882
1.5.	87927859	51289626	18459212	18102706	40045310	23201004	8323995	8888538	47482549	28088622	10135217	9213168
1.6.	316789	187746	64715	46046	140167	82694	27069	17589	176622	105052	37646	28457

1. Urban and rural population – Stadt-und Landbevölkerung – Gorodskoe i sel'skoe naselenie
   of which – darunter – v tom čisle:
1.1. Gainfully employed population – beschäftigte Bevölkerung – zanjatoe naselenie
1.2. Persons engaged in private agricultural subsidiary enterprises – Beschäftigte i.d.privaten landwirtschaftlichen Nebenbetrieben – zanjatye v ličnom podsobnom sel'skom chozjajstve
1.3. Persons living on state welfare (pensioners and others) – von der Staatsfürsorge lebende Personen (Rentner u.a.) – lica, nachodjaščiesja na obespečenii gosudarstva (pensionery i drugie)
1.4. Scholars – Stipendiaten – stipendiaty
1.5. Dependants of single persons – abhängige Familienmitglieder einzelner Personen – iždivency otdel'nych lic
1.6. Persons with other means of income, not indicated by them –
     Personen mit anderen, von ihnen nicht angegebenen Einkommens-Quellen –
     Lica imejuščie drugie istočniki sredstv suščestvovanija i ne ukazavšie istočnik

437

7.4 Social Structure / Soziale Struktur

	Both sexes-beide Geschlechter-Oba pola				Males-Männer-Mužčiny				Females-Frauen-Ženščiny			
	A.	B.	C.	D.	A.	B.	C.	D.	A.	B.	C.	D.
2.	135330189	89247466	42676887	3228191	62677636	43626203	17888621	1123559	72652553	45621263	24788266	2104632
2.1.	70900220	45911714	24367480	502440	35490325	25338321	9858017	277418	35409895	20573393	14509463	225022
2.2.	221183	155877	13522	48276	17137	11275	882	4240	204046	144602	12640	44036
2.3.	15896027	10852294	3427701	1603645	5794361	3984862	1431304	374556	10101666	6867432	1996397	1229089
2.4.	3160628	1433698	1322042	403616	1479848	670251	603282	205575	1680780	763447	718760	198041
2.5.	4496338	30771508	13496104	662884	19814114	13568117	5974886	259601	25149224	17203391	7521218	403283
2.6.	188793	122375	50038	7330	81851	53377	20250	2169	106942	68993	29788	5161
3.	106105824	47683315	11874847	46233360	48504629	23343584	5389302	19686732	57601195	24339731	6485545	26546628
3.1.	44303856	20409508	6250385	17397398	22338129	11370462	2696143	8217539	21965727	9039046	3554242	9179859
3.2.	1602316	761722	53084	780620	144737	52725	2043	88433	1457579	708997	51041	692187
3.3.	16745183	5755613	535042	10446543	5129524	2162649	305512	2657983	11615659	3592964	229530	7788560
3.4.	361952	172983	58551	130261	202727	95544	29676	77420	159225	77439	28875	52841
3.5.	42964521	20518118	4963108	17439822	20631196	9632887	2349109	8629937	22333325	10885231	2613999	8809885
3.6.	127996	65371	14677	38716	58316	29317	6819	15420	69680	36054	7858	23296

RSFSR

	A.	B.	C.	D.	A.	B.	C.	D.	A.	B.	C.	D.
1.	129941212	79617464	31528248	18634111	59160721	38460469	13021671	7636144	70780491	41156995	18506577	10997967
1.1.	64818232	39902049	18425442	6379093	32240036	21781667	7190367	3245181	32578196	18120382	11235075	3133912
1.2.	669185	410895	21936	232265	42266	22327	867	18113	626919	388568	21069	214152
1.3.	18600875	10724363	2578953	5288348	5865234	3667996	1096268	1098352	12735641	7056367	1482685	4189996
1.4.	1955205	943397	812243	199010	880192	421711	361312	96935	1075013	521686	451131	102075
1.5.	43747702	27539677	9658447	6520444	20068785	12524462	4360336	3172772	23678917	15015215	5298111	3347672
1.6.	150013	97083	31027	14951	64208	42306	12521	4791	85805	54777	18506	10160

2. Urban population - Stadtbevölkerung - Gorodskoe naselenie
2.1. Gainfully employed population - beschäftigte Bevölkerung - zanjatoe naselenie
2.2. Persons engaged in private agricultural subsidiary enterprises - Beschäftigte i.d.privaten landwirtschaftlichen Nebenbetrieben - zanjatye v ličnom podsobnom sel'skom chozjajstve
2.3. Persons living on state welfare (pensioners and others) - von der Staatsfürsorge lebende Personen (Rentner u.a.) - lica, nachodjaščiesja na obespečenii gosudarstva (pensionery i drugie)
2.4. Scholars - Stipendiaten - stipendiaty
2.5. Dependants of single persons - abhängige Familienmitglieder einzelner Personen - iždivency otdel'nych lic
2.6. Persons with other means of income, not indicated by them - Personen mit anderen, von ihnen nicht angegebenen Einkommens-Quellen - Lica imejuščie drugie istočniki sredstv suščestvovanija i ne ukazavšie istočnik

3. Rural population - Landbevölkerung - Sel'skoe naselenie
3.1. - 3.6. see above - siehe oben

Social Structure 7.4
Soziale Struktur

	Both sexes-beide Geschlechter-Oba pola				Males-Männer-Mužčiny				Females-Frauen-Ženščiny			
	A.	B.	C.	D.	A.	B.	C.	D.	A.	B.	C.	D.
2.	80631371	53725406	25506889	1339420	36930897	26078725	10465382	373332	43700474	27646681	15041507	966088
2.1.	43732720	28603799	14964863	127487	21525027	15580840	5850444	88683	22207693	13022959	9114419	38804
2.2.	69948	54440	3637	10549	4660	3376	243	766	65288	51064	3394	9783
2.3.	10152113	7064212	2236707	845813	3465813	2410486	903673	150193	6686300	4653726	1333034	694974
2.4.	1781297	846279	783442	151244	787870	370460	347916	69282	993427	475819	435526	81962
2.5.	24799331	17092957	7492965	201733	11105730	7685310	3352893	63653	13693601	9407647	4140072	138080
2.6.	95962	63719	25275	3240	41797	28253	10213	755	54165	35466	15062	2485
3.	49309841	25892058	6021359	17294691	22229824	12381744	2556289	7262812	27080017	13510314	3465070	10031879
3.1.	21085512	11298250	3460579	6251606	10715009	6200827	1339923	3156498	10370503	5097423	2120656	3095108
3.2.	599237	356455	18299	221716	37606	18951	624	17347	561631	337504	17675	204369
3.3.	8448762	3660151	342246	4443181	2399421	1257510	192595	948159	6049341	2402641	149651	3495022
3.4.	173908	97118	29001	47766	92322	51251	13396	27653	81586	45867	15605	20113
3.5.	18948371	10446720	2165482	6318711	8963055	4839152	1007443	3109119	9985316	5607568	1158039	3209592
3.6.	54051	33364	5752	11711	22411	14053	2308	4036	31640	19311	3444	7675

Ukrainskaja SSR

	A.	B.	C.	D.	A.	B.	C.	D.	A.	B.	C.	D.
1.	47055852	23429542	9281475	14230270	21284158	11519051	4006364	5727633	25771694	11910491	5275111	8502637
1.1.	23270653	12059267	5400180	5725250	11528128	6644352	2280308	2585834	11742525	5414915	3119872	3139416
1.2.	529219	196279	10652	320418	56963	16591	518	39358	472256	179688	10134	281060
1.3.	7398839	2707335	742838	3945568	2543872	1168722	350269	1023401	4854967	1538613	392569	2922167
1.4.	660607	286309	227936	146131	326208	145123	108212	72762	334399	141186	119724	73369
1.5.	15136464	8146749	2888676	4083608	6802338	3530183	1262590	2002619	8334126	4616566	1626086	2080989
1.6.	60070	33603	11193	9295	26649	14080	4467	3659	33421	19523	6726	5636
2.	25545650	16697867	7711579	1093887	11823177	8107735	3308203	398657	13722473	8590132	4403376	695230
2.1.	13388366	8683567	4432525	241523	6751648	4753761	1877171	116721	6636718	3929806	2555354	124802
2.2.	84241	54627	3517	25389	5580	3269	153	1990	78661	51358	3364	23399
2.3.	3187587	2038320	661734	485876	1288328	856609	300216	130816	1899259	1181711	361518	355060
2.4.	598239	264917	220613	112519	293340	133660	104507	55083	304899	131257	116106	57436
2.5.	8249611	5632429	2384018	226940	3469083	2350922	1022602	93659	4780528	3281507	1361416	133281
2.6.	37606	24007	9172	1640	15198	9514	3554	388	22408	14493	5618	1252
3.	21510202	6731675	1569896	13136383	9460981	3411316	698161	5328976	12049221	3320359	871735	7807407
3.1.	9882287	3375700	967655	5483727	4776480	1890591	403137	2469113	5105807	1485109	564518	3014614
3.2.	444978	141652	7135	295029	51383	13322	365	37368	393595	128330	6770	257661
3.3.	4211252	669015	81104	3459692	1255544	312113	50053	892585	2955708	356902	31051	2567107
3.4.	62368	21392	7323	33612	32868	11463	3705	17679	29500	9929	3618	15933
3.5.	6886853	2514320	504658	3856668	3333255	1179261	239988	1908960	3553598	1335059	264670	1947708
3.6.	22464	9596	2021	7655	11451	4566	913	3271	11013	5030	1108	4384

7.4 Social Structure / Soziale Struktur

	Both sexes-beide Geschlechter-Oba pola				Males-Männer-Mužčiny				Females-Frauen-Ženščiny			
	A.	B.	C.	D.	A.	B.	C.	D.	A.	B.	C.	D.
Belorusskaja SSR												
1.	8992190	4700161	1738519	2536091	4129064	2281744	776521	1065771	4863126	2418417	961998	1470320
1.1.	4299658	2319374	994231	972805	2106810	1230314	428776	444575	2192848	1089060	565455	528230
1.2.	83293	45651	2023	35369	8431	3375	95	4912	74862	42276	1928	30457
1.3.	1324474	574864	89694	659176	443885	211711	45497	186355	880589	363153	44197	472821
1.4.	134575	53592	44455	36503	62328	25262	19668	17394	72247	28330	24787	19109
1.5.	3142585	1702710	606572	830962	1504407	809481	281919	412101	1638178	893229	324653	418861
1.6.	7605	3970	1544	1276	3203	1601	566	434	4402	2369	978	842
2.	3890580	2457684	1301929	126103	1826626	1199560	578399	47588	2063954	1258124	723530	78515
2.1.	2101672	1349107	739840	9460	1030834	704220	320385	5729	1070838	644887	419455	3731
2.2.	6526	4626	368	1442	693	540	19	113	5833	4086	349	1329
2.3.	365767	223792	73824	67747	144148	86952	35302	21767	221619	136840	38522	45980
2.4.	117810	46198	42760	28836	53416	21435	18772	13205	64394	24763	23988	15631
2.5.	1294936	831623	444062	18436	596059	385565	203527	6728	698877	446058	240535	11708
2.6.	3869	2338	1075	182	1476	848	394	46	2393	1490	681	136
3.	5101610	2242477	436590	2409988	2302438	1082184	198122	1018183	2799172	1160293	238468	1391805
3.1.	2197986	970267	254391	963345	1075976	526094	108391	438846	1122010	444173	146000	524499
3.2.	76767	41025	1655	33927	7738	2835	76	4799	69029	38190	1579	29128
3.3.	958707	351072	15870	591429	299737	124759	10195	164588	658970	226313	5675	426841
3.4.	16765	7394	1695	7667	8912	3827	896	4189	7853	3567	799	3478
3.5.	1847649	871087	162510	812526	908348	423916	78392	405373	939301	447171	84118	407153
3.6.	3736	1632	469	1094	1727	753	172	388	2009	879	297	706
Uzbekskaja SSR												
1.	11773869	5358748	2345927	3997722	5732096	2750015	1134011	1833047	6041773	2608733	1211916	2164675
1.1.	4238002	1938959	973330	1267614	2211336	1172399	495466	534545	2026666	766560	477864	733069
1.2.	55701	24375	3664	26965	6990	2978	224	3627	48711	21397	3440	23338
1.3.	1009162	399358	88597	519798	412055	176828	38703	195851	597107	222530	49894	323947
1.4.	162680	63616	60785	37896	98177	38344	32049	27560	64503	25272	28736	10336
1.5.	6283480	2920655	1213962	2138556	2991135	1353289	564597	1068481	3292345	1567366	649365	1070075
1.6.	24844	11785	5589	6893	12403	6177	2972	2983	12441	5608	2617	3910
2.	4297953	2725168	1375430	175260	2076961	1383067	603419	85221	2220992	1342101	772011	90039
2.1.	1756197	1059661	643991	37520	947589	650840	277476	17130	808608	408821	366545	20390
2.2.	7935	4685	851	2057	1049	567	84	327	6886	4118	767	1730
2.3.	331045	227226	71644	31494	141303	97147	30247	13574	189742	130079	41397	17920
2.4.	139168	56066	55829	26932	81636	33243	28904	19290	57532	22823	26925	7642

Social Structure 7.4
Soziale Struktur

	Both sexes-beide Geschlechter-Oba pola				Males-Männer-Mužčiny				Females-Frauen-Ženščiny			
	A.	B.	C.	D.	A.	B.	C.	D.	A.	B.	C.	D.
2.5.	2052138	1370759	599551	76505	899650	597782	265036	34524	1152488	772977	334515	41981
2.6.	11470	6771	3564	752	5734	3488	1672	376	5736	3283	1892	376
3.	7475916	2633580	970497	3822462	3655135	1366948	530592	1747826	3820781	1266632	439905	2074636
3.1.	2481805	879298	329339	1230094	1263747	521559	217990	517415	1218058	357739	111349	712679
3.2.	47766	19690	2813	24908	5941	2411	140	3300	41825	17279	2673	21608
3.3.	678117	172132	16953	488304	270752	79681	8456	182277	407365	92451	8497	306027
3.4.	23512	7550	4956	10964	16541	5101	3145	8270	6971	2449	1811	2694
3.5.	4231342	1549896	614411	2062051	2091485	755507	299561	1033957	2139857	794389	314850	1028094
3.6.	13374	5014	2025	6141	6669	2689	1300	2607	6705	2325	725	3534
Kazachskaja SSR												
1.	13009272	8854938	3056672	1074330	6265985	4433409	1337959	490515	6743287	4421529	1718713	583815
1.1.	5492078	3639432	1519851	313919	2927805	2116953	638199	170123	2564273	1522479	881652	143796
1.2.	105222	81273	7181	16258	6759	4874	198	1567	98463	76399	6983	14691
1.3.	1153301	834899	125484	192043	485884	366977	63129	55514	667417	467922	62355	136529
1.4.	184837	98147	73902	12714	84936	46680	30811	7415	99901	51467	43091	5299
1.5.	6055522	4188923	1325956	537916	2752947	1892662	603975	255295	3302575	2296261	721981	282621
1.6.	18312	12264	4298	1480	7654	5263	1647	601	10658	7001	2651	879
2.	6512238	4496772	1930885	74443	3139425	2300698	813037	24097	3372813	2196074	1117848	50346
2.1.	3128810	2073404	1041289	6539	1663861	1242764	415896	4416	1464949	830640	625393	2123
2.2.	13363	10980	1048	1108	1025	780	67	154	12338	10200	981	954
2.3.	557344	423750	95877	37083	242024	188167	45283	8418	315320	235583	50594	28665
2.4.	157424	80652	67272	9426	69314	36638	27442	5204	88110	44014	39830	4222
2.5.	2645660	1901504	722650	20045	1159169	829478	323328	5845	1486491	1072026	399322	14200
2.6.	9637	6482	2749	242	4032	2871	1021	60	5605	3611	1728	182
3.	6497034	4358166	1125787	999887	3126560	2132711	524922	466418	3370474	2225455	600865	533469
3.1.	2363268	1566028	478562	307380	1263944	874189	222303	165707	1099324	691839	256259	141673
3.2.	91859	70293	6133	15150	5734	4094	131	1413	86125	66199	6002	13737
3.3.	595957	411149	29607	154960	243860	178810	17846	47096	352097	232339	11761	107864
3.4.	27413	17495	6630	3288	15622	10042	3369	2211	11791	7453	3261	1077
3.5.	3409862	2287419	603306	517871	1593778	1063184	280647	249450	1816084	1224235	322659	268421
3.6.	8675	5782	1549	1238	3622	2392	626	541	5053	3390	923	697
Gruzinskaja SSR												
1.	4674591	2185731	1163779	1307630	2195490	1102759	518595	569674	2479101	1082972	645184	737956
1.1.	2101734	956780	608736	521575	1090852	569129	283443	235007	1010882	387651	325293	286568

441

7.4 Social Structure / Soziale Struktur

	Both sexes-beide Geschlechter-Oba pola				Males-Männer-Mužčiny				Females-Frauen-Ženščiny			
	A.	B.	C.	D.	A.	B.	C.	D.	A.	B.	C.	D.
1.2.	62154	21912	3316	36769	8644	2189	358	6066	53510	19723	2958	30703
1.3.	543746	206767	79353	257322	197060	85395	31237	80324	346686	121372	48116	176998
1.4.	46135	14701	25065	6329	25131	8577	12435	4096	21004	6124	12630	2233
1.5.	1911434	980738	444972	483842	869361	435067	190086	243444	1042073	545671	254886	240398
1.6.	9388	4833	2337	1793	4442	2402	1036	737	4946	2431	1301	1056
2.	2210973	1272206	875742	56508	1032535	626021	378734	25953	1178438	646185	497008	30555
2.1.	1035524	558775	457263	15001	551529	332853	209475	8217	483995	225922	247788	6784
2.2.	6287	4175	582	1445	1067	633	146	277	5220	3542	436	1168
2.3.	221477	133259	66607	21343	85185	53314	24346	7432	136292	79945	42261	13911
2.4.	37576	11582	23497	2462	19747	6607	11579	1543	17829	4975	11918	919
2.5.	904319	560997	325877	16109	372296	230986	132395	8406	532023	330011	193482	7703
2.6.	5790	3418	1916	148	2711	1628	793	78	3079	1790	1123	70
3.	2463618	913525	288037	1251122	1162955	476738	139861	543721	1300663	436787	148176	707401
3.1.	1066210	398005	151473	506574	539323	236276	73968	226790	526887	161729	77505	279784
3.2.	55867	17737	2734	35324	7577	1556	212	5789	48290	16181	2522	29535
3.3.	322269	73508	12746	235979	111875	32081	6891	72892	210394	41427	5855	163087
3.4.	8559	3119	1568	3867	5384	1970	856	2553	3175	1149	712	1314
3.5.	1007115	419741	119095	467733	497065	204081	57691	235038	510050	215660	61404	232695
3.6.	3598	1415	421	1645	1731	774	243	659	1867	641	178	986

Azerbajdžanskaja SSR

	A.	B.	C.	D.	A.	B.	C.	D.	A.	B.	C.	D.
1.	5116525	2662635	1188076	1253528	2483631	1346408	571693	562276	2632894	1316227	616383	691252
1.1.	1774737	914485	486630	364556	986293	563884	258534	162050	788444	350601	228096	202506
1.2.	61423	24301	7108	29737	6103	1839	251	3944	55320	22462	6857	25793
1.3.	438229	214037	50700	173141	155814	84138	20524	50981	282415	129899	30176	122160
1.4.	64095	27552	27294	9209	39325	17047	15112	7139	24770	10505	12182	2070
1.5.	2771249	1478534	614786	675491	1292954	677757	276504	337607	1478295	800777	338282	337884
1.6.	6792	3726	1558	1394	3142	1743	768	555	3650	1983	790	839
2.	2549597	1643091	840564	60093	1247303	834458	382265	29012	1302294	808633	458299	31081
2.1.	994337	597655	380592	12252	571827	381783	183627	5721	422510	215872	196965	6531
2.2.	7126	4495	984	1471	815	492	62	208	6311	4003	922	1263
2.3.	221425	158932	45805	16463	89208	64294	18241	6557	132217	94638	27564	9926
2.4.	59750	25897	26439	7378	36325	15903	14604	5795	23425	9994	11835	1583
2.5.	1262878	853481	385568	22232	547162	370734	165159	10648	715716	482747	220409	11684
2.6.	4081	2631	1176	177	1966	1252	572	83	2115	1379	604	94

442

Social Structure 7.4
Soziale Struktur

	Both sexes-beide Geschlechter-Oba pola				Males-Männer-Mužčiny				Females-Frauen-Ženščiny			
	A.	B.	C.	D.	A.	B.	C.	D.	A.	B.	C.	D.
3.	2566928	1019544	347512	1199435	1236328	511950	189428	533264	1330600	507594	158084	660171
3.1.	780400	316830	106038	352304	414466	182101	74907	156329	365934	134729	31131	195975
3.2.	54297	19806	6124	28266	5288	1347	189	3736	49009	18459	5935	24530
3.3.	216804	55105	4895	156658	66606	19844	2283	44424	150198	35261	2612	112234
3.4.	4345	1655	855	1831	3000	1144	508	1344	1345	511	347	487
3.5.	1508371	625053	229218	653159	745792	307023	111345	326959	762579	318030	117873	326200
3.6.	2711	1095	382	1217	1176	491	196	472	1535	604	186	745
Litovskaja SSR												
1.	3118941	1684664	605643	816822	1462850	827832	261702	368905	1656091	856832	343941	447917
1.1.	1531249	833930	365002	324137	787024	469079	151992	163592	744225	364851	213010	160545
1.2.	62835	42820	474	19456	7875	4179	35	3641	54960	38641	439	15815
1.3.	383249	171682	22760	187802	146658	71118	10789	64301	236591	100564	11971	123501
1.4.	59357	25186	15091	19042	28008	12377	6703	8909	31349	12809	8388	10133
1.5.	1073380	606558	200966	264664	489159	269501	91585	127678	584221	337057	109381	136986
1.6.	8871	4488	1350	1721	4126	1578	598	784	4745	2910	752	937
2.	1557731	1021170	496228	36466	733683	501549	215839	15119	824048	519621	280389	21347
2.1.	850719	547562	298357	2392	429616	300666	126753	1728	421103	246896	171604	664
2.2.	3451	3184	60	189	426	377	3	46	3025	2807	57	143
2.3.	124703	88534	19812	15916	48727	33729	9077	5751	75976	54805	10735	10165
2.4.	48728	21340	14029	13325	21919	10143	6042	5715	26809	11197	7987	7610
2.5.	525718	357694	163079	4430	231256	155705	73619	1780	294462	201989	89460	2650
2.6.	4412	2856	891	214	1739	929	345	99	2673	1927	546	115
3.	1561210	663494	109415	780356	729167	326283	45863	353786	832043	337211	63552	426570
3.1.	680530	286368	66645	321745	357408	168413	25239	161864	323122	117955	41406	159881
3.2.	59384	39636	414	19267	7449	3802	32	3595	51935	35834	382	15672
3.3.	258546	83148	2948	171886	97931	37389	1712	58550	160615	45759	1236	113336
3.4.	10629	3846	1062	5717	6089	2234	661	3194	4540	1612	401	2523
3.5.	547662	248864	37887	260234	257903	113796	17966	125898	289759	135068	19921	134336
Moldavskaja SSR												
1.	3569846	1295839	497073	1768791	1669166	652202	214328	799505	1900680	643637	282745	969286
1.1.	1788606	682266	300705	800926	868443	371578	126099	369298	920163	310688	174606	431628
1.2.	34782	9402	438	24638	4010	887	55	2956	30772	8515	383	21682
1.3.	345131	85000	27214	232681	124862	36999	12655	75110	220269	48001	14559	157571
1.4.	58765	17706	12786	28257	28023	8497	4932	14582	30742	9209	7854	13675

443

7.4 Social Structure / Soziale Struktur

	Both sexes-beide Geschlechter-Oba pola				Males-Männer-Mužčiny				Females-Frauen-Ženščiny			
	A.	B.	C.	D.	A.	B.	C.	D.	A.	B.	C.	D.
1.5.	1338608	499673	155190	681334	642119	233579	70262	337194	696489	266094	84928	344140
1.6.	3954	1792	740	955	1709	662	325	365	2245	1130	415	590
2.	1123512	672353	356795	91679	525339	331764	151957	40795	598173	340589	204838	50884
2.1.	597768	365737	210603	19990	295505	197619	88458	9156	302263	168118	122145	10834
2.2.	3789	2010	134	1567	347	207	17	92	3442	1803	117	1475
2.3.	99539	53056	23587	22799	42822	22873	10511	9403	56717	30183	13076	13396
2.4.	47986	14278	11727	21969	21250	6294	4380	10568	26736	7984	7347	11401
2.5.	372160	235957	110542	25165	164515	104316	48330	11524	207645	131641	61812	13641
2.6.	2270	1315	602	189	900	455	261	52	1370	860	341	137
3.	2446334	623486	140278	1677112	1143827	320438	62371	758710	1302507	303048	77907	918402
3.1.	1190838	316529	90102	780936	572938	173959	37641	360142	617900	142570	52461	420794
3.2.	30993	7392	304	23071	3663	680	38	2864	27330	6712	266	20207
3.3.	245592	31944	3627	209882	82040	14126	2144	65707	163552	17818	1483	144175
3.4.	10779	3428	1059	6288	6773	2203	552	4014	4006	1225	507	2274
3.5.	966448	263716	45048	656169	477604	129263	21932	325670	488844	134453	23116	330499
3.6.	1684	477	138	766	809	207	64	313	875	270	74	453

Latvijskaja SSR

	A.	B.	C.	D.	A.	B.	C.	D.	A.	B.	C.	D.
1.	2351903	1331971	600027	413523	1073060	648165	244270	179002	1278843	683806	355757	234521
1.1.	1258382	729741	363868	160189	626543	400199	141572	83802	631839	329542	222296	76387
1.2.	25816	13923	486	11343	3316	1380	21	1904	22500	12543	465	9439
1.3.	361686	191888	45915	123057	128610	72569	17957	37926	233076	119319	27958	85131
1.4.	35195	14744	14889	5504	18117	7813	7597	2699	17078	6931	7292	2805
1.5.	666546	379006	174104	113053	294456	165013	76830	52529	372090	213993	97274	60524
1.6.	4278	2669	765	377	2018	1191	293	142	2260	1478	472	235
2.	1463872	930863	502447	27542	669067	451718	206093	10532	794805	479145	296354	17010
2.1.	850351	538134	305719	4597	415432	290582	120946	3549	434919	247552	184773	1048
2.2.	995	828	31	121	128	117	5	3	867	711	26	118
2.3.	178203	123721	39295	14653	61356	43019	14793	3456	116847	80702	24502	11197
2.4.	29167	12034	13951	3147	14809	6259	7028	1518	14358	5775	6923	1629
2.5.	402319	254313	142797	4926	176013	110895	63077	1981	226306	143418	79720	2945
2.6.	2837	1833	654	93	1329	846	244	25	1508	987	410	73
3.	888031	401108	97580	385981	403993	196447	38177	168470	484038	204661	59403	217511
3.1.	408031	191607	58149	155592	211111	109617	20626	80253	196920	81990	37523	75339
3.2.	24821	13095	455	11222	3188	1263	16	1901	21633	11832	439	9321

444

Social Structure 7.4
Soziale Struktur

	Both sexes-beide Geschlechter-Oba pola				Males-Männer-Mužčiny				Females-Frauen-Ženščiny			
	A.	B.	C.	D.	A.	B.	C.	D.	A.	B.	C.	D.
3.3.	183483	68167	6620	108404	67254	29550	3164	34470	116229	38617	3456	73934
3.4.	6028	2710	938	2357	3308	1554	569	1181	2720	1156	369	1176
3.5.	264227	124693	31307	108127	118443	54118	13753	50548	145784	70575	17554	57579
3.6.	1441	836	111	279	689	345	49	117	752	491	62	162
Kirgizskaja SSR												
1.	2933732	1517173	573585	833711	1402186	753375	259581	386785	1531546	763798	314004	446926
1.1.	1123774	602328	261791	252430	579566	338837	115515	123715	544208	263491	146276	128715
1.2.	20642	9735	1413	9415	1950	753	44	1118	18692	8982	1369	8297
1.3.	281304	134375	24611	122170	113167	59862	12444	40798	168137	74513	12167	81372
1.4.	39126	15366	14528	9220	18575	7320	6226	5021	20551	8046	8302	4199
1.5.	1465176	753119	270558	439858	687373	345652	125068	215925	777803	407467	145490	223933
1.6.	3710	2250	684	618	1555	951	284	208	2155	1299	400	410
2.	1095444	724127	333586	35190	514626	356965	141597	15351	580818	367162	191989	19839
2.1.	489867	314225	169829	4125	250494	178565	69066	2500	239373	135660	100763	1625
2.2.	2079	1520	208	309	270	198	4	42	1809	1322	204	267
2.3.	97768	67710	18448	11519	42408	29777	8792	3815	55360	37933	9656	7704
2.4.	34861	13363	13444	8042	16103	6109	5754	4232	18758	7254	7690	3810
2.5.	468807	325922	131211	11041	204547	141784	57807	4704	264260	184138	73404	6337
2.6.	2062	1387	446	154	804	532	174	58	1258	855	272	96
3.	1838288	793046	239999	798521	887560	396410	117984	371434	950728	396636	122015	427087
3.1.	633907	288103	91962	248305	329072	160272	46449	121215	304835	127831	45513	127090
3.2.	18563	8215	1205	9106	1680	555	40	1076	16883	7660	1165	8030
3.3.	183536	66665	6163	110651	70759	30085	3652	36983	112777	36580	2511	73668
3.4.	4265	2003	1084	1178	2472	1211	472	789	1793	792	612	389
3.5.	996369	427197	139347	428817	482826	203868	67261	211221	513543	223329	72086	217596
3.6.	1648	863	238	464	751	419	110	150	897	444	128	314
Tadžikskaja SSR												
1.	2899317	1171877	528298	1189529	1426928	614770	265227	545135	1471389	557107	263071	644394
1.1.	1003906	421381	219341	356679	551634	271435	118337	160929	452272	149935	101004	195750
1.2.	67645	17743	5063	44582	3302	719	132	2411	64343	17024	4931	42171
1.3.	222148	67172	17707	137052	93680	30382	9269	53921	128468	36790	8438	83131
1.4.	37444	14133	12660	10629	25970	9181	7443	9324	11474	4952	5217	1305
1.5.	1560334	648966	272523	637363	749137	301774	129556	317186	811197	347192	142967	320177
1.6.	6840	2493	1004	3224	3205	1279	490	1364	3635	1214	514	1860

445

7.4 Social Structure / Soziale Struktur

	Both sexes-beide Geschlechter-Oba pola				Males-Männer-Mužčiny				Females-Frauen-Ženščiny			
	A.	B.	C.	D.	A.	B.	C.	D.	A.	B.	C.	D.
2.	1073506	708799	317083	44671	526361	359120	142290	24412	547145	349679	174793	20259
2.1.	431530	269931	152467	7226	234610	164454	65979	4019	196920	105477	86488	3207
2.2.	9525	6128	1242	1963	520	319	35	137	9005	5809	1207	1826
2.3.	71953	47551	13704	10618	32688	20570	6720	5346	39265	26981	6984	5272
2.4.	33826	12857	12173	8774	23080	8144	7144	7770	10746	4713	5029	1004
2.5.	524816	371150	136977	15961	234656	165113	62217	7057	290160	206037	74760	8904
2.6.	1856	1182	520	129	807	520	195	83	1049	662	325	46
3.	1824811	463078	211215	1144858	900567	255650	122937	520723	924244	207428	88278	624135
3.1.	572376	151439	66874	349453	317024	106981	52358	156910	255352	44458	14516	192543
3.2.	58120	11615	3821	42619	2782	400	97	2274	55338	11215	3724	40345
3.3.	150195	19621	4003	126434	60992	9812	2549	48575	89203	9809	1454	77859
3.4.	3618	1276	487	1855	2890	1037	299	1554	728	239	188	301
3.5.	1035518	277816	135546	621402	514481	136661	67339	310129	521037	141155	68207	311273
3.6.	4984	1311	484	3095	2398	759	295	1281	2586	552	189	1814

Armjanskaja SSR

	A.	B.	C.	D.	A.	B.	C.	D.	A.	B.	C.	D.
1.	2492616	1446098	604553	427133	1217463	734756	283583	196755	1275153	711342	320970	230378
1.1.	980149	551735	285383	132644	526844	324583	138285	62852	453296	227152	147098	69792
1.2.	21225	9500	1334	8807	1930	799	69	934	19295	8701	1265	7873
1.3.	206276	114936	26504	64005	76286	46173	10649	19246	129990	68763	15855	44759
1.4.	38444	13671	20037	4652	21588	7768	10771	2991	16856	5903	9266	1661
1.5.	1239712	752194	269797	215946	587339	353228	123229	110136	652373	398966	146568	105810
1.6.	6819	4062	1498	1079	3476	2205	580	596	3343	1857	918	483
2.	1472723	953006	484216	29628	721546	484929	221185	14493	751177	468077	263031	15135
2.1.	618152	372549	235261	6339	338790	223927	110344	4178	279362	148622	124917	2161
2.2.	2559	1592	433	382	274	173	32	52	2285	1419	401	330
2.3.	113324	78671	23893	10116	45378	32909	9252	3060	67946	45762	14641	7056
2.4.	34571	12086	19146	3255	19095	6736	10195	2106	15476	5350	8951	1149
2.5.	700113	485518	204318	9434	315992	219751	90917	5053	384121	265767	113401	4381
2.6.	4004	2590	1165	102	2017	1433	445	44	1987	1157	720	58
3.	1019893	493092	120337	397505	495917	249827	62398	182262	523976	243265	57939	215243
3.1.	361988	179186	50122	126305	188054	100656	27941	58674	173934	78530	22181	67631
3.2.	18666	7908	901	8425	1656	626	37	882	17010	7282	864	7543
3.3.	92952	36265	2611	53889	30908	13264	1397	16186	62044	23001	1214	37703
3.4.	3873	1585	891	1397	2493	1032	576	885	1380	553	315	512

Social Structure
Soziale Struktur 7.4

	Both sexes-beide Geschlechter-Oba pola				Males-Männer-Mužčiny				Females-Frauen-Ženščiny			
	A.	B.	C.	D.	A.	B.	C.	D.	A.	B.	C.	D.
3.5.	539599	266676	65479	206512	271347	133477	32312	105083	268252	133199	33167	101429
3.6.	2815	1472	333	977	1459	772	135	552	1356	700	198	425

Turkmenskaja SSR

	A.	B.	C.	D.	A.	B.	C.	D.	A.	B.	C.	D.
1.1.	2152534	860366	479778	800549	1059540	448703	234955	373765	1092994	411663	244823	426784
1.1.	800529	330107	194930	264541	435803	213418	101697	119002	364726	116689	93233	145539
1.2.	14691	4774	1312	8550	1812	306	32	1461	12879	4468	1280	7089
1.3.	159428	56128	15251	87933	63977	23188	7290	33438	95451	32940	7961	54495
1.4.	27384	9358	11691	6292	17566	5902	6639	4986	9818	3456	5052	1306
1.5.	1147948	458883	255916	432496	539186	205349	118943	214591	608762	253534	136973	217905
1.6.	2554	1116	678	737	1196	540	354	287	1358	576	324	450
2.	1028429	654572	345910	24047	509400	336545	158288	13977	519029	318027	187622	10070
2.1.	419143	256347	153773	5622	237564	162859	70662	3689	181579	93488	83111	1933
2.2.	2884	2228	401	208	187	141	6	33	2697	2087	395	175
2.3.	67561	48059	13760	5670	29152	19368	6459	3298	38409	28691	7301	2372
2.4.	25057	8859	11260	4897	15529	5459	6311	3722	9528	3400	4949	1175
2.5.	512372	338214	166222	7614	226307	148308	74621	3222	286065	189906	91601	4392
2.6.	1412	865	494	36	661	410	229	13	751	455	265	23
3.	1124105	205794	133868	776502	550140	112158	76667	359788	573965	93636	57201	416714
3.1.	381386	73760	41157	258919	198239	50559	31035	115313	183147	23201	10122	143606
3.2.	11807	2546	911	8342	1625	165	26	1428	10182	2381	885	6914
3.3.	91867	8069	1491	82263	34825	3820	831	30140	57042	4249	660	52123
3.4.	2327	499	431	1395	2037	443	328	1264	290	56	103	131
3.5.	635576	120669	89694	424882	312879	57041	44322	211369	322697	63628	45372	213513
3.6.	1142	251	184	701	535	130	125	274	607	121	59	427

Estonskaja SSR

	A.	B.	C.	D.	A.	B.	C.	D.	A.	B.	C.	D.
1.	1354613	813574	360081	177811	619927	396129	147463	75379	734686	417445	212618	102432
1.1.	722396	439399	218445	63480	361337	240956	85570	34452	361059	198443	132875	29028
1.2.	9666	5016	206	4324	1523	804	26	661	8143	4212	180	3663
1.3.	213362	125103	27162	60092	72841	45453	10136	17021	140521	79650	17026	43071
1.4.	18731	9203	7031	2489	8431	4193	3048	1182	10300	5010	3983	1307
1.5.	387719	233241	106787	47173	174614	104007	48515	21980	213105	129234	58272	25193
1.6.	2739	1612	450	253	1181	716	168	83	1558	896	282	170

447

7.4 Social Structure / Soziale Struktur

	both sexes-beide Geschlechter-Oba pola				Males-Männer-Mužčiny				Females-Frauen-Ženščiny			
	A.	B.	C.	D.	A.	B.	C.	D.	A.	B.	C.	D.
2.	876610	564382	297604	13254	400690	273349	121933	5020	475920	291033	175671	8234
2.1.	505064	321261	181108	2367	245999	172589	71335	1982	259065	148673	109773	385
2.2.	475	359	26	76	96	86	6	—	379	273	20	76
2.3.	106218	75501	23004	7161	35821	25648	8392	1670	70397	49853	14612	5491
2.4.	15168	7290	6460	1410	6415	3161	2704	542	8753	4129	3756	868
2.5.	248160	158990	86667	2213	111679	71468	39358	817	136481	87522	47309	1396
2.6.	1525	981	339	27	680	398	138	9	845	583	201	18
3.	478003	249192	62477	164557	219237	122780	25530	70359	258766	126412	36947	94198
3.1.	217332	118138	37337	61113	115338	68368	14235	32470	101994	49770	23102	28643
3.2.	9191	4657	180	4248	1427	718	20	661	7764	3939	160	3587
3.3.	107144	49602	4158	52931	37020	19805	1744	15351	70124	29797	2414	37580
3.4.	3563	1913	571	1079	2016	1032	344	640	1547	881	227	439
3.5.	139559	74251	20120	44960	62935	32539	9157	21163	76624	41712	10963	23797
3.6.	1214	631	111	226	501	318	30	74	713	313	81	152

Social Structure
Soziale Struktur 7.5

7.5 SOCIAL STRUCTURE OF THE POPULATION OF THE UNION REPUBLICS (in percentage)
SOZIALE STRUKTUR DER BEVÖLKERUNG DER UNIONSREPUBLIKEN (in Prozent)
SOCIAL'NAJA STRUKTURA NASELENIJA SOJUZNYCH RESPUBLIK (v procentach)
1 9 3 9

Republics – Republiken – Respublika	Total population – Gesamtbevölkerung – Vse naselenie				Main nation – Hauptnation – Korennaja nacional'nost'			
	Workers and employees Arbeiter u. Angestellte Rabočie i služaščie	Workers Arbeiter Rabočie	Employees Angestellte Služaščie	Collect. farmers Kolchos- bauern Kolchoz- niki	Other social groups Andere sozia- le Gruppen Drugie social' nye gruppy	Workers and employees Arbeiter u. Angestellte Rabočie i služaščie	Workers Arbeiter Rabočie	Employees Angestellte Služaščie	Collect. farmers Kolchos- bauern Kolchoz- niki	Other social groups Andere sozia- le Gruppen Drugie social' nye gruppy
SSSR	50.2	32.5	17.7	47.2	2.6	--	--	--	--	--
RSFSR	53.6	35	18.6	43.9	2.5	56.9	38.2	18.7	38.5	4.6
Ukrainskaja SSR	49.8	32.6	17.2	48.7	1.5	42.4	29.3	13.1	54.6	3.0
Belorusskaja SSR	36.4	21.9	14.5	57.2	6.4	31.5	20.7	10.8	60.4	8.1
Gruzinskaja SSR	36.7	19.5	17.2	52.7	10.6	29.4	12.4	17.0	58.2	12.4
Azerbajdžan- skaja SSR	41.7	25.1	16.6	54.2	4.1	21.7	12.2	9.5	70.1	8.2
Armjanskaja SSR	32.2	17.6	14.6	64.1	3.7	41.3	21.5	19.7	52.5	6.2
Uzbekskaja SSR	32.2	19.3	12.9	64.9	2.9	16.5	11.1	5.4	79.6	3.9
Turkmenskaja SSR	40.6	25.2	15.4	56.3	3.1	17.7	11.7	6.1	77.2	5.1
Tadžikskaja SSR	23.1	12.9	10.2	72.5	4.4	14.4	8.7	5.7	79.2	6.4
Kazachskaja SSR	51.2	33.8	17.4	47.5	1.3	33.6	25.6	8.0	60.8	5.6
Kirgizskaja SSR	33.7	21.3	12.4	62.2	4.1	12.1	7.5	4.6	83.8	4.1

449

7.6 Social Structure / Soziale Struktur

7.6 SOCIAL STRUCTURE OF THE POPULATION OF THE UNION REPUBLICS (in percentage)
SOZIALE STRUKTUR DER BEVÖLKERUNG DER UNIONSREPUBLIKEN (in Prozent)
SOCIAL'NAJA STRUKTURA NASELENIJA SOJUZNYCH RESPUBLIK (v procentach)
1 9 5 9

Republics – Republiken	Total population – Gesamtbevölkerung – Vse naselenie			Main nation – Hauptnation – Korennaja nacional'nost'			
	Workers and employees Arbeiter u. Angestellte Rabočie i služaščie	Workers Arbeiter Rabočie	Employees Angestellte Služaščie	Collective farmers a.o. Kolchosbauern u.a. Kolchozniki i.pr.	Workers and employees Arbeiter u. Angestellte Rabočie i služaščie	Workers-Arbeiter-Rabočie: Total Insg. Vsego / Industrial workers Industriearbeiter v promyšlennosti	Employees Angestellte Služaščie	Collective farmers a.o. Kolchosbauern u.a. Kolchozniki i.pr.

Republics	W+E	W	E	CF	W+E	Total	Ind.	E	CF
RSFSR	76	54	22	24	76	54	23	22	24
Ukrainskaja SSR	58	41	17	42	47	34	15	13	53
Belorusskaja SSR	51	35	16	49	43	31	11	12	57
Uzbekskaja SSR	57	40	17	43	35	27	4	8	65
Kazachskaja SSR	79	58	21	21	60	44	6	16	40
Gruzinskaja SSR	56	32	24	44	45	22	10	23	55
Azerbajdžanskaja SSR	57	35	22	43	39	24	8	15	51
Litovskaja SSR	56	40	16	44	48	34	12	14	52
Moldavskaja SSR	32	21	11	68	17	13	4	4	83
Latvijskaja SSR	73	51	22	27	65	46	19	19	35
Kirgizskaja SSR	58	40	18	42	30	22	4	8	70
Tadžikskaja SSR	46	30	16	54	26	18	4	8	74
Armjanskaja SSR	62	40	22	38	60	38	17	22	40
Turkmenskaja SSR	57	37	21	42	31	22	5	9	69
Estonskaja SSR	79	55	24	21	73	51	19	22	27
Total: U.S.S.R. 1959 Insg.: UdSSR 1959 Itogo: po SSSR 1959 g.	68	48	20	32					
1939 (for comparison – zum Vergleich – dlja sravnenija)	50	32	18	50					

450

8. SCIENCE – WISSENSCHAFT – NAUKA

8.1 ACADEMY OF SCIENCES OF THE USSR, ACADEMIES OF SCIENCES OF THE UNION REPUBLICS AND BRANCH ACADEMIES
AKADEMIE DER WISSENSCHAFTEN DER UdSSR, AKADEMIEN DER WISSENSCHAFTEN DER UNIONSREPUBLIKEN UND BRANCHENAKADEMIEN
AKADEMIJA NAUK SSSR, AKADEMII NAUK SOJUZNYCH RESPUBLIK I OTRASLEVYE AKADEMII
(end of 1975 – Stand: Ende 1975)

Academies of Sciences of – Akademien der Wissenschaften der Akademii Nauk	A. Year of foundation – Gründungsjahr – God osnovanija	B. Number of full and corresponding members – Zahl der ordentlichen u. korrespondierenden Mitglieder – Čislo dejstvitel'nych členov i členov-korrespondentov	C. Number of scientific institutions of the academy – Zahl d. wissenschaftlichen Institutionen der Akademie – Čislo naučnych učreždenij prinadležaščich akademii	D. Number of scientific staff of these institutions (not counting persons occupying several posts simultaneously) – Zahl d.wissenschaftl.Mitarbeiter dieser Institutionen (ohne Personen, die mehrere Posten zugleich bekleiden) – Čislo naučnych rabotnikov etich učreždenij (bez sovmestitelej)	E. of which – davon – iz nich Doctors of sciences – Doktoren der Wissenschaften – Doktora nauk	F. Candidates of sciences – Kandidaten der Wissenschaften – Kandidaty nauk
SSSR	1724	678	246	41,836	3,633	18,553
Ukrainskaja SSR	1919	282	76	12,102	822	5,465
Belorusskaja SSR	1928	131	33	4,640	173	1,263
Uzbekskaja SSR	1943	96	31	3,699	172	1,524
Kazachskaja SSR	1945	132	33	3,731	177	1,493
Gruzinskaja SSR	1941	109	40	5,493	332	1,733
Azerbajdžanskaja SSR	1945	90	32	4,222	244	1,685
Litovskaja SSR	1941	39	12	1,534	53	707
Moldavskaja SSR	1961	37	19	883	56	492
Latvijskaja SSR	1946	52	16	1,760	68	702
Kirgizskaja SSR	1954	44	19	1,434	60	526
Tadžikskaja SSR	1951	42	19	1,213	47	476
Armjanskaja SSR	1943	90	31	2,835	170	898

8.1 Science / Wissenschaft

	A.	B.	C.	D.	E.	F.
Turkmenskaja SSR	1951	49	16	866	35	393
Estonskaja SSR	1946	44	16	949	56	500
Academy of Arts of the USSR – Akademie der Künste der UdSSR – Akademija chodožestv SSSR	1947	130	5	386	18	134
All-Union V.I.Lenin Academy of Agricultural Sciences – V.I.Lenin-Unionsakademie für Agrarwissenschaften – Vsesojuznaja akademija sel'skochozjajstvennych nauk imeni V.I.Lenina	1929	211	166	10,339	429	5,133
Academy of Medical Sciences of the USSR – Akademie der Medizinischen Wissenschaften der UdSSR – Akademija medicinskich nauk SSSR	1944	271	40	5,480	862	3,201
Academy of Pedagogical Sciences of the USSR – Akademie der Pädagogischen Wissenschaften der UdSSR – Akademija pedagogičeskich nauk SSSR	1943	131	14	1,711	122	749
Academy of Communal Economy of the RSFSR – Akademie für Kommunalwirtschaft der RSFSR – Akademija kommunal'nogo chozjajstva RSFSR	1931	--	5	427	10	216

8.2 SCIENTIFIC CENTERS OF THE ACADEMY OF SCIENCES - WISSENSCHAFTLICHE ZENTREN DER AKADEMIE DER WISSENSCHAFTEN - NAUČNYE CENTRY AKADEMIJ NAUK
(end of 1975 - Stand: Ende 1975)

	A. Number of scientific institutions - Zahl der wissenschaftlichen Institutionen - Čislo naučnych učreždenij	B. Number of scientific staff (not counting persons occup. several posts simultaneously) Zahl der wissenschaftlichen Mitarbeiter (ohne Personen, die mehrere Posten zugleich bekleiden) - Čislo naučnych rabotnikov v nich (bez sovmestitelej)	C. of which - davon - of which - iz nich Doctors of sciences - Doktoren d.Wissenschaften - doktora nauk	D. Candidates of sciences - Kandidaten d.Wissenschaften - kandidaty nauk
Siberian Department of the Academy of Sciences of the USSR - Sibirische Abteilung der Akademie der Wissenschaften der UdSSR - Sibirskoe otdelenie Akademii nauk SSSR Prospekt Nauki 21, Novosibirsk; Chairman-Vorsitzender-predsedatel': G.I.MARČUK	51	6,234	397	3,043
Branches - Filialen - Filialy: Buriat - Burjatische - Burjatskij ul. Fabričnaja 6, Ulan-Ude; Chairman of the presidium-Vorsitzender des Präsidiums - Predsedatel' prezidiuma: M.V.MOCHOSOEV	4	264	12	142
East Siberian - Ostsibirische - Vostočno-Sibirskij ul. Lenina 5, Irkutsk 33; Chairman-Vorsitzender-predsedatel': V.B.SOČAVA	9	1,045	47	462
Jakutsk - Jakutische - Jakutskij ul. Petrovskogo 36, Jakutsk; Chairman-Vorsitzender-predsedatel': N.V.ČERSKIJ	6	512	19	213

Science 8.2
Wissenschaft

453

8.2 Science / Wissenschaft

	A.	B.	C.	D.
Scientific Centers of the Academy of Sciences of the USSR – Wissenschaftliche Zentren der Akademie der Wissenschaften der UdSSR – Naučnye centry Akademii Nauk SSSR:				
Far Eastern – Fernost – Dal'nevostočnyj ul. Leninskaja 50, Vladivostok Chairman-Vorsitzender-predsedatel': N.A.ŠILO	18	1,912	71	759
Urals – Ural – Ural'skij ul. Pervomajskaja 91, Sverdlovsk Chairman-Vorsitzender-predsedatel': S.V.VONSOVSKIJ	15	1,718	97	683
Branches of the Academy of Sciences of the USSR – Filialen der Akademie der Wissenschaften der UdSSR – Filialy Akademii nauk SSSR:				
Bashkir – Baschkirische – Baškirskij, ul. K.Marksa 6, Ufa Chairman-Vorsitzender-predsedatel': S.R.RAFIKOV	8	475	26	214
Daghestan – Dagestanische – Dagestanskij ul. Gadžieva 45, Machačkala; Chairman-Vorsitzender-predsedatel': K.I.AMIRCHANOV	4	352	12	137
Karelian – Karelische – Karelskij ul. Puškinskaja 11, Petrozavodsk; Chairman-Vorsitzender-predsedatel': V.A.SOKOLOV	8	347	16	179
Kola – Kol'skij Murmanskaja oblast, Apatity, ul. Fersmana 14 Chairman-Vorsitzender-predsedatel': G.J.GORBUNOV	8	768	12	220
Komi ul. Kommunističeskaja 24, Komi ASSR, Syktyvkar; Chairman-Vorsitzender-predsedatel': V.P.PODOPLELOV	4	288	8	113
Kazan – Kazanskij, ul. Lobačevskogo 2/31, Kazan Chairman-Vorsitzender: M.M.ZARIPOV	5	504	27	258
Karakalpaks Branch of the Academy of Sciences of the Uzbek SSR – Karakalpakische Filiale der Akademie der Wissenschaften der Usbekischen SSR – Karakalpaksij filial Akademii nauk Uzbekskoj SSR	3	182	8	120

Science
Wissenschaft 8.

Organizational Chart of the Academy of Sciences of the U.S.S.R.

GENERAL ASSEMBLY OF THE ACADEMY OF SCIENCES OF THE U.S.S.R.
GENERALVERSAMMLUNG DER AKADEMIE DER WISSENSCHAFTEN DER UdSSR
OBŠČEE SOBRANIE AKADEMII NAUK SSSR

PRESIDIUM OF THE ACADEMY OF SCIENCES OF THE U.S.S.R.
PRÄSIDIUM DER AKADEMIE DER WISSENSCHAFTEN DER UdSSR
PRESIDIUM AKADEMII NAUK SSSR

Sections

- **SECTION OF PHYSICAL-TECHNICAL AND MATHEMATICAL SCIENCES**
  SEKTION DER PHYSIKOTECHNISCHEN U. MATHEMATISCHEN WISSENSCHAFTEN
  SEKCIJA FIZIKO-TECHNIČESKICH I MATEMATIČESKICH NAUK

- **SECTION OF CHEMISTRY, CHEMICAL TECHNOLOGY AND BIOLOGY**
  SEKTION DER CHEMIKO-TECHNOLOG. U. BIOLOGISCHEN WISSENSCHAFTEN
  SEKCIJA CHIMIKO-TECHNOLOGIČESKICH I BIOLOGIČESKICH NAUK

- **SECTION OF EARTH SCIENCES**
  SEKTION DER WISSENSCHAFTEN ÜBER DIE ERDKUGEL
  SEKCIJA NAUK O ZEMLE

- **SECTION OF SOCIAL SCIENCES**
  SEKTION DER GESELLSCHAFTSWISSENSCHAFT.
  SEKCIJA OBŠČESTVENNYCH NAUK

Each section has:
- SCIENTIFIC COUNCILS ON PROBLEMS, COMMISSIONS, SCIENTIFIC SOCIETIES — WISSENSCHAFTL. RÄTE FÜR PROBLEME, KOMMISSIONEN, WISSENSCHAFTL. GESELLSCHAFTEN — NAUČNYE SOVETY PO PROBLEMAM, KOMISSII, NAUČNYE OBŠČESTVA

DEPARTMENTS — ABTEILUNGEN — OTDELENIJA

- GENERAL & TECHNICAL CHEMISTRY — ALLGEMEINE U. TECHN. CHEMIE — OBŠČEJ I TECHNIČESKOJ CHIMII
- PHYSICAL CHEMISTRY & TECHNOLOGY OF INORGANIC MATERIALS — PHYSIKO-CHEMIE UND TECHNOLOGIE D. ANORGANISCHEN MATERIAL. — FIZIKO-CHIMII I TECHNOLOGII NEORGANIČESKICH MATERIAL.
- BIOCHEMISTRY, BIOPHYSICS & CHEMISTRY OF PHYSIOLOGICALLY ACTIVE COMP. — BIOCHEMIE, BIOPHYSIK U. CHEMIE D. PHYSIOLOGISCH AKTIVEN VERBINDUNGEN — BIOCHIMII, BIOFIZIKI I CHIMII FIZIOLOGIČESKI AKTIVNYCH SOEDINENIJ
- PHYSIOLOGY — PHYSIOLOGIE — FIZIOLOGII
- GENERAL BIOLOGY — ALLGEMEINE BIOLOGIE — OBŠČEJ BIOLOGII
- GEOLOGY, GEOPHYSICS AND GEOCHEMISTRY — GEOLOGIE, GEOPHYSIK U. GEOCHEMIE — GEOLOGII, GEOFIZIKI I GEOCHIMII
- OCEANOLOGY AND ATMOSPHERIC PHYSICS — MEERESKUNDE, GEOGRAPHIE & PHYSIK D. ATMOSPH. — OKEANOLOGII, GEOGRAFII I FIZIKI ATMOSFERY

- INSTITUTES AND OTHER SCIENTIFIC INSTITUTIONS — INSTITUTE U. ANDERE WISS. INSTITUTIONEN — INSTITUTY I DRUGIE NAUČNYE UČREŽDENIJA
- SCIENTIFIC COUNCILS IN THE DEPARTMENTS — WISSENSCHAFTL. RÄTE BEI DEN ABTEILUNGEN — NAUČNYE SOVETY PRI OTDELENIJACH

DEPARTMENTS — ABTEILUNGEN — OTDELENIJA

- MATHEMATICS — MATHEMATIK — MATEMATIKI
- GENERAL PHYSICS AND ASTRONOMY — ALLG. PHYSIK U. ASTRONOMIE — OBŠČEJ FIZIKI I ASTRONOMII
- NUCLEAR PHYSICS — KERNPHYSIK — JADERNOJ FIZIKI
- PHYSICAL & TECHNICAL PROBLEMS OF ENERGY — PHYSIKO-TECHNISCHE PROBLEME D. ENERGETIK — FIZIKO-TECHNIČESKICH PROBLEM ENERGETIKI
- MECHANICS AND CONTROL PROCESSES — MECHANIK U. STEUERUNGSPROZESSE — MECHANIKI I PROCESSOV UPRAVLEN.
- HISTORY — GESCHICHTE — ISTORII
- PHILOSOPHY AND LAW — PHILOSOPHIE UND RECHT — FILOSOFII I PRAVA
- ECONOMICS — WIRTSCHAFT — EKONOMIKI
- LITERATURE & LINGUISTICS — LITERATUR U. SPRACHE — LITERATURY I JAZYKA

- INSTITUTES AND OTHER SCIENTIFIC INSTITUTIONS — INSTITUTE U. ANDERE WISS. INSTITUTIONEN — INSTITUTY I DRUGIE NAUČNYE UČREŽDENIJA
- SCIENTIFIC COUNCILS IN THE DEPARTMENTS — WISSENSCHAFTL. RÄTE BEI DEN ABTEILUNGEN — NAUČNYE SOVETY PRI OTDELENIJACH

SIBERIAN DEPARTMENT OF THE ACADEMY OF SCIENCES OF THE U.S.S.R.
SIBIRISCHE ABTEILUNG DER AKADEMIE DER WISSENSCHAFTEN DER UdSSR
SIBIRSKOE OTDELENIE AKADEMII NAUK SSSR

- BRANCHES OF THE SIBERIAN DEPARTMENT OF THE ACADEMY OF SCIENCES OF THE U.S.S.R. — FILIALEN DER SIBIRISCHEN ABTEILUNG DER AKADEMIE DER WISSENSCHAFTEN DER UdSSR — FILIALY SIBIRSKOGO OTDELENIJA AKADEMII NAUK SSSR
- INSTITUTES AND OTHER SCIENTIFIC INSTITUTIONS — INSTITUTE U. ANDERE WISSENSCH. INSTITUTIONEN — INSTITUTY I DRUGIE NAUČNYE UČREŽDENIJA
- JOINT SCIENTIFIC COUNCILS BY SCIENCE BRANCHES, SCIENTIFIC COUNCILS ON PROBLEMS, COMMISSIONS — VEREINIGTE WISS. RÄTE NACH WISSENSCH. ZWEIGEN, WISS. RÄTE FÜR PROBLEME, KOMMISSIONEN — OB'EDINENNYE UČENYE SOVETY PO OTRASLJAM NAUK, NAUČNYE SOVETY PO PROBLEMAM, KOMISSII

SCIENTIFIC CENTERS AND BRANCHES OF THE ACADEMY OF SCIENCES OF THE U.S.S.R.
WISSENSCHAFTLICHE ZENTREN UND FILIALEN DER AKADEMIE DER WISSENSCHAFTEN DER UdSSR
NAUČNYE CENTRY I FILIALY AKADEMII NAUK SSSR

- INSTITUTES AND OTHER SCIENTIFIC INSTITUTIONS — INSTITUTE U. ANDERE WISS. INSTITUTIONEN — INSTITUTY I DRUGIE NAUČNYE UČREŽDENIJA

Other Bodies

- SCIENTIFIC COUNCILS ON PROBLEMS, COMMISSIONS, SCIENTIFIC SOCIETIES — WISS. RÄTE F. PROBLEME, KOMMISSIONEN, WISS. GESELLSCHAFTEN — NAUČNYE SOVETY PO PROBLEMAM, KOMISSII, NAUČNYE OBŠČESTVA
- SECTION OF APPLIED PROBLEMS — SEKTION DER ANGEWANDTEN PROBLEME — SEKCIJA PRIKLADNYCH PROBLEM
- INSTITUTES & OTH. SCIENTIFIC INSTITUTIONS — INSTITUTE U.A. WISSENSCHAFTL. INSTITUTIONEN — INSTITUTY I DRUGIE NAUČN. UČREŽDENIJA
- COUNCIL ON COORDINATION OF SCIENTIFIC ACTIVITIES OF ACADEMIES OF THE UNION REPUBLICS — RAT F.D. KOORDINIERUNG D. WISS. TÄTIGKEIT D. AKADEMIEN D. WISSENSCHAFTEN D. UNIONSREPUBLIKEN — SOVET PO KOORDINACII NAUČNOJ DEJATEL'NOSTI AKADEMIJ NAUK SOJUZNYCH RESPUBLIK
- EDITORIAL & PUBLISHERS' BOARD — REDAKTIONS- U. VERLAGSKOLLEGIUM — REDAKCIONNO-IZDATEL'SKIJ SOVET
- PUBLISHING HOUSE — VERLAG IZDATEL'STVO "NAUKA"
- PERMANENT EXHIBITION OF WORKS OF THE USSR ACADEMY OF SCIENCES ON EXHIBITION OF ACHIEVEMENTS OF THE NATIONAL ECONOMY — STÄNDIGE AUSSTELLUNG D. ARBEITEN D. AKADEMIE DER WISSENSCHAFTEN D. UdSSR AUF D. AUSSTELLUNG D. ERRUNGENSCHAFTEN D. VOLKSWIRTSCHAFT — POSTOJANNAJA VYSTAVKA RABOT AKADEMII NAUK SSSR NA VYSTAVKE DOSTIŽENIJ NARODNOGO CHOZJAJSTVA

8.3 Science
Wissenschaft

8.3 PERSONNEL COMPOSITION OF THE ACADEMY OF SCIENCES OF THE USSR
PERSONELLE ZUSAMMENSETZUNG DER AKADEMIE DER WISSENSCHAFTEN DER UdSSR
SOSTAV AKADEMII NAUK SSSR

Presidium - Präsidium - Prezidia
Leninskij Prospekt 14, Moskva V-71

President-Präsident-Prezident: ALEKSANDROV, A.P.

Vice-Presidents -
Vize-Präsidenten -
Vice-Prezidenty: FEDOSEEV, P.N.
KOTELNIKOV, V.A.
LOGUNOV, A.A.
MARČUK, G.I. (also Chairman, Siberian Department - glz.Vorsitzender der Sibirischen Abteilung)
OVČINNIKOV, Ju.A.
SIDORENKO, A.V.
VELICHOV, E.P.

Chief Learned Secretary -
Wissenschaftl.Generalsekretär -
Glavnyj učenyj sekretar': SKRJABIN, G.K.

Presidium members -
Mitglieder des Präsidiums -
Členy prezidiuma:

BAEV, A.A.	BASOV, N.G.
GOBOLJUBOV, N.N.	VONSOVSKIJ, S.V.
BRECHOVSKICH, L.M.	GLEBOV, I.A.
GILJAROV, M.S.	INOZEMCEV, M.N.
EGOROV, A.G.	KAPICA, A.P.
ŽAVORONKOV, N.M.	KAPICA, P.L.
ŽUKOV, E.M.	LAVRENTEV, M.A.
KOSTJUK, P.G.	MELNIKOV, N.V.
MARKOV, M.A.	NESMEJANOV, A.N.
PETROV, B.N.	PATON, B.E.
PROCHOROV, A.M.	PILJUGIN, N.A.
SOKOLOV, B.S.	POSPELOV, P.N.
STYRIKOVIČ, M.A.	SADYKOV, A.S.
FEDORENKO, N.P.	SEMENOV, N.N.
CHRAPČENKO, M.B.	TROFIMUK, A.A.
EMANUEL, N.M.	TUČKEVIČ, V.M.
AMBARCUMJAN, V.A.	ŠILO, N.N.

Sections and Departments - Sektionen und Abteilungen - Sekcii i otdelenija

Section of Physical-Technical and Mathematical Sciences -
Sektion der physikalisch-technischen und mathematischen Wissenschaften -
Sekcija fiziko-techničeskich i matematičeskich nauk
    Chairman: LOGUNOV, A.A.

   Department of Mathematics - Abteilung für Mathematik -
   Otdelenie matematiki
      Academician-Secretary - Wissenschaftl.Sekretär -
      Akademik-Sekretar': BOGOLJUBOV, N.N.

456

Science
Wissenschaft 8.3

Department of General Physics and Astronomy -
Abteilung für allgemeine Physik und Astronomie -
Otdelenie obščej fiziki i astronomii
Academician-Secretary-Wissenschaftl.Sekretär-
Akademik-Sekretar':   PROCHOROV, A.M.

Department of Physical and Technical Problems of Energy -
Abteilung für physikalisch-technische Probleme der Energetik -
Otdelenie fiziko-techničeskich problem energetiki
Academician-Secretary-Wissenschaftl.Sekretär-
Akademik-Sekretar':   STYRIKOVIČ, M.A.

Department of Mechanics and Control Processes -
Abteilung für Mechanik und Steuerungsprozesse -
Otdelenie mechaniki i processov upravlenija
Academician-Secretary-Wissenschaftl.Sekretär-
Akademik-Sekretar':   PETROV, B.N.

Section of Chemistry, Chemical Technology and Biology -
Sektion der chemisch-technologischen und biologischen Wissenschaften -
Sekcija chimiko-technologičeskich i biologičeskich nauk
Chairman: OVČINNIKOV, Ju.A.

Department of General and Technical Chemistry -
Abteilung für allgemeine und technische Chemie -
Otdelenie obščej i techničeskoj chimii
Academician-Secretary-Wissenschaftl.Sekretär-
Akademik-Sekretar':   EMANUEL, N.M.

Department of Physical Chemistry and Technology of Inorganic Materials -
Abteilung für physikalische Chemie und Technologie anorganischer Stoffe -
Otdelenie fiziko-chimii i technologii neorganičeskich materialov
Academician-Secretary-Wissenschaftl.Sekretär-
Akademik-Sekretar':   ŽAVORONKOV, N.M.

Department of Biochemistry, Biophysics and Chemistry of Physiologically
Active Compounds - Abteilung für Biochemie, Biophysik und Chemie physio-
logisch aktiver Verbindungen - Otdelenie biochimii, biofiziki i chimii
fiziologičeski aktivnych soedinenij
Academician-Secretary-Wissenschaftl.Sekretär-
Akademik-Sekretar':   BAEV, A.A.

Department of Physiology - Abteilung für Physiologie - Otdelenie fiziologii
Academician-Secretary-Wissenschaftl.Sekretär-
Akademik-Sekretar':   KOSTJUK, P.G.

Department of General Biology - Abteilung für allgemeine Biologie -
Otdelenie obščej biologii
Academician-Secretary-Wissenschaftl.Sekretär-
Akademik-Sekretar':   GILJAROV, M.S.

Section of Earth Sciences - Sektion der Erdwissenschaften - Sekcija nauk i Zemle
Chairman: SIDORENKO, A.V.

Department of Geology, Geophysics and Geochemistry -
Abteilung für Geologie, Geophysik und Geochemie -
Otdelenie geologii, geofiziki i geochimii
Academician-Secretary-Wissenschaftl.Sekretär-
Akademik-Sekretar':   SOKOLOV, B.S.

8.3 Science / Wissenschaft

Department of Oceanology, Atmospheric Physics and Geography -
Abteilung für Ozeanologie, physische Atmosphäre und Geographie -
Otdelenie okeanologii, fiziki atmosfery i geografii
  Academician-Secretary-Wissenschaftl.Sekretär-
  Akademik-Sekretar':   BRECHOVSKICH, L.M.

Section of Social Sciences - Sektion der Gesellschaftswissenschaften -
Sekcija obščestvennych nauk
  Chairman: FEDOSEEV, P.N.

Department of History - Abteilung für Geschichte -
Otdelenie istorii
  Academician-Secretary-Wissenschaftl.Sekretär-
  Akademik-Sekretar':   ŽUKOV, E.M.

Department of Philosophy and Law -
Abteilung für Philosophie und Recht -
Otdelenie filosofii i prava
  Academician-Secretary-Wissenschaftl.Sekretär-
  Akademik-Sekretar'   EGOROV, A.G.

Department of Economics - Abteilung für Wirtschafts-
wissenschaften - Otdelenie ekonomiki
  Academician-Secretary-Wissenschaftl.Sekretär-
  Akademik-Sekretar'   FEDORENKO, N.P.

Department of Literature and Linguistics -
Abteilung für Literatur und Sprache -
Otdelenie literatury i jazyka
  Academician-Secretary-Wissenschaftl.Sekretär-
  Akademik-Sekretar'   STEPANOV, G.V.

Members and Corresponding Members - Mitglieder u.korrespondierende Mitglieder -
členy i členy korrespondenty

Name	Date of Birth / Geburtsdatum	Special Branch / Fachgebiet

Section of Physical-Technical and Mathematical Sciences -
Sektion der physikalisch-technischen u.mathematischen Wissenschaften

a) Members-Mitglieder:

ALEKKSANDROV, A.D.	22.7.(4.8.)1912	Mathematician-Mathematiker
ALEKKSANDROV, A.P.	31.1.(13.2.)1903	Physicist-Physiker
ALEKSANDROV, P.S.	25.4.(7.5.)1896	Mathematician-Mathematiker
BARMIN, V.P.	4.(17.)3.1909	Specialist for mechanics - Spezialist für Mechanik
BASOV, N.G.	14.12.1922	Physicist-Physiker
BELJAEV, S.T.	27.10.1923	Nuclear physicist-Kernphysiker
BERG, A.I.	29.10.(10.11.)1893	Specialist for radio-engineering - Spezialist für Radiotechnik
BOGOLJUBOV, N.N.	8.(21.)8.1909)	Mathematician-Mathematiker
BOROVIK-ROMANOV, A.S.	18.3.1920	Physicist, Astronomer - Physiker, Astronom
BRUEVIČ, N.G.	31.10.(12.11.)1896	Specialist for mechanics - Spezialist für Mechanik
BUNKIN, B.V.	16.7.1922	Physicist,Specialist for radio-engineering - Physiker, Spezialist für Radiotechnik
CELIKOV, A.I.	7.(20.)4.1904	Specialist for mechanics - Spezialist für Mechanik

Science
Wissenschaft 8.3

ČELOMEJ, V.N.	17.(30.)6.1914	Specialist for mechanics - Spezialist für Mechanik
ČERENKOV, P.A.	15.(28.)7.1904	Nuclear physicist-Kernphysiker
CHARITON, J.B.	14.(27.)2.1904	Physicist-Physiker
CHOCHLOV, R.V.	15.7.1926	Specialist for radio-engineering - Spezialist für Radiotechnik
CHRISTIANOVIČ, S.A.	27.10.(9.11.)1908	Specialist for mechanics - Spezialist für Mechanik
DEVJATKOV, N.D.	29.3.(11.4.)1907	Specialist for electrical and radio engineering - Spezialist für Elektro- und Radiotechnik
DIKUŠIN, V.I.	26.7.(8.8.)1902	Specialist for mechanical engineering - Spezialist für Maschinenbau
DOLLEŽAL', N.A.	15.(27.)10.1899	Specialist for mechanics - Spezialist für Mechanik
FADDEEV, L.D.	1934	Mathematician-Mathematiker
FLEROV, G.N.	17.2.(2.3.)1913	Nuclear physicist-Kernphysiker
FRANK, I.M.	10.(23.)10.1908	Physicist-Physiker
GAPONOV-GRECHOV, A.V.	7.6.1926	Physicist,Specialist f.radio-engineering Physiker,Spezialist f.Radiotechnik
GINZBURG, V.L.	21.9.(4.10.)1916	Physicist-Physiker
GLEBOV, I.A.		Energetician-Energetiker
GLUŠKO, V.P.	20.8.(2.9.)1908	Specialist for thermics - Spezialist für Wärmetechnik
GLUŠKOV, V.M.	24.8.1923	Mathematician-Mathematiker
GRUŠIN, P.D.	15.(28.)1.1906	Specialist for mechanics - Spezialist für Mechanik
ISANIN, N.N.	9.(22.)4.1904	Specialist for ship-building - Spezialist für Schiffbau
IŠLINSKIJ, A.J.	24.7.(6.8.)1913	Specialist for mechanics - Spezialist für Mechanik
JAKOVLEV, A.S.		Aircraft constructor-Flugzeugkonstrukteur
JANENKO, N.N.	22.5.1921	Spec.f.mechanics - Spez.f.Mechanik
KADOMCEV, B.B.	9.11.1928	Physicist-Physiker
KANTOROVIČ, L.V.	6.(19.)1.1912	Mathematician-Mathematiker
KAPICA, P.L.	26.6.(8.7.)1894	Physicist-Physiker
KELDYŠ, L.V.		Physicist-Physiker
KIKOIN, I.K.	15.(28.)3.1908	Physicist-Physiker
KIRILLIN, V.A.	7.(20.)1.1913	Specialist for thermics-Wärmetechniker
KOBZAREV, J.B.	25.11.(8.12.)1905	Specialist for radio-engineering - Spezialist für Radiotechnik
KOČINA, P.J.	1.(13.)5.1899	Mathematician-Mathematikerin
KOLMOGOROV, A.N.		Mathematician-Mathematiker
KOTEL'NIKOV, V.A.	24.8.(6.9.)1908	Specialist for radio-engineering - Spezialist für Radiotechnik
KRASOVSKIJ, N.N.	7.9.1924	Spec.f.mechanics - Spez.f.Mechanik
KUZNECOV, N.D.	10.(23.)6.1911	Specialist for control operations - Spezialist für Steuerungsprozesse
KUZNECOV, V.I.	14.(27.)4.1913	Spec.f.mechanics - Spez.f.Mechanik
LAVRENT'EV, M.A.	6.(19.)11.1900	Mathematician-Mathematiker
LEONTOVIČ, M.A.	22.2.(7.3.)1903	Physicist-Physiker
LIFŠIC, I.M.	31.12.1916(13.1.1917)	Physicist -Physiker
LJUL'KA, A.M.	10.(23.)3.1908	Energetician,constructor of aircraft engines - Energetiker,Konstrukteur von Flugzeugtriebwerken
LOGUNOV, A.A.	30.12.1926	Nuclear physicist,Kernphysiker
MAKAREVSKIJ, A.I.	3.(16.)4.1904	Specialist for construction of airplanes- Spezialist für Flugzeugbau
MAKEEV, V.P.		Spec.f.mechanics - Spez.f.Mechanik

459

8.3 Science / Wissenschaft

MARDŽANIŠVILI, K.K.	13.(26.)8.1903	Mathematician-Mathematiker
MARKOV, M.A.	30.4.(13.5.)1908	Physicist-Physiker
MELENT'EV, L.A.	26.11.(9.12.)1908	Energetician-Energetiker
MIGDAL, A.B.	26.2.(11.3.)1911	Physicist-Physiker
MIKULIN, A.A.	2.(14.)2.1895	Constructor of airplanes – Flugzeugkonstrukteur
MIŠIN, V.P.	5.(18.)1.1917	Spec.f.mechanics – Spez.f.Mechanik
NIKOL'SKIJ, S.M.	17.(30.)4.1905	Mathematician-Mathematiker
NOVOŽILOV, V.V.	18.5.1910	Spec.f.mechanics – Spez.f.Mechanik
OBRAZCOV, I.F.	28.7.1920	Spec.f.mechanics – Spez.f.Mechanik
OBREIMOV, I.V.	8.3.1894	Physicist-Physiker
PETROV, B.N.	26.2.(11.3.)1913	Specialist for control operations– Spezialist für Steuerungsprozesse
PETROV, G.I.	18.(31.)5.1912	Spec.f.mechanics – Spez.f.Mechanik
PILJUGIN, N.A.	5.(18.)5.1908	Specialist f.automation & telemechani Spezialist f.Automation u.Telemechan
POGORELOV, A.V.	1919	Mathematician-Mathematiker
PONTEKORVO, B.M.	22.8.1913	Physicist-Physiker
PONTRJAGIN, L.S.	21.8.(3.9.)1908	Mathematician-Mathematiker
POPKOV, V.I.	21.1.(3.2.)1908	Specialist for electrical engineering Spezialist für Elektrotechnik
PROCHOROV, A.M.	11.7.1916	Physicist-Physiker
PROCHOROV, J.V.	15.12.1929	Mathematician-Mathematiker
RABOTNOV, J.N.	11.(24.)2.1914	Spec.f.mechanics – Spez.f.Mechanik
SACHAROV, A.D.	21.5.1921	Physicist-Physiker
SAMARSKIJ, A.A.	1919	Mathematician-Mathematiker
ŠČUKIN, A.N.	9.(22.)7.1900	Specialist for radio-engineering – Spezialist für Radiotechnik
SEDOV, L.I.	1.(14.)11.1907	Specialist f.mechanics & hydromechan Spezialist f.Mechanik u.Hydromechan
ŠEJNDLIN, A.E.	22.8.(4.9.)1916	Spec.f.energetics – Spez.f.Energetik
SEMENICHIN, V.S.	27.1.(9.2.)1918	Spec.f.mechanics – Spez.f.Mechanik
SEMENOV, N.N.	3.(15.)4.1896	Physicist, physical chemist – Physiker, Physikochemiker
SEVERNYJ, A.B.	28.4.(11.5.)1913	Astronomer – Astronom
SKOBEL'CYN, D.V.	12.(24.)11.1892	Physicist – Physiker
SKRINSKIJ, A.N.	15.1.1936	Physicist – Physiker
SOBOLEV, S.L.	23.9.(6.10.)1908	Mathematician, Spec.f.mechanics – Mathematiker, Spez.f.Mechanik
STRUMINSKIJ, V.V.	16.(29.)4.1914	Spec.f.mechanics – Spez.f.Mechanik
STYRIKOVIČ, M.A.	3.(16.)11.1902	Spec.f.thermics – Spez.f.Wärmetechni
SVIŠČEV, G.P.		Spec.f.mechanical engineering – Spez.f.Maschinenbau
TICHONOV, A.N.	17.(30.)10.1906	Mathematician – Mathematiker
TRAPEZNIKOV, V.A.	15.(28.)11.1905	Specialist for automation – Spezialist für Automation
TUČKEVIČ, V.M.	16.(29.)12.1904	Physicist – Physiker
VAJNŠTEIN, B.K.		Physicist, Spec.f.crystallography – Physiker, Spez.f.Kristallographie
VELICHOV, E.P.	2.2.1935	Physicist – Physiker
VERNOV, S.N.	28.6.(11.7.)1910	Nuclear physicist – Kernphysiker
VINOGRADOV, I.M.	2.(14.)9.1891	Mathematician– Mathematiker
VLADIMIROV, V.S.	9.1.1923	Mathematician– Mathematiker
VONSOVSKIJ, S.V.	20.8.(2.9.)1910	Physicist – Physiker
VORONOV, A.A.	15.(28.)11.1910	Spec.f.mechanics – Spez.f.Mechanik
VUL, B.M.	9.(22.)5.1903	Physicist, Astronomer – Physiker, Astronom
ZABABACHIN, E.I.	3.(16.)1.1917	Physicist – Physiker
ZEL'DOVIČ, J.B.	23.2.(8.3.)1914	Physicist – Physiker
ŽURKOV, S.N.	16.(29.)5.1905	Physicist – Physiker

Science
Wissenschaft 8.3

b) Corresponding members - korrespondierende Mitglieder:

ABDULLAEV, G.M.B.o.	20.8.1918	Physicist - Physiker
ABRIKOSOV, A.A.	25.6.1928	Physicist - Physiker
ALEKSANDROV, K.S.	9.1.1931	Physicist - Physiker
ALEKSEEVSKIJ, N.E.	10.(23.)5.1912	Physicist - Physiker
ALFEROV, Ž.I.	15.3.1930	Physicist - Physiker
ALICHANJAN, A.I.		Physicist - Physiker
ALTŠULER, S.A.		Physicist - Physiker
AMIRCHANOV, Ch.I.	9.(22.)4.1907	Physicist - Physiker
AVDUEVSKIJ, V.S.	28.7.1920	Spec.f.mechanics - Spez.f.Mechanik
BABAEV, J.N.	21.5.1928	Nuclear physicist - Kernphysiker
BABEBKO, K.I.		Specialist f.control operations - Spezialist f.Steuerungsprozesse
BABUŠKIN, M.N.		Specialist f.control operations - Spezialist f.Steuerungsprozesse
BACHRACH, L.D.	22.7.1921	Physicist - Physiker
BALDIN, A.M.	26.2.1926	Nuclear physicist - Kernphysiker
BARKOV, L.M.	24.10.1928	Nuclear physicist - Kernphysiker
BELJAKOV, R.A.		Specialist f.mechanical engineering - Spezialist f.Maschinenbau
BELOCERKOVSKIJ, O.M.	29.8.1925	Spec.f.mechanics - Spez.f.Mechanik
BICADZE, A.V.	9.(22.)5.1916	Mathematician - Mathematiker
BJUŠGENS, G.S.	3.(16.)9.1916	Spec.f.mechanics - Spez.f.Mechanik
BLINOVA, E.N.		Geophysicist - Geophysikerin
BLOCHINCEV, D.I.	29.12.1907(11.1.1908)	Physicist - Physiker
BOGOMOLOV, A.F.	20.5.1918	Physicist - Physiker
BOJARČUK, A.A.		Astrophysicist - Astrophysiker
BOLOTIN, V.V.		Spec.f.mechanics - Spez.f.Mechanik
BOLŠEV, L.N.		Mathematician - Mathematiker
BORISEVIČ, N.A.	21.9.1923	Physicist, Spec.f.optics - Physiker, Spezialist f. Optik
BOROVKOV, A.A.	6.3.1931	Mathematician - Mathematiker
BUNKIN, F.V.		Physicist - Physiker
BURCEV, V.S.		Specialist f.control operations - Spezialist f.Steuerungsprozesse
BUSLENKO, N.P.	15.2.1922	Mathematician - Mathematiker
BUŠUEV, K.D.	10.(23.)5.1914	Spec.f.mechanics - Spez.f.Mechanik
ČERNYJ, G.G.		Spec.f.mechanics - Spez.f.Mechanik
ČERSKIJ, N.V.	20.1.(2.2.)1905	Spec.f.mechanics - Spez.f.Mechanik
ČERTOK, B.E.	1.3.1912	Spec.f.mechanics - Spez.f.Mechanik
CHALATNIKOV, I.M.		Physicist - Physiker
CHIMIČ, G.L.	22.10.(4.11.)1908	Specialist f.mechanical engineering - Spezialist f.Maschinenbau
CHLOPKIN, N.S.		Energetician - Energetiker
CHRENOV, K.K.	13.(25.)2.1894	Specialist for electric welding - Spezialist f.Elektroschweißen
ČUCHANOV, Z.F.	8.(21.)10.1912	Technol.chemist-Chemiker-Technologe
ČUDAKOV, A.E.	16.6.1921	Nuclear physicist - Kernphysiker
CYPKIN, J.Z.		Specialist f.control operations - Spezialist f.Steuerungsprozesse
DELONE, B.N.		Mathematician - Mathematiker
DEMIRČAN, K.S.		Energetician - Energetiker
DENISJUK, J.N.	27.7.1927	Physicist, specialist for optics - Physiker, Spezialist für Optik
DŽELEPOV, B.S.	29.11.(12.12.)1910	Physicist - Physiker
DŽELEPOV, V.P.	30.3.(12.4.)1913	Physicist - Physiker
DZJALOŠINSKIJ, I.E.		Physicist - Physiker
EMELJANOV, I.J.		Nuclear energetician - Atomenergetiker
EMEL'JANOV, S.V.	18.5.1929	Spec.f.mechanics - Spez.f.Mechanik
ENEEV, T.M.	23.9.1924	Spec.f.mechanics - Spez.f.Mechanik

8.3 Science / Wissenschaft

ERŠOV, A.P.	19.4.1931	Mathematician - Mathematiker
ERŠOV, J.L.	1.5.1940	Mathematician - Mathematiker
FADDEEV, D.K.	17.(30.)6.1907	Mathematician - Mathematiker
FEJNBERG, E.L.	14.(27.)6.1912	Nuclear physicist - Kernphysiker
FEOFILOV, P.P.	31.3.(13.4.)1915	Physicist - Physiker
FEOKTISTOV, L.P.	14.2.1928	Nuclear physicist - Kernphysiker
FRADKIN, E.S.	24.2.1924	Nuclear physicist - Kernphysiker
FRIŠ, S.E.		Physicist, Specialist for optics - Physiker, Spezialist für Optik
FROLOV, K.V.		Specialist f.mechanical engineering - Spezialist für Maschinenbau
GALICKIJ, V.M.		Nuclear physicist - Kernphysiker
GALIN, L.A.	15.(28.)9.1912	Mathematician - Mathematiker
GAVRILOV, M.A.	29.10.(11.11.)1903	Specialist for automatic control - Spezialist f.automatische Steuerung
GELFAND, I.M.	20.8.(2.9.)1913	Mathematician - Mathematiker
GLEBOV, I.A.		Specialist f.energetic mechanic.engin.- Spezialist f.energet.Maschinenbau
GODUNOV, S.K.		Mathematician - Mathematiker
GONČAR, A.A.		Mathematician - Mathematiker
GOR'KOV, L.P.	14.6.1929	Physicist - Physiker
GOVORUN, N.N.	18.3.1930	Mathematician - Mathematiker
GRIBOV, V.N.	23.3.1930	Nuclear physicist - Kernphysiker
GRIGOLJUK, E.I.	13.12.1923	Spec.f.mechanics - Spez.f.Mechanik
GRINBERG, G.A.	3.(16.)6.1900	Physicist,Mathematician - Physiker, Mathematiker
GUREVIČ, I.I.	30.7.(13.7.)1912	Nuclear physicist - Kernphysiker
IEVLEV, V.M.	15.5.1926	Spec.f.thermodynamics and mechanics - Spez.f.Wärmephysik und Mechanik
IL'JUŠIN, A.A.	7.(20.)1.1911	Spec.f.aerodynamics-Spez.f.Aerodynamik
IVANOV, V.K.	18.9.(1.10.)1908	Mathematician - Mathematiker
JABLONSKIJ, S.V.	6.12.1924	Mathematician - Mathematiker
KAGAN, J.M.	6.7.1928	Physicist - Physiker
KARDAŠEV, N.S.		Astrophysicist - Astrophysiker
KISUNKO, G.V.	20.7.1918	Specialist f.radio-engineering - Spezialist f.Radiotechnik
KONOPATOV, A.D.		Energetician - Energetiker
KOSTENKO, M.V.	15.(28.)12.1912	Spec.f.energetics - Spez.f.Energetik
KOSTRIKIN, A.I.		Mathematician - Mathematiker
KOVALEV, N.N.	9.(22.)2.1908	Spec.f.mechanics - Spez.f.Mechanik
KOZLOV, V.J.	15.(28.)6.1914	Mathematician - Mathematiker
KOZYREV, B.M.	21.4.(4.5.)1905	Physicist - Physiker
KRASOVSKIJ, A.A.	10.4.1921	Spec.f.mechanics - Spez.f.Mechanik
KRAT, V.A.	8.(21.)7.1911	Astronomer - Astronom
KRUŽILIN, G.N.	24.5.(6.6.)1911	Spec.f.thermics - Spez.f.Wärmetechnik
KURBATOV, L.N.		Physicist - Physiker
KUTATELADZE, S.S.	5.(18.)7.1914	Energetician - Energetiker
LAVRENTEV, M.M.	2.7.1932	Mathematician - Mathematiker
LAVROV, S.S.	12.3.1923	Spec.f.mechanics - Spez.f.Mechanik
LEONTEV, A.F.	14.3.1917	Mathematician - Mathematiker
LIDORENKO, N.S.	20.3.(2.4.)1916	Specialist f.electrical engineering - Spezialist f.Elektrotechnik
LIFŠIC, E.M.	8.(21.)2.1915	Physicist - Physiker
LJUSTERNIK, L.A.	31.12.1899	Mathematician - Mathematiker
LOBAŠEV, V.M.	29.7.1934	Nuclear physicist - Kernphysiker
LUPANOV, O.B.	2.6.1932	Mathematician - Mathematiker
LUR'E, A.I.	6.(19.)7.1901	Physicist, Specialist f.mechanics - Physiker, Spezialist f.Mechanik
MAKAROV, I.M.		Specialist f.control operations - Spezialist f.Steuerungsprozesse

Science
Wissenschaft 8.3

MALMEJSTER, A.K.	5.(18.)10.1911	Spec.f.mechanics – Spez.f.Mechanik
MALYŠEV, N.A.		Energetician – Energetiker
MARKOV, A.A.	9.(22.)9.1903	Mathematician – Mathematiker
MATROSOV, V.M.		Specialist f.control operations – Spezialist f.Steuerungsprozesse
MELNIKOV, N.P.		Specialist f.mechanical and metal constructions – Spezialist f.Baumechanik u.Metallkonstruktionen
MELNIKOV, O.A.	20.3.(2.4.)1912	Astronomer – Astronom
MELNIKOV, V.A.		Mathematician – Mathematiker
MENŠOV, D.E.	6.(18.)4.1892	Mathematician – Mathematiker
MERGELJAN, S.N.	19.5.1928	Mathematician – Mathematiker
MEŠČERJAKOV, M.G.	4.(17.)9.1910	Physicist – Physiker
MIGULIN, V.V.	27.6.(10.7.)1911	Physicist – Physiker
MIŠČENKO, E.F.		Specialist f.control operations – Spezialist f.Steuerungsprozesse
MOISEEV, N.N.	10.(23.)8.1917	Spec.f.mechanics – Spez.f.Mechanik
MOLODENSKIJ, M.S.	3.(16.)6.1909	Geophysicist, spec.f.gravimetrics – Geophysiker, Spez.f.Gravimetrie
MUSTEL, E.R.	21.5.(3.6.)1911	Astronomer, astrophysicist – Astronom, Astrophysiker
NAUMOV, A.A.	14.(27.)1.1916	Nuclear physicist – Kernphysiker
NAUMOV, B.N.		Specialist f.control operations – Spezialist f.Steuerungsprozesse
NEGIN, E.A.		Spec.f.mechanics – Spez.f.Mechanik
NESTERICHIN, J.E.	10.10.1930	Physicist – Physiker
NOVIKOV, I.I.	15.(28.)1.1916	Spec.f.thermics – Spez.f.Wärmetechnik
NOVIKOV, S.P.	20.3.1938	Mathematician – Mathematiker
OCHOCIMSKIJ, D.E.	26.2.1921	Mathematician, specialist f.mechanics – Mathematiker, Spezialist f.Mechanik
OKUN, L.B.	7.7.1929	Nuclear physicist – Kernphysiker
OSIPJAN, J.A.	5.2.1931	Physicist – Physiker
OVSJANNIKOV, L.V.	22.4.1919	Spec.f.mechanics – Spez.f.Mechanik
PAVLOV, I.M.	10.(23.)6.1900	Spec.f.metallurgy – Spez.f.Metallurgie
PETROV, A.P.	19.8.(1.9.)1910	Spec.f.transportation – Spez.f.Transportwesen
PETROV, G.N.	22.4.(4.5.)1899	Specialist f.electrical engineering – Spezialist f.Elektrotechnik
PETROV, V.V.	9.(22.)9.1912	Specialist f.automatic control – Spezialist f.Regeltechnik
PETUCHOV, B.S.		Energetician – Energetiker
PISTOLKORS, A.A.	28.9.(10.10.)1896	Specialist f.radio-engineering – Spezialist f.Radiotechnik
PITAEVSKIJ, L.P.		Physicist – Physiker
POLIKANOV, S.M.		Nuclear physicist – Kernphysiker
POPOV, E.P.	1.(14.)2.1914	Spec.f.mechanics – Spez.f.Mechanik
POPYRIN, L.S.		Energetician – Energetiker
POSPELOV, G.S.	12.(25.)5.1914	Spec.f.mechanics – Spez.f.Mechanik
PROKOŠKIN, J.D.		Nuclear physicist – Kernphysiker
PUGAČEV, V.S.	12.(25.)3.1911	Spec.f.mechanics – Spez.f.Mechanik
RABINOVIČ, I.M.		Specialist f.mechanical construction – Spezialist für Baumechanik
RAUŠENBACH, B.V.	5.(18.)1.1915	Spec.f.mechanics – Spez.f.Mechanik
RAZIN, N.V.	13.(26.)4.1904	Hydroenergetician – Hydroenergetiker
REBANE, K.K.		Physicist – Physiker
RESETNEV, M.F.		Specialist f.mechanical engineering – Spezialist f.Maschinenbau
RIZNIČENKO, J.V.	15.(28.)9.1911	Physicist – Physiker
RJAZANSKIJ, M.S.	23.3.(5.4.)1909	Specialist for radio-engineering – Spezialist für Radiotechnik

Science
Wissenschaft

RJUTOV, D.D.		Nuclear physicist - Kernphysiker
RUDENKO, J.N.		Energetician - Energetiker
RUMJANCEV, V.V.	19.7.1921	Spec.f.mechanics - Spez.f.Mechanik
RUSANOV, V.V.		Mathematician - Mathematiker
RYTOV, S.M.	20.6.(3.7.)1908	Physicist, Spec.f.radio-engineering - Physiker, Spez.f.Radiotechnik
RŽANOV, A.V.	9.4.1920	Specialist f.radio-engineering - Spezialist f.Radiotechnik
SAFAREVIČ, I.R.	3.6.1923	Mathematician - Mathematiker
SALNIKOV, A.I.	27.4.(10.5.)1905	Physicist - Physiker
SARVIN, J.V.	24.6.1919	Physicist - Physiker
SIDOROV, V.A.	19.10.1930	Nuclear physicist - Kernphysiker
SIFOROV, V.I.	18.(31.)5.1904	Specialist f.radio-engineering - Spezialist f.Radiotechnik
SIRKOV, D.V.	3.3.1928	Physicist - Physiker
SIRŠOV, A.I.	8.8.1921	Mathematician - Mathematiker
ŠKLOVSKIJ, I.S.	18.6.(1.7.)1916	Astronomer, astrophysicist - Astronom, Astrophysiker
SMOLENSKIJ, G.A.	10.(23.)6.1910	Physicist - Physiker
SOBOLEV, V.V.	20.8.(2.9.)1915	Astronomer - Astronom
SOKOLOVSKIJ, V.V.	4.(17.)10.1912	Spec.f.mechanics - Spez.f.Mechanik
SOLOUCHIN, R.I.	19.11.1930	Spec.f.mechanics - Spez.f.Mechanik
SPIVAK, P.E.	11.(24.)3.1911	Nuclear physicist - Kernphysiker
STEPANOV, V.E.	1.(14.)12.1913	Astronomer, physicist - Astronom, Physiker
SUBBOTIN, V.I.	12.12.1919	Physicist, thermal physicist - Physiker, Wärmephysiker
SUR, J.S.	7.(20.)4.1908	Physicist - Physiker
TATARSKIJ, V.I.		Physicist - Physiker
TICHOMIROV, V.V.	10.(23.)12.1912	Spec.f.radio-engineering & electronics- Spez.f.Radiotechnik u.Elektronik
TIMOFEEV, P.V.	12.(25.)6.1902	Spec.f.radio-engineering & electronics- Spez.f.Radiotechnik u.Elektronik
TROICKIJ, V.S.	12.(25.)3.1913	Physicist, Astronomer - Physiker, Astronom
TRUTNEV, J.A.	2.11.1927	Nuclear physicist - Kernphysiker
VAJNŠTEIN, L.A.	6.12.1920	Radiation physicist - Strahlenphysiker
VALIEV, K.A.	15.1.1931	Physicist - Physiker
VANIČEV, A.P.	29.7.(11.8.)1916	Spec.f.energetics - Spez.f.Energetik
VASILEV, O.F.	1.8.1925	Spec.f.mechanics - Spez.f.Mechanik
VAVILOV, A.A.		Specialist f.control operations - Spezialist f.Steuerungsprozesse
VELIKANOV, D.P.	12.(25.)10.1908	Specialist f.motor transportation - Spezialist f.Autotransport
VITUŠKIN, A.G.		Mathematician - Mathematiker
VLADIMIRSKIJ, V.V.	20.7.(2.8.)1915	Physicist - Physiker
VOJCECHOVSKIJ, B.V.	25.1.1922	Specialist f.hydromechanics - Spezialist f.Hydromechanik
VOROVIČ, I.I.	21.6.1920	Spec.f.mechanics - Spez.f.Mechanik
ZACEPIN, G.T.	15.(28.)5.1917	Nuclear physicist - Kernphysiker
ZACHARČENJA, B.P.		Physicist - Physiker
ŽELTUCHIN, N.A.	31.10.(13.11.)1915	Specialist f.mechanics and thermics - Spezialist f.Mechanik u.Wärmetechnik
ŽIMERIN, D.G.	12.(25.)10.1906	Energetician - Energetiker
ZOLOTOV, E.V.	29.4.1922	Mathematician - Mathematiker
ZOREV, N.N.		Specialist f.mechanical engineering - Spezialist f.Maschinenbau
ZUEV, V.E.	29.1.1925	Physicist - Physiker
ŽUKOV, M.F.	24.8.(6.9.)1917	Specialist for aerodynamics - Spezialist f.Aerodynamik
ZVEREV, M.S.	3.(16.)4.1903	Astronomer, astrophysicist - Astronom, Astrophysiker

Section of Chemistry, Chemical Technology and Biology -
Sektion der chemisch-technologischen und biologischen Wissenschaften

a) Members-Mitglieder:

AGEEV, N.V.	17.(30.)6.1903	Chemist,metallurgist-Chemiker,Metallurg
ALIMARIN, I.P.	29.8.(11.9.)1903	Chemist - Chemiker
ARBUZOV, B.A.	4.11.1903	Organic chemist - organischer Chemiker
BAEV, A.A.	28.12.1903(10.1.1904)	Biologist,medical spec.-Biologe,Mediziner
BELJAEV, D.K.	4.(17.)7.1917	Biologist, geneticist-Biologe,Genetiker
BELOV, A.F.	15.(28.)3.1906	Specialist for metallurgy - Spezialist für Metallurgie
BOČVAR, A.A.		Spec.f.metallurgy - Spez.f.Metallurgie
BORESKOV, G.K.	7.(20.)4.1907	Physical chemist - Physikochemiker
BRAUNŠTEJN, A.E.	13.(26.)5.1902	Biochemist - Biochemiker
ČAJLACHJAN, M.Ch.	8.(21.)3.1902	Plant physiologist - Pflanzenphysiologe
ČERNIGOVSKIJ, V.N.	16.2.(1.3.)1907	Physiologist - Physiologe
CICIN, N.V.	6.(18.)12.1898	Botanist - Botaniker
DEVJATYCH, G.G.	14.12.1918	Chemist - Chemiker
DOLGOPLOSK, B.A.	31.10.(13.11.)1905	Organic chemist - organischer Chemiker
DUBININ, M.M.	19.12.1900(1.1.1901)	Physical chemist - Physikochemiker
DUBININ, N.P.	22.12.1906(4.1.1907)	Biologist,geneticist-Biologe,Genetiker
EMANUEL, N.M.	18.9.(1.10.)1915	Physical chemist - Physikochemiker
ENGELGARDT, V.A.	21.11.(3.12.)1894	Biochemist - Biochemiker
ENIKOLOPOV, N.S.		Chemist - Chemiker
FOKIN, A.V.	13.(26.)8.1912	Organic chemist - organischer Chemiker
GAZENKO, O.G.		Physiologist - Physiologe
GERASIMOV, I.P.	26.11.(9.12.)1905	Physical geographer-Physikogeograph
GILJAROV, M.S.	9.(22.)2.1912	Zoologist - Zoologe
IMŠENECKIJ, A.A.	26.12.1904(8.1.1905)	Microbiologist - Mikrobiologe
KABAČNIK, M.I.	27.8.(9.9.)1908	Organic chemist - organischer Chemiker
KIŠKIN, S.T.	17.(30.)5.1906	Spec.f.mechanics - Spez.f.Mechanik
KNUNJANC, I.L.	22.5.(4.6.)1906	Organic chemist - organischer Chemiker
KOČEŠKOV, K.A.	30.11.(12.12.)1894	Organic chemist - organischer Chemiker
KOLOSOV, M.N.	11.5.1927	Biochemist - Biochemiker
KOLOTYRKIN, J.M.	1.(14.)11.1910	Physical chemist - Physikochemiker
KONDRATEV, V.N.	19.1.(1.2.)1902	Chemist, physical chemist - Chemiker, Physikochemiker
KORŠAK, V.V.		Chemist - Chemiker
KOSTJUK, P.G.	20.8.1924	Physiologist, medical specialist - Physiologe, Mediziner
KRASNOVSKIJ, A.A.		Biochemist, biophysicist - Biochemiker, Biophysiker
KREPS, E.M.	19.4.(1.5.)1899	Physiologist - Physiologe
KURDJUMOV, G.V.	1.(14.)2.1902	Metallo-physicist - Metallophysiker
KURSANOV, A.L.	26.10.(8.11.)1902	Plant physiologist and biochemist - Pflanzenphysiologe und -biochemiker
LASKORIN, B.N.		Technological chemist - Chemiker-Technologe
LAVRENKO, E.M.	11.(23.)2.1900	Geographical botanist - Geobotaniker
LIVANOV, M.N.	7.(20.)10.1907	Physiologist - Physiologe
MIŠUSTIN, E.N.	9.(22.)2.1901	Microbiologist - Mikrobiologe
NESMEJANOV, A.N.	28.8.(9.9.)1899	Chemist - Chemiker
NIKOLSKIJ, B.P.	1.(14.)10.1900	Physical chemist - Physikochemiker
NOVOSELOVA, A.V.	11.(24.)3.1900	Chemist - Chemikerin
OPARIN, A.I.	18.2.(2.3.)1894	Biologist, biochemist - Biologe, Biochemiker
OVČINNIKOV, J.A.	2.8.1934	Chemist - Chemiker
PATON, B.E.	27.11.1918	Spec.f.metallurgy - Spez.f.Metallurgie
PETRJANOV-SOKOLOV,I.V.	5.(18.)6.1907	Physical chemist - Physikochemiker

8.3 Science / Wissenschaft

PETROVSKIJ, B.V.	14.(27.)6.1908	Surgeon – Chirurg
POSTOVSKIJ, I.J.	4.(16.)3.1898	Chemist – Chemiker
RAZUVAEV, G.A.	11.(23.)8.1895	Organic chemist – organischer Chemiker
REMESLO, V.N.		Geneticist – Genetiker
REUTOV, O.A.	5.9.1920	Chemist – Chemiker
RYKALIN, N.N.	14.(27.)9.1903	Spec.f.metallurgy – Spez.f.Metallurgie
SADOVSKIJ, V.D.	24.7.(6.8.)1908	Chemist – Chemiker
SADYKOV, A.S.	2.(15.)11.1913	Organic chemist – organischer Chemiker
SAGDEEV, R.Z.	26.12.1932	Physicist – Physiker
SEVERIN, S.E.	8.(21.)12.1901	Biochemist – Biochemiker
SOKOLOV, V.E.	1.2.1928	Zoologist – Zoologe
SPICYN, V.I.	12.(25.)4.1902	Chemist – Chemiker
SPIRIN, A.S.	4.9.1931	Biochemist – Biochemiker
TACHTADŽJAN, A.L.	28.5.(10.6.)1910	Botanist – Botaniker
TANANAEV, I.V.	22.5.(4.6.)1904	Chemist – Chemiker
VOLFKOVIČ, S.I.	11.(23.)10.1896	Chemist – Chemiker
VOROŽCOV, N.N.		Organic chemist – organischer Chemiker
ŽAVORONKOV, N.M.	25.7.(7.8.)1907	Chemist – Chemiker
ŽUKOV, A.B.	24.7.(6.8.)1901	Biologist – Biologe
ŽUKOV, B.P.	30.10.(12.11.)1912	Chemist – Chemiker

b) Corresponding members – korrespondierende Mitglieder:

ALEKIN, O.A.	10.(23.)8.1908	Chemist, hydrochemist – Chemiker, Hydrochemiker
ALESKOVSKIJ, V.B.	21.5.(3.6.)1912	Physical chemist – Physikochemiker
ANDRIJAŠEV, A.P.	19.8.1910	Zoologist – Zoologe
ASRATJAN, E.A.	31.5.1903	Physiologist – Physiologe
BAGDASARJAN, Ch.S.	18.11.1908	Physical chemist – Physikochemiker
BAŠKIROV, A.N.	9.(22.)12.1903	Chemist – Chemiker
BECHTEREVA, N.P.	7.7.1924	Physiologist, neurosurgeon – Physiologin, Neurochirurgin
BELECKAJA, I.P.		Chemist – Chemikerin
BEREZIN, I.V.	9.8.1923	Physical chemist – Physikochemiker
BERGELSON, L.D.	28.8.1918	Biochemist, organic chemist – Biochemiker, organischer Chemiker
BOKIJ, G.B.	26.9.(9.10.)1909	Physical chemist – Physikochemiker
BOLŠAKOV, K.A.	11.(24.)12.1906	Chemist – Chemiker
BUKIN, V.N.	15.(27.)1.1899	Biochemist – Biochemiker
BUSLAEV, J.A.	22.11.1929	Physical chemist – Physikochemiker
BUTENKO, R.G.		Biologist – Biologin
CHESIN-LURJE, R.B.		Biochemist – Biochemiker
CHOCHLOV, A.S.	23.6.(6.7.)1916	Biochemist – Biochemiker
ČIBISOV, K.V.	17.2.(1.3.)1897	Chemist – Chemiker
ČMUTOV, K.V.	8.(21.)3.1902	Physical chemist – Physikochemiker
ČUFAROV, G.I.	1.(14.)11.1900	Physical chemist – Physikochemiker
CVETKOV, V.N.	3.(16.)2.1910	Organic chemist-organischer Chemiker
DANILOV, S.N.	25.12.1888(6.1.1889)	Organic chemist-organischer Chemiker
DERJAGIN, B.V.	27.7.(9.8.)1902	Physical chemist- Physikochemiker
EICHFELD, J.H.	13.(25.)1.1893	Biologist, botanist – Biologe, Botaniker
ELJAKOV, G.B.	13.9.1929	Organic chemist-organischer Chemiker
ELJUTIN, V.P.	26.2.(-1.3.)1907	Spec.f.metallurgy – Spez.f.Metallurgie
EMELJANOV, V.S.	30.1.(12.2.)1901	Spec.f.metallurgy – Spez.f.Metallurgie
EVSTRATOV, V.F.		Chemist – Chemiker
EVSTIGNEEVA, R.P.		Chemist – Chemikerin
FEDOROV, A.A.	24.11.(7.12.)1906	Biologist – Biologe
FEDOROV, A.A.	17.(30.)10.1908	Botanist – Botaniker
FOMIN, V.V.	12.(25.)1.1909	Chemist – Chemiker
FREJDLINA, R.Ch.	7.(20.)9.1906	Organic chemist-organische Chemikerin
FRIDLJANDER, J.N.		Physicist-chemist – Physiker-Chemiker
GALAZIJ, G.I.	5.3.1922	Botanist – Botaniker

Science
Wissenschaft 8.3

Name	Date	Field
GELD, P.V.	7.(20.)12.1911	Chemist - Chemiker
GEORGIEV, G.P.	4.2.1933	Biologist - Biologe
GERASIMOV, J.I.	10.(23.)9.1903	Physical chemist - Physikochemiker
GERŠUNI, G.V.	21.7.(3.8.)1905	Medical specialist, physiology - Mediziner, Physiologie
GOLDANSKIJ, V.I.	18.6.1923	Physical chemist - Physikochemiker
GORLENKO, M.V.		Biologist - Biologe
GOVYRIN, V.A.		Physiologist - Physiologe
GUTYRJA, V.S.		Chemist - Chemiker
ISAEV, A.S.		Biologist - Biologe
IVANICKIJ, G.R.		Biologist - Biologe
IVANOV, V.T.		Chemist - Chemiker
IVANOV, V.E.	9.(22.)11.1908	Physical chemist - Physikochemiker
JAGODIN, G.A.		Chemist - Chemiker
JUNUSOF, S.J.	5.(18.)3.1909	Organic chemist-organischer Chemiker
KABANOV, V.A.	15.1.1934	Organic chemist-organischer Chemiker
KAFAROV, V.V.	5.(18.)6.1914	Chemist - Chemiker
KARAMJAN, A.I.	2.(15.)3.1908	Physiologist, medical specialist - Physiologe, Mediziner
KARAVAEV, N.M.		Chemist - Chemiker
KARPAČEV, S.V.	11.(24.)2.1906	Electro-chemist - Elektrochemiker
KAZANSKIJ, V.B.		Physical chemist - Physikochemiker
KAZARNOVSKIJ, I.A.	17.(29.)9.1890	Chemist - Chemiker
KIRPIČNIKOV, P.A.		Chemist - Chemiker
KNORRE, D.G.	28.7.1926	Chemist - Chemiker
KOČETKOV, N.K.	5.(18.)5.1915	Chemist, biochemist - Chemiker, Biochemiker
KOLESNIKOV, B.P.	17.(30.)5.1909	Specialist for forestry - Spezialist für Forstwesen
KOLOSOV, N.G.	17.(29.)4.1897	Histologist - Histologe
KONTRIMAVIČUS, V.L.	22.1.1930	Helminthologist (worm researcher) - Helminthologe (Wurmforscher)
KOPTJUG, V.A.	9.6.1931	Organic chemist-organischer Chemiker
KOTON, M.M.	16.(29.)12.1908	Chemist - Chemiker
KOVALSKIJ, A.A.	28.8.(10.9.)1906	Chemist - Chemiker
KOVDA, V.A.	16.(29.)12.1904	Soil scientist - Bodenkundler
KRETOVIČ, V.L.	14.(27.)1.1907	Biochemist - Biochemiker
KRUŠINSKIJ, L.V.		Biologist - Biologe
KUNAEV, A.M.		Physical chemist - Physikochemiker
KURSANOV, D.N.	1.(13.)4.1899	Organic chemist-organischer Chemiker
KUZIN, A.M.	17.(30.)5.1906	Radio-biologist - Radiobiologe
KUZNECOV, S.I.	4.(17.)11.1900	Microbiologist - Mikrobiologe
LAPIN, P.I.		Biologist - Biologe
LEGASOV, V.A.		Chemist - Chemiker
LEVIČ, V.G.	17.(30.)3.1917	Physical chemist - Physikochemiker
LEVKOEV, I.I.	19.11.(2.12.)1909	Chemist - Chemiker
MALININ, A.J.		Physical chemist - Physikochemiker
MALJUSOV, V.A.	21.6.(4.7.)1913	Chemist - Chemiker
MAMAEV, V.P.	30.11.1925	Chemist - Chemiker
MATULIS, J.J.	19.(31.)3.1899	Physical chemist - Physikochemiker
MEJSEL, M.N.	28.9.(11.10.)1901	Microbiologist - Mikrobiologe
MICHAJLOV, B.M.	21.3.(3.4.)1906	Organic chemist - organischer Chemiker
MINAČEV, Ch.M.	11.(24.)12.1908	Organic chemist - organischer Chemiker
MOLČANOV, A.A.	19.8.(1.9.)1902	Botanist - Botaniker
MOLIN, J.N.		Chemist - Chemiker
NAMETKIN, N.S.	3.(16.)8.1916	Organic chemist - organischer Chemiker
NEKRASOV, B.V.	6.(18.)9.1899	Chemist - Chemiker
NESMEJANOV, A.N.	2.(15.)1.1911	Chemist - Chemiker
NEUNYLOV, B.A.	20.9.(3.10.)1908	Biologist - Biologe
NIČIPOROVIČ, A.A.	30.10.(11.11.)1899	Physiologist - Physiologe

8.3 Science / Wissenschaft

NIKOLAEV, G.A.	4.(17.)1.1903	Specialist for welding - Spezialist für Schweißen
NIKOLSKIJ, G.V.	23.4.(6.5.)1910	Zoologist, ichthyologist - Zoologe, Ichthyologe
NOVIKOV, S.S.		Chemist - Chemiker
PETROV, A.A.	13.(26.)3.1913	Organic chemist-organischer Chemiker
PETROVSKIJ, G.T.		Physical chemist - Physikochemiker
PIRUZJAN, L.A.		Physiologist - Physiologe
PJAVČENKO, N.I.	18.11.(1.12.)1902	Soil scientist, geobotanist - Bodenkundler, Geobotaniker
PLATE, N.A.		Chemist - Chemiker
PORAJ-KOŠIC, M.A.		Chemist - Chemiker
PRAVEDNIKOV, A.N.		Chemist - Chemiker
PROKOFEV, M.A.	5.(18.)11.1910	Biochemist - Biochemiker
PUDOVIK, A.N.	2.(15.)3.1916	Organic chemist-organischer Chemiker
RAFIKOV, S.R.	6.(19.)4.1912	Chemist - Chemiker
RAKITIN, J.V.	23.4.(5.5.)1911	Botanist, plant physiologist - Botaniker, Pflanzenphysiologe
REIMERS, F.E.	12.(25.)7.1904	Plant physiologist - Pflanzenphysiologe
REŠETNIKOV, F.G.		Physical chemist - Physikochemiker
ROJTBAK, A.I.	17.2.1919	Physiologist - Physiologe
ROMANKOV, P.G.	4.(17.)1.1904	Chemist - Chemiker
RYŽIKOV, K.M.	13.(26.)9.1912	Biologist, helminthologist - Biologe, Helminthologe
RYŽKOV, V.L.	18.(30.)6.1896	Biologist, botanist - Biologe, Botaniker
SAMOJLOV, A.G.		Physical chemist - Physikochemiker
SAVICKIJ, E.M.	17.(30.)1.1912	Physical chemist - Physikochemiker
SKRJABIN, G.K.	4.(17.)9.1917	Biochemist, microbiologist - Biochemiker, Mikrobiologe
SKULAČEV, V.P.		Biochemist - Biochemiker
SLINKO, M.G.	2.(15.)9.1914	Chemist, physical chemist - Chemiker, Physikochemiker
SLYK, A.A.	1.11.1928	Botanist, plant physiologist - Botaniker, Pflanzenphysiologe
SOKOLOV, A.V.	25.7.(6.8.)1898	Agrochemist - Agrochemiker
ŠOSTAKOVIČ, M.F.	24.5.(6.6.)1905	Chemist - Chemiker
ŠPAK, V.S.	7.(20.)2.1909	Chemist - Chemiker
STRUNNIKOV, V.A.		Biologist - Biologe
ŠULC, M.M.		Physical chemist - Physikochemiker
ŠVEJKIN, G.P.		Chemist - Chemiker
SVETOVIDOV, A.N.	21.10.(3.11.)1903	Zoologist, ichthyologist - Zoologe, Ichthyologe
TALROZE, V.L.	15.4.1922	Physical chemist - Physikochemiker
TATARINOV, L.P.		Biologist - Biologe
TERSKOV, I.A.	11.9.1918	Physicist, biophysicist - Physiker, Biophysiker
TORGOV, I.V.	2.(15.)2.1912	Chemist - Chemiker
TROŠIN, A.S.	10.(23.)10.1912	Biologist, cytologist - Biologe, Zytologe
TUMANOV, I.I.	19.6.(1.7.)1894	Botanist, plant physiologist - Botaniker, Pflanzenphysiologe
TURPAEV, T.M.	20.10.1918	Physiologist - Physiologe
UGOLEV, A.M.	9.3.1926	Physiologist, medical specialist Physiologe, Mediziner
VATOLIN, N.A.	13.11.1926	Spec.f.metallurgy - Spez.f.Metallurgie
VDOVENKO, V.M.	23.12.1906(5.1.1907)	Radiochemist - Radiochemiker
VINBERG, G.G.		Biologist - Biologe
VOLKENŠTEJN, M.V.	10.(23.)10.1912	Biochemist - Biochemiker

Science
Wissenschaft 8.3

VOLOBUEV, V.R.	12.(25.)7.1909	Soil scientist, agrochemist - Bodenkundler, Agrochemiker
VORONIN, L.G.	22.7.(4.8.)1908	Physiologist - Physiologe
VORONKOV, M.G.	6.12.1921	Chemist - Chemiker
ZAJMOVSKIJ, A.S.	26.9.(9.10.)1905	Spec.f.metallurgy - Spez.f.Metallurgie
ZAMARAEV, K.I.		Physical chemist - Physikochemiker
ZAVARZIN, G.A.		Physiologist - Physiologe
ŽDANOV, J.A.	20.8.1919	Organic chemist-organischer Chemiker
ZEFIROV, A.P.	12.(25.)3.1907	Chemist, spec.f.metallurgy of rare and precious metals - Chemiker, Spez.f. Metallurgie seltener u.kostbarer Metalle
ŽIRMUNSKIJ, A.V.	15.10.1921	Biologist - Biologe
ZOLOTOV, J.A.	4.10.1932	Chemist - Chemiker

Section of Earth Sciences - Sektion der Erdwissenschaften

a) Members - Mitglieder:

AMBARCUMJAN, V.A.	5.(18.)9.1908	Astrophysicist - Astrophysiker
BELOV, N.V.	14.12.1891	Geochemist - Geochemiker
BRECHOVSKICH, L.M.	23.4.(6.5.)1917	Physicist, oceanologist - Physiker, Ozeanologe
ČUCHROV, F.V.	2.(15.)7.1908	Geochemist - Geochemiker
DORODNICYN, A.A.	19.11.(2.12.)1910	Geophysicist - Geophysiker
FEDOROV, E.K.	28.3.(10.4.)1910	Geophysicist - Geophysiker
JANŠIN, A.L.	15.(28.)3.1911	Geologist - Geologe
KORŽINSKIJ, D.S.	1.(13.)9.1899	Geologist, petrologist, mineralogist - Geologe, Petrograph, Mineraloge
KOSYGIN, J.A.	2.(22.)1.1911	Geologist - Geologe
KRYLOV, A.P.	1.(14.)8.1904	Geologist - Geologe
KUZNECOV, J.A.	6.(19.)4.1903	Geologist - Geologe
KUZNECOV, V.A.	30.3.(12.4.)1906	Geologist, geographer - Geologe, Geograph
MARČUK, G.I.	8.6.1925	Physicist - Physiker
MARKOV, K.K.	7.(20.)5.1905	Oceanologist, geophysicist, geographer - Ozeanologe, Geophysiker, Geograph
MELNIKOV, N.V.	15.(28.)2.1909	Mining specialist - Bergbaufachmann
MENNER, V.V.	11.(24.)11.1905	Geologist, palaeontologist - Geologe, Paläontologe
MICHAJLOV, A.A.	14.(26.)4.1888	Astronomer, gravimetric specialist - Astronom, Spezialist f.Gravimetrie
NALIVKIN, D.V.	13.(25.)8.1889	Geologist, palaeontologist - Geologe, Paläontologe
OBUCHOV, A.M.	5.5.1918	Geophysicist - Geophysiker
PEJVE, A.V.	27.1.(9.2.)1909	Geologist - Geologe
SADOVSKIJ, M.A.	24.10.(6.11.)1904	Geophysicist - Geophysiker
SIDORENKO, A.V.	6.(19.)10.1917	Geologist - Geologe
ŠILO, N.A.	25.3.(7.4.)1913	Geologist - Geologe
SMIRNOV, V.I.	18.(31.)1.1910	Geologist - Geologe
SOBOLEV, V.S.	17.(30.)5.1908	Petrologist, mineralogist - Petrograph, Mineraloge
SOČAVA, V.B.	7.(20.)6.1905	Geographer - Geograph
SOKOLOV, B.S.	27.3.(9.4.)1914	Geologist, geographer - Geologe, Geograph
ŠULEJKIN, V.V.	1.(13.)1.1895	Geophysicist - Geophysiker
TROFIMUK, A.A.	3.(16.)8.1911	Petrogeologist - Erdölgeologe

8.3 Science / Wissenschaft

b) Corresponding members - korrespondierende Mitglieder:

Name	Date	Field
AGOŠKOV, M.I.	30.10.(12.11.)1905	Mining specialist - Bergbauspezialist
ALEKSEEV, A.S.	12.10.1928	Geophysicist - Geophysiker
AVSJUK, G.A.	16.(29.)12.1906	Hydrogeologist - Hydrogeologe
BABAEV, A.G.		Geographer - Geograph
BARSUKOV, V.L.		Geochemist - Geochemiker
BELOUSOV, V.V.	17.(30.)10.1907	Geologist - Geologe
BEZRUKOV, P.L.	20.1.(2.2.)1909	Oceanologist - Ozeanologe
BOGORODSKIJ, V.V.	22.4.1919	Oceanologist - Ozeanologe
BUDYKO, M.I.	20.1.1920	Geophysicist - Geophysiker
BULANŽE, J.D.	28.7.(10.8.)1911	Geologist, Geophysicist - Geologe, Geophysiker
BULAŠEVIĆ, J.P.	28.6.(11.7.)1911	Geophysicist - Geophysiker
ČEPIKOV, K.R.	12.(25.)12.1900	Geologist - Geologe
CHAIN, V.E.	13.(26.)2.1914	Geologist, geophysicist - Geologe, Geophysiker
CHITAROV, N.I.	3.(16.)10.1903	Geochemist - Geochemiker
CHOMENTOVSKIJ, A.S.	11.(24.)3.1908	Geologist - Geologe
ČINAKAL, N.A.		Mining specialist - Bergbauspezialist
CYTOVIĆ, N.A.	13.(26.)5.1900	Geologist - Geologe
DOKUKIN, A.V.		Geologist - Geologe
FEDOTOV, S.A.	19.3.1931	Geophysicist - Geophysiker
FLORENSOV, N.A.	15.(28.)1.1909	Geologist - Geologe
FOTIADI, E.E.	10.(23.)1.1907	Geologist, geophysicist - Geologe, Geophysiker
GORBUNOV, G.I.	13.10.1918	Geologist - Geologe
GUBIN, I.E.		Geologist - Geologe
ILIČEV, V.I.		Hydrologist - Hydrologe
IVANOV, S.N.	3.(16.)2.1911	Geologist - Geologe
IZRAEL, J.A.		Physicist - Physiker
KAPICA, A.P.	9.7.1931	Geologist, geomorphologist - Geologe, Geomorphologe
KONDRATEV, K.J.	14.6.1920	Meteorologist - Meteorologe
KOTLJAKOV, V.M.		Hydrologist - Hydrologe
KRASNYJ, L.I.	22.3.(4.4.)1911	Geologist - Geologe
KRATC, K.O.	16.6.1914	Mineralogist, petrologist - Mineraloge, Petrograph
KROPOTKIN, P.N.	11.(24.)11.1910	Geologist, geophysicist - Geologe, Geophysiker
KURBATKIN, G.P.		Physicist - Physiker
LISICYN, A.P.		Geophysicist - Geophysiker
LOMOV, B.F.		Physicist - Physiker
LUČICKIJ, I.V.	23.4.1912	Geophysicist - Geophysiker
MAGNICKIJ, V.A.	30.5.(12.6.)1915	Geophysicist - Geophysiker
MELNIKOV, P.I.	6.(19.)6.1908	Geophysicist - Geophysiker
MILANOVSKIJ, E.E.		Geologist - Geologe
MONIN, A.S.	2.7.1921	Oceanologist - Ozeanologe
MURATOV, M.V.	29.2.(13.3.)1908	Geologist - Geologe
NALIVKIN, V.D.	17.(30.)4.1915	Geologist - Geologe
NESTEROV, I.I.		Geologist - Geologe
ODINCOV, M.M.	23.10.(5.11.)1911	Geologist - Geologe
OVČINNIKOV, L.N.	26.9.(9.10.)1913	Geologist - Geologe
PARIJSKIJ, N.N.	17.(30.)9.1900	Geophysicist - Geophysiker
PUŠČAROVSKIJ, J.M.		Geologist - Geologe
PUZYREV, N.N.	9.(22.)11.1914	Geophysicist - Geophysiker
RADKEVIČ, E.A.	29.11.(12.12.)1908	Geologist - Geologin
RONOV, A.B.	3.(16.)12.1913	Geochemist - Geochemiker
RŽEVSKIJ, V.V.	23.7.1919	Mining specialist - Bergbauspezialist

Science
Wissenschaft 8.3

SAKS, V.N.	9.(22.)4.1911	Geologist, geographer-Geologe,Geograph
SAVARENSKIJ, E.F.	5.(18.)7.1911	Geologist, geophysicist - Geologe, Geophysiker
ŠEMJAKIN, E.I.		Mining specialist - Bergbauspezialist
SERGEEV, E.M.	10.(23.)3.1914	Hydrogeologist - Hydrogeologe
SOLONENKO, V.P.	2.(15.)11.1916	Geophysicist - Geophysiker
SOLOVEV, S.L.	12.4.1930	Spec.f.seismology,geophysics,hydrophysics- Spez.f.Seismologie,Geophysik,Hydrophysik
SPIVAKOVSKIJ, A.O.	17.(29.)1.1888	Mining specialist - Bergbauspezialist
ŠVECOV, P.F.		Geologist, hydrogeologist - Geologe, Hydrogeologe
TAUSON, L.V.	14.(27.)10.1917	Geochemist - Geochemiker
TIMOFEEV, P.P.		Geologist - Geologe
TREŠNIKOV, A.F.		Geographer - Geograph
TUGARINOV, A.I.	27.1.(12.3.)1917	Geochemist - Geochemiker
VARENCOV, M.I.	7.(20.)1.1902	Geologist - Geologe
VASSOEVIČ, N.B.	17.(30.)3.1902	Geologist - Geologe
VOROPAEV, G.V.		Hydrologist - Hydrologe
ŽARIKOV, V.A.	20.9.1926	Mineralogist - Mineraloge

Section of Social Sciences - Sektion der Gesellschaftswissenschaften

a) Members - Mitglieder:

AGANBEGJAN, A.G.	8.10.1932	Economic scientist-Wirtschaftswissen- schaftler
ALEKSEEV, M.P.	24.5.(5.7.)1896	Literary scientist - Literaturwissenschaftler
ARBATOV, G.A.	19.5.1923	Economic scientist - Wirtschaftswissenschaftler
BELODED, I.K.	16.(29.)8.1906	Linguistic scientist - Sprachwissenschaftler
BORKOVSKIJ, V.I.	6.(19.)1.1900	Linguistic scientist - Sprachwissenschaftler
BROMLEJ, J.V.		Historian - Historiker
CHAČATUROV, T.S.	23.9.(6.10.)1906	Economic scientist - Wirtschaftswissenschaftler
CHRAPČENKO, M.B.	8.(21.)11.1904	Literary scientist, critic - Literaturwissenschaftler, Kritiker
DRUŽININ, N.M.	1.(13.)1.1886	Historian - Historiker
EFIMOV, A.N.	3.(16.)7.1908	Economic scientist - Wirtschaftswissenschaftler
EGOROV, A.G.	25.10.1920	Philosopher - Philosoph
FEDORENKO, N.P.	15.(28.)4.1917	Economic scientist - Wirtschaftswissenschaftler
FEDOSEEV, P.N.	9.(22.)8.1908	Philosopher - Philosoph
ILIČEV, L.F.		Philosopher - Philosoph
INOZEMCEV, N.N.	4.4.1921	Economic scientist - Wirtschaftswissenschaftler
KEDROV, B.M.	27.11.(10.12.)1903	Philosopher, historian - Philosoph, Historiker
KONONOV, A.N.	14.(27.)10.1906	Orientalist-turkologist - Orientalist-Türkologe
KONSTANTINOV, F.V.	8.(21.)2.1901	Philosopher - Philosoph
KOROSTOVCEV, M.A.		Orientalist
LEONOV, L.M.	7.(19.)5.1899	Writer - Schriftsteller
LICHAČEV, D.S.	15.(28.)11.1906	Literary scientist - Literaturwissenschaftler
MINC, I.I.	22.1.(3.2.)1896	Historian - Historiker
MITIN, M.B.	22.6.(5.7.)1901	Philosopher - Philosoph
NAROČNICKIJ, A.L.	3.(16.)2.1907	Historian - Historiker
NEČKINA, M.V.	12.(25.)2.1901	Historian - Historikerin

Science
Wissenschaft

NEKRASOV, N.N.	18.6.(1.7.)1906	Economic scientist - Wirtschaftswissenschaftler
OKLADNIKOV, A.P.	3.(16.)10.1908	Historian, archaeologist - Historiker, Archäologe
PIOTROVSKIJ, B.B.	1.(14.)2.1908	Archaeologist, orientalist - Archäologe, Orientalist
PONOMAREV, B.N.	4.(17.)1.1905	Historian - Historiker
POSPELOV, P.N.	7.(19.)6.1898	Historian - Historiker
RUMJANCEV, A.M.	3.(16.)2.1905	Economic scientist - Wirtschaftswissenschaftler
RYBAKOV, B.A.	21.5.(3.6.)1908	Historian, archaeologist - Historiker, Archäologe
SOLOCHOV, M.A.	11.(24.)5.1905	Writer - Schriftsteller
ŽUKOV, E.M.	23.10.1907	Historian - Historiker

b) Corresponding members - korrespondierende Mitglieder:

AFANASEV, V.G.	18.11.1922	Philosopher - Philosoph
AKSENENOK, G.A.	5.(18.)11.1910	Jurist
ANČISKIN, A.I.		Economic scientist - Wirtschaftswissenschaftler
ARCICHOVSKIJ, A.V.	13.(26.)12.1902	Archaeologist - Archäologe
ASIMOV, M.S.		Philosopher - Philosoph
AVANESOV, R.I.	1.(14.)2.1902	Linguistic scientist - Sprachwissenschaftler
AVRORIN, V.A.	10.(23.)12.1907	Linguistic scientist - Sprachwissenschaftler
BARCHUDAROV, S.G.		Linguistic scientist - Sprachwissenschaftler
BAZANOV, V.G.	14.(27.)10.1911	Literary scientist - Literaturwissenschaftler
BELČIKOV, N.F.	4.(16.)11.1890	Literary scientist - Literaturwissenschaftler
BERDNIKOV, G.P.		Literary scientist - Literaturwissenschaftler
BLAGOJ, D.D.	28.1.(9.2.)1893	Literary scientist - Literaturwissenschaftler
BOGOLJUBOV, M.N.	11.(24.)1.1918	Linguistic scientist - Sprachwissenschaftler
BOGOMOLOV, O.T.	20.8.1927	Economic scientist - Wirtschaftswissenschaftler
BUDAGOV, R.A.	23.8.(5.9.)1910	Philologist-Specialist in Romance languages - Philologe-Romanist
BUNIČ, P.G.	25.10.1929	Economic scientist - Wirtschaftswissenschaftler
BUŠMIN, A.S.	2.(15.)10.1910	Literary scientist - Literaturwissenschaftler
ČAGIN, B.A.	10.(22.)3.1899	Philosopher - Philosoph
ČCHIKVADZE, V.M.	19.12.1911(1.1.1912)	Jurist
ČECHARIN, E.M.		Jurisprudent - Rechtswissenschaftler
DESNICKAJA, A.V.	10.(23.)8.1912	Linguistic & literary scientist - Sprach-u.Literaturwissenschaftler
FEDORENKO, N.T.	9.(22.)11.1912	Philologist,literary scientist-Sinolog. Philologe,Literaturwiss.-Sinologe
FILIN, F.P.	23.2.(7.3.)1908	Linguistic scientist - Sprachwissenschaftler
FROLOV, I.T.		Philosopher - Philosoph
GATOVSKIJ, L.M.	13.(26.)7.1903	Economic scientist - Wirtschaftswissenschaftler
GVIŠIANI, D.M.	24.12.1928	Philosopher - Philosoph

Science 8.3
Wissenschaft

IOVČUK, M.T.	6.(19.)11.1908	Philosopher - Philosoph
JANIN, V.L.	6.2.1929	Historian, Archaeologist - Historiker, Archäologe
JARCEVA, V.N.	21.10.(3.11.)1906	Philologist, linguistic scientist - Philologin, Sprachwissenschaftlerin
KAPUSTIN, E.I.		Economic scientist - Wirtschaftswissenschaftler
KARAKEEV, K.G.	25.10.(7.11.)1913	Historian - Historiker
KERIMOV, D.A.A.o.	18.7.1923	Jurist
KIM, G.F.		Orientalist
KIM, M.P.	12.(25.)5.1908	Historian - Historiker
KOVALČENKO, I.D.	26.11.1923	Historian - Historiker
KOZLOV, G.A.	22.1.(4.2.)1901	Economic scientist - Wirtschaftswissenschaftler
KRUŠANOV, A.I.	1.6.1921	Historian - Historiker
KRUŽKOV, V.S.	3.(16.)6.1905	Philosopher - Philosoph
KUDRJAVCEV, V.N.		Jurisprudent - Rechtswissenschaftler
KUKIN, D.M.	10.(23.)5.1908	Historian - Historiker
LOMIDZE, G.I.	15.(28.)7.1914	Literary scientist - Literaturwissenschaftler
MARKOV, D.F.	10.(23.)10.1913	Literary scientist - Literaturwissenschaftler
MIKULINSKIJ, S.R.		Historian of science - Historiker der Wissenschaften
MILEJKOVSKIJ, A.G.	2.(15.)1.1911	Economic scientist - Wirtschaftswissenschaftler
NOTKIN, A.I.		Economic scientist - Wirtschaftswissenschaftler
OJZERMAN, T.I.	1.(14.)5.1914	Philosopher - Philosoph
OLDEROGGE, D.A.	23.4.(6.5.)1903	Linguistic scientist (Africanist) - Sprachwissenschaftler (Afrikanist)
OMELJANOVSKIJ, M.E.	6.(19.)1.1904	Philosopher - Philosoph
PAŠKOV, A.I.	2.(15.)11.1900	Economic scientist - Wirtschaftswissenschaftler
PAŠUTO, V.T.		Historian - Historiker
PLOTNIKOV, K.N.	11.(24.)5.1907	Economic scientist - Wirtschaftswissenschaftler
POLJAKOV, J.A.	18.10.1921	Historian - Historiker
PRIMAKOV, E.M.		Economic scientist - Wirtschaftswissenschaftler
REIZOV, B.G.	19.10.(1.11.)1902	Literary scientist - Literaturwissenschaftler
RJABUŠKIN, T.V.	17.(30.)12.1914	Economic scientist - Wirtschaftswissenschaftler
RUTENBURG, V.I.		Historian - Historiker
RUTKEVIČ, M.N.	19.9.(2.10.)1917	Philosopher - Philosoph
SAMSONOV, A.M.	26.12.1907(8.1.1908)	Historian - Historiker
ŠANIDZE, A.G.	14.(26.)2.1887	Philologist (Armenian, Georgian) - Philologe (Armenist, Grusinist)
SATALIN, S.S.		Economic scientist - Wirtschaftswissenschaftler
ŠČERBINA, V.R.		Literary scientist - Literaturwissenschaftler
SEREBRENNIKOV, B.A.	21.1.(6.3.)1915	Linguistic scientist - Sprachwissenschaftler
SERGEEV, M.A.		Economic scientist - Wirtschaftswissenschaftler
SIDOROV, A.A.	1.(13.)6.1891	Art historian - Kunsthistoriker
SLADKOVSKIJ, M.I.	8.(21.)11.1906	Economic scientist - Wirtschaftswissenschaftler
SOLODOVNIKOV, V.G.	8.3.1918	Economic scientist - Wirtschaftswissenschaftler

8.3 Science / Wissenschaft

SOROKIN, G.M.	10.(23.)2.1910	Economic scientist - Wirtschaftswissenschaftler
SPIRKIN, A.G.		Philosopher - Philosoph
STEPANJAN, C.A.	19.12.1910(1.1.1911)	Philosopher - Philosoph
STEPANOV, G.V.		Linguistic scientist - Sprachwissenschaftler
STROGOVIČ, M.S.		Jurisprudent - Rechtswissenschaftler
TICHVINSKIJ, S.L.	1.9.1918	Historian - Historiker
TIMOFEEV, L.I.	23.12.1903(5.1.1904)	Literary scientist - Literaturwissenschaftler
TIMOFEEV, T.T.	30.11.1928	Economic scientist - Wirtschaftswissenschaftler
TRAPEZNIKOV, S.P.		Historian - Historiker
TRUBAČEV, O.N.		Linguistic scientist - Sprachwissenschaftler
TRUCHANOVSKIJ, V.G.	2.(15.)7.1914	Historian - Historiker
TUNKIN, G.I.		Jurisprudent - Rechtswissenschaftler
UDALCOVA, Z.V.		Historian - Historikerin
VINOGRADOV, V.A.	2.7.1921	Economic scientist - Wirtschaftswissenschaftler
VOLOBUEV, P.V.	1.1.1923	Historian - Historiker
ZASLAVSKAJA, T.I.	9.9.1927	Economic scientist - Wirtschaftswissenschaftler
ŽILIN, P.A.	20.2.(5.3.)1913	Historian - Historiker

Honorary Members - Ehrenmitglieder:

CHVOLSON, O.D.	4.12.1852 - 11.5.1934	Physicist - Physiker
EGOROV, D.F.	10.(22.)12.1869 - 10.9.1931	Mathematician - Mathematiker
GAMALEJA, N.F.	5.(17.)2.1859 - 29.3.1949	Microbiologist - Mikrobiologe
GLAZENAP, S.P.	13.(25.)9.1848 - 12.4.1937	Astronomer - Astronom
GORJAČKIN, V.P.	17.(29.)1.1868 - 21.9.1935	Spec.f.agricultural machines - Spez.f.Landwirtschaftsmaschinen
GRAVE, D.A.	25.8.(6.9.)1863 - 19.12.1939	Mathematician - Mathematiker
ILINSKIJ, M.A.	1.(13.)11.1856 - 18.11.1941	Organic chemist, spec.f.synthetic colours - organ.Chemiker, Spez.f. synthetische Farben
KABLUKOV, I.A.	21.8.(2.9.)1857 - 5.5.1942	Physical chemist - physikalischer Chemiker
KAREEV, N.I.	24.11.(6.12.)1850 - 18.2.1931	Historian - Historiker
KIŽNER, N.M.	27.11.(9.12.)1867 - 28.11.1935	Organic chemist - organischer Chemiker
KNIPOVIČ, N.M.	6.4.1862 - 23.2.1939	Zoologist, Hydrobiologist - Zoologe, Hydrobiologe
KOROLENKO, V.G.	15.(27.)7.1853 - 25.12.1921	Writer - Schriftsteller
KRUPSKAJA, N.K.	14.(26.)2.1869 - 27.2.1939	Theorist of the Marxist pedagogics - Theoretikerin d.marxist.Pädagogik
MENZBIR, M.A.	23.10.1855-10.10.1935	Zoologist - Zoologe
MIČURIN, I.V.	15.(27.)10.1855 - 7.7.1935	Biologist, selector - Biologe, Selektionär
MOROZOV, N.A.	25.6.(12.7.)1854 - 30.7.1946	Chemist,Astronomer,Culture historian, writer - Chemiker,Astronom,Kulturhistoriker,Schriftsteller

Science
Wissenschaft 8.3

PAVLOVA, M.V.	15.(27.)6.1854 – 23.12.1938	Palaeontologist – Paläontologin
PEKARSKIJ, E.K.	13.(25.)10.1858 – 29.6.1934	Linguistic scientist, ethnographer – Sprachwissenschaftler, Ethnograph
SOKALSKIJ, J.M.	5.(17.)10.1856 – 26.3.1940	Geographer, Oceanologist – Geograph, Ozeanologe
STALIN (DŽUGAŠVILI), I.V.	9.(21.)12.1879 – 5.3.1953	Soviet state and party functionary – Sowjet. Staats-und Parteifunktionär
SUCHOV, V.G.	5.(17.)8.1854 – 2.2.1939	Spec.f.petrol technology, thermics, mechanical construction – Spez.f. Erdöltechnik,Wärmetechnik,Baumechanik
TAGANCEV, N.S.	19.2.(3.3.)1843 – 21.3.1923	Jurist, criminal investigator – Jurist, Kriminalist
VINOGRADSKIJ, S.N.	1.(13.)9.1856 – 24.2.1953	Microbiologist – Mikrobiologe

Foreign Members – Ausländische Mitglieder:

AKABORI, S. (Japan)	20.10.1900	Biochemist – Biochemiker
ALFVEN, H. (Sweden-Schweden)	30.5.1908	Spec.f.electronics, astrophysicist – Spez.f.Elektronik, Astrophysiker
AMALDI, E. (Italy-Italien)	5.9.1908	Physicist – Physiker
AUBOINE, J. (France-Frankreich)	1928	Geologist, tectonist – Geologe, Tektoniker
BACO, Z.M. (Belgium-Belgien)	31.12.1903	Biologist, Physiologist – Biologe, Physiologe
BALEVSKI, A.T. (Bulgaria-Bulgarien)	15.4.1910	Spec.f.mechanics & mechanical engineerg.– Spez.f.Mechanik u.Maschinenbau
BERGSTRÖM, S. (Sweden – Schweden)	1916	Biochemist, medical specialist – Biochemiker, Mediziner
BIRCH, A. (Australia-Australien)	1915	Organic chemist – Organischer Chemiker
BLAŠKOVIČ, D. (Czechoslovakia-CSSR)	2.8.1913	Microbiologist – Mikrobiologe
BLOUT, E. (USA)	1919	Biochemist – Biochemiker
BROGLIE, L.V.prince de (France-Frankreich)	15.8.1892	Physicist – Physiker
CAYA, S. (Japan)	21.12.1898	Physicist – Physiker
CHAIN, E. (Great Britain-Großbritannien)	1906	Biochemist – Biochemiker
CHAN DAY NGIA (Vietnam)	13.9.1913	Specialist for mechanics – Spezialist für Mechanik
CORNU, A. (France-Frankr)	9.8.1888	Philosopher – Philosoph
ČUBRILOVIČ, V. (Yugoslavia-Jugoslawien)	1897	Historian – Historiker
DASKALOV, C.S. (Bulgaria-Bulgarien)	1903	Geneticist – Genetiker
DIRAC, P.A.M. (Great Britain-Großbritannien)	8.8.1902	Physicist – Physiker
DRESCH, J. (France-Frankreich)	30.11.1905	Geographer – Geograph
EIGEN, M. (West Germany-BRD)	1927	Physical chemist – Physikochemiker
GANOVSKI, S.C. (Bulgaria-Bulgarien)	1897	Philosopher – Philosoph
GO MO-ZO (China)	16.11.1892	Historian,writer,literary scientist, state functionary – Historiker,Schriftsteller,Literaturwiss.,Staatsfunktionär
GROSZKOWSKI, J. (Poland-Polen)	21.3.1898	Physicist, spec.f.electronics – Physiker, Spez.f.Elektronik

8.3 Science / Wissenschaft

GUSTAFSON, T. (Sweden - Schweden)	1911	Embryologist - Embryologe
GYLLENBERG, H. (Finland - Finnland)	1924	Microbiologist - Mikrobiologin
HAGENMULLER, P. (France - Frankreich)	1921	Chemist - Chemiker
HARTKE, W. (East Germany - DDR)	1.3.1907	Philologist, Historian - Philologe, Historiker
HASAN, N. (India-Indien)	1921	Historian - Historiker
HODGKIN, A. (Great Britain-Großbritannien)	1914	Physiologist - Physiologe
HODGKIN, D.M.C. (Great Britain-Großbritannien)	1910	Molecular biologist - Molekularbiologin
ILIEV, L.G. (Bulgaria - Bulgarien)	1913	Mathematician - Mathematiker
JABŁOŃSKI, H. (Poland - Polen)	27.12.1909	Historian - Historiker
KHORANA, H.G. (USA)	9.1.1922	Organic chemist - organ.Chemiker
KLAESSEN, St. (Sweden - Schweden)	1917	Physical chemist - Physikochemiker
KLARE, H. (DDR)	12.5.1909	Chemist - Chemiker
KOTARBIŃSKI, T. (Poland - Polen)	31.3.1886	Philosopher - Philosoph
KOTARI, D.S. (India-Indien)	1906	Astrophysicist - Astrophysiker
KOŽEŠNIK, J. (Czechoslovakia - CSSR)	8.6.1907	Mathematician, spec.f.mechanics - Mathematiker, Spez.f.Mechanik
KRYSTANOV, L. (Bulgaria - Bulgarien)	15.11.1908	Geophysicist, meteorologist - Geophysiker, Meteorologe
KUCZINSKI, J. (East Germany - DDR)	1904	Economic scientist - Wirtschaftswissenschaftler
KURATOWSKI, K. (Poland - Polen)	2.2.1896	Mathematician - Mathematiker
LERAY, J. (France - Frankreich)	7.11.1906	Mathematician - Mathematiker
LI SYN GI (Korea)	1905	Chemist - Chemiker
MARINELLO, V.Z. (Cuba-Kuba)	1919	Medical specialist - Mediziner
MARK, H.F. (USA)	3.5.1895	Physical chemist-Physikochemiker
MATEEV, E.G. (Bulgaria - Bulgarien)	1920	Economic scientist - Wirtschaftswissenschaftler
MOTHES, K. (East Germany - DDR)	3.11.1900	Biochemist, pharmacologist, plant physiol.- Biochemiker, Pharmakologe, Pflanzenphys.
MURGULESCU, I. (Romania - Rumänien)	27.1.1902	Physical chemist - Physikochemiker
NADŽAKOV, G.S. (Bulgaria - Bulgarien)	26.12.1896	Physicist - Physiker
NAŁĘCZ, M. (Poland-Polen)	1922	Spec.in cybernetics - Kybernetiker
NATTA, G. (Italy-Italien)	26.2.1903	Chemist - Chemiker
NEEL, L.E.F. (France - Frankreich)	22.11.1904	Physicist - Physiker
NGUEN, K.T. (Vietnam)	1907	Historian - Historiker
OCHOA, S. (USA)	24.9.1906	Biochemist - Biochemiker
OORT, J.H. (Netherlands-Niederlande)	28.4.1900	Astronomer - Astronom
PAL, L. (Hungary-Ungarn)	1925	Physicist - Physiker
PAULING, L.C. (USA)	28.2.1901	Chemist, physicist-Chemiker, Physiker
PAVLOV, T. (Bulgaria - Bulgarien)	14.2.1890	Philosopher, literary critic - Philosoph, Literaturkritiker
PEK NAM UN (Korea)	17.3.1894	Historian, economic scientist - Historiker, Wirtschaftswissenschaft.
PRELOG, V. (Switzerland - Schweiz)	23.7.1906	Chemist - Chemiker

Science
Wissenschaft 8.3

RIENÄCKER, G. (DDR)	13.5.1904	Chemist – Chemiker
REINHOLD, O. (DDR)	1925	Economic scient.-Wirtschaftswiss.
RODGERS, J. (USA)	1914	Geologist – Geologe
RYLE, M., Sir	27.9.1918	Radioastronomer – Spezialist für
(Great Britain-Großbritannien)		Radioastronomie
SALAM, A. (Pakistan)	29.1.1926	Physicist – Physiker
SAVIĆ, P.	10.1.1909	Physical chemist –
(Yugoslavia-Jugoslawien)		Physikochemiker
SEABORG, G.T. (USA)	19.4.1912	Chemist,physicist,spec.f.radiochemistry, nuclear chemistry and physics – Chemiker,Physiker, Spez.f.Radiochemie, Kernchemie und -physik
SHIRENDEV, B.	15.5.1912	Historian, state functionary –
(Mongolia – Mongolei)		Historiker, Staatsfunktionär
SIEGBAHN, K.M.G.	3.12.1886	Physicist – Physiker
(Sweden – Schweden)		
SIRACKY, A. (CSSR)	1900	Philosopher – Philosoph
SIŠKA, K. (CSSR)	19.3.1906	Medical spec.,surgeon-Mediziner,Chirurg
ŠORM, F. (CSSR)	28.2.1913	Organic chemist – organ. Chemiker
STEENBECK, M. (DDR)	21.3.1904	Physicist – Physiker
STENSJÖ, E.H.O.	2.10.1891	Palaeozoologist – Paläozoologe
(Sweden – Schweden)		
STOMMEL, H. (USA)	1920	Ozeanologist – Ozeanologe
SZABO, I. (Hungary-Ungarn)	1912	Jurisprudent-Rechtswissenschaftler
SZENT-GYÖRGYI, A. (USA)	16.9.1893	Biochemist – Biochemiker
SZENTÁGOTHAI, J.	1912	Physiologist, histologist –
(Hungary – Ungarn)		Physiologe, Histologe
SZÖKEFALVI-NADY, B.	29.7.1913	Mathematician – Mathematiker
(Hungary – Ungarn)		
THIESSEN, P.A. (DDR)	6.4.1899	Physical chemist – Physikochemiker
TITEICA, G.Ș.	27.3.1908	Physicist – Physiker
(Romania – Rumänien)		
TOMONAGA, S.-i. (Japan)	31.3.1906	Physicist – Physiker
TRZEBIATOWSKI, W.	1906	Chemist – Chemiker
(Poland – Polen)		
VENKATARAMAN, K.(India-Indien)		Organic chemist – organ.Chemiker
WEISSKOPF, V.F. (USA)	1908	Nuclear physicist – Kernphysiker
WOODWARD, R. (USA)	1917	Biochemist – Biochemiker
YUKAWA, H. (Japan)	23.1.1907	Physicist – Physiker
ZERVAS, L.	1902	Chemist (peptide and albumen) –
(Greece – Griechenland)		Chemiker (Peptid und Eiweiß)
ZOUBEK, V. (CSSR)	1903	Geologist – Geologe

Females – Frauen

a) Members – Mitglieder:

   3 from a total of 234 (Mathematician, chemist, historian) –
   3 von insgesamt 234 (Mathematikerin, Chemikerin, Historikerin)

b) Corresponding Members – korrespondierende Mitglieder:

   11 from a total of 487(3 chemist, 1 geophysicist, physiologist, biologist, geo-
                        logist, linguistic & literary scientist, linguistic
                        scientist, historian, economic scientist) –
   11 von insgesamt 487 (3 Chemikerinnen, 1 Geophysikerin, Physiologin, Biologin,
                        Geologin, Sprach-u.Literaturwiss., Sprachwiss., Histo-
                        rikerin, Wirtschaftswiss.)

477

8.3.1 Science
Wissenschaft

8.3.1
USSR BRANCH ACADEMIES - ZWEIG-AKADEMIEN DER UdSSR - OTRASLEVYE AKADEMII SSSR

USSR Academy of Medical Sciences - Akademie der Medizinischen Wissenschaften der UdSSR - Akademija medicinskich nauk SSSR
  Soljanka, 14, Moskva
  (founded - gegründet 1944)
    on 1/1/1977: 103 members, 150 corresponding members, 26 foreign members;
        41 scientific institutes -
    zum 1.1.1977: 103 Mitglieder, 150 korrespondierende Mitglieder, 26 ausländische Mitglieder; 41 wissenschaftliche Forschungsinstitute
    President - Präsident   - BLOCHIN, N.N.
    Vice Presidents-Vizepräsidenten - CERNUCH, A.M.   PAVLOV, A.S.
    Acting Vice President -   DEBOV, S.S.
    Amt. Vizepräsident   - VOLKOV, M.V.
    Academic Secretary-Akad. Sekretär- SIDORENKO, G.I.

USSR Academy of Pedagogical Sciences - Akademie der Pädagogischen Wissenschaften der UdSSR - Akademija pedagogičeskich nauk SSSR
  Poljanka, 58, Moskva
  (founded 1966 as successor to the Academy of Pedagogical Sciences of the RSFSR, founded 1943 - 1966 gegründet als Nachfolger der Akademie der Pädagogischen Wissenschaften der RSFSR, gegründet 1943)
    on 1/1/1977: 51 members, 76 corresponding members; 4 branches, 13 scientific research institutes, 14 experimental schools, 2 boarding-schools, National Scientific Pedagogical K.D.Ushinsky Library, Institute for further education of teachers of pedagogical sciences at universities and pedagogical institutes -
    zum 1.1.1977: 51 Mitglieder, 76 korrespondierende Mitglieder; 4 Filialen, 13 wissenschaftl.Forschungsinstitute, 14 experimentelle Schulen, 2 Schulinternate, Staatl.Wissenschaftl.Pädagogische K.D.Ušinskij-Bibliothek, Institut zur Erhöhung der Qualifikation der Lehrer für pädagogische Fächer an Universitäten und pädagogischen Hochschulen
    President - Präsident   - STOLETOV, V.N.
    Vice Presidents-Vizepräsidenten - CHRIPKOVA, A.G.   PETROVSKIJ, A.V.
                                     KONDAKOV, M.I.
    Academic Secretary-Akad.Sekretär - PROTCENKO, I.F.

V.I.Lenin All-Union Academy of Agricultural Sciences - V.I.Lenin-Unionsakademie für Agrarwissenschaften - Vsesojuznaja Akademija sel'skochozjajstvennych nauk imeni V.I.Lenina
  Bol. Charitonevskij pereulok, 21, Moskva
  (founded - gegründet 1929)
    on 1/1/1977: 1 honorary member, 98 members, 106 corresponding members, 37 foreign members
    President - Präsident   - VAVILOV, P.P.
    Vice Presidents-Vizepräsidenten - ERNST, L.K.   ŠATILOV, I.S.
                                     KUZMENKO, I.V.   SINJAGIN, I.I.
                                     PANNIKOV, V.D.
    Academic Secretary-Akad.Sekretär - MUROMCEV, G.S.

USSR Academy of Arts - Akademie der Künste der UdSSR - Akademija chudožestv SSSR
  Kropotkinskaja ulica, 21, Moskva
  (founded - gegründet 1947)
    on 1/1/1977: 48 members, 78 corresponding members, 11 honorary members
    zum 1.1.1977: 48 Mitglieder, 78 korrespondierende Mitglieder, 11 Ehrenmitglieder
    President - Präsident   - TOMSKIJ, N.V.
    Vice Presidents-Vizepräsidenten - KEMENOV, V.S.   REŠETNIKOV, F.P.
    Academic Secretary-Akad.Sekretär - SYSOEV, P.M.

8.3.2 ACADEMIES OF SCIENCES OF THE UNION REPUBLICS
AKADEMIEN DER WISSENSCHAFTEN DER UNIONSREPUBLIKEN
AKADEMII NAUK SOJUZNYCH RESPUBLIK

	President-Präsident
Academy of Sciences of the Ukrainian SSR - Akademie der Wissenschaften der Ukrainischen SSR ul. Vladimirskaja, 54, Kiev	- PATON, B.E.
Academy of Sciences of the Belorussian SSR - Akademie der Wissenschaften der Belorussischen SSR Leninskij prosp. 66, Minsk	- BORISEVIČ, N.A.
Academy of Sciences of the Uzbek SSR - Akademie der Wissenschaften der Usbekischen SSR ul. Kujbyševa, 15, Taškent	- SADYKOV, A.S.
Academy of Sciences of the Kazakh SSR - Akademie der Wissenschaften der Kasachischen SSR ul. Ševčenko, 28, Alma-Ata	- KUNAEV, A.M.
Academy of Sciences of the Georgian SSR - Akademie der Wissenschaften der Grusinischen SSR ul. Dzeržinskogo, 8, Tbilisi	- CHARADZE, E.
Academy of Sciences of the Azerbaidzhan SSR - Akademie der Wissenschaften der Aserbaidschanischen SSR Kommunističeskaja ul., 10, Baku	- ABDULLAEV, G.B.
Academy of Sciences of the Lithuanian SSR - Akademie der Wissenschaften der Litauischen SSR ul. K. Poželos, 2/8, Vilnius	- MATULIS, Ju.Ju.
Academy of Sciences of the Moldavian SSR - Akademie der Wissenschaften der Moldauischen SSR prosp. Lenina, 1, Kišinev	- ZUČENKO, A.A.
Academy of Sciences of the Latvian SSR - Akademie der Wissenschaften der Lettischen SSR Riga, ul. Turgeneva 19	- MALMEJSTER, A.K.
Academy of Sciences of the Kirghiz SSR - Akademie der Wissenschaften der Kirgisischen SSR Puškinskaja ul., 78, Frunze	- KARAKEEV, K.K.
Academy of Sciences of the Tadzhik SSR - Akademie der Wissenschaften der Tadschikischen SSR Dušanbe	- ASIMOV, M.S.
Academy of Sciences of the Armenian SSR - Akademie der Wissenschaften der Armenischen SSR ul. Abovjana, 61, Erevan	- AMBARCUMJAN, V.A.
Academy of Sciences of the Turkmen SSR - Akademie der Wissenschaften der Turkmenischen SSR Komsomol'skaja ul., 31, Aschabad	- BABAEV, A.G.
Academy of Sciences of the Estonian SSR - Akademie der Wissenschaften der Estnischen SSR Kochtu ul., 6, Tallin	- REBANE, K.K.

8.4 Science / Wissenschaft

8.4 LIST OF INSTITUTES - VERZEICHNIS DER INSTITUTE

a) Section of Physical-Technical and Mathematical Sciences -
Sektion der physikalisch-technischen u.mathematischen Wissensch.:

Department of General Physics and Astronomy -
Abteilung für allgemeine Physik und Astronomie:

Acoustics Institute - Akustisches Institut - Akustičeskij institut,
ul. Televidenija, 4, Moskva

Astronomical Council - Astronomischer Rat - Astronomičeskij sovet,
ul. Vavilova, 34, Moskva

Central Astronomical Observatory Pulkovo - Astronomisches Hauptobservatorium
Pulkovo - Glavnaja astronomičeskaja observatorija-Pulkovskaja observatorija,
GAO, Pulkovo bliz Leningrada

Crimean Astro-Physical Observatory - Astrophysikalisches Observatorium auf
der Krim -Krymskaja astrofizičeskaja observatorija, KAO, Partizanskoe

Special Astro-Physical Observatory - Astrophysikalisches Spezialobservatorium -
Special'naja astrofizičeskaja observatorija

Institute of Terrestrial Magnetism, Radio Research and the Ionosphere -
Institut für Erdmagnetismus, die Ionosphäre und die Ausbreitung von Radiowellen - Institut zemnogo magnetizma, ionosfery i rasprostranenija radiovoln,
IZMIRAN, Akademgorodok, Podolsky oblast

Institute of Precision Mechanics and Computing Equipment - Institut für
Feinmechanik und Rechentechnik - Institut točnoj mechaniki i vyčislitel'noj
techniki, ITOČMECh, Leninskij prosp., 51, Moskva

Institute of Solid State Physics - Institut für Festkörperphysik -
Institut fiziki tverdogo tela, ul.Radio, 23/29, Moskva

Institute of High-Pressure Physics - Institut für Hochdruckphysik -
Institut fiziki vysokich davlenij, IFVD, Akademgorodok, Podolskogo rajona

Leningrad Institute of Nuclear Physics - Institut für Kernphysik Leningrad -
Leningradskij institut jadernoj fiziki, Leningrad

Institute of Cosmic Rays - Institut für kosmische Forschungen - Institut
kosmičeskich issledovanij, Profsojuznaja ul.,88, Moskva

Institute of Crystallography - Institut für Kristallographie -
Institut kristallografii, IK, Leninskij prosp.,59, Moskva

Institute of Physical Problems - Institut für physikalische Probleme -
Institut fizičeskich problem im. S.I.Vavilova, IFP,
Vorobevskoe šosse,2, Moskva

Institute of Radio Engineering - Institut für Radiotechnik - Radiotechničeskij
institut, ul.8 Marta, 10-12, Moskva

Institute of Radio Engineering and Electronics - Institut für Radiotechnik
und Elektronik - Institut radiotechniki i elektroniki,
Prosp.Karla Marksa,18, Moskva

Institute of Spectroscopy - Institut für Spektroskopie - Institut spektroskopii

Institute of Theoretical Astronomy - Institut für theoretische Astronomie -
Institut teoretičeskoj astronomii, ITA, linija Mendeleeva,1, Leningrad, V.O.

Science
Wissenschaft 8.4

L.D.Landau Institute of Theoretical Physics - Institut für theoretische
Physik, L.D.Landau-Institut - Institut teoretičeskoj fiziki im. L.D.Landau,
ITF, pos.Černogolovka, Noginskogo rajona,Moskovskoj oblasti

P.N.Lebedev Physical Institute - Physikalisches Institut, P.N.Lebedev-Institut
Fizičeskij institut im. P.N.Lebedeva, FIAN, Leninskij prosp.,53, Moskva

Physical Laboratory - Physikalisches Laboratorium - Fizičeskaja laboratorija,
Vorobevskoe šosse,2, Moskva

A.F.Ioffe Physical-Technical Institute - Physikalisch-technisches Institut,
A.F.Joffe-Institut - Fiziko-techničeskij institut im. A.F.Joffe, LFTI,
Politechničeskaja ul.,2, Leningrad

Kazan Physical-Technical Institute - Physikalisch-technisches Institut
Kazan - Kazanskij fiziko-techničeskij institut, Kazan

Department of Nuclear Physics - Abteilung für Kernphysik

Department of Mathematics - Abteilung für Mathematik:

Institute of Applied Mathematics - Institut für angewandte Mathematik -
Institut prikladnoj matematiki,Miusskaja ploščad',4, Moskva

V.A.Steklov Institute of Mathematics - Mathematisches Institut, V.A.Steklov-
Institut - Matematičeskij institut im. V.A.Steklova, MIAN,
ul. Vavilova,42, Moskva

Leningrad Department - Abteilung Leningrad - Leningradskoe otdelenie,
Fontanka,25, Leningrad

Computing Center - Rechenzentrum - Vyčislitel'nyj centr ,
ul.Vavilova,40, Moskva

Department of Mechanics and Control Processes - Abteilung für Mechanik und
Regelungsprozesse:

Institute of Problems of Information Transmission - Institut für Probleme
der Informationsübertragung - Institut problem peredači informacii, IPPI,
Aviamotornaja ul.,8, korpus 2, Moskva

Institute of Problems of Mechanics - Institut für Probleme der Mechanik -
Institut problem mechaniki, Leningradskij prosp.,7, Moskva

Institute of Operating Problems - Institut für Probleme der Steuerung -
Institut problem upravlenija, Profsojuznaja ul.,81, Moskva

Department of Physical and Technical Problems of Energetics -
Abteilung für physikalisch-technische Probleme der Energetik:

Institute of Electromechanics - Institut für Elektromechanik - Institut
elektromechaniki, IEM, Dvorcovaja naberežnaja,18, Leningrad

Institute of High Temperature - Institut für hohe Temperaturen - Institut
vysokich temperatur, Krasnokazarmennaja ul.,17, korpus A, Moskva

b) **Section of Chemistry, Chemical Technology and Biology - Sektion
der chemisch-technologischen und biologischen Wissenschaften:**

Department of General Biology - Abteilung für allgemeine Biologie:

V.L.Komarov Botanical Institute - Botanisches Institut, V.L.Komarov-Institut -
Botaničeskij institut im. V.L.Komarova, ul.Popova,2, Leningrad

Experimental Scientific Research Station - Wissenschaftliche Versuchs-
station - Naučno-opytnaja stancija, Otradnoe, Priozerskij rajon

Great Botanical Garden - Großer Botanischer Garten - Glavnyj botaničeskij
sad, GBS, Botaničeskaja ul.,4, Moskva

481

8.4 Science / Wissenschaft

Laboratory of Helminthology - Helminthologisches Laboratorium - Laboratorija gel'mintologii, Leninskij prosp.,33, Moskva

Institute of General Genetics - Institut für allgemeine Genetik - Institut obščej genetiki, Profsojuznaja ul.,7, korpus 1, Moskva

Institute of Biology of Inland Waters - Institut für die Biologie von Binnengewässern - Institut biologii vnutrennich vod, p/o Borok, Nekouzskogo rajona, jaroslavskoj oblasti

Institute of Developmental Biology - Institut für Entwicklungsbiologie - Institut biologii razvitija im. N.K.Kol'cova, ul.Vavilova,26, Moskva

Institute of Forestry - Institut für Forstwesen - Institut lesovedenija, s.Uspenskoe, Odincovskogo rajona, Moskovskoj oblasti

Institute of Genetics - Institut für Genetik - Institut genetiki, IGEN, Leninskij prosp.,33, Moskva

Paleontological Institute - Paläontologisches Institut - Paleontologičeskij institut, PIN, Leninskij prosp.,33, Moskva

Zoological Institute - Zoologisches Institut - Zoologičeskij institut, ZIN Universitetskaja naberežnaja,1, Leningrad

Department of General and Technical Chemistry - Abteilung für allgemeine und technische Chemie:

Institute of Chemistry - Institut für Chemie - Institut chimii, ul.Artelnaja,11/15, Gorkij

Institute of Chemical Physics - Institut für chemische Physik - Institut chimičeskoj fiziki, IChF, Vorobevskoe šosse,2b, Moskva

Branch-Filiale-Filial: pos.Černogolovka, Noginskogo rajona, Moskovskoj oblast

Laboratory of Anisotropical Structures - Laboratorium für anisotrope Strukturen - Laboratorija anizotropnych struktur, Kolobovskij per.,1/6, Mosk

Institute of Electro-Chemistry - Institut für Elektrochemie - Institut elektrochimii, IELAN, Leninskij prosp.,31, Moskva

Institute of Elementary Organic Compounds - Institut für elementare organische Verbindungen - Institut elementoorganičeskich soedinenij , IEOS, ul.Vavilova,28, Moskva

Institute of Macro-Molecular Compounds - Institut für hochmolekulare Verbindungen - Institut vysokomolekuljarnych soednineij, Bol'šoj prosp.,31,Leningra

N.D.Zelinsky Institute of Organic Chemistry - Institut für organische Chemie, N.D.Zelinskij-Institut - Institut organičeskoj chimii im.N.D.Zelinskogo, IOChAN, Leninskij prosp.,47, Moskva

A.E.Arbuzov Institute of Organic and Physical Chemistry - Institut für organische und physikalische Chemie, A.E.Arbuzov-Institut - Institut organičeskoj i fizičeskoj chimii im. A.E.Arbuzova, ul.Arbuzova,8, Kazan 83

A.V.Topchiev Institute of Oil Chemical Synthesis - Institut für petrochemische Synthese, A.V.Topčiev-Institut - Institut neftechimičeskogo sinteza im. A.V.Topčieva, INChS, Leninskij prosp.,29, Moskva

Institute of Physical Chemistry - Institut für physikalische Chemie - Institut fizičeskoj chimii, IFCh, Leninskij prosp.,31, Moskva

Department of Biochemistry, Biophysics and Chemistry of Physiologically Active Compounds - Abteilung für Biochemie, Biophysik und die Chemie physiologisch aktiver Verbindungen:

A.N.Bakh Institute of Biochemistry - Institut für Biochemie, A.N.Bach-Institu Institut biochimii im. A.N.Bacha, InBi, Leninskij prosp.,33, Moskva

Kazan Biological Institute - Institut für Biologie, Kazan' - Kazanskij
institut biologii, ul. Lobačevskogo,2/31, Kazan

M.M.Šemjakin Institute of Chemistry of Natural Compounds - Institut für die
Chemie der Naturstoffverbindungen, M.M.Šemjakin-Institut - Institut chimii
prirodnych soedinenij im. M.M.Šemjakina, IChPS, ul.Vavilova,32, Moskva

Institute of Microbiology - Institut für Mikrobiologie - Institut
mikrobiologii, INMI, Profsojuznaja ul.,7a, Moskva

Institute of Molecular Biology - Institut für Molekularbiologie -
Institut molekuljarnoj biologii, ul.Vavilova,32, Moskva

K.A.Timiryazev Institute of Plant Physiology - Institut für Pflanzen-
physiologie, K.A.Timirjazev-Institut - Institut fiziologii rastenij im.
K.A.Timirjazeva, Leninskij prosp., 33, Moskva

Institute of Cytology - Institut für Zytologie - Institut citologii,
prosp.Maklina, 32, Leningrad

Scientific Center of Biological Research - Wissenschaftliches Zentrum für
biologische Forschungen - Naučnyj centr biologičeskich issledovanij

   Institute of Biochemistry and Physiology of Microorganisms -
   Institut für Biochemie und Physiologie der Mikroorganismen -
   Institut biochimii i fiziologii mikroorganizmov, g.Puščino

   Institute of Biological Physics - Institut für biologische Physik -
   Institut biologičeskoj fiziki, Akademgorodok, Puščino

Institute of Agrochemistry and Soil Science - Institut für Agrochemie und
Bodenkunde - Institut agrochimii i počvovedenija, Serpukov, Puščino

Institute of Albumen - Institut für Eiweiß - Institut belka, Puščino

Institute of Photosynthesis - Institut für Photosynthese - Institut foto-
sinteza, Akademgorodok, Puščino

Special Construction Office for the Construction of Biological Devices -
Spezialkonstruktionsbüro für den Bau biologischer Apparaturen -
SKB biologičeskogo priborostroenija, Puščino

Department of Physical Chemistry and Technology of Inorganic Materials -
Abteilung für physikalische Chemie und Technologie anorganischer Stoffe:

N.S.Kurnakov Institute of General and Inorganic Chemistry - Institut für
allgemeine und anorganische Chemie, N.S.Kurnakov-Institut - Institut obščej
i neorganičeskoj chimii im. N.S.Kurnakova, IONCh, Leninskij prosp.,31, Moskva

I.V.Grebenshchikov Institute of Chemistry of Silicates - Institut für Chemie
der Silikate, I.V.Grebenščikov-Institut - Institut chimii silikatov im.
I.V.Grebenščikova, IChS, naberežnaja Makarova, 2, Leningrad

A.A.Baikov Institute of Metallurgy - Institut für Metallurgie, A.A.Bajkov-
Institut - Institut metallurgii im. A.A.Bajkova, IMet,
Leninskij prosp., 49, Moskva

Institute of New Chemical Problems - Institut für neue chemische Probleme -
Institut novych chimičeskich problem, Leninskij prosp., 14, Moskva

Department of Physiology - Abteilung für Physiologie:

   I.M.Sechenov Institute of Evolutionary Physiology and Biochemistry -
   Institut für Evolutionsphysiologie und Biochemie, I.M.Sečenov-Institut -
   Institut evoljucionnoj fiziologii i biochimii im. I.M.Sečenova,
   prosp. M.Toreza, 52, Leningrad

   Institute of Higher Nervous Activity and Neurophysiology - Institut für
   höhere Nerventätigkeit und Neurophysiologie - Institut vysšej nervnoj
   dejatel'nosti i nejrofiziologii, IVNDiNF, Pjatnickaja ul., 48, Moskva

8.4 Science
Wissenschaft

I.P.Pavlov Institute of Physiology - Institut für Physiologie, I.P.Pavlov-Institut - Institut fiziologii im. I.P.Pavlova, nabereznaja Makarova, 6, Leningrad

c) Section of Earth Sciences - Sektion der Erdwissenschaften

Institute of Geology - Geologisches Institut - Geologičeskij institut, GIN, Pyževskij per., 7, Moskva

A.A.Skochinsky Institute of Mining - Institut für Bergbau, A.A.Skočinskij-Institut - Institut gornogo dela im. A.A.Skočinskogo, IGD, stancija Panki, Moskva

Institute of the Geology and Mining of Fuel - Institut für die Geologie und die Förderung von Brennstoffen - Institut geologii i razrabotki gorjučich iskopaemych, ul. Fersmana, 50, Moskva

Institute of Geology and Precambrian Geochronology - Institut für die Geologie und Geochronologie des Präkambriums - Institut geologii i geochronologii dokembrija, nabereznaja Makarova, 2, Leningrad

Institute of the Geology of Ore Deposits, Petrography, Mineralogy and Geochemistry - Institut für die Geologie von Erzvorkommen, Petrographie, Mineralogie und Geochemie - Institut geologii rudnych mestoroždenija, petrografii, mineralogii i geochimii, IGEM, Staromonetnyj per.,35, Moskva

Institute of Experimental Mineralogy - Institut für experimentelle Mineralogie - Institut eksperimental'noj mineralogii, Noginskij naučnyj centr

V.I.Vernadsky Institute of Geochemistry and Analytical Chemistry - Institut für Geochemie und analytische Chemie, V.I.Verdnadskij-Institut - Institut geochimii i analitičeskoj chimii im. V.I.Vernadskogo, GEOChI, Vorobevskoe šosse, 47a, Moskva

Institute of Geography - Institut für Geographie - Institut geografii, IGAN, Staromonetnyj per., 29, Moskva

Institute of Limnology - Institut für Limnologie - Institut ozerovedenija, nabereznaja Makarova, 2, Leningrad

Institute of Mineralogy, Geochemistry and Crystallochemistry of Rare Elements - Institut für Mineralogie, Geochemie und Kristallchemie seltener Elemente - Institut mineralogii, geochimii i kristallochimii redkich elementov, IMGRE, Sadovničeskaja nabereznaja, 71, Moskva

Institute of Atmospheric Physics - Institut für die Physik der Atmosphäre - Institut fiziki atmosfery, IFA, Pyževskij per., 3, Moskva

O.Y.Schmidt Institute of Earth Physics - Institut für die Physik der Erde, O.Ju.Šmidt-Institut - Institut fiziki Zemli im. O.Ju.Šmidta, IFZ, B.Gruzinskaja ul., 10, Moskva

Institute of Water Problems - Institut für Wasserfragen - Institut vodnych problem, Sadovaja-Černogrjazskaja ul., 13/3, Moskva

A.E.Fersman Mineralogical Museum - Mineralogisches Museum, A.E.Fersman-Museum - Mineralogičeskij muzej im. A.E.Fersmana, Leninskij prosp.,14/16, Moskva

P.P.Shirshov Institute of Oceanology - Ozeanologisches Institut, P.P.Širšov-Institut - Institut okeanologii im. P.P.Širšova, IOAN, Letnjaja ul., 1, Ljublino

Science 8.4
Wissenschaft

All-Union Research Institute of Mineralogical Raw Materials and Prospecting –
Unionsforschungsinstitut für die wirtschaftliche Nutzung mineralischer Rohstoffe und geologische Erkundung – Vsesojuznyj naučno-issledovatel'skij institut ekonomiki mineral'nogo syr'ja i geologorazvedočnych rabot, VIEMS, ul. Volodarskogo, 38, Moskva

d) Section of Social Sciences – Sektion der Gesellschaftswissenschaften

Institute of the International Working-Class Movement – Institut der internationalen Arbeiterbewegung – Institut meždunarodnogo rabočego dviženija, Kolpačnyj per., 9a, Moskva

Institute of Concrete Social Research – Institut für konkrete soziale Forschungen – Institut konkretnych social'nych issledovanij, Novočeremuškinskaja ul., 46, Moskva

Institute of Information and Fundamental Library on Social Sciences –
Institut für wissenschaftliche Information und Fundamentalbibliothek der Gesellschaftswissenschaften – Institut naučnoj informacii i Fundamental'naja biblioteka po obščestvennym naukam, ul. Frunze, 11/11, Moskva

Department of History – Abteilung für Geschichte:

Archive of the Academy of Sciences of the U.S.S.R. – Archiv der Akademie der Wissenschaften der UdSSR – Archiv Akademii nauk SSSR, AAN, Moskva

N.N.Miklukho-Maklay Institute of Ethnography – Ethnographisches Institut, N.N.Miklucho-Maklaj-Institut – Institut etnografii im. N.N.Miklucho-Maklaja, ul. Dmitrija Ul'janova, 19, Moskva

Institute of General History – Institut für allgemeine Geschichte – Institut vseobščej istorii, ul. Dmitrija Ul'janova, 19, Moskva

Institute of Archaeology – Institut für Archäologie – Institut archeologii, IA, ul. Dmitrija Ul'janova, 19, Moskva

Institute of History of the U.S.S.R. – Institut für Geschichte der UdSSR – Institut istorii SSSR, ul. Dmitrija Ul'janova, 19, Moskva

Institute of Oriental Studies – Institut für Orientalistik – Institut vostokovedenija, Armjanskij per., 2, Moskva

Institute of Slavonic and Balkan Studies – Institut für Slawistik und Balkanistik – Institut slavjanovedenija i balkanistiki, Trubnikovskij per., 30a, Moskva

Laboratory for Preservation and Restoration of Documents – Laboratorium für die Konservierung und Restaurierung von Dokumenten – Laboratorija konservacii i restavracii dokumentov, LKRD, Leningrad

Petr-Velikij Museum of Anthropology and Ethnography – Museum für Anthropologie und Ethnographie, Petr-Velikij-Museum – Muzej antropologii i etnografii im. Petra Velikogo, Universitetskaja naberežnaja, 3, Leningrad

Department of Literature and Linguistics – Abteilung für Literatur und Sprache:

Institute of Russian Language – Institut für die russische Sprache – Institut russkogo jazyka, IRJaz, Volchonka, 18/2, Moskva

Institute of Russian Literature (Pushkin House) – Institut für russische Literatur (Puškin-Haus) – Institut russkoj literatury (Puškinskij dom), naberežnaja Makarova, 4, Leningrad

G.Ibraghimov Institute of Language, Literature and History – Institut für Sprache, Literatur und Geschichte, G.Ibragimov-Institut – Institut jazyka, literatury i istorii im. G.Ibragimova, Ul. Lobačevskogo, 2/31, Kazan

Institute of Linguistic Studies – Institut für Sprachwissenschaft – Institut jazykoznanija, IJaz, ul. Marksa i Engel'sa, 1/14, Moskva

8.4 Science / Wissenschaft

A.M.Gorky Institute of World Literature - Institut für Weltliteratur, A.M.Gorkij-Institut - Institut mirovoj literatury im. A.M.Gor'kogo, IMLI, ul. Vorovskogo, 25a, Moskva

Faculty of Foreign Languages - Lehrstuhl für Fremdsprachen - Kafedra inostrannych jazykov, Moskva

L.N.Tolstoy State Literature Museum - Staatliches literarisches L.N.Tolstoj-Museum - Gosudarstvennyj literaturnyj muzej L.N.Tolstogo, Kropotkinskaja ul., Moskva

Department of Philosophy and Law - Abteilung für Philosophie und Recht:

Institute of History of Natural Science and Engineering - Institut für Geschichte der Naturwissenschaft und der Technik - Institut istorii estestvoznanija i techniki, IIEsTech, Staropanskij per., 1/5, Moskva

Institute of State and Law - Institut für Staat und Recht - Institut gosudarstva i prava, InPrav, ul. Frunze, 10, Moskva

Faculty of Philosophy - Lehrstuhl für Philosophie - Kafedra filosofii, Leningrad

Philosophical Institute - Philosophisches Institut - Institut filosofii, Volchonka, 14, Moskva

Department of Economics - Abteilung für Wirtschaftswissenschaften:

Africa Institute - Afrika-Institut - Institut Afriki, Starokonjušennyj per., 16, Moskva

Institute of the Far East - Institut für den Fernen Osten - Institut Dal'nego Vostoka, ul. Kržižanovskogo, 14, korp.2, Moskva

Institute of the U.S.A. - Institut für die Vereinigten Staaten von Amerika - Institut Soedinennych Statov Ameriki, Chlebnyj per., 2/3, Moskva

Institute of Economics of the International Socialist System - Institut für die Wirtschaft des sozialistischen Weltsystems - Institut ekonomiki mirovoj socialističeskoj sistemy, IEMSS, Novočeremuškinskaja ul., 46, Moskva

Institute of Latin America - Institut für Lateinamerika - Institut Latinskoj Ameriki, B.Ordynka, 21, Moskva

Institute of World Economics and International Relations - Institut für Weltwirtschaft und internationale Beziehungen - Institut mirovoj ekonomiki i meždunarodnych otnošenij, IMEMO, Jaroslavskaja ul., 13, Moskva

Institute of Economics - Institut für Wirtschaftswissenschaften - Institut ekonomiki, IE, Volchonka, 14, Moskva

Central Economic Mathematical Institute - Zentrales wirtschaftswissenschaftlich-mathematisches Institut - Central'nyj ekonomiko-matematičeskij institut, CEMI, Leninskij prosp., 14, Korpus 7, Moskva

e) <u>Siberian Department - Sibirische Abteilung</u>

Novosibirsk:
Institute of Automation and Electrical Measuring - Institut für Automatik und Elektrometrie - Institut avtomatiki i elektrometrii, Akademgorodok, Novosibirsk

Institute of Semiconductor Physics - Institut für Halbleiterphysik - Institut fiziki poluprovodnikov, Akademgorodok, Novosibirsk

Institute of Hydrodynamics - Institut für Hydrodynamik - Institut gidrodinamiki, Akademgorodok, Novosibirsk

Institute of Nuclear Physics - Institut für Kernphysik - Institut jadernoj fiziki, Akademgorodok, Novosibirsk

Institute of Theoretical and Applied Mechanics - Institut für theoretische
und angewandte Mechanik - Institut teoretičeskoj i prikladnoj mechaniki,
ITiPM, Akademgorodok, Novosibirsk

Institute of Transport and Energy - Institut für Transportwesen und Energetik -
Transportno-energetičeskij institut, TEI, Akademgorodok, Novosibirsk

Institute of Thermophysics - Institut für Wärmephysik - Institut teplofiziki
Akademgorodok, Novosibirsk

Institute of Mathematics - Institut für Mathematik - Institut matematiki,
Akademgorodok, Novosibirsk

Computing Center - Rechenzentrum - Vyčislitel'nyj centr, Akademgorodok, Novos.

Institute of Biology - Biologisches Institut - Biologičeskij institut,
ul. Frunze, 23a, Novosibirsk

Institute of Inorganic Chemistry - Institut für anorganische Chemie -
Institut neorganičeskoj chimii, Akademgorodok, Novosibirsk

Institute of Soil Science and Agrochemistry - Institut für Bodenkunde und
Agrochemie - Institut počvovedenija i agrochimii, Sovetskaja 18, Novosibirsk

Institute of Chemical Kinetics and Combustion - Institut für chemische
Kinetik und Verbrennungstechnik - Institut chimičeskoj kinetiki i gorenija,
Akademgorodok, Novosibirsk

Institute of Catalysis - Institut für Katalyse - Institut kataliza,
Akademgorodok, Novosibirsk

Institute of Organic Chemistry - Institut für organische Chemie - Institut
organičeskoj chimii, Akademgorodok, Novosibirsk

Institute of Physiology - Institut für Physiologie - Institut fiziologii,
Zolotodolinskaja, 75, Novosibirsk

Institute of Cytology and Genetics - Institut für Zytologie und Genetik -
Institut citologii i genetiki, Akademgorodok, Novosibirsk

Experimental Station of the Institutes of Biology - Versuchsbetrieb der biologischen Institute - Eksperimental'noe chozjajstvo, Novosibirsk

Central Siberian Botanical Garden - Zentraler sibirischer botanischer
Garten - Central'nyj Sibirskij botaničeskij sad, Novosibirsk

Institute of Mining - Institut für Bergbau - Institut gornogo dela,
Akademgorodok, Novosibirsk

Institute of the Physical and Chemical Foundations of Mineral Processing -
Institut für die physikalisch-chemischen Grundlagen der Verarbeitung von
mineralischen Grundstoffen - Institut fiziko-chimičeskich osnov pererabotki
mineral'nogo syr'ja, ul. Dzeržinskogo, 18, Novosibirsk

Institute of Geology and Geophysics - Institut für Geologie und Geophysik -
Institut geologii i geofiziki, Akademgorodok, Novosibirsk

Institute of History, Philology and Philosophy - Institut für Geschichte,
Philologie und Philosophie - Institut istorii, filologii i filosofii,
Akademgorodok, Novosibirsk

Institute of Economics and Management of Industrial Production - Institut für
Ökonomie und Organisation der Industrieproduktion - Institut ekonomiki i
organizacii promyšlennogo proizvodstva, IEiOPP, Akademgorodok, Novosibirsk

Faculty of Foreign Languages - Lehrstuhl für Fremdsprachen - Kafedra
inostrannych jazykov, Akademgorodok, Novosibirsk

Faculty of Philosophy - Lehrstuhl für Philosophie - Kafedra filosofii,
Novosibirsk

8.4 Science
Wissenschaft

State Public Scientific and Technical Library of the Siberian Department's Presidium - Staatliche öffentliche wissenschaftlich-technische Bibliothek beim Präsidium der Sibirischen Abteilung - Gosudarstvennaja publičnaja naučno-techničeskaja biblioteka, GPNTB, pri Prezidiume SO AN SSSR, ul. Voschod, 15, Novosibirsk

Publishing House of the Siberian Department - Verlag der Sibirischen Abteilung - Izdatel'stvo Sibirskogo otdelenija AN SSSR, Novosibirsk

Irkutsk:
Institute for the Study of the Earth Crust - Institut für die Erforschung der Erdrinde - Institut zemnoj kory, ul. Favorskogo, 1, Irkutsk

Institute of Fuel Chemistry - Institut für Brennstoffchemie - Institut chimii topliv

Institute for the Geography of Siberia and the Far East - Institut für die Geographie Sibiriens und des Fernen Ostens - Institut geografii Sibiri i Dal'nego Vostoka, Vuzovskaja nabereznaja, 36, Irkutsk

Institute of Energy - Institut für Energetik - Energetičeskij institut, ul. Lermontova, 130, Irkutsk

Institute of Geochemistry - Institut für Geochemie - Institut geochimii, ul. Favorskogo, 1, Irkutsk

Irkutsk Institute of Organic Chemistry - Institut für organische Chemie-Irkutsk - Irkutskij institut organičeskoj chimii, ul. Favorskogo, 1, Irkutsk

Institute of Terrestrial Magnetism, the Ionosphere and Radio Wave Propagation - Institut zur Erforschung des Erdmagnetismus, der Ionosphäre und der Ausbreitung von Radiowellen - Institut zemnogo magnetizma, ionosfery i rasprostranenija radiovoln, ul. Lenina, 5, Irkutsk

Institute of Limnology - Limnologisches Institut - Limnologičeskij institut, Irkutsk

Siberian Institute of Plant Physiology and Biochemistry - Sibirisches Institut für die Physiologie und die Biochemie der Pflanzen - Sibirskij institut fiziologii i biochimii rastenij, ul. Lenina, 5, Irkutsk

Jakutsk:
Institute of Frozen Soils - Institut für Frostbodenkunde - Institut merzlotovedenija

Ionospheric Station - Ionosphärenstation - Ionosfernaja stancija

Station for the Continued Registration of the various Components of the Cosmic Radiation - Station für die kontinuierliche Registrierung der verschiedenen Komponenten der kosmischen Strahlung - Stancija nepreryvnoj registracii različnych komponentov kosmičeskogo izlučenija

Krasnojarsk:
V.N.Sukachev Institute of Forestry and Timber - Forst- und Holzinstitut, V.N.Sukačev-Institut - Institut lesa i drevesiny im. V.N.Sukačeva, Prospekt Mira, 53, Krasnojarsk

Institute of Geology and Geophysics - Institut für Geologie und Geophysik - Institut geologii i geofiziki

L.V.Kirensky Institute of Physics - Institut für Physik, L.V.Kirenskij-Institut - Institut fiziki im. L.V.Kirenskogo, Krasnojarsk

Others - Andere:
Institute of Atmosphere Optics - Institut für die Optik der Atmosphäre - Institut optiki atmosfery, ul. Gercena, 8, Tomsk

Institute of Oil Chemistry - Institut für Petrochemie - Institut chimii nefti, Kooperativnyj per., 5, Tomsk

Science
Wissenschaft 8.4

Branches of the Siberian Department - Filialen der Sibirischen Abteilung:

East Siberian Branch - Ostsibirische Filiale - Vostočno-Sibirskij filial, ul. Lenina, 5, Irkutsk

  Department of Economics and Geography - Abteilung für Wirtschaftswissenschaften und Geographie - Otdel ekonomiki i geografii

  Institute of Chemistry - Institut für Chemie - Institut chimii

  Institute of Electro-Chemistry - Institut für Elektrochemie - Institut elektrochimii

  Institute of the Synthesis of Oil Chemistry and Coal Chemistry - Institut für petrochemische und kohlechemische Synthese - Institut nefte- i uglechimičeskogo sinteza

Yakutsk Branch - Filiale Jakutsk - Jakutskij filial, ul. Petrovskogo, 36, Jakutsk

  Department of Energy - Abteilung für Energetik - Otdel energetiki

  Department of Economics - Abteilung für Wirtschaftswissenschaften - Otdel ekonomiki

  Yakutsk Institute of Biology - Biologisches Institut Jakutsk - Jakutskij biologičeskij institut

  Botanical Garden - Botanischer Garten - Botaničeskij sad

  Geophysical Observatory - Geophysikalisches Observatorium - Geofizičeskaja observatorija

  Institute of Geology - Institut für Geologie - Institut geologii

  Institute of Space Physics Research and Aeronomics - Institut für kosmophysikalische Forschungen und Aeronomie - Institut kosmofizičeskich issledovanij i aeronomii

  Institute of Physical and Chemical Problems of the North - Institut für physikalisch-technische Probleme des Nordens - Institut fiziko-techničeskich problem Severa

  Institute of Linguistics, Literature and History - Institut für Sprache, Literatur und Geschichte - Institut jazyka, literatury i istorii

  Laboratory of Forestry and Plant Reserves - Laboratorium für Forsten und Pflanzenbestand - Laboratorija lesa i rastitel'nych resursov

  Laboratory of Cosmic Radiation - Laboratorium für kosmische Strahlung - Laboratorija kosmičeskich lučej

V.L.Komarov Far Eastern Branch - Fernöstliche Filiale, V.L.Komarov-Filiale - Dal'nevostočnyj filial im. V.L.Komarova, Leninskaja ul., 50, Vladivostok

  Department of Economic and Sociological Research - Abteilung für wirtschaftswissenschaftliche und soziologische Forschungen - Otdel ekonomičeskich i sociologičeskich issledovanij

  Bolshe-Chechcirski Reservation - Bol'še-Chechcirskij Naturschutzgebiet - Bol'še-Chechcirskij zapovednik

  Botanical Garden - Botanischer Garten - Botaničeskij sad

  Department of Chemistry - Chemische Abteilung - Chimičeskij otdel

  Far Eastern Institute of Geography - Fernöstliches Institut für Geographie - Dal'nevostočnyj institut geografii

  V.L.Komarov Mountain Taiga Station - Gebirgstaiga-Station, V.L.Komarov-Station - Gorno-taežnaja stancija im. V.L.Komarova

489

8.4 Science
Wissenschaft

Geophysical Observatory - Geophysikalisches Observatorium - Geofizičeskaja observatorija

Laboratory of Automation - Laboratorium für Automatisierung - Laboratorija avtomatizacii

Laboratory of Water Problems and Geochemistry of the Far Eastern Province - Laboratorium für den Wasserhaushalt und die Geochemie der Landschaft des Fernen Ostens - Laboratorija vodnogo balansa i geochimii landšafta Dal'nego Vostoka

Laboratory of Geography and Cartography - Laboratorium für Geographie und Kartographie - Laboratorija geografii i kartografii

Chingan Reservation - Naturschutzgebiet Cingan - Činganskij zapovednik

Komsomol Reservation - Naturschutzgebiet Komsomol'sk - Komsomol'skij zapovednik

Zeja Reservation - Naturschutzgebiet Zeja - Zejskij zapovednik

Buryat Branch - Burjatische Filiale - Burjatskij filial, Fabričnaja 6, Ulan-Ude

Buryat Institute of Social Sciences - Burjatisches Institut für Gesellschaftswissenschaften - Burjatskij institut obščestvennych nauk

Buryat Institute of Natural Sciences - Burjatisches Institut für Naturwissenschaften - Burjatskij institut estestvennych nauk

Complex Scientific Research Institute Kamchatka - Komplexes wissenschaftliches Forschungsinstitut Kamčatka - Kamčatskij kompleksnyj institut

Transbaikal Complex Scientific Research Institute - Transbajkalisches komplexes wissenschaftliches Forschungsinstitut - Zabajkal'skij kompleksnyj naučno-issledovatel'skij institut

f) Scientific Centers of the Academy of Sciences of the U.S.S.R. - Wissenschaftszentren der Akademie der Wissenschaften der UdSSR

Far Eastern Scientific Center - Wissenschaftszentrum Fernost - Dal'nevostočnyj naučnyj centr

Institute of Biology and Soil Science - Institut für Biologie und Bodenkunde - Biologo-počvennyj institut, Vladivostok

Far Eastern Institute of Geology - Fernöstliches geologisches Institut - Dal'nevostočnyj geologičeskij institut, Vladivostok

Fundamental Library - Fundamentalbibliothek - Fundamental'naja biblioteka, Vladivostok

Institute of Automation and Control Processes with Computinger Center - Institut für Automatik und Steuerungsprozesse mit Rechenzentrum - Institut avtomatiki processov upravlenija s Vyčislitel'nym centrom, Vladivostok

Institute of Biologically Active Substances - Institut für biologisch aktive Stoffe - Institut biologičeski aktivnych veščestv, Vladivostok

Institute of Chemistry - Institut für Chemie - Institut chimii, Vladivostok

Institute of History, Archaeology and Ethnography of the Far Eastern Peoples - Institut für Geschichte, Archäologie und Ethnographie der Völker des Fernen Ostens - Institut istorii, archeologii i etnografii narodov Dal'nego Vostoka, Vladivostok

Institute of Marine Biology - Institut für Meeresbiologie - Institut biologii morja

Institute of Tectonics and Geophysics - Institut für Tektonik und Geophysik - Institut tektoniki i geofiziki, Chabarovsk

Science
Wissenschaft 8.4

Institute of Vulcanology - Institut für Vulkanologie - Institut vulkanologii, Petropavlovsk/Kamčatka

Institute of Economic Research - Institut für wirtschaftswissenschaftliche Forschungen - Institut ekonomičeskich issledovanij, Chabarovsk

Khabarovsk Complex Scientific Research Institute - Komplexes wissenschaftliches Forschungsinstitut Chabarovsk - Chabarovskij kompleksnyj naučno-issledovatel'skij institut

Sakhalin Complex Scientific Research Institute - Komplexes wissenschaftliches Forschungsinstitut Sachalin - Sachalinskij kompleksnyj naučno-issledovatel'skij institut, Novo-Aleksandrovsk

North-Eastern Complex Scientific Research Institute - Nordöstliches komplexes wissenschaftliches Forschungsinstitut - Severo-Vostočnyj kompleksnyj naučno-issledovatel'skij institut, Magadan

Pacific Institute of Geography - Pazifisches Institut für Geographie - Tichookeanskij institut geografii, Vladivostok

Urals Scientific Center - Wissenschaftszentrum Ural - Ural'skij naučnyj centr

Department of Polymer Physics - Abteilung für Physik der Polymere - Otdel fiziki polimerov, Perm'

Department of Physical and Technical Problems of Energetics - Abteilung für physikalisch-technische Probleme der Energetik - Otdel fiziko-techničeskich problem energetiki

Institute of Mining-Geology - Bergbau-geologisches Institut - Gorno-geologičeskij institut, Sverdlovsk

Botanical Garden - Botanischer Garten - Botaničeskij sad

Fundamental Library - Fundamentalbibliothek - Fundamental'naja biblioteka, Sverdlovsk

Institute of Mining - Institut für Bergbau - Institut gornogo dela

Institute of Chemistry - Institut für Chemie - Institut chimii, Sverdlovsk

Institute of Electrochemistry - Institut für Elektrochemie - Institut elektrochimii, Sverdlovsk

Institute of Geology and Geochemistry - Institut für Geologie und Geochemie - Institut geologii i geochimii

Institute of Geophysics - Institut für Geophysik - Institut geofiziki

Institute of Mathematics and Mechanics - Institut für Mathematik und Mechanik - Institut matematiki i mechaniki, Sverdlovsk

Institute of Metal Physics - Institut für Metallphysik - Institut fiziki metallov, IFM, ul. S.Kovalevskoj, 13, Sverdlovsk

Institute of Metallurgy - Institut für Metallurgie - Institut metallurgii, ul. Mamina-Sibirjaka, Sverdlovsk

Institute of Plant and Animal Ecology - Institut für die Ökologie der Pflanzen und der Tiere - Institut ekologii rastenij i životnych, Sverdlovsk

Institute of Economics - Institut für Wirtschaftswissenschaften - Institut ekonomiki

V.I.Lenin Ilmen State Reservation - Naturschutzgebiet Il'men'-See, V.I. Lenin-Naturschutzgebiet - Il'menskij zapovednik im. V.I.Lenina

Salekhard Station - Station Salechard - Salechardskij stacionar

8.4 Science / Wissenschaft

g) Branches of the Academy of Sciences of the U.S.S.R. -
   Filialen der Akademie der Wissenschaften der UdSSR

   Bashkir Branch - Filiale Baškirien - Baškirskij filial, Ufa

   Department of Biochemistry and Citochemistry - Abteilung für Biochemie
   und Zytochemie - Otdel biochimii i citochimii

   Department of Physics and Mathematics (with computing center) -
   Abteilung für Physik und Mathematik (mit Rechenzentrum) -
   Otdel fiziki i matematiki s vyčislitel'nym centrom

   Department of Economic Studies - Abteilung für wirtschaftswissenschaftliche Forschungen - Otdel ekonomičeskich issledovanij

   Institute of Biology - Institut für Biologie - Institut biologii

   Institute of Chemistry - Institut für Chemie - Institut chimii

   Institute of Geology - Institut für Geologie - Institut geologii

   Institute of History, Linguistics and Literature - Institut für Geschichte,
   Sprache und Literatur - Institut istorii, jazyka i literatury

   Daghestan Branch - Filiale Dagestan - Dagestanskij filial, Machačkala

   Department of Biology - Abteilung für Biologie - Otdel biologii

   Department of Biological Foundations of Fauna - Abteilung für die
   Erforschung des Pflanzenbestandes - Otdel rastitel'nych resursov

   Department of Economics - Abteilung für Wirtschaftswissenschaften -
   Otdel ekonomiki

   Institute of Geology - Institut für Geologie - Institut geologii

   Institute of History, Linguistics and Literature - Institut für Geschichte,
   Sprache und Literatur - Institut istorii, jazyka i literatury im. G.Cadasy

   Institute of Physics - Institut für Physik - Institut fiziki

   Karelian Branch - Filiale Karelien - Karel'skij filial, Petrozavodsk

   Department of Water Problems - Abteilung für wasserwirtschaftliche
   Probleme - Otdel vodnych problem

   Department of Economics - Abteilung für Wirtschaftswissenschaften -
   Otdel ekonomiki

   Institute of Forestry - Forstinstitut - Institut lesa

   Institute of Biology - Institut für Biologie - Institut biologii

   Institute of Ore Mining - Institut für Erzbergbau - Gornometallurgičeskij
   institut

   Institute of Geology - Institut für Geologie - Institut geologii

   Petrozavodsk Institute of Linguistics, Literature and History -
   Institut für Sprache, Literatur und Geschichte - Petrozavodsk -
   Petrozavodskij institut jazyka, literatury i istorii

   S.M.Kirov Kola Branch - Filiale Kola, S.M.Kirov-Filiale - Kol'skij filial
   im. S.M.Kirova, Kirov

   Department of Economic Research - Abteilung für wirtschaftswissenschaftliche Forschungen - Otdel ekonomičeskich issledovanij

   Murmansk Marine Biological Institute - Biologisches Meeresinstitut
   Murmansk - Murmanskij morskoj biologičeskij institut

Science 8.4
Wissenschaft

Institute of Geology - Geologisches Institut - Geologičeskij institut

Institute of Chemistry and Technology of Rare Elements and Minerals - Institut für Chemie und Technologie seltener Elemente und mineralischer Rohstoffe - Institut chimii i technologii redkich elementov i mineral'nogo syr'ja

Institute of Ore Mining - Institut für Erzbergbau - Gornometallurgičeskij institut

Laboratory of Energetics - Laboratorium für Energetik - Laboratorija energetiki

Polar Alpine Botanical Garden - Polarer alpiner botanischer Garten - Poljarno-al'pijskij botaničeskij sad

Polar Institute of Geophysics - Polares geophysikalisches Institut - Poljarnyj geofizičeskij institut, Murmansk

Komi Branch - Komi-Filiale - Komi filial, Syktyvkar

Department of Economics - Abteilung für Wirtschaftswissenschaften - Otdel ekonomiki

Institute of Biology - Institut für Biologie - Institut biologii

Institute of Geology - Institut für Geologie - Institut geologii

Institute of Linguistics, Literature and History - Institut für Sprache, Literatur und Geschichte - Institut jazyka, literatury i istorii

Laboratory for Radiobiology - Laboratorium für Strahlenbiologie - Laboratorija radiobiologii

8.5 Science / Wissenschaft

8.5 NUMBER OF PERSONS ENGAGED IN THE SCIENTIFIC FIELD - ZAHL DER IM WISSENSCHAFTLICHEN BEREICH TÄTIGEN PERSONEN - ČISLENNOST' NAUČNYCH RABOTNIKOV

(end-of-year figures; in thousands - zum Jahresende; in Tsd. - na konec goda; tys.)

Year Jahr Gody	Total number of persons working in scientific field (incl. scientific-pedagogical cadres of universities) - im wissenschaftl. Bereich Tätige insg. (einschl.wissenschaftlich-pädagogische Kader der Hochschulen) - Vsego naučnych rabotnikov (vključaja naučno-pedagogičeskie kadry vuzov)	Doctors of sciences - Doktoren der Wissenschaften - doktora nauk	Candidates of sciences - Kandidaten der Wissenschaften - kandidaty nauk	Full or corresponding members of the Academy, professors - Ordentliche oder korrespondierende Mitglieder d.Akademie, Professoren Akademiki, členy-korrespondenty, professora	Assistant professors - Dozenten - docenty	Senior scientific collaborators - Ältere wissenschaftl.Mitarbeiter - staršie naučnye sotrudniki	Junior scientific collaborators and assistants - Jüngere wissenschaftl.Mitarbeiter und Assistenten - mladšie naučnye sotrudniki i assistenty
1950	162.5	8.3	45.5	8.9	21.8	11.4	19.6
1951	170.2	8.4	49.3	8.7	22.4	12.1	18.7
1952	179.1	8.4	53.8	8.6	23.4	12.4	19.0
1953	191.9	8.5	59.5	8.5	24.7	12.9	19.8
1954	210.2	9.0	69.2	8.8	26.8	14.0	16.2
1955	223.9	9.5	78.0	9.0	28.6	14.6	17.1
1956	239.9	9.8	85.7	9.1	30.4	15.6	17.8
1957	261.6	10.0	87.2	9.4	31.6	16.7	21.3
1958	284.0	10.3	90.0	9.6	32.7	17.2	23.6
1959	310.0	10.5	94.0	9.7	34.3	18.4	26.3
1960	354.2	10.9	98.3	9.9	36.2	20.3	26.7
1961	404.1	11.3	102.5	10.3	38.2	21.0	28.7
1962	524.5	11.9	108.7	11.0	40.6	23.8	45.0
1963	566.0	12.7	115.2	11.4	42.9	25.8	47.9
1964	612.0	13.7	123.9	12.0	46.0	27.2	48.2
1965	664.6	14.8	134.4	12.5	48.6	28.7	48.9
1966	712.4	16.6	152.4	13.6	52.8	30.2	47.6
1967	770.0	18.3	169.3	14.7	56.9	32.4	46.3
1968	822.9	20.0	186.4	15.9	60.9	35.1	48.0
1969	883.4	21.8	205.4	16.9	64.9	37.3	48.4
1970	927.7	23.6	224.5	18.1	68.6	39.0	48.8
1971	1002.9	26.1	249.2	19.5	73.2	42.4	49.2
1972	1056.0	28.1	269.5	20.6	77.0	45.4	47.5
1973	1108.5	29.8	288.3	21.6	80.5	47.8	47.1
1974	1169.7	31.7	309.5	22.5	84.4	50.7	46.4
1975	1223.4	32.3	326.8	22.9	87.9	53.3	45.0
1976							
1977							

Science 8.5.1
Wissenschaft 8.5.2

8.5.1 NUMBER OF PERSONS ENGAGED IN THE SCIENTIFIC FIELD BY NATIONALITY
ZAHL DER IM WISSENSCHAFTLICHEN BEREICH TÄTIGEN PERSONEN NACH NATIONALITÄT
ČISLENNOST' NAUČNYCH RABOTNIKOV PO NACIONAL'NOSTJAM SOJUZNYCH RESPUBLIK

(end-of-year figures - zum Jahresende - na konec goda)

	1950			1975		
	Total Insg. Vsego	Doctors of sciences Doktoren d. Wissensch. doktora nauk	Candidates of sciences Kandidaten d. Wissensch. kandidaty nauk	Total Insg. Vsego	Doctors of sciences Doktoren d. Wissensch. doktora nauk	Candidates of sciences Kandidaten d. Wissensch. kandidaty nauk
Total- Insg.- Vsego	162,508	8,277	45,530	1,223,428	32,264	326,767
Russkie	98,948	4,948	26,101	818,246	18,158	195,957
Ukraincy	14,692	415	3,731	134,243	3,196	38,076
Belorusy	2,713	93	692	26,501	557	7,070
Uzbeki	845	27	242	16,062	476	6,383
Kazachi	739	19	181	11,463	276	4,045
Gruziny	4,263	301	1,573	22,673	1,240	7,482
Azerbajd- žancy	1,932	80	565	16,826	805	6,684
Litovcy	1,213	37	96	11,230	273	4,183
Moldavane	126	2	36	3,565	83	1,493
Latyši	1,468	57	188	7,469	192	2,307
Kirgizy	94	1	14	2,708	70	955
Tadžiki	168	5	32	3,235	93	1,219
Armjane	3,864	246	1,302	26,777	1,175	8,005
Turkmeny	128	6	38	2,549	64	1,173
Estoncy	1,235	63	198	5,829	221	2,185

8.5.2 NUMBER OF PERSONS ENGAGED IN THE SCIENTIFIC FIELD BY UNION REPUBLICS
ZAHL DER IM WISSENSCHAFTLICHEN BEREICH TÄTIGEN PERSONEN NACH UNIONSREPUBLIKEN
ČISLENNOST' NAUČNYCH RABOTNIKOV PO SOJUZNYM RESPUBLIKAM

(end-of-year figures - zum Jahresende - na konec goda)

	1940	1950	1960	1970	1975
SSSR	98,315	162,508	354,158	927,709	1,223,428
RSFSR	61,872	111,699	242,872	631,111	838,473
Ukrainskaja SSR	19,304	22,363	46,657	129,781	171,478
Belorusskaja SSR	2,227	2,629	6,840	21,863	31,020
Uzbekskaja SSR	3,024	4,541	10,329	25,244	30,835
Kazachskaja SSR	1,727	3,305	9,623	26,802	32,011
Gruzinskaja SSR	3,513	4,843	9,137	20,160	24,941
Azerbajdžanskaja SSR	1,933	3,364	7,226	17,082	21,280
Litovskaja SSR	633	1,402	3,320	8,978	12,538
Moldavskaja SSR	180	745	1,999	5,695	7,309
Latvijskaja SSR	1,128	2,184	3,348	8,895	12,024
Kirgizskaja SSR	323	841	2,315	5,867	7,131
Tadžikskaja SSR	353	715	2,154	5,067	6,629
Armjanskaja SSR	1,067	2,000	4,275	12,808	17,138
Turkmenskaja SSR	487	656	1,836	3,649	4,634
Estonskaja SSR	544	1,221	2,227	4,707	5,987

8.5.3 Science / Wissenschaft

8.5.3 NUMBER OF FEMALES ENGAGED IN THE SCIENTIFIC FIELD, BY UNION REPUBLICS
ZAHL DER IM WISSENSCHAFTLICHEN BEREICH TÄTIGEN FRAUEN NACH UNIONSREPUBLIKEN
ČISLENNOST' ŽENŠČIN V SOSTAVE NAUČNYCH RABOTNIKOV PO SOJUZNYM RESPUBLIKAM

(end-of-year figures - zum Jahresende - na konec goda)

	1960 Total Insg. Vsego	1960 Doctors of sciences Doktoren d. Wissensch. doktora nauk	1960 Candidates of sciences Kandidaten d. Wissensch. kandidaty nauk	1975 Total Insg. Vsego	1975 Doctors of sciences Doktoren d. Wissensch. doktora nauk	1975 Candidates of sciences Kandidaten d. Wissensch. kandidaty nauk
SSSR	128,730	1,149	28,761	488,306	4,485	94,013
RSFSR	90,731	875	20,711	341,418	3,114	63,327
Ukrainskaja SSR	15,417	132	3,627	61,949	590	12,121
Belorusskaja SSR	2,583	17	520	12,612	71	2,498
Uzbekskaja SSR	3,680	24	683	11,581	88	2,689
Kazachskaja SSR	3,456	11	536	13,161	117	2,862
Gruzinskaja SSR	3,103	35	809	10,227	156	2,231
Azerbajdžanskaja SSR	2,443	13	400	7,958	86	1,697
Litovskaja SSR	1,062	1	169	4,815	42	1,221
Moldavskaja SSR	682	3	139	2,677	22	724
Latvijskaja SSR	1,336	7	295	5,137	54	1,113
Kirgizskaja SSR	869	5	158	3,087	33	682
Tadžikskaja SSR	772	4	105	2,587	18	539
Armjanskaja SSR	1,279	13	376	6,805	65	1,309
Turkmenskaja SSR	673	3	103	1,827	12	416
Estonskaja SSR	644	6	130	2,465	17	584

Science 8.5.4
Wissenschaft

8.5.4 NUMBER OF ASPIRANTS - ZAHL DER ASPIRANTEN - CISLENNOST' ASPIRANTOV
(end-of-year figures - zum Jahresende - na konec goda)

Year Jahr Gody	Total number of aspirants - Aspiranten, insg. Vsego aspirantov	at scientific institutions (without universities) - in wissenschaftl. Institutionen (ohne Hochschulen) - v naučnych učreždenijach (bez vuzov)	of which-davon-iz nich		at universities - an Hochschulen - v vysšich učebnych zavedenijach	of which-davon iz nich	
			not pursuing an occupation - ohne Ausübung einer berufl. Tätigkeit. s otryvom ot proizvodstva	besides pursuing an occupation - neben Ausübung einer berufl. Tätigkeit - bez otryva ot proizvodstva		not pursuing an occupation - ohne Ausübung einer berufl. Tätigkeit - s otryvom ot proizvodstva	besides pursuing an occupation - neben Ausübung einer berufl. Tätigkeit - bez otryva ot proizvods.
1940	16,863	3,694	2,919	775	13,169	11,506	1,663
1950	21,905	9,418	6,944	2,474	12,487	11,199	1,288
1951	24,845	10,253	7,293	2,960	14,592	12,738	1,854
1952	26,704	11,004	7,623	3,381	15,700	13,534	2,166
1953	29,162	11,946	7,993	3,953	17,216	14,379	2,837
1954	30,841	12,773	8,485	4,288	18,068	14,644	3,424
1955	29,362	12,588	8,145	4,443	16,774	13,212	3,562
1956	25,495	11,408	7,160	4,248	14,087	10,592	3,495
1957	22,236	10,155	6,016	4,139	12,081	8,756	3,325
1958	23,084	10,756	6,528	4,228	12,328	9,004	3,324
1959	28,644	13,048	7,861	5,187	15,596	10,752	4,844
1960	36,754	16,348	9,515	6,833	20,406	13,463	6,943
1961	47,560	20,494	11,308	9,186	27,066	17,367	9,699
1962	61,809	25,475	13,584	11,891	36,334	23,130	13,204
1963	73,105	29,808	15,312	14,496	43,297	27,583	15,714
1964	83,271	33,749	16,737	17,012	49,522	31,191	18,331
1965	90,294	36,882	17,765	19,117	53,412	33,344	20,068
1966	93,755	38,729	18,427	20,302	55,026	34,509	20,517
1967	96,779	40,536	18,934	21,602	56,243	35,314	20,929
1968	98,139	41,594	19,126	22,468	55,545	35,892	20,653
1969	99,532	42,522	19,131	23,391	57,010	36,472	20,538
1970	99,427	42,518	18,725	23,793	56,909	36,299	20,610
1971	99,308	42,311	17,842	24,469	56,997	35,997	21,000
1972	98,945	41,693	16,903	24,790	57,252	35,598	21,654
1973	98,860	41,220	15,579	25,641	57,640	34,123	23,517
1974	96,939	40,369	14,163	26,206	56,570	31,194	25,376
1975	95,675	39,969	13,052	26,917	55,706	28,805	26,901
1976							
1977							

8.5.5 Science / Wissenschaft

8.5.5 NUMBER OF ASPIRANTS BY UNION REPUBLICS – ZAHL DER ASPIRANTEN NACH UNIONSREPUBLIKEN – ČISLENNOST' ASPIRANTOV PO SOJUZNYM RESPUBLIKAM

(end-of-year figures – zum Jahresende – na konec goda)

Year Jahr Gody	A. Total number of aspirants / Aspiranten, insg. / Vsego aspirantov	B. at scientific institutions (without universities – in wissenschaftl. Institutionen (ohne Hochschulen) / v naučnych učreždenijach (bez vuzov)	C. not pursuing an occupation – ohne Ausübung einer berufl. Tätigkeit s otryvom ot proizvodstva	D. besides pursuing an occupation – neben Ausübung einer berufl. Tätigkeit – bez otryva ot proizvodstva	E. at universities – an Hochschulen – v vysšich učebnych zavedenijach	F. not pursuing an occupation – ohne Ausübung einer berufl. Tätigkeit s otryvom ot proizvodstva	G. besides pursuing an occupation – neben Ausübung einer berufl. Tätigkeit bez otryva ot proizv.
RSFSR							
1960	24,578	10,348	4,907	5,441	14,230	9,366	4,864
1970	67,619	28,412	10,637	17,775	39,207	25,469	13,738
1975	65,728	26,952	8,057	18,895	38,776	21,817	16,959
Ukrainskaja SSR							
1960	4,536	1,478	1,040	438	3,058	1,901	1,157
1970	13,513	4,675	2,479	2,196	8,838	5,145	3,693
1975	12,955	4,489	1,768	2,721	8,466	3,486	4,980
Belorusskaja SSR							
1960	985	627	460	167	358	255	103
1970	2,739	1,329	620	709	1,410	818	592
1975	3,055	1,424	541	883	1,631	604	1,027
Uzbekskaja SSR							
1960	1,432	940	727	213	492	337	155
1970	3,197	1,636	1,037	599	1,561	983	578
1975	3,001	1,546	577	969	1,455	615	840
Kazachskaja SSR							
1960	879	511	350	161	368	273	95
1970	2,485	1,090	613	477	1,395	862	533
1975	2,557	1,061	397	664	1,496	667	829
Gruzinskaja SSR							
1960	804	382	299	83	422	255	167
1970	1,427	746	478	268	681	493	188
1975	1,176	627	224	403	549	250	299
Azerbajdžanskaja SSR							
1960	1,044	573	534	39	471	336	135
1970	1,991	1,315	756	559	676	429	247
1975	1,718	1,128	435	693	590	207	383
Litovskaja SSR							
1960	332	173	115	18	159	127	32
1970	1,041	435	269	166	606	381	225
1975	914	406	160	246	508	183	325
Moldavskaja SSR							
1960	201	96	74	22	105	78	27
1970	767	449	300	149	318	219	99
1975	655	387	145	242	268	104	164

Science 8.5.5
Wissenschaft 8.5.6

Year Jahr Gody	A.	B.	C.	D.	E.	F.	G.
Latvijskaja SSR							
1960	237	156	127	29	81	67	14
1970	908	328	214	114	580	374	206
1975	833	286	111	175	547	233	314
Kirgizskaja SSR							
1960	279	183	143	40	96	71	25
1970	721	506	328	178	215	127	88
1975	560	380	135	245	180	91	89
Tadžikskaja SSR							
1960	454	304	245	59	150	106	44
1970	648	349	243	106	299	228	71
1975	600	309	125	184	291	117	174
Armjanskaja SSR							
1960	364	206	168	38	158	112	46
1970	1,180	585	367	218	595	405	190
1975	897	422	179	243	475	237	238
Turkmenskaja SSR							
1960	291	193	141	52	98	87	11
1970	632	414	212	202	218	161	57
1975	572	337	114	223	235	92	143
Estonskaja SSR							
1960	338	178	145	33	160	92	68
1970	559	249	172	77	310	205	105
1975	454	215	84	131	239	102	137

8.5.6 NUMBER OF FEMALE ASPIRANTS - ZAHL DER FRAUEN-ASPIRANTEN -
ČISLENNOST' ŽENŠČIN-ASPIRANTOV

(end-of-year figures - zum Jahresende - na konec goda)

Year Jahr Gody	Total number of female aspirants Frauen-Aspiranten,insg. Vsego Ženščin- aspirantov	of which educated - davon ausgebildet - v tomčisle obučavšichsja	
		at scientific institutions (without universities) in wissenschaftlichen Institutionen (ohne Hochschulen) v naučnych učreždenijach (bez vuzov)	at universities an Hochschulen v vysšich učebnych zavedenijach
1950	8,588	3,575	5,013
1960	8,405	3,625	4,780
1970	28,012	11,864	16,148
1975	27,021	10,950	16,071

499

8.5.7 Science / Wissenschaft

8.5.7 BREAKDOWN OF ASPIRANTS BY NATIONALITIES RESP. ETHNIC ORIGIN
AUFTEILUNG DER ASPIRANTEN NACH NATIONALITÄT BZW. ETHNISCHER ABSTAMMUNG
ČISLENNOST' ASPIRANTOV PO NACIONAL'NOSTJAM SOJUZNYCH I AVTONOMNYCH RESPUBLIK I AVTONOMNYCH OBLASTEJ

(end-of-year figures - zum Jahresende - na konec goda)

1 9 7 5

Total number of aspirants -
Aspiranten insg. -
Vsego aspirantov   95,675

Russkie	59,120	Kabardincy	84
Ukraincy	11,863	Kalmyki	61
Belorusy	2,634	Karakalpaki	90
Uzbeki	2,628	Karely	21
Kazachi	2,011	Komi, Komi-permjaki	70
Gruziny	1,638	Marijcy	52
Azerbajdžancy	1,820	Mordva	152
Litovcy	1,056	Narodnosti Dagestana	499
Moldavane	565	Osetiny	234
Latyši	615	Tatary	1,419
Kirgizy	446	Tuvincy	11
Tadžiki	502	Udmurty	51
Armjane	2,036	Čečency	89
Turkmeny	450	Čuvaši	247
Estoncy	480	Jakuty	122
Abchazy	34	Adygejcy	39
Balkarcy	30	Altajcy	23
Baškiry	259	Evrei	2,841
Burjaty	299	Karačaevcy	32
Inguši	28	Chakasy	17
		Čerkesy	27

Science
Wissenschaft

SCHEME OF THE STATE SYSTEM OF SCIENTIFIC-TECHNICAL INFORMATION
SCHEMA DES STAATLICHEN SYSTEMS DER WISSENSCHAFTLICH-TECHNISCHEN INFORMATION
SCHEMA GOSUDARSTVENNOJ SISTEMY NAUČNO-TECHNIČESKOJ INFORMACII

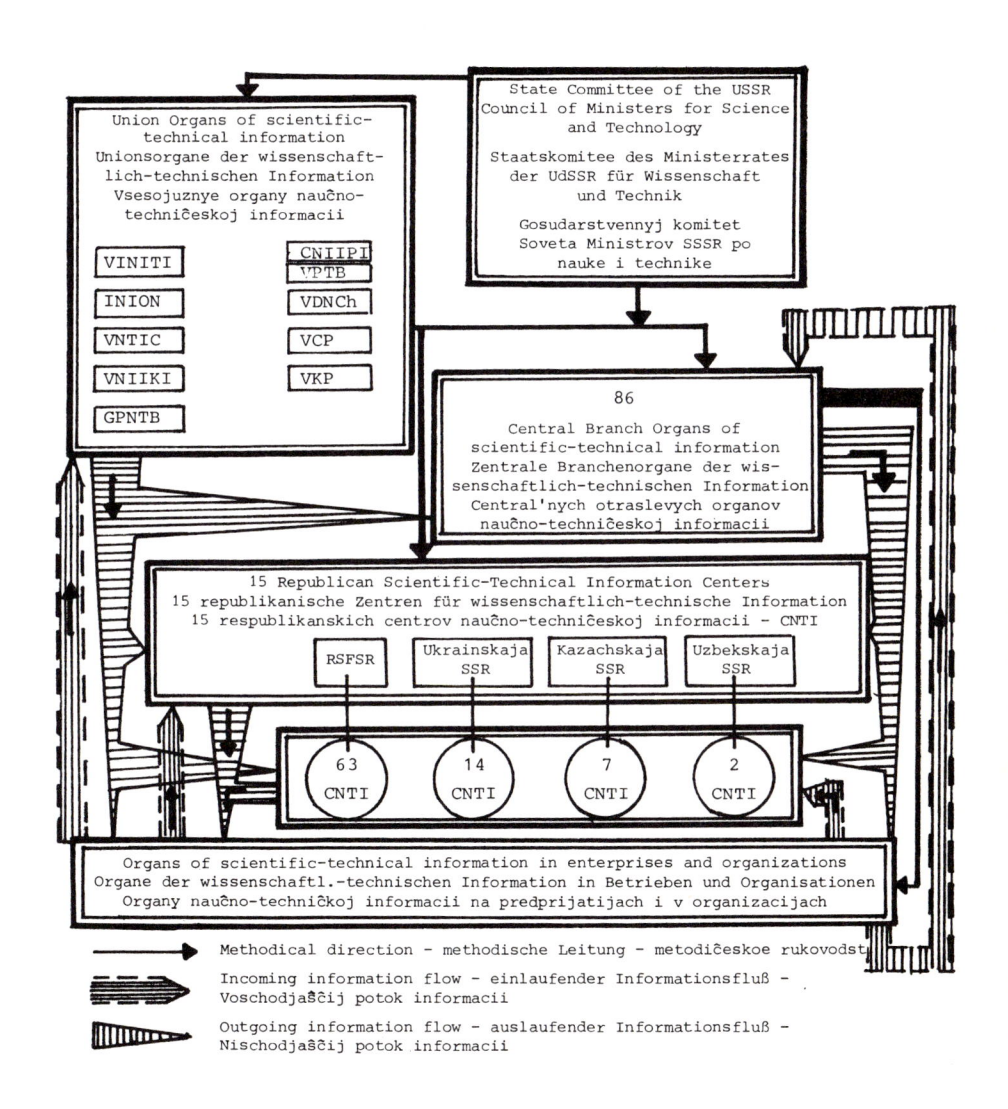

State Committee of the USSR Council of Ministers for Science and Technology

Staatskomitee des Ministerrates der UdSSR für Wissenschaft und Technik

Gosudarstvennyj komitet Soveta Ministrov SSSR po nauke i technike

Union Organs of scientific-technical information
Unionsorgane der wissenschaftlich-technischen Information
Vsesojuznye organy naučno-techničeskoj informacii

- VINITI
- INION
- VNTIC
- VNIIKI
- GPNTB
- CNIIPI
- VPTB
- VDNCh
- VCP
- VKP

86 Central Branch Organs of scientific-technical information
Zentrale Branchenorgane der wissenschaftlich-technischen Information
Central'nych otraslevych organov naučno-techničeskoj informacii

15 Republican Scientific-Technical Information Centers
15 republikanische Zentren für wissenschaftlich-technische Information
15 respublikanskich centrov naučno-techničeskoj informacii - CNTI

| RSFSR | Ukrainskaja SSR | Kazachskaja SSR | Uzbekskaja SSR |

- 63 CNTI
- 14 CNTI
- 7 CNTI
- 2 CNTI

Organs of scientific-technical information in enterprises and organizations
Organe der wissenschaftl.-technischen Information in Betrieben und Organisationen
Organy naučno-techničkoj informacii na predprijatijach i v organizacijach

→ Methodical direction - methodische Leitung - metodičeskoe rukovodstvo
▶ Incoming information flow - einlaufender Informationsfluß - Voschodjaščij potok informacii
◁ Outgoing information flow - auslaufender Informationsfluß - Nischodjaščij potok informacii

Science
8.6 Wissenschaft

8.6 SCIENTIFIC AND TECHNICAL INFORMATION
WISSENSCHAFTLICH-TECHNISCHE INFORMATION
NAUČNO-TECHNIČESKAJA INFORMACIJA

Union Organs of Scientific and Technical Information -
Unionsorgane der wissenschaftlich-technischen Information

CNIIPI — Central Scientific Research Institute for Patent Information and Technical-Economic Research of the State Committee of the USSR Council of Ministers for Inventions and Discoveries - Zentrales Wissenschaftliches Forschungsinstitut für Patentinformation und technisch-wirtschaftliche Forschungen des Staatskomitees des Ministerrates der UdSSR für Erfindungen und Entdeckungen - Central'nyj naučno-issledovatel'skij institut patentnoj informacii i techniko-ekonomičeskich issledovanij Gosudarstvennogo komiteta Soveta Ministrov SSSR po delam izobretenij i otkrytij
Raušskaja naberežnaja, 4, Moskva

GPNTB — State Public Scientific and Technical Library of the State Committee of the USSR Council of Ministers for Science and Technology - Öffentliche Wissenschaftlich-Technische Staatsbibliothek des Staatskomitees des Ministerrates der UdSSR für Wissenschaft und Technik - Gosudarstvennaja publičnaja naučno-techničeskaja biblioteka Gosudarstvennogo komiteta Soveta Ministrov SSSR po nauke i technike
Kuzneckij most, 12, Moskva

INION — Institute of Scientific Information on Social Sciences of the USSR Academy of Sciences - Institut für Wissenschaftliche Information über gesellschaftliche Wissenschaften der Akademie der Wissenschaften der UdSSR - Institut naučnoj informacii po obščestvennym naukam Akademii Nauk SSSR
ul. Krasikova, 28/45, Moskva

VCP — All-Union Center for Translations of Scientific and Technical Literature and Documentation of the State Committee of the USSR Council of Ministers for Science and Technology and of the USSR Academy of Sciences - Unionszentrum für Übersetzungen der wissenschaftlich-technischen Literatur und Dokumentation des Staatskomitees des Ministerrates der UdSSR für Wissenschaft und Technik und der Akademie der Wissenschaften der UdSSR - Vsesojuznyj centr perevodov naučno-techničeskoj literatury i dokumentacii Gosudarstvennogo komiteta Soveta Ministrov SSSR po nauke i technike i Akademii nauk SSSR
ul. Kržižanovskogo, 14, Moskva

VDNCh — Exhibition of the Achievements of the USSR Economy - Ausstellung der Errungenschaften der Volkswirtschaft d.UdSSR - Vystavka dostiženij narodnogo chozjajstva SSSR
prospekt Mira, Moskva

VINITI - All-Union Institute of Scientific and Technical Information of the State Committee of the USSR Council of Ministers for Science and Technology and of the USSR Academy of Sciences - Unionsinstitut für Wissenschaftliche und Technische Information des Staatskomitees des Ministerrates der UdSSR für Wissenschaft und Technik und derAkademie der Wissenschaften der UdSSR - Vsesojuznyj institut naučnoj i techničeskoj informacii Gosudarstvennogo komiteta Soveta Ministrov SSSR po nauke i technike i Akademii nauk SSSR
ul. Baltijskaja, 14, Moskva

VKP - All-Union Chamber of Books of the State Committee of the USSR Council of Ministers for Publishing Houses, Printing Plants and the Book Trade - Unions-Buchkammer des Staatskomitees des Ministerrates der UdSSR für Verlagswesen, Polygraphie und Buchhandel - Vsesojuznaja knižnaja palata Gosudarstvennogo komiteta Soveta Ministrov SSSR po delam izdatel'stv, poligrafii i knižnoj torgovli
Kremlevskaja naberežnaja, 1/9, Moskva

VNIIKI - All-Union Scientific Research Institute of Technical Information, Classification and Coding of the State Committee of the USSR Council of Ministers for Standards - Wissenschaftliches Unionsforschungsinstitut für technische Information, Klassifizierung und Kodierung des Staatskomitees des Ministerrates der UdSSR für Normen - Vsesojuznyj naučno-issledovatel'skij institut techničeskoj informacii, klassifikacii i kodirovanija Gosudarstvennogo komiteta standartov Soveta Ministrov SSSR
ul. Ščuseva, 4, Moskva

VNTIC - All-Union Scientific and Technical Information Center of the State Committee of the USSR Council of Ministers for Science and Technology - Wissenschaftlich-Technisches Unionsinformationszentrum des Staatskomitees des Ministerrates der UdSSR für Wissenschaft und Technik - Vsesojuznyj naučno-techničeskij informacionnyj centr Gosudarstvennogo komiteta Soveta Ministrov SSSR po nauke i technike
ul. Smol'naja, 14, Moskva

VPTB - All-Union Patent-Technical Library - Patent-technische Unionsbibliothek - Vsesojuznaja patentno-techničeskaja biblioteka
Berežkovskaja naberežnaja, 24, Moskva

9. EDUCATION – BILDUNGSWESEN – OBRAZOVANIE

EDUCATIONAL SYSTEM OF THE U.S.S.R.
BILDUNGSSYSTEM DER UdSSR
SISTEMA OBRAZOVANIJA V SSSR

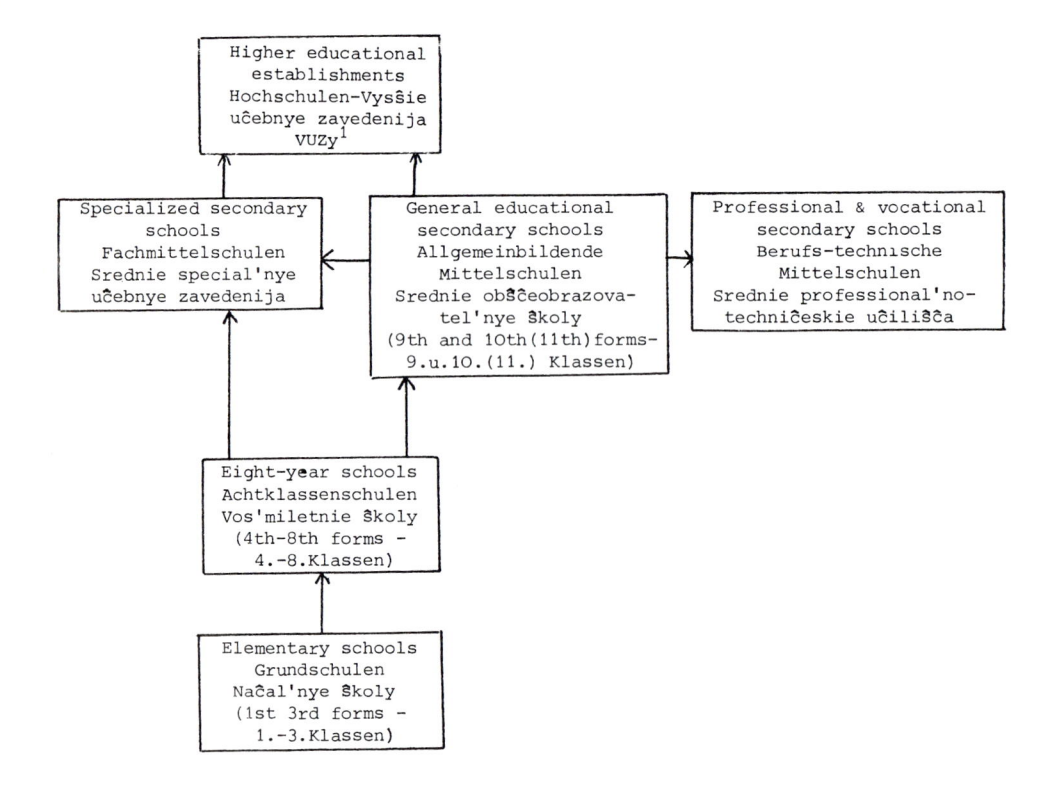

```
                    ┌─────────────────────┐
                    │ Higher educational  │
                    │   establishments    │
                    │ Hochschulen-Vysšie  │
                    │ učebnye zavedenija  │
                    │        VUZy[1]      │
                    └─────────────────────┘
                              ▲
        ┌─────────────────────┼─────────────────────┐
┌──────────────────────┐ ┌──────────────────────┐ ┌──────────────────────────┐
│Specialized secondary │ │ General educational  │ │Professional & vocational │
│       schools        │ │  secondary schools   │ │    secondary schools     │
│  Fachmittelschulen   │◄│   Allgemeinbildende  │►│   Berufs-technische      │
│ Srednie special'nye  │ │    Mittelschulen     │ │     Mittelschulen        │
│  učebnye zavedenija  │ │ Srednie obščeobrazova│ │ Srednie professional'no- │
└──────────────────────┘ │    tel'nye školy     │ │ techničeskie učilišča    │
            ▲            │(9th and 10th(11th)   │ └──────────────────────────┘
            │            │ forms- 9.u.10.(11.)  │
            │            │      Klassen)        │
            │            └──────────────────────┘
            │                       ▲
            └───────────┬───────────┘
                 ┌──────────────────────┐
                 │  Eight-year schools  │
                 │  Achtklassenschulen  │
                 │  Vos'miletnie školy  │
                 │   (4th-8th forms -   │
                 │     4.-8.Klassen)    │
                 └──────────────────────┘
                            ▲
                 ┌──────────────────────┐
                 │  Elementary schools  │
                 │     Grundschulen     │
                 │   Načal'nye školy    │
                 │   (1st 3rd forms -   │
                 │     1.-3.Klassen)    │
                 └──────────────────────┘
```

---

[1] VUZ = general term for universities, polytechnic, industrial and branch institutes, higher military secondary schools, conservatories etc. – VUZen als Oberbegriff für Universitäten, polytechnische, Industrie- und Brancheninstitute, Höhere Militärlehranstalten, Konservatorien u.a.

9.1 NUMBER OF PUPILS AND STUDENTS BY TYPES OF EDUCATION — ZAHL DER SCHÜLER UND STUDENTEN NACH SCHULARTEN —
CISLENNOST' UCASCICHSJA PO VIDAM OBUCENIJA
(at the beginning of the school year, in thousands — zu Beginn des Schuljahres, in Tsd. —
na načalo učebnogo goda, tysjac čelovek)

Education
Bildungswesen 9.1

	1914/15	1950/51	1960/61	1970/71	1971/72	1972/73	1973/74	1974/75	1975/76
Total — Insgesamt — Vsego	10,588	48,770	52,693	79,634	80,287	80,985	85,552	89,841	92,605
in general educational schools — in allgemeinbildenden Schulen — v obščeobrazovatel'nych školach	9,656	34,752	36,187	49,193	48,937	48,857	48,533	48,088	47,594
in professional-vocational and FZU-schools — in berufstechnischen Lehranstalten u.FZU-Schulen — v professional'no-techničeskich učebnych zavedenijach i školach FZU[1]	106	882	1,141	2,591	2,717	2,910	3,065	3,250	3,381
of which—davon—iz nich:									
in professional-vocational secondary schools — in berufs-technischen Mittelschulen — v srednich professional'no-techničeskich učilišč.	—	—	—	180	295	468	691	953	1,216
in technical schools — in technischen Lehranstalten — v techničeskich učilišcach	—	—	174	191	229	265	317	364	408
in specialized secondary schools — in Fachmittelschulen — v srednich special'nych učebnych zavedenijach	54	1,298	2,060	4,388	4,421	4,438	4,448	4,478	4,525
at higher educational establishments — an Hochschulen — v vysšich učebnych zavedenij	127	1,247	2,396	4,581	4,597	4,630	4,671	4,751	4,854
those who learned new trades and took refresher courses at enterprises,institutions, organizations,collective farms and other educational establishments — erlernten neue Berufe und qualifizierten sich in Betrieben, Institutionen,Organisationen,Kolchosen oder anderen Ausbildungsstätten — obučališ'novym professijam i povyšali svoju kvalifikaciju na predprijatijach, v učreždenijach, organizacijach i kolchozach, a takže byli ochvačeny drugimi vidami obučenija	645	10,591	10,909	18,881	19,615	20,150	24,835	29,274	32,251

[1] FZU-School: factory school — FZU-Schule: Betriebsschule — Školach FZU: fabrično-zavodskoe učilišče

9.2 Education / Bildungswesen

9.2 GENERAL EDUCATIONAL DAY SCHOOLS BY UNION REPUBLICS — ALLGEMEINBILDENDE TAGESSCHULEN NACH UNIONSREPUBLIKEN — DNEVNYE OBŠČEOBRAZOVATEL'NYE ŠKOLY PO SOJUZNYM RESPUBLIKAM

(at the beginning of the school year — zu Beginn des Schuljahres — na načalo učebnogo goda)

Year Jahr Gody	A. Total number of schools — Schulen insg. — vsego škol	of which — darunter — v tom čisle				F. Total number of pupils, in thou. — Schüler insg., in Tsd. — Čislennost' učaščichsja, vsego, tys.	of which in — darunter in — v tom čisle v				K. Number of teachers, in thousands — Zahl der Lehrer, in Tsd. — Čislennost' učitelej, tys.
		B. Elementary schools — Grundschulen — načal'nych	C. Eight-year schools — Achtklassenschulen — nepolnych srednich škol	D. Secondary schools — Mittelschulen — srednich	E. Schools for physically and mentally disturbed children — Schulen für geistig u. körperlich behinderte Kinder — Škol dlja detej s defektami umstvennogo i fizičeskogo razvitija		G. Elementary schools — Grundschulen — načal'nych	H. Eight-year schools — Achtklassenschulen — nepolnych srednich škol	I. Secondary schools — Mittelschulen — srednich škol	J. Schools for physically and mentally disturbed children — Schulen für geistig u. körperlich behinderte Kinder — Školach dlja detej s defektami umstvennogo i fizičeskogo razvitija	

SSSR

1. in towns and rural areas — in Städten u. auf dem Lande — v gorodach i sel'skich mestnostjach

1940/41	191,545	125,894	45,745	18,811	1,095	34,784	9,786	12,525	12,199	274	1,216
1945/46	186,853	131,625	41,687	12,836	705	26,094	9,430	9,558	7,021	85	1,043
1970/71	174,645	74,481	53,848	44,226	2,090	45,448	2,349	12,502	30,235	362	2,510
1975/76	149,486	47,869	47,748	51,466	2,403	42,611	1,037	8,731	32,406	437	2,583

2. in towns — in Städten — v gorodach

1940/41	21,501	6,903	4,831	8,887	880	10,778	1,370	2,182	7,118	108	374
1945/46	18,393	7,156	4,646	6,129	462	7,908	1,453	2,064	4,329	62	281
1970/71	33,243	4,018	8,577	19,307	1,341	23,069	425	4,012	18,373	259	1,127

3. in rural areas — auf dem Lande — v sel'skich mestnostjach

1940/41	170,044	118,991	40,914	9,924	215	24,006	8,416	10,343	5,081	166	842
1945/46	168,460	124,469	37,041	6,707	243	18,186	7,977	7,494	2,692	23	762
1970/71	141,402	70,463	45,271	24,919	749	22,379	1,924	8,490	11,862	103	1,383
1975/76	116,988	45,710	40,979	29,488	811	20,266	878	6,201	13,068	119	1,416

Education
Bildungswesen 9.2

Year Jahr Gody	A.	B.	C.	D.	E.	F.	G.	H.	I.	J.	K.
RSFSR											
1. 1940/41	113,880	80,958	22,221	9,932	769	20,229	6173.5	6,785	7,179	91	700
1945/46	113,453	85,896	20,523	6,698	336	15,018	5,826	5,079	4,071	42	615
1970/71	96,934	47,483	26,945	21,164	1,342	23,235	1,450	6,371	15,185	229	1,232
1975/76	80,097	30,710	23,394	24,476	1,517	20,176	608	4,030	15,274	263.5	1,173
2. 1940/41	12,511	4,629	2,375	4,872	635	6,619	955	1,230	4,362	72	221
1945/46	11,218	5,032	2,607	3,316	263	5,026	1,079	1,300	2,610	37	176
1970/71	19,013	2,727	4,851	10,572	863	13,018	306	2,356	10,189	167	607
1975/76	18,274	1,525	3,815	11,923	1,011	12,023	115	1,445	10268.5	194	598
3. 1940/41	101,369	76,329	19,846	5,060	134	13,610	5,219	5,555	2,817	19	479
1945/46	102,235	80,864	17,916	3,382	73	9,992	4,747	3,779	1,461	5	439
1970/71	77,921	44,756	22,094	10,592	479	10,217	1,144	4,015	4,996	62	625
1975/76	61,823	29,185	19,579	12,553	506	8,153	493	2,585	5,006	69	575
Ukrainskaja SSR											
1. 1940/41	30,881	15,310	10,957	4,435	179	6,687	1,177	2,846	2,592	72	251
1945/46	28,470	17,365	8,467	2,321	317	5,050	1,569	2,176	1,268	37	182
1970/71	27,558	8,700	11,206	7,279	373	7,565	249	2,573	4,676	67	453
1975/76	23,809	5,271	10,140	8,024	374	7,080	130	1,924	4,954	72	455
2. 1940/41	4,564	981	1,267	2,171	145	2,183	154	511	1,499	19	83
1945/46	3,456	1,021	1,059	1,223	153	1,431	189	435	787	20	50
1970/71	6,359	670	1,956	3,473	260	4,071	37	850	3,135	49	214
1975/76	5,978	285	1,578	3,856	259	4,014	15	571	3,375	53	220
3. 1940/41	26,317	14,329	9,690	2,264	34	4,504	1,023	2,335	1,093	53	168
1945/46	25,014	16,344	7,408	1,098	164	3,619	1,380	1,741	481	17	132
1970/71	21,199	8,030	9,250	3,806	113	3,494	212	1,723	1,541	18	239
1975/76	17,831	4,986	8,562	4,168	115	3,066	115	1,353	1,579	19	235
Belorusskaja SSR											
1. 1940/41	11,844	8,312	2,562	934	36	1,691	590	618	480	3	56
1945/46	10,915	8,910	1,641	353	11	1,337	749.8	391	194	2	40
1970/71	10,725	5,919	2,538	2,193	75	1,730	133	393	1,191	13	107
1975/76	8,492	3,822	2,240	2,346	84	1,586	65	284	1221.5	16	109

9.2 Education / Bildungswesen

Year Jahr Gody	A.	B.	C.	D.	E.	F.	G.	H.	I.	J.	K.
2. 1940/41	761	88	234	423	16	359	12	81	264	2	13
1945/46	454	92	124	227	11	214	18.9	54	139	2	7
1970/71	903	25	111	726	41	735	2	39	686	8	37
1975/76	960	24	75	810	51	769	1	23	735	10.5	42
3. 1940/41	11,083	8,224	2,328	511	20	1,332	578	537	216	1	43
1945/46	10,461	8,818	1,517	126	—	1,123	730.9	337	55	—	33
1970/71	9,822	5,894	2,427	1,467	34	995	131	354	505	5	70
1975/76	7,532	3,798	2,165	1,536	33	817	64	261	486.5	6	67

Uzbekskaja SSR

Year	A.	B.	C.	D.	E.	F.	G.	H.	I.	J.	K.
1. 1940/41	4,875	2,686	1,687	493	9	1,271	361	568	320.5	22	36
1945/46	4,523	2,014	2,009	498	2	920	190	487	242	1	34
1970/71	6,940	1,014	2,516	3,369	41	3,116	76	708	2,323	9	161
1975/76	7,292	605	2,340	4,283	64	3,545	25	587	2,917	15.6	206
2. 1940/41	520	112	174	229	5	283	28	79	172	4	9
1945/46	448	92	170	185	1	192	17	58	117	0.3	7
1970/71	1,062	24	200	811	27	957	3	102	846	6	46
1975/76	1,242	14	139	1,041	48	1,096	1	58	1,025	12	58
3. 1940/41	4,355	2,574	1,513	264	4	988	333	489	148	18	27
1945/46	4,075	1,922	1,839	313	1	728	173	429	125.4	0.4	27
1970/71	5,878	990	2,316	2,558	14	2,159	73	606	1,477	3	115
1975/76	6,050	591	2,201	3,242	16	2,449	24	529	1,892	4	148

Kazachskaja SSR

Year	A.	B.	C.	D.	E.	F.	G.	H.	I.	J.	K.
1. 1940/41	7,790	5,289	1,770	698	33	1,138	297	419	419	3	44
1945/46	7,869	5,437	1,708	714	10	792	252	250	289	1	40
1970/71	9,262	3,562	2,974	2,677	49	3,019	152	819	2,038	10	158
1975/76	8,533	2,486	2,589	3,380	78	3,051	80.2	575	2,379	17	176
2. 1940/41	823	339	174	279	31	352	51	79	218.5	3	11
1945/46	821	355	174	282	10	272	48	55	168	1	10
1970/71	1,782	259	520	966	37	1,327	39	262	1,018	8	60
1975/76	1,722	122	376	1,162	62	1,306	15	151	1,126	14	65
3. 1940/41	6,967	4,950	1,596	419	2	786	245.5	340	200.6	0.1	33
1945/46	7,048	5,082	1,534	432	—	520	204	195	121	—	30
1970/71	7,480	3,303	2,454	1,711	12	1,692	113	557	1,020	2	98
1975/76	6,811	2,364	2,213	2,218	16	1,745	65	424	1,253	3	111

Education 9.2
Bildungswesen

Year Jahr Gody	A.	B.	C.	D.	E.	F.	G.	H.	I.	J.	K.
Gruzinskaja SSR											
1. 1940/41	4,511	2,441	1,283	759	28	743	121	231	389	2	30
1945/46	4,114	2,168	1,186	756	4	593	99	175	319	0.3	35
1970/71	4,204	1,548	1,121	1,520	15	986	38	162	784	2	75
1975/76	3,952	1,247	1,034	1,655	16	953	21.5	130	800	2	81
2. 1940/41	378	53	55	256	14	194	5	14	174	1	8
1945/46	342	53	40	246	3	163	6.6	9	147	0.3	8
1970/71	671	42	57	560	12	449	2	13	432	2	29
1975/76	695	32	57	593	13	450	1	12	436	1	31
3. 1940/41	4,133	2,388	1,228	503	14	549	116	217	215	1	22
1945/46	3,772	2,115	1,146	510	1	430	92	166	172	0.0	27
1970/71	3,533	1,506	1,064	960	3	537	36	149	352	0.3	46
1975/76	3,257	1,215	977	1,062	3	503	20.5	118	364	1	50
Azerbajdžanskaja SSR											
1. 1940/41	3,575	1,668	1,240	654	13	655	102	229	322	2	22
1945/46	3,258	1,492	1,290	470	6	487	90	199	197	1	19
1970/71	4,343	1,221	1,821	1,287	14	1,356	66	470	817	3	71
1975/76	4,137	648	1,805	1,664	20	1,476	21	402	1,048	5	92
2. 1940/41	365	72	94	187	12	210	14	42	152	2	7
1945/46	322	77	86	153	6	155	18	34	102	1	5
1970/71	821	65	319	423	14	603	11	167	422	3	31
1975/76	855	31	278	526	20	633	2	120	506	5	38
3. 1940/41	3,210	1,596	1,146	467	1	445	88	187	170	0.1	15
1945/46	2,936	1,415	1,204	317	--	332	72	165	95	--	14
1970/71	3,522	1,156	1,502	864	--	753	55	303	395	--	40
1975/76	3,282	617	1,527	1,138	--	843	19	282	542	--	54
Litovskaja SSR											
1. 1940/41	2,829	2,723	39	67	--	376	335	6	35	--	9
1945/46	3,243	2,966	185	92	--	305	235	26	44	--	9
1970/71	3,611	2,297	793	493	28	539	64	118	352	5	33
1975/76	2,672	1,388	714	530	40	552	27.8	106	409	9	34
2. 1940/41	361	212	45	36	--	120	81	4	34.5	--	4
1945/46	292	206	13	73	--	85	44	3	38	--	3
1970/71	387	39	58	265	25	300	8	20	268	4	16
1975/76	406	15	47	309	35	341	0.8	15	317	8.2	18

9.2 Education / Bildungswesen

Year Jahr Gody	A.	B.	C.	D.	E.	F.	G.	H.	I.	J.	K.
3. 1940/41	2,468	2,450	16	2	–	256	254	2	0.5	–	5
1945/46	2,951	2,760	172	19	–	220	191	23	6	–	6
1970/71	3,224	2,258	735	228	3	239	56	98	84	1	17
1975/76	2,266	1,373	667	221	5	211	27	91	92	0.6	16
Moldavskaja SSR											
1. 1940/41	1,839	1,463	288	88	–	437	233	88	44	72	10
1945/46	1,825	1,461	300	64	–	353	217.6	106	29	–	9
1970/71	1,828	315	739	735	39	734	16	210	502	6	41
1975/76	1,676	159	630	837	50	701	6	144	542	9	44
2. 1940/41	178	88	34	56	–	59	17	11	28.4	3	2
1945/46	132	62	23	47	–	37	10	7	20	–	1
1970/71	299	20	69	196	14	199	2	30	164	3	11
1975/76	304	8	51	229	16	205	1	17	183	4	12
3. 1940/41	1,661	1,375	254	32	–	378	216	77	16	69	8
1945/46	1,693	1,399	277	17	–	316	208	99	9	–	8
1970/71	1,529	295	670	539	25	535	14	180	338	3	30
1975/76	1,372	151	579	608	34	496	5	127	359	5	32
Latvijskaja SSR											
1. 1940/41	1,586	679	821	67	19	238	44	167	25	1.5	9
1945/46	1,448	476	870	96	6	221	28	151	42	0.4	9
1970/71	1,113	227	578	265	43	323	9	113	195	6	23
1975/76	941	65	522	300	54	329	3	94	224	8	24
2. 1940/41	296	22	198	62	14	95	3	67	24	1	4
1945/46	226	12	136	72	6	79	1	44	34	0.4	3
1970/71	339	18	110	199	12	223	4	43	174	2	14
1975/76	341	5	91	226	18	235	2	32	198	3	14
3. 1940/41	1,290	657	623	5	5	143	41	100	1	0.5	5
1945/46	1,222	464	734	24	–	142	27	107	8	–	6
1970/71	774	209	468	66	31	100	5	70	21	4	9
1975/76	600	59	431	74	36	94	1	62	26	5	10
Kirgizskaja SSR											
1. 1940/41	1,645	841	643	159	2	329	78	153	95	3	11
1945/46	1,537	639	689	207	2	223	45	98	80	0.1	12

510

Education
Bildungswesen 9.2

Year Jahr Gody	A.	B.	C.	D.	E.	F.	G.	H.	I.	J.	K.
1970/71	1,668	368	562	723	15	737	25	164	545	3	39
1975/76	1,618	217	503	878	20	797	11.1	134	647	5	46
2. 1940/41	119	30	35	52	2	62	7	16	39	0.2	2
1945/46	122	32	34	54	2	49	8	10	31	0.1	2
1970/71	268	15	61	185	7	236	2	33	199	2	11
1975/76	274	5	48	212	9	235	0.5	21	211	3	12
3. 1940/41	1,526	811	608	107	--	267	71	137	56	3	9
1945/46	1,415	607	655	153	--	174	37	88	49	--	10
1970/71	1,400	353	501	538	8	501	23	131	346	1	28
1975/76	1,344	212	455	666	11	562	10.6	113	436	2	34

Tadžikskaja SSR

	A.	B.	C.	D.	E.	F.	G.	H.	I.	J.	K.
1. 1940/41	2,628	1,745	815	66	2	304	131	135	38	0.4	13
1945/46	2,881	1,995	788	97	1	240	89	113	38	0.0	13
1970/71	2,889	1,169	809	902	9	748	48	151	547	2	41
1975/76	2,768	845	806	1,106	11	901	26	149.4	723	2.4	53
2. 1940/41	127	53	31	41	2	46	9	10	27	0.3	2
1945/46	135	47	33	54	1	40	6	8	26	0.0	2
1970/71	357	54	55	243	5	247	4	20	222	1	12
1975/76	383	46	55	276	6	282	2	18	260	1.5	15
3. 1940/41	2,501	1,692	784	25	--	258	122	125	11	0.1	11
1945/46	2,746	1,948	755	43	--	200	83	105	12	--	11
1970/71	2,532	1,115	754	659	4	501	44	131	325	1	29
1975/76	2,385	799	751	830	5	619	24.1	131.4	463	1	38

Armjanskaja SSR

	A.	B.	C.	D.	E.	F.	G.	H.	I.	J.	K.
1. 1940/41	1,155	255	572	325	3	327	14	115	198	0.1	11
1945/46	1,173	254	615	300	4	252	13	100	139	0.2	12
1970/71	1,338	103	493	729	13	628	4	96	526	2	35
1975/76	1,366	62	420	861	23	632	1.6	68	558	4	42
2. 1940/41	135	20	21	91	3	83	2	7	74.1	0.1	3
1945/46	163	27	33	99	4	76	2	10	64	0.2	3
1970/71	433	9	79	334	11	331	1	20	308	2	19
1975/76	483	5	63	394	21	344	0.1	14	326	4	22

9.2 Education / Bildungswesen

Year Jahr Gody	A.	B.	C.	D.	E.	F.	G.	H.	I.	J.	K.
3. 1940/41	1,020	235	551	234	—	244	12	108	124	—	8
1945/46	1,010	227	582	201	—	176	11	90	75	—	9
1970/71	905	94	414	395	2	297	3	76	218	0.2	16
1975/76	883	57	357	467	2	288	1.5	54	232	0.2	20
Turkmenskaja SSR											
1. 1940/41	1,254	421	737	94	2	240	28	161	49	2	9
1945/46	1,089	296	676	115	2	178	18	116	44	0.1	9
1970/71	1,479	313	414	746	6	539	13	84	441	1	28
1975/76	1,546	256	320	960	10	640	8	53	577	2	34
2. 1940/41	179	31	81	66	1	69	2	29	37	0.6	3
1945/46	157	46	60	51	—	49	5	19	25	0.0	2
1970/71	352	40	66	240	6	231	2	21	207	1	12
1975/76	380	38	45	287	10	267	2	12	251	2	13
3. 1940/41	1,075	390	656	28	1	171	26	132	12	1	6
1945/46	932	250	616	64	2	129	13	97	19	0.0	7
1970/71	1,127	273	348	506	—	308	11	63	234	—	16
1975/76	1,166	218	275	673	—	373	6	41	326	—	21
Estonskaja SSR											
1. 1940/41	1,253	1,103	110	40	—	119	102	4	13	—	5
1945/46	1,055	256	740	55	4	125	9	91	25	0.2	5
1970/71	753	242	339	144	28	193	6	70	113	4	13
1975/76	587	88	291	166	42	192	2.4	51	132	7	14
2. 1940/41	184	112	35	37	—	44	30	2	12	—	2
1945/46	105	2	54	47	2	40	1	18	21	0.1	2
1970/71	197	11	65	114	7	142	2	36	103	1	8
1975/76	201	3	51	134	13	145	0.6	21	120.5	3	9
3. 1940/41	1,069	991	75	3	—	75	72	2	0.6	—	3
1945/46	950	254	686	8	2	85	8	73	4	0.1	3
1970/71	556	231	274	30	21	51	4	34	10	3	5
1975/76	386	85	240	32	29	47	1.8	30	11.9	3.7	5

512

Education 9.3
Bildungswesen

9.3
GRADUATES FROM GENERAL EDUCATIONAL SCHOOLS OF ALL TYPES BY UNION REPUBLICS
ABSOLVENTEN AUS DEN ALLGEMEINBILDENDEN SCHULEN ALLER ARTEN NACH UNIONSREPUBLIKEN
VYPUSK UČAŠČICHSJA IZ OBŠČEOBRAZOVATEL'NYCH ŠKOL VSECH VIDOV PO SOJUZNYM RESPUBLIKAM

(in thousands - in Tsd. - tysjac čelovek)

Year Jahr Gody	Graduates from eight-year schools Absolventen aus den Achtklassenschulen okončili nepolnuju srednjuju školu		Graduates from secondary schools Absolventen aus den Mittelschule okončili polnuju srednjuju školu	
	Total Insg. vsego	day schools Tagesschulen dnevnuju školu	Total Insg. vsego	day schools Tagesschulen dnevnuju školu
SSSR				
1940	1,860	1,794	303	277
1950	1,491	1,360	284	228
1970	4,661	4,251	2,581	1,968
1975	5,201	4,951	3,564	2,716
RSFSR				
1960	1,281	1,117	519	319
1970	2,575	2,314	1,288	995
1975	2,628	2,490	1,717	1,307
Ukrainskaja SSR				
1960	536	490	252	180
1970	812	763	536	371
1975	880	850	693	475
Belorusskaja SSR				
1960	101	92	46	34
1970	181	167	104	82
1975	193	189	151	119
Uzbekskaja SSR				
1960	96	92	58	45
1970	245	233	178	140
1975	363	352	273	228
Kazachskaja SSR				
1960	93	84	42	29
1970	269	238	144	114
1975	354	326	222	175
Gruzinskaja SSR				
1960	48	45	29	23
1970	85	79	60	50
1975	105	100	75	65
Azerbajdžanskaja SSR				
1960	44	39	26	18
1970	104	96	66	50
1975	161	148	103	81
Litovskaja SSR				
1960	30	27	13	10
1970	51	46	22	17
1975	64	60	35	23
Moldavskaja SSR				
1960	31	25	10	7
1970	74	69	34	26
1975	85	83	59	43

9.3 Education / Bildungswesen

Year Jahr Gody	Graduates from eight-year schools / Absolventen aus den Achtklassenschulen / okončili nepolnuju srednjuju školu — Total Insg. vsego	day schools Tagesschulen dnevnuju školu	Graduates from secondary schools / Absolventen aus d.Mittelschulen / okončili polnuju srednjuju školu — Total Insg. vsego	day schools Tagesschulen dnevnuju školu
Latvijskaja SSR				
1960	25	23	11	8
1970	33	30	15	11
1975	36	35	21	15
Kirgizskaja SSR				
1960	21	19	12	8
1970	64	60	38	31
1975	84	80	58	48
Tadžikskaja SSR				
1960	25	23	10	8
1970	56	53	33	28
1975	89	86	56	50
Armjanskaja SSR				
1960	21	19	11	8
1970	50	46	31	26
1975	75	71	47	41
Turkmenskaja SSR				
1960	17	16	9	7
1970	43	40	23	20
1975	63	61	42	37
Estonskaja SSR				
1960	14	13	7	5
1970	19	17	9	7
1975	21	20	12	9

Education 9.4
Bildungswesen

9.4 PERCENTAGE OF FEMALES IN RELATION TO TOTAL NUMBER OF TEACHERS AT GENERAL
EDUCATIONAL DAY SCHOOLS - ANTEIL DER FRAUEN AN DER GESAMTZAHL DER LEH-
RER DER ALLGEMEINBILDENDEN TAGESSCHULEN - ČISLENNOST' ŽENŠČIN V SOSTAVE
UČITELEJ DNEVNYCH OBŠČEOBRAZOVATEL'NYCH ŠKOL

(At schools of the USSR Ministries of Education and of Transport; at the beginning
of the school year - in den Schulen der Ministerien für Volksbildung und Verkehrswesen der UdSSR; zu Beginn des Schuljahres - po školam Ministerstva prosveščenija
i Ministerstva putej soobščenija SSSR; na načalo učebnogo goda)

	Number of female teachers (without persons practising several occupations) Zahl der Lehrerinnen(ohne Personen mit mehreren Tätigkeiten) Čislennost' ženščin-učitelej (bez sovmestitelej) '000 - Tsd. - tys.	% in relation to total number of teachers % im Verhältnis zur Gesamtzahl der Lehrer V % k obščej čislennosti učitelej
All teachers (incl.principals) - Alle Lehrer (einschl.Schulleiter) - Vse učitelja (vkl.rukovoditelej škol):		
1950/51	999	70
1960/61	1,312	70
1970/71	1,669	71
1975/76	1,692	71
1976/77	1,673	70
of which-darunter-v tom čisle:		
Principals of elementary schools - Direktoren der Grundschulen - Direktora načal'nych škol	0.3	83
Principals of eight-year schools - Direktoren der Achtklassenschulen - Direktora vos'miletnich škol	15	33
Principals of secondary schools - Direktoren der Mittelschulen - Direktora srednich škol	16	30
Vice-principals of eight-year schools - Stellv.Direktoren d.Achtklassenschulen - Zamestiteli direktorov vos'miletnich škol	16	60
Vice-principals of secondary schools - Stellv.Direktoren der Mittelschulen - Zamestiteli direktorov srednich škol	77	66
Teachers of 1-10(11) forms, without teacher-principals - Lehrer der 1-10(11) Klassen, ohne Lehrer-Schulleiter - Učitelja 1-10 (11) klassov, krome učitelej-rukovoditelej škol	1,443	79
Teachers of music,singing,drawing, technical drawing,phys.educ.,manual work - Lehrer für Musik,Gesang,Zeichnen,techn.Zeichnen,Turnen u.Werken - Učitelja muzyki,penija,risovanija, čerčenija,fizkul'tury i po trudu	106	35

515

9.5 Education / Bildungswesen

**9.5 NUMBER OF TEACHERS AT GENERAL EDUCATIONAL DAY SCHOOLS BY JOBS,
ZAHL DER LEHRER AN ALLGEMEINBILDENDEN TAGESSCHULEN NACH
ČISLENNOST' UČITELEJ DNEVNYCH OBŠČEOBRAZOVATEL'NYCH ŠKOL PO ZANIMAEMYM**

(at the beginning of the school year 1975/76 - zu Beginn des

	Teachers, total (without) persons practising several functions), '000 Lehrer insg.(ohne Personen, die mehrere Funktionen zugleich ausüben), Tsd. Vsego učitelej (bez somestitelej), tys.	of which with – Higher education Hochschulbildung vysšee	Education – Schul- Teacher colleges & equivalent educational institutions – Lehrerinstitute und gleichgestellte Lehranstalten – v ob'eme učitel'skic institutov i učebnyc zavedenij, priravnennych k nim
	A.	B.	C.
SSSR			
1. Teachers, total - Lehrer insg. - vse učitelja	2399.3	64.3	8.6
of which-darunter:			
2. Principals of elementary schools-Direktoren der Grundschulen-direktora načal'nych škol	0.3	44.4	7.9
3. Principals of eight-year schools-Direktoren der Achtklassenschulen-direktora vos'miletnich škol	47.5	95.9	3.7
4. Principals of secondary schools-Direktoren der Mittelschulen-direktora srednich škol	51.3	99.6	0.4
5. Vice-principals of eight-year schools-stellv.Direktoren d.Achtklassenschulen-zamestiteli direktorov vos'miletnich škol	29.3	92.7	5.3
6. Vice-principals of secondary schools-stellv.Direktoren d.Mittelschulen-zamestiteli direktorov srednich škol	114.3	97.1	1.9
7. Teachers of 1-10(11) forms, without teacher-principals-Lehrer der 1-10(11)Klassen, außer Lehrer-Schulleiter - učitelja 1-10(11)klassov, krome učitelej-rukovoditelej škol	1848.1	65.4	9.8

1 USSR: at schools of the USSR Ministries of Education and of Transport- UdSSR: in SSSR: po školam Ministerstva prosveščenija i Ministerstva putej soobščenija SSSR - in den Schulen des Ministeriums für Volksbildung der UdSSR - po školam Ministerstva

Education 9.5
Bildungswesen

EDUCATION AND DURATION OF THEIR PEDAGOGICAL OCCUPATION
POSTEN, BILDUNG UND DAUER IHRER PÄDAGOGISCHEN TÄTIGKEIT
DOLŽNOSTJAM, UROVNJU OBRAZOVANIJA I STAŽU PEDAGOGIČESKOJ RABOTY[1]

Schuljahres 1975/76 - na načalo 1975/76 učebnogo goda)

davon mit - iz nich imejut (in %)			Duration of pedagogical occupation-Dauer d.pädagogischen Tätigkeit-staž pedag.raboty		
bildung - obrazovanie					
Secondary pedagogical education - Mittlere pädagogische Ausbildg.- srednee pedagogičeskoe	Specialized secondary educ.(non-pedagogical) & gen.secondary educ. Mittlere Fachausbildung (nicht pädagogisch) u.allgemeine mittl.Schulbildung- srednee special'noe (ne pedagogičeskoe) i srednee obščee	Incomplete secondary education - nicht abgeschlossene Mittelschulbildung - ne imejut polnogo srednego obrazovanija	up to 5 yrs. bis 5 Jahre do 5 let	5-25 yrs. 5-25 J. ot 5 do 25 let	25 yrs. & more 25 J. u.mehr 25 let i bolee
D.	E.	F.	G.	H.	I.
21.0	5.9	0.2	20.7	58.8	20.5
47.4	0.3	--	1.2	36.5	62.3
0.4	0.0	--	6.9	58.6	34.5
--	--	--	2.6	56.9	40.5
1.7	0.3	--	10.4	67.1	22.5
0.8	0.2	--	8.6	68.5	22.9
22.2	2.6	0.0	20.6	58.5	20.9

den Schulen der Ministerien für Volksbildung und für Verkehrswesen der UdSSR -
Union Republics: at schools of the USSR Ministry of Education - Unionsrepubliken:
prosveščenija SSSR

9.5 Education / Bildungswesen

	A.	B.	C.	D.	E.	F.	G.	H.	I.
8. Teachers of music, singing, drawing, technical drawing, phys.educ., manual work - Lehrer für Musik, Gesang, Zeichnen, techn. Zeichnen, Turnen u. Werken - učitelja muzyki, penija, risovanija, čerčenija, fiz'kultury i po trudu	308.5	32.5	6.5	29.5	29.8	1.7	31.7	57.0	11.3
RSFSR									
1.	1061.7	60.7	8.4	24.6	5.9	0.4	20.5	57.5	22.0
2.	0.3	41.6	8.0	50.0	0.4	--	1.4	37.1	61.5
3.	23.0	95.6	4.0	0.4	0.0	--	9.0	56.3	34.7
4.	23.7	99.8	0.2	--	--	--	3.3	56.3	40.4
5.	12.3	92.2	6.0	1.7	0.1	--	11.7	65.2	23.1
6.	51.6	96.9	2.0	0.9	0.2	--	9.5	68.0	22.5
7.	806.9	61.8	9.7	26.3	2.2	0.0	20.0	57.2	22.8
8.	143.9	27.3	5.6	33.4	30.8	2.9	32.7	54.9	12.4
Ukrainskaja SSR									
1.	413.4	71.5	6.4	17.4	4.7	0.0	15.4	60.8	23.8
2.	0.0	44.5	22.2	33.3	--	--	--	22.2	77.8
3.	10.1	99.9	0.1	--	--	--	4.1	57.8	38.1
4.	8.0	100.0	--	--	--	--	1.6	55.6	42.8
5.	5.3	100.0	0.0	--	--	--	6.1	66.7	27.2
6.	17.9	99.9	0.1	--	--	--	6.6	67.4	26.0
7.	317.2	73.7	7.3	18.3	0.7	--	14.9	60.3	24.8
8.	54.9	37.7	6.1	24.7	31.3	0.2	26.6	62.1	11.3
Belorusskaja SSR									
1.	99.4	64.5	9.8	20.3	5.3	0.1	18.2	57.0	24.8
3.	2.3	96.6	3.4	--	--	--	9.4	58.6	32.0
4.	2.3	100.0	0.0	--	--	--	3.8	57.7	38.5
5.	0.9	94.0	5.8	0.2	--	--	14.2	64.2	21.6
6.	5.0	98.4	1.3	0.3	0.0	--	12.2	63.6	24.2
7.	76.1	65.4	11.6	20.2	2.8	0.0	16.9	56.5	26.6
8.	12.8	32.0	5.7	37.0	24.7	0.6	32.4	57.1	10.5
Uzbekskaja SSR									
1.	197.2	71.2	10.5	14.6	3.7	0.0	26.8	61.8	11.4
2.	0.0	100.0	--	--	--	--	--	100.0	--
3.	2.3	98.0	1.9	0.1	--	--	4.5	71.9	23.6
4.	4.3	99.5	0.5	--	--	--	2.3	63.2	34.5
5.	2.3	95.4	4.1	0.4	0.1	--	9.3	76.5	14.2
6.	10.5	96.8	2.3	0.5	0.4	--	7.9	74.9	17.2
7.	155.9	72.1	11.4	14.4	2.1	--	28.1	60.9	11.0
8.	21.9	42.4	11.0	28.7	17.8	0.1	35.7	58.8	5.5
Kazachskaja SSR									
1.	163.3	56.3	9.4	23.0	11.0	0.3	25.5	60.0	14.5
2.	0.0	42.1	10.5	47.4	--	--	--	42.1	57.9
3.	2.5	86.7	10.5	2.3	0.5	--	4.7	63.9	31.4
4.	3.3	97.3	2.7	--	--	--	1.8	62.3	35.9
5.	2.3	77.9	11.2	8.4	2.5	--	11.8	69.0	19.2
6.	7.9	91.1	5.0	3.0	0.9	--	9.6	72.7	17.1
7.	127.7	56.7	10.3	25.1	7.9	0.0	25.9	59.7	14.4
8.	19.6	26.6	6.3	25.3	39.5	2.3	37.5	54.4	8.

Education 9.5
Bildungswesen

	A.	B.	C.	D.	E.	F.	G.	H.	I.
Gruzinskaja SSR									
1.	76.8	73.5	10.4	11.9	4.2	--	15.5	58.8	25.7
2.	0.0	50.0	--	50.0	--	--	--	--	100.0
3.	1.0	98.6	1.2	0.2	--	--	4.1	51.6	44.3
4.	1.6	100.0	--	--	--	--	0.9	45.5	53.6
5.	0.7	98.6	1.4	--	--	--	5.5	60.6	33.9
6.	3.5	99.3	0.6	0.1	--	--	5.3	61.8	32.9
7.	60.7	74.1	11.2	12.4	2.3	--	15.8	58.6	25.6
8.	9.3	51.0	12.0	17.4	19.6	--	22.5	61.9	15.6
Azerbajdžanskaja SSR									
1.	85.5	63.7	10.0	22.1	4.2	0.0	26.5	56.5	17.0
2.	0.0	100.0	--	--	--	--	--	--	100.0
3.	1.8	95.9	3.4	0.7	--	--	5.7	62.2	32.1
4.	1.6	99.9	0.1	--	--	--	1.6	58.0	40.4
5.	1.5	93.3	5.0	1.6	0.1	--	13.8	64.2	22.0
6.	3.1	96.9	1.9	0.8	0.4	--	9.7	64.6	25.7
7.	68.3	64.0	11.3	24.0	0.7	--	27.4	55.9	16.7
8.	9.2	33.6	6.5	26.3	33.3	0.3	36.1	55.7	8.2
Litovskaja SSR									
1.	30.2	56.1	14.3	21.0	8.5	0.1	18.1	62.6	19.3
3.	0.7	79.6	20.4	--	--	--	4.5	67.0	28.5
4.	0.5	97.5	2.5	--	--	--	0.8	60.5	38.7
5.	0.6	84.7	15.3	--	--	--	17.2	69.7	13.1
6.	1.3	97.8	2.2	--	--	--	7.1	72.8	20.1
7.	23.7	53.1	15.7	24.1	7.1	0.0	18.2	62.5	19.3
8.	3.4	45.1	9.9	18.1	26.3	0.6	27.2	57.8	15.0
Moldavskaja SSR									
1.	40.0	65.9	7.4	20.6	6.0	0.1	19.1	65.0	15.9
3.	0.6	97.9	2.1	--	--	--	7.6	68.9	23.5
4.	0.8	99.9	0.1	--	--	--	3.5	63.1	33.4
5.	0.5	96.0	3.4	0.6	--	--	12.6	69.0	18.4
6.	1.8	98.4	1.3	0.3	--	--	8.2	71.3	20.5
7.	31.5	67.5	8.4	21.1	3.0	0.0	18.9	65.3	15.8
8.	4.8	29.5	5.6	33.3	30.5	1.1	29.3	59.7	11.0
Latvijskaja SSR									
1.	20.0	64.6	11.6	14.7	9.0	0.1	17.3	60.0	22.7
2.	0.0	100.0	--	--	--	--	--	50.0	50.0
3.	0.5	91.4	8.6	--	--	--	1.3	63.1	35.6
4.	0.3	99.7	0.3	--	--	--	0.7	58.2	41.1
5.	0.5	91.8	7.4	0.8	--	--	3.5	74.6	21.9
6.	0.8	96.4	3.2	0.1	0.3	--	3.4	71.9	24.7
7.	14.6	65.4	13.2	15.8	5.6	--	17.6	59.2	23.2
8.	3.3	42.5	8.9	18.8	29.3	0.5	25.0	58.6	16.4
Kirgizskaja SSR									
1.	43.9	63.9	9.8	20.6	5.6	0.1	27.0	58.4	14.6
2.	0.0	66.7	--	33.3	--	--	--	66.7	33.3
3.	0.5	99.4	0.4	0.2	--	--	5.8	70.1	24.1
4.	0.9	100.0	--	--	--	--	2.2	69.0	28.8
5.	0.5	97.9	2.1	--	--	--	10.5	75.0	14.5
6.	2.2	98.7	0.9	0.3	0.1	--	8.1	74.1	17.8
7.	34.0	65.5	11.1	21.1	2.3	--	27.3	57.5	15.2
8.	5.8	31.0	8.4	31.0	29.1	0.5	38.6	53.6	7.8

519

9.5 Education / Bildungswesen

	A.	B.	C.	D.	E.	F.	G.	H.	I.
Tadžikskaja SSR									
1.	50.2	62.1	9.6	18.7	9.5	0.1	27.5	58.3	14.2
3.	0.8	94.5	5.0	0.5	--	--	7.4	68.7	23.9
4.	1.1	99.7	0.3	--	--	--	1.4	66.7	31.9
5.	0.7	86.5	9.9	2.4	1.2	--	12.5	72.1	15.4
6.	2.6	93.9	4.5	1.2	0.4	--	7.5	74.4	18.1
7.	40.0	61.6	10.7	20.8	6.9	0.0	29.0	56.9	14.1
8.	5.0	32.8	5.9	20.0	40.6	0.7	37.3	55.4	7.3
Armjanskaja SSR									
1.	40.2	69.2	7.4	17.1	6.3	0.0	27.2	52.8	20.0
3.	0.4	95.9	3.4	0.7	--	--	6.7	43.7	49.6
4.	0.9	99.8	0.2	--	--	--	2.7	39.5	57.8
5.	0.3	93.1	5.2	1.4	0.3	--	16.8	48.5	34.7
6.	1.8	98.1	0.8	0.5	0.6	--	8.1	53.0	38.9
7.	31.8	69.8	8.3	17.0	4.9	--	28.2	53.1	18.7
8.	5.0	46.6	5.7	29.1	18.6	0.0	34.4	53.7	11.9
Turkmenskaja SSR									
1.	32.0	68.1	9.2	16.6	6.0	0.1	27.6	55.7	16.7
2.	0.0	100.0	--	--	--	--	--	--	100.0
3.	0.3	94.9	4.5	0.6	--	--	8.0	65.0	27.0
4.	0.9	99.3	0.7	--	--	--	2.3	55.7	42.0
5.	0.3	91.7	6.9	0.7	0.7	--	11.3	74.5	14.2
6.	2.0	97.2	2.1	0.6	0.1	--	8.2	66.5	25.3
7.	26.0	66.5	10.3	18.0	5.2	0.0	29.4	54.7	15.9
8.	2.5	43.8	7.1	25.2	22.7	1.2	38.4	54.0	7.6
Estonskaja SSR									
1.	11.4	65.1	8.8	18.4	7.3	0.4	16.3	65.4	18.3
2.	0.0	100.0	--	--	--	--	--	--	100.0
3.	0.3	80.7	13.1	3.8	2.4	--	1.0	52.4	46.6
4.	0.2	98.2	1.8	--	--	--	--	48.5	51.5
5.	0.3	81.8	12.4	4.7	1.1	--	2.2	75.2	22.6
6.	0.4	93.7	3.7	1.9	0.7	--	4.0	68.9	27.1
7.	8.3	65.1	10.0	19.1	5.7	0.1	15.4	67.3	17.3
8.	1.9	51.2	4.0	24.9	18.0	1.9	29.1	57.9	13.0

Education 9.6
Bildungswesen

9.6 NUMBER OF TEACHERS OF THE UPPER FORMS AT GENERAL EDUCATIONAL DAY SCHOOLS BY
SUBJECTS AND EDUCATION (INCLUDING INSTRUCTING PRINCIPALS)
ZAHL DER LEHRER DER OBEREN KLASSEN DER ALLGEMEINBILDENDEN TAGESSCHULEN NACH
FÄCHERN UND BILDUNG (EINSCHLIESSLICH UNTERRICHTENDE SCHULLEITER)
ČISLENNOST' UČITELEJ STARŠICH KLASSOV DNEVNYCH OBŠČEOBRAZOVATEL'NYCH ŠKOL
POSPECIAL'NOSTJAM I OBRAZOVANIJU (VKLJUČAJA RUKOVODITELEJ ŠKOL, VED.PREPODAVANIE)

(at the beginning of the school year 1975/76 - zu Beginn des Schuljahres 1975/76 -
na načalo 1975/76 učebnogo goda)

	Teachers, total of 4-10(11) forms (without persons with several functions) - Lehrer der 4-10(11)Klassen insg.(ohne Personen mit mehreren Funktionen) - Vsego učitelej 4-10(11)klassov (bez sovmestitelej) '000 - Tsd. - tys.	Education-Schulbildung-obrazovanie(%)		
		Higher education - Hochschulbildung vysšee	Teacher colleges and equivalent educational establishments - Lehrerinstitute u.gleichgestellte Lehranstalten - v obl'eme učitel'skich institutov i učebnych zavedenij, priravnennych k nim	Complete & incomplete secondary education - abgeschlossene u.nicht abgeschlossene Mittelschulbildung - srednee i ne imejut polnogo srednego obrazovanija
Russian language & literature - Russische Sprache u.Literatur - Russkogo jazyka i literatury:				
at schools with Russian language of instruction - in Schulen mit russischer Unterrichtssprache - v školach s obučeniem na russkom jazyka	225.7	83.9	10.6	5.5
at schools with non-Russian language of instruction - in Schulen mit nichtrussischer Unterrichtssprache - v školach s obučeniem na nerusskom jazyka	114.5	76.3	12.1	11.6
Native language (except Russian) and literature - Muttersprache(ohne Russisch) und Literatur - Rodnogo jazyka (krome russkogo) i literatury	144.0	81.7	11.6	6.7
History - Geschichte - istorii	172.6	86.6	8.7	4.7
Physics - Physik - fiziki	123.9	89.9	6.3	3.8
Mathematics-Mathematik-matematiki	320.2	81.3	12.3	6.4
Chemistry - Chemie - chimii	86.5	92.0	4.6	3.4
Geography - Geographie - geografii	105.1	83.9	9.7	6.4
Biology - Biologie - biologii	113.0	82.0	11.3	6.7
Foreign languages - Fremdsprachen - inostrannych jazykov	177.4	88.3	5.2	6.5

521

9.7 Education / Bildungswesen

9.7 GENERAL EDUCATIONAL EVENING (SHIFT) SCHOOLS IN THE UNION REPUBLICS
ALLGEMEINBILDENDE ABEND(SCHICHT-)SCHULEN IN DEN UNIONSREPUBLIKEN
VEČERNIE (SMENNYE) OBŠČEOBRAZOVATEL'NYE ŠKOLY PO SOJUZNYM RESPUBLIKAM

(at the beginning of the school year - zu Beginn des Schuljahres -
na načalo učebnogo goda)

Year Jahr Gody	Number of schools Zahl der Schulen Čislo škol	Number of pupils Zahl der Schüler Čislo učaščichsja '000-Tsd.-tys.	of which in-darunter in-v tom čis. 1-8 forms 1.-8. Klassen 1-8 klassach	9-10(11)forms 9.-10.(11.)Klassen 9-10(11)klassach
	A.	B.	C.	D.
SSSR				
1950/51	20.465	1.438	1.246	192
1960/61	25.229	2.770	1.709	1.061
1970/71	15.116	3.745	903	2.842
1975/76	14.736	4.983	453	4.530
RSFSR				
1950/51	9.610	788	680	108
1960/61	12.083	1.663	1.071	592
1970/71	6.836	2.049	604	1.445
1975/76	6.739	2.780	279	2.501
Ukrainskaja SSR				
1950/51	4.906	292	251	41
1960/61	6.643	566	325	241
1970/71	2.233	849	85	764
1975/76	1.871	983	40	943
Belorusskaja SSR				
1950/51	948	57	49	8
1960/61	1.412	90	56	34
1970/71	521	123	21	102
1975/76	361	136	5	131
Uzbekskaja SSR				
1950/51	1.188	54	49	5
1960/61	1.101	63	29	34
1970/71	2.239	154	27	127
1975/76	2.261	213	18	195
Kazachskaja SSR				
1950/51	363	30	25	5
1960/61	852	100	59	41
1970/71	885	207	73	134
1975/76	1.071	296	45	251
Gruzinskaja SSR				
1950/51	520	24	19	5
1960/61	364	36	20	16
1970/71	361	48	13	35
1975/76	388	53	9	44
Azerbajdžanskaja SSR				
1950/51	603	38	33	5
1960/61	596	52	28	24
1970/71	753	83	20	63
1975/76	432	149	22	127

Education
Bildungswesen 9.7

	A.	B.	C.	D.
Litovskaja SSR				
1950/51	144	15	11	4
1960/61	213	38	25	13
1970/71	148	33	12	21
1975/76	117	70	5	65
Moldavskaja SSR				
1950/51	1.119	69	68	1
1960/61	750	47	32	15
1970/71	327	56	10	46
1975/76	361	94	4	90
Latvijskaja SSR				
1950/51	109	14	10	4
1960/61	134	26	15	11
1970/71	65	29	7	22
1975/76	73	34	2	32
Kirgizskaja SSR				
1950/51	272	14	13	1
1960/61	215	17	9	8
1970/71	180	34	8	26
1975/76	156	61	7	54
Tadžikskaja SSR				
1950/51	226	13	12.5	0.7
1960/61	325	22	13	9
1970/71	189	24	6	18
1975/76	408	35	5	30
Armjanskaja SSR				
1950/51	245	17	15	2
1960/61	275	19	10	9
1970/71	167	23	7	16
1975/76	200	33	6	27
Turkmenskaja SSR				
1950/51	139	6	5	0.7
1960/61	180	12	6	6
1970/71	160	17	5	12
1975/76	247	23	3	20
Estonskaja SSR				
1950/51	73	7	5	2
1960/61	86	19	11	8
1970/71	52	16	5	11
1975/76	51	23	3	20

9.8 Education / Bildungswesen

9.8 PERMANENT PREPARATORY EDUCATIONAL ESTABLISHMENTS IN THE UNION REPUBLICS
STÄNDIGE VORSCHULEINRICHTUNGEN IN DEN UNIONSREPUBLIKEN
POSTOJANNYE DOŠKOL'NYE UČREŽDENIJA PO SOJUZNYM RESPUBLIKAM

(end-of-year figures - zum Jahresende - na konec goda)

Year Jahr Gody	Number of permanent preparatory educational establishments - Zahl der ständigen Vorschuleinrichtungen - Čislo postojannych doškol'nych učreždenij		Number of children, '000 Zahl der Kinder, Tsd. V nich detej, tys.	
	Total Insg. Vsego	Kindergarten & nursery schools - Kindergärten u.-krippen - detskich sadov i jaslej-sadov	Total Insg. Vsego	in kindergarten & nursery schools - in Kindergärten u.-krippen-v detskich sadach i jasljach-sadach
A.	B.	C.	D.	E.

SSSR
1. in towns and rural areas -
in Städten u.a.dem Lande -
v gorodach i sel'skich mestnostjach

1940	46.031	23.999	1.953	1.172
1950	45.251	25.624	1.788	1.169
1960	70.584	43.569	4.428	3.115
1970	102.730	83.134	9.281	8.100
1975	115.173	99.392	11.523	10.470

2. in towns - in Städten - v gorodach

1940	23.651	14.427	1.422	906
1950	26.290	17.055	1.380	958
1960	43.346	28.632	3.565	2.550
1970	61.516	49.008	7.380	6.396
1975	64.484	53.575	8.980	8.067

3. in rural areas - auf dem Lande -
v sel'skich mestnostjach

1940	22.380	9.572	531	266
1950	18.961	8.569	408	211
1960	27.238	14.937	863	565
1970	41.214	34.126	1.901	1.704
1975	50.689	45.817	2.543	2.403

RSFSR
1.
1940	29.855	15.409	1.266	752
1950	30.153	17.775	1.239	830
1960	47.610	30.123	3.038	2.150
1970	65.032	51.676	5.666	4.845
1975	68.702	57.698	6.681	5.930

2.
1940	14.888	9.234	919	583
1950	17.402	11.534	961	675
1960	28.999	19.324	2.447	1.747
1970	39.403	30.907	4.543	3.856
1975	40.538	32.947	5.366	4.712

3.
1940	14.967	6.175	347	169
1950	12.751	6.241	278	155
1960	18.611	10.799	591	402.5
1970	25.629	20.769	1.123	989
1975	28.164	24.751	1.315	1.218

Education 9.8
Bildungswesen

A.	B.	C.	D.	E.		A.	B.	C.	D.	E.
Ukrainskaja SSR										
1. 1940	6.904	3.384	319	172	2. 1940	536	301	25	15
1950	5.165	2.839	213	141	1950	809	458	36	22
1960	9.299	5.283	589	399.4	1960	1.518	929	119	81
1970	16.509	13.257	1.574	1.391	1970	2.759	2.329	375	338
1975	20.164	17.707	2.038	1.886	1975	2.966	2.603	466	435
2. 1940	4.432	2.426	257	147	3. 1940	536	252	12	6
1950	4.070	2.476	205	136	1950	521	233	10	5
1960	6.620	4.153	516	359.9	1960	1.755	934	51	32
1970	9.992	7.874	1.277	1.126	1970	3.075	2.820	189	180
1975	10.659	8.947	1.603	1.472	1975	3.611	3.443	243	236
3. 1940	2.472	958	62	25	Gruzinskaja SSR				
1950	2.175	836	46	20	1. 1940	977	664	48	39
1960	2.679	1.130	73.5	39.5	1950	850	514	33	24
1970	6.517	5.383	297	265	1960	1.062	669	58	46
1975	9.505	8.760	435	414	1970	1.784	1.417	116	105
					1975	1.938	1.621	143	133
Belorusskaja SSR										
1. 1940	1.316	823	64	45.5	2. 1940	504	342	34	28
1950	732	425	29	20	1950	511	340	26	20
1960	1.373	877	98	70	1960	641	437	48	40
1970	2.430	2.062	274	247	1970	936	745	86	79
1975	2.968	2.668	373	348	1975	965	796	105	98
2. 1940	902	541	54	37.7	3. 1940	473	322	14	11
1950	523	336	25	18	1950	339	174	7	4
1960	996	651	88	63	1960	421	232	10	6
1970	1.658	1.385	246	221	1970	848	672	30	26
1975	1.864	1.627	329	306	1975	973	825	38	35
3. 1940	414	282	10	7.8	Azerbajdžanskaja SSR				
1950	209	89	4	2	1. 1940	1.298	909	57	44
1960	377	226	10	7.3	1950	850	539	31	22
1970	772	677	28	26	1960	1.006	668	53	40
1975	1.104	1.041	44	42	1970	1.600	1.250	111	100
					1975	1.725	1.433	127	118
Uzbekskaja SSR										
1. 1940	2.215	780	74	34	2. 1940	579	388	35	27
1950	2.182	757	66	30	1950	655	431	28	20
1960	2.964	1.426	173	110	1960	796	544	48	37
1970	3.353	2.827	348	311	1970	1.075	915	98	90
1975	5.194	4.873	561	532	1975	1.136	1.006	111	105
2. 1940	657	399	37	23	3. 1940	719	521	21.5	17
1950	765	493	35	23	1950	195	108	3	2
1960	1.164	793	102	73	1960	210	124	5	3
1970	1.735	1.451	248	220	1970	525	335	13	10
1975	2.035	1.792	332	307	1975	589	427	16	13
3. 1940	1.558	381	37	11	Litovskaja SSR				
1950	1.417	264	31	7	1. 1940	253	249	14	13
1960	1.800	633	71	37	1950	253	197	8	6.5
1970	1.618	1.376	100	91	1960	419	298	21	16
1975	3.159	3.081	229	225	1970	794	714	80	76
					1975	936	881	119	116
Kazachskaja SSR										
1. 1940	1.072	553	37	21	2. 1940	190	186	12	11
1950	1.330	691	46	27	1950	214	160	7	5.8
1960	3.273	1.863	170	113	1960	377	262	20	15.4
1970	5.834	5.149	564	518	1970	567	490	74	70
1975	6.577	6.046	709	671	1975	644	591	110	107

9.8 Education
Bildungswesen

A.	B.	C.	D.	E.	A.	B.	C.	D.	E.
3. 1940	63	63	2	2	Tadžikskaja SSR				
1950	39	37	1	0.7	1. 1940	325	103	8	3
1960	42	36	1	1	1950	338	150	10	5
1970	227	224	6	6	1960	370	252	32	23.3
1975	292	290	9	9	1970	508	445	68	62
Moldavskaja SSR					1975	594	543	87	82
1. 1940	106	58	5	3	2. 1940	129	59	5	2
1950	220	112	7	4	1950	179	95	7	4
1960	442	263	28	19.8	1960	280	187	28	20
1970	901	825	91	85	1970	375	318	60	54
1975	1.780	1.728	188	183	1975	410	363	75	70
2. 1940	79	50	4	3	3. 1940	196	44	3	1
1950	109	65	5	3	1950	159	55	3	1
1960	252	162	21	15.3	1960	90	65	4	3.3
1970	455	398	69	64	1970	133	127	8	8
1975	533	487	103	98	1975	184	180	12	12
3. 1940	27	8	1	0.3	Armjanskaja SSR				
1950	111	47	2	1	1. 1940	376	286	18	14.5
1960	190	101	7	4.5	1950	344	238	13	10
1970	446	427	22	21	1960	498	416	33	30
1975	1.247	1.241	85	85	1970	892	874	90	89
Latvijskaja SSR					1975	1.012	998	111	110
1. 1940	97	87	6	5.5	2. 1940	206	143	13	9.7
1950	232	154	10	7	1950	240	171	10	8
1960	438	305	26	20	1960	360	300	28	25
1970	756	672	72	67	1970	579	564	70	69
1975	831	757	91	86	1975	628	614	87	86
2. 1940	87	78	6	5.2	3. 1940	170	143	5	4.8
1950	213	138	10	7	1950	104	67	3	2
1960	361	246	24	18	1960	138	116	5	5
1970	569	489	64	59	1970	313	310	20	20
1975	602	530	78	73	1975	384	384	24	24
3. 1940	10	9	0.3	0.3	Turkmenskaja SSR				
1950	19	16	0.3	0.3	1. 1940	936	502	25	16
1960	77	59	2	2	1950	1.017	463	27	15
1970	187	183	8	8	1960	952	544	52	35
1975	229	227	13	13	1970	848	684	78	69
Kirgizskaja SSR					1975	998	861	102	94
1. 1940	197	101	7	4	2. 1940	273	144	12	7
1950	297	170	10	7	1950	263	145	11	6
1960	533	338	36	26	1960	395	243	30.5	21
1970	845	718	90	81	1970	498	385	57	50
1975	1.056	956	119	111	1975	538	447	77	71
2. 1940	103	63	5	3	3. 1940	663	358	13	9
1950	155	104	7	5	1950	754	318	16	9
1960	306	214	27	20.3	1960	557	301	21	14
1970	488	406	63	55	1970	350	299	21	19
1975	517	447	77	70	1975	460	414	25	23
3. 1940	94	38	2	1					
1950	142	66	3	2					
1960	227	124	9	6					
1970	357	312	27	26					
1975	539	509	42	41					

Education 9.8
Bildungswesen 9.9

A.	B.	C.	D.	E.	A.	B.	C.	D.	E.
Estonskaja SSR					1960	281	187	19	14
1. 1940	104	91	5	5	1970	427	352	50	45
1950	208	127	8	5.4	1975	449	378	61	57
1960	345	244	21	16	3. 1940	18	18	1	1
1970	644	564	59	54	1950	26	18	0.5	0.3
1975	698	622	74	70	1960	64	57	2	2
2. 1940	86	73	4	4	1970	217	212	9	9
1950	182	109	7	5.1	1975	249	244	13	13

9.9
NUMBER OF OTHER EDUCATIONAL INSTITUTIONS OF THE USSR MINISTRY OF EDUCATION
ZAHL DER AUSSERSCHULISCHEN EINRICHTUNGEN DES MINISTERIUMS FÜR VOLKSBILDUNG DER UdSSR
ČISLO VNEŠKOL'NYCH DETSKICH UČREŽDENIJ MINISTERSTVA PROSVEŠČENIJA SSSR

(end-of-year figures - zum Jahresende - na konec goda)

Year Jahr Gody	Pioneer and Pupils Palaces & Houses Pionier-u.Schüler- paläste u.häuser Dvorcy,doma pione- rov i škol'nikov	Stations of Young Technicians Stationen der Jungtechniker Stancii junych technikov	Stations of Young Naturalists Stationen d.jungen Naturforscher Stancii junych naturalistov	Excursion and Tou- rist Stations Ausflugs-und Tou- ristenstationen Ekskursionno - tu- ristskie stancii
1950	1.297	417	231	66
1960	3.142	324	269	147
1965	3.404	381	285	184
1966	3.497	399	293	176
1967	3.577	424	295	163
1968	3.687	463	305	161
1969	3.773	535	326	168
1970	3.857	589	337	169
1971	3.940	660	379	174
1972	4.040	720	413	177
1973	4.154	799	454	186
1974	4.285	899	525	197
1975	4.392	985	584	202

9.10 Education
Bildungswesen

9.10 MUSIC, ART AND BALLET SCHOOLS OF THE USSR MINISTRY OF CULTURE
IN THE UNION REPUBLICS
MUSIK-, KUNST- UND BALLETTSCHULEN DES KULTURMINISTERIUMS
DER UdSSR IN DEN UNIONSREPUBLIKEN
DETSKIE MUZYKAL'NYE, CHUDOŽESTVENNYE I CHOREOGRAFIČESKIE ŠKOLY
MINISTERSTVA KUL'TURY SSSR PO SOJUZNYM RESPUBLIKAM

(at the beginning of the school year - zu Beginn des Schuljahres -
na načalo učebnogo goda)

	Number of schools - Zahl der Schulen - Čislo škol				Number of pupils, '000 - Zahl der Schüler, Tsd. - Čislo učaščichsja, tys.			
	1960/61	1965/66	1970/71	1975/76	1960/61	1965/66	1970/71	1975/76
SSSR	1,750	2,829	4,510	6,109	314.9	488.9	761.5	1079.5
RSFSR	1,001	1,695	2,756	3,729	161.2	241.8	387.6	553.6
Ukrainskaja SSR	276	413	696	939	62.3	98.0	154.4	226.2
Belorusskaja SSR	93	120	161	227	17.5	24.4	30.3	42.6
Uzbekskaja SSR	44	100	159	211	9.6	19.4	34.9	54.0
Kazachskaja SSR	43	78	154	262	8.5	19.9	34.2	50.6
Gruzinskaja SSR	80	105	123	151	20.7	27.3	33.6	38.3
Azerbajdžanskaja SSR	38	52	84	97	8.0	12.1	18.2	22.5
Litovskaja SSR	29	42	64	70	4.2	6.4	10.7	14.3
Moldavskaja SSR	19	37	56	76	3.6	5.7	10.8	14.0
Latvijskaja SSR	39	42	46	52	4.0	5.0	6.7	8.6
Kirgizskaja SSR	13	29	43	57	1.9	5.1	7.4	9.6
Tadžikskaja SSR	6	26	32	61	1.6	5.5	6.5	10.5
Armjanskaja SSR	39	44	66	97	6.3	9.7	15.0	22.7
Turkmenskaja SSR	9	21	42	44	2.6	4.7	6.3	6.0
Estonskaja SSR	21	25	28	36	2.9	3.9	4.9	6.0

10. PRINTING AND PUBLISHING — DRUCK- UND VERLAGSWESEN — PEČAT'

10.1
PUBLICATION OF BOOKS AND BROCHURES IN THE LANGUAGES OF THE NATIONALITIES OF THE USSR AND FOREIGN LANGUAGES IN 1976
PUBLIKATION VON BÜCHERN UND BROSCHÜREN IN DEN SPRACHEN DER VÖLKER DER UdSSR UND DER VÖLKER DES AUSLANDS IM JAHRE 1976
VYPUSK KNIG I BROŠJUR NA JAZYKACH NARODOV SSSR I NARODOV ZARUBEŽNYCH STRAN V 1976 G.

	Publications, total Veröffentlichungen insg. Vse izdanija		of which translated davon übersetzte v tom čisle perevodnye		
	Number of books, brochures, printed units Zahl d.Bücher u.Broschüren, Druckeinheiten Čislo knig i brošjur,pečat-nych edinic	Edition, 'OOO copies Auflage, Tsd.Exempl. Tiraž, tys.ekz.	Number of books, brochures, printed units Zahl d.Bücher u.Broschüren, Druckeinheiten Čislo knig i brošjur,pečat-nych edinic	Edition, 'OOO copies Auflage, Tsd.Exempl. Tiraž, tys.ekz.	Number of language from which translations were made Zahl d.Sprachen, aus denen über-setzt wurde Čislo jazykov, s kotorych sdelan perevod
	A.	B.	C.	D.	E.
Total - Insg. - Vsego	84,304	1,744,515	8,208	281,980	108
In the languages of the USSR peoples- In den Sprachen d. Völker der UdSSR- Na jazykach narodov SSSR	80,713	1,666,009	5,581	235,770	108
of which-darun-ter-v tom čisle:					
Russian - Russisch - na russkom	66,126	1,412,897	2,023	132,544	102
Ukrainian - Ukrainisch - na ukrainskom	2,495	104,156	349	37,560	45
Belorussian - Belorussisch - na belorusskom	417	9,167	112	3,436	17
Uzbek - Usbekisch - na uzbekskom	909	24,036	305	10,820	28
Kazakh - Kasachisch - na kazachskom	661	13,297	201	5,332	20
Georgian - Georgisch - na gruzinskom	1,509	13,269	245	4,054	24
Azerbaidzhan - Aserbaidschanisch- na azerbajžanskom	804	9,292	211	4,784	19
Lithuanian - Litauisch - na litovskom	1,156	14,610	247	6,131	36

10.1 Druck-u.Verlagswesen

	A.	B.	C.	D.	E.
Moldavian - Moldauisch - na moldavskom	591	7,478	287	4,464	25
Latvian - Lettisch - na latyšskom	1,097	12,166	251	6,590	25
Kirghiz - Kirgisisch - na kirgizskom	417	4,395	191	2,534	21
Tadzhik - Tadschikisch - na tadžikskom	371	3,910	148	2,234	7
Armenian - Armenisch - na armjanskom	831	8,809	236	4,527	20
Turkmenian - Turkmenisch - na turkmenskom	207	3,838	74	1,880	3
Estonian - Estnisch - na estonskom	1,556	13,780	350	5,828	37
Abasinian - Abasinisch - na abazinskom	12	15	--	--	--
Abkhazian - Abchasisch - na abchazskom	62	96	10	13	3
Adegeyish - Adygeisch - na adygejskom	21	43	2	2	1
Altayish - Altaiisch - na altajskom	22	44	4	10	1
Balkar - Balkarisch - na balkarskom	25	39	3	3	1
Bashkir - Baschkirisch - na baškirskom	119	992	27	323	2
Buryat - Burjatisch - na burjatskom	35	116	4	5	1
In the languages of the Dagestan peoples - In den Sprachen der Völker Dagestans - na jazykach narodov Dagestana:					
Avark - Awarisch - na avarskom	29	194	7	48	1
Dargin - Darginisch - na darginskom	27	116	6	33	1
Kumuk - Kumykisch - na kumykskom	34	124	5	18	2
Lakish - Lakisch - na lakskom	14	29	2	3	1
Lesgian - Lesginisch - na lezginskom	34	124	8	28	1
Tabasaran - Tabasarnisch - na tabasaranskom	12	27	2	2	1
Dungan - Dunganisch - na dunganskom	4	5	--	--	--
Jewish - Jiddisch - na evrejskom	7	10	1	2	1
Inghushian - Inguschisch - na ingušskom	20	75	4	8	1
Kabardian - Kabardinisch - na kabardinskom	31	153	3	6	1
Kalmyk - Kalmückisch - na kalmyckom	26	45	4	6	2
Karakalpak - Karakalpakisch - na karakalpaks.	102	673	46	402	5
Karachayish - Karatschaierisch - na karačaevskom	14	43	--	--	--
Komi - na jazyke komi	23	81	--	--	--
Komi and Permyak - Komi-Permjakisch - na komi-permjackom	9	20	--	--	--
Krim-Tatar - Krimtatarisch - na krymsko-tatarskom	15	32	2	6	1
Kurdish - Kurdisch - na kurdskom	7	23	--	--	--
Karelian - Karelisch - na karelskom	1	2	--	--	--
Mari - na marijskom	38	171	6	22	1
Mari (mountain dialect) - Mari (Bergdialekt) - na marijskom (gornoe narečie)	15	30	2	2	1
Mordvinian-Moksha - Mordwinisch-Mokša - na mordovskom-mokša	24	45	3	3	1
Mordvinian-Ersa - Mordwinisch-Ersa - na mordovskom-erzja	19	36	2	4	1
Nogaish - Nogaisch - na nogajskom	12	14	--	--	--
Ossetian - Ossetinisch - na osetinskom	89	235	13	14	4
In the languages of the Northern peoples - In den Sprachen der nördlichen Völker - na jazykach narodov Severa:					
Neneish - Neneisch - na neneckom	2	7	--	--	--
Chukchish - Tschukotisch - na čukotskom	4	6	4	6	1
Evenk - Ewenkisch - na evenkijskom	2	6	--	--	--
Tatar - Tatarisch - na tatarskom	214	3,249	66	1,263	5
Tatish - Tatisch - na tatskom	2	2	--	--	--
Tuvinian - Tuwinisch - na tuvinskom	47	283	17	119	4

Druck-u.Verlagswesen 10.1

	A.	B.	C.	D.	E.
Udmurt - Udmurtisch - na udmurtskom	33	108	1	3	1
Udegeish - Udegeisch - na udegejskom	1	7	--	--	--
Uyghur - Ujgurisch - na ujgurskom	87	255	45	153	3
Khakas - Chakasisch - na chakasskom	5	14	2	6	1
Circassian - Tscherkessisch - na čerkesskom	4	4	--	--	--
Chechenish - Tschetschenisch - na čečenskom	24	220	5	12	1
Chuvash - Tschuwaschisch - na čuvašskom	93	1,119	13	177	2
Yakut - Jakutisch - na jakutskom	83	856	28	315	3
in several languages of the USSR peoples - in mehreren Sprachen der Völker der UdSSR - na neskol'kich jazykach narodov SSSR	39	289	4	35	3
Dictionaries (in several languages) - Wörterbücher (in mehreren Sprachen) - slovari (na neskol'kich jazykach)	24	832	--	--	--
In languages of foreign peoples - In Sprachen der Völker des Auslands - Na jazykach narodov zarubežnych stran	3,591	78,506	2,627	46,210	24
of which-darunter-v tom čisle:					
English - Englisch - na anglijskom	1,263	26,799	914	11,589	17
Arabic - Arabisch - na arabskom	129	2,279	128	2,257	7
Afghan - Afghanisch - na amcharskom	4	26	4	26	1
Amharian - Amharisch - na amcharskom	14	223	14	223	3
Bulgarian - Bulgarisch - na bolgarskom	20	929	18	927	3
Hungarian - Ungarisch - na vengerskom	83	1,597	66	1,051	5
Vietnamese - Vietnamesisch - na v'etnamskom	27	731	26	731	1
Dutch - Niederländisch - na gollandskom	12	54	12	54	3
Greek - Griechisch - na grečeskom	3	87	2	77	1
Danish - Dänisch - na datskom	8	112	8	112	2
In languages of Indian peoples - in den Sprachen der Völker Indiens - na jazykach narodov Indii:					
Bengali	33	578	32	378	4
Gujarat - Gudsharati - gudžarati	8	48	8	48	4
Malajalami	16	379	16	379	2
Marathi - Maratchi	8	30	8	30	3
Punjab - Pendshabi - pendžabi	14	122	14	122	3
Tamil - Tamilisch - tamil'skom	17	131	15	130	2
Telug - Telugu	18	123	18	123	3
Urdu	20	125	20	125	2
Hindi - chindi	26	392	26	392	3
Kashmiri - Kaschmiri - Kašmiri	6	31	6	31	1
Orissa - Orija - orja	1	5	1	5	1
Indonesian - Indonesisch - na indonezijskom	10	127	10	127	5
Spanish - Spanisch - na ispanskom	326	10,934	306	10,100	10
Italian - Italienisch - na ital'janskom	39	416	39	416	4
Chinese - Chinesisch - na kitajskom	10	40	9	39	2
Korean - Koreanisch - na korejskom	9	54	9	54	1
Latin - Lateinisch - na latinskom	27	65	--	--	--
Malay - Malaiisch - na malajskom	4	13	4	13	1
Mongolian - Mongolisch - na mongol'skom	18	149	18	149	1
German - Deutsch - na nemeckom	400	12,690	205	4,632	12
Nepalese - Nepalesisch - na nepal'skom	9	120	9	120	2
Norwegian - Norwegisch - norvežskom	7	47	7	47	1
Persian - Persisch - na persidskom	30	279	24	270	5
Polish - Polnisch - na pol'skom	77	2,332	58	2,284	5
Portuguese - Portugiesisch - na portugal'skom	30	806	28	805	1

531

10.1
10.1.1 Druck-u.Verlagswesen

	A.	B.	C.	D.	E.
Romanian - Rumänisch - na rumynskom	28	559	28	559	3
Serbocroatic - Serbokoratisch - na serbskochorvatskom	17	249	16	244	1
Singalese - Singalesisch - na singal'skom	13	180	13	180	1
Slovak - Slowakisch - na slovackom	23	455	23	455	4
Slovenian - Slowenisch - na slovenskom	1	1	--	--	--
Somali	3	30	3	30	1
Kisuaheli - na suachili	10	21	10	21	2
Turkish - Türkisch - na tureckom	1	100	1	100	1
Finnish - Finnisch - na finskom	45	236	37	215	4
French - Französisch - na francuzskom	431	7,699	301	4,747	11
Hausa - Hausa - na chausa	8	7	8	7	1
Czech - Tschechisch - na češskom	31	833	30	818	5
Swedish - Schwedisch - na švedskom	22	262	21	247	4
Japanese - Japanisch - na japonskom	25	86	23	85	2
In several languages of foreign peoples - In mehreren Sprachen der Völker des Auslands - na neskol'kich jazykach narodov zarubež-nych stran	105	929	30	626	4
Dictionaries (in several languages) - Wörterbücher (in mehreren Sprachen) - slovari (na neskol'kich jazykach)	101	3,976	--	--	--
Esperanto	1	10	1	10	1

10.1.1 In the Union Republics - in den Unionsrepubliken - po sojuznym respublikam:

RSFSR
Total - Insg. - Vsego	54,440	1,374,942	3,991	158,588	103
Russian - Russisch - na russkom	50,509	1,296,107	1,466	113,213	102
In languages of other USSR peoples - in Sprachen anderer Völker der UdSSR - na drugich jazykach narodov SSSR	1,205	8,675	249	2,454	13
In languages of foreign peoples - in Sprachen der Völker des Auslands - na jazykach narodov zarubežnych stran	2,726	70,160	2,276	42,921	22

Ukrainskaja SSR
Total - Insg. - Vsego	9,110	159,368	669	45,771	46
Ukrainian - Ukrainisch - na ukrainskom	2,494	104,154	348	37,558	45
Russian - Russisch - na russkom	6,252	50,460	130	6,519	9

Belorusskaja SSR
Total - Insg. - Vsego	2,489	34,769	161	6,953	21
Belorussian - Belorussisch - na belorusskom	416	9,167	111	3,436	17
Russian - Russisch - na russkom	2,002	24,547	22	2,883	8

Uzbekskaja SSR
Total - Insg. - Vsego	1,980	33,182	370	12,349	30
Uzbek - Usbekisch - na uzbekskom	897	23,986	297	10,777	27
Russian - Russisch - na russkom	944	8,026	25	1,164	5

Kazachskaja SSR
Total - Insg. - Vsego	1,922	23,499	277	7,667	22
Kazakh - Kasachisch - na kazachskom	660	13,295	200	5,331	20
Russian - Russisch - na russkom	1,162	9,797	24	2,123	3

Druck-u.Verlagswesen 10.1.1

	A.	B.	C.	D.	E.
Gruzinskaja SSR					
Total - Insg. - Vsego	2,311	16,043	312	4,706	26
Georgian - Georgisch - na gruzinskom	1,508	13,269	244	4,054	24
Russian - Russisch - na russkom	642	2,106	35	570	3
Azerbajdžanskaja SSR					
Total - Insg. - Vsego	1,263	11,552	246	5,053	19
Azerbaidzhan - Aserbaidschanisch - na azerbajžanskom	798	9,283	209	4,781	17
Russian - Russisch - na russkom	426	1,988	22	227	2
Litovskaja SSR					
Total - Insg. - Vsego	1,476	17,001	313	7,102	35
Lithuanian - Litauisch - na litovskom	1,155	14,610	246	6,131	34
Russian - Russisch - na russkom	244	2,051	34	866	1
Moldavskaja SSR					
Total - Insg. - Vsego	1,557	13,486	303	6,147	26
Moldavian - Moldauisch - na moldavskom	574	7,341	282	4,440	25
Russian - Russisch - na russkom	964	5,829	21	1,707	4
Latvijskaja SSR					
Total - Insg. - Vsego	2,168	15,134	332	7,889	26
Latvian Lettisch - na latyšskom	1,095	12,164	250	6,590	25
Russian - Russisch - na russkom	981	2,388	59	1,034	1
Kirgizskaja SSR					
Total - Insg. - Vsego	897	7,872	198	3,505	24
Kirghiz - Kirgisisch - na kirgizskom	416	4,395	190	2,534	21
Russian - Russisch - na russkom	468	3,421	8	971	3
Tadžikskaja SSR					
Total - Insg. - Vsego	784	5,150	160	2,331	8
Tadzhik - Tadschikisch - na tadžikskom	369	3,909	147	2,234	7
Russian - Russisch - na russkom	397	1,185	6	54	1
Armjanskaja SSR					
Total - Insg. - Vsego	1,165	10,231	242	4,589	21
Armenian - Armenisch - na armjanskom	812	8,732	228	4,484	20
Russian - Russisch - na russkom	304	1,265	11	101	1
Turkmenskaja SSR					
Total - Insg. - Vsego	506	4,518	77	1,993	4
Turkoman - Turkmenisch - na turkmenskom	206	3,838	73	1,880	3
Russian - Russisch - na russkom	281	598	3	113	1
Estonskaja SSR					
Total - Insg. - Vsego	2,236	17,768	557	7,337	38
Estonian - Estnisch - na estonskom	1,555	13,780	349	5,828	37
Russian - Russisch - na russkom	550	3,129	157	999	1

533

10.2
10.3 Druck-u.Verlagswesen

10.2 BOOKS AND BOOKLETS IN RUSSIAN AND IN OTHER LANGUAGES OF USSR PEOPLES
BÜCHER UND BROSCHÜREN IN RUSSISCHER SPRACHE UND IN SPRACHEN ANDERER
VÖLKER DER UdSSR
KNIGI I BROŠJURY NA RUSSKOM JAZYKE I JAZYKACH DRUGICH NARODOV SSSR

(in percent - in Prozent - v procentach)

Year Jahr Gody	in Russian in russischer Sprache na russkom jazyke	in languages of other USSR peoples in Sprachen anderer Völker der UdSSR na jazykach drugich narodov SSSR
1928	72.4	25.4
1940	75.0	23.3
1950	70.8	27.3
1956	73.5	24.0
1960	63.0	37.0
1971	76.0	24.0
1973	77.0	23.0
1975	77.5	22.5
1976	78.4	21.6

10.3 BOOK PRODUCTION BY SUBJECTS
BUCHPRODUKTION IN THEMATISCHER AUFTEILUNG
VYPUSK KNIŽNOJ PRODUKCII PO TEMATIČESKIM RAZDELAM

	A. Number of books, brochures, printed units - Zahl d.Bücher u.Broschü- ren, Druckeinheiten - Čislo knig i brošjur, pečatnych edinic	B. Edition, '000 copies - Auflage, Tsd.Exemplare - Tiraž, tys.eks.	C. Number of sheets, in '000 Druckbogenabzüge, Tsd. - Pečatnych listov- ottiskov, tys.	D. Average edition per book or brochure, '000 copies Durchschnittl.Auflage pro Buch u.Broschüre,Tsd.Exemp. Srednij tiraž odnoj knigi i brošjury, tys.eks.	E. Average number of pages per book and brochure,in sheets Durchschnittl.Umfang pro Buch u.Broschüre,Druckbogen Srednij obëm odnoj knigi i brošjury,pečatnych listov
Total-Insg.-Vsego:					
1940	45,830	462,203	2,848,300	10.1	6.2
1950	43,060	820,529	6,980,341	19.0	8.5
1965	76,101	1,279,268	12,994,519	16.8	10.2
1970	78,875	1,309,648	13,953,541	16.6	10.7
1971	85,463	1,581,263	16,836,488	18.5	10.6
1975	83,439	1,671,782	17,601,688	20.0	10.5
1976	84,304	1,744,515	18,256,561	20.7	10.5
Political and economical literature - politische u. sozial-ökonomische Litera- tur - političeskaja i so- cial'no-ekonomičeskaja literatura:					
1940	7,432	88,233	533,539	11.9	6.0
1950	7,353	216,792	1,381,879	29.5	6.4

534

	A.	B.	C.	D.	E.
1965	10,083	189,786	1,867,439	18.8	9.8
1970	11,541	228,844	2,359,746	19.8	10.3
1971	12.593	276,901	2,694,791	22.0	9.7
1975	11,878	253,927	2,739,326	21.4	10.8
1976	11,423	288,085	3,024,086	25.2	10.5

Natural sciences & mathematics - Naturwissenschaften u.Mathematik - Estestvennye nauki,matematika:

	A.	B.	C.	D.	E.
1940	3,639	58,795	533,124	16.2	9.1
1950	3,382	103,316	1,052,132	30.5	10.2
1965	7,067	188,552	2,166,539	26.7	11.5
1970	7,350	177,343	2,453,887	24.1	13.8
1971	8,164	188,804	2,635,513	23.1	14.0
1975	9,217	200,708	2,608,853	21.8	13.0
1976	10,262	199,489	2,629,898	19.4	13.2

Technology, industry, transport, communications,municipal services - Technik,Industrie,Transport,Post- u.Fernmeldewesen,Kommunalwesen - Technika,promyšlennost',transport, svjaz', kommunal'noe delo:

	A.	B.	C.	D.	E.
1940	12,236	35,265	156,455	2.9	4.4
1950	12,062	65,531	393,114	5.4	6.0
1965	27,021	141,989	1,234,533	5.3	8.7
1970	29,271	139,060	1,189,795	4.8	8.6
1971	30,106	188,906	1,568,384	6.3	8.3
1975	28,484	175,844	1,564,455	6.2	8.9
1976	28,065	166,493	1,442,823	5.9	8.7

Agriculture - Landwirtschaft - Sel'skoe chozjajstvo:

	A.	B.	C.	D.	E.
1940	4,127	23,909	116,047	5.8	4.9
1950	4,793	43,139	222,698	9.0	5.2
1965	6,101	37,386	264,103	6.1	7.1
1970	5,664	36,034	276,905	6.4	7.7
1971	5,850	37,019	304,324	6.3	8.2
1975	6,857	41,365	383,828	6.0	9.3
1976	6,620	41,303	383,314	6.2	9.3

Trade,procurement,public catering - Handel,Beschaffungen,öffentliche Verpflegung - Torgovlja,zagotovki, obščestvennoe pitanie:

	A.	B.	C.	D.	E.
1940	765	5,458	10,975	7.1	2.0
1950	577	25,264	106,830	43.8	4.2
1965	905	14,228	137,224	15.7	9.6
1970	862	13,376	107,232	15.5	8.0
1971	909	10,384	98,793	11.4	9.5
1975	721	10,242	88,202	14.2	8.6
1976	750	12,850	115,949	17.1	9.0

Health, medicine - Gesundheitswesen, Medizin - Zdravoochranenie, medicina:

	A.	B.	C.	D.	E.
1940	2,236	13,456	46,022	6.0	3.4
1950	1,977	21,834	133,408	11.0	6.1
1965	3,404	44,398	280,826	13.0	6.3
1970	3,314	24,198	195,717	7.3	8.1

10.3 Druck-u.Verlagswesen

	A.	B.	C.	D.	E.
1971	3,492	30,753	242,915	8.8	7.9
1975	3,385	32,285	293,716	9.5	9.1
1976	3,222	30,523	298,043	9.5	9.8
Physical culture, sports - Körperkultur, Sport - Fizkul'tura, sport:					
1940	487	3,149	9,511	6.5	3.0
1950	519	6,849	24,718	13.2	3.6
1965	659	11,686	60,482	17.7	5.2
1970	636	10,970	72,616	17.2	6.6
1971	665	12,601	82,527	18.9	6.5
1975	649	10,333	79,569	15.9	7.7
1976	613	11,536	87,540	18.8	7.6
Culture, education, science - Kultur, Bildung, Wissenschaft - Kul'tura, prosveščenie, nauka:					
1940	3,358	19,301	56,347	5.7	2.9
1950	2,370	24,732	153,332	10.4	6.2
1965	4,002	42,213	335,268	10.5	7.9
1970	3,667	46,659	410,827	12.7	8.8
1971	4,070	54,344	540,317	13.4	9.9
1975	4,217	64,315	542,587	15.3	8.4
1976	4,312	63,802	578,682	14.8	9.1
Linguistics - Sprachwissenschaft - Jazykoznanie:					
1940	1,492	66,709	512,249	44.7	7.7
1950	1,273	77,416	861,118	60.8	11.1
1965	2,267	106,720	1,356,047	47.1	12.7
1970	2,273	111,768	1,516,182	49.2	13.6
1971	2,622	123,374	1,786,461	47.1	14.5
1975	2,256	99,830	1,383,250	44.3	13.9
1976	2,430	107,306	1,418,072	44.2	13.2
Science of literature - Literaturwissenschaft - Literaturovedenie:					
1940	744	17,351	275,341	23.3	15.9
1950	587	21,960	499,112	37.4	22.7
1965	1,084	32,368	560,163	29.9	17.3
1970	1,078	38,185	724,707	35.4	19.0
1971	1,276	53,559	987,949	42.0	18.4
1975	1,488	53,110	980,001	35.7	18.5
1976	1,464	48,339	847,967	33.0	17.5
Belles lettres - Belletristik - Chudožestvennaja literatura:					
1940	3,603	46,648	237,179	12.9	5.1
1950	4,688	178,892	1,902,259	38.2	10.6
1965	7,257	411,749	4,148,519	56.7	10.1
1970	6,847	416,463	3,942,706	60.8	9.5
1971	7,860	514,642	4,787,092	65.5	9.3
1975	7,818	650,513	5,936,729	83.2	9.1
1976	8,075	697,247	6,434,203	86.3	9.2

Druck-u.Verlagswesen 10.3

	A.	B.	C.	D.	E.
Russian literature - Russische Literatur - Russkaja literatura:					
1940	1,848	30,848	143,605	16.7	4.7
1950	2,762	136,520	1,438,296	49.4	10.5
1965	3,348	280,589	2,666,334	83.8	9.5
1970	2,814	286,788	2,561,556	101.9	8.9
1971	3,361	364,748	3,137,017	108.5	8.6
1975	3,721	464,308	3,823,782	124.8	8.2
1976	3,802	496,983	4,045,413	130.8	8.1
Literature of other USSR peoples- Literatur d.anderen Völker der UdSSR - Literatura drugich narodov SSSR:					
1940	1,407	10,700	54,516	7.6	5.1
1950	1,585	25,799	257,715	16.3	10.0
1965	3,071	75,758	668,927	24.7	8.8
1970	3,282	90,151	706,753	27.5	7.8
1971	3,687	101,953	849,964	27.7	8.3
1975	3,345	122,432	1,080,375	36.6	8.8
1976	3,472	118,679	1,055,840	34.2	8.9
Literature of foreign peoples - Literatur der Völker d.Auslands - Literatura narodov zarubežnych stran:					
1940	348	5,100	39,058	14.7	7.7
1950	341	16,573	206,248	48.6	12.4
1965	838	55,402	813,258	66.1	14.7
1970	751	39,524	674,397	52.6	17.1
1971	812	47,941	800,111	59.0	16.7
1975	752	63,773	1,032,572	84.8	16.2
1976	801	81,585	1,332,950	101.9	16.3
Art - Kunst - Iskusstvo:					
1940	1,338	7,534	21,016	5.6	2.8
1950	936	7,363	39,884	7.9	5.4
1965	1,860	21,708	190,933	11.7	8.8
1970	1,727	21,509	225,574	12.5	10.5
1971	2,363	27,614	288,428	11.7	10.4
1975	1,806	24,461	243,159	13.5	9.9
1976	1,729	25,529	257,783	14.8	10.1
Printing and publishing, library trade - Druck-u.Verlagswesen, Bücherkunde,Bibliothekswesen - Pečat', knigovedenie, bibliotečnoe delo, bibliografija:					
1940	1,095	4,214	9,944	3.8	2.4
1950	1,314	4,892	15,958	3.7	3.3
1965	2,528	14,626	128,900	5.8	8.8
1970	2,776	9,949	77,563	3.6	7.8
1971	3,484	16,220	148,172	4.7	9.1
1975	2,531	15,160	100,058	6.0	6.6
1976	3,270	14,478	108,323	4.4	7.5

10.4 Druck-u.Verlagswesen

10.4 PUBLICATION OF LITERATURE (BOOKS AND BROCHURES)
PUBLIKATION VON LITERATUR (BÜCHER UND BROSCHÜREN)
VYPUSK LITERATURY (KNIG I BROŠJUR) PO

	Total - Insgesamt - Vsego			
	Number of books and brochures, printed units Zahl d.Bücher u.Broschüren, Druckeinheiten Čislo knig i brošjur, pečatnych edinic	Edition, '000 copies Auflage, Tsd.Exempl. Tiraž, tys.eks.	Sheets, in thousands Druckbogenabzüge,Tsd. Pečatnych listovottiskov, tys.	Average edition per book or brochure,'000 copies Durchschnittl. Auflage pro Buch und Broschüre, Tsd. Exemplare Srednij tiraž odnoj knigi i brošjury, tys.eks.
	A.	B.	C.	D.
Marxism-Leninism - Marxismus-Leninismus - Marksizm-Leninizm	601	25,611	336,612	42.6
CPSU - KPdSU - KPSS	1,464	60,261	506,037	41.2
History of the CPSU - Geschichte der KPdSU - istorija KPSS	358	6,103	81,803	17.0
Lenin Communist Youth Association of the USSR - Leninscher Kommunistischer Jugendverband der UdSSR - VLKSM - Vsesojuznyj Leninskij Kommunističeskij Sojuz Molodeži	290	11,364	54,793	39.2
Philosophy-Philosophie- Filosofija	1,298	24,079	285,446	18.6
History-Geschichte-Istorija	1,545	57,485	949,818	37.2
History of the USSR - Geschichte der UdSSR - istorija SSSR	922	40,329	669,016	43.7
Economic sciences - Wirtschaftswissenschaften - Ekonomičeskie nauki	325	2,350	41,350	7.2
International relations,political & economic foreign status - internationale Beziehungen, politische u.Wirtschaftslage des Auslands - Meždunarodnye otnošenija,političeskoe i ekonomičeskoe položenie zarubežnych stran	1,040	22,425	221,601	21.6
Communist structure of the USSR - Kommunistischer Aufbau d.UdSSR - Kommunističeskoe stroitel'stvo SSSR	1,467	24,050	167,104	16.4

Druck-u.Verlagswesen 10.4

DIVIDED BY SUBJECTS FOR THE YEAR 1976
IN THEMATISCHER AUFTEILUNG IM JAHRE 1976
TEMATIČESKIM RAZDELAM V 1976 G.

Average number of pages per book and brochure, in sheets Durchschnittl. Umfang pro Buch u.Broschüre, Druckbogen Srednij obém odnoj knigi i brošjury, pečatnych listov E.	Literature of group "A" – Literatur der Gruppe "A" – literatura gruppy "A"				
	Number of books and brochures, printed units Zahl d.Bücher u.Broschüren, Druckeinheiten Čislo knig i brošjur, pečatnych edinic F.	Edition, '000 copies Auflage, Tsd.Exempl. Tiraž, tys.eks. G.	Sheets, in thousands Druckbogenabzüge, Tsd. Pečatnych listovottiskov, tys. H.	Average edition per book or brochure,'000 copies Durchschnittl. Auflage pro Buch und Broschüre, Tsd.Exemplare Srednij tiraž odnoj knigi i brošjury, tys.eks. I.	Average number of pages per book & brochure, in sheets Durchschnittl. Umfang pro Buch u.Broschüre, Druckbogen Srednij obém odnoj knigi i brošjury, pečatnych listov J.
13.1	582	25,576	336,561	43.9	13.2
8.4	1,100	59,032	503,660	53.7	8.5
13.4	288	5,994	81,534	20.8	13.6
4.8	218	10,850	53,560	49.8	4.9
11.9	1,009	23,070	282,336	22.9	12.2
16.5	1,394	56,904	947,889	40.8	16.7
16.6	852	40,023	668,057	47.0	16.7
17.6	248	2,250	40,953	9.1	18.2
9.9	845	21,981	220,193	26.0	10.0
6.9	1,127	21,971	160,297	19.5	7.3

10.4 Druck-u.Verlagswesen

	A.	B.	C.	D.
Planung,Statistik,Organisation d.Leitung - Planirovanie, učet, organizacija upravlenija	845	5,288	49,444	6.3
Finances - Finanzen - Financy	158	1,412	11,850	8.9
Labor - Arbeit - Trud	673	25,161	123,320	37.4
State and Law - Staat und Recht - Gosudarstvo i pravo	1,497	22,887	224,984	15.3
- Wehrwesen - Voennoe delo	1,986	30,426	315,292	15.3
Natural sciences, mathematics - Naturwissenschaften, Mathematik - Estestvennye nauki, matematika	10,262	199,489	2,629,898	19.4
Mathematics-Mathematik-matematika	1,398	80,041	1,061,183	57.3
Astronomy, geodesy - Astronomie, Geodäsie - astronomija,geodezija	268	4,186	51,941	15.6
Mechanics,physics - Mechanik, Physik - mechanika, fizika	2,598	28,216	452,928	10.9
Chemical sciences - chemische Wissenschaften - chimičeskie nauki	899	17,720	253,605	19.7
Geology - Geologie - geologija	2,722	6,930	68,320	2.5
Geography - Geographie - geografija	689	23,813	282,962	34.6
Biological sciences, general problems - biologische Wissenschaften, allgemeine Fragen - biologičeskie nauki, obščie voprosy	586	7,242	113,332	12.4
Botany - Botanik - botanika	320	4,863	77,536	15.2
Zoology - Zoologie - zoologija	253	4,399	56,658	17.4
Physiology - Physiologie-fiziologija	267	5,571	92,877	20.9
Technology,industry - Technik,Industrie - technika, promyšlennost'	23,205	122,656	994,261	5.3
General industrial problems - allgemeine Fragen d.Industrie - obščie voprosy promyšlennosti	1,222	5,359	47,679	4.4
General technical disciplines - allgemeine techn.Disziplinen - obščetechničeskie discipliny	685	9,135	106,808	13.3
Standards,technical quality regulations - Standards, technische Gütevorschriften - standarty, techničeskie uslovija	6,395	37,451	58,250	5.9
Construction-Bauwesen stroitel'noe delo	3,032	19,869	196,433	6.6
Power industry - Energiewirtschaft - energetika	3,748	16,810	234,163	4.5
Mining - Bergbau - gornoe delo	1,595	4,496	36,232	2.8
Metallurgy - Metallurgie - metallurgija	789	2,059	21,733	2.6
Technology of metals - Technologie der Metalle - technologija metallov	883	3,848	50,794	4.4
Machine building - Maschinenbau - mašinostroenie	1,311	7,184	87,489	5.5

Druck-u.Verlagswesen 10.4

E.	F.	G.	H.	I.	J.
9.4	449	4,513	46,147	10.1	10.2
8.4	91	904	10,116	9.9	11.2
4.9	402	23,597	120,862	58.7	5.1
9.8	1,075	21,795	219,065	20.3	10.1
10.4	1,806	29,301	311,110	16.2	10.6
13.2	6,388	193,828	2,603,895	30.3	13.4
13.3	1,030	78,274	1,051,452	76.0	13.4
12.4	173	4,132	51,723	23.9	12.5
16.1	1,023	27,151	448,809	26.5	16.5
14.3	590	17,025	251,132	28.9	14.8
9.9	1,700	6,238	63,887	3.7	10.2
11.9	586	23,046	280,279	39.3	12.2
15.6	402	7,068	112,510	17.6	15.9
15.9	259	4,715	76,998	18.2	16.3
12.9	232	4,365	56,500	18.8	12.9
16.7	198	5,511	92,617	27.8	16.8
8.1	7,284	55,285	804,462	7.6	14.6
8.9	478	3,912	41,491	8.2	10.6
11.7	321	7,250	97,822	22.6	13.5
1.6	7	497	10,391	71.0	20.9
9.9	1,164	10,081	145,072	8.7	14.4
13.9	1,961	13,163	214,886	6.7	16.3
8.1	711	1,972	23,630	2.8	12.0
10.6	377	1,355	17,226	3.6	12.7
13.2	393	2,993	48,475	7.6	16.2
12.2	588	5,174	80,172	8.8	15.5

10.4 Druck-u.Verlagswesen

	A.	B.	C.	D.
Chemical industry – chemische Industrie – chimičeskaja promyšlennost'	1,472	2,970	34,997	2.0
Timber and wood processing industry – Holz-u.holzbearbeitende Industrie – lesnaja i derevoobrabatyvajuščaja promyšlennost'	513	1,658	15,270	3.2
Light industry – Leichtindustrie – legkaja promyšlennost'	740	7,486	63,554	10.1
Food industry – Nahrungsmittelindustrie – piščevaja promyšlenn	713	2,853	34,076	4.0
Agriculture – Landwirtschaft – Sel'skoe chozjajstvo	6,620	41,303	383,314	6.2
General problems – allgemeine Fragen – obščie voprosy	1,275	9,140	75,132	7.2
Mechanization & electrification, agricultural machine building – Mechanisierung u.Elektrifizierung, Landwirtschaftsmaschinenbau – mechanizacija i elektrifikacija, sel'skochozjajstvennoe mašinos.	1,085	8,378	94,426	7.7
Plant cultivation – Pflanzenzucht – rastenievodstvo	2,309	12,877	122,508	5.6
Forestry – Forstwirtschaft – lesnoe chozjajstvo	375	1,426	12,235	3.8
Cattle breeding – Viehzucht – životnovodstvo	1,043	6,476	48,279	6.2
Hunting, fishing – Jagd, Fischereiwesen-ochota,rybolovstvo	286	1,570	15,611	5.5
Veterinary sciences – Veterinärwesen – veterinarija	247	1,436	15,123	5.8
Transport, transport machine building – Transport, Transportmaschinenbau – Transport, transportnoe mašinostr.	3,407	30,210	303,716	8.9
Railway transport – Eisenbahntransport – železnodoržnyj transport	513	3,825	44,801	7.5
City and highway transport – Stadt-u.schienenloser Verkehr – gorodskoj i bezrel'sovyj transport	950	17,859	163,397	18.8
Water transport – Wassertransport – vodnyj transport	784	2,919	41,056	3.7
Air transport – Luftverkehr – vozdušnyj transport	731	2,151	19,586	2.9
Space travel – Raumschiffahrt – kosmonavtika	109	2,349	24,961	21.6
Communications, radio technics – Post-u.Fernmeldewesen, Radiotechnik – Svjaz', radiotechnika	942	11,268	124,833	12.0
Trade, procurement, public catering – Handel,Beschaffungen,öffentl.Verpflegung – Torgovlja, zagotovki, obščestvennoe pitanie	750	12,850	115,949	17.1
Communal services – Kommunalwesen – Kommunal'noe delo	511	2,359	20,013	4.6
Health, medicine – Gesundheitswesen, Medizin – Zdravoochranenie,medicina	3,222	30,523	298,043	9.5

542

Druck-u.Verlagswesen 10.4

E.	F.	G.	H.	I.	J.
11.8	550	2,152	31,908	3.9	14.8
9.2	223	1,157	13,360	5.2	11.5
8.5	264	3,618	48,879	13.7	13.5
11.9	239	1,921	30,463	8.0	15.9
9.3	3,543	32,423	346,090	9.2	10.7
8.2	718	7,351	66,441	10.2	9.0
11.3	500	5,915	78,321	11.8	13.2
9.5	1,278	10,618	116,635	8.3	11.0
8.6	220	1,072	11,187	4.9	10.4
7.5	538	4,886	43,823	9.1	9.0
9.9	135	1,410	14,996	10.4	10.6
10.5	154	1,171	14,687	7.6	12.5
10.1	1,767	21,422	251,278	12.1	11.7
11.7	299	2,057	30,734	6.9	14.9
9.1	388	12,484	134,998	32.2	10.8
14.1	431	2,282	36,215	5.3	15.9
9.1	450	1,672	16,758	3.7	10.0
10.6	80	2,296	24,616	28.7	10.7
11.1	528	9,237	109,889	17.5	11.9
9.0	322	7,792	89,736	24.2	11.5
8.5	145	1,840	18,024	12.7	9.8
9.8	1,960	26,826	289,623	13.7	10.8

10.4
10.5 Druck-u.Verlagswesen

	A.	B.	C.	D.
Physical culture, sports – Körperkultur,Sport – Fizkul'tura, sport	613	11,536	87,540	18.8
Culture, education, science – Kultur, Bildung, Wissenschaft – Kul'tura, prosveščenie, nauka	4,312	63,802	578,682	14.8
Linguistics – Sprachwissenschaft – Jazykoznanie	2,430	107,306	1,418,072	44.2
Science of literature – Literaturwissenschaft – Literaturovedenie	1,464	48,339	847,967	33.0
Belles lettres – Belletristik – Chudožestvennaja literatura	8,075	697,247	6,434,203	86.3
Art – Kunst – Iskusstvo	1,729	25,529	257,783	14.8
Atheism, science & religion, religion – Atheismus, Wissenschaft u.Religion, Religion – Ateizm, nauka i religija, religija	220	5,712	51,727	26.0
Printing and publishing, library trade – Druck-u.Verlagswesen, Bücherkunde,Bibliothekswesen – Pečat', knigovedenie, bibliotečnoe delo, bibliografija	3,270	14,478	108,323	4.4
Library science – Bibliothekswesen – bibliotečnoe delo, bibliografija	586	2,147	14,180	3.7
Bibliographic indices – bibliographische Verzeichnisse – bibliografičeskie ukazateli	1,900	2,897	20,791	1.5
General reference-books, encyclopedia – Allgemeine Nachschlagwerke, Enzyklopädien – Spravočniki obščego charaktera, enciklopedii	83	7,109	314,586	85.7

10.5 PUBLICATION OF BOOKS AND BROCHURES
PUBLIKATION VON BÜCHERN UND BROSCHÜREN
VYPUSK KNIG I BROŠJUR PO TEMA-

	Books – Bücher – Knigi			
	Number of books, printed units Zahl d.Bücher, Druckeinheiten Cislo knig,pečatnych edinic	Edition, '000 copies Auflage, Tsd.Exempl. Tiraž, tys.eks.	Sheets, in thousands Druckbogenabzüge,Tsd. Pečatnych listov-ottiskov, tys.	Average edition per book, in thousands Durchschnittl. Auflage pro Buch,Tsd.Exemp Srednij tiraž odnoj knigi, tys.eks.
	A.	B.	C.	D.
Total – Insg. – Vsego	52,915	1,222,680	17,254,972	23.1
Political & economical literature – politische u.sozialökonomische Literatur – političeskaja i social'noekonomičeskaja literatura	8,405	233,906	2,915,481	27.8

E.	F.	G.	H.	I.	J.
7.6	335	9,823	81,490	29.3	8.3
9.1	1,951	51,224	520,190	26.3	10.2
13.2	2,036	103,579	1,404,684	50.9	13.6
17.5	1,322	47,881	846,926	36.2	17.7
9.2	8,072	697,238	6,434,195	86.4	9.2
10.1	1,148	23,587	251,685	20.5	10.7
9.1	160	5,419	46,128	33.9	8.5
7.5	555	3,326	31,053	6.0	9.3
6.6	150	1,363	11,334	9.1	8.3
7.2	215	840	9,799	3.9	11.7
44.3	66	7,070	314,412	107.1	44.5

DIVIDED BY SUBJECTS FOR THE YEAR 1976
IN THEMATISCHER AUFTEILUNG IM JAHRE 1976
TIČESKIM RAZDELAM V 1976 G.

	Booklets - Broschüren - Brošjury				
Average number of pages per book, in sheets Durchschnittl. Umfang pro Buch, Druckbogen Srednij obem odnoj knigi, pečatnych listov	Number of brochures, printed units Zahl der Broschüren,Druckeinheiten Čislo brošjur, pečatnych edinic	Edition, '000 copies Auflage, Tsd.Exempl. Tiraž, tys.eks.	Number of sheets, in thousands Druckbogenabzüge,Tsd. Pečatnych listov-ottiskov, tys.	Average edition per brochure, '000 copies Durchschnittl. Auflage pro Broschüre, Tsd.Exemplare Srednij tiraž odnoj brošjuri tys.eks.	Average number of pages per brochure, in sheets Durchschnittl. Umfang pro Broschüre, Druckbogen Srednij obem odnoj brošjuri, pečatnych listov
E.	F.	G.	H.	I.	J.
14.1	31,389	521,835	1,001,589	16.6	1.9
12.5	3,018	54,179	108,605	18.0	2.0

10.5 Druck-u.Verlagswesen

	A.	B.	C.	D.
Natural sciences, mathematics - Naturwissenschaften, Mathematik - Estestvennye nauki, matematika	7,426	193,190	2,617,019	26.0
Technology, industry, transport, communications, municipal services - Technik, Industrie, Transport, Post- u.Fernmeldewesen, Kommunalwesen - Technika, promyšlennost', transport, svjaz', kommunal'noe delo	13,220	100,553	1,332,904	7.6
Agriculture - Landwirtschaft - Sel'skoe chozjajstvo	4,182	31,223	364,692	7.5
Trade, procurement, public catering - Handel, Beschaffungen, öffentliche Verpflegung - Torgovlja, zagotovki, obščestvennoe pitanie	382	8,977	109,631	23.5
Health, medicine - Gesundheitswesen, Medizin - Zdravoochranenie, medicina	1,936	23,442	286,461	12.1
Physical culture, sports - Körperkultur, Sport - Fizkul'tura, sport	400	9,610	83,282	24.0
Culture, education, science - Kultur, Bildung, Wissenschaft - Kul'tura, prosveščenie, nauka	2,636	52,444	552,471	19.9
Linguistics - Sprachwissenschaft - Jazykoznanie	2,241	103,738	1,409,019	46.3
Science of literature - Literaturwissenschaft - Literaturovedenie	1,299	46,283	843,089	35.6
Belles lettres - Belletristik - Chudožestvennaja literatura	6,388	352,089	5,768,741	55.1
Art - Kunst - Iskusstvo	1,132	21,345	249,645	18.9
Printing and publishing, library trade - Druck- u.Verlagswesen, Bücherkunde, Bibliothekswesen - Pečat', knigovedenie, bibliotečnoe delo, bibliografija	1,505	10,454	99,810	6.9

Druck-u.Verlagswesen 10.5

E.	F.	G.	H.	I.	J.
13.5	2,836	6,299	12,879	2.2	2.0
13.3	14,845	65,940	109,919	4.4	1.7
11.7	2,438	10,080	18,622	4.1	1.8
12.2	368	3,873	6,318	10.5	1.6
12.2	1,286	7,081	11,582	5.5	1.6
8.7	213	1,926	4,258	9.0	2.2
10.5	1,676	11,358	26,211	6.8	2.3
13.6	189	3,568	9,053	18.9	2.5
18.2	165	2,056	4,878	12.5	2.4
16.4	1,687	345,158	665,462	204.6	1.9
11.7	597	4,184	8,138	7.0	1.9
9.5	1,765	4,024	8,513	2.3	2.1

10.6 Druck-u.Verlagswesen

10.6   PUBLICATION OF BOOKS AND BROCHURES BY SUBJECTS
PUBLIKATION VON BÜCHERN UND BROSCHÜREN NACH THEMATIK
VYPUSK KNIG I BROŠJUR PO CELEVOMU NAZNAČENIJU

	Number of books and brochures, printed units - Zahl d.Bücher u.Broschüren, Druckeinheiten - Čislo knig i brošjur, pečatnych edinic A.	Edition, '000 copies - Auflage, Tsd.Exemplare - Tiraž, tys.eks. B.	Number of sheets, in '000 - Druckbogenabzüge, Tsd. - Pečatnych listov-ottiskov, tys. C.	Average edition per book and brochure, in '000 copies - Durchschnittl.Auflage pro Buch u.Broschüre,Tsd.Exempl. Srednij tiraž odnoj knigi i brošjury, tys.eks. D.	Average number of pages per book and brochure,in sheets- Durchschnittl.Umfang pro Buch u.Broschüre,Druckbogen- Srednij obém odnoj knigi i brošjury, pečatnych listov E.
Total - Insg. - Vsego:					
1940	45,830	462,203	2,848,300	10.1	6.2
1950	43,060	820,529	6,980,341	19.0	8.5
1965	76,101	1,279,268	12,994,519	16.8	10.2
1970	78,875	1,309,648	13,953,541	16.6	10.7
1971	85,463	1,581,263	16,836,488	18.5	10.6
1975	83,439	1,671,782	17,601,688	20.0	10.5
1976	84,304	1,744,515	18,256,561	20.7	10.5
Political mass literature - Politische Massenliteratur - Massovaja političeskaja literatura:					
1940	3,360	63,849	261,044	19.0	4.1
1950	4,120	139,355	515,407	33.8	3.7
1965	4,177	98,351	667,759	23.5	6.8
1970	4,610	138,820	1,170,422	30.1	8.4
1971	5,016	184,038	1,444,184	36.7	7.8
1975	5,056	161,835	1,199,157	32.0	7.4
1976	4,411	174,760	1,311,200	39.6	7.5
Scientific literature - Wissenschaftliche Literatur - Naučnaja literatura:					
1940	4,514	11,517	124,870	2.6	10.8
1950	2,989	16,623	369,774	5.6	22.2
1965	7,291	12,844	264,131	1.8	20.6
1970	11,403	19,774	331,086	1.7	16.7
1971	13,059	23,598	404,344	1.8	17.1
1975	17,559	35,670	583,097	2.0	16.3
1976	18,903	37,677	639,272	2.0	17.0
Popular-science literature - Populärwissenschaftl.Literatur - Naučno-populjarnaja literatura:					
1940	1,145	12,779	30,231	11.2	2.4
1950	1,919	39,304	143,256	20.5	3.6
1965	2,214	59,984	470,074	27.1	7.8
1970	1,907	50,560	475,147	26.5	9.4
1971	2,222	66,338	683,617	29.9	10.3
1975	2,308	77,915	722,437	33.8	9.3
1976	2,379	81,745	739,983	34.4	9.1

Druck-u.Verlagswesen 10.6

	A.	B.	C.	D.	E.
Instructions - Instruktionen - Proizvodstvennaja i instruktivnaja literatura:					
1940	14,017	76,819	215,663	5.5	2.8
1950	13,495	100,463	451,035	7.4	4.5
1965	28,529	173,812	1,231,217	6.1	7.1
1970	28,221	151,940	1,093,122	5.4	7.2
1971	28,849	204,075	1,422,090	7.1	7.0
1975	26,764	175,979	1,284,951	6.6	7.3
1976	25,922	180,657	1,362,342	7.0	7.5
Official instructions and normatives - Offizielle Instruktionen u.Normativen - Instruktivno-oficial'naja i normativnaja literatura:					
1940	5,428	41,170	110,941	7.6	2.7
1950	6,465	40,997	81,211	6.3	2.0
1965	9,108	69,992	243,348	7.7	3.5
1970	10,374	53,634	203,235	5.2	3.8
1971	10,750	86,942	312,280	8.1	3.6
1975	9,309	60,911	176,027	6.5	2.9
1976	9,059	64,638	211,253	7.1	3.3
Textbooks - Lehrbücher - Učebnaja literatura:					
1940	5,965	164,286	1,579,291	27.5	9.6
1950	4,850	211,939	2,757,822	43.7	13.0
1965	11,206	376,198	4,944,457	33.6	13.1
1970	8,446	372,005	5,545,543	44.0	14.9
1971	9,407	417,722	6,364,995	44.4	15.2
1975	10,231	397,308	5,995,320	38.8	15.1
1976	10,727	394,470	5,948,220	36.8	15.1
for general educational schools - für allgemeinbildende Schulen - dlja obščeobrazovatel'noj školy:					
1940	2,162	125,493	1,241,033	58.0	9.9
1950	2,216	189,275	2,419,455	85.4	12.8
1965	2,606	310,699	3,908,698	119.2	12.6
1970	2,483	313,667	4,367,262	126.3	13.9
1971	2,693	345,246	4,881,405	128.2	14.1
1975	2,427	321,249	4,585,027	132.4	14.3
1976	2,444	321,171	4,663,754	131.4	14.5
for universities - für Hochschulen - dlja vysšej školy:					
1940	2,019	9,740	163,507	4.8	16.8
1950	1,452	9,099	182,561	6.3	20.1
1965	5,668	36,594	621,490	6.5	17.0
1970	4,316	32,084	693,266	7.4	21.6
1971	4,938	38,719	827,818	7.8	21.4
1975	5,855	39,057	778,578	6.7	19.9
1976	6,242	36,819	737,282	5.9	20.0
Program and methodical literature - Programm- und methodische Literatur - Programmnaja i metodičeskaja literatura:					
1940		5,484	20,176	55,390	3.7	2.7
1950		5,881	33,829	146,547	5.8	4.3

549

10.6 Druck-u.Verlagswesen

	A.	B.	C.	D.	E.
1965	8,482	63,830	357,513	7.5	5.6
1970	11,205	77,706	502,859	6.9	6.5
1971	12,398	79,713	618,820	6.4	7.8
1975	8,266	78,200	589,905	9.5	7.5
1976	7,435	84,571	645,135	11.4	7.6
Belles lettres (without children's books) - Belletristik (ohne Kinderbücher) - Chudožestvennaja literatura (bez detskoj):					
1940	2,568	20,975	161,939	8.2	7.7
1950	3,285	113,079	1,506,091	34.4	13.3
1965	5,045	223,213	3,194,965	44.2	14.3
1970	4,608	166,281	2,703,878	36.1	16.3
1971	5,104	187,681	3,125,876	36.8	16.7
1975	5,061	221,894	4,015,533	43.8	18.1
1976	5,137	236,626	4,368,929	46.1	18.5
Literature for children - Literatur für Kinder - Literatura dlja detej:					
1940	1,734	35,134	117,158	20.3	3.
1950	1,697	72,977	448,468	43.0	6.
1965	2,595	205,264	1,164,177	79.1	5.
1970	2,540	265,996	1,410,419	104.7	5.
1971	3,077	344,013	1,818,480	111.8	5.
1975	3,031	448,675	2,139,105	148.0	4.
1976	3,215	478,826	2,251,258	148.9	4.
of which belles lettres - davon Belletristik - iz nee chudožestvennaja literatura:					
1940	1,462	32,426	105,015	22.2	3.
1950	1,418	66,216	399,485	46.7	6.
1965	2,212	188,536	953,554	85.2	5.
1970	2,239	250,182	1,238,828	111.7	5.
1971	2,756	326,961	1,661,216	118.6	5.
1975	2,757	428,619	1,921,196	155.5	4.
1976	2,938	460,621	2,065,274	156.8	4.
Official documentary and reference-books - Offizielle Dokumentar- und Nachschlagwerke - Oficial'no-dokumental'naja i spravočnaja literatura:					
1940	4,477	18,998	64,413	4.2	3.
1950	4,035	43,140	190,332	10.7	4.
1965	6,351	57,986	590,043	9.1	10.
1970	5,416	43,847	452,145	8.1	10
1971	5,920	49,480	732,097	8.4	14
1975	4,627	53,550	759,658	11.6	14
1976	5,700	54,736	730,205	9.6	13

Druck-u.Verlagswesen 10.7

10.7 PUBLICATION OF PERIODICALS AND SERIALIZED LITERATURE (WITHOUT NEWSPAPERS)
PUBLIKATION VON PERIODISCHEN UND FORTSETZUNGSPUBLIKATIONEN (OHNE ZEITUNGEN)
VYPUSK PERIODIČESKICH I PRODOLŽAJUŠČICHSJA IZDANIJ (BEZ GAZET)

	A. Number of publications - Zahl der Publikationen - Čislo izdanij	B. Number of issues - Zahl der Nummern - Čislo nomerov	C. Total number of pages of all publications, in sheets - Umfang aller Publikationen, Druckbogen - Ob'em vsech izdanij, pečatnych listov	D. Annual edition, '000 copies - Jahresauflage, Tsd.Exempl. - Godovoj tiraž, tys.eks.	E. Number of sheets, '000 - Druckbogenabzüge, Tsd. - Pečatnych listov-ottiskov, tys.	F. Average circulation per issue, in '000 copies - Durchschnittl.Auflage pro Nummer, Tsd.Exempl. - Srednij razovyj tiraž odnogo nomera, tys.eks.
Total - Insg. - Vsego:						
1940	1,822	16,219	60,000	245,408	1,019,066	15.1
1950	1,408	11,605	46,833	181,282	754,119	15.6
1965	3,846	33,718	187,373	1,547,625	7,472,141	45.9
1970	5,969	48,346	278,950	2,675,013	13,688,296	55.3
1971	5,967	46,772	270,802	2,572,268	13,224,941	55.0
1975	4,726	49,482	241,747	3,080,189	15,677,190	62.2
1976	4,860	52,243	249,290	3,107,085	16,040,187	59.5
Journals - Zeitschriften - Žurnaly:						
1940	673	7,299	31,572	190,236	920,228	26.1
1950	430	4,934	25,350	136,665	663,334	27.7
1965	1,044	11,513	96,328	1,088,375	6,368,913	94.5
1970	1,204	13,121	115,259	1,995,295	11,483,744	152.1
1971	1,208	13,118	115,191	1,966,443	11,367,879	149.9
1975	1,334	14,437	127,489	2,310,233	13,484,957	160.0
1976	1,350	14,722	131,864	2,320,189	13,774,344	157.6
"Serialized pulp novels - "Roman-Zeitung" - "Roman-Gazeta"[1]:						
1970	1	24	239	52,800	536,800	2200.0
1971	1	24	244	36,000	366,000	1500.0
1975	1	24	245	37,500	382,813	1562.5
1976	1	24	240	38,323	383,232	1596.8

[1]
up to and incl. 1966 was listed under "books and brochures" -
bis einschl.1966 unter der Rubrik "Bücher und Broschüren" geführt -
po 1966 (vključitel'no) učityvalas' v razdele "Knigi i brošjury"

10.7 Druck-u.Verlagswesen

	A.	B.	C.	D.	E.	F.
Notebooks for Agitators - Notizbücher des Agitators - Bloknoty agitatora:						
1940	9	140	200	7,537	9,158	53.8
1950	113	1,974	2,924	27,643	43,028	14.0
1965	74	1,727	2,713	34,240	83,680	19.8
1970	62	1,472	2,195	31,884	50,472	21.7
1971	59	1,403	2,216	27,881	47,073	19.9
1975	44	1,044	1,693	18,683	30,428	17.9
1976	41	968	1,510	17,218	27,172	17.8
Collections - Sammelbände - Sborniki[1]:						
1940	591	1,080	10,479	2,196	14,891	2.0
1950	632	1,162	12,155	2,444	24,513	2.1
1965	1,316	3,067	37,430	8,649	98,031	2.8
1970	2,306	6,008	67,301	12,986	138,345	2.2
1971	2,294	5,939	63,588	12,889	145,184	2.2
1975	261	712	5,952	10,312	100,955	14.5
1976	245	705	6,162	10,727	112,791	15.2
Bulletins - Bjulleteni:						
1940	488	7,025	10,244	27,143	33,889	3.9
1950	233	3,535	6,404	14,530	23,244	4.1
1965	1,412	17,411	50,902	416,361	921,517	23.9
1970	2,396	27,721	93,956	582,048	1,478,935	21.0
1971	2,405	26,288	89,563	529,055	1,298,805	20.1
1975	3,086	33,265	106,368	703,461	1,678,037	21.1
1976	3,223	35,824	109,514	720,628	1,742,648	20.1

All-Union Copyright Agency
Unionsagentur für Autorenrechte·
Vsesojuznoe Agenstvo po Avtorskim Pravam
Bol'šaja Bronnaja, 6A, Moskva

---

[1] Since 1975 "Papers, scientific notes" and other similar literature without specific periodical characteristics are being listed under the heading "Books and Brochures" -
ab 1975 werden "Arbeiten, wissenschaftliche Notizen" und andere analogische Herausgaben ohne bestimmten Periodikacharakter unter der Rubrik "Bücher und Broschüren" geführt -
S 1975 g. "Trudy, učenye zapiski" i drugie analogičnye izdanija, ne imejuščie opredelennoj pereodičnosti vypuska, učteny v razdele "Knigi i brošjury".

10.8 PUBLICATION OF PERIODICALS AND SERIALS (WITHOUT NEWSPAPERS) IN THE
LANGUAGES OF THE MAIN NATIONALITIES OF THE USSR FOR THE YEAR 1976
PUBLIKATION VON PERIODISCHEN UND FORTSETZUNGSPUBLIKATIONEN (OHNE ZEITUNGEN)
IN DEN SPRACHEN DER HAUPTNATIONEN DER UdSSR IM JAHRE 1976
VYPUSK PERIODIČESKICH I PRODOLŽAJUŠČICHSJA IZDANIJ (BEZ GAZET) NA JAZYKACH
KORENNYCH NACIJ SSSR V 1976 G.

	A. Number of publications – Zahl der Publikationen – Čislo izdanij	B. Number of issues – Zahl der Nummern – Čislo nomerov	C. Total number of pages of all publications, in sheets – Umfang aller Herausgaben, Druckbogen – Ob'em vsech izdanij, pečatnych listov	D. Single edition, '000 copies Einzelauflage, Tsd.Exempl. – Razovyj tiraž, tys.eks.	E. Annual edition, '000 copies Jahresauflage, Tsd.Exempl. – Godovoj tiraž, tys.eks.	F. Number of sheets, in '000 Druckbogenabzüge, Tsd. – Pečatnych listov-ottiskov, tys.
In the languages of the USSR peoples – in den Sprachen der Völker der UdSSR – Na jazykach narodov SSSR	4,656	50,482	239,872	183,880	3,061,254	15,712,976
a) of which journals – darunter Zeitschriften – v tom čisle žurnaly	1,255	13,606	124,587	154,380	2,277,736	13,456,726
in Russian – in Russisch – na russkom	3,909	42,035	202,639	151,251	2,429,212	13,606,446
a)	941	9,930	101,194	129,050	1,896,032	11,798,082
in Ukrainian – in Ukrainisch – na ukrainskom	109	1,327	7,163	10,321	203,037	741,171
a)	63	692	5,589	9,112	158,922	648,953
in Belorussian – in Belorussisch – na belorusskom	30	324	1,898	1,582	30,233	92,281
a)	17	150	1,311	1,066	16,237	62,892
in Uzbek – in Usbekisch – na uzbekskom	32	450	1,987	4,975	101,707	290,004
a)	19	229	1,350	3,867	54,045	238,030
in Kazakh – in Kasachisch – na kazachskom	28	390	1,615	2,011	25,923	138,448
a)	14	155	992	1,717	19,968	122,046
in Georgian – in Georgisch – na gruzinskom	68	590	2,875	1,447	25,828	50,734
a)	24	254	1,534	930	13,389	40,595
in Azerbaidzhan – in Aserbaidschanisch – na azerbajdžanskom	65	614	2,661	1,699	34,893	84,341
a)	22	240	1,479	1,068	14,847	59,661

10.8
10.9 Druck-u.Verlagswesen

	A.	B.	C.	D.	E.	F.
in Lithuanian - in Litauisch - na litovskom	105	922	4,377	2,651	43,733	215,745
a)	23	297	1,939	1,746	23,896	133,994
in Moldavian - in Moldauisch- na moldavskom	17	255	1,078	965	26,880	63,637
a)	12	154	776	633	9,815	29,394
in Latvian - in Lettisch - na latysskom	47	649	2,676	1,965	48,278	155,147
a)	19	248	1,452	1,325	19,090	99,836
in Kirghiz - in Kirgisisch - na kirgizskom	21	283	889	534	8,983	27,587
a)	9	120	612	449	5,588	24,232
in Tadzhik - in Tadschikisch - na tadžikskom	14	268	951	633	14,133	30,200
a)	8	120	575	498	7,564	23,458
in Armenian - in Armenisch - na armjanskom	58	680	3,101	905	18,008	56,985
a)	21	258	1,656	588	7,027	33,986
in Turkoman - in Turkmenisch - na turkmenskom	13	233	545	495	11,133	17,852
a)	8	108	443	352	4,449	14,682
in Estonian - in Estnisch - na estonskom	75	770	2,437	953	19,602	55,503
a)	18	250	1,463	619	8,660	44,216

10.9 PUBLICATION OF PERIODICALS AND SERIALS (WITHOUT NEWSPAPERS) BY SUBJECTS FOR THE YEAR 1976
PUBLIKATION VON PERIODISCHEN UND FORTSETZUNGSPUBLIKATIONEN (OHNE ZEITUNGEN) IN THEMATISCHER AUFTEILUNG IM JAHRE 1976
VYPUSK PERIODIČESKICH I PRODOLŽAJUŠČICHSJA IZDANIJ (BEZ GAZET) PO TEMATIČESKIM RAZDELAM V 1976 G.

	A. Number of publications - Zahl der Veröffentlichungen - Čislo izdanij	B. Number of iss. - Zahl d.Nummern - Čislo nomerov	C. Single edition, '000 copies - Einzelauflage, Tsd.Exempl. - Razovyj tiraž, tys.eks.	D. Annual edition, '000 copies - Jahresauflage, Tsd.Exempl. - Godovoj tiraž, tys.eks.	E. Number of sheets,'000- Druckbogen-abzüge, Tsd. - Pečatnych list-
Political & social-economical literature - politische und sozial-ökonomische Literatur - političeskaja i social'no-ekonomičeskaja literatura:					
1. Total publications - alle Publikationen - vse izdanija	627	7,798	52,865	774,735	4,512,120
2. Journals - Zeitschriften - žurnaly	245	3,032	49,436	715,393	4,365,908

Druck-u.Verlagswesen 10.9

	A.	B.	C.	D.	E.
3. Notebooks for Agitators - Notizbücher des Agitators - Bloknoty agitatora	41	968	669	17,218	27,172
4. Collections - Sammelbände - Sborniki	23	83	155	343	3,992
5. Bulletins - Bjulleteni	318	3,715	2,605	41,781	115,048
Defense - Wehrwesen - Voennoe delo:					
1.	63	670	3,157	57,965	342,098
2.	29	442	3,037	57,402	339,215
5.	34	228	120	563	2,883
Natural sciences, mathematics - Naturwissenschaften, Mathematik - Estestvennye nauki, matematika:					
1.	506	4,952	10,654	124,147	1,213,670
2.	224	1,943	10,261	121,566	1,200,762
4.	45	100	116	309	3,337
5.	237	2,909	277	2,272	9,571
Technology,industry,transport,communications, municipal services - Technik, Industrie, Transport, Post- u.Fernmeldewesen, Kommunalwesen - Technika, promyšlennost', transport, svjaz', kommunal'noe delo:					
1.	1,586	18,101	20,545	442,998	1,482,887
2.	255	2,630	10,065	106,404	759,321
4.	45	141	295	1,586	13,273
5.	1,286	15,330	10,185	335,008	710,293
Agriculture - Landwirtschaft - Sel'skoe chozjajstvo:					
1.	271	2,696	5,673	63,631	383,804
2.	122	1,386	5,124	58,997	371,601
4.	5	12	207	225	2,649
5.	144	1,298	342	4,409	9,554
Trade,procurement ,public catering - Handel, Beschaffungen, öffentliche Verpflegung - Torgovlja, zagotovki, obščestvennoe pitanie:					
1.	58	673	1,595	18,513	89,788
2.	12	125	936	11,643	74,517
5.	46	548	659	6,870	15,271
Health, medicine - Gesundheitswesen, Medizin - Zdravoochranenie, medicina:					
1.	196	1,797	15,361	179,746	889,850
2.	109	1,082	15,076	178,043	885,695
4.	6	10	8	15	133
5.	81	705	277	1,688	4,022
Physical culture, sport - Körperkultur, Sport - Fizkul'tura, sport:					
1.	56	583	5,507	115,219	366,920
2.	10	124	3,561	42,749	220,951
4.	9	22	393	620	4,528
5.	37	437	1,553	71,850	141,441

10.9 Druck-u.Verlagswesen

	A.	B.	C.	D.	E.
Culture, education, science – Kultur, Bildung, Wissenschaft – Kul'tura, prosveščenie, nauka:					
1.	166	1,384	9,685	102,885	758,199
2.	71	744	8,657	87,505	709,752
4.	19	64	164	603	3,628
5.	76	576	864	14,777	44,819
Linguistics, comparative literature – Sprach- und Literaturwissenschaft – Jazykoznanie, literaturovedenie:					
1.	45	222	397	2,470	26,823
2.	25	153	274	2,076	20,878
4.	15	47	116	354	5,774
5.	5	22	7	40	171
Belles lettres – Belletristik – Chudožestvennaja literatura:					
1.	223	2,383	50,961	981,952	5,267,069
2.	161	2,090	45,527	844,968	4,377,841
Serialized pulp novels – "Roman-Zeitung" – "Roman-Gazeta"	1	24	1,597	38,323	383,232
4.	56	176	1,857	4,902	52,482
5.	5	93	1,980	93,759	453,514
Art – Kunst – Iskusstvo:					
1.	132	2,116	7,729	199,564	470,213
2.	34	405	3,985	73,004	283,864
4.	13	24	330	1,597	21,440
5.	85	1,687	3,414	124,963	164,909
Atheism, science & religion, religion – Atheismus, Wissenschaft u.Religion, Religion – Ateizm, nauka i religija, religija:					
1.	12	94	655	7,742	66,605
2.	11	93	655	7,742	66,601
5.	1	1	0	0	4
Printing and publishing, library trade – Druck-u. Verlagswesen, Bücherkunde, Bibliothekswesen – Pečat', knigovedenie, bibliotečnoe delo, bibliografija:					
1.	849	8,077	1,901	24,656	111,144
2.	14	160	607	7,246	56,361
4.	7	22	33	162	1,445
5.	828	7,895	1,261	17,248	53,338
Publications with other subjects – Publikationen mit gemischter Thematik – Izdanija smešannoj tematiki:					
1.	70	697	887	10,862	58,99
2.	28	313	421	5,451	41,07
4.	2	4	6	11	11
5.	40	380	460	5,400	17,81

Druck-u.Verlagswesen 10.10

	A.	B.	C.	D.	E.
Published from the total number of publications - aus der Gesamtzahl der Publikationen wurden herausgegeben - iz obščego čisla izdanij vyšlo:					
for children - für Kinder - dlja detej	46	494	23,573	280,354	1,007,653
of which journals-darunter Zeitschriften-v tom čisle žurnaly	40	466	23,131	277,240	1,000,865
for the youth - für die Jugend - dlja molodeži	37	492	17,281	242,056	1,674,105
of which journals-darunter Zeitschriften-v tom čisle žurnaly	27	348	16,330	238,483	1,634,567
for women - für Frauen - dlja ženščin (journals-Zeitschriften-žurnaly)	42	428	27,496	323,082	1,764,261

10.10 PUBLICATION OF PERIODICALS AND SERIALS (WITHOUT NEWSPAPERS) BY DESTINATION FOR THE YEAR 1976
PUBLIKATION VON PERIODISCHEN UND FORTSETZUNGSPUBLIKATIONEN (OHNE ZEITUNGEN) NACH ZIELBESTIMMUNG IM JAHRE 1976
VYPUSK PERIODIČESKICH I PRODOLŽAJUSČICHSJA IZDANIJ (BEZ GAZET) PO CELEVOMU NAZNAČENIJU V 1976 G.

	A. Number of publications - Zahl der Publikationen - Cislo izdanij	B. Number of issues - Zahl der Nummern - Cislo nomerov	C. Single edition, '000 copies - Einzelauflage, Tsd.Exempl. - Razovyj tiraž, tys.eks.	D. Annual edition, '000 copies - Jahresauflage, Tsd.Exempl. - Godovoj tiraž, tys.eks.	E. Number of sheets, in '000 - Druckbogenabzüge, Tsd. - Pečatnych listov-ottiskov, tys.
Total - Insgesamt - Vsego	4,860	52,243	187,572	3,107,085	16,040,187
Mass publications - Massenpublikationen - Massovye izdanija	661	8,947	111,246	1,901,842	10,055,323
of which journals - darunter Zeitschriften-v tom č.žurnaly	387	5,216	98,437	1,617,426	8,843,412
of which-davon-iz nich: Party organs - Parteiorgane - partijnye	54	1,076	9,343	183,585	1,401,031
satirical and humorous - satirische u.humoristische - satiričeskie i jumorističeskie	22	457	11,827	342,398	911,707
Scientific publications - Wissenschaftliche Publikationen - Naučnye izdanija	493	3,165	1,914	15,608	209,382

10.10 Druck-u.Verlagswesen

	A.	B.	C.	D.	E.
of which journals - darunter Zeitschriften - v tom čisle žurnaly	375	2,914	1,652	15,008	202,691
Scientific information - Wissenschaftliche Informationspublikationen - Naučno-informacionnye izdanija	1,122	12,452	2,022	22,048	226,823
of which journals - darunter Zeitschriften - v tom čisle žurnaly	158	1,902	485	6,619	168,492
Popular-science publications - Populärwissenschaftl.Publikationen - Naučno-populjarnye izdanija	63	578	34,573	410,440	2,667,172
of which journals - darunter Zeitschriften - v tom čisle žurnaly	48	521	34,332	408,775	2,650,307
Scientific practical and production-technological publications - Wissenschaftliche praxis-und produktionsbezogene Publikationen - Naučno-praktičeskie i proizvodstvennye izdanija	1,357	14,187	19,169	238,075	1,430,994
of which journals - darunter Zeitschriften - v tom čisle žurnaly	317	3,527	16,065	209,441	1,328,851
Instructional and methodical publications - Instruktions- und methodische Publikationen - Instruktivno-metodičeskie izdanija	170	1,034	7,692	68,901	618,058
of which journals - darunter Zeitschriften - v tom čisle žurnaly	46	453	6,603	61,264	564,928
Official documentary publications - Offizielle Dokumentarpublikationen - Oficial'no-dokumental'nye izdanija	87	1,458	1,096	26,853	51,311
Reference works - Nachschlagpublikationen - Spravočnye izdanija	889	10,205	9,795	422,637	777,144
of which journals - darunter Zeitschriften - v tom čisle žurnaly	4	48	94	1,127	12,334
Publications with other subjects - Publikationen anderer Thematik - Izdanija drugich razdelov	18	217	65	681	3,980
of which journals - darunter Zeitschriften - v tom čisle žurnaly	15	141	54	529	3,329

10.11 PUBLICATION OF NEWSPAPERS BY TYPES - PUBLIKATION VON ZEITUNGEN NACH TYPEN - VYPUSK GAZET PO TIPAM

	A. Number of publications - Zahl der Herausgaben - Cislo izdanij	B. Number of issues - Zahl der Nummern - Cislo nomerov	C. Single edition, '000 copies - Einzelauflage, Tsd.Exempl. - Razovyj tiraž, tys.eks.	D. Annual edition, '000 copies - Jahresauflage, Tsd.Exempl. - Godovoj tiraž, tys.eks.	E. Average edition per newspaper, '000 copies - Durchschnittl.Auflage pro Zeitung, Tsd.Exempl. - Srednij razovyj tiraž odnoj gazety, tys.eks.
Total - Insgesamt - Vsego:					
1940	8,806	946,681	38,355	7,528,062	4.4
1950	7,831	812,792	35,964	6,997,947	4.6
1965	7,687	777,439	103,030	23,072,627	13.4
1970	8,694	935,832	140,716	31,175,836	16.2
1971	7,863	923,505	145,463	32,431,663	18.5
1975	7,985	871,799	168,033	37,975,649	21.0
1976	7,844	878,804	168,994	38,457,593	21.5
All-union papers - Unionszeitungen - Svesojuznye:					
1940	46	7,065	8,769	2,158,340	191.3
1950	23	4,663	9,423	2,311,798	408.6
1965	23	4,185	45,161	11,899,243	1963.5
1970	28	4,874	62,364	16,232,309	2227.3
1971	28	4,872	64,189	16,710,505	2292.5
1975	29	4,875	75,970	19,570,514	2619.7
1976	29	4,835	76,103	19,735,681	2624.2
Republican papers - Republikanische Zeitungen - Respublikanskie:					
1940	135	22,029	5,284	1,064,392	39.3
1950	137	21,466	4,819	1,075,874	35.1
1965	154	26,071	18,728	3,763,350	121.6
1970	153	26,022	23,831	4,103,606	155.8
1971	152	25,972	24,345	4,270,148	160.2
1975	156	26,844	26,277	4,744,378	168.4
1976	156	26,947	26,174	4,802,715	167.8
Krai, Oblast and District papers - Krai-, Oblast- und Kreiszeitungen - Kraevye, oblastnye i okružnye:					
1940	321	67,622	6,978	1,749,728	21.7
1950	310	66,547	7,349	1,820,661	23.7
1965	258	58,590	12,855	3,405,839	49.8
1970	284	63,493	18,696	4,892,479	65.8
1971	286	65,393	19,814	5,164,579	69.3
1975	309	70,198	23,884	6,194,744	77.3
1976	312	71,191	24,187	6,304,705	77.5

10.11 Druck-u.Verlagswesen

	A.	B.	C.	D.	E.
Papers of the autonomous republics and oblasts - Zeitungen der autonomen Republiken u.Oblaste - Avtonomych respublik i oblastej:					
1940	119	23,437	1,197	280,517	10.1
1950	71	15,351	838	201,675	11.8
1965	95	20,660	2,231	555,206	23.5
1970	93	19,995	3,203	778,940	34.4
1971	93	19,946	3,494	842,610	37.6
1975	95	20,462	4,123	1,002,850	43.4
1976	95	20,495	4,188	1,019,751	44.1
City papers - Stadtzeitungen - Gorodskie[1]:					
1940	251	62,639	1,802	398,347	7.2
1950	346	60,382	1,493	315,149	4.3
1965	566	101,069	6,820	1,491,736	12.1
1970	617	120,614	10,723	2,483,484	17.4
1971	614	118,738	11,429	2,612,781	18.6
1975	655	127,877	14,840	3,400,043	22.7
1976	657	128,671	15,125	3,476,240	23.0
Rayon papers - Rayonzeitungen - Rajonnye:1940	3,502	486,251	8,647	1,430,213	2.5
1950	4,193	355,773	6,903	609,602	1.6
1965	2,388	317,011	11,302	1,587,044	4.7
1970	2,825	436,011	14,596	2,261,810	5.2
1971	2,858	434,136	16,125	2,415,952	5.6
1975	2,899	449,012	17,310	2,692,575	6.0
1976	2,907	451,669	17,517	2,732,541	6.0
Local papers - Lokalzeitungen - Nizovye[2]:1940	4,432	277,638	5,678	446,525	1.2
1950	2,751	288,610	5,139	663,188	1.8
1965	2,769	228,193	4,908	354,489	1.8
1970	3,251	242,209	6,268	406,325	1.9
1971	2,847	237,990	5,321	402,301	1.9
1975	2,932	154,907	4,922	356,572	1.7
1976	2,965	158,843	5,113	372,891	1.7
Kolkhoz papers - Kolchoszeitungen - Kolchoznye:					
1965	1,434	21,660	1,025	15,720	0.7
1970	1,443	22,614	1,035	16,883	0.7
1971	985	16,458	746	12,787	0.8
1975	910	17,624	707	13,973	0.8
1976	723	16,153	587	13,069	0.8

1 including papers published jointly by city and rayon organizations - einschl. der von Stadt-und Rayonsorganisationen gemeinsam herausgegebenen Zeitungen - Vključaja gazety, izdavaemye sovmestno gorodskimi i rajonnymi organizacijami

2 With large circulation, without kolkhoz papers - Mit großer Auflage, ohne Kolchoszeitungen - Mnogotiražnye, krome kolchoznych

10.12 PUBLICATION OF NEWSPAPERS IN THE LANGUAGES OF THE NATIONALITIES OF THE
USSR AND FOREIGN LANGUAGES IN 1976
PUBLIKATION VON ZEITUNGEN IN DEN SPRACHEN DER VÖLKER DER UdSSR UND DES
AUSLANDS IM JAHRE 1976
VYPUSK GAZET NA JAZYKACH NARODOV SSSR I NARODOV ZARUBEŽNYCH STRAN V 1976 G.

	Number of publications – Zahl der Publikationen – Cislo izdanij	Number of issues – Zahl der Nummern – Cislo nomerov	Single edition, '000 copies – Einzelauflage, Tsd.Exempl. – Razovyj tiraž, tys.eks.	Annual edition, '000 copies – Jahresauflage, Tsd.Exempl. – Godovoj tiraž, tys.eks.
In the languages of the USSR peoples – In den Sprachen d.Völker d.UdSSR – Na jazykach narodov SSSR	7,823	875,497	167,921	38,366,467
Russian-Russisch-na russkom	4,978	558,024	128,564	31,040,498
Ukrainian-Ukrainisch-na ukrainskom	1,392	112,171	16,129	2,924,035
Belorussian-Belorussisch-na belorusskom	128	19,934	1,669	280,988
Uzbek-Usbekisch-na uzbekskom	178	25,621	3,533	710,172
Kazakh-Kasachisch-na kazachskom	157	25,692	1,769	328,513
Georgian-Georgisch-na gruzinskom	123	14,954	2,714	578,264
Aserbaidzhan-Aserbaidschanisch-na azerbajdžanskom	101	13,245	2,295	412,684
Lithunian-Litauisch-na litovskom	89	10,889	1,822	348,254
Moldavian-Moldauisch-na moldavskom	68	7,917	1,212	213,566
Latvian-Lettisch-na latyšskom	54	6,690	1,070	218,551
Kirgiz-Kirgisisch-na kirgizskom	57	7,278	743	128,680
Tadshik-Tadschikisch-na tadžikskom	49	6,413	848	148,949
Armenian-Armenisch-na armjanskom	84	10,434	1,530	248,760
Turkmenian-Turkmenisch-na turkmenskom	14	2,174	606	115,108
Estonian-Estnisch-na estonskom	29	4,346	1,000	212,876
In languages of foreign peoples – In Sprachen der Völker des Auslands – Na jazykach narodov zarubežnych stran	21	3,307	1,073	91,126
English-Englisch-na anglijskom	2	104	566	29,431
Arabian-Arabisch-na arabskom	1	52	81	4,196
Hungarian-Ungarisch-na vengerskom	5	929	64	15,540
Greek-Griechisch-na grečeskom	1	259	4	1,036
Spanish-Spanisch-na ispanskom	1	52	27	1,420
Korean-Koreanisch-na korejskom	2	513	18	4,668
German-Deutsch-na nemeckom	3	416	187	14,619
Polish-Polnisch-na pol'skom	4	774	55	15,661
Finnish-Finnisch-na finskom	1	156	9	1,326
French-Französisch-na francuzskom	1	52	62	3,229

11. STANDARD OF LIVING, SOCIAL SECURITY
LEBENSSTANDARD, SOZIALFÜRSORGE
ZIZNENNYJ UROVEN', SOCIAL'NOE OBESPEČENIE

11.1 INCOME OF THE POPULATION - EINKOMMEN DER BEVÖLKERUNG DOCHOFY NASELENIJA

11.1.1 GROWTH OF THE REAL INCOME OF THE POPULATION (PER CAPITA)
WACHSTUM DES REALEINKOMMENS DER BEVÖLKERUNG (PRO KOPF DER BEVÖLKERUNG)
ROST REAL'NYCH DOCHODOV NASELENIJA (NA DUŠU NASELENIJA)

Year Jahr Gody	in percent in Prozent v procentach	Year Jahr Gody	in percent in Prozent v procentach
1970	5.2	1974	4.2
1971	4.5	1975	4.2
1972	4.0	1976	3.7
1973	5.0	1977	3.5

11.1.2 AVERAGE MONTHLY WAGES AND SALARIES OF WORKERS AND EMPLOYEES IN THE NATIONAL ECONOMY - DURCHSCHNITTLICHER MONATSLOHN DER ARBEITER UND ANGESTELLTEN IN DER VOLKSWIRTSCHAFT - SREDNEMESJAČNAJA ZARABOTNAJA PLATA RABOČICH I SLUŽAŠČICH V NARODNOM CHOZJAJSTVE
(Rubles - Rubel - rublej)

Year Jahr Gody	Average monthly wage and salary with allowances and benefits from social consumer funds Durchschnittl.Monatslohn zuzüglich Zahlungen u.Leistungen aus d.gesellschaftl.Konsumationsfonds Srednemesjačnaja zarabotnaja plata s dobavleniem vyplat i l'got iz obščestvennych fondov potreblenija A.	Average monthly wage and salary Durchschnittl. Monatslohn Srednemesjačnaja denežnaja zarabotnaja plata B.
1940	40.6	33.1
1946	62.4	48.1
1950	82.4	64.2
1955	91.8	71.8
1960	107.7	80.6
1965	129.2	96.5
1970	164.5	122.0

Standard of living, social security 11.1.2
Lebensstandard, Sozialfürsorge 11.1.3

	A.	B.
1971	169.8	125.9
1972	175.4	130.2
1973	182.6	134.9
1974	190.9	141.1
1975	198.9	145.8
1976	206.3	151.4
1977 (planned-geplant)	211	154.5

11.1.3 AVERAGE MONTHLY WAGES AND SALARIES OF WORKERS AND EMPLOYEES BY BRANCHES OF THE NATIONAL ECONOMY - DURCHSCHNITTLICHER MONATSLOHN DER ARBEITER UND ANGESTELLTEN NACH VOLKSWIRTSCHAFTSZWEIGEN - SREDNEMESJAČNAJA DENEŽNAJA ZARABOTNAJA PLATA RABOČICH I SLUŽAŠČICH PO OTRASLJAM NARODNOGO CHOZJAJSTVA
(Rubles - Rubel - rublej)

	1940	1965	1970	1975	1976
In the national economy, total - In der Volkswirtschaft insg. - Vsego po narodnomu chozjajstvu	33.1	96.5	122.0	145.8	151.4
Industry (industry-production staff) - Industrie (Industrie-Produktionspersonal)- Promyšlennost' (promyšlenno-proizvodstvennyj personal)	34.1	104.2	133.3	162.2	169.5
Workers-Arbeiter-rabočie	32.4	101.7	130.6	160.9	168.2
Engineers and techn.specialists - ingenieur-technische Kader - inženerno-techničeskie rabotniki	69.6	148.4	178.0	199.2	205.8
Employees-Angestellte-služaščhie	36.0	85.8	111.6	131.3	139.2
Agriculture - Landwirtschaft - Sel'skoe chozjajstvo	23.3	75.0	101.0	126.8	134.6
State farms, inter-farm enterprises, subsidiary and other agricultural enter- prises - Sowchosen, zwischenwirtschaft- liche Landwirtschaftsbetriebe, Nebenwirt- schaften u.a.landwirtschaftl.Produk- tionsbetriebe - sovchozy, mežchozjajst- vennye sel'skochozjajstvennye predprija- tija,podsobnye i pročie proizvodstvennye sel'skochozjajstvennye predprijatija	22.0	74.6	100.9	126.7	134.7
Workers-Arbeiter-rabočie	20.7	72.4	98.5	124.7	133.1
Agronomical,zoo-technical,veterinary, engineering and techn. professions - agronomische,zootechnische,tierärzt- liche u.ingenieur-technische Kader - agronomičeskie,zootechničeskie,vete- rinarnye i inženerno-techničeskie rabotniki	50.4	138.4	164.3	179.4	182.9
Employees-Angestellte-služaščie	31.1	82.3	95.6	114.0	119.1
Transport	34.8	106.0	136.7	173.5	181.8
Railway - Eisenbahn - železnodoržnyj	34.2	98.7	123.4	158.1	159.9

11.1.3 Standard of living, social security
Lebensstandard, Sozialfürsorge

	1940	1965	1970	1975	1976
Water transport-Wassertransport-vodnyj	41.2	135.1	169.5	212.8	220.0
Automobile, municipal electrical and other transport; loading & unloading organizations- Automobil-, städtischer Elektro-u.a. Transport; Be-u.Entladeorganisationen - Avtomobil'nyj, gorodskoj električeskij i pročij transport; pogruzočno-razgruzočnye organizacii	34.5	107.5	140.3	177.1	187.7
Communications-Post-u.Fernmeldewesen-Svjaz'	28.2	74.2	96.8	123.6	133.7
Construction - Bauwesen - stroitel'stvo	36.3	111.9	149.9	176.8	181.0
Construction and assembling work - Bau-und Montagearbeiten - Stroitel'no-montažnye raboty	34.0	112.4	153.0	181.1	185.2
Workers - Arbeiter - raboče	31.1	108.4	148.5	180.3	185.3
Engineers and techn. specialists - ingenieur-technische Kader - inženerno-techničeskie rabotniki	75.3	160.7	200.0	207.0	205.5
Employees - Angestellte - služaščie	45.8	102.4	136.8	145.8	145.6
Trade, public catering, material & technical supply and sale, procurements - Handel, öffentl.Verpflegung, materiell-technische Versorgung u.Absatz, Beschaffungen - Torgovlja,obščestvennoe pitanie,material'no-techničeskoe snabženie i sbyt,zagotovki	25.0	75.2	95.1	108.7	112.3
Housing and municipal services, consumer services - Wohnungs-u.Kommunalwirtschaft, Dienstleistungen für die Bevölkerung - Žiliščno-kommunal'noe chozjajstvo, bytovoe obsluživanie naselenija	26.1	72.0	94.5	109.0	112.7
Health, physical culture, social security - Gesundheitswesen, Körperkultur, Sozialfürsorge - Zdravoochranenie, fizkul'tura i social'noe obespečenie	25.5	79.0	92.0	102.3	104.0
Education - Volksbildung - prosveščenie	33.1	96.1	108.3	126.9	128.0
Culture - Kultur - kul'tura	22.3	67.3	84.8	92.2	93.2
Art - Kunst - Iskusstvo	39.1	78.2	94.8	103.1	103.3
Science and scientific services - Wissenschaft u.wissenschaftl.Dienstleistungen - Nauka i naučnoe obsluživanie	47.1	120.6	139.5	157.5	161.6
Banking and State Insurance - Banken u.staatliche Versicherung - Kreditovanie i gosudarstvennoe strachov.	33.4	86.3	111.4	133.8	134.2
Administration of state and economics, cooperative and social organizations - Staats-u.Wirtschaftsverwaltung, Verwaltung d.genossenschaftl.u.gesellschaftlichen Organisationen - Apparat organov gosudarstvennogo i chozjajstvennogo upravlenija, organov upravlenija kooperativnych i obščestvennych organizacij	39.0	105.9	122.2	130.6	132.4

Standard of living, social security 11.1.4
Lebensstandard, Sozialfürsorge 11.1.5
11.1.6

11.1.4 GROWTH OF THE MONTHLY WAGES AND SALARIES OF WORKERS AND EMPLOYEES
WACHSTUM DES DURCHSCHNITTLICHEN MONATSLOHNES DER ARBEITER U. ANGESTELLTEN
ROST SREDNEMESJAČNOJ DENEŽNOJ ZARABOTNOJ PLATY RABOČICH I SLUŽAŠČICH

Year Jahr Gody	Rubles Rubel rublej	As a percentage of the previous year In Prozent gegenüber dem Vorjahr V procentach k predydnšćemu godu
1970	122	4
1971	126	3.3
1972	130.3	3.5
1973	135	3.7
1974	140.7	4.3
1975	146	3.5
1976	151	3.4
1977	155	2.6

11.1.5 AVERAGE MONTHLY WAGE AND SALARY IN THE NATIONAL ECONOMY AND IN
BRANCHES WITH HIGHEST AND LOWEST WAGE AND SALARY BRACKET
DURCHSCHNITTLICHER MONATSLOHN IN DER VOLKSWIRTSCHAFT UND IN DEN
ZWEIGEN MIT HÖCHSTER UND NIEDRIGSTER LOHNSTUFE
SREDNEMESJAČNAJA ZARABOTNAJA PLATA V NARODNOM CHOZJAJSTVE I V OTRASLJACH
S VYSŠIM I NIZŠIM EE UROVNEM

Year Jahr Gody	Average monthly wage & salary Durchschnittl. Monatslohn Srednemesjačnaja zarabotnaja plata (Rub.)	Lowest wage & salary bracket-niedrigste Lohnstufe-nizšij uroven'		Highest wage & salary bracket-höchste Lohnstufe-vysšij uroven'	
		Rub.	in % to average wage & salary in % zum Durchschnittslohn	Rub.	in % to lowest wage and salary bracket in % zur niedrigsten Lohnstufe
1950	64.2	38.3	60.0	93.7	245.0
1965	96.5	67.3	70.0	116.8	174.0
1975	145.8	92.2	63.0	176.8	192.0

11.1.6 CORRELATION BETWEEN AVERAGE AND MINIMUM WAGE AND SALARY
VERHÄLTNIS ZWISCHEN DURCHSCHNITTS- UND MINIMALLOHN
SOOTNOŠENIE SREDNEJ I MINIMAL'NOJ ZARABOTNOJ PLATY

Year Jahr Gody	Average wage and salary Durchschnittslohn Srednjaja zarabotnaja plata (Rub.) A.	Minimum wage and salary Minimallohn Minimal'naja zarabotnaja plata (Rub.) B.	Difference between average and minimum wage and salary Unterschied zwischen Durchschnitts- und Minimallohn Raznost' meždu srednej i minimal'noj zarabotnoj platoj (Rub.) C.	Correlation between average and minimum wage and salary Verhältnis zwischen Durchschnitts-und Minimallohn Otnošenie srednej zarabotnoj platy k minimal'noj (%) D.
1946 end of - Ende - Konec	48.1	22	26.1	219
1956	75.2	22	53.2	342

11.1.6
11.1.7 Standard of living, social security
11.1.8 Lebensstandard, Sozialfürsorge

	A.	B.	C.	D.
Beginning of - Anfang - Načalo 1957	75.2	27	48.2	278
End of - Ende - Konec 1964	93.6	27	66.6	347
Beginning of - Anfang - Načalo 1965	93.6	40	53.6	234
End of - Ende - Konec 1967	108.7	40	68.7	272
Beginning of - Anfang - Načalo 1968	108.7	60	48.7	181
End of - Ende - Konec 1975	148.4	60	88.6	248
1979 (planned - geplant)	165	70	95	236

11.1.7 GROWTH OF PAY OF KOLKHOZ WORKERS
WACHSTUM DER ENTLOHNUNG DER KOLCHOSBAUERN
ROST OPLATY TRUDA KOLCHOZNIKOV
(in percentage - in Prozent - v procentach)

Year Jahr Gody	%	Year Jahr Gody	%
1970	6.8	1974	5.0
1971	3.0	1975	3.0
1972	4.7	1976	6.0
1973	5.9	1977	4.3

11.1.8 SHARE OF INCOME FROM PRIVATE FARMING OF TOTAL INCOME
OF INDUSTRIAL AND KOLKHOZ WORKERS
ANTEIL DES EINKOMMENS AUS PRIVATEN NEBENWIRTSCHAFTEN
AM EINKOMMEN DER INDUSTRIEARBEITER UND KOLCHOSBAUERN
UDEL'NYJ VES DOCHODOV OT LIČNOGO PODSOBNOGO CHOZJAJSTVA
V DOCHODACH RABOČICH PROMYŠLENNOSTI I KOLCHOZNIKOV
(in percentage - in Prozent - v procentach)

	1940	1965	1970	1975
Workers - Arbeiter - RaboČie	11.4	2.0	1.5	1.0
Collective farmers - Kolchosbauern - Kolchozniki	50.0	40.6	35.8	29.0

11.1.9
ALLOWANCES AND BENEFITS FOR THE POPULATION OUT OF THE PUBLIC CONSUMER FUNDS
ZAHLUNGEN UND LEISTUNGEN FÜR DIE BEVÖLKERUNG AUS DEN ÖFFENTLICHEN BEDARFSFONDS
VYPLATY I L'GOTY, POLUČENNYE NASELENIEM IZ OBŠČESTVENNYCH FONDOV POTREBLENIJA
('000 mill. rubles - Mrd. Rubel)

	1940	1965	1970	1975	1976
Allowances and benefits, total - Zahlungen und Leistungen insg. - Vyplaty i l'goty vsego	4.6	41.9	63.9	90.1	95.0
Education (free schooling, cultural enlightenment) - Bildungswesen (unentgeltliche Schulbildung, kulturelle Aufklärungsarbeit) - Prosveščenie (besplatnoe obrazovanie, kul'turno-prosvetitel'naja rabota)	2.0	13.2	18.7	25.1	26.2
Health and physical culture (free medical care, cures in sanitariums and reconvalescent homes, physical education etc.) - Gesundheitswesen und Körperkultur (unentgeltliche ärztliche Hilfe, Betreuung in Sanatorien u. Kurheimen, körperliche Erziehung u.a.) - Zdravoochranenie i fizičeskaja kul'tura (besplatnaja medicinskaja pomošč', sanatorno-kurortnoe obsluživanie, fizičeskoe vospitanie i.d.)	1.0	6.9	10.0	12.9	13.6
Social security and social insurance - Sozialfürsorge und Sozialversicherung - Social'noe obespečenie i social'noe strachovanie	0.9	14.4	22.8	34.6	36.9
Pensions - Renten - Pensii	0.3	10.6	16.2	24.4	25.8
Financial aid - Unterstützungen - Posobija	0.5	3.5	6.1	9.2	9.9
State expenditures for maintenance of public housing (in cases where low rents do not cover maintenance) - Ausgaben des Staates für die Instandhaltung des Wohnfonds (in Fällen, wo sie nicht durch niedrige Mieten gedeckt wird) - Raschody gosudarstva na soderžanie žiliščnogo fonda (v časti, nepokryvaemoj nizkoj kvartirnoj platoj)	0.1	2.3	3.4	4.9	5.2
Allowances and benefits per capita, rubles - Zahlungen und Leistungen pro Kopf der Bevölkerung, Rubel - Vyplaty i l'goty na dušu naselenija, rublej	24	182	263	354	370

11.1.10 Standard of living, social security
11.1.11 Lebensstandard, Sozialfürsorge

11.1.10 GROWTH OF ALLOWANCES AND BENEFITS FOR THE POPULATION OUT OF THE PUBLIC CONSUMER FUNDS - WACHSTUM DER ZAHLUNGEN UND LEISTUNGEN FÜR DIE BEVÖLKERUNG AUS DEN ÖFFENTLICHEN BEDARFSFONDS - ROST VYPLAT I L'GOT NASELENIJU IZ OBSCESTVENNYCH FONDOV POTREBLENIJA

Year / Jahr / Gody	'000 mill.rubles / Mrd. Rubel / Mrd. Rublej	Percentage in relation to previous year / In Prozent gegenüber dem Vorjahr
1970	64	7.3
1971	68.6	7.4
1972	73	6.4
1973	78	6.1
1974	83	6.4
1975	90	8.4
1976	94.5	5.0
1977	99.5	4.5

11.1.11 BASKET OF CONSUMER GOODS FOR MAY 1976, IN WORK UNITS
LEBENSMITTELKORB FÜR MAI 1976, IN ARBEITSEINHEITEN

Item / Ware	Kgs	Washington	Moscow / Moskau	Munich / München	London	Paris
		(Minutes of worktime - Arbeitsminuten)				
Flour - Mehl	1.0	6	30	8	9	9
Bread - Brot	6.0	126	78	132	60	108
Noodles - Nudeln	2.0	46	54	58	56	28
Beef - Rindfleisch	1.0	66	144	115	147	166
Pork - Schweinefleisch	1.5	75	206	137	161	180
Minced beef - Rinderhack	1.0	34	208	58	76	100
Sausages - Würste	1.0	71	158	67	60	84
Cod - Kabeljau	1.0	49	56	52	98	113
Fish fingers - Fischstäbchen	0.5	22	44	21	39	50
Sugar - Zucker	4.0	36	260	48	60	52
Butter	0.5	23	130	31	29	39
Margarine	0.2	6	26	5	7	7
Milk (liters) - Milch (Liter)	10.0	70	210	90	110	80
Cheese - Käse	1.0	89	216	71	72	84
Eggs, cheapest, pieces - Eier, billigste, Stck.	17	15	111	27	19	39
Potatoes - Kartoffeln	9.0	72	63	72	207	117
Cabbage - Kohl	2.0	12	216	34	26	36
Carrots - Karotten	0.5	5	36	6	5	3
Tomatoes - Tomaten	0.5	9	108	12	24	14
Apples - Äpfel	1.0	25	50	10	20	12
Tea - Tee	0.1	9	75	29	6	18
Beer (liters) - Bier (Liter)	3.0	39	96	12	69	21
Gin/vodka (liters) - Gin/Wodka (Liter)	1.0	96	837	90	296	210
Cigarettes (units) - Zigaretten (Stck.)	120	60	138	108	162	48

Standard of living, social security 11.1.11
Lebensstandard, Sozialfürsorge 11.2.1

Item Ware	Washington	Moscow Moskau	Munich München	London	Paris
(Hours of worktime - Arbeitsstunden)					
Weekly basket, as above - Wöchentlicher Korb, wie oben	17.7	59.2	21.6	30.3	27.0
Rent, monthly - Miete,monatlich	46.5	9.9	32.0	48.5	35.6
Color TV - Farbfernseher	85.6	780.0	191.5	221.6	327.3
(Months of worktime - Arbeitsmonate)					
Fiat 131/Zhiguli VAZ-2101	6.9	37.5	7.7	11.1	10.6

(Keith Bush, Retail Prices in Moscow and four Western Cities in May 1976, Osteuropa, Wirtschaft, No.2/1977, p.125)

11.2 HOUSING CONSTRUCTION - WOHNUNGSBAU - ŽILIŠČNOE STROITEL'STVO

11.2.1 NUMBER OF NEWLY BUILT APARTMENT HOUSES - FERTIGGESTELLTE WOHNHÄUSER - VVOD V DEJSTVIE ŽILYCH DOMOV
(Total useful floor-space, mill.sq.m. - Gesamte Nutzfläche der Wohnhäuser, Mio m² - Millionov m² obščej (poleznoj) ploščadi žilišč)

	Total - Insgesamt - Vsego A.	By state & co-operative enterprises & organizations & by housing co-operatives - von staatl.u.genossen-schaftl.Betrieben u.Organisationen u.Wohnungsbaugenossenschaften - Gosudarstvennymi i kooperativnymi predprijatijami i organizacijami i žilkooperaciej B.	By workers & employees at their own expense & with the help of state credits - von Arbeitern u.Angestell-ten aus eigenen Mitteln u.mit Hilfe staatl.Kredite - Rabočimi i služaš-čimi za svoj sčet i s pomoščju gosudarstvennogo kredita C.	In collective farms(by collective farms,collective farmers & by rural intellectuals - in Kolchosen (von Kolchosen,Kolchosbauern u.ländlicher Intelligenz-v kolchozach(kolchozami, kolchoznikami i sel'skoj intellig.) D.
1918-1977 Total-Insg.-Vsego	3199.1	1807.8	544.5	846.8
1918-1928	203.0	23.7	27.5	151.8
First Five-Year Plan - Erster Fünfjahrplan - Pervaja pjatiletka (1929-1932)	56.9	32.6	7.6	16.7
Second Five-Year Plan - Zweiter Fünfjahrplan - Vtoraja pjatiletka (1933-1937)	67.3	37.2	7.1	23.0

11.2.1 Standard of living, social security
11.2.2 Lebensstandard, Sozialfürsorge

	A.	B.	C.	D.
Three and a half years of Third Five-Year Plan (1938 - first half of 1941) - Dreieinhalb Jahre des Dritten Fünfjahrplanes (1938 - 1.Halbjahr 1941) - Tri s polovinoj goda tretej pjatiletki (1938 - pervoe polugodie 1941 g.)	81.7	34.4	10.9	36.4
Four and a half years (July 1,1941-January 1,1946)- Viereinhalb Jahre (1.Juli 1941-1.Januar 1946) - Četyre s polovinoj goda (s 1.ijulja 1941 do 1 janvarja 1946)	102.5	41.3	13.6	47.6
Fourth Five-Year Plan - Vierter Fünfjahrplan - Četvertaja pjatiletka (1946-1950)	200.9	72.4	44.7	83.8
Fifth Five-Year Plan - Fünfter Fünfjahrplan - Pjataja pjatiletka (1951-1955)	240.5	113.0	65.1	62.4
Sixth Five-Year Plan - Sechster Fünfjahrplan - Šestaja pjatiletka (1956-1960)	474.1	224.0	113.8	136.3
Seventh Five-Year Plan - Siebenter Fünfjahrplan - Sed'maja pjatiletka (1961-1965)	490.6	300.4	94.0	96.2
1965	97.6	63.2	16.1	18.3
Eighth Five-Year Plan - Achter Fünfjahrplan - Vos'maja pjatiletka (1966-1970)	518.5	352.5	72.8	93.2
1970	106.0	76.6	13.0	16.4
Ninth Five-Year Plan - Neunter Fünfjahrplan - Devjataja pjatiletka (1971-1975)	544.8	407.3	64.3	73.2
1971	107.6	78.7	13.0	15.9
1972	106.7	79.4	12.5	14.8
1973	110.5	82.9	13.2	14.4
1974	110.1	83.0	13.0	14.1
1975	109.9	83.3	12.6	14.0
1976	106.2	82.7	11.4	12.1
1977	112.1	86.3	11.7	14.1

11.2.2   MUNICIPAL HOUSING FUND - STÄDTISCHER WOHNUNGSFONDS -
                    GORODSKOJ ŽILIŠČNYJ FOND

(end-of-year figures; mill.sq.m. of total useful floor-space - zum Jahresende; Mio m² der gesamten Nutzfläche der Wohnhäuser - na konec goda; millionov m² obščej (poleznoj) ploščadi žilišč)

	1917	1940	1965	1970	1975	1976
Municipal housing fund, total - Städtischer Wohnungsfonds, insg. - Ves' gorodskoj žiliščnyj fond	185	421	1,238	1,529	1,867	1,932
socialized - verstaatlicht - obobščestvlennyj	27	267	806	1,072	1,385	1,446
private property - im Privatbesitz - v ličnoj sobstvennosti	158	154	432	457	482	486

Standard of living, social security 11.2.3
Lebensstandard, Sozialfürsorge 11.3.1

11.2.3 HOUSING FUNDS OF THE CAPITALS OF THE UNION REPUBLICS
WOHNUNGSFONDS DER HAUPTSTÄDTE DER UNIONSREPUBLIKEN
ŽILIŠČNYJ FOND STOLIC SOJUZNYCH RESPUBLIK

(end-of-year figures; '000 sq.m. of total useful floor-space - zum Jahresende; Tsd.m² der gesamten Nutzfläche der Wohnhäuser - na konec goda; tysjač m² obščej (poleznoj) ploščadi žilišč)

	1940	1965	1970	1975	1976
Moskva	28,165	78,537	97,713	117,030	120,679
Kiev	6,660	16,390	21,264	27,200	28,212
Minsk	1,804	6,915	10,051	14,052	14,729
Taškent	4,025	9,674	11,350	15,316	16,019
Alma-Ata	1,320	6,010	7,730	9,770	10,149
Tbilisi	4,609	7,891	9,772	12,242	12,690
Baku	5,830	11,020	13,061	14,970	15,434
Vilnius	...	3,296	4,467	5,616	5,715
Kišinev	...	2,909	3,936	5,453	5,715
Riga	...	8,494	9,970	11,676	11,928
Frunze	568	3,032	3,986	4,935	5,093
Dušanbe	457	2,703	3,440	4,351	4,487
Erevan	1,350	5,722	7,368	9,365	9,771
Ašchabad	806	2,063	2,495	2,889	3,042
Tallin	...	4,025	4,966	6,084	6,306

11.3 RETAIL TRADE — EINZELHANDEL — ROZNIČNAJA TORGOVLJA

11.3.1 RETAIL STORES AND SALES FLOOR SPACE OF STATE AND COOPERATIVE ORGANIZATIONS IN THE UNION REPUBLICS
EINZELHANDELSBETRIEBE UND VERKAUFSFLÄCHE DER LÄDEN DER STAATLICHEN UND GENOSSENSCHAFTLICHEN ORGANISATIONEN IN DEN UNIONSREPUBLIKEN
PREDPRIJATIJA ROZNIČNOJ TORGOVLI I TORGOVAJA PLOŠČAD' MAGAZINOV GOSUDARSTVENNYCH I KOOPERATIVNYCH ORGANIZACIJ PO SOJUZNYN RESPUBLIKAM
(end of 1977 - Ende 1977 - na konec 1977 goda)

	Number of enterprises, '000 Zahl der Betriebe, Tsd. Čislo predprijatij, tys.			Selling area of the shops,'000 sq.m. Verkaufsfläche der Läden, Tsd.m² Torgovaja ploščad' magazinov,tys.m²		
	Total — Insgesamt — Vsego	in the cities — i.d.Städten — v gorodskich poselenijach	in the country — auf dem Lande v sel'skoj mestnosti	Total — Insgesamt — Vsego	in the cities — i.d.Städten — v gorodskich poselenijach	in the country — auf dem Lande v sel'skoj mestnosti
	A.	B.	C.	D.	E.	F.
SSSR	695.5	360.6	334.9	42182.1	26914.3	15267.8
RSFSR	359.5	186.8	172.7	23403.0	15321.7	8081.3
Ukrainskaja SSR	146.9	79.2	67.7	8484.4	5509.0	2975.4
Belorusskaja SSR	24.6	10.4	14.2	1689.4	976.6	712.8
Uzbekskaja SSR	33.4	15.5	17.9	1634.5	821.7	812.8
Kazachskaja SSR	41.3	17.4	23.9	2292.3	1204.1	1088.2

11.3.1 Standard of living, social security
11.3.2 Lebensstandard, Sozialfürsorge

	A.	B.	C.	D.	E.	F.
Gruzinskaja SSR	15.4	9.1	6.3	766.0	519.1	246.9
Azerbajdžanskaja SSR	17.2	10.3	6.9	612.7	487.2	125.5
Litovskaja SSR	7.4	4.5	2.9	508.9	362.5	146.4
Moldavskaja SSR	10.2	4.0	6.2	529.9	270.1	259.8
Latvijskaja SSR	7.0	4.7	2.3	446.0	323.0	123.0
Kirgizskaja SSR	7.6	3.2	4.4	382.6	186.5	196.1
Tadžikskaja SSR	7.2	3.6	3.6	378.5	223.4	155.1
Armjanskaja SSR	7.0	4.9	2.1	437.4	296.2	141.2
Turkmenskaja SSR	6.1	3.8	2.3	324.6	195.3	129.3
Estonskaja SSR	3.9	2.4	1.5	254.5	180.5	74.0

11.3.2 COMMUNAL CATERING ORGANIZATIONS AND NUMBER OF AVAILABLE
PLACES IN THE UNION REPUBLICS
BETRIEBE DER GEMEINSCHAFTSVERPFLEGUNG UND ZAHL DER DORT VORHANDENEN
PLÄTZE IN DEN UNIONSREPUBLIKEN
PREDPRIJATIJA OBSČESTVENNOGO PITANIJA I ČISLO MEST V NICH PO
SOJUZNYM RESPUBLIKAM
(end of 1977 - Ende 1977 - na konec 1977 goda)

	Number of enterprises, '000 Zahl der Betriebe, Tsd. Čislo predprijatij, tys.			Number of seats, '000 Zahl der Plätze, Tsd. Čislo mest, tys.		
	Total - Insgesamt - Vsego	in the cities - i.d.Städten - v gorodskich poselenijach	in the country - auf dem Lande - v sel'skoj mestnosti	Total - Insgesamt - Vsego	in the cities - i.d.Städten - v gorodskich poselenijach	in the country - auf dem Lande - v sel'skoj mestnosti
SSSR	286.2	196.7	89.5	15138.6	12134.7	3003.9
RSFSR	148.9	110.9	38.0	8255.6	7018.1	1237.5
Ukrainskaja SSR	54.7	37.1	17.6	3074.8	2402.4	672.4
Belorusskaja SSR	10.5	6.2	4.3	581.2	408.2	173.0
Uzbekskaja SSR	16.4	7.5	8.9	655.4	390.1	265.3
Kazachskaja SSR	14.8	9.0	5.8	636.1	450.0	186.1
Gruzinskaja SSR	7.1	4.5	2.6	284.3	218.8	65.5
Azerbajdžanskaja SSR	8.1	5.1	3.0	295.4	233.1	62.3
Litovskaja SSR	3.3	2.3	1.0	214.7	172.7	42.0
Moldavskaja SSR	3.8	2.0	1.8	204.6	126.6	78.0
Latvijskaja SSR	3.0	2.2	0.8	226.9	171.2	55.7
Kirgizskaja SSR	3.1	1.7	1.4	127.0	88.2	38.8
Tadžikskaja SSR	3.7	2.2	1.5	135.1	103.9	31.2
Armjanskaja SSR	3.6	2.4	1.2	187.3	144.0	43.3
Turkmenskaja SSR	2.7	1.6	1.1	101.2	76.5	24.7
Estonskaja SSR	1.9	1.4	0.5	125.4	97.3	28.1

Standard of living, social security
Lebensstandard, Sozialfürsorge 11.3.3

11.3.3 SELF-SERVICE SHOPS - SELBSTBEDIENUNGSLÄDEN - MAGAZINY SAMOOBSLUŽIVANIJA
(end of 1977 - Ende 1977 - na konec 1977 goda)

	A. Number of shops - Zahl der Läden - Cislo magazinov	B. Turnover in the 4th quart. - Warenumsatz im IV.Quartal - Tovarooborot za IV kvartal	\multicolumn{2}{c}{Percentage of self-service shops - Prozentualer Anteil der Selbstbedienungsläden - Magaziny samoobsluživanija v % ko vsem magazinam}
			C. Number of shops / Zahl der Läden / Cislo magazinov	D. Turnover / Warenumsatz / Tovarooborot
State trade - Staatlicher Handel - Gosudarstvennaja torgovlja:				
Food stores - Lebensmittelgeschäfte - Prodovol'stvennye magaziny	35,912	6894.8	35.1	42.9
of which-darunter-v tom čisle:				
with universal assortment - mit universellem Warensortiment - s universal'nym assortimentom tovarov	6,613	3509.6	6.5	21.8
bread-shops - Brotgeschäfte - chlebnye	9,158	550.0	8.9	3.4
dairies - Milchgeschäfte - moločnye	1,074	159.4	1.0	1.0
fruit & vegetable shops - Obst- und Gemüseläden - plodoovoščnye	4,402	386.5	4.3	2.4
others-andere-pročie	14,665	2072.9	14.4	14.3
Department stores - Warenhäuser - Neprodovol'stvennye magaziny	31,881	9950.1	48.0	62.7
of which-darunter-v tom čisle:				
department stores - Kaufhäuser - univermagi	588	2731.3	0.9	17.2
shoe-shops - Schuhgeschäfte - obuvi	2.074	527.5	3.1	3.3
clothing shops - Bekleidungsgeschäfte - odežby	2.263	1061.2	3.4	6.7
household articles shops - Haushaltswarengeschäfte - chozjajstvennye	4.088	484.5	6.2	3.4
bookshops - Buchhandlungen - knižnye	5.176	152.2	7.8	1.0

573

11.3.3 Standard of living, social security
11.3.4 Lebensstandard, Sozialfürsorge

	A.	B.	C.	D.
mixed - gemischte - Smešannye magaziny	1.854	237.7	9.3	20.4
Co-operative societies - Konsumgenossenschaften - Potrebitel'skaja kooperacija:				
Food stores - Lebensmittelgeschäfte - Prodovol'stvennye magaziny	60.321	3786.2	60.9	67.5
Department stores - Warenhäuser - Neprodovol'stvennye magaziny	77.915	5095.2	80.7	85.2
Mixed shops (articles of daily use) - Gemischte Läden (Waren des täglichen Gebrauchs) - Smešannye magaziny (tovarov povsednevnogo sprosa)	58.138	2068.6	52.9	61.6

11.3.4 GROWTH IN TRADE TURNOVER AND RETAIL OUTLETS
WACHSTUM DES WARENUMSATZES UND DES HANDELSNETZES IM EINZELHANDEL
ROST ROZNICNOGO TOVAROOBOROTA I TORGOVOJ SETI

	1940	1965	1970	1975	1976
Retail trade turnover of the state and co-operative trade (in comparable prices; as a percentage of 1940) - Einzelhandelsumsatz des staatlichen und genossenschaftlichen Handels (in Vergleichspreisen; in % zu 1940) - Rozničnyj tovarooborot gosudarstvennoj i kooperativnoj torgovli (v sopostavimych cenach; v % k 1940 g.)	100	423	628	854	893
Trade turnover per capita (in comparable prices; in percentage of 1940) - Handelsumsatz pro Kopf der Bevölkerung (in Vergleichspreisen; in % zu 1940) - Tovarooborot na dušu naselenija (v sopostavimych cenach; v % k 1940 g.)	100	358	505	656	680
of which in rural areas-darunter auf dem Lande - v tom čisle v sel'skich mestnostj.	100	396	601	828	854
Per 10,000 of the population - auf 10.000 der Bevölkerung entfielen - na 10.000 čelovek naselenija prichodilos':					
retail trade - Einzelhandelsbetriebe - predprijatij rozničnoj torgovli	21	28	28	27	27
selling area of the shops, sq.m. - Verkaufsfläche in den Läden, m^2 - torgovoj ploščadi v magazinych, m^2	620	1,066	1,290	1,537	1,579
public catering enterprises - Betriebe der Gemeinschaftsverpflegung - predprijatij obščestvennogo pitanija	4	8	10	11	11
number of seats in public catering enterprises - Zahl der Plätze i.d.Betrieben der Gemeinschaftsverpflegung - čislo posadočnych mest na predprijatijach obščestvennogo pit.	112	295	411	537	560

574

11.3.5 PROVISION OF CITY AND RURAL POPULATION WITH DURABLE CONSUMER AND HOUSEHOLD GOODS
VERSORGUNG DER STADT- UND LANDBEVÖLKERUNG MIT LANGLEBIGEN KULTUR- UND HAUSHALTSGÜTERN
OBESPEČENNOST' GORODSKOGO I SEL'SKOGO NASELENIJA PREDMETAMI KUL'- TURNO-BYTOVOGO NAZNAČENIJA DLITEL'NOGO POL'ZOVANIJA
(end-of-year figures - zum Jahresende - na konec goda)

	Per 100 families je 100 Familien na 100 semej				Per 1,000 of the population je 1.000 der Bevölkerung na 1000 čelovek naselenija			
	1965	1970	1975	1976	1965	1970	1975	1976
Clocks and watches of all types - Uhren aller Art - Časy vsech vidov	319	411	455	470	885	1,193	1,319	1,362
Radio sets and radiograms - Rundfunkempfänger und Musiktruhen - Radiopriemniki i radioly	59	72	79	81	165	199	230	235
TV sets - Fernsehempfänger - Televizory	24	51	74	77	68	143	215	223
Photo cameras - Photoapparate - Fotoapparaty	24	27	27	27	67	77	77	78
Refrigerators - Haushaltskühlschränke - Cholodil'niki	11	32	61	67	29	89	178	194
Washing machines - Haushaltswaschmaschinen - Stiral'nye maš.	21	52	65	67	59	141	189	195
Vacuum cleaners - elektrische Staubsauger - Elektropylesosy	7	12	18	20	18	31	52	58
Motorcycles and scooters - Motorräder und -roller - Motocikly i motorollery	6	7	8	9	17	21	25	26
Bicycles and mopeds - Fahrräder und Mopeds - Velosipedy i mopedy	48	50	54	53	134	145	156	153
Sewing machines - Haushaltsnähmaschinen - Švejnye mašiny	52	56	61	62	144	161	178	181

11.4.1 Standard of living, social security
       Lebensstandard, Sozialfürsorge

11.4 HEALTH - GESUNDHEITSWESEN - ZDRAVOOCHRANENIE

11.4.1 BASIC INDICATORS OF THE DEVELOPMENT OF HEALTH SERVICES
GRUNDKENNZIFFERN DER ENTWICKLUNG DES GESUNDHEITSWESENS
POKAZATELI RAZVITIJA ZDRAVOOCHRANENIJA

	1940	1950	1960	1975
Expenses for health and physical culture from the state budget (mill.rubles) - Ausgaben für Gesundheitswesen und Körperkultur aus dem Staatsbudget (Mio Rubel) - Raschody na zdravoochranenie i fizičeskuju kul'turu iz gosudarstvennogo bjudžeta (mln.rub.)	903.5	2162.6	4841.0	11469.9
Medical staff - medizinische Kader - Medicinskie kadry:				
Number of doctors of all special branches,'000 - Zahl der Ärzte aller Fachrichtungen, Tsd. Čislennost' vračej vsech special'nostej,tys.	155.3	265.0	431.7	834.1
Number of doctors per 10,000 of the population - Zahl der Ärzte pro 10.000 der Bevölkerung - Čislo vračej na 10.000 naselenija	7.9	14.6	20.0	32.6
Number of paramedical staff, in '000 - Zahl des mittleren medizinischen Personals,Tsd.- Čislennost' srednich medicinskich rabotnikov,tys.	472.0	719.4	1388.3	2515.1
Number of paramedical staff, per 10,000 population - Zahl des mittleren medizinischen Personals pro 10.000 der Bevölkerung - Čislo srednich medicinskich rabotnikov na 10.000 naselenija	24.0	39.6	64.2	98.4
Medical education - medizinische Ausbildung - medicinskoe obrazovanie:				
Number of higher medical educational establishments incl. university faculties - Zahl der höheren medizinischen Lehranstalten einschl.Fakultäten an den Universitäten - Čislo vysšich medicinskich učebnych zavedenij, vključaja fakul'tety universitetov	72	76	85	92
Number of students ('000) - Zahl der Studenten (Tsd.) - Čislo studentov (tys.)	116.0	105.5	175.0	318.9
doctors trained there ('000) - dort ausgebildete Ärzte (Tsd.) - Vypusk vračej (tys.)	16.4	19.5	28.2	47.5
Number of secondary medical educational establishments - Zahl der mittleren medizinischen Lehranstalten - Čislo srednich medicinskich učebnych zavedenij	990	565	498	632
Number of pupils ('000) - Zahl der Schüler (Tsd.) - Čislo učaščichsja (tys.)	222.8	112.8	170.2	397.4

Standard of living, social security 11.4.1
Lebensstandard, Sozialfürsorge

	1940	1950	1960	1975
Paramedical staff trained there, in '000 - dort ausgebildetes mittleres mediz.Personal (Tsd.) - Vypusk rednich medicinskich rabotnikov (tys.)	84.05	51.7	62.3	131.3

Hospital and dispensary care -
Krankenhaus-und ambulant-poliklinische Betreuung -
Bol'ničnaja i ambulatorno-polikliničeskaja pomošč':

Number of hospital beds ('000) - Zahl der Krankenhausbetten (Tsd.) - Čislo bol'ničnych koek (tys.)	790.9	1010.7	1739.2	3009.2
Number of hospitals ('000) - Zahl der Krankenanstalten (Tsd.) - Čislo bol'ničnych učreždenij (tys.)	13.8	18.3	26.7	24.3
Number of hospital beds per 10,000 of the population - Zahl der Krankenhausbetten pro 10.000 d.Bevölkerung - Čislo bol'ničnych koek na 10.000 naselenija	40.2	55.7	80.4	117.8
Number of medical facilities for outpatient treatment (in '000) - Zahl der medizinischen Einrichtungen für ambulant-poliklinische Betreuung (Tsd.) - Čislo vračebnych učreždenij,okazyvajuščich ambulatorno-polikliničeskuju pomošč' (tys.)	36.8	36.2	39.3	35.6

Number of visits at medical-therapeutical
facilities of the USSR Ministry of Health -
Zahl der Besuche der medizinischen therapeutisch-
prophylaktischen Einrichtungen des Ministeriums für
Gesundheitswesen der UdSSR - Čislo poseščenij do
vračebnych lečebno-profilaktičeskich učreždenij
Ministerstva zdravoochranenija SSSR:

ambulant (mill.-Mio) - na ambulantnom prieme(mln.)	513.1	630.0	1044.3	1969.5
House calls (mill.) - Hausbesuche (Mio) - na domu (mln.)	35.4	48.3	84.9	138.8
Number of specialized dispensary establishments - Zahl der spezialisierten dispensarischen Einrichtungen- Čislo specializirovannych dispansernych učreždenij	1284	1748	2787	3003

Cure and sanitarium treatment - Kurbetreuung -
Sanatorno-kurortnaja pomošč:

Number of boarding sanitariums and pensions with medical treatment (for children and adults) - Zahl der Ganztagssanatorien und Pensionen mit Heilbehandlung (für Erwachsene und Kinder) - Čislo sanatoriev kruglosutočnogo prebyvanija i pansionatov s lečeniem (dlja vzroslych i detej)	1838	2070	2106	2350
of which for children - darunter für Kinder - v tom čisle dlja detej	957	1027	1106	1219
Number of beds ('000) - Zahl der Betten (Tsd.) - Čislo koek (tys.)	240	255	325	504
of which for children ('000) - darunter für Kinder (Tsd.) - v tom čisle dlja detej (tys.)	95	95	120	162

Sanitary-epidemiological services -
Sanitär-epidemiologischer Dienst -
Sanitarno-epidemiologičeskaja služba:

11.4.1 Standard of living, social security
Lebensstandard, Sozialfürsorge

	1940	1950	1960	1975
Number of sanitary-epidemiological stations - Zahl der sanitär-epidemiologischen Stationen - Čislo sanitarno-epidemiologičeskich stancij	1943	5756	4843	4754
Number of doctors of the sanitary anti-epidemical group ('000) - Zahl der Ärzte der sanitär-antiepidemischen Gruppe (Tsd.) - Čislo vračej sanitarno-protivoepidemičeskoj gruppy (tys.)	12.5	21.9	31.4	49.1
Number of paramedical staff in sanitary-epidemiological sector ('000) - Zahl des mittleren medizinischen Personals der sanitär-antiepidemischen Fachrichtung (Tsd.) - Čislo srednich medicinskich rabotnikov sanitarno-protivoepidemičeskogo profilja (tys.)	25.6	45.5	80.6	140.7
Therapeutic-prophylactic care of women and children - Therapeutisch-prophilaktische Betreuung von Frauen und Kindern - Lečebno-profilaktičeskaja pomošč' ženščinam i detjam:				
Number of gynecologists and accoucheurs ('000) - Zahl der Frauenärzte und Geburtshelfer (Tsd.) - Čislo vračej akušerov-ginekologov (tys.)	10.6	16.6	28.7	49.6
Number of midwives ('000) - Zahl der Geburtshelferinnen u.Hebammen (Tsd.) - Čislo feldšeric-akušerok i akušerok (tys.)	80.9	108.5	215.5	329.3
Number of beds (in hospitals and maternity homes) for pregnant women and women in childbed ('000) - Zahl der Betten (in Kranken-und Entbindungsstationen) für Schwangere und Wöchnerinnen (Tsd.) - Čislo koek (vračebnych i ekušerskich) dlja beremennych i rožčenic (tys.)	147.1	143.0	213.4	223.6
Number of gynecological beds ('000) - Zahl der gynäkologischen Betten (Tsd.) - Čislo ginekologičeskich koek (tys.)	33.6	42.2	91.3	169.4
Number of children's specialists ('000) - Zahl der Kinderärzte (Tsd.) - Čislo vračej-pediatrov (tys.)	19.4	32.1	58.9	96.3
Number of maternity consultations, children's policlinics and dispensaries (independent or attached to other institutions, '000) - Zahl der Frauenberatungsstellen, Kinderpolikliniken und -ambulatorien (selbständige oder anderen Institutionen angehörende, Tsd.) - Čislo ženskich konsultacij, detskich poliklinik i ambulatorij (samostojatel'nych i vchodjaščich v sostav drugich učreždenij, tys.)	8.6	11.3	16.4	22.1
Number of hospital beds for children ('000) - Zahl der Krankenhausbetten für Kinder (Tsd.) - Čislo bol'ničnych koek dlja detej (tys.)	89.7	133.1	260.1	529.3
Number of children attending regular pre-school children's facilities ('000) - Zahl der Kinder, die ständige vorschulische Kindereinrichtungen besuchen (Tsd.) - Čislo detej, posešČajuščich postojannye detskie doškol'nye učreždenija, tys.	1953	1788	4428	11523

Standard of living, social security 11.4.1
Lebensstandard, Sozialfürsorge 11.4.2

	1940	1950	1960	1975
Pharmaceutical care - Pharmazeutische Betreuung - Aptečnaja pomošč:				
Number of pharmacies ('000) - Zahl der Apotheken (Tsd.) - Čislo aptek (tys.)	11.1	12.3	15.3	25.4
Number of pharmacists with university education ('000) - Zahl der Pharmazeuten mit Hochschulbildung (Tsd.) - Čislo farmacevtov s vysšim obrazovaniem (tys.)	9.5	12.2	26.5	61.9
Number of pharmacists with secondary education ('000) - Zahl der Pharmazeuten mit Mittelschulbildung (Tsd.) - Čislo farmacevtov so srednim obrazovaniem (tys.)	36.2	44.9	74.3	145.5

11.4.2 NUMBER OF DOCTORS OF ALL SPECIAL BRANCHES BY UNION REPUBLICS
ZAHL DER ÄRZTE ALLER FACHRICHTUNGEN NACH UNIONSREPUBLIKEN
ČISLENNOST' VRAČEJ VSECH SPECIAL'NOSTEJ PO SOJUZNYM RESPUBLIKAM

	Total number of doctors (in '000) Gesamtzahl der Ärzte (in Tsd.) Obščee čislo vračej (v tys.)				Number of doctors per 10,000 of the population Zahl der Ärzte pro 10.000 der Bevölkerung Čislo vračej na 10.000 naselenija			
	1940	1965	1970	1975	1940	1965	1970	1975
SSSR	155.3	554.2	668.4	834.1	7.9	23.9	27.4	32.6
RSFSR	90.8	315.5	378.4	468.9	8.2	24.8	29.0	34.8
Ukrainskaja SSR	35.3	110.6	131.0	157.1	8.4	24.3	27.6	32.0
Belorusskaja SSR	5.2	18.9	23.4	28.3	5.7	21.8	25.8	30.2
Uzbekskaja SSR	3.2	17.7	24.4	35.4	4.7	17.0	20.1	25.1
Kazachskaja SSR	2.7	22.5	28.8	39.2	4.3	18.7	21.8	27.3
Gruzinskaja SSR	4.9	15.8	17.1	20.4	13.3	35.0	36.2	41.1
Azerbajdžanskaja SSR	3.3	11.0	13.1	16.5	10.0	23.8	25.0	28.9
Litovskaja SSR	2.0	6.4	8.7	11.3	6.7	21.5	27.4	34.2
Moldavskaja SSR	1.1	6.0	7.4	10.1	4.2	17.9	20.5	26.2
Latvijskaja SSR	2.5	7.1	8.5	9.8	13.2	31.2	35.6	39.2
Kirgizskaja SSR	0.6	5.0	6.2	8.2	3.8	19.1	20.7	24.4
Tadžikskaja SSR	0.6	3.8	4.7	7.2	4.1	15.0	15.9	20.6
Armjanskaja SSR	1.0	6.0	7.3	9.8	7.5	26.7	28.8	34.8
Turkmenskaja SSR	1.0	4.1	4.8	6.6	7.6	21.2	21.4	25.7
Estonskaja SSR	1.1	3.8	4.6	5.3	10.0	29.5	33.1	36.8

11.4.3 Standard of living, social security
11.4.4 Lebensstandard, Sozialfürsorge

11.4.3 NUMBER OF WOMAN DOCTORS OF ALL SPECIAL BRANCHES
ZAHL DER ÄRZTINNEN ALLER FACHRICHTUNGEN
ČISLENNOST' ŽENŠČIN-VRAČEJ VSECH SPECIAL'NOSTEJ

(end-of-year figures - zum Jahresende - na konec goda)

	1940	1950	1960	1975	1976
in thousands - in Tausend - v tysjačach	96.3	408.9	479.6	583.5	600.6
in percentage to total of doctors - in Prozent zur Gesamtzahl der Ärzte - v % k obščej čislennosti vračej	62	74	72	70	69

11.4.4 NUMBER OF MEDICAL FACILITIES FOR AMBULANT TREATMENT
ZAHL DER MEDIZINISCHEN EINRICHTUNGEN FÜR AMBULANT-POLIKLINISCHE
ÄRZTLICHE BETREUUNG
ČISLO MEDICINSKICH UČREŽDENIJ, OKAZYVAJUŠČICH VRAČEBNUJU AMBULA-
TORNO-POLIKLINIČESKUJU POMOŠČ'

	All authorities Alle Behörden Vse vedomstva		System of the USSR Ministry of Health- System des Ministeriums für Gesund- heitswesen der UdSSR - Sistema Mini- sterstva zdravoochranenija SSSR	
	1970	1975[1]	1970	1975[1]
SSSR	37,360	35,641	35,013	33,329
RSFSR	19,903	18,903	18,417	17,430
Ukrainskaja SSR	6,417	5,870	6,031	5,480
Belorusskaja SSR	1,493	1,357	1,430	1,292
Uzbekskaja SSR	1,767	1,848	1,746	1,799
Kazachskaja SSR	2,220	2,202	2,071	2,088
Gruzinskaja SSR	1,392	1,345	1,341	1,291
Azerbajdžanskaja SSR	1,075	1,044	1,025	985
Litovskaja SSR	484	429	471	416
Moldavskaja SSR	428	480	414	466
Latvijskaja SSR	405	367	384	347
Kirgizskaja SSR	343	341	336	332
Tadžikskaja SSR	371	389	365	382
Armjanskaja SSR	457	487	445	473
Turkmenskaja SSR	323	338	304	319
Estonskaja SSR	282	241	233	229

[1] Reduction of the number of establishments by consolidation -
Verringerung der Zahl der Einrichtungen durch Zusammenlegung -
Snizenie čisla učreždenij ob'jasnjaetsja ich ukrupleniem

Standard of living, social security
Lebensstandard, Sozialfürsorge
11.4.5

11.4.5 GROWTH IN NUMBER OF HOSPITALS AND HOSPITAL BEDS
WACHSTUM DES NETZES DER KRANKENANSTALTEN UND DES BETTENKONTINGENTS
ROST SETI BOL'NIČNYCH UČREŽDENIJ I KOEČNOGO FONDA

	1940	1960	1970	1975[1]
Number of hospitals ('000) - Zahl der Krankenanstalten (Tsd.) - Čislo bol'ničnych učreždenij (tys.)	13.8	26.7	26.2	24.3
Number of hospital beds ('000) - Zahl der Krankenhausbetten (Tsd.) - Čislo bol'ničnych koek (tys.)	790.9	1739.2	2663.3	3009.2
Number of hospital beds per 10,000 of the population - Zahl der Krankenhausbetten pro 10.000 der Bevölkerung - Čislo bol'ničnych koek na 10.000 naselenija	40.2	80.4	109.2	117.8

[1] Reduction of the number of hospitals by consolidation and disbandment of smaller hospitals - Verringerung der Zahl der Krankenanstalten durch Zusammenlegung und Auflösung kleiner Krankenhäuser - Nekotoroe umen'šenie čisla bol'ničnych učreždenij svjazano s ich ukrupleniem i likvidaciej melkich bol'nic

Note: Besides the hospitals of the USSR Ministry of Health there are special clinics for top functionaries of the Party, the Government, the USSR Ministry of Defense, the Committee for State Security and other agencies. These clinics are under the supervision of the IV. Main Administration of the USSR Council of Ministers. Besides psychiatric clinics there are special psychiatric clinics where - according to reports of Amnesty International - countless Soviet citizens are being "cured" of their political views. There are also so-called "Platnye polikliniki" (Paying Polyclinics) where Soviet citizens are treated for a nominal official fee. All persons holding the honorary title of "Hero of the Soviet Union" are treated in these medical centers and hospitals which are administered by the USSR Ministry of Defense, the Committee for State Security of the USSR Council of Ministers and the USSR Ministry of the Interior, in their respective home towns, depending on where they have served.

Anmerkung: Außerhalb des Netzes der Krankenanstalten des Ministeriums für Gesundheitswesen der UdSSR bestehen Sonderkliniken für Spitzenfunktionäre der Partei, der Staatsapparate, des Verteidigungsministeriums der UdSSR, des Komitees für Staatssicherheit u.a. Behörden. Sie werden von der IV. Hauptverwaltung des Ministerrates der UdSSR verwaltet. Neben psychiatrischen Kliniken bestehen psychiatrische Spezialkliniken, in welchen nach Berichten von Amnesty International viele Sowjetbürger aufgrund ihrer politischen Anschauungen "geheilt" werden. Auch gibt es sogenannte "Platnye polikliniki", in denen von den Bürgern für die ärztliche Behandlung ein geringer offizieller Tarif erhoben wird. Alle Inhaber des Ehrentitels "Held der Sowjetunion" werden an ihrem Wohnort in Polikliniken und Lazaretten (Krankenhäusern) des Verteidigungsministeriums der UdSSR, des Komitees für Staatssicherheit beim Ministerrat der UdSSR und des Innenministeriums der UdSSR behandelt, je nachdem, wo sie gedient haben.

12. PUBLIC ORGANIZATIONS
GESELLSCHAFTLICHE ORGANISATIONEN
OBŠČESTVENNYE ORGANIZACII

12.1 LIST OF LEADING PUBLIC ORGANIZATIONS
VERZEICHNIS DER WICHTIGSTEN GESELLSCHAFTLICHEN ORGANISATIONEN
SPISOK VAŽNEJŠYCH OBŠČESTVENNYCH ORGANIZACII

I. Trade Unions - Gewerkschaften   Professional'nye Sojuzy

II. All-Union Leninist Young Communist League -
Leninscher Kommunistischer Jugendverband -
Vsesojuznyj Leninskij Kommunističeskij Sojuz Molodeži (Komsomol)

III. Consumers' Cooperatives - Genossenschaftliche Vereinigungen -
Kooperativnye ob'edinenija

   Agricultural Cooperative (collective farms) -
   Landwirtschaftliche Genossenschaft (Kolchosen) -
   Sel'skochozjajstvennaja kooperacija (kolchozy)

   Consumers' Cooperative - Konsumgenossenschaft -
   Potrebitel'skaja kooperacija

   Housing Construction Cooperative - Wohnungsbaugenossen-
   schaft - Žiliščno-stroitel'naja kooperacija

IV. Social-political organizations -
Gesellschaftspolitische Organisationen -
Obščestvenno-političeskie organizacii

   Soviet Peace Committee - Sowjetisches Friedenskomitee -
   Sovetskij komitet zaščity mira

   Committee of Soviet Women - Komitee sowjetischer Frauen -
   Komitet sovetskich ženščin

   USSR Committee of Youth Organizations - Komitee der Jugendorganisationen der UdSSR - Komitet molodežnych organizacij SSSR

   Soviet Committee of War Veterans - Sowjetisches Komitee der
   Kriegsveteranen - Sovetskij komitet veteranov vojny

   Union of Soviet Societies for Friendship and Cultural
   Relations with Foreign Countries - Verband der sowjetischen
   Gesellschaften für Freundschaft und kulturelle Verbindungen
   mit dem Ausland - Sojuz sovetskich obščestv družby i kul'-
   turnoj svjazi s zarubežnymi stranami

   Soviet Committee for Solidarity with Asian and African
   Countries - Sowjetisches Komitee für Solidarität mit den
   Ländern Asiens und Afrikas - Sovetskij komitet solidarnosti
   stran Azii i Afriki

V. Scientific, scientific-technical and academic training
societies - Wissenschaftliche, wissenschaftlich-technische und
wissenschaftlich bildende Gesellschaften - Naučnye, naučno-
techničeskie i naučno-prosvetitel'nye obščestva

   All-Union Society for Knowledge - Unionsgesellschaft
   "Znanie" - Vsesojuznoe obščestvo "Znanie"

Public organizations
Gesellschaftl.Organisationen 12.1

Scientific-technical societies - Wissenschaftlich-technische Gesellschaften - Naučno-techničeskie obščestva

All-Union Society of Inventors and Innovators - Unionsgesellschaft der Erfinder und Rationalisatoren - Vsesojuznoe obščestvo izobretatelej i racionalizatorov - VOIR

All-Union Scientific-Medical Societies - Wissenschaftlich-medizinische Unionsgesellschaften - Vsesojuznye naučno-medicinskie obščestva

Society of Philosophers - Philosophen-Gesellschaft - Obščestvo filosofov

VI. Sports and defense societies - Sport- und Verteidigungsgesellschaften - Sportivnye i oboronnye obščestva

Voluntary Sports Societies - Freiwillige Sportgesellschaften - Dobrovol'nye sportivnye obščestva

All-Union Voluntary Society for the Promotion of the Army, Aviation and Navy - Freiwillige Gesellschaft zur Zusammenarbeit mit Armee, Luftwaffe und Flotte - Dobrovol'noe obščestvo sodejstvija armii, aviacii i flotu - DOSAAF

Society of Hunters and Anglers - Gesellschaft der Jäger und Angler - Obščestvo ochotnikov i rybolovov

River and shore patrol societies - Wasserwachtgesellschaften - Obščestva spasanija na vodach - OSVOD

VII. Cultural instructive societies - Kulturell bildende Gesellschaften - Kul'turno-prosvetitel'nye obščestva

Societies for the Protection of Nature - Naturschutzgesellschaften - Obščestva ochrany prirody

Societies for the Protection of Monuments - Gesellschaften für Denkmalschutz - Obščestva ochrany pamjatnikov istorii i kul'tury

Theatre societies - Theatergesellschaften - Teatral'nye obščestva

Choral societies - Chorgesellschaften - Chorovye obščestva

VIII. Creative unions - Schöpferische Verbände - Tvorčeskie sojuzy

USSR Writers' Union - Schriftstellerverband der UdSSR - Sojuz pisatelej SSSR

USSR Journalists' Union - Journalistenverband der UdSSR - Sojuz žurnalistov SSSR

USSR Artists' Union - Kunstmalerverband der UdSSR - Sojuz chudožnikov SSSR

USSR Composers' Union - Komponistenverband der UdSSR - Sojuz kompozitorov SSSR

USSR Cinema Workers' Union - Verband der Filmschaffenden der UdSSR - Sojuz rabotnikov kinematografii SSSR

USSR Architects' Union - Architektenverband der UdSSR - Sojuz architektorov SSSR

IX. Others - Andere - Pročie

Union of Societies of the Red Cross and Red Crescent of the USSR - Verband der Gesellschaften des Roten Kreuzes und des Roten Halbmondes der UdSSR - Sojuz obščestv Krasnogo Kresta i Krasnogo Polumesjaca SSSR

12.1 Public organizations
12.2.1 Gesellschaftl.Organisationen

Voluntary Fire-Brigade - Freiwillige Feuerwehr - Dobrovol'noe požarnoe obŝĉestvo

Philatelists' Society - Philatelisten-Gesellschaft - Obŝĉestvo filatelistov

12.2 TRADE UNIONS - GEWERKSCHAFTEN - PROFESSIONAL'NYE SOJUZY

12.2.1 NUMBER OF TRADE UNION MEMBERS AT USSR TRADE UNION CONGRESSES
ZAHL DER GEWERKSCHAFTSMITGLIEDER ZU GEWERKSCHAFTSKONGRESSEN DER UdSSR
ĈISLO ĈLENOV PROFESSIONAL'NYCH SOJUZOV K S'EZDAM PROFSOJUZOV SSSR
(in thousands - in Tausend - tys.ĉelovek)

Congress Kongress S'ezd	Date - Datum - data	Number of members Mitgliederzahl Ĉislo ĉlenov
I	January-Januar-Janvar' 1918	2,638.8
II	January-Januar-Janvar' 1919	3,422.0
III	April - Aprel' 1920	4,227.0
IV	May - Mai - Maj 1921	8,485.8
V	September - Sentjabr' 1922	5,100.0[1]
VI	November - Nojabr' 1924	6,400.0
VII	December - Dezember - Dekabr' 1926	9,236.0
VIII	December - Dezember - Dekabr' 1928	11,000.0
IX	April - Aprel' 1932	16,500.0
X	April - Aprel' 1949	28,500.0
XI	June - Juni - Ijun' 1954	40,420.0
XII	March - März - Mart 1959	52,780.0
XIII	October - Oktober - Oktjabr' 1963	68,175.6
XIV	February - Februar - Fevral' 1968	86,130.0
XV	March - März - Mart 1972	98,022.0
XVI	March - März - Mart 1977	113,500.0

---

[1] Decrease in membership due to change from obligatory to voluntary membership -
Verringerung der Mitgliederzahl im Zusammenhang mit dem Übergang von der Pflicht- zur freiwilligen Mitgliedschaft.

Public organizations 12.2.2
Gesellschaftl.Organisationen 12.2.3
12.2.4

12.2.2 CHAIRMEN OF THE ALL-UNION CENTRAL COUNCIL OF TRADE UNIONS
VORSITZENDE DES UNIONSZENTRALRATES DER GEWERKSCHAFTEN
PREDSEDATELI VSESOJUZNOGO CENTRAL'NOGO SOVETA PROFESSIONAL'NYCH SOJUZOV

ZINOVEV, G.E.	January-March - Januar-März 1918	1936	liquidated - liquidiert
TOMSKIJ, M.P.	March-März 1918 - 1929	1936	suicide-Selbstmord
SVERNIK, N.M.	1930-1944 and/und 1953-1956	1970	died-gestorben
KUZNECOV, V.V.	1944-1953		
GRIŠIN, V.V.	1956-1967		
SELEPIN, A.N.	1967-1975	1975	discharged - abgesetzt
SIBAEV, A.I.	1976-		

12.2.3 ALL-UNION CENTRAL COUNCIL OF TRADE UNIONS
UNIONSZENTRALRAT DER GEWERKSCHAFTEN
VSESOJUZNYJ CENTRAL'NYJ SOVET PROFESSIONAL'NYCH SOJUZOV
(August 1, 1978 - Stand v. 1.8.1978)

Address-Adresse: Leninskij prospekt, 42, Moskva

Chairman - Vorsitzender -
Predsedatel' — SIBAEV, A.I.

Deputy - Stellvertreter -
Zamestitel'predsedatelja — PROCHOROV, V.I.

Secretaries - Sekretäre -
Sekretari
— BIRJUKOVA, A.P.   SALAEV, S.A.
  BOGATIKOV, V.F.   UŠAKOV, A.P.
  MACKJAVIČIUS, K.Ju.   VIKTOROV, A.V.
  PIMENOV, P.T.   VLADYČENKO, I.M.
       ZEMIJANNIKOVA, L.A.

Chairwoman of the Auditing Commission -
Vorsitzende der Revisionskommission -
Predsedatel' revizionnoj — GUGINA, E.F.

12.2.4 CCs OF THE BRANCH TRADE UNIONS - ZKs DER BRANCHENGEWERKSCHAFTEN -
CK OTRASLEVYCH PROFESSIONAL'NYCH SOJUZOV
(January 1, 1977 - Stand v. 1.1.1977)

Trade Union - Gewerkschaft - Professional'nyj sojuz	Chairman - Vorsitzender - Predsedatel'
Aircraft and defense industry - Flugzeug- und Verteidigungsindustrie - rabočich aviacionnoj i oboronnoj promyšlennosti Leninskij prospekt, 42, Moskva	— KAREV, A.T.
Civil aviation - zivile Luftfahrt - aviacionnych rabotnikov ul. Kržižanovskogo, 20/30, Moskva	— ZUEV, V.A.

585

12.2.4 Public organizations
Gesellschaftl.Organisationen

Trade Union – Gewerkschaft – Professional'nyj sojuz	Chairman – Vorsitzender – Predsedatel'
Motor transport and road construction – Kraftverkehr und Straßenwesen – rabočich avtomobil'nogo transporta i šossejnych dorog ul. Krživanovskogo, 20/30, Moskva	– KONNOV, V.K.
Geological prospecting – geologische Schürfarbeiten – rabočich geologorazvedočnych rabot ul. Krživanovskogo, 20/30, Moskva	– KURZIN, L.N.
State trade enterprises and cooperative societies – Staatshandelsbetriebe und Konsumgenossenschaften – rabotnikov gosudarstvennoj torgovli i potrebitel' skoj kooperacii Leninskij prospekt, 42, Moskva	– SALAUROVA, A.G.
State institutions – staatliche Institutionen – rabotnikov gosudarstvennych učreždenij Leninskij prospekt, 42, Moskva	– MAKEEV, G.A.
Railway transport – Eisenbahntransport – rabočich železnodoroznogo transporta Sad.Spasskaja, 21, Moskva	– KOVALEV, N.I.
Culture – Kultur – rabotnikov kul'tury Leninskij prospekt, 42, Moskva	– PAŠKOV, M.V.
Timber, paper and wood processing industry – Holz-, Papier- und holzbearbeitende Industrie – rabočich lesnoj, bumažnoj i derevoobrabatyvajuščej promyšlennosti Leninskij prospekt, 42, Moskva	– BELIKOV, B.A.
Mechanical engineering industry – Maschinenbauindustrie – rabočich mašinostroenija Leninskij prospekt, 42, Moskva	– DRAGUNOV, N.V.
Public health – Gesundheitswesen – medicinskich rabotnikov Leninskij prospekt, 42, Moskva	– NOVAK, L.I.
Local industry, municipal and consumer services – lokale Industrie, Kommunal- und Dienstleistungsbetriebe – rabočich mestnoj promyšlennosti i kommunal'nobytovych predprijatij Leninskij prospekt, 42, Moskva	– SOROKINA, G.P.
Metallurgical industry – Metallindustrie – rabočich metallurgičeskoj promyšlennosti Leninskij prospekt, 42, Moskva	– KOSTJUKOV, I.I.
High-sea and inland navigation – Hochsee- und Binnenschiffahrt – rabočich morskogo i rečnogo flota Leninskij prospekt, 42, Moskva	– PETRIKEEV, V.I.
Petrol, chemical and gas industry – Erdöl-, chemische und Gasindustrie – rabočich neftjanoj, chimičeskoj i gazovoj promyšlennosti Leninskij prospekt, 42, Moskva	– SVETCOV, N.P.
Food industry – Nahrungsmittelindustrie – rabočich piščevoj promyšlennosti Leninskij prospekt, 42, Moskva	– MATROSOVA, N.L.

Public organizations 12.2.4
Gesellschaftl.Organisationen 12.2.5

Trade Union - Gewerkschaft - Professional'nyj sojuz	Chairman - Vorsitzender - Predsedatel'

Schools, universities and scientific institutions -
Schul- und Hochschulwesen und wissenschaftliche
Institutionen - rabotnikov prosveščenija, vysšej
školy i naučnych učreždenij
    Leninskij prospekt, 42, Moskva — JANUŠKOVSKAJA, T.P.

Radio and electronic industry - Radio- und elektronische
Industrie - rabočich radio- i elektronnoj promyšlennosti
    Golutvinskij p., 3, Moskva — IVANOV, V.I.

Communications - Post- und Fernmeldewesen - rabotnikov svjazi
    ul. Vavilova, 68, Moskva — KANAEVA, A.M.

Agriculture and registration organs -
Landwirtschaft und Erfassungsorgane - rabočich i
služaščich sel'skogo chozjajstva i zagotovok
    Leninskij prospekt, 42, Moskva — SKURATOV, I.F.

Construction and construction materials industry -
Bauwesen und Baustoffindustrie - rabočich stroitel'stva
i promyšlennosti stroitel'nych materialov
    Leninskij prospekt, 42, Moskva — LANSIN, I.A.

Shipbuilding industry - Schiffsbauindustrie -
rabočich sudostroitel'noj promyšlennosti
    Moskva — BURIMOVIČ, A.G.

Textile and light industry - Textil- und Leichtindustrie -
rabočich tekstil'noj i legkoj promyšlennosti
    Leninskij prospekt, 42, Moskva — DOLŽENKOVA, M.G.

Coal industry - Kohlenindustrie -
rabočich ugol'noj promyšlennosti
    Leninskij prospekt, 42, Moskva — EFREMENKO, E.I.

Power plants and electrical engineering industry -
Kraftwerke und elektrotechnische Industrie -
rabočich elektrostancij i elektrotechničeskoj promyšlennosti
    Leninskij prospekt, 42, Moskva — SIMOČATOV, N.P.

12.2.5 TRADE UNION COUNCILS OF THE UNION REPUBLICS - GEWERKSCHAFTSRÄTE DER UNIONSREPUBLIKEN - SOVETY PROFSOJUZOV SOJUZNYCH RESPUBLIK

Republic-Republik- Respublika A.	Chairman-Vorsitzender- Predsedatel' B.	Number of members (in millions) Mitgliederzahl (in Millionen) Čislo členov (mln. čelovek) 1.1.1977 C.
Ukrainskaja SSR	SOLOGUB, V.A.	22.0
Belorusskaja SSR	POLOZOV, N.N.	4.2
Uzbekskaja SSR	MACHMUDOVA, N.M.	3.5
Kazachskaja SSR	MUKAŠEV, S.M.	5.8
Gruzinskaja SSR	MOSAŠVILI, T.I.	2.0
Azerbajdžanskaja SSR	GUSEJNOVA, Z.I.	1.7
Litovskaja SSR	FERENSAS, A.A.	1.5

12.2.5 Public organizations
12.2.6 Gesellschaftl.Organisationen
12.3.1

A.	B.	C.
Moldavskaja SSR	PETRIK, P.P.	1.5
Latvijskaja SSR	ZITMANIS, A.K.	1.3
Kirgizskaja SSR	ABAKIROV, E.	1.0
Tadžikskaja SSR	CHAJDAROV, A.	0.8
Armjanskaja SSR	SAAKJAN, L.G.	1.2
Turkmenskaja SSR	CARYEV, M.A.	0.6
Estonskaja SSR	LENCMAN, L.N.	0.7

12.2.6
SOCIETIES AND ORGANIZATIONS WORKING UNDER THE GUIDANCE OF TRADE UNIONS
UNTER DER LEITUNG DER GEWERKSCHAFTEN TÄTIGE GESELLSCHAFTEN UND ORGANISATIONEN
POD RUKOVODSTVOM PROFSOJUZOV RABOTAJUŠCIE OBŠČESTVA I ORGANIZACII

Scientific-technical societies - Wissenschaftlich-technische Gesellschaften - Naučno-techničkie obščestva - NTO

All-Union Society of Inventors and Innovators - Unionsgesellschaft der Erfinder und Rationalisatoren - Vsesojuznoe obščestvo izobretatelej i racionalizatorov-VOIR

Voluntary sports societies - Freiwillige Sportgesellschaften - Dobrovol'nye sportivnye obščestva - DSO

Organizations for tourism and excursions - Organisationen für Tourismus und Exkursionen - Turistsko-ekskursionnye organizacii

12.3 ALL-UNION LENINIST YOUNG COMMUNIST LEAGUE
LENINSCHER KOMMUNISTISCHER JUGENDVERBAND - KOMSOMOL
VSESOJUZNYJ LENINSKIJ KOMMUNISTIČESKIJ SOJUZ MOLODEŽI - VLKSM

12.3.1 NUMBER OF MEMBERS AT KOMSOMOL CONGRESSES - ZAHL DER MITGLIEDER
ZU KOMSOMOLKONGRESSEN - ČISLENNOST' VLKSM K S'EZDAM KOMSOMOLA

Congress Kongress S'ezd	Date - Datum - Data	Number of members Mitgliederzahl Čislo členov
I	October-Oktober-Oktjabr' 1918	22,100
II	February-Februar-Fevral' 1919	96,096
III	October-Oktober-Oktjabr' 1920	482,342
IV	September-Sentjabr' 1921	475,000
V	October-Oktober-Oktjabr' 1922	303,944
VI	July-Juli-Ijul' 1924	702,000
VII	March-März-Mart 1926	1,750,000
VIII	May-Mai-Maj 1928	1,960,000
IX	January-Januar-Janvar' 1931	2,897,000

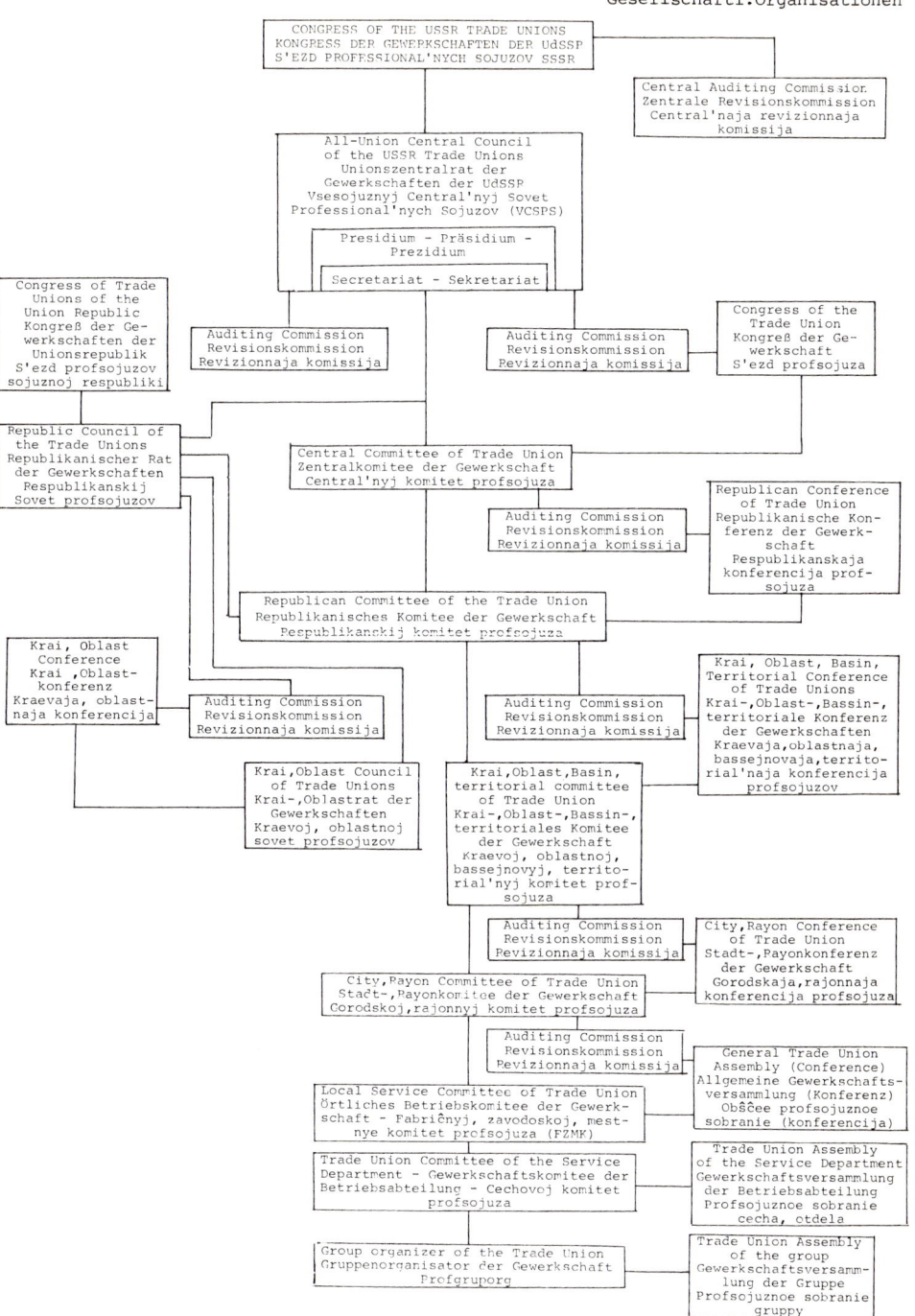

Public Organizations
Gesellschaftl. Organisationen

```
CONGRESS OF THE USSR TRADE UNIONS
KONGRESS DER GEWERKSCHAFTEN DER UdSSR
S'EZD PROFESSIONAL'NYCH SOJUZOV SSSR
```

- Central Auditing Commission / Zentrale Revisionskommission / Central'naja revizionnaja komissija

All-Union Central Council of the USSR Trade Unions
Unionszentralrat der Gewerkschaften der UdSSR
Vsesojuznyj Central'nyj Sovet Professional'nych Sojuzov (VCSPS)

- Presidium – Präsidium – Prezidium
- Secretariat – Sekretariat

Auditing Commission / Revisionskommission / Revizionnaja komissija

Auditing Commission / Revisionskommission / Revizionnaja komissija

Congress of Trade Unions of the Union Republic / Kongreß der Gewerkschaften der Unionsrepublik / S'ezd profsojuzov sojuznoj respubliki

Congress of the Trade Union / Kongreß der Gewerkschaft / S'ezd profsojuza

Republic Council of the Trade Unions / Republikanischer Rat der Gewerkschaften / Respublikanskij Sovet profsojuzov

Central Committee of Trade Union
Zentralkomitee der Gewerkschaft
Central'nyj komitet profsojuza

Auditing Commission / Revisionskommission / Revizionnaja komissija

Republican Conference of Trade Union / Republikanische Konferenz der Gewerkschaft / Pespublikanskaja konferencija profsojuza

Republican Committee of the Trade Union
Republikanisches Komitee der Gewerkschaft
Respublikanskij komitet profsojuza

Krai, Oblast Conference / Krai-, Oblastkonferenz / Kraevaja, oblastnaja konferencija

Auditing Commission / Revisionskommission / Revizionnaja komissija

Auditing Commission / Revisionskommission / Revizionnaja komissija

Krai, Oblast, Basin, Territorial Conference of Trade Unions / Krai-, Oblast-, Bassin-, territoriale Konferenz der Gewerkschaften / Kraevaja, oblastnaja, bassejnovaja, territorial'naja konferencija profsojuzov

Krai, Oblast Council of Trade Unions / Krai-, Oblastrat der Gewerkschaften / Kraevoj, oblastnoj sovet profsojuzov

Krai, Oblast, Basin, territorial committee of Trade Union
Krai-, Oblast-, Bassin-, territoriales Komitee der Gewerkschaft
Kraevoj, oblastnoj, bassejnovyj, territorial'nyj komitet profsojuza

Auditing Commission / Revisionskommission / Revizionnaja komissija

City, Rayon Conference of Trade Union / Stadt-, Rayonkonferenz der Gewerkschaft / Gorodskaja, rajonnaja konferencija profsojuza

City, Rayon Committee of Trade Union
Stadt-, Rayonkomitee der Gewerkschaft
Gorodskoj, rajonnyj komitet profsojuza

Auditing Commission / Revisionskommission / Revizionnaja komissija

General Trade Union Assembly (Conference) / Allgemeine Gewerkschaftsversammlung (Konferenz) / Obščee profsojuznoe sobranie (konferencija)

Local Service Committee of Trade Union
Örtliches Betriebskomitee der Gewerkschaft – Fabričnyj, zavodskoj, mestnye komitet profsojuza (FZMK)

Trade Union Committee of the Service Department
Gewerkschaftskomitee der Betriebsabteilung
Cechovoj komitet profsojuza

Trade Union Assembly of the Service Department / Gewerkschaftsversammlung der Betriebsabteilung / Profsojuznoe sobranie cecha, otdela

Group organizer of the Trade Union
Gruppenorganisator der Gewerkschaft
Profgruporg

Trade Union Assembly of the group / Gewerkschaftsversammlung der Gruppe / Profsojuznoe sobranie gruppy

12.3.1 Public organizations
12.3.2 Gesellschaftl.Organisationen

Congress Kongress S'ezd	Date - Datum - Data	Number of members Mitgliederzahl Čislo členov
X	March-März-Mart 1936	3,981,777
XI	April-Aprel' 1949	9,283,289
XII	March-März-Mart 1954	18,825,327
XIII	April-Aprel' 1958	18,092,538
XIV	April-Aprel' 1962	19,400,000
XV	May-Mai-Maj 1966	23,050,700
XVI	May-Mai-Maj 1970	27,028,301
XVII	April-Aprel' 1974	33,760,000
XVIII	April-Aprel' 1978	35,600,000 (1.1.1977)

12.3.2   CC OF USSR KOMSOMOL - ZK DES KOMSOMOL DER UdSSR - CK VLKSM
(August 1, 1978 - Stand v. 1.8.1978)

First Secretary - Erster Sekretär - Pervyj sekretar'	- PASTUCHOV, B.N.	
Secretaries and members of the bureau - Sekretäre und Mitglieder des Büros - Sekretari i členy bjuro	- DEREVJANKO, A.P. GRIGOREV, V.V. GUSEJNOV, V.A. FEDULOVA, A.V. FILIPPOV, D.N.	MIŠIN, V.M. NOVOŽILOVA, Z.G. OCHROMIJ, D.A. ŽUGANOV, A.V.
Members of the bureau - Mitglieder des Büros - Členy bjuro	- BORCOV, A.G. GAFURZANOV, E.G. GANIČEV, V.N. GLEBOV, V.S. JANAEV, G.I. KOLJAKIN, A.N.	KORNIENKO, A.I. LYSENKO, I.E. SIDORIK, V.G. SULTANOV, K.S. VOLČICHIN, V.G.
Candidates of the bureau - Kandidaten des Büros - Kandidaty v členy bjuro	- ANDRIANOV, N.E. BALTRUNAS, V.S. GROŠEV, V.P. KATUNIN, V.A.	KULEŠOV, S.P. PLATONOV, K.M. ROGATIN, B.N.
Chairman of the Central Auditing Committee - Vorsitzender der Zentralen Revisionskommission - Predsedatel' Central'noj revizionnoj komissii	- ARSENTEV, V.B.	

Public organizations 12.3.3
Gesellschaftl.Organisationen 12.3.4

12.3.3 CCs OF THE KOMSOMOL OF THE UNION REPUBLICS - ZKs DES KOMSOMOL DER UNIONSREPUBLIKEN - CK DES LKSM SOJUZNYCH RESPUBLIK

Republic Republik Respublika	First Secretary Erster Sekretär Pervyj Sekretar'	Number of members Mitgliederzahl Cislennost'členov (1.1.1977)
Ukrainskaja SSR	KORNIENKO, A.I.	5,962,920
Belorusskaja SSR	PLATONOV, K.M.	1,280,274
Uzbekskaja SSR	GAFURŽANOV, E.	1,721,923
Kazachskaja SSR	SULTANOV, K.S.	1,704,077
Gruzinskaja SSR	SARTAVA, Ž.K.	634,424
Azerbajdžanskaja SSR	GUSEJNOV, V.A.	700,110
Litovskaja SSR	BALTRUNAS, V.S.	365,829
Moldavskaja SSR	GUCU, I.T.	505,272
Latvijskaja SSR	PLAUDE, A.K.	281,350
Kirgizskaja SSR	RYSMENDIEV, A.A.	387,475
Tadžikskaja SSR	SATOROV, A.	324,896
Armjanskaja SSR	KOTANDŽJAN, G.S.	401,700
Turkmenskaja SSR	ISANKULIEV, O.I.	315,395
Estonskaja SSR	TOOME, J.Ch.	145,773

12.3.4
NUMBER OF CPSU MEMBERS AND CANDIDATES WITHIN THE KOMSOMOL ("Party Core")
ZAHL DER IM KOMSOMOL TÄTIGEN MITGLIEDER UND KANDIDATEN DER KPdSU ("Parteikern")
KOLIČESTVO ČLENOV I KANDIDATOV KPSS RABOTAJUŠČICH V KOMSOMOLE ("Partijnoe jadro")
(as of January 1 of the corresponding year - zum 1. Januar des
jeweiligen Jahres - na 1 janvarja sootvetstvujuščego goda)

1966	268,240
1967	267,328
1968	310,152
1969	388,348
1970	460,638
1971	549,662
1978	1,100,000

12.3.5 Public organizations
12.4 Gesellschaftl. Organisationen

12.3.5 ALL-UNION PIONEERS ORGANIZATION - UNIONSPIONIERORGANISATION - VSESOJUZNAJA PIONERSKAJA ORGANIZACIJA

Chairwoman - Vorsitzende: FEDULOVA, A.V.

Number of members - Mitgliederzahl 1970: 23 million-Millionen

Organ: "Pionerskaja pravda" as well as the organs of the pioneers organizations in the 15 union republics - sowie Organe der Pionierorganisationen in den 15 Unionsrepubliken

12.4 NUMBER OF MEMBERS OF SOME VOLUNTARY ALL-UNION SOCIETIES MITGLIEDERZAHL EINIGER FREIWILLIGER UNIONSGESELLSCHAFTEN ČISLENNYJ SOSTAV NEKOTORYCH VSESOJUZNYCH DOBROVOL'NÝCH OBŠČESTV (1965 - 1976)

Year Jahr God	NTO of USSR[1] NTO der UdSSR NTO SSSR ('000-Tsd.-tys.)	VOIR[2]	"Znaniye" "Znanie" ('000-Tsd.-tys.)	SOKK and KP[3] SOKK und KP SOKK i KP
1965	2477.4	3,580,048	1460.8	61,108,701
1966	2781.5	4,063,542	1637.3	65,573,881
1967	3059.3	4,451,607	1823.5	69,931,804
1968	3354.1	4,781,863	1980.7	75,358,889
1969	3644.9	5,080,715	2088.1	78,541,681
1970	4104.8	5,437,881	2187.9	81,829,718
1971	4752.8	5,781,528	2318.9	84,484,904
1972	5424.7	6,204,973	2457.1	87,151,138
1973	5965.0	6,536,702	2596.0	89,199,382
1974	6469.5	7,026,893	2705.3	91,216,309
1975	7012.2	7,607,126	2855.2	93,178,961
1976	7542.6	8,336,931	2979.3	94,976,471

[1] NTO - USSR Scientific-Technical Society - Wissenschaftlich-Technische Gesellschaft der UdSSR - Naučno-Techničeskoe obščestvo SSSR
[2] VOIR - All-Union Society of Inventors and Innovators - Unionsgesellschaft der Erfinder und Rationalisatoren - Vsesojuznoe obščestvo izobretatelej i racionalizatorov
[3] SOKK KP - Union of Societies of the Red Cross and Red Crescent of the USSR - Verband der Gesellschaften des Roten Kreuzes und des Roten Halbmondes der UdSSR - Sojuz obščestv Krasnogo kresta i Krasnogo polumesjaca

12.5
ADDITIONAL INFORMATION ON SOME PUBLIC ORGANIZATIONS
ZUSÄTZLICHE INFORMATIONEN ÜBER EINIGE GESELLSCHAFTL.ORGANISATIONEN

All-Union Society for Knowledge - Unionsgesellschaft "Znanie" -
Vsesojuznoe obščestvo "Znanie"
    Centr, Prosp. Serova, 4, Moskva
    founded - gegründet 1947
    Chairman - Vorsitzender: BASOV, N.G.
    on 1/1/1977 - z.1.1.1977: number of members - Mitgliederzahl: 3,130,400
    number of basic organizations - Zahl der Grundorganisationen: 146,869

All-Union Voluntary Society for the Promotion of the Army, Aviation & Navy -
Freiwillige Gesellschaft zur Zusammenarbeit mit Armee, Luftwaffe und Flotte -
Dobrovol'noe obščestvo sodejstvija armii, aviacii i flotu (DOSAAF)
    founded - gegründet 1951
    Chairman of the CC - Vorsitzender des ZK: POKRYŠKIN, A.I. (Marshal of the
        Air Force - Marschall der Luftwaffe)
    on 1/1/1977 - z.1.1.1977: number of members - Mitgliederzahl:
        above 80 million - über 80 Millionen
    number of basic organizations - Zahl der Grundorganisationen: 330,000
    Organs - Organe: Newspaper - Zeitung: "Sovetskij patriot"
    Journals - Zeitschriften: "Voennye znanija", "Krylja Rodiny", "Radio",
    "Za rulem"

Committee of Soviet Women - Komitee sowjetischer Frauen -
Komitet sovetskich ženščin
    founded - gegründet 1941
    Chairwoman - Vorsitzende: NIKOLAEVA-TEREŠKOVA, V.V. (cosmonaut,female-Kosmonautin)
    Organ: "Sovetskaja ženščina"

Committee of Youth Organizations of the USSR - Komitee der Jugendorganisationen
der UdSSR - Komitet molodežnych organizacij SSSR (KMO SSSR)
    founded - gegründet 1956
    Chairman - Vorsitzender: JANAEV, G.I.
    Organ: "Vestnik KMO SSSR"

Soviet Committee for European Security and Cooperation - Sowjetisches Komitee
für europäische Sicherheit und Zusammenarbeit - Sovetskij Komitet za evropejskuju
bezopasnost' i sotrudničestvo
    founded - gegründet 1971
    Chairman - Vorsitzender: SITIKOV, A.P.
    Organ: "Informacionnyj bjulleten'"

Soviet Committee for Solidarity with Asian and African Countries -
Sowjetisches Komitee für Solidarität mit den Ländern Asiens und Afrikas -
Sovetskij komitet solidarnosti stran Azii i Afriki (SKSSAA)
    Kropotkinskaja ul., 10, Moskva
    founded - gegründet 1956
    Chairman - Vorsitzender: IBRAGIMOV, M.A.
Soviet Committee of War Veterans - Sowjetisches Komitee der Kriegsveteranen -
Sovetskij komitet veteranov vojny
    founded - gegründet 1956
    Chairman - Vorsitzender: BATOV, P.I. (Army General - Armeegeneral)

Soviet Association for International Law - Sowjetische Gesellschaft für internationales Recht - Sovetskaja associacija meždunarodnogo prava
    founded - gegründet 1957
    Chairman - Vorsitzender: TUNKIN, G.I.

12.5 Public organizations
Gesellschaftl.Organisationen

number of members - Mitgliederzahl 1976: above 360 - über 360
Organ: "Sovetskij ežegodnik meždunarodnogo prava"

Soviet Peace Committee - Sowjetisches Friedenskomitee - Sovetskij komitet zaščity mira
  Kropotkinskaja ul., 10, Moskva
  founded - gegründet 1949
  Chairman - Vorsitzender: TICHONOV, N.S.
  Organ: "Vek XX i mir"

Soviet Sociological Association - Sowjetische Soziologische Gesellschaft - Sovetskaja Sociologičeskaja Associacija
  founded - gegründet 1958

Union Council of Collective Farms - Unionsrat der Kolchosen - Sojuznyj Sovet Kolchozov
  Chairman - Vorsitzender: MESJAC, V.K. (USSR Minister of Agriculture - Landwirtschaftsminister der UdSSR)

Union of Societies of the Red Cross and Red Crescent of the USSR - Verband der Gesellschaften des Roten Kreuzes und des Roten Halbmondes der UdSSR - Sojuz obščestv Krasnogo Kresta i Krasnogo Polumesjaca SSSR (SOKK i KP SSSR)
  Pervyj Čeremuškinskij Prosp., 5, Moskva
  founded - gegründet 1925
  Chairman - Vorsitzender: BALTIJSKIJ, V.A.
  Number of basic organizations - Zahl der Grundorganisationen 1976: 410
  Organ: "Sovetskij Krasnyj Krest"

Union of Soviet Societies for Friendship and Cultural Relations with Foreign Countries - Verband der sowjetischen Gesellschaften für Freundschaft und kulturelle Verbindungen mit dem Ausland - Sojuz sovetskich obščestv družby i kul'turnoj svjazi s zarubežnymi stranami (SOD)
  Prosp. Kalinina, 14, Moskva
  founded - gegründet 1958
  Chairwoman - Vorsitzende: KRUGLOVA, Z.M.
  Organs - Organe: "Moskovaskie novosti", "Kul'tura i žizn'"

USSR Union of Architects - Architektenverband der UdSSR - Sojuz architektorov SSSR
  ul. Ščuseva, 3, Moskva
  founded - gegründet 1932
  First Secretary - Erster Sekretär: ORLOV, G.M.
  Number of members on 1/1/1977 - Mitgliederzahl z. 1.1.1977: 13,903
  Organ: "Architektura SSSR"

USSR Union of Artists - Kunstmalerverband der UdSSR - Sojuz chudožnikov SSSR
  Gogolevskij bul'var, 10, Moskva
  Chairman - Vorsitzender: PONOMAREV, N.A.
  First Secretary - Erster Sekretär: SALACHOV, T.T.
  Number of members on 1/1/1977 - Mitgliederzahl z. 1.1.1977: 15,390
  Organs - Organe: "Tvorčestvo", "Dekorativnoe iskusstvo", "Iskusstvo"
  Publishing house - Verlag: "Sovetskij chodožnik"

USSR Union of Cinema Workers - Verband der Filmschaffenden der UdSSR - Sojuz rabotnikov kinematografii SSSR
  Vasilevskaja ul., 13, Moskva
  founded - gegründet 1965
  First Secretary - Erster Sekretär: KULIDŽANOV, L.A.
  Number of members on 1/1/1977 - Mitgliederzahl z. 1.1.1977: 5,267
  Organs - Organe: "Iskusstvo kino", "Sovetskij ekran"

USSR Union of Composers - Komponistenverband der UdSSR - Sojuz kompozitorov SSSR
  ul. Neždanavoj, 8/10, Moskva
  founded - gegründet 1932
  First Secretary - Erster Sekretär: CHRENNIKOV, T.N.
  Number of members on 1/1/1977 - Mitgliederzahl z. 1.1.1977: 1,997
  Organs - Organe: "Sovetskaja muzyka", "Muzykal'naja žizn'"

USSR Union of Journalists - Journalistenverband der UdSSR -
Sojuz žurnalistov SSSR
  Prospekt Mira, 30, Moskva
  founded - gegründet 1959
  Chairman - Vorsitzender: AFANASEV, V.G.
  Number of members - Mitgliederzahl 1976: above - über 60,000
  Organs - Organe: "Za rubežom", "Žurnalist", "Sovetskoe foto",
                   "Demokratičeskij žurnalist", "Informacionnyj vestnik"

USSR Union of Writers - Schriftstellerverband der UdSSR - Sojuz pisatelej SSSR
  ul. Vorovskogo, 52, Moskva
  founded - gegründet 1932
  First Secretary - Erster Sekretär: MARKOV, G.M.
  Number of members on 1/1/1977 - Mitgliederzahl z. 1.1.1977: 7,955
  Publishing houses - Verlage: "Literaturnaja gazeta", "Sovetskij pisatel'"
  Organs - Organe: "Literaturnaja gazeta"
  Journals - Zeitschriften: "Novyj Mir", "Znamja", "Družba narodov",
                            "Voprosy literatury", "Literaturnoe obozrenie",
                            "Detskaja literatura", "Inostrannaja literatura",
                            "Junost'", "Sovetskaja literatura", "Teatr",
                            "Sovetskaja rodina", "Zvezda", "Koster"

13. RELIGION — RELIGIJA

13.1
Council for Religious Affairs at the USSR Council of Ministers -
Rat für Religiöse Angelegenheiten beim Ministerrat der UdSSR -
Sovet po delam religij pri Soveta Ministrov SSSR

Smolenskij Bul'var, 11/2, Moskva
Chairman - Vorsitzender: KUROEDOV, V.A.

(In the 15 union republics: Councils at the Councils of Ministers
of the Union Republics - in den 15 Unionsrepubliken: Räte bei
den Ministerräten der Unionsrepubliken)

13.2 GENERAL DATA - ALLGEMEINE DATEN - OBŠČIE SVEDENIJA

	1917	1976
Number of churches - Zahl der Kirchen:		
Orthodox churches - orthodoxe Kirchen	77,676[1]	7,500
Catholic churches - katholische Kirchen	4,200[1]	ca. 1,000
Islam mosques - islamische Moscheen	24,500	ca. 1,000
Old Believers' churches - Kirchen der Altgläubigen	1,500	300
Synagogues - Synagogen	5,000	ca. 200
Sects - Sekten	--	4,000

	1977
Number of Orthodox priests - Zahl der orthodoxen Pfarrer	5,900
Number of rabbis - Zahl der Rabbiner	ca. 50
Number of believers - Zahl der Gläubigen[2]	approx. 20 to 25% of the grown-up urban and rural population - ca. 20-25% der erwachsenen Stadt- und Landbevölkerung
Number of all religions and denominations - Zahl aller Religionen und Richtungen	48
Number of religious sects - Zahl der religiösen Sekten of which 60% loyal to the Soviet regime - davon 60% dem sowjetischen Regime loyal	4,000
Number of illegal sects - Zahl der illegalen Sekten	1,200

---

[1] for - für 1939
[2] according to official data - nach offiziellen Angaben

13.3 THE RUSSIAN ORTHODOX CHURCH
DIE RUSSISCH-ORTHODOXE KIRCHE
RUSSKAJA PRAVOSLAVNAJA CERKOV'

Administrative formation - Administrative Gliederung:

      4 exarchies - Exarchien - Ekzarchata
     76 eparchies - Eparchien - Eparchij
     11 vicarages - Vikariate - Vikariatstv

Included are the eparchies and vicarages united in the three patriarchal exarchies abroad - Western Europe, Central Europe, Central and South America. In the Soviet Union there exist 2 theological academies, 3 seminaries and 16 monasteries. Publications: "Zhurnal Moskovskoy Patriarchy" (in Russian and English), theological papers, religious literature and church-calendars; in the Ukraine: "Pravoslavny visnyk". -
Darunter auch die in den drei patriarchalischen Exarchien im Ausland - Westeuropa, Mitteleuropa, Zentral- und Südamerika - vereinigten Eparchien und Vikariate. In der Sowjetunion gibt es 2 Geistliche Akademien, 3 Seminare und 16 Klöster. Publikationen: "Žurnal Moskovskoj Patriarchii" (in russischer und englischer Sprache), theologische Arbeiten, religiöse Literatur und Kirchenkalender; in der Ukraine: "Pravoslavnyj visnyk".

The Patriarch of Moscow and All Russia - Patriarch von Moskau und ganz Rußland:

        PIMEN (S.M. Izvekov)

Metropolitans, Resident Members of the Holy Synod -
Metropoliten, Ständige Mitglieder des Heiligen Synods:

                                 Metropolitan of - Metropolit von
NIKODIM   (B.G.Rotov)   Leningrad and/und Novgorod (died 9/5/1978 -
                                                      gestorben 5.9.1978)
FILARET   (M.A.Denisenko)   Kiev and Galicia - Kiev und Galizien
ALEKSIJ   (A.M.Ridiger)   Tallinn and Estonia - Tallinn und Estland
IUVENALIJ (V.K.Pojarkov)   Kruticy and/und Kolomna

Metropolitans - Metropoliten:

PALLADIJ   (Serstjannikov)   Orel and/und Brjansk
FILARET   (K.V.Vachromeev)   Berlin and Central Europe - Berlin und Mitteleuropa
IOANN   (D.A.Razumov)   Pskov and/und Porchov
ANTONIJ   (A.Blum)   Suroga
IOANN   (K.N.Vendland)   Jaroslavl and/und Rostov
SERGIJ   (S.V.Petrov)   Kherson and/und Odessa
NIKOLAJ   (E.N.Jurik)   Lvov and/und Ternopol
ANTONIJ   (A.S.Melnikov)   Minsk and Belorussia - Minsk und Belorußland

Archbishops - Erzbischöfe:
                                 Archbishop of - Erzbischof von
ALEKSIJ   (A.E.van der Mensbrugge) Düsseldorf
ALEKSIJ   (V.A.Konoplev)   Kalinin and/und Kašir
ANTONIJ   (O.I.Vakarik)   Černigov and/und Nežin
DAMJAN   (D.G.Marčuk)   Volhynia and Rovno - Wolhynien und Rovno
GERMOGEN   (G.V.Orechov)   Krasnodar and/und Kuban
IONAFAN   (I.M.Kopalovič)   Kišinev and Moldavia/und Moldau
IOSIF   (I.M.Savraš)   Ivano-Frankovsk and/und Kolomyja
IRENEJ   (I.V.Zuzemil)   Baden and Bavaria/und Bayern
KASSIAN   (S.N.Jaroslavskij) Kostroma and/und Galič
LEONID   (L.K.Poljakov)   Riga and Latvia/und Lettland

13.3 Religion

		Archbishop of - Erzbischof von
LEONTIJ	(L.F.Bondar)	Orenburg and/und Buzuluk
LEONTIJ	(I.A.Gudimov)	Simferopol and Crimea / und Krim
MIKHAIL	(M.A.Čub)	Tambov and/und Mičurinsk
NIKODIM	(N.S.Rusnak)	Charkov and/und Bogoduchov
NIKOLAJ	(O.N.Syčkovskij)	Perm and/und Solikamsk
NIKOLAJ	(N.V.Kutepov)	Gorkij and/und Arzamas
PITIRIM	(K.V.Nečaev)	Volokolamsk
PLATON	(V.P.Udovenko)	Argentina and South America - Argentinien und Südamerika
VARFOLOMEJ	(N.N.Gandorovskij)	Taškent and Central Asia / und Mittelasien
VASILIJ	(Krivošein)	Brussels and Belgium - Brüssel und Belgien
VLADIMIR	(V.S.Kotljarov)	Vladimir and/und Suzdal
VLADIMIR	(V.M.Sabodan)	Dmitrov

Bishops - Bischöfe:		Bishop of - Bischof von
AGATHANGEL	(A.M.Savvin)	Vinnica and/und Braclav
AMVROSIJ	(A.P.Sčurov)	Ivanovo and/und Kinešma
ANATOLIJ	(E.V.Kuznecov)	Zvenigorod
ANTONIJ	(A.M.Savgorodnij)	Stavropol and/und Baku
CHRISANT	(Ja.A.Čepil)	Kirov and/und Slobodskoj
CHRIZOSTOM	(G.F.Martyškin)	Kursk and/und Belgorod
DAMASKIN	(A.I.Bodryj)	Vologda and/und Velikij Ustijug
FEODOSIJ	(M.N.Dikun)	Poltava and/und Kremenčug
FEODOSIJ	(I.I.Procjuk)	Smolensk and/und Vjazma
GEDEON	(A.N.Dokukin)	Novosibirsk and/und Barnaul
GERMAN	(G.E.Timofeev)	Tula and/und Belev
HIOB	(D.Ja.Tyvonjuk)	Zarajsk
IAKOV	(Akkersdaik)	The Hague and Netherlands - Den Haag und Niederlande
IOANN	(I.M.Snyčev)	Kuibyšev and/und Syzran
IOANN	(V.N.Bodnarčuk)	Zitomir and/und Ovruč
IOASAF	(V.S.Ovsjannikov)	Rostov and/und Novočerkassk
IRENEJ	(I.P.Seredni)	Ufa and/und Sterlitamak
KIRILL	(Gundjaev)	Vyborg
KLIMENT	(A.A.Perestjuk)	Sverdlovsk and/und Kurgan
MAKARIJ	(L.N.Svistun)	Head of the delegation of the Moscow Patriarchate in Geneva - Leiter der Vertretung des Patriarchats Moskau in Genf
MARK	(Savykin)	Ladoga
MAKSIM	(B.Krocha)	Omsk and/und Tjumen
MELITON	(M.D.Solovev)	Tichvin
MELKHISEDEK	(V.M.Lebedev)	Penza and/und Saransk
MICHAIL	(M.N.Mudjugin)	Astrakhan and/und Enotaevka
NIKOLAJ	(P.Sajama)	Možajsk
NIKON	(N.V.Fomičev)	Kaluga and/und Borovsk
PANTELEJMON	(S.A.Mitrjukovskij)	Kazan and/und Marijsk
PIMEN	(P.V.Chmelevskij)	Saratov and/und Volgograd
PJOTR	(P.l'Huillier)	Korsun
SAVVA	(A.P.Babinec)	Mukačevo and/und Uzgorod
SERAFIM	(V.I.Rodinov)	Zürich
SERAFIM	(Gačkovskij)	Alma Ata and Kazakhstan/und Kasachstan
SERAPION	(N.S.Fadeev)	Irkutsk and/und Čita
SIMON	(S.M.Novikov)	Rjazan and/und Kasimov
VARLAAM	(A.T.Iljuščenko)	Černovcy and/und Bukovina
VARNAVA	(Kedrov)	Čeboksary and Chuvashia/und Tschuwaschien
VIKTORIN	(V.V.Beljaev)	Vilnius and Lithuania/und Litauen
SEVASTJAN	(S.Ja.Pilipčuk)	Kirovograd and/und Nikolaev

Religion
13.4
13.5
13.6
13.7

13.4 THE GEORGIAN ORTHODOX CHURCH
DIE GEORGISCHE ORTHODOXE KIRCHE
GRUZINSKAJA PRAVOSLAVNAJA CERKOV'

Patriarch-Catholicos of All Georgia -
Katholikos, Patriarch von ganz Georgien -
Katolikos-Patriarch vseja Gruzii   - IL'JA

Residence - Residenz: Tbilisi

1 theological seminary - 1 Geistliches Seminar in Mocheta

13.5 THE ARMENIAN GREGORIAN CHURCH
DIE ARMENISCH-GREGORIANISCHE KIRCHE
ARMJANO-GRIGORIANSKAJA CERKOV'

Supreme Patriarch-Catholicos of All Armenians -
Katholikos, Patriarch aller Armenier -
Verchovnyj Patriarch-katolikos vsech armjan   - VAZGEN I.
                                              (since-seit 1955)
Residence - Residenz: Ečmiadzin near-bei Erevan

1 theological academy - 1 Geistliche Akademie

13.6 THE OLD BELIEVERS - DIE ALTGLÄUBIGEN - STAROVERCY

Consists of three independent lines - besteht aus drei selbständigen Richtungen:

Cerkov' belokrinickogo soglasija
  (Head: Archbishop of Moscow and All Russia -
   Oberhaupt: Erzbischof von Moskau und ganz Rußland)
Cerkov' beglopopovskogo soglasija
  (Head: Archbishop of Novozybkov, Moscow and All Russia -
   Oberhaupt: Erzbischof von Novozybkov, Moskau und ganz Rußland)
Cerkov' bespopovskogo tolka
  (rejects the ecclesiastical hierarchy, works independently and
   is united in the Lithuanian SSR by the Supreme Council of the
   Old Believers - lehnt die kirchliche Hierarchie ab, ist selb-
   ständig tätig und in der Litauischen SSR durch den Obersten
   Rat der Altgläubigen vereinigt)

13.7 ISLAM - MOSLEMS - ISLAM

Consists of two lines: Sunnites (in the central asiatic republics, Kazakhstan, Transcaucasia, the·Autonomous Republics of North Caucasus and Volga district, and in various districts of the RSFSR) and Shiites (in the Azerbaidžan SSR). There exist four independent ecclesiastical boards of the Moslems: in Central Asia and Kazakhstan (Taškent); in the European part of the USSR and Siberia (Ufa); in the North Caucasus (Buinaksk, Daghestan); and in Transcaucasia (Baku); a theological college in Taškent. -

Besteht aus zwei Richtungen: Sunniten (in den mittelasiatischen Republiken, Kasachstan, Transkaukasien, in den Autonomen Republiken des Nordkaukasus und des Wolgagebietes und in verschiedenen Gebieten

13.7
13.8
13.9 Religion
13.10
13.11   der RSFSR) und Schiiten (in der Aserbaidschanischen SSR). Es
            bestehen vier selbständige kirchliche Verwaltungen der Moslems:
            in Mittelasien und Kasachstan (Taŝkent); im europäischen Teil der
            UdSSR und in Sibirien (Ufa); im Nordkaukasus (Buinaksk, Dagestan)
            und in Transkaukasien (Baku); Geistliche Hochschule in Taŝkent.

13.8 THE ROMAN CATHOLIC CHURCH - DIE RÖMISCH-KATHOLISCHE KIRCHE - RIMSKO-KATOLIČESKAJA CERKOV'

To be found mostly in the Western Ukraine and Western Belorussia, Moldavia, in the Baltic republics and some parts of the Russian Federation. There is no single administrative center. It has a vicarage, seven dioceses, and parishes. -

Ist hauptsächlich in den westlichen Gebieten der Ukraine und Belorußlands, in Moldau, in den baltischen Republiken und in einigen Teilen der RSFSR verbreitet. Ein einheitliches Glaubenszentrum ist nicht vorhanden. Es gibt ein Vikariat, 7 Diözesen und Gemeinden.

13.9 THE EVANGELICAL LUTHERAN CHURCH - DIE EVANGELISCH-LUTHERISCHE KIRCHE - EVANGELIČESKO-LJUTERANSKAJA CERKOV'

Members of the Church are to be found in the Baltic republics. There are three independent Consistories. The Latvian and Estonian congregations are headed by Archbishops, the Lithuanian congregation by the President of the Consistory. -

Im Baltikum tätig; es bestehen drei unabhängige Konsistorien. In der Lettischen und Estnischen SSR werden diese von Erzbischöfen, in der Litauischen SSR vom Präsidenten des Konsistoriums geleitet.

13.10   THE EVANGELICAL CHRISTIANS-BAPTISTS DIE CHRISTLICH-EVANGELISCHEN BAPTISTEN CERKOV' EVANGEL'SKICH CHRISTIAN-BAPTISTOV

Headed by the National Council of Evangelical Christians-Baptists - geleitet vom Unionsrat der christlich - evangelischen Baptisten - Vsesojuznyj sovet evangel'skich christian-baptistov (Moskva);
Chairman - Vorsitzender: IL'JA IVANOV;
Organ: "Bratskij vestnik" (Fraternal Information Sheet - Brüderliches Informationsblatt), Moskva.

13.11   JUDAISM - MOSAISCHE GLAUBENSGEMEINSCHAFTEN - IUDAIZM

To be found mostly among the Jewish population in the Russian Federation, Ukraine, Belorussia, Georgia, and some other rayons of the country. Each synagogue operates autonomously. -

Ist hauptsächlich unter der jüdischen Bevölkerung in der RSFSR, Ukraine, Belorußland, Georgien und in einigen anderen Rayons des Landes verbreitet. Jede Synagoge arbeitet autonom.

Religion 13.12
13.13
13.14

13.12 BUDDHISM - BUDDHISMUS - BUDDIZM

Believers are to be found in the Buryat, Kalmyk and Tuva autonomous republics and some parts of the Chita and Irkutsk regions of the Russian Federation. They are headed by the Central Theological Board of Buddhists of the USSR. A theological school in Ulan-Ude. -

Die Anhänger dieses Glaubensbekenntnisses leben in der Burjatischen, Kalmückischen und Tuwinischen ASSR und in einigen Teilen der Gebiete Čita und Irkutsk (RSFSR). Sie werden von der Zentralen Geistlichen Verwaltung der Buddhisten in der UdSSR geleitet. Geistliche Schule in Ulan-Ude.

13.13 OTHER DENOMINATIONS - ANDERE KONFESSIONEN - DRUGIE OBOZNAČENIJA

The Reformed Church in Transcarpathia (Ukraine) -
Die Reformierte Kirche in Transkarpatien (Ukraine) -
Reformatskaja cerkov' v Transkarpatskoj oblasti

The Methodist Church in Estonia -
Die Methodistische Kirche in Estland -
Metodistskaja cerkov' v Estonii

The Seventh-Day Adventists -
Die Adventisten des Siebenten Tages -
Adventisty sed'mogo dnja

Molokani - Molokanen - Molokane

Mennonites - Mennoniten - Mennonity

13.14 MOST IMPORTANT ILLEGAL CHURCHES AND SECTS
WICHTIGSTE ILLEGALE KIRCHEN UND SEKTEN
VAŽNEJŠIE NELEGAL'NYE CERKVI I SEKTY

The True Orthodox Church -
Die Wahre Orthodoxe Kirche -
Istinno-pravoslavnaja cerkov'

The Greek-Catholic Church (Western Ukraine) -
Die Griechisch-Katholische Kirche (Westukraine) -
Greko-katoličeskaja cerkov'

The Ukrainian Autonomous Orthodox Church (groups of believers) -
Die Ukrainische Autonome Orthodoxe Kirche (Gruppen von Anhängern) -
Ukrainska avtonomna pravoslavna cerkva

The Evangelical Christians-Baptists -
Die Christlich-Evangelischen Baptisten -
Evangel'skie christiane-baptisty - EChB (Initiativniki)

(schismed in the early sixties from the legal church of the Evangelical Christians-Baptists. Organ: "Bjulleten' Soveta rodstvennikov uznikov Evangel'skich christian-baptistov" - The Council's Bulletin for relatives of Evangelical Christians-Baptists' prisoners -. In 1971 there was founded the Council of Churches ("Sovet Cerkvi EChB") but not recognized by the government. -

601

13.14 Religion

Anfang der 60er Jahre abgespaltet von der legalen Kirche der
Christlich-Evangelischen Baptisten. Organ: Bulletin des
Rates für Verwandte von Christlich-Evangelischen Baptisten-
Häftlingen. 1971 wurde der Rat der Kirchen (EChB) gegründet,
jedoch von der Regierung nicht anerkannt.)

Church of the True and Free Seventh-Day Adventists -
Kirche der Wahren, Freien Adventisten des Siebenten Tages -
Cerkov' vernych svobodnych adventistov sed'mogo dnja

   (schismed from the legal denomination of the Seventh Day
   Adventists - abgespaltet von der legalen Glaubensgemein-
   schaft der Adventisten des Siebenten Tages)

Pentecostals - Pentakosten - Pjatidesjatniki

Innocentives - Inokentivzen - Inokentivci
   (Moldavian republic - SSR Moldau)

Moroshkoves - Moroschkovzen - Moroŝkivci

Jehova's Witnesses - Zeugen Jehovas - Svideteli Ehovy
   (Organ: "Storoẑevaja baŝnja" - watch-tower - Wachturm)

14. MISCELLANEOUS INFORMATION-DIVERSES

14.1 SOVIET ANTHEM - HYMNE DER SOWJETUNION

Great Russia has united forever	Von Rußland, dem großen, auf ewig verbündet,
The indestructible alliance of free republics,	ragt hoch der Sowjetrepubliken Bastion.
Long live the united powerful Soviet Union	Es lebe, vom Willen der Völker gegründet,
Created by the will of the people.	die einig' und mächtige Sowjetunion!
Glory! Our free fatherland,	Dir, freies Vaterland, Ehre und Ruhm gebührt!
A reliable stronghold of peoples friendship,	Freundschaft der Völker hast fest du gefügt.
The party of Lenin - the national strength	Uns führt des Volkes Kraft, Lenins Partei uns führt
Leads us to the triumph of communism.	zum Kommunismus, zu unserem Sieg.
The sun of freedom shone upon us through storms,	Die Sonne der Freiheit durch dunkles Gewölk drang,
And great Lenin lighted up the way to us,	und Lenin, der große, erhellte den Pfad,
He elevated the people to the just cause	entflammte zum Kampf für die Freiheit der Völker,
And inspired us to work and to feats.	beseelt uns zum Schaffen, beschwingt uns zur Tat.
Glory! Our free fatherland,	Dir, freies Vaterland, Ehre und Ruhm gebührt!
A reliable stronghold of peoples' friendship	Freundschaft der Völker hast fest du gefügt.
The party of Lenin - the national strength	Uns führt des Volkes Kraft, Lenins Partei uns führt
Leads us to the triumph of communism.	zum Kommunismus, zu unserem Sieg.
The future of our country we see	Wir schmieden den Sieg unsrer hehren Ideen,
In the victory of the immortal ideas of communism;	in ihm wir erblicken die Zukunft des Lands.
And we will always be selflessly loyal	Das Banner der ruhmreichen Heimat, es wehe,
To the red banner of our glorious fatherland.	wir schwören ihm Treue mit Herz und mit Hand.
Glory! Our free fatherland,	Dir, freies Vaterland, Ehre und Ruhm gebührt!
A reliable stronghold of peoples friendship	Freundschaft der Völker hast fest du gefügt.
The party of Lenin - the national strength	Uns führt des Volkes Kraft, Lenins Partei uns führt
Leads us to the triumph of communism.	zum Kommunismus, zu unserem Sieg.

14.2 Miscellaneous Information
14.3 Diverses

14.2 TERRITORIAL EXPANSION AFTER THE SECOND WORLD WAR
TERRITORIALE AUSDEHNUNG NACH DEM ZWEITEN WELTKRIEG

Nov.1,1939: The Western Ukraine was annexed by the Soviet Union;
March 12,1940: The Karelian isthmus and the town of Vyborg, the western and northern shore of Lake Ladoga and islands in the Gulf of Finland, a region in the Northeast, east of Merkjärvi, and parts of the peninsulas of the Barents Sea (Rybačij, Srednij polu ostrov) were annexed by the Soviet Union;
Sept.19,1944: The Finnish part of Petsamo was incorporated with the Soviet Union;
June 28,1940: Bessarabia and the Northern Bukovina were annexed by the Soviet Union;
Aug.3,1940: The Lithuanian SSR was annexed by the Soviet Union;
Aug.5.1940: The Latvian SSR was annexed by the Soviet Union;
Aug.6,1940: The Estonian SSR was annexed by the Soviet Union;
Oct.13,1940: The Tuva People's Republic was incorporated with the Soviet Union;
June 29,1945: The Carpathian Ukraine (until then part of Czechoslovakia) was annexed by the Soviet Union.

1.11.1939: Anschluß der Westukraine an die Sowjetunion;
12.3.1940: Anschluß der Karelischen Landenge mit der Stadt Vyborg, des West- und Nordufers des Ladoga-Sees und Inseln im Finnischen Golf, ein Gebiet im Nordosten östlich von Merkjärvi und Teile der Halbinseln der Barents-See (der Fischer- und der Mittleren Halbinsel Finnlands) an die Sowjetunion;
19.9.1944: Eingliederung des finnischen Gebiets von Petsamo an die Sowjetunion;
28.6.1940: Anschluß Bessarabiens und der Nordbukowina an die Sowjetunion;
3.8.1940: Anschluß der Litauischen SSR an die Sowjetunion;
5.8.1940: Anschluß der Lettischen SSR an die Sowjetunion;
6.8.1940: Anschluß der Estnischen SSR an die Sowjetunion;
13.10.1940: Eingliederung der Tuwinischen Volksrepublik an die Sowjetunion;
29.6.1945: Anschluß der Karpato-Ukraine (bisher Tschechoslowakei) an die Sowjetunion.

14.3 THE BOUNDARIES OF THE USSR - DIE STAATSGRENZE DER UdSSR

In the northwest the Soviet Union borders on Norway and Finland, in the west on Poland, Czechoslovakia, Hungary and Romania, in the south on Turkey, Iran, Afghanistan, China and the Mongolian People's Republic, and in the southeast on Korea. The total length of the Soviet border is more than 60,000 km, of which 43,000 km are water and 17,000 national boundaries.
The Soviet Union borders on three oceans: the Atlantic, the Arctic and the Pacific Ocean, and on 12 seas: the Black Sea, the Sea of Azov, the Baltic Sea, the White Sea, the Barents Sea, the Kara Sea, the Laptev Sea, the East Siberian Sea, the Chukchi Sea, the Bering Sea, the Sea of Okhotsk and the Sea of Japan.

Im Nordwesten grenzt die UdSSR an Norwegen und Finnland, im Westen an Polen, die Tschechoslowakei, Ungarn und Rumänien, im Süden an die Türkei, Iran, Afghanistan, China und die Volksrepublik Mongolei, im Südosten an Korea. Die Gesamtlänge der sowjetischen Staatsgrenze beträgt über 60.000 km, davon 43.000 km Wasser- und 17.000 km Landgrenze.

Die Sowjetunion grenzt an drei Ozeane: Atlantik, Nördliches Eismeer und Pazifik; 12 Meere und Seen: Schwarzes Meer, Asowsches Meer, Ostsee, Weißes Meer, Barents-See, Karisches Meer, Laptev-See, Ostsibirische See, Tschuktschen-See, Bering-See, Ochotskisches Meer und Japanische See.

Others 14.4
Diverses 14.5
14.6

14.4 THE BIGGEST MOUNTAINS - DIE HÖCHSTEN BODENERHEBUNGEN

Name of the peak Name des Gipfels	Range of mountains Gebirgsmassiv	Altitude Höhe ü.M. (in m)
Pik Kommunizma	Pamirs - Pamir	7,495
Pik Pobedy	Tien Shan - Tjan' Šan'	7,439
Pik Lenina	Transalay mountain - Transalai-Gebirge	7,134
Pik Korženevskoj	Pamirs - Pamir	7,105
Pik Chan-Tengri	Tien Shan - Tjan' Šan'	6,995
Elbrus	Great Caucasus - Großkaukasus	5,633
Dych-Tau	Great Caucasus - Großkaukasus	5,198
Kazbek	Great Caucasus - Großkaukasus	5,047
Belucha	Altai	4,506
Aragac	Small Caucasus - Kleinkaukasus	4,095
Munku-Sardyk	East-Sayan - Ost-Sajan	3,492
Pobeda	Chersky mountain - Čerskij-Gebirge	3,147
Burun-Šibertuj	Daur mountain - Daur Gebirge	2,523
Sochondo	Borshchvochny mountain - Borščvočnyj-Gebirge	2,508
Golec Skalistyj	Kalar mountain - Kalar-Gebirge	2,467
Verchnij Zub	Kuzneckij-Alatau	2,178
Tardoki-Jani	Sichote-Alin'	2,078
Goverla	East Carpathian Mountains - Ostkarpaten	2,061

14.5 VOLCANOES - VULKANE

Name of the volcano Name des Vulkans	Range of mountains Gebirgsmassiv	Altitude Höhe ü.M. (in m)
Ključevaja sopka	Kamchatka Peninsula - Halbinsel Kamčatka	4,750
Tolbačik	Kamchatka Peninsula - Halbinsel Kamčatka	3,682
Korjakskaja sopka	Kamchatka Peninsula - Halbinsel Kamčatka	3,456
Šiveluč	Kamchatka Peninsula - Halbinsel Kamčatka	3,283
Sopka Županova	Kamchatka Peninsula - Halbinsel Kamčatka	2,929
Avačinskaja sopka	Kamchatka Peninsula - Halbinsel Kamčatka	2,751
Alaid	Kurile Islands, Atlasov Island - Kurilleninseln, Atlasov-Insel	2,339
Mutnovskaja sopka	Kamchatka Peninsula - Halbinsel Kamčatka	2,323

14.6 THE PRINCIPAL RIVERS - DIE WICHTIGSTEN FLÜSSE

Name of the river Name des Flusses	Length (in km) Länge (in km)
Amur (with Shilka and Onon - mit Šilka und Onon)	4,350
Lena	4,320
Enissej (with-mit Bij-Chem)	4,130
Ob (with-mit Katun')	4,070
Volga	3,460

14.6 Others
14.7 Diverses

Name of the river Name des Flusses	Length (in km) Länge (in km)
Syr-Darya (with-mit Naryn)	2,850
Amu-Darja (with-mit Pjandžem,Vachandarja,Vachdžiry)	2,600
Ural	2,530
Dnepr	2,280
Kolyma	2,150
Don	1,950
Indigirka	1,790
Pečora	1,790
Kura	1,510
Dnestr	1,410
North Dune - Nord-Düne (with-mit Suchona)	1,300
Jana (with-mit Dulgalach)	1,070
Selenga (with-mit Ider)	1,020
West Dune - West-Düne	1,020
Mezen'	966
Kuban'	906
Neman	854
Terek	626
Onega	416
Neva	74

14.7   THE BIGGEST LAKES - DIE GRÖSSTEN SEEN

Name of the lake Name des Sees	Area in sq.km Fläche in km²	Altitude Höhe ü.M. (in m)	Deepest point Tiefster Punkt (in m)
Caspian Sea - Kaspisches Meer	395,000	28	980
Aral	65,500	53	68
Baikal	30,500	455	1,741
Ladoga	17,700	4	225
Balchaš	17,400	339	26
Onega	9,610	33	110
Issyk-Kul	6,130	1,609	702
Chanka	4,400	69	10
Peipus (with-mit Pskov)	3,560	30	14
Čany	2,600	105	10
Ilmen (maximum and minimum extent - Maximal- und Minimalausdehnung)	2,330/660	19	5
Alakol	2,070	340	47
Zajsan	1,800	386	8
Sevan	1,410	1,914	99
White lake - Weißsee	1,120	111	11
Imandra	880	128	67
Teleckoe	230	436	325

14.8 THE PRINCIPAL PENINSULAS - DIE WICHTIGSTEN INSELN

Name of the peninsula Name der Insel	Area in sq.km Fläche in km²	Sea - Meer
Novaja Zemlja	82,600	Barents and Kara Seas - Barents- und Karskoe-Seen
Severnyj ostrov	48,200	
Južnyj ostrov	33,200	
Sachalin	76,400	Sea of Okhotsk-Ochotskisches M.
Novosibirskie ostrova	38,400	Laptev and East Siberian Seas - Laptev- und Ostsibirische Seen
Kotelnyj	12,000	
Zemlja Bunge	7,220	
Novaja Sibir'	6,460	
Bol'šoj Ljachovskij	5,240	
Fadeevskij	4,970	
Severnaja Zemlja	37,560	Laptev and Kara Seas - Laptev- und Karskoe-Seen
Oktjabrskoj Revoljucii	14,170	
Bolševik	11,440	
Komsomolec	9,260	
Pioner	1,600	
Zemlja Franca Josifa	16,500	Barents Sea - Barents-See
Zemlja Georga	2,900	
Zemlja Vilčeka	1,980	
Ostrov Greem Bell	1,700	
Zemlja Aleksandry	1,130	
Kuril'skie ostrova	10,010	Pacific Ocean - Stiller Ozean
Vrangelja	7,270	East Siberian and Chukchi Seas - Ostsibirische u. Khukotskoe-See
Kolguev	5,250	Barents Sea - Barents-See
Vajgač	3,250	Kara Sea - Karskoe-See
Sarema	2,650	Baltic Sea - Ostsee
Karaginskij	2,120	Bering Sea - Bering-See
Ajon	2,040	East Siberian Sea - Ostsibirische See
Bolšoj Šantar	2,000	Okhotsk Sea - Ochotskisches Meer
Belyj	1,910	Kara Sea - Karskoe-See
Dickson	26	Kara Sea - Karskoe-See

14.9 ECONOMY - WIRTSCHAFT

14.9.1 Official Exchange Rate of the Ruble (March 1978)
Offizieller Rubelkurs (März 1978)

Country - Land	Currency - Währung	Rate of exchange Umrechnungskurs
Afghanistan	100 Afghani-Afghanen	1.66
Algeria - Algerien	100 Dinar	17.02
Albania - Albanien	100 Lek	18.00
Argentina - Argentinien	100 Pesetas	0.10
Australia - Australien	100 Dollar	78.04
Austria - Österreich	100 Schilling	4.70
Belgium - Belgien	100 Franc	2.17
Burma - Birma	100 Kyat	10.00
Bulgaria - Bulgarien	100 Lev	76.92
Canada - Kanada	100 Dollar	61.42
China	100 Yuan	45.00

14.9.1 Others / Diverses

Country - Land	Currency - Währung	Rate of exchange Umrechnungskurs
Cuba - Kuba	1 Peso	0.90
Czechoslovakia -- Tschechoslowakei	100 Koruna	12.50
Denmark - Dänemark	100 Krone	12.22
Egypt - Ägypten	1 Pound	1.75
Ethiopia - Äthiopien	100 Dollar	36.00
Finland - Finnland	100 Markka	16.45
France - Frankreich	100 Franc	14.31
Germany, Federal Republic of Deutsche Bundesrepublik	100 Deutsche Mark	33.88
German Democratic Republic - DDR	100 Mark	40.50
Ghana	1 Cedi	0.61
Greece - Griechenland	100 Drachma	1.95
Guinea	100 syli	3.18
Hungary - Ungarn	100 Forint	7.67
Iceland - Island	100 Króna	0.27
India - Indien	100 Rupee	8.50
Indonesia - Indonesien	1000 Rupiah	1.80
Iran	100 Rial	0.97
Iraq - Irak	1 Dinar	2.31
Italy - Italien	1000 Lira	0.80
Japan	1000 Yen	2.87
Korea	100 Won	74.93
Kuwait - Kuweit	1 Dinar	2.48
Lebanon - Libanon	100 Pound	23.35
Libya - Libyen	1 Dinar	2.38
Malaysia	100 Dollar	29.13
Mali	1000 Franc	1.42
Mexico - Mexiko	100 Peso	3.01
Mongolia - Mongolei	100 Tugrik	22.50
Morocco - Marokko	100 Dirham	16.05
Nepal	100 Rupee	5.53
Netherlands - Niederlande	100 Guilder	31.52
New Zealand - Neuseeland	100 Dollar	70.96
Norway - Norwegen	100 Krone	12.93
Pakistan	100 Rupee	7.54
Poland - Polen	100 Zloty	22.50
Portugal	100 Escudo	1.72
Romania - Rumänien	100 Leu	15.00
Singapore - Singapur	100 Dollar	29.59
Somalia	100 Shilling	10.97
Spain - Spanien	100 Peseta	0.87
Sudan	1 Pound	2.01
Sweden - Schweden	100 Krona	14.96
Switzerland - Schweiz	100 Franc	38.04
Sri Lanka	100 Rupee	4.50
Syria - Syrien	100 Pound	17.56
Tunisia - Tunesien	1 Dinar	1.63
Turkey - Türkei	100 Pound	3.61
United Kingdom - Großbritannien	1 Pound	1.34
USA	100 Dollar	68.48
Uruguay	100 Peso	12.75
Yemen Arab Republic - Arabische Republik Jemen	100 Riyal	16.06
Yemen, People's Democratic Republic of - VR Jemen	1 Dinar	2.16
Yugoslavia - Jugoslawien	100 Dinar	3.74

Others 14.9.2
Diverses 14.9.3
14.9.4

14.9.2 Five-Year Plans - Fünfjahrpläne

1st Five-Year Plan -	I. Fünfjahrplan	1929-1932
2nd Five-Year Plan -	II. Fünfjahrplan	1933-1937
3rd Five-Year Plan -	III. Fünfjahrplan	1938-1942 [1]
4th Five-Year Plan -	IV. Fünfjahrplan	1946-1950
5th Five-Year Plan -	V. Fünfjahrplan	1951-1955
6th Five-Year Plan -	VI. Fünfjahrplan	1956-1960 [2]
Seven-Year Plan -	Siebenjahrplan	1959-1965
8th Five-Year Plan -	VIII. Fünfjahrplan	1966-1970
9th Five-Year Plan -	IX. Fünfjahrplan	1971-1975
10th Five-Year Plan -	X. Fünfjahrplan	1976-1980

14.9.3 Wheat Imports - Weizenimporte ('000 tons - Tsd. t)

Country - Land	1973	1974	1975	1976
Argentina - Argentinien		206.2	810.1	961
Hungary - Ungarn		117.8	674.6	20
Canada - Kanada	3,534.8	410.5	2,196.8	2,038
USA	9,847.9	1,323.0	3,811.9	2,052

14.9.4 Mineral Oil and Mineral Oil Products Exports ('000 tons) Export von Erdöl und Erdölprodukten (Tsd. t)

Country - Land	1973	1974	1975	1976
Total - Insgesamt	118,300	116,200	130,350	148,514
Afghanistan	165	193	149	149
Austria - Österreich	1,250	970	1,327	1,513
Belgium - Belgien	1,673	1,752	1,255	2,082
Bulgaria - Bulgarien	9,322	10,855	11,553	11,868
Cuba - Kuba	7,435	7,643	8,060	8,809
Czechoslovakia - Tschechoslowakei	14,340	14,836	15,965	17,233
Cyprus - Zypern	122	106	206	257
Denmark - Dänemark	633	703	1,178	1,632
Egypt - Ägypten	352	229	231	226
Finland - Finnland	10,028	9,173	8,768	9,620
France - Frankreich	5,348	1,360	3,307	5,729
Germany, Federal Republic of- Bundesrepublik Deutschland	5,849	6,340	7,634	7,132
Germany, Democratic Republic- DDR	12,985	14,424	14,952	16,766

[1] In the war years 1942-46 only annual, quarterly and monthly reports were published -
In den Kriegsjahren 1942-1946 gab es nur Jahres-, Quartal- und Monatspläne.

[2] The Seven-Year Plan was voted on before the end of the Sixth Five-Year Plan upon the initiative of N.S. Khrushchev at the XXI. Party Congress (1959) on the grounds that a number of major economic ventures needed a longer period of time in order to be realized. The Seven-Year Plan is not reflected in this statistic. -

Auf dem XXI.Parteitag (1959) wurde auf Initiative von N.S.Chruŝĉev vor Ablauf des VI.Fünfjahrplanes der Siebenjahrplan beschlossen, mit der Begründung, eine Reihe wichtiger Wirtschaftsvorhaben benötigten eine längere Zeitspanne für deren Realisierung. In der Statistik wird der Siebenjahrplan nicht berücksichtigt.

14.9.4 Others
14.9.5 Diverses
14.9.6

Country - Land	1973	1974	1975	1976
Ghana	614	309	144	250
Great Britain - Großbritannien	834	918	1,503	4,051
Greece - Griechenland	797	1,032	1,888	1,948
Guinea	85	82	62	81
Hungary - Ungarn	6,294	6,729	7,535	8,435
Iceland - Island	468	460	448	417
India - Indien	477	1,009	1,207	1,113
Ireland - Irland	183	118	176	155
Italy - Italien	8,652	6,788	6,883	11,982
Japan	2,023	1,241	1,320	1,773
Korea	585	942	1,110	1,061
Morocco - Marokko	943	647	649	665
Mongolia - Mongolei	323	347	364	415
Netherlands - Niederlande	3,220	2,975	3,090	2,674
Norway - Norwegen	603	279	283	218
Poland - Polen	12,336	11,855	13,271	14,073
Somalia	75	113	118	136
Spain - Spanien	510	1,351	1,724	2,002
Sweden - Schweden	3,216	3,027	3,450	2,729
Switzerland - Schweiz	658	779	960	942
Vietnam	230	293	403	439
Yugoslavia - Jugoslawien	3,891	3,790	4,444	4,858

14.9.5 Natural gas export - Export von Erdgas
(mill.cu.m. - Mio m^3)

Country - Land	1973	1974	1975	1976
Total	6,832	14,039	19,333	25,780
Austria - Österreich	1,622	2,106	1,883	2,785
Bulgaria - Bulgarien	--	--	1,185	2,229
Czechoslovakia - Tschechoslowakei	989	1,094	3,694	4,287
Finland - Finnland	--	--	719	870
Germany, Federal Republic of - Bundesrepublik Deutschland	353	2,145	3,898	3,976
Germany, Democratic Republic- DDR	--	--	3,302	3,369
Italy - Italien	--	790	2,342	3,720
Poland - Polen	1,709	2,117	2,509	2,549

14.9.6
Share of Agricultural Production of Private Subsidiary Enterprises
Anteil der privaten Nebenwirtschaften an der landwirtschaftl.Produktion

Sowing area - Ackerbaufläche:	3.3 %	(3.4 mill.hectares-ha)
Pasture-ground - Weide:	0.3 %	(0.2 mill.hectares-ha)
Potatoes - Kartoffeln:	23 %	
Livestock and poultry - Vieh u.Geflügel:	11 %	
Wool - Wolle:	7 %	
Eggs - Eier:	7 %	
Milk - Milch:	5 %	
Vegetables - Gemüse:	5 %	

Others 14.10
Diverses 14.11
14.12

14.10 OTHER ORGANIZATIONS AND INSTITUTIONS OF CPSU CC
WEITERE ORGANISATIONEN UND INSTITUTIONEN DES ZK DER KPdSU

Institute of Marxism-Leninism of CPSU CC
Institut des Marxismus-Leninismus beim ZK der KPdSU
Institut Marksizma-Leninizma pri CK KPSS
   Tretij Sel'skochozjajstvennyj Pereulok, 4, Moskva

Higher Party School of CPSU CC
Parteihochschule des ZK der KPdSU
Vysŝaja Ordena Lenina Partijnaja Ŝkola pri CK KPSS (VPŜ)
   Miusskaja Ploŝĉad', 6, Moskva
   Tel.: 251 39 33

Institute of Social Sciences of CPSU CC
Institut für Gesellschaftswissenschaften des ZK der KPdSU
Institut Obŝĉestvennych Nauk pri CK KPSS

Academy of Social Sciences of CPSU CC
Akademie für Gesellschaftswissenschaften des ZK der KPdSU
Akademija Obŝĉestvennych Nauk pri CK KPSS
   Sadovaja-Kudrinskaja, 9, Moskva

Party High School for Correspondence Courses of the CC of the CPSU
Parteifernhochschule des ZK der KPdSU
Zaoĉnaja Partijnaja vysŝaja ŝkola pri CK KPSS
   Leningradskij prospekt, 17, Moskva
   Tel.: 250 03 42

14.11 PRESS AGENCIES - PRESSEAGENTUREN

USSR Telegraph Agency - TASS
Telegraphen-Agentur der UdSSR - TASS
Telegrafnoe Agentstvo Sovetskogo Sojuza - TASS
   Tverskoj Bul'var, 10, Moskva

Press Agency "Novosti" - APN
Presseagentur "Novosti" - APN
Agentstvo Peĉati "Novosti" - APN
   Puŝkinskaja Plosĉad', 2, Moskva
   Tel.: 299 00 03

14.12 USSR ORDERS - ORDEN DER UdSSR

Order of Lenin - Leninorden - Orden Lenina (since 4/6/1930-seit 6.4.1930)

Order of the October Revolution - Orden der Oktoberrevolution -
  Orden Oktjabrskoj Revoljucii (since 10/31/1967-seit 31.10.1967)

Order of Victory - Siegesorden   Orden "Pobeda"
  (since 11/8/1943 - since 8.11.1943)

Order of Red Banner - Orden des Roten Banners - Orden "Krasnoe znamja"
  (since 9/16/1918 - seit 16.9.1918)

14.12 Others
Diverses

Order of Suvorov - Suvorov-Orden - Orden Suvorova
(since 7/29-1942 - seit 29.7.1942)
1st, 2nd and 3rd class - I., II. und III. Klasse

Order of Ushakov - Uŝakov-Orden - Orden Uŝakova
(since 3/3/1944 - seit 3.3.1944)
1st and 2nd class - I. und II. Klasse

Order of Kutuzov - Kutuzov-Orden - Orden Kutuzova
(1st and 2nd class since 7/29-1942 - I. und II.Klasse seit 29.7.1942;
3rd class since 2/8/1943 - III. Klasse seit 8.2.1943)

Order of Nakhimov - Nachimov-Orden - Orden Nachimova
(since 3/3/1944 - seit 3.3.1944)
1st and 2nd class - I. und II. Klasse

Order of Bogdan Khmelnitsky - Bogdan-Chmelnickij-Orden -
Orden Bogdana Chmelnickogo (since 10/10/1943 - seit 10.10.1943)
1st, 2nd and 3rd class - I., II. und III. Klasse

Order of Aleksandr Nevsky - Aleksandr Nevskij Orden -
Orden Aleksandra Nevskogo (since 7/29 1942 - seit 29.7.1942)

Order of the Patriotic War - Orden des Vaterländischen Krieges -
Orden Otečestvennoj vojny (since 5/20/1942 - seit 20.5.1942)
1st and 2nd class - I. und II. Klasse

Order of the Red Banner of Labour - Orden des Roten Arbeitsbanners -
Orden "Trudovoe Krasnoe Znamja" (since 9/7/1928 - seit 7.9.1928)

Order of Friendship between Nations - Orden der Völkerfreundschaft -
Orden Družby narodov (since 12/17/1972 - seit 17.12.1972)

Order of the Red Star - Orden des Roten Sterns - Orden "Krasnaja zvezda"
(since 4/6/1930 - seit 6.4.1930)

Order "Honorary Badge" - Orden "Ehrenabzeichen" - Orden "Znak početa"
(since 11/25-1935 - seit 25.11.1935)

Order of Glory - Orden des Ruhmes - Orden slavy
(since 11/8/1943 - seit 8.11.1943)
1st, 2nd and 3rd class - I., II. und III. Klasse

Order of Labor Glory - Orden des Arbeitsruhmes - Orden trudovoj slavy
(since 1/18/1974 - seit 18.1.1974)
1st, 2nd and 3rd class - I., II. und III. Klasse

Order of the Heroic Mother - Orden "Mutter-Heldin" -
Orden "Mat'-geroinja" (since 7/8/1944 - seit 8.7.1944)

Order of Mother's Glory - Orden "Mutterruhm" - Orden
"Materinskaja slava" (since 7/8/1944 - seit 8.7.1944)
1st, 2nd and 3rd class - I., II. und III. Klasse

Others 14.13.1
Diverses 14.13.2
14.13.3

14.13 SOME CULTURAL INSTITUTIONS - EINIGE KULTURELLE INSTITUTIONEN

14.13.1 Libraries - Bibliotheken
(end-of-year figures - zum Jahresende)

	1960	1975
Total - Insgesamt (in thousands - in Tsd.)	382	350
Scientific, technical and professional libraries - Wissenschaftliche, technische und Fachbibliotheken (in thousands - in Tsd.)	50	65

14.13.2 Public Libraries in the Union Republics
Öffentliche Bibliotheken in den Unionsrepubliken
(end-of-year figures - zum Jahresende)

	Number of libraries Zahl der Bibliotheken (in thousands-in Tsd.)		Number of books and journals Zahl der Bücher u.Zeitschriften (in thousands-in Tsd.)	
	1960	1975	1960	1975
SSSR	135,721	131,354	845,183	1541,179
RSFSR	69,107	62,248	483,672	867,455
Ukrainskaja SSR	32,642	26,881	190,074	320,448
Belorusskaja SSR	7,300	7,153	28,810	70,822
Uzbekskaja SSR	3,316	6,302	17,968	39,857
Kazachskaja SSR	6,140	9,061	28,870	82,878
Gruzinskaja SSR	3,170	3,858	14,628	25,696
Azerbajdžanskaja SSR	2,494	3,479	14,732	26,702
Litovskaja SSR	2,389	2,661	12,780	21,799
Moldavskaja SSR	1,650	2,030	11,050	17,890
Latvijskaja SSR	1,998	1,418	11,037	17,964
Kirgizskaja SSR	1,060	1,542	5,761	12,430
Tadžikskaja SSR	884	1,412	4,962	9,385
Armjanskaja SSR	1,142	1,324	7,304	11,763
Turkmenskaja SSR	1,188	1,271	5,604	7,222
Estonskaja SSR	1,241	714	7,931	8,868

14.13.3 Number of Theatres in the Union Republics
Zahl der Theater in den Unionsrepubliken
(end-of-year figures - zum Jahresende)

	1960	1975			
		Total Insg.	Opera and ballet Oper und Ballett	Drama, Comedy and Music Drama, Komödie u.Musik	Children's and youth theatres Kinder-und Jugendtheater
		A.	B.	C.	D.
SSSR	502	570	42	373	155
RSFSR	288	313	20	196	97
Ukrainskaja SSR	68	77	6	44	27
Belorusskaja SSR	11	14	1	9	4
Uzbekskaja SSR	20	26	2	20	4
Kazachskaja SSR	19	28	1	25	2

14.13.3 Others
14.13.4 Diverses
14.13.5

	1960	1975			
		A.	B.	C.	D.
Gruzinskaja SSR	20	23	1	18	4
Azerbajdžanskaja SSR	12	14	1	11	2
Litovskaja SSR	11	11	2	7	2
Moldavskaja SSR	5	7	1	4	2
Latvijskaja SSR	11	10	1	7	2
Kirgizskaja SSR	8	7	1	5	1
Tadžikskaja SSR	6	11	1	8	2
Armjanskaja SSR	11	14	1	10	3
Turkmenskaja SSR	6	6	1	4	1
Estonskaja SSR	9	9	2	5	2

14.13.4 Circuses - Zirkusse (end-of-year figures - zum Jahresende)

	1960	1975
Total - insgesamt	80	94
Stationary circuses - ständige Zirkusse	46	56
Travelling circuses - Wanderzirkusse	14	18

14.3.5 Number of Museums in the Union Republics
Zahl der Museen in den Unionsrepubliken
(end-of-year figures - zum Jahresende)

	1960	1975
SSSR	929	1,295
RSFSR	492	646
Ukrainskaja SSR	132	154
Belorusskaja SSR	38	56
Uzbekskaja SSR	14	31
Kazachskaja SSR	25	37
Gruzinskaja SSR	68	81
Azerbajdžanskaja SSR	18	41
Litovskaja SSR	38	37
Moldavskaja SSR	12	36
Latvijskaja SSR	24	64
Kirgizskaja SSR	7	7
Tadžikskaja SSR	4	7
Armjanskaja SSR	22	35
Turkmenskaja SSR	4	11
Estonskaja SSR	31	52

ALA Reference Book of the Year 1978:

Who's Who in the Socialist Countries
A biographical encyclopedia of 10,000 leading personalities in 16 communist countries. Edited by Borys Lewytzkyj and Juliusz Stroynowski. 1978. XVI, 736 pages. Cloth DM 198.00.
ISBN 3-7940-3193-8

Who's Who in the Socialist Countries is a pioneering work in its field and the only reference work of its kind in scope and comprehensiveness. For the first time ever some 10,000 biographies of the leadership of 16 communist countries have been collected into one volume. The result of extensive research by two distinguished communist-affairs analysts, it covers the world of politics, science, economics, literature, religion and the arts.

Each biography contains full name, date and place of birth, nationality, education, party affiliation, political activities, present and former positions held, decorations, orders and prizes as well as publications.

There are over 4,000 listings for the Soviet Union alone, including all major changes in the Politburo and the Central Committee of the Communist Party which occurred following the XXVth Party Congress in February 1976. The section on Communist China takes into account the changes following the death of Chairman Mao, and extensive material on Poland, Czechoslovakia and the German Democratic Republic offer the latest information available to Western observers.

The 16 territories covered are: The Soviet Union, the German Democratic Republic, Poland, Czechoslovakia, Romania, Bulgaria, Hungary, Yugoslavia, Albania, Mongolia, China, North Korea, Vietnam, Laos, Cambodia and Cuba.

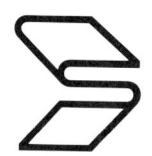

K · G · SAUR   München · New York · London · Paris

Bibliography of Social Research in the Soviet Union (1960–1970)
Compiled by Sergej Woronitzin. 1973. 215 pages. Cloth DM 48.00. ISBN 3-7940-3650-6. In German and English.

This bibliography includes approximately 700 selected books and essays on the theoretical and practical aspects of social research in the USSR which were published in Russian or Ukrainian in the Soviet Union between 1960 and 1970.

Selection was made on the basis of significance of the information contained in the individual works, whereby the greatest value was attached to empirically gathered data. In order to facilitate use of the bibliography, translations in German and English are given with the original title, occasionally these translation also offer a brief explanation of the contents of a particular work. For the scientist interested in empirical data, tables of such data found in the works are indicated with a notation.

The bibliography consists of three main parts: compilations, theoretical and methodical foundations, and results of practical social research. The last part is divided into 15 sections according to individual fields of research.

Christine Kunze

Journalismus in der UdSSR

This publication explores the responsibilities and functions of Soviet journalists with special consideration given to the structure of the mass media in the USSR and examination of the profession in the periodical Zhurnalist. = Dortmunder Beiträge zur Zeitungsforschung, Vol. 27. 1978. 342 pages. Paperback DM 28,–.
ISBN 3-7940-2527-X. In German.

Christine Kunze studied the original sources and in her extensive analysis of Soviet journalism, she thoroughly evaluates the Soviet Journalists' Association. Kunze portrays the journalistic profession against the background of a brief description of the media system. She emphasizes education and advanced training. The appendix includes documents on the development of journalism in the USSR as well as the by-laws of the Journalists' Association. (1959, 1966, and 1971)

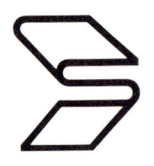

K · G · SAUR   München · New York · London · Paris